What experts are saying about The PDR Family Guide to Prescription Drugs

"Superbly written and understandable by those we wish to help—our patients and their families. In addition to providing drug information in an easily readable format, this book also serves to educate about major illnesses, such as heart disease. Any patient or family member of a patient should have ready access to this book. It is informative, useful and a pleasure to read."

Edwin C. Cadman, M.D.
Ensign Professor and Chairman
Department of Internal Medicine
Yale University School of Medicine

"As individuals increasingly empower themselves in a variety of areas in our society, so too are they requiring more information and input into their own medical care decisions. This book is a great resource for the patient in his or her dialogue with the physician."

Joseph R. Cruse, M.D.
Founding Medical Director
The Betty Ford Center

"A valuable and timely adjunct in this age of consumer education, patient rights, and quality health care for all. . . . The PDR Family Guide, written in clear, understandable terms with easily accessible cross references, will provide an efficient way for consumers to know more about their prescribed medications, side effects, and interactions with food or other medications."

Roberta S. Abruzzese, Ed.D., R.N., F.A.A.N.
Editor, *Decubitus: The Journal of Skin Ulcers*

"An excellent supplement to the education that should occur during every health care visit. The Guide allows people to find answers when and where they need them—any time of the day or night in their own home."

Barbara P. Yawn, M.D., M.S.
Associate Professor of Clinical Family Medicine and Community Health
University of Minnesota

"An easy-to-read guide to medications, side effects, and efficacy. . . . Now one can get understandable medical information which can help keep health costs down, yet give patients a fine comfort level with the medicines they take."

Leon G. Smith, M.D., F.A.C.P.
Director of Medicine
Saint Michael's Medical Center

Other Books and Products
from Medical Economics Data

Physicians' Desk Reference®
PDR Guide to Drug Interactions,
  Side Effects, Indications™
PDR For Nonprescription Drugs®
PDR For Ophthalmology®
PDR® Drug I.D. System
Pocket PDR™ (Handheld Electronic Database)
PDR Library on CD-ROM™
PDR Drug Interactions and Side Effects
  Diskettes with Indications™

Medical Device Register™
MDR™ International Edition
Directory of Hospital Personnel™
HMO/PPO Directory™
Directory of Healthcare Group Purchasing
  Organizations™
Directory of U.S. Nursing Homes and
  Nursing Home Chains™
Product Development Directory™
Product SOS™ (FDA Problem Reports)
Breast Implant Problem Reports™

Red Book®
MicREData
The Red Book® Database

THE PDR®
FAMILY GUIDE
TO PRESCRIPTION DRUGS™

MEDICAL ECONOMICS DATA   **MONTVALE, NEW JERSEY**

Publisher's Note

The information contained in this book is based on product labeling published in the 1993 edition of Physicians' Desk Reference®, supplemented with facts from other sources the publisher believes reliable. While diligent efforts have been made to assure the accuracy of this information, the book does not list every possible action, adverse reaction, interaction, and precaution; and all information is presented without guarantees by the authors, consultants, and publisher, who disclaim all liability in connection with its use.

This book is intended only as a reference for use in an ongoing partnership between doctor and patient in the vigilant management of drug therapy. It is not a substitute for a doctor's professional judgement, and serves only as a reminder of concerns that may need discussion. All readers are urged to consult with a physician before beginning or discontinuing use of any prescription drug.

Brand names listed in this book are intended to represent only the more commonly used products. Inclusion of a brand name does not signify endorsement of the product, absence of a name does not imply a criticism or rejection of the product. The publisher is not advocating the use of any product described in this book, does not warrant or guarantee any of these products, and has not performed any independent analysis in connection with the product information contained herein.

ISBN: 1-56363-020-6 (Medical Economics Data). Manufactured in the United States of America.

Officers of Medical Economics Data Inc.: President and Chief Executive Officer: Norman R. Snesil; Executive Vice President: Mark L. Weinstein; Senior Vice President and Chief Financial Officer: J. Crispin Ashworth; Senior Vice President of Business Development: Stephen J. Sorkenn; Vice President of Product Management: Curtis B. Allen; Vice President, Sales and Marketing: Thomas F. Rice; Vice President of Operations: John R. Ware; Vice President of Information Systems and Services; Edward J. Zecchini

X

Contents

Contributors and Consultants iv
Foreword...v
How to Use this Book................................vii

Part I: Drug Profiles **1**

Part II: Disease Overviews **711**
1. New Hope for Heart Patients.............711
2. Defusing High Blood Pressure............721
3. Coping with Arthritis.........................725
4. Osteoporosis, Back Pain, and Other
    Bone Disorders 731
5. Digestive Disorders, Minor
    and Major...737
6. Defeating the Dangers of
    Respiratory Disease 743
7. Cancer: Improving the Odds
    of a Cure...749
8. New Answers for Pain 759
9. Overcoming Emotional and
    Psychological Problems.....................763
10. OB/GYN Disorders:
    Causes and Treatments 773
11. Birth Control:
    More Options than Ever....................781
12. Handling Familiar
    Childhood Infections 787
13. Ear, Nose, and Throat Disorders........791

14. Relief for Common Allergies 797
15. Dealing with Skin Problems................801
16. Correcting Glandular Disorders 807
17. Counterattacking Major Infections.....813
18. Overcoming Kidney Disease 819
19. Bringing Urinary Disorders
    under Control 825
20. Dealing with Liver Disease 829
21. Facing Up to Sexually
    Transmitted Disease..........................833
22. The Facts about AIDS 841
23. Keeping Diabetes under Control........847
24. Correcting Disorders
    in the Blood 853
25. Relief for Troubled Feet 857
26. Drugs and the Elderly.........................861

Part III Color Photo Section **865**

Appendix 1: Safe medication use 867
Appendix 2: Sugar-free products 869
Appendix 3: Alcohol-free products...........873
Appendix 4: Drugs that may cause
    a reaction to sunlight 876
Appendix 5: Poison control centers 879
Sources 883
Disease and Disorder Index 899
General Index...914

The PDR® Family Guide to Prescription Drugs™

Editorial Director: David W. Sifton
Pharmaceutical Director: Mukesh Mehta, RPh

Text: Healthy Mind Press Inc.: Lawrence D. Chilnick; Regina C. Vengrow; Janet S. Chilnick

Assistant Editors: Ann Ben Larbi; Deborah Epstein; Beret R. Erway; Kris Hallam; Barbara A. Klink; Jayne Jacobson; Theresa Maria O'Neill; MaryJane A. Pantaleo, RN; Sarah G. Terzides

Pharmaceutical Consultants: Paula R. Ajmera, RPh; John Benz, RPh; Brian Cohan, RPh; Bill Doutré, PharmD; Barbara L. Fuhrman, PharmD; Kim Hulko, RPh; Nancy Jacoby, RPh; David R. Shahan, PharmD; Susan Smolinske, RPh; Sharon Vandenberg RPh; Cheryl Voight, PharmD

Editorial Production: Marjorie Duffy, Director of Production; Carrie Williams, Assistant Director of Production; Mildred Schumacher, Format Editor

Creative Director: Gregory Thomas
Art Director: Robert Hartman
Illustrations: Christopher Wikoff, MAMS

Special Acknowledgments: Doreen Adams; James Barron; Michele Barth; Robin Bartlett; Laurie Blumas, RPh; Matthew J. Connell, RPh; Geraldine Connelly; Lindsay DeVane, Pharm D; Marilyn Devroye; Susan Galis; Korey Halsch; Kimberly Hiller; Elizabeth Karst; Margaret McCaffrey; Steve Michel; Dan Montopoli; Bonny Redlich; Bart Rubenstein; A. Michael Velthaus

Product Development Manager: Karen B. Sperber
Senior Vice President of Business Development: Stephen J. Sorkenn

Foreword

Doctors can prescribe and pharmacists dispense, but ultimately it is the patient who manages the way a medicine is taken. Once back home, only the patient can assure that the right doses are administered at the right times, and that the prescribed course of therapy is completed as planned. Likewise, if a side effect or drug interaction develops, it is often the patient who first calls attention to it.

Medical treatment is, of necessity, a partnership—and for it to succeed, both doctor and patient must keep the other informed. The doctor must tell how and why to use a particular drug, what benefits to expect from it, and what significant problems it might cause. By the same token, it's up to the patient to make certain that the doctor knows of the allergies, prior reactions, and pre-existing conditions that could interfere with the doctor's plan.

The PDR Family Guide to Prescription Drugs is offered as an aid in this ongoing collaboration. It serves first as a reminder of the basic instructions and caveats that all too often are forgotten by the time a patient leaves the doctor's office. But just as importantly, it attempts to highlight the problems and conditions that might call for a review of your prescription—facts you must be sure your doctor knows in order to assure the safest, most effective treatment possible.

For almost 50 years, Physicians' Desk Reference has been providing this type of information to doctors in a detailed, technical format approved by the Food and Drug Administration for use by health care professionals. Now, to meet the needs of alert modern consumers, the publishers of PDR have sifted this enormous collection of data for the key facts of greatest concern to the patient, stripped them of medical shorthand and technical terminology, and arranged them in a standard format designed for maximum convenience and ease of use.

Almost all the information you'll find in the Family Guide's consumer drug profiles has been extracted from PDR itself. When necessary, however, information has been added from other sources—in particular, the publisher's Computerized Clinical Information System, used in hospitals throughout the nation. Generally, this extra information describes uses for a drug that are still awaiting formal FDA approval, or supplies instructions meant specifically for the patient, such as how to make up a missed dose.

Finally, to give you added perspective, the book includes a series of chapters that provide a general overview of many common ailments and the ways they can be treated today. As with the drug profiles, these chapters are designed to supplement the information you receive from your doctor, and to aid you in discussing your treatment.

Modern drug therapy is a vast and complicated field—so complicated that, for many questions about medicines, the answer varies with each patient. The PDR Family Guide gives you general guidelines for safe drug use; but only your doctor, evaluating the unique details of your case, can give you the exact instructions best suited for you. Our goal in this book is simply to alert you to the most pertinent questions to ask, and to help clarify your doctor's answers—in short, to give you the tools you need to supervise your own medical care as effectively as possible. We wish you good health.

Robert W. Hogan, M.D.
Chairman, Board of Medical Consultants

How to Use this Book

Modern medicines spare us all an incredible amount of suffering. If you doubt it, imagine a world without antibiotics to cure infections, analgesics to alleviate pain, or any of the many drugs we use to ease stiff joints and help weakened hearts.

But today's potent medicines are not without their risks. For certain people, at certain times, some drugs can cause problems. And for all people, misusing a medication is an invitation to trouble. The purpose of this book is to alert you to those times and those conditions which should make you wary, and to help you use all of your medications safely and effectively.

This book is not a substitute for a doctor's advice. Only a doctor can weigh all the diverse aspects of your condition and choose the treatment most likely to meet your needs. What we hope this book can do, however, is help you sort out the facts and questions that deserve further discussion. Your doctor, after all, can respond only to the problems and concerns you mention. And a seemingly

unimportant question could turn out to be a crucial aspect of your particular case.

The book is divided into two major parts. In the first section, you'll find profiles of the more frequently prescribed medications. The second section gives you an overview of common diseases and disorders, and the types of treatments to expect.

The Drug Profiles

The profiles in this section are designed to give you detailed information on the nation's most frequently prescribed prescription drugs, plus a few widely used over-the-counter medications. Though the section covers more than 1,000 products, it is not all-inclusive. If you do not find a profile for a particular prescription you've received, you shouldn't be concerned. There are a number of specialized yet valuable drugs in current use that have been omitted here due to lack of space.

Most prescription products have two names—a generic chemical name and a manufacturer's brand name. Both are listed alphabetically in this book, with a profile of the drug appearing under the more familiar of the two. In most instances, that means the brand name. In a few cases—such as insulin, for example—the generic name heads the profile. In either case, the drug's other name gives you a cross-reference to the profile.

If there is more than one brand of a drug, you'll usually find the profile under the name that's most frequently prescribed. For example, information on amoxicillin can be found in the profile of Amoxil, the nation's leading brand. Other brands of amoxicillin, such as Wymox and Polymox, are cross-referenced to the Amoxil entry.

The drug profiles are divided into 10 sections. Here's what you'll find in each.

Why is this drug prescribed?

This section provides an overview of the major diseases and disorders for which the drug is generally given. It names each basic problem, but does not go into technical details. For instance, the information here will confirm that a particular antibiotic is used to fight, say, upper respiratory tract infections. The section does not, however, attempt to list all the specific germs that the antibiotic is capable of eliminating.

Most important fact about this drug

Highlighted here is one key point—out of the dozens found in a typical profile—that is especially worthwhile to remember. We've placed it here for the sake of emphasis. Never regard this section as a definitive summary of the drug.

How should you take this medication?

Some drugs should never be taken with meals. Others must be. This section details such special instructions including how and when to take the medication, and any dietary restrictions that may apply.

What side effects may occur?

Shown here are the potential side effects that the manufacturer has listed in the drug's FDA-approved product labeling. Virtually any drug will occasionally cause an unwanted reaction. However, even the most common of these reactions is generally seen in only a small minority of patients. For that reason, presence of a long list of possible side effects does not mean that the drug is unusually dangerous or trouble-prone. In fact, your odds of experiencing even one of these effects are typically very low; and they are listed here merely as an extra precaution in the unlikely event that one does occur. Not listed are the few side effects that can be detected only by a physician or by analysis in a laboratory.

Why should this drug not be prescribed?

A few drugs are known to be harmful under certain specific conditions, which are detailed here—the most common being hypersensitivity to the drug itself. If you think one of these restrictions applies to you, you should alert your doctor immediately. If you're correct, he or she may decide to use an alternative treatment.

Special warnings about this medication

This cautionary information is presented as a double check. If it includes any problems or conditions that your doctor may be unaware of, be sure to bring them to his or her attention. Chances are that no change in treatment will be called for; but it's worth making sure. In any event, do not take this information as a signal to change your dosage or discontinue the drug without consulting your doctor. Such a change might well do more harm than good.

Possible food and drug interactions when taking this medication

In this section you'll find a list of specific drugs—and types of drugs—that have been known to interact with the medicine being profiled. Generally, the list includes a few examples of each type. However, it is far from inclusive. If you're not certain whether a medication you're taking falls into one of these categories, be sure to check with your doctor or pharmacist. Pharmacies are now required to advise you of possible interactions if you so request.

Remember, too, that the chances of an interaction—and its intensity if one occurs—vary from person to person. In many cases, the benefits of the two medicines may outweigh the results of an interaction. Don't stop taking either drug without first consulting your doctor.

Special information if you are pregnant or breastfeeding

Very few medicines have been definitely proved safe for use during pregnancy. On the other hand, only a handful are known to be inevitably harmful. Most drugs fall in-between, in a gray area where no harm has been reported, but neither has safety been conclusively proved. With many of these drugs, the small theoretical risk they pose may be overshadowed by your need for treatment.

This section will tell you whether a drug has been confirmed safe, is known to be dangerous, or is part of that large group about which scientists are not really sure. If you are pregnant or planning a pregnancy,

and one of your medicines falls into this questionable category, the best thing to do is check with your doctor immediately. He or she can tell you whether your need for the medicine outweighs any possible risk.

Recommended dosage

Shown here are excerpts of the dosage guidelines your doctor uses. They generally present a range of doses recommended for typical cases, and sometimes include a recommended maximum. The information is presented as a convenient double-check in case you suspect a misunderstanding or a typographical error on your prescription label. It is not useful for determining an exact dosage yourself. The dose that's best for you depends on numerous factors—such as your age, weight, physical condition, and response to the drug—that can be properly evaluated only by your doctor.

Overdosage

As another safety measure, this section lists, when available, the signs of an overdose. Treatment is usually quite complex, and requires specialized medical training; so we have not attempted to summarize it here. If the symptoms listed in this section lead you to suspect an overdose, your best response is to seek emergency attention immediately.

The Disease Overviews

Though each drug profile gives you a thorough rundown on a particular medication, none of the profiles addresses the larger question of alternative therapies. To accomplish that, this second major section presents a series of very brief, highly condensed surveys of major health problems and the treatments currently used to combat them. Only generally accepted treatments are included, and none is described in detail. The aim is merely to give you insight into the problem itself, and to brief you on the range of treatments your doctor has at his or her disposal.

When reviewing this material, it's important to remember that every drug and every treatment has specific benefits and drawbacks, and that your doctor must weigh these against the unique details of your personal physical condition when prescribing a medication. It's more than likely that your prescription is the best—and in some cases, the only—remedy that's right for you. But if you have reason to suspect that it's not working as intended, you shouldn't hesitate to ask your doctor about it. If one of the alternatives mentioned here is appropriate for you, he or she may decide it's time to try it.

The Disease and Disorder Index

To quickly identify drugs available for a particular problem, you can turn to this special index. Arranged alphabetically by ailment, it lists all the alternatives profiled in the book. (You'll also find a regular general index nearby.)

The Color Photo Section

It's wise to keep all your prescription medications in their original bottles or vials. However, if they do somehow get mixed up, you may find this section helpful for sorting them out. It includes actual-size photographs of the leading products discussed in the book. Because some of the more common generic alternatives are shown along with the brand-name drugs, the section is arranged by each drug's generic name.

Manufacturers occasionally change the color and shape of a product, so if a prescription does not match the photo shown here, do check with your pharmacist, but don't automatically assume there's been a mistake.

The Appendices

For ready reference in case of emergency, you'll find a directory of regional poison control centers near the back cover of the book. Also found nearby is a set of tips for safe medication use, as well as lists of drugs that meet certain special conditions, such as those that are sugar or alcohol free, and those that may make you unusually sensitive to light. These lists include prescription and over-the-counter products, and are not limited to brands mentioned in the drug profiles. On the other hand, they are not all-inclusive; so even if a medication fails to appear on a particular list, there's still a chance it may qualify. Check with your pharmacist to be sure.

The Doctor-Patient Partnership

Although doctors today can often work miracles with advanced technology and sophisticated medicines, they still need the help of the patient to make most treatments work. No matter how potent the medication, it can still prove worthless if you fail to take it properly. Likewise, if you react badly to a drug, or have a condition that makes it dangerous, there is nothing any doctor can do about it unless you report the problem.

This book is offered as an aid in this cooperative effort with your doctor. We hope it suggests the right questions to ask, while allaying any unwarranted concerns you might have. Most of all, we hope it helps in some small way to make all of your treatments as effective as can be.

PART ONE

Drug Profiles

Brand name:

A/T/S

See Erythromycin, Topical, page 242.

Brand name:

ACCUTANE

Generic name: Isotretinoin

Why is this drug prescribed?

Accutane, a chemical cousin of vitamin A, is prescribed for the treatment of severe, disfiguring cystic acne that has not cleared up in response to milder medications such as antibiotics. It works on the oil glands within the skin, shrinking them and diminishing their output. You take Accutane by mouth every day for several months, then stop. The antiacne effect can last even after you have finished your course of medication.

Most important fact about this drug

Because Accutane can definitely cause severe birth defects, including mental retardation and physical malformations, a woman *must not* become pregnant while taking it. If you are a woman of childbearing age, your doctor will ask you to sign a detailed consent form before you start taking Accutane. If you accidentally become pregnant while taking the medication, you should immediately consult your doctor to explore the option of having an abortion.

How should you take this medication?

Take Accutane exactly as prescribed by your doctor. The capsules come in strengths of 10, 20, and 40 milligrams. Take the medication with food or milk. A typical schedule is one capsule twice a day, every day for 15 to 20 weeks. Depending on your reaction to Accutane, your doctor may need to adjust the dosage upward or downward.

If you respond quickly and very well (total cyst count reduced by more than 70 percent), the doctor may take you off Accutane even before the 15 or 20 weeks are up.

After you finish taking Accutane, there should be at least a two-month "rest period" during which you are off the drug. This is because your acne may continue to get better even though you are no longer taking the medication. Once the two months are up, if your acne is still severe, your doctor may want to give you a second course of Accutane.

You may experience worsening of acne during the initial period of the treatment. This does not indicate failure, and is not a reason to stop therapy.

Avoid consumption of alcoholic beverages.

Read the patient information leaflet available with the product.

Do not crush the capsules.

Do not take Vitamin A supplements while taking Accutane.

Accutane may cause sensitivity to sunlight. Avoid prolonged exposure to the sun.

What side effects may occur?

Side effects cannot be anticipated. If any develop or change in intensity, inform your doctor as soon as possible. Only your doctor can determine if it is safe for you to continue taking Accutane.

■ *Common side effects may include:*
Conjunctivitis (pinkeye)
Dry or fragile skin
Dry, cracked lips

Dry mouth
Dry nose
Itching
Joint pains
Nosebleed

■ *Less common side effects may include:*
Bowel inflammation and pain, chest pain,
decreased night vision, decreased
tolerance to contact lenses, depression,
fatigue, headache, nausea, vomiting,
peeling palms or soles, rash, skin infections,
stomach discomfort, sunburn-sensitive
skin, thinning hair, urinary discomfort,
vision problems

Why should this drug not be prescribed?

You should not take Accutane if you are
sensitive to or have ever had an allergic
reaction to parabens, the preservative used
in the capsules.

If you are a woman of childbearing age, you
should not take Accutane if you think
there is a possibility you might get pregnant
during the treatment, or if you are unable
to keep coming back to the doctor for
monthly checkups, including pregnancy
testing.

Special warnings about this medication

When you first start taking Accutane,
it is possible that your acne will get
worse before it starts to get better.

If you are a woman of childbearing age and
you are considering taking Accutane,
you will be given both spoken and written
warnings about the importance of
avoiding pregnancy during the treatment. You
will be asked to sign a consent form
noting that:

■ Accutane is a powerful, "last resort"
medication for severe acne;
■ You must not take Accutane if you are
pregnant or may become pregnant
during treatment;
■ If you get pregnant while taking Accutane,
your baby will be at high risk for
birth defects;
■ If you take Accutane, you must use
effective birth control from 1 month
before the start of treatment through 1
month after the end of treatment;
■ You must test negative for pregnancy
within 2 weeks before starting
Accutane, and you must start Accutane
on the second or third day of your
menstrual period;
■ You may participate in a program that
includes an initial free pregnancy test
and birth control counseling session;
■ If you get pregnant, you must immediately
stop taking Accutane and see your
doctor regarding the option of abortion:
■ You have read and understood the
Accutane patient brochure and asked
your doctor any questions you had;
■ You are not currently pregnant and do
not plan to become pregnant for at
least 30 days after you finish taking
Accutane;
■ You have been invited to participate in a
survey of women being treated with
Accutane.

Some people taking Accutane, including some
who simultaneously took tetracycline, have
experienced headache, nausea, and visual
disturbances caused by increased pressure
within the skull. See a doctor immediately if
you have these symptoms; if the doctor
finds swelling of the optic nerve at the back
of your eye, you must stop taking Accutane
at once and see a neurologist for further care.

Be careful driving at night.

Some people taking Accutane have
had problems regulating their blood
sugar level.

You should not donate blood during your therapy with Accutane and for at least a month after you stop taking it.

Possible food and drug interactions when taking this medication

While taking Accutane, do not take vitamin supplements containing vitamin A. Accutane and vitamin A are chemically related; taking them together is like taking an overdose of vitamin A.

Special information if you are pregnant or breastfeeding

Accutane causes birth defects; do not use it while pregnant. Nursing mothers should not take Accutane because of the possibility of passing the drug on to the baby via breast milk.

Recommended dosage

The recommended dosage range for Accutane is 0.5 to 2 milligrams per kilogram (2.2 pounds) of body weight, divided into two doses daily, for 15 to 20 weeks.

It is recommended that for most patients the starting dose of Accutane be 0.5 to 1 milligram per kilogram per day.

Patients whose disease is very severe or is primarily on the body may have to take up to the maximum recommended dose—2 milligrams per kilogram per day.

If after a period of 2 months or more off therapy, severe cystic acne persists, your doctor may prescribe a second course of therapy.

Overdosage

Any medication taken in excess can have serious consequences. If you suspect an overdose, seek medical attention immediately.

Overdosage of Accutane, like overdosage of vitamin A, can cause headache, vomiting, facial flushing, dry, cracked lips, abdominal pain, dizziness, incoordination and clumsiness.

Generic name:

ACEBUTOLOL HYDROCHLORIDE

See Sectral, page 569.

Generic name:

ACETAMINOPHEN

See Tylenol, page 661.

Generic name:

ACETAMINOPHEN WITH CODEINE

See Tylenol with Codeine, page 662.

Generic name:

ACETAZOLAMIDE SODIUM

See Diamox, page 190.

Brand name:

ACHROMYCIN V CAPSULES

Generic name: Tetracycline hydrochloride
Other brand name: Sumycin

Why is this drug prescribed?

Achromycin V, a "broad-spectrum" antibiotic, is used to treat bacterial infections such as Rocky Mountain spotted fever, typhus fever, and tick fevers; upper respiratory infections such as strep throat; pneumonia; gonorrhea; amoebic infections; and urinary tract infections caused by bacteria such as E. coli, streptoccocus, Shigella, staphylococcus, and chlamydia. It is also used to help treat severe acne and to treat trachoma (a chronic eye infection), and conjunctivitis (pink-eye). Tetracycline is often an alternative drug for people who are allergic to penicillin.

Most important fact about this drug
Tetracycline should not be used during the last half of pregnancy or in children under the age of 8. It may damage developing teeth and cause permanent discoloration.

How should you take this medication?
Achromycin V should be taken exactly as prescribed by your doctor. Be sure to use the entire prescription.

The liquid form of tetracycline should be stored in the refrigerator. Do not freeze. Shake well before using and check the expiration date.

Do not use outdated Achromycin V. Outdated tetracycline is highly toxic to the kidneys.

Do not take antacids containing aluminum, calcium, or magnesium (e.g., Mylanta, Maalox) while taking this medication. They will affect the absorption of the drug.

Take Achromycin V 1 hour before or 2 hours after meals. Foods, milk, and some dairy products affect absorption of the drug.

Achromycin V should be continued for at least 24 to 48 hours after your symptoms have subsided.

What side effects may occur?
Side effects cannot be anticipated. If any occur or change in intensity, inform your doctor as soon as possible. Only your doctor can determine if it is safe for you to continue taking Achromycin V.

■ *More common side effects may include:*
Blurred vision and headache (in adults), bulging soft spot (in infants), diarrhea, difficult or painful swallowing, extreme allergic reactions, genital or anal sores or rash, hives, inflammation of large bowel, inflammation of the tongue, increased sensitivity to light, loss of appetite, nausea, rash, swelling due to fluid accumulation, vomiting

■ *Less common or rare side effects may include:*
Anemia, blood disorders, liver poisoning, peeling, inflamed skin

Why should this drug not be prescribed?
Do not take this medication if you are sensitive to or have ever had an allergic reaction to Achromycin V or any other tetracycline medication.

Special warnings about this medication
If you have kidney disease, your doctor should prescribe a lower than customary dose of Achromycin V and carefully monitor your kidney function while you are taking the medication.

Tetracycline drugs can make you more prone to sunburn when you are in sunlight or ultraviolet light. Take appropriate precautions.

Some adults may develop a headache and blurred vision while taking tetracycline, and infants may develop a bulging soft spot. Contact your doctor if you experience or notice these symptoms. They usually disappear soon after the medication is stopped.

As with other antibiotics, use of this medication may cause other infections to develop. Contact your doctor if this occurs.

If you are taking Achromycin V over an extended period of time, your doctor should perform blood, kidney, and liver tests periodically.

Possible food and drug interactions when taking this medication

If Achromycin V is taken with certain other drugs, the effects of either could be increased, decreased, or altered. It is especially important to check with your doctor before combining Achromycin V with the following:

Antacids containing aluminum, calcium, or magnesium
Blood thinners (Coumadin, Panwarfin)
Oral contraceptives
Penicillin

Special information
if you are pregnant or breastfeeding

Achromycin V is not recommended for use during pregnancy. It can affect the development of the unborn child's bones and teeth. If you are pregnant or plan to become pregnant, inform your doctor immediately. Achromycin V appears in breast milk and may affect a nursing infant. If this medication is essential to your health, your doctor may recommend that you stop breastfeeding until your treatment is finished.

Recommended dosage

Your doctor will adjust your dose on the basis of the condition to be treated, your age and risk factors such as kidney problems.

Use of this drug should continue for at least 24 to 48 hours after symptoms and fever have subsided. For a streptococcal infection, doses should be taken for at least 10 days.

ADULTS

For most infections, the usual daily dose is 1 to 2 grams divided into 2 or 4 equal doses, depending on severity.

For treatment of brucellosis
The usual dose is 500 milligrams 4 times daily for 3 weeks; the drug should be accompanied by streptomycin.

For treatment of syphilis
A total of 30 to 40 grams, divided into equal doses over a period of 10 to 15 days, should be taken.

Gonorrhea patients sensitive to penicillin can take tetracycline, starting with 1.5 grams, followed by 0.5 gram every 6 hours for 4 days, to a total dosage of 9 grams.

For urethral, endocervical, or rectal infection in adults caused by Chlamydia trachomatis
The usual dose is 500 milligrams, 4 times a day for at least 7 days.

CHILDREN 8 YEARS OF AGE AND ABOVE

The usual daily dose is 10 to 20 milligrams per pound of body weight divided into 2 or 4 equal doses.

Overdosage

Any medication taken in excess can have serious consequences. Seek medical attention immediately if you suspect an overdose of Achromycin V.

Brand name:

ACLOVATE

Generic name: Alclometasone dipropionate

Why is this drug prescribed?

Aclovate, a synthetic steroid medication of the cortisone family, is spread on the skin to relieve certain types of itchy rashes, including psoriasis. It can be bought in cream or ointment form.

Most important fact about this drug

Although the drug in Aclovate is intended to act only on the skin where it is applied, some of it does get absorbed through the skin and into the bloodstream. Try to minimize such absorption. Unless your doctor specifically instructs otherwise, do not use waterproof coverings, such as adhesive bandages, diapers, or plastic pants on top of Aclovate, as they will increase the drug's absorption.

How should you use this medication?

Use Aclovate exactly as prescribed by your doctor and only to treat the condition for which your doctor prescribed it. The usual procedure is to spread a thin film of Aclovate cream or ointment over the rash and massage gently until the medication disappears. Do this 2 or 3 times a day.

For areas of deep-seated, persistent rash, your doctor may recommend a thick layer of Aclovate cream or ointment topped with waterproof bandaging, to be left in place for 1 to 4 days. If necessary, this procedure may be repeated 3 or 4 times. Do not use bandaging at all, however, unless your doctor so advises.

What side effects may occur?

Side effects cannot be anticipated. If any develop or change in intensity, inform your doctor as soon as possible. Only your doctor can determine if it is safe for you to continue taking Aclovate.

■ *Common side effects include:*
Abnormally excessive growth of hair, acne-like pimples, allergic rash, burning, dryness, infected hair follicles, infection, irritation, itching, maceration (sponginess), pale (depigmented) spots, prickly heat, rash around the mouth, redness, skin inflammation, stretch marks on skin

Why should this drug not be prescribed?

Do not use Aclovate if you are sensitive to or have ever had an allergic reaction to alclometasone dipropionate (the active ingredient) or other corticosteriods, or to any of the oils, waxes, alcohols, or other chemicals in the cream or ointment.

Special warnings about this medication

Aclovate is for external use only. Do not let the cream or ointment get into your eyes.

If you use Aclovate over large areas of skin for prolonged periods of time, the amount of hormone absorbed into your bloodstream may eventually lead to Cushing's syndrome: a moon-faced appearance, fattened neck and truck, and purplish streaks on the skin. Children, because of their relatively larger ratio of skin surface to body weight, are particularly susceptible to overabsorption of hormone from Aclovate.

Possible food and drug interactions when taking this medication

Check with your doctor before combining Aclovate with other more potent steroids, since this could lead to undesirably large amounts of hormone circulating in your bloodstream.

Special information if you are pregnant or breastfeeding

Drug absorbed from Aclovate cream or ointment into the bloodstream may find its way across the placenta and into an unborn child's blood, or it may seep into breast milk. To avoid any possible harm to your child, use Aclovate very sparingly—and only with your doctor's permission—if you are pregnant or nursing a baby.

Recommended dosage

Apply a thin film of Aclovate cream or ointment to the affected skin areas 2 or 3 times daily; massage gently until the medication disappears.

Bandages that block out air may be used to control psoriasis and other severe skin rashes.

To prevent evaporation of Aclovate from the skin, use an airtight bandage as follows:

1. Cover the affected area with a thick layer of Aclovate cream or ointment and a light gauze dressing, then cover the area with a pliable plastic film.
2. Seal the edges to the normal skin by adhesive tape or other means.
3. Leave the dressing in place 1 to 4 days and repeat the procedure 3 or 4 times as needed. With this method of treatment, marked improvement is often seen in a few days. If an infection develops, the use of airtight bandages should be discontinued, and your doctor will recommend an alternative treatment.

Overdosage

Any medication taken in excess can have serious consequences. If you suspect an overdose, seek medical attention immediately.

In a child, an overdose of Aclovate may cause increased pressure within the skull leading to bulging fontanelles (in infants), headache, and nausea or vomiting. If this happens, see a doctor without delay.

Over the long term, overuse of Aclovate can interfere with a child's normal growth and development.

Brand name:

ACTIGALL

Generic name: Ursodiol

Why is this drug prescribed?

Actigall is used to help dissolve certain kinds of gallstones. If you suffer from gallstones but do not want to undergo surgery to remove them, or if age or infirmity make you a poor candidate for surgery, Actigall treatment may be a good alternative.

Most important fact about this drug

Actigall is not a quick remedy. It takes months of Actigall therapy to dissolve gallstones; and there is a possibility of incomplete dissolution and recurrence of stones. Your doctor will weigh Actigall against alternative treatments and recommend the best one for you.

Actigall is most effective if your gallstones are small or "floatable" (i.e., high cholesterol content). In addition, your gallbladder must still be functioning properly.

How should you take this medication?

Actigall should be taken exactly as prescribed by your doctor; otherwise the gallstones may dissolve slowly or not dissolve at all. During treatment, you should have periodic ultrasound exams to see if your stones are dissolving.

What side effects may occur?

Side effects cannot be anticipated. If any develop or change in intensity, inform your doctor as soon as possible. Only your doctor can determine if it is safe for you to continue taking Actigall.

■ *Side effects may include:*
Abdominal pain, anxiety, appetite loss, back pain, constipation, cough, depression, dry skin, fatigue, gas, hair thinning, headache, hives, indigestion, itching, metallic taste, mild, temporary diarrhea, muscle and joint pain, nausea, rash, runny nose, severe pain in the upper right side of the abdomen, sleep disorders, sweating, vomiting

Why should this drug not be prescribed?

Do not take this medication if you are sensitive to or have ever had an allergic reaction to ursodiol (ursodeoxycholic acid) or to other bile acids.

Actigall will not dissolve certain types of gallstones. If your doctor tells you that your gallstones are calcified cholesterol stones, radio-opaque stones, or radiolucent bile pigment stones, you are not a candidate for treatment with Actigall.

Also, if you have biliary tract problems or certain liver and pancreas diseases, your doctor may not be able to prescribe Actigall.

Special warnings about this medication

Although Actigall is not known to cause liver damage, it is theoretically possible in some people with a particular body chemistry. Thus, your doctor should check the levels of liver enzymes in your blood before you start to take Actigall and again while you are taking it.

Possible food and drug interactions when taking this medication

If Actigall is taken with certain other drugs, the effects of either could be increased, decreased, or altered. It is especially important to check with your doctor before combining Actigall with the following:

Aluminum-based antacid medications (Alu-Cap, Alu-Tab, Rolaids, and others)
Birth control pills
Certain cholesterol-lowering medications, such as cholestyramine (Questran) and colestipol (Colestid)
Estrogens (Premarin and others)
Lipid-lowering medications (Atromid-S and others)

Special information
if you are pregnant or breastfeeding

If you are pregnant or plan to become pregnant, inform your doctor immediately. So far there is no evidence that Actigall can harm an unborn baby; but to be safe, the medication is not recommended during pregnancy. Caution is needed during breastfeeding; it is not known whether Actigall taken by a nursing mother passes into her breast milk.

Recommended dosage

The recommended dose for Actigall treatment of radiolucent gallbladder stones is 8 to 10 milligrams per kilogram (2.2 pounds) per day divided into 2 or 3 doses.

Overdosage

Although there have been no reports of overdose with Actigall, the most likely symptom of severe overdose would be diarrhea. Since any medication taken in excess can have serious consequences, you should seek medical attention immediately if you suspect an Actigall overdose.

Generic name:

ACYCLOVIR

See Zovirax, page 704.

Brand name:

ADALAT

See Procardia, page 505.

Brand name:

ADAPIN

See Sinequan, page 581.

Brand name:

ADVIL

See Motrin, page 393.

Brand name:

AEROBID

Generic name: Flunisolide

Why is this drug prescribed?

AeroBid, an anti-inflammatory steroid, is a cortisone-like metered-dose aerosol system prescribed for patients who need long-term treatment to control the symptoms of bronchial asthma.

Most important fact about this drug

Steroid medications suppress the activity of the adrenal glands. Deaths due to adrenal insufficiency have occurred in asthmatic patients during and after transfer from steroid tablets to such aerosol steroids as AeroBid Inhaler.

If your doctor has reduced your dosage or has discontinued your treatment with a form of steroid medication, such as tablets, that affects the whole body as opposed to specific parts or organs (systemic corticosteroids) and has transferred you to treatment with AeroBid Inhaler, you should carry a warning card indicating that you may need supplemental systemic corticosteroid treatment during periods of stress or a severe asthma attack not responsive to bronchodilators.

How should you take this medication?

AeroBid Inhaler is not used as a broncho-dilator (a drug that widens the airways in the lungs) and is not for rapid relief of bronchial asthma attacks.

Take this medication at regular intervals, exactly as prescribed by your doctor. Taking doses higher than your doctor has prescribed may impair the function of your adrenal glands.

If you are also using a bronchodilator inhalant, it should be used before the AeroBid inhalant to derive the best effects from this drug. Use of the two inhalers should be separated by several minutes.

To help reduce hoarseness and dry mouth, rinse with water or mouthwash after each use.

Illustrated instructions for use are available with the product.

What side effects may occur?

Side effects cannot be anticipated. If any develop or change in intensity, inform your doctor as soon as possible. Only your doctor can determine if it is safe for you to continue taking AeroBid.

■ *More common side effects may include:*
Cold symptoms
Diarrhea
Flu
Headache
Nasal congestion
Nausea
Sore throat
Unpleasant taste
Upset stomach
Vomiting

■ *Less common side effects may include:*
Abdominal pain, chest congestion, chest pain, cough, decreased appetite, dizziness, ear infection, fever, heartburn, hoarseness, irritability, itching, loss of smell or taste, menstrual disturbances, nasal discharge, nervousness, phlegm, pounding heartbeat, rash, runny nose, shakiness, sinus congestion, sinus drainage, sinus infection, sinus inflammation, sneezing, swelling due to fluid retention, wheezing, yeastlike fungal infection

■ *Rare side effects may include:*
Acne, anxiety, blurred vision, chest tightness, chills, constipation, depression, dry throat, earache, excessive restlessness, eye

discomfort, eye infection, faintness, fatigue, gas, general feeling of illness, head stuffiness, high blood pressure, hives, inability to fall or stay asleep, increased appetite, indigestion, inflammation of the tongue, laryngitis, moodiness, mouth irritation, nasal irritation, nosebleed, numbness, pneumonia, rapid heart rate, shortness of breath, sinus discomfort, sluggishness, sweating, throat irritation, vertigo, weakness, weight gain

Why should this drug not be prescribed?

AeroBid should not be used if your asthma can be controlled with bronchodilators and other non-steroid medications.

This medication should not be used if you require only occasional corticosteroid treatment for asthma. It is not for treatment of prolonged, severe asthma attacks where more intensive measures are required.

AeroBid should not be used for the treatment of non-asthmatic bronchitis.

If you are allergic or sensitive to AeroBid or other steroid drugs, advise your doctor before using this medication.

Special warnings about this medication

A patient's asthma should be reasonably stable before treatment with AeroBid Inhaler is started. AeroBid should be started in combination with a patient's usual maintenance dose of systemic or oral steroid. After approximately 1 week, gradual withdrawal of the systemic steroid should be started by reducing the daily or alternate daily dose. A slow rate of withdrawal is very important, as some patients have experienced systemic steroid withdrawal symptoms such as joint and/or muscular pain, fatigue, and depression.

This medication is not useful when rapid relief of asthma symptoms is needed.

Transfer of patients from steroid tablet therapy to AeroBid Inhaler may produce allergic conditions that were previously controlled by steroid tablet therapy. These include rhinitis (inflammation of the mucous membrane of the nose), conjunctivitis (pink-eye), and eczema.

Patients treated with AeroBid should be carefully observed by their doctor for any evidence of adverse effects such as the suppression of bone growth in children. Postoperative patients or patients experiencing extreme stress should also be closely monitored.

The use of AeroBid may cause a yeastlike fungal infection of the mouth, pharynx (throat), or larynx (voice box). If you suspect a fungal infection, notify your doctor. Treatment with antifungal medication may be necessary.

Since the contents of this inhalant are under pressure, do not puncture the container and do not use or store the medication near heat or an open flame. Exposure to temperatures above 120 degrees may cause the container to explode.

Possible food and drug interactions when taking this medication

Inhaled corticosteroids such as AeroBid are not recommended for long-term use with alternate-day prednisone treatment.

Special information if you are pregnant or breastfeeding

The effects of AeroBid during pregnancy have not been adequately studied. If you are pregnant or plan to become pregnant, inform your doctor immediately. It is not known whether AeroBid appears in breast milk. If this medication is essential to your health, your doctor may advise you to discontinue breastfeeding your baby until your treatment with this medication is finished.

Recommended dosage

The AeroBid Inhaler system is for oral inhalation only.

ADULTS

The recommended starting dose is 2 inhalations twice daily, in the morning and evening, for a total daily dose of 1 milligram. The daily dose should not exceed 4 inhalations twice a day, for a total daily dose of 2 milligrams.

When AeroBid is used long term at 2 milligrams per day, periodic monitoring by your doctor is recommended.

CHILDREN

For children 6 to 15 years of age, 2 inhalations may be administered twice daily, for a total daily dose of 1 milligram.

Long-term use of AeroBid in children should be monitored by your doctor for effects on growth and adrenal gland function.

The safety and effectiveness of this drug have not been established in children under 6 years of age.

Overdosage

Any medication taken in excess can have serious consequences. If you suspect an overdose, seek emergency medical treatment immediately.

Generic name:

ALBUTEROL SULFATE

See Proventil, page 518.

Generic name:

ALCLOMETASONE DIPROPIONATE

See Aclovate, page 5.

Brand name:

ALDACTAZIDE

Generic ingredients: Spironolactone, Hydrochlorothiazide
Other brand name: Spirozide

Why is this drug prescribed?

Aldactazide is used in the treatment of high blood pressure and other conditions that require the elimination of excess fluid (water) from the body. These conditions include congestive heart failure, cirrhosis of the liver, and kidney disease. Aldactazide combines two diuretic drugs that help your body produce and eliminate more urine. Spironolactone, one of the ingredients, helps to minimize the potassium loss that can be caused by the hydrochlorothiazide component.

Most important fact about this drug

This medication should be used only if your doctor has determined that the precise amount of each ingredient in Aldactazide meets your specific needs.

How should you take this medication?

Take Aldactazide exactly as prescribed by your doctor. Stopping Aldactazide suddenly could cause your condition to worsen.

If you forget to take a dose, take it as soon as you remember. If it is almost time for your next dose, skip the one you missed and go back to your regular schedule. Never take two doses at the same time.

What side effects may occur?

Side effects cannot be anticipated. If any develop or change in intensity, inform your doctor as soon as possible. Only your doctor can determine if it is safe for you to continue taking Aldactazide.

■ *Side effects may include:*
Abdominal cramps, breast development in males, change in potassium levels leading to symptoms like dry mouth, excessive thirst, weak or irregular heartbeat, muscle pain or cramps, deepening of the voice, diarrhea, dizziness, dizziness on rising, drowsiness, excessive hairiness, fever, headache, hives, inflammation of blood vessels or lymph vessels, inflammation of the pancreas, irregular menstruation, lack of coordination, loss of appetite, mental confusion, muscle spasms, nausea, postmenopausal bleeding, rash, red or purple spots on skin, restlessness, sensitivity to light, sexual dysfunction, sluggishness, stomach bleeding, stomach inflammation, stomach ulcers, tingling or pins and needles, vertigo, vomiting, weakness, yellow eyes and skin, yellow vision

Why should this drug not be prescribed?

Aldactazide should not be used if you have acute kidney disease or liver failure, have difficulty urinating or are unable to urinate or have high potassium levels in your blood.

If you are sensitive to or have ever had an allergic reaction to spironolactone, hydrochlorothiazide or similar drugs, or if you are sensitive to other sulfonamide-derived drugs, you should not take this medication. Make sure your doctor is aware of any drug reactions you may have experienced.

Special warnings about this medication

Potassium supplements (including salt substitutes) or other potassium-sparing diuretics should not be used while taking Aldactazide, unless specifically recommended by your doctor.

If you are taking an ACE inhibitor medication such as Vasotec, this drug should be used with extreme caution.

If you have liver disease or collagen vascular disease (lupus erythematosus), Aldactazide should be used with caution.

Excessive sweating, dehydration, severe diarrhea or vomiting could cause you to lose too much water and cause your blood pressure to become too low. Be careful when exercising and in hot weather.

Notify your doctor or dentist that you are taking Aldactazide if you have a medical emergency, and before you have surgery or dental treatment.

Possible food and drug interactions when taking this medication

If Aldactazide is taken with certain other drugs, the effects of either could be increased, decreased, or altered. It is especially important to check with your doctor before combining Aldactazide with the following:

ACE inhibitors such as Vasotec
Antigout medications such as Zyloprim
Digoxin (Lanoxin)
Glucocorticoids such as Prednisone
Indomethacin (Indocin)
Insulin or oral antidiabetic drugs such as
    Micronase
Lithium
Loop diuretics (Lasix)
Norepinephrine (Levophed)
Potassium-sparing diuretics such as Midamor
Potassium supplements
Tubocurarine

Special Information
If you are pregnant or breastfeeding

The effects of Aldactazide during pregnancy have not been adequately studied. If you are pregnant or plan to become pregnant, inform your doctor immediately. Aldactazide appears in breast milk and could affect a nursing infant. If this medication is essential to your health, your doctor may advise you to discontinue breastfeeding until your treatment is finished.

Recommended dosage

ADULTS

For Congestive Heart Failure, Cirrhosis, Nephrotic Syndrome (kidney disorder)
The usual dosage is 100 milligrams each of spironolactone and hydrochlorothiazide daily, taken as a single dose or in divided doses. Dosage may range from 25 milligrams to 200 milligrams of each ingredient daily, depending on the individual needs of the patient.

High Blood Pressure
The usual dose is 50 milligrams to 100 milligrams each of spironolactone and hydrochlorthiazide daily, in a single dose or in divided doses.

CHILDREN

The usual dose of Aldactazide should provide 0.75 milligram to 1.5 milligrams of spironolactone per pound of body weight.

ELDERLY

Dosage should be determined by the particular needs of the elderly patient.

Aldactazide is supplied in tablets containing 25 milligrams of spironolactone and 25 milligrams of hydrochlorothiazide and in tablets containing 50 milligrams of each ingredient.

Overdosage

Any medication taken in excess can cause symptoms of overdose. If you suspect an overdose, seek medical attention immediately.

There is no information on specific signs of Aldactazide overdose.

Brand name:

ALDACTONE

Generic name: Spironolactone

Why is this drug prescribed?

Aldactone is a diuretic and high blood pressure medication. It is used in the diagnosis and treatment of hyperaldosteronism, a condition in which the adrenal gland secretes too much aldosterone (a hormone that regulates the body's salt and potassium levels.) It is also used in treating other conditions that require the elimination of excess fluid (water) from the body. These conditions include congestive heart failure, high blood pressure, cirrhosis of the liver, kidney disease and unusually low potassium levels in the blood. When used for high blood pressure, Aldactone can be used alone or with other high blood pressure medications. Aldactone causes increased amounts of sodium and water to be eliminated, without potassium loss.

Most important fact about this drug

If you have high blood pressure, you must take Aldactone regularly for it to be effective. Even if you are feeling well, you need the medication to maintain control of your blood pressure.

How should you take this medication?

Take Aldactone exactly as prescribed by your doctor. Stopping Aldactone suddenly could cause your condition to worsen.

If you forget to take a dose, take it as soon as you remember. If it is almost time for your next dose, skip the one you missed and go back to your regular schedule. Never take two doses at the same time.

What side effects may occur?

Side effects cannot be anticipated. If any develop or change in intensity, inform your doctor as soon as possible. Only your doctor can determine if it is safe for you to continue taking Aldactone.

■ *Side effects may include:*
Abdominal cramps, breast development in males, change in potassium levels leading to symptoms like dry mouth, excessive thirst, weak or irregular heartbeat, muscle pain or cramps, deepening of voice, diarrhea, drowsiness, excessive hairiness, fever, headache, hives, irregular menstruation, lack of coordination, lethargy, mental confusion, postmenopausal bleeding, sexual dysfunction, skin eruptions, stomach bleeding, stomach inflammation, ulcers, vomiting

Why should this drug not be prescribed?

You should not take Aldactone if you have kidney disease, an inability to urinate, difficulty urinating, or high potassium levels in your blood.

Special warnings about this medication

Potassium supplements or other potassium-sparing diuretics such as Maxzide should not be used while taking Aldactone, unless specifically indicated by your doctor.

ACE inhibitors (Vasotec, Capoten) used for blood pressure and heart failure, should not be taken while using Aldactone.

If you are taking Aldactone, your kidney function should be given a complete assessment and should continue to be monitored.

If you have liver disease, this medication should be used with caution.

Excessive sweating, dehydration, severe diarrhea or vomiting could cause you to lose too much water and cause your blood pressure to become too low. Be careful when exercising and in hot weather.

Notify your doctor or dentist that you are taking Aldactone if you have a medical emergency, and before you have surgery or dental treatment.

Possible food and drug interactions when taking this medication

If Aldactone is taken with certain other drugs, the effects of either could be increased, decreased, or altered. It is especially important to check with your doctor before combining Aldactone with the following:

ACE inhibitors (Vasotec, Capoten)
Digoxin (Lanoxin)
Indomethacin (Indocin)
Norepinephrine (Levophed)
Other diuretics
Other high blood pressure medications

Special information
if you are pregnant or breastfeeding

The effects of Aldactone during pregnancy have not been adequately studied. If you are pregnant or plan to become pregnant, inform your doctor immediately. Aldactone appears in breast milk and could affect a nursing infant. If this medication is essential to your health, your doctor may advise you to discontinue breastfeeding until your treatment with this medication is finished.

Recommended dosage

ADULTS

Primary Hyperaldosteronism
Initial dosages of this medication are used

to determine the presence of primary hyperaldosteronism (too much secretion of the adrenal hormone aldosterone). Patients can be tested with this medication over either a long or a short period of time.

In the long test, the patient takes 400 milligrams per day for 3 to 4 weeks. If potassium levels and blood pressure are corrected with this dosage in this time period, your physician may assume you have this condition.

In the short test, the patient receives 400 milligrams per day for 4 days. A laboratory test is performed to compare potassium levels while on Aldactone and after the medication is stopped. Your doctor may then make a diagnosis.

After the diagnosis of primary hyperaldosteronism is made and confirmed by more tests, the usual dose is 100 to 400 milligrams per day, prior to surgery. In patients who are not good candidates for surgery, this drug is given over the long term at the lowest effective dose.

Adult Edema (Congestive Heart Failure, Cirrhosis of the Liver or Kidney Disorders)
The usual starting dosage is 100 milligrams daily in either a single or divided dose. However, daily doses as low as 25 milligrams and as high as 200 milligrams may be given.

Your doctor may choose to adjust your dosage after an initial 5-day trial period or add another diuretic medication to this one.

Essential Hypertension
The usual starting dosage is 50 to 100 milligrams daily in a single dose or divided into smaller doses. This medication can be given with another diuretic or with other high blood pressure medications that has a more direct effect on the kidneys.

It may take up to 2 weeks before the full effect of this medication is seen. Dosage can then be adjusted according to your response.

Hypokalemia (Potassium Loss)
Daily dosages of 25 milligrams to 100 milligrams may by used when potassium loss caused by the effects of a diuretic cannot be treated by a potassium supplement.

CHILDREN

Edema (Swelling Due to Water Retention)
The usual starting dosage is 1.5 milligrams per pound of body weight daily in a single or smaller dose.

Aldactone comes in tablets containing 25 milligrams, 50 milligrams, or 100 milligrams of spironolactone.

Overdosage

Any medication taken in excess can cause symptoms of overdose. If you suspect an overdose, seek medical attention immediately.

No specific information or signs of Aldactone overdose is available.

Brand name:

ALDOMET

Generic name: Methyldopa

Why is this drug prescribed?
Aldomet is used to treat high blood pressure. It is effective when used alone or with other high blood pressure medications.

Most important fact about this drug
Aldomet must be taken regularly for it to be effective. Continue taking it even if you are feeling well. Your high blood pressure will return if you stop.

How should you take this medication?

Take this medication exactly as prescribed by your doctor.

Try not to miss any doses. Do not stop taking the drug without your doctor's knowledge.

Drowsiness may occur when dosage is increased. If your doctor increases the amount of Aldomet you take, start the new dosage in the evening.

If you miss a dose of this medicine, take it as soon as you remember. If it is almost time for your next dose, skip the one you missed and go back to your regular schedule. Never take two doses at the same time.

What side effects may occur?

Side effects cannot be anticipated. If any develop or change in intensity, inform your doctor as soon as possible. Only your doctor can determine if it is safe for you to continue taking Aldomet.

■ *More common side effects may include:*
Drowsiness during first few weeks of
  therapy
Fluid retention or weight gain
Headache
Weakness

■ *Less common or rare side effects may include:*
Anemia, Bell's palsy (paralysis of the face, making it look distorted), bloating, blood disorders, breast development in males, breast enlargement, changes in menstruation, chest pain, congestive heart failure, constipation, decreased mental ability, decreased sex drive, depression, diarrhea, dizziness when standing up, dry mouth, fever, gas, hepatitis, impotence, inflammation of the large intestine, inflammation of the pancreas, inflammation of the salivary glands, involuntary movements, joint pain, lightheadedness, liver

disorders, milk production, muscle pain, nasal stuffiness, nausea, nightmares, parkinsonism (tremors, shuffling walk, stooped posture, muscle weakness), rash, slow heartbeat, sore or "black" tongue, tingling or pins and needles, vomiting, yellow eyes and skin

Why should this drug not be prescribed?

If you have liver disease or cirrhosis, or if you have taken Aldomet before and developed liver disease, do not take this medication.

If you are sensitive to or have ever had an allergic reaction to Aldomet, or if you are taking the oral suspension form of Aldomet and have ever had an allergic reaction to sulfites, you should not take this medication.

Special warnings about this medication

Before you begin taking Aldomet, your doctor should perform a complete study of your liver function, and it should be monitored periodically thereafter.

Aldomet can cause liver disorders. You may develop a fever, jaundice (yellow eyes and skin), or both, usually within the first 2 to 3 months of therapy. If either of these symptoms occurs, stop taking Aldomet and contact your doctor immediately. If the fever and/or jaundice were caused by the medication, your liver function should gradually return to normal.

If you have a history of liver disease, this medication should be used with caution.

Hemolytic anemia, a blood disorder in which red blood cells are destroyed, can develop with long-term use of Aldomet, and blood counts should be done periodically thereafter.

Aldomet can cause water retention or weight gain in some people. A diuretic will usually relieve these symptoms.

If you have asthma and are taking the liquid form of Aldomet, you could have an allergic reaction to the sulfite component of the liquid.

If you are a dialysis patient and are taking Aldomet for high blood pressure, your blood pressure may rise after your dialysis treatments.

Aldomet can cause you to become drowsy or less alert, especially during the first few weeks of therapy or when dosage levels are increased. If it affects you this way, driving or operating heavy machinery or participating in any hazardous activity that requires full mental alertness is not recommended.

Notify your doctor or dentist that you are taking Aldomet if you have a medical emergency, and before you have surgery or dental treatment.

Possible food and drug interactions when taking this medication

If Aldomet is taken with certain other drugs, the effects of either could be increased, decreased, or altered. It is especially important to check with your doctor before combining Aldomet with the following:

Anesthetics
Lithium (Eskalith)
Other high blood pressure drugs

Special information
if you are pregnant or breastfeeding

The use of Aldomet during pregnancy appears to be relatively safe. However, if you are pregnant or plan to become pregnant, inform your doctor immediately. Aldomet appears in breast milk and could affect a nursing infant. If this medication is essential to your health, your doctor may advise you to discontinue breastfeeding until your treatment is finished.

Recommended dosage

ADULTS

The usual starting dose is 250 milligrams, 2 or 3 times per day in the first 48 hours of treatment. Your doctor may increase or decrease your dose over the next few days to achieve the correct blood pressure.

To reduce the effect of any sedation the medication may cause, dosage increases will usually be given in the evening.

The usual maintenance dosage is 500 milligrams to 2 grams per day divided into 2 to 4 doses. The maximum dose is usually 3 grams. Some people may be told by their doctor to take the entire daily dose at bedtime.

Your doctor will also adjust your dosage of Aldomet when it is given in combination with certain other high blood pressure drugs.

If it is given with a non-thiazide high blood pressure medicine, the initial dosage should be limited to 500 milligrams daily divided into small doses.

Dosages will be adjusted, and other high blood pressure drugs may be added, during the first few months of treatment with Aldomet. Patients with reduced kidney function may require smaller doses. Older patients who are prone to fainting spells due to arterial disease may also require smaller doses.

CHILDREN

The usual starting dose is 10 milligrams per 2.2 pounds of body weight daily, divided into 2 to 4 doses. Doses will be adjusted until blood pressure is normal. The maximum daily dose is usually 65 milligrams per 2.2 pounds of body weight or 3 grams, whichever is less.

ELDERLY

Dosages of this drug should be adjusted to each individual patient's needs. Lower doses may be prescribed by your doctor.

Overdosage

Any medication taken in excess can cause symptoms of overdose. If you suspect an overdose, seek medical attention immediately.

The symptoms of Aldomet overdose may include:
Bloating, constipation, diarrhea, dizziness, extreme drowsiness, gas, light-headedness, nausea, severely low blood pressure, slow heartbeat, vomiting, weakness

Generic name:

ALLOPURINOL

See Zyloprim, page 705.

Generic name:

ALPRAZOLAM

See Xanax, page 689.

Brand name:

ALTACE

Generic name: Ramipril

Why is this drug prescribed?

Altace is used in the treatment of high blood pressure. It is effective when used alone or when combined with other high blood pressure medications, especially thiazide-type diuretics. Altace works by preventing the conversion of a chemical in your blood called Angiotensin I into a more potent substance that increases salt and water retention in your body. It also enhances blood flow in your circulatory system. It is a member of the group of drugs called ACE inhibitors.

Most important fact about this drug

Since blood pressure drops gradually, it may take several weeks for the full effect of Altace to occur.

How should you take this medication?

Altace works best when taken on an empty stomach, one hour before or two hours after a meal.

Take this medication exactly as prescribed by your doctor.

If you forget to take a dose, take it as soon as you remember. If it is almost time for your next dose, skip the one you missed and go back to your regular schedule. Never take two doses at the same time.

What side effects may occur?

Side effects cannot be anticipated. If any develop or change in intensity, inform your doctor as soon as possible. Only your doctor can determine if it is safe for you to continue taking Altace.

■ *More common side effects may include:*
Cough
Dizziness
Fatigue
Headache
Nausea
Vomiting
Weakness

■ *Less common or rare side effects may include:*
Abdominal pain, angina pectoris, anxiety, change in taste, changes in kidney function, chest pain, constipation, convulsions, depression, diarrhea, difficulty swallowing, dry mouth, fluid retention, hearing loss, heart attack,

impotence, inability to sleep, indigestion, inflammation of the stomach and intestines, irregular heartbeat, itching, joint pain or inflammation, labored breathing, lightheadedness, loss of appetite, low blood pressure, memory loss, nervousness, nosebleed, rash, ringing in ears, skin inflammation, skin sensitivity to light, sleepiness, sudden loss of strength or fainting, tingling or pins and needles, tremors, vertigo, very rapid heartbeat, vision changes, weight gain

Why should this drug not be prescribed?

If you are sensitive to or have ever had an allergic reaction to Altace or similar drugs, or if you have a history of swelling in the mouth or throat, you should not take this medication. Make sure that your doctor is aware of any drug reactions that you have experienced.

Special warnings about this medication

If you develop chest pain, palpitations or other heart effects, swelling of the face, around your lips, tongue or throat or difficulty swallowing, swelling of arms and legs or sore throat and fever, you should contact your doctor immediately. You may have a serious illness or need emergency treatment.

If you are taking Altace your kidney function should be given a complete assessment, and should continue to be monitored.

Altace should be used with caution if you have liver disease.

If you are taking high doses of diuretics and Altace, you may develop excessively low blood pressure.

Do not use salt substitutes containing potassium without consulting your doctor.

Altace may cause you to become drowsy or less alert, especially if you are also taking a water pill (diuretic) at the same time. If it has this effect on you, driving or operating dangerous machinery or participating in any hazardous activity that requires full mental alertness is not recommended.

Dehydration, excessive sweating, severe diarrhea or vomiting could deplete your body's fluids, causing your blood pressure to drop dangerously.

Possible food and drug interactions when taking this medication

If Altace is taken with certain other drugs, the effects of either could be increased, decreased, or altered. It is especially important to check with your doctor before combining Altace with the following:

Diuretics such as Hydrochlorothiazide
Lithium
Potassium-sparing diuretics such as
   Triamterene, Amiloride, Spironolactone
Potassium supplements (salt substitutes)

Special information if you are pregnant or breastfeeding

Altace can cause birth defects, prematurity and death to the fetus and newborn. If you are pregnant or plan to become pregnant and are taking Altace, contact your doctor immediately to discuss the potential hazard to your unborn child. Altace may appear in breast milk and could affect a nursing infant. If this medication is essential to your health, your doctor may advise you to discontinue breastfeeding until your treatment is finished.

Recommended dosage

ADULTS

For patients not on diuretics, the usual starting dose is 2.5 milligrams, taken 1 time a day. After blood pressure is adjusted, dosage should be 2.5 to 20 milligrams a day in a single dose or in 2 equal doses.

Diuretic use should, if possible, be stopped before using Altace. If not, your physician may give an initial dose under his supervision before any further medication is prescribed.

Patients with kidney disorders must be carefully monitored, and dosages will be adjusted to the individual patient's needs, depending on his or her level of kidney function.

CHILDREN

The safety and effectiveness of Altace in children have not been established.

ELDERLY

Dosage should be determined by the particular needs of the elderly patient.

Overdosage

Any medication taken in excess can cause symptoms of overdose. If you suspect an overdose, seek medical attention immediately.

A sudden drop in blood pressure is likely to be the primary effect of an Altace overdose.

Brand name:

ALUPENT

Generic name: Metaproterenol sulfate
Other brand name: Metaprel

Why is this drug prescribed?

Alupent is a bronchodilator prescribed for the prevention and relief of bronchial asthma and bronchial spasms (wheezing) associated with bronchitis and emphysema. Alupent Inhalation Solution is also used to treat acute asthmatic attacks in children 6 years of age and older.

Most important fact about this drug

Alupent's effects last up to 6 hours; therefore, it should not be used more frequently than your doctor recommends.

Increasing the number of doses can be dangerous and may actually make symptoms of asthma worse. Fatalities have occurred with excessive use of this medication.

If the dose your doctor recommends does not provide relief of your symptoms or if your symptoms become worse, seek medical attention immediately.

How should you take this medication?

Take this medication exactly as prescribed by your doctor.

What side effects may occur?

Side effects cannot be anticipated. If any develop or change in intensity, inform your doctor as soon as possible. Only your doctor can determine if it is safe for you to continue taking Alupent.

- *Side effects may include:*
  Cough, dizziness, exaggerated asthma symptoms, headache, high blood pressure, increased heart rate, nausea, nervousness, rapid, strong heartbeat, stomach upset, throat irritation, tremors, vomiting

Side effects can occur when a new container is used, even though the patient has had no trouble with the medication in the past. Replacing the container may solve the problem.

Why should this drug not be prescribed?

If you are sensitive to or have ever had an allergic reaction to Alupent or similar drugs, you should not take this medication. Make sure that your doctor is aware of any drug reactions that you have experienced.

Unless you are directed to do so by your doctor, do not take this medication if you have an irregular, rapid heart rate.

Special warnings about this medication

When taking Alupent, you should not use other inhaled medications (called *sympathomimetics*) before checking with your doctor. Only your doctor can determine the sufficient amount of time between inhaled medications.

A single dose of nebulized Alupent used to treat an acute attack of asthma may not completely stop the attack.

Consult with your doctor before using this medication if you have a heart or convulsive disorder (e.g., epilepsy) high blood pressure, hyperthyroidism or diabetes mellitus.

Possible food and drug interactions when taking this medication

If Alupent is taken with certain other drugs, the effects of either could be increased, decreased, or altered. It is especially important to check with your doctor before combining Alupent with the following:

MAO inhibitors (Nardil)
Other beta adrenergic aerosol bronchodilators (Ventolin, Proventil)
Tricyclic antidepressants (Elavil)

Special information if you are pregnant or breastfeeding

The effects of Alupent during pregnancy have not been adequately studied. If you are pregnant or plan to become pregnant, inform your doctor immediately. It is not known whether Alupent appears in breast milk. If this medication is essential to your health, your doctor may advise you to stop nursing your baby until your treatment is finished.

Recommended dosage

ADULTS

Inhalation Aerosol Dosage
The usual single dose is 2 to 3 inhalations. Inhalation should usually not be repeated more often than about every 3 to 4 hours. Total dosage per day should not exceed 12 inhalations.

Inhalation Solution
Treatment usually need not be repeated more often than every 4 hours to relieve acute attacks of bronchospasm.

As part of a total treatment program for chronic breathing disorders, the inhalation solution may be taken 3 to 4 times per day, as determined by your doctor.

Inhalation Solution 5%
Inhalation solution is given by oral inhalation with the aid of a hand-bulb nebulizer or an intermittent positive pressure breathing (IPPB) apparatus. The usual single daily dose with the nebulizer is 10 inhalations. However, a single dose of 5 to 15 inhalations can be taken, as determined by your doctor.

The usual single daily dose with the IPPB is 0.3 milliliter diluted in approximately 2.5 milliliters of saline solution. The dosage range is 0.2 to 0.3 milliliters, as determined by your doctor.

Inhalation Solution 0.4% and 0.6% Unit-Dose Vials
Inhalation solution unit-dose vial is administered by oral inhalation using an intermittent positive pressure breathing apparatus. The usual adult dose is 1 vial per treatment.

Syrup
The usual dose is 2 teaspoonfuls, 3 or 4 times a day.

Tablets
The usual dose is 20 milligrams taken 3 or 4 times per day.

CHILDREN

Inhalation Aerosol Dosage
Alupent Inhalation Aerosol is not recommended for use in children under 12 years of age.

Inhalation solution
For children aged 6 to 12 years, the usual single dose is 0.1 milliliter, given by oral inhalation with a nebulizer. Dosage can be increased to 0.2 milliliter.

Syrup
The usual dose for children 6 to 9 years of age or weighing under 60 pounds is 1 teaspoonful, 3 or 4 times a day.

The usual dose for children over 9 years of age or weighing over 60 pounds is 2 teaspoonfuls, 3 or 4 times a day.

Experience in children under the age of 6 is limited. However, a daily dose of 1.3 to 2.6 milligrams per 2.2 pounds of body weight is usually well tolerated.

Tablets
The usual dose for children 6 to 9 years of age or weighing under 60 pounds is 10 milligrams taken 3 or 4 times a day.

The usual dose for children over 9 years of age or weighing over 60 pounds is 20 milligrams taken 3 or 4 times a day.

Tablets are not recommended for use in children under 6 years of age.

Overdosage
If you suspect an overdose, seek medical attention immediately.

Symptoms of Alupent overdose may include:
Dizziness, dry mouth, fatigue, general feeling of bodily discomfort, headache, high or low blood pressure, inability to fall or stay asleep, irregular heartbeat, nausea, nervousness, rapid, strong heartbeat, severe, suffocating chest pain, tremors

Generic name:

AMANTADINE HYDROCHLORIDE

See *Symmetrel,* page 595.

Generic name:

AMCINONIDE

See *Cyclocort,* page 148.

Generic name:

AMILORIDE HYDROCHLORIDE WITH HYDROCHLOROTHIAZIDE

See *Moduretic,* page 388.

Generic name:

AMITRIPTYLINE HYDROCHLORIDE

See *Elavil,* page 226.

Generic name:

AMOXAPINE

See *Asendin,* page 38.

Generic name:

AMOXICILLIN

See *Amoxil,* page 23.

Generic name:

AMOXICILLIN/CLAVULANATE POTASSIUM

See Augmentin, page 47.

Brand name:

AMOXIL

Generic name: Amoxicillin
Other brand names: Larotid, Polymox,
Trimox, Wymox

Why is this drug prescribed?
Amoxil, an antibiotic, is used to treat a wide variety of infections, including: gonorrhea, middle ear infections, skin infections, upper and lower respiratory tract infections, genitourinary tract infections.

Most important fact about this drug
Amoxil should not be taken by people who are allergic to penicillin or cephalosporin antibiotics (for example, Ceclor), since serious reactions—even death—can result.

Anyone experiencing adverse reactions to Amoxil—such as fever, skin rash, joint pain, and/or swollen lymph nodes, should stop taking it. If you experience these symptoms, you should not take Amoxil unless your doctor feels it is the only treatment for your condition.

How should you take this medication?
Amoxil can be taken with or without food.

What side effects may occur?
Side effects cannot be anticipated. If any develop or change in intensity, inform your doctor as soon as possible. Only your doctor can determine if it is safe for you to continue taking Amoxil.

■ *Side effects may include:*
Agitation, anemia, anxiety, changes in behavior, confusion, diarrhea, dizziness, hives, hyperactivity, insomnia, nausea, rash, vomiting

Why should this drug not be prescribed?
You should not use Amoxil if you are allergic to penicillin or cephalosporin antibiotics, for example, Ceclor.

Special warnings about this medication
If you have ever had asthma, hives, hay fever, or other allergies, consult with your doctor before taking Amoxil.

You should stop using Amoxil if you experience reactions such as bruising, fever, skin rash, itching, joint pain, swollen lymph nodes, and/or sores on the genitals. If these reactions occur, stop taking Amoxil unless your doctor advises you to continue.

For infections such as strep throat, it is important to take Amoxil for the entire amount of time your doctor has prescribed. Even if you feel better, you need to continue taking Amoxil. If you stop taking Amoxil before your treatment time is complete, you may get other infections, such as glomerulonephritis (a kidney infection) or rheumatic fever.

If you are diabetic, be aware that Amoxil may cause a *false positive* Clinitest (urine glucose test) result to occur. You should consult with your doctor about using different tests while taking Amoxil.

Before taking Amoxil, tell your doctor if you have ever had asthma, colitis (inflammatory bowel disease), diabetes, or kidney or liver disease.

Possible food and drug interactions when taking this medication
If Amoxil is taken with certain other drugs, the effects of either could be increased,

decreased, or altered. It is especially important to check with your doctor before combining Amoxil with the following:

Chloramphenicol (Chloromycetin)
Erythromycin
Oral contraceptives
Probenecid (Benemid)
Tetracyclines

Special information
if you are pregnant or breastfeeding

Amoxil should be used during pregnancy only when clearly needed. If you are pregnant or plan to become pregnant, inform your doctor immediately. Since Amoxil may appear in breast milk you should consult your doctor if you plan to breastfeed your baby.

Recommended dosage

Dosages will be determined by the type of infection being treated.

ADULTS

For Ear, Nose, Throat, Skin, and Genitourinary Infections
The usual dosage is 250 milligrams, taken every 8 hours.

For Infections of the Lower Respiratory Tract
The usual dosage is 500 milligrams, taken every 8 hours.

For Gonorrhea
The usual dosage is 3 grams in a single oral dose.

For Gonococcal Infections Such as Acute, Uncomplicated Anogenital and Urethral Infections
3 grams as a single oral dose.

CHILDREN

Children weighing over 44 pounds should follow the recommended adult dose schedule.

Children weighing under 44 pounds should have their dosage determined by their weight.

Dosage of Pediatric Drops:
Use the dropper provided with the medication to measure all doses.

For All Indications Except Infections of the Lower Respiratory Tract
Under 13 pounds:
  0.75 milliliter every 8 hours.
13 to 15 pounds:
  1 milliliter every 8 hours.
16 to 18 pounds:
  1.25 milliliters every 8 hours.

Infections of the Lower Respiratory Tract
Under 13 pounds:
  1.25 milliliters every 8 hours.
13 to 15 pounds:
  1.75 milliliters every 8 hours.
16 to 18 pounds:
  2.25 milliliters every 8 hours.

Children weighing more than 18 pounds should take the oral liquid. The required amount of suspension should be placed directly on the child's tongue for swallowing. It can also be added to formula, milk, fruit juice, water, ginger ale, or cold drinks. The preparation should be taken immediately. To be certain the child is getting the full dose of medication, make sure he or she drinks the entire preparation.

ELDERLY

Elderly patients should use Amoxil cautiously.

Overdosage

Any medication taken in excess can cause symptoms of overdose. If you suspect an overdose, seek medical attention immediately.

Symptoms of Amoxil overdose may include:
Diarrhea
Nausea
Stomach cramps
Vomiting

Brand name:

ANAFRANIL

Generic name: Clomipramine hydrochloride

Why is this drug prescribed?

Anafranil, a chemical cousin of tricyclic antidepressant medications such as Tofranil and Elavil, is used to treat people who suffer from obsessions and compulsions.

An obsession is a disturbing idea, image, or urge that keeps coming to mind despite the person's efforts to ignore or forget it—for example, a preoccupation with avoiding contamination.

A compulsion is an irrational action that the person knows is senseless but feels driven to repeat again and again—for example, hand-washing perhaps dozens or even scores of times throughout the day.

Most important fact about this drug

Many men who take Anafranil find that the drug makes them impotent or unable to ejaculate. However, their relief at the freedom from obsessive thoughts and/or compulsive behaviors may lead them to stick with the drug, at least for a limited time.

How should you take this medication?

Anafranil may cause your skin to become more sensitive to sunlight. Avoid prolonged exposure to sunlight.

This medicine may cause dry mouth. Using sugarless gum, hard candy, or bits of ice may bring relief from this side effect.

Avoid alcoholic beverages while taking Anafranil.

Anafranil may be taken with food to avoid stomach upset.

What side effects may occur?

Side effects cannot be anticipated. If any develop or change in intensity, inform your doctor as soon as possible. Only your doctor can determine if it is safe for you to continue taking Anafranil.

The most significant risk is that of seizures (convulsions). Drowsiness, confusion, nausea, and vomiting are common. Men are likely to experience problems with sexual function. Unwanted weight gain is a potential problem for many people who take Anafranil, although a small number of patients actually lose weight.

■ *Other side effects may include:*
Abnormal thinking, abnormality in walking, acne, agitation, anxiety, appetite loss, back pain, chest pain, chills, confusion, constipation, coughing, depression, diarrhea, difficulty breathing, difficulty urinating, dizziness, double vision, dreaming abnormality, drowsiness, dry mouth, dry skin, earache, eye pain, fast heartbeat, fatigue, feelings of unreality, fever, gas, genital itching, headache, hives, hot flushes, impotence, increased appetite, increased sweating, indecisiveness, irritability, itching, memory problems, menstrual pain and disorders, muscle jerks, muscle twitching, nausea, nervousness, numbness, rash, refusal or inability to speak, ringing in the ears, "runny" nose, sex-drive changes, sleeplessness, sleep disturbances, sore throat, speech disturbances, stomach pain, stomach upset, suicidal ideation, taste changes, teeth grinding, tingling, tremor, urinary problems, vertigo, vision problems, vomiting, weakness, yawning

Why should this drug not be prescribed?

Do not take this medication if you are sensitive or have ever had an allergic reaction to a tricyclic antidepressant, such as Tofranil, Elavil and others.

Do not take Anafranil if you are taking, or have taken within the past 14 days, a monoamine oxidase inhibitor (MAO inhibitor) antidepressant such as Parnate, Nardil, or Marplan. Combining Anafranil with one of these medications could lead to fever, seizures, coma, and even death.

Do not take Anafranil if you have recently had a heart attack.

Special warnings about this medication

If you have narrow-angle glaucoma, increased pressure inside the eyeball, or urinary retention problems, Anafranil could make these conditions worse. Use Anafranil with caution if your kidney function is abnormal.

If you have a tumor of the adrenal medulla, this medication could cause your blood pressure to rise suddenly and dangerously.

Because Anafranil poses a possible risk of seizures, and because it may impair mental or physical ability to perform complicated tasks, your doctor will probably warn you to take special precautions if you need to operate complicated machinery while taking the medication. Note that your risk of seizures is increased:

If you ever had a seizure in the past;
If you have a history of brain damage or alcoholism; or
If you are taking another medication hat might predispose you to seizures.

Patients with manic-depressive illness (a condition of extreme mood swings) may develop increased manic symptoms while taking Anafranil. Patients with unrecognized schizophrenia may develop an acute psychotic episode. As with Tofranil, Elavil, and other tricyclic antidepressants, an overdose of Anafranil can be fatal. Do not be surprised if your doctor prescribes only a small quantity of Anafranil at a time.

This is standard procedure to minimize the risk of overdose.

Before having any kind of surgery involving the use of general anesthesia, tell your doctor or dentist that you are taking Anafranil. You may be advised to discontinue the drug temporarily.

When it is time to stop taking Anafranil, do not stop abruptly. Taper off gradually over a period of days to avoid withdrawal symptoms such as dizziness, nausea, vomiting, headache, malaise, fever, sleep problems, irritability or worsening emotional or mental problems.

Possible food and drug interactions when taking this medication

If Anafranil is taken with certain other drugs, the effects of either could be increased, decreased, or altered. It is especially important to check with your doctor before combining Anafranil with the following:

Alcohol
Anticholinergic drugs such as Donnatal, Cogentin, and Bentyl
Certain blood pressure drugs such as Esmelin, Catapress, and others
Cimetidine (Tagamet)
Digoxin (Lanoxin)
Fluoxetine (Prozac)
Haloperidol (Haldol)
Methylphenidate (Ritalin)
Monoamine oxidase inhibitors such as Nardil, Parnate, and others
Psychoactive drugs such as Thorazine, Valium
Thyroid medications such as Synthroid
Warfarin (Coumadin)

Special information if you are pregnant or breastfeeding

If you are pregnant or plan to become pregnant, inform your doctor immediately.

Anafranil should not be used during pregnancy unless absolutely necessary;

some babies born to women who took Anafranil have had withdrawal symptoms such as jitteriness, tremors, and seizures.

Anafranil does make its way into breast milk. Your doctor may advise you to stop breastfeeding while you are taking Anafranil.

Recommended dosage
Your doctor may ask you to take Anafranil with meals to avoid stomach upset.

ADULTS

The usual recommended initial dose is 25 milligrams daily. This dosage may be increased by your doctor to 100 milligrams during the first 2 weeks. During this period you will be asked to take this drug in divided doses with meals. The maximum daily dosage is 200 milligrams. After the dose has been determined, your doctor may direct you to take one single dose at bedtime with meals, to avoid daytime sedation.

CHILDREN

The usual recommended initial dose is 25 milligrams daily. The dose may be increased by your doctor to a maximum of 100 milligrams or 3 milligrams per 2.2 pounds of body weight per day, whichever is smaller.

Overdosage
An overdose of Anafranil may be lethal. If you suspect an Anafranil overdose, seek medical attention immediately.

Early signs and symptoms of Anafranil overdose may include:
Agitation, coma, convulsions, delirium, drowsiness, grimacing, hyperactive reflexes, loss of coordination, restlessness, rigid muscles, staggering gait, stupor, sweating, writhing

Other signs and symptoms of overdosage may include shallow breathing, low blood

pressure, shock, bluish skin color, dilated pupils, fever, vomiting, and urine retention. There is a danger of heart malfunction and even, in rare cases, cardiac arrest.

Brand name:

ANAPROX

Generic name: Naproxen sodium

Why is this drug prescribed?
Anaprox, a nonsteroidal anti-inflammatory drug, is used to relieve mild to moderate pain and menstrual cramps. It is also prescribed for relief of the inflammation, swelling, stiffness and joint pain associated with rheumatoid arthritis, osteoarthritis (the most common form of arthritis) and juvenile arthritis, ankylosing spondylitis (spinal arthritis), tendinitis, bursitis, acute gout and other types of pain.

Most important fact about this drug
You should have frequent check-ups with your doctor if you take Anaprox regularly. Ulcers or internal bleeding can occur without warning.

How should you take this medication?
Your doctor may ask you to take Anaprox with food or an antacid to avoid stomach upset.

Take this medication exactly as prescribed by your doctor.

If you are using Anaprox for arthritis, it should be taken regularly.

If you forget to take a dose, take it as soon as you remember. If it is almost time for your next dose, skip the one you missed and go back to your regular schedule. Never take two doses at the same time.

What side effects may occur?
Side effects cannot be anticipated. If any develop or change in intensity, inform

your doctor as soon as possible. Only your doctor can determine if it is safe for you to continue taking Anaprox.

■ *More common side effects may include:*
Abdominal pain, bruising, constipation, diarrhea, dizziness, drowsiness, headache, hearing changes, heartburn, indigestion, inflammation of the mouth, itching, lightheadedness, nausea, rapid heartbeat, red or purple spots on the skin, ringing in ears, shortness of breath, skin eruptions, sweating, swelling due to fluid retention, thirst, vertigo, vision changes

■ *Less common or rare side effects may include:*
Abdominal bleeding, anemia, black stools, blood in the urine, change in dream patterns, changes in hearing, chills and fever, colitis, congestive heart failure, depression, hair loss, inability to concentrate, inability to sleep, inflammation of the lungs, kidney failure, menstrual problems, muscle weakness and/or pain, peptic ulcer, skin inflammation due to sensitivity to light, skin rashes, vomiting, vomiting blood, yellow skin and eyes.

Why should this drug not be prescribed?
If you are sensitive to or have ever had an allergic reaction to Anaprox, aspirin, or similar drugs, or if you have had asthma attacks caused by aspirin or other drugs of this type, you should not take this medication. Make sure that your doctor is aware of any drug reactions that you have experienced.

Special warnings about this medication
Peptic ulcers and bleeding can occur without warning.

This drug should be used with caution if you have kidney or liver disease. It can cause liver inflammation in some people.

Do not take aspirin or any other anti-inflammatory medications while taking Anaprox, unless your doctor tells you to do so.

Anaprox contains sodium. If you are on a low sodium diet, discuss this with your doctor.

Use with caution if you have heart disease or high blood pressure. This drug can increase water retention.

If you are taking Anaprox for an extended period of time, your doctor should check your blood for anemia.

Anaprox prolongs bleeding time. If you are taking blood-thinning medication, this drug should be used with caution.

Anaprox may cause vision problems. If you experience any changes in your vision, inform your doctor.

Anaprox may cause you to become drowsy or less alert; therefore, driving or operating dangerous machinery or participating in any hazardous activity that requires full mental alertness is not recommended.

Possible food and drug interactions when taking this medication
If Anaprox is taken with certain other drugs, the effects of either could be increased, decreased, or altered. It is especially important to check with your doctor before combining Anaprox with the following:

Aspirin
Beta-blockers including blood pressure drugs such as Tenormin
Blood thinners such as Coumadin
Lithium (Lithobid)
Loop diuretics such as Lasix
Hydantoins such as Dilantin

Methotrexate
Naproxen in other forms such as Naprosyn
Oral antidiabetic agents such as Micronase
Probenecid (Benemid)

Special information
if you are pregnant or breastfeeding
The effects of Anaprox during pregnancy have
not been adequately studied. If you are
pregnant or plan to become pregnant, inform
your doctor immediately. Anaprox appears
in breast milk and could affect a nursing
infant. If this medication is essential to
your health, your doctor may advise you to
discontinue breastfeeding until your
treatment with this medication is finished.

Recommended dosage
Anaprox is available in 275-milligram
tablets and, as Anaprox DS, in
double-strength 550-milligram tablets.

ADULTS

Mild to Moderate Pain, Menstrual Cramps,
Acute Tendinitis and Bursitis
The starting dose is 550 milligrams followed
by 275 milligrams every 6 to 8 hours.
The total daily dose should not exceed 1,375
milligrams.

Rheumatoid Arthritis, Osteoarthritis, and
Ankylosing Spondylitis
The starting dose is 275 milligrams or 550
milligrams 2 times a day (morning and
evening). Doses can be adjusted by your
physician for maximum benefit. Symptoms
should improve within 2 to 4 weeks.

Acute Gout
The starting dose is 825 milligrams, followed
by 275 milligrams every 8 hours, until
symptoms subside.

CHILDREN

Juvenile Arthritis
The usual daily dosage is a total of 10

milligrams per 2.2 pounds. Dosage should
not exceed 15 milligrams per 2.2 pounds per
day.

The safety and effectiveness of Anaprox
has not been established in children under
2 years of age.

ELDERLY

Dosage should be determined by the particular
needs of the elderly patient.

Overdosage
Any medication taken in excess can cause
symptoms of overdose. If you suspect an
overdose, seek medical attention immediately.

The symptoms of Anaprox overdose may
include:
Drowsiness
Heartburn
Indigestion
Nausea or Vomiting

Brand name:

ANASPAZ

See Levsin, page 316.

Brand name:

ANDROID

Generic name: Methyltestosterone

Why is this drug prescribed?
Android, a synthetic male sex hormone sold
in tablet form, is given to help develop
and/or maintain male sex characteristics in
boys and men who, for some reason, are
not producing enough of the hormone on
their own. A relatively short course of
Android is sometimes used to try to trigger
pubertal changes in boys whose puberty
seems delayed. Android may also be given

to women who have certain advanced, inoperable forms of breast cancer.

Most important fact about this drug
Because of potentially serious adverse health effects, Android is *not* recommended as a treatment for athletes who want to enhance their physique and/or improve their performance.

An adult man taking Android should report too frequent or persistent erections to his doctor immediately.

An adult woman should report any hoarseness, acne, or changes in the menstrual cycle.

How should you take this medication?
Take Android exactly as prescribed by your doctor. The tablets, which come in strengths of 10 and 25 milligrams, may be either swallowed or dissolved in the cheek.

Android Buccal Tablets (those dissolved between the gum and the cheek) should *not* be swallowed. Avoid eating, drinking or smoking while the tablet is in place.

What side effects may occur?
Side effects cannot be anticipated. If any develop or change in intensity, inform your doctor as soon as possible. Only your doctor can determine if it is safe for you to continue taking Android.

In men, possible adverse effects include breast development, annoyingly frequent and persistent erections, and (at high dosage) decreased sperm count.

In women, possible adverse effects include irregular menstrual periods, deepened voice, and enlarged clitoris.

Elderly males risk enlarged prostate or prostate cancer.

■ *Other possible side effects include:*
  Acne, allergic reactions, anxiety, bloating,

depression, excess body hair, headache, itching, burning, or tingling skin, jaundice, male-pattern baldness, nausea, sex-drive changes (increase or decrease)

Why should this drug not be prescribed?
Do not take Android if you are sensitive to or have ever had an allergic reaction to a synthetic male hormone.

Men with breast or prostate cancer should not take Android.

Women should not take Android during pregnancy, since the drug may masculinize the genitals of a female fetus.

Special warnings about this medication
Extreme caution is needed when giving Android to a child. If taken for too long by a boy who has not yet reached puberty, the drug may prematurely arrest bone development so that the youngster never reaches full height. For safety's sake, any young boy being treated with Android should have X-rays of the wrist and hand every 6 months so the doctor can monitor his bone growth.

Women taking Android should be alert for signs of virilization: acne, deepened voice, enlarged clitoris, increased hairiness, and irregular menstrual periods. If the drug is not discontinued promptly while such changes are still mild, the masculinizing effects may be permanent.

Patients who already have heart, kidney, or liver disease may risk fluid accumulation and congestive heart failure.

Possible food and drug interactions when taking this medication
If Android is taken with certain other drugs, the effects of either could be increased, decreased, or altered. It is especially important to check with your doctor before combining Android with the following:

The blood thinners (Coumadin, Dicumarol, and others)

Insulin

The antiarthritis and antigout medication oxyphenbutazone (Oxalid, Tandearil)

With any of these, you may need a reduced dosage while taking Android.

Special Information
if you are pregnant or breastfeeding

If you become pregnant while taking Android, notify your doctor immediately. If the unborn baby is a girl, the drug may cause her to develop certain sexual abnormalities: enlargement of the clitoris, formation of a pseudo-scrotum, and malformation of the vagina. These fetal abnormalities are especially likely if Android is taken during the first 3 months of pregnancy. It is not known whether Android is excreted in breast milk. If this medication is essential to your health, your doctor may advise you to stop breastfeeding until your treatment with Android is finished.

Recommended dosage

The dosage prescribed by your doctor is determined by the age, sex, and diagnosis of the patient, response to the drug, and other factors. The following are only general guidelines.

Treatment of delayed puberty in males
The suggested daily dosage is 5 to 25 milligrams daily for a limited time, usually 4 to 6 months.

For androgen replacement therapy in men
The suggested daily dosage is 10 to 50 milligrams daily in oral form.

For androgen therapy in female breast cancer
The usual daily dose is 50 to 200 milligrams in oral form.

Overdosage

Although no specific overdosage information is available for Android, any medication taken in excess can have serious consequences. If you suspect an overdose, seek medical attention immediately.

Brand name:

ANEXSIA

See Vicodin, page 678.

Brand name:

ANSAID

Generic name: Flurbiprofen

Why is this drug prescribed?

Ansaid, a nonsteroidal anti-inflammatory drug, is used to relieve the inflammation, swelling, stiffness and joint pain associated with rheumatoid arthritis and osteoarthritis (the most common form of arthritis). It is also used in the treatment of other types of pain.

Most important fact about this drug

You should have frequent check-ups with your doctor if you take Ansaid regularly. Ulcers or internal bleeding can occur without warning.

How should you take this medication?

Your doctor may ask you to take Ansaid with food or an antacid.

Take this medication exactly as prescribed by your doctor.

If you are using Ansaid for arthritis, it should be taken regularly.

If you forget to take a dose, take it as soon as you remember. If it is almost time for your next dose, skip the one you missed and go back to your regular schedule. Never take two doses at the same time.

What side effects may occur?

Side effects cannot be anticipated. If any develop or change in intensity, inform your doctor as soon as possible. Only your doctor can determine if it is safe for you to continue taking Ansaid.

■ *More common side effects may include:*
Abdominal bleeding, abdominal pain, anxiety, changes in liver function, constipation, depression, diarrhea, dizziness, gas, headache, heartburn, inflammation of the nose, indigestion, loss of memory, nausea, nervousness, rash, ringing in ears, sleepiness, stomach upset, swelling due to fluid retention, tremors, trouble sleeping, urinary tract infection, vision changes, vomiting, weakness, weight changes

■ *Less common or rare side effects may include:*
Altered sense of smell, anemia, asthma, blood in the urine, bloody diarrhea, chills and fever, confusion, heart failure, hepatitis, high blood pressure, hives, inflammation of the eyelids, inflammation of the mouth and tongue, inflammation of the stomach, itching, kidney failure, lack of coordination, nosebleed, peptic ulcer, pins and needles, rash, reduced white blood cells, sensitivity of skin to light, skin inflammation, swelling of throat, twitching, vomiting blood, welts, yellow eyes and skin

Why should this drug not be prescribed?

If you are sensitive to or have ever had an allergic reaction to Ansaid, aspirin, or similar drugs, or if you have had asthma attacks caused by aspirin or other drugs of this type, you should not take this medication. Make sure that your doctor is aware of any drug reactions that you have experienced.

Special warnings about this medication

Peptic ulcers and bleeding can occur without warning.

This drug should be used with caution if you have kidney or liver disease. It can cause liver inflammation in some people.

Do not take aspirin or any other anti-inflammatory medications while taking Ansaid, unless your doctor tells you to do so.

Ansaid can cause vision problems. If you experience a change in your vision, inform your doctor. Blurred and/or decreased vision have occurred while taking this medication.

Ansaid prolongs bleeding time. If you are taking blood-thinning medication, this drug should be taken with caution.

This drug can increase water retention if you have heart disease or high blood pressure. Use with caution.

Ansaid may cause you to become drowsy or less alert; therefore, driving or operating dangerous machinery or participating in any hazardous activity that requires full mental alertness is not recommended.

Possible food and drug interactions when taking this medication

If Ansaid is taken with certain other drugs, the effects of either could be increased, decreased, or altered. It is especially important to check with your doctor before combining Ansaid with the following:

Aspirin
Beta-blockers such as Inderal, Tenormin
Blood thinners such as Coumadin
Cimetidine (Tagamet)
Loop diuretics such as Lasix, Bumex
Methotrexate

Special information
if you are pregnant or breastfeeding

The effects of Ansaid during pregnancy have not been adequately studied. If you are pregnant or plan to become pregnant, inform your doctor immediately. Ansaid appears in breast milk and could affect a nursing infant. If this medication is essential to your health, your doctor may advise you to discontinue breastfeeding until your treatment is finished.

Recommended dosage

ADULTS

Rheumatoid Arthritis or Osteoarthritis:
The usual starting dosage is a total of 200 to 300 milligrams a day, divided into 2, 3 or 4 smaller doses (usually 3 or 4 for rheumatoid arthritis.) Doses should be tailored to each patient; however, no single dose should be greater than 100 milligrams and total dosage should not exceed 300 milligrams a day.

CHILDREN

The safety and effectiveness of Ansaid have not been established in children.

ELDERLY

Dosage should be determined by the particular needs of the elderly patient.

Overdosage

Any medication taken in excess can cause symptoms of overdose. If you suspect an overdose, seek medical attention immediately.

The symptoms of Ansaid overdose may include:
Agitation, change in pupil size, coma, disorientation, dizziness, double vision, drowsiness, headache, nausea, semi-consciousness, shallow breathing, stomach pain

Brand name:

ANSPOR

See Velosef, page 676.

Generic name:

ANTIPYRINE AND BENZOCAINE IN GLYCERIN

See Auralgan, page 48.

Brand name:

ANTIVERT

Generic name: Meclizine hydrochloride

Why is this drug prescribed?

Antivert, an antihistamine, is prescribed for the management of nausea, vomiting, and dizziness associated with motion sickness.

Antivert may also be prescribed for the management of vertigo (a spinning sensation or a feeling that the ground is tilted) due to diseases affecting the vestibular system (the bony labyrinth of the ear, which contains the organs of equilibrium that affect your sense of balance).

Most important fact about this drug

Antivert may cause you to become drowsy or less alert; therefore, driving a car or operating dangerous machinery is not recommended.

How should you take this medication?

Take this medication exactly as prescribed by your doctor.

What side effects may occur?

Side effects cannot be anticipated. If any develop or change in intensity, inform your doctor as soon as possible. Only your doctor can determine if it is safe for you to continue taking Antivert.

■ *More common side effects may include:*
Drowsiness
Dry mouth

■ *Rare side effects may include:*
Blurred vision

Why should this drug not be prescribed?
If you are sensitive to or have ever had an allergic reaction to meclizine hydrochloride or similar drugs, do not take this drug. Make sure that your doctor is aware of any drug reactions that you have experienced.

Special warnings about this medication
If you have asthma, glaucoma, or an enlarged prostate gland, check with your doctor before using Antivert.

Possible food and drug interactions when taking this medication
Antivert may intensify the effects of alcohol. Do not drink alcohol while taking this medication.

Special information
If you are pregnant or breastfeeding
Studies regarding the use of Antivert in pregnant women do not indicate that this drug increases the risk of abnormalities. However, if you are pregnant or plan to become pregnant, inform your doctor before using Antivert. Check with him, too, if you are breastfeeding your baby.

Recommended Dosage

ADULTS

Motion Sickness
For protection against motion sickness, the usual starting dose of 25 to 50 milligrams should be taken 1 hour before traveling. The dose may be repeated every 24 hours for the duration of the journey.

Vertigo
The recommended dosage is 25 to 100 milligrams per day, divided into equal, smaller doses as determined by your doctor.

CHILDREN

The safety and effectiveness of Antivert have not been established in children under 12 years of age.

Overdosage
Any medication taken in excess can have serious consequences. If you suspect an overdose, seek emergency medical treatment immediately.

Brand name:

ARMOUR THYROID

Generic name: Natural thyroid hormones T_3 and T_4

Why is this drug prescribed?
Armour Thyroid may be prescribed if you have an underactive thyroid gland that is not producing enough hormone. This medication may also be given to treat various forms of goiter. Alternatively, if your doctor suspects that you might have an overactive thyroid gland, Armour Thyroid may be used in a suppression test to diagnose this condition.

Most important fact about this drug
Although Armour Thyroid will speed up your metabolism, it is not effective as a weight-loss drug and should not be used for that purpose. Too much Armour Thyroid may cause life-threatening side effects, especially if you are also taking appetite suppressants.

How should you take this medication?
Take Armour Thyroid exactly as prescribed by your doctor. There is no "typical" dosage; the amount you need to take will depend on how much thyroid hormone

your body is able to produce. Take no more or less than the amount your doctor prescribes. Take your dose at the same time every day for consistent effect.

Do not change brands of medication without consulting your doctor.

If you are taking Armour Thyroid to compensate for an underactive thyroid gland, you will probably need to take the medication indefinitely.

What side effects may occur?
Side effects are rare when Armour Thyroid is taken at the correct dosage. However, taking too much medication or increasing the dosage too quickly may lead to over-stimulation of the thyroid gland.

■ *Symptoms of overstimulation may include:* Changes in appetite, diarrhea, fever, headache, increased heart rate, irritability, nausea, nervousness, sleeplessness, sweating, weight loss

Although children treated with Armour Thyroid may initially lose some hair, the hair loss is temporary.

Why should this drug not be prescribed?
You should not take Armour Thyroid if:

You have ever had an allergic reaction to this drug; your thyroid gland is overactive; or your adrenal glands are not making enough corticosteroid hormone.

Special warnings about this medication
If you are elderly, particularly if you suffer from angina (chest pain due to a heart condition), Armour Thyroid should be prescribed at a lower dosage, and your doctor should schedule frequent checkups.

Armour Thyroid tends to aggravate symptoms of diabetes mellitus, diabetes insipidus, and underactive adrenal glands.

If you take medication to treat any of these disorders, your dosage of that medication will probably need to be adjusted once you start taking Armour Thyroid.

Possible food and drug interactions when taking this medication
If you take Armour Thyroid with certain other drugs, the effect of either drug could be increased, decreased, or altered. It is especially important to check with your doctor before combining Armour Thyroid with the following:

Antidiabetic drugs (Diabinese, Glucotrol)
Blood thinners (Coumadin, Dicumarol)
Cholestyramine (Questran)
Colestipol (Colestid)
Estrogen preparations (including some birth
    control pills)
Insulin

Special information if you are pregnant or breastfeeding
If you need to take Armour Thyroid because of a thyroid hormone deficiency, you may continue using the medication during pregnancy. Once your baby is born, you may breastfeed while continuing treatment with Armour Thyroid.

Recommended dosage
ADULTS

Your doctor will tailor the dosage of Armour Thyroid to meet your individual requirements, taking into consideration the status of your thyroid gland and any other medical conditions you may have.

Overdosage
An overdose of Armour Thyroid will speed up all of the body's vital processes, causing physical and mental hyperactivity, increased appetite, excessive sweating, chest pain, increased pulse rate, palpitations,

nervousness, intolerance to heat, and possibly tremors or a rapid heartbeat.

Brand name:

ARTANE

Generic name: Trihexyphenidyl hydrochloride

Why is this drug prescribed?
Artane is used, in conjunction with other drugs, for the relief of certain symptoms of Parkinson's disease, a brain disorder that causes muscle tremor, stiffness, and weakness. It is also used to control certain reactions induced by antipsychotic drugs such as Thorazine and Haldol. Artane works by relaxing the muscles.

Most important fact about this drug
Artane is not a cure for Parkinson's disease; it merely minimizes and reduces the frequency of symptoms such as tremors.

How should you take this medication?
Take Artane exactly as prescribed by your doctor. You may take it either before meals or after meals, whichever you find more comfortable. Your doctor will probably start you on a small amount and increase the dosage gradually.

If the medication makes your mouth feel dry, try chewing gum, sucking mints, or simply sipping water.

Artane comes in tablets or as a liquid to be swallowed. With either the tablets or the liquid, you will probably need to take 3 or 4 doses a day.

Once you are stabilized on the dosage that is best for you, your doctor may switch you to sustained-release capsules ("Sequels") which are to be taken only once or twice a day.

Elderly patients are highly sensitive to drugs like Artane. They should use it with caution.

Artane can reduce the body's ability to perspire, one of the key ways it prevents overheating. Avoid excess sun or exercise that would ordinarily cause excessive sweating.

What side effects may occur?
Side effects cannot be anticipated. If any develop or change in intensity, inform your doctor as soon as possible. Only your doctor can determine if it is safe for you to continue taking Artane.

■ *Common side effects may include:*
Blurry vision
Dry mouth
Nausea
Nervousness

These side effects, which appear in 30 to 50 percent of all people who take Artane, tend to be mild. They may disappear as your body gets used to the drug; if they persist, your doctor may want to lower your dosage slightly.

■ *Other potential side effects include:*
Agitation, bowel obstruction, confusion, constipation, delusions, difficulty urinating, dilated pupils, disturbed behavior, drowsiness, hallucinations, headache, rapid heartbeat, rash, vomiting, weakness

Why should this drug not be prescribed?
Do not take Artane if you are known to be excessively sensitive to it or if you have ever had an allergic reaction to it or to other antiparkinsonian medications.

Tardive dyskinesia is a syndrome of involuntary facial movements that sometimes develops in people who take antipsychotic medications. Artane should not be given for tardive dyskinesia; it will not help, and it may make the condition worse.

Special warnings about this medication

Older people—especially over age 60—can be very sensitive to this drug and must be monitored carefully.

Be sure to tell your doctor if you have any of the following conditions, since Artane could make them worse:

Enlarged prostate
Gastrointestinal obstructive disease
Glaucoma
Urinary tract obstructive disease

It is important to stick to the prescribed dosage; taking larger amounts "for kicks" could lead to an overdose.

Your doctor should watch you carefully if you have heart, liver, or kidney disease or high blood pressure, and should check your eyes frequently. You should also be watched for the development of any allergic reactions.

Possible food and drug interactions when taking this medication

If you take Artane simultaneously with levodopa (Larodopa) or with an antipsychotic medication (Haldol, Stelazine, Navane, others), your doctor may need to adjust your dosage of Artane, the other medication, or possibly both. You will need close medical monitoring while the dosages are being adjusted.

Special information if you are pregnant or breastfeeding

No specific information is available concerning the use of Artane during pregnancy or breastfeeding. If you are pregnant or plan to become pregnant while taking Artane, inform your doctor immediately.

Recommended dosage

All dosages should be individualized.

The dose should be low to start with and then be increased gradually, especially in patients over 60 years of age.

ADULTS

Parkinson's Disease
The usual starting dose, in tablet or elixir form, is 1 milligram on the first day.

After the first day, the dose may be increased by 2 milligrams at intervals of 3 to 5 days, until a total of 6 to 10 milligrams is given daily.

The total daily dose will depend upon what is found to be the most effective level. For many patients, 6 to 10 milligrams is most effective. Some patients, however, may require a total daily dose of 12 to 15 milligrams.

Drug-induced Parkinsonism
The size and frequency of the dose of Artane needed to control tremors and muscle rigidity that results from commonly used tranquilizers must be determined by trial and error.

The total daily dosage usually ranges between 5 and 15 milligrams, although, in some cases, symptoms have been satisfactorily controlled on as little as 1 milligram daily.

Your doctor may start you on 1 milligram of Artane a day. If symptoms are not controlled in a few hours, the dose may be slowly increased until satisfactory control is achieved.

Use of Artane with Levodopa
When Artane is used at the same time as levodopa, the usual dose of each may need to be reduced. Careful adjustment is necessary, depending on side effects and degree of symptom control. Artane dosage of 3 to 6 milligrams daily, divided into equal doses, is usually adequate.

Artane Tablets and Elixir
The total daily intake of Artane tablets or elixir is tolerated best if divided into 3 doses and taken at mealtimes. High doses (more than 10 milligrams daily) may be divided into 4 parts, with 3 doses administered at mealtimes and the fourth at bedtime.

Artane Sequels (Controlled-Release Form)
Sustained-release Sequels are usually used only after the patient has been stabilized on one of the other dosage forms.

The usual recommended daily dosage is 5 milligrams after breakfast with an additional 5 milligrams taken 12 hours later.

Overdosage
Overdosage with Artane may cause agitation, delirium, disorientation, hallucinations, or psychotic episodes. If you suspect an overdose of Artane, seek medical attention immediately.

Brand name:

ASENDIN

Generic name: Amoxapine

Why is this drug prescribed?
Asendin, an antidepressant with a mild sedative effect, relieves the symptoms of depression with or without anxiety or agitation. Antidepressants can improve mood, appetite, and sleep, and increase mental alertness and physical activity.

Most important fact about this drug
In some people, continued use of this type of medication has caused tardive dyskinesia, a condition characterized by involuntary movements or twitches of facial and body muscles. Although the problem is more common in the elderly, especially elderly women, it can affect anyone taking this type of

medication. Your doctor should discuss the benefits and risks of Asendin before starting treatment.

Relief of symptoms usually occurs within 2 weeks, but can take as few as 4 to 7 days.

How should you take this medication?
Asendin should be taken exactly as prescribed by your doctor.

What side effects may occur?
Side effects cannot be anticipated. If any develop or change in intensity, inform your doctor as soon as possible. Only your doctor can determine if it is safe for you to continue taking Asendin.

■ *More common side effects may include:*
Anxiety, blurred vision, confusion, constipation, difficulty sleeping, dizziness, drowsiness, dry mouth, excessive appetite, excitement, fatigue, fluid retention, headache, increased perspiration, lack of muscle coordination, nausea, nervousness, nightmares, pounding heartbeat, restlessness, skin rash, tremors, weakness

■ *Less common side effects may include:*
Abdominal pain, blood disorders, breast enlargement and excessive or spontaneous flow of milk in women, diarrhea, difficulty urinating, dilation of the pupils of the eye, disorientation, disturbed concentration, drug fever, extremely high body temperature, fainting, gas, high blood pressure, hives, impotence, incoordination, increased or decreased sex drive, itching, low blood pressure, menstrual irregularity, numbness, painful ejaculation, peculiar taste, rapid heartbeat, ringing in the ears, seizures, sensitivity to light, stuffy nose, teary eyes, tingling or pins and needles in arms and legs, upset stomach, vomiting, weight gain or loss

Why should this drug not be prescribed?

Asendin should not be used if you are taking an antidepressant classified as an MAO inhibitor, including such drugs as Nardil and Parnate. Also, do not take Asendin if you are recovering from a heart attack, or if you are sensitive to or have ever had an allergic reaction to amoxapine or dibenzoxazepine medications.

Special warnings about this medication

Remember that Asendin may cause the facial and body twitching known as tardive dyskinesia. Your doctor should prescribe the smallest dose for the shortest duration that achieves the desired results.

Neuroleptic malignant syndrome (NMS) has occurred in people using Asendin. NMS is characterized by extremely high body temperature, rigid muscles, altered mental state, and irregular pulse, blood pressure, and heartbeat. Report any of these symptoms to your doctor immediately.

Asendin should be used with care if you have a history of urinary retention, angle-closure glaucoma, increased eye pressure, or heart disease.

Extreme caution should be used if you have a seizure disorder or a history of seizure disorder.

Asendin can cause heart attack or stroke.

In certain people Asendin may cause an exaggeration of particular symptoms. For instance, manic-depressives may experience a shift to the manic phase; schizophrenics may develop increased symptoms of psychosis. If you experience such changes, your doctor may need to reduce your dosage or prescribe a tranquilizer.

Antidepressants can cause allergic reactions such as skin rashes or "drug fever" in some people. This usually occurs during the first few days of treatment. If these symptoms develop, the medication should be discontinued.

Asendin may cause you to become drowsy or less alert. Be careful driving, operating machinery or appliances, or doing any activity that requires full mental alertness until you know how you react on Asendin.

Possible food and drug interactions when taking this medication

Asendin may increase the effects of alcohol. Do not drink alcohol while taking this medication.

If Asendin is taken with certain other drugs, the effects of either could be increased, decreased, or altered. It is especially important to check with your doctor before combining Asendin with the following:

Albuterol (Ventolin, Proventil)
Anticholinergics such as Bentyl
Barbiturates/sedatives such as Phenobarbital
    and Seconal
Cimetidine (Tagamet)
MAO inhibitors (antidepressant drugs such
    as Nardil and Marplan)
Other central nervous system depressants such
    as Percocet and Halcion

Special information if you are pregnant or breastfeeding

Although the effects of Asendin during pregnancy have not been adequately studied, stillbirths and decreased birth weight have appeared in animal studies. Asendin should be used only if the potential benefits outweigh the potential risks. If you are pregnant or plan to become pregnant, inform your doctor immediately. Asendin appears in breast milk and could affect a nursing infant. If this medication is essential to your health, your doctor may advise you to stop breastfeeding until your treatment is finished.

Recommended dosage

Effective dosages of Asendin may vary from one patient to another.

ADULTS

The usual starting dosage is 50 milligrams 2 or 3 times daily. If you tolerate the drug well, your doctor may increase the dosage to 100 milligrams 2 or 3 times daily by the end of the first week. Increases above 300 milligrams daily should be made only if that dose has proved ineffective during a trial period of at least 2 weeks.

When the effective dosage is established, the drug may be taken in a single dose (not to exceed 300 milligrams) at bedtime.

CHILDREN

Safety and effectiveness have not been established in children under the age of 16.

ELDERLY

In general, lower dosages are recommended for the elderly. Recommended starting dosage of Asendin is 25 milligrams 2 or 3 times daily. If no intolerance is observed, dosage may be increased by the end of the first week to 50 milligrams 2 or 3 times daily.

Overdosage

Any medication taken in excess can have serious consequences. If you suspect an overdose, seek medical treatment immediately.

Symptoms of Asendin overdose may include:
Coma
Convulsions
Kidney failure
Status epilepticus

Generic name:

ASPIRIN

Brand names: Empirin, Ecotrin, Genuine Bayer

Why is this drug prescribed?

Aspirin is an anti-inflammatory pain medication (analgesic) that is used to relieve headaches, toothaches, and minor aches and pains, and to reduce fever. It also temporarily relieves the minor aches and pains of arthritis, muscle aches, colds, flu, and menstrual discomfort. In some patients, a small daily dose of aspirin may be used to ensure sufficient blood flow to the brain and prevent stroke. Aspirin may also be taken to decrease recurrence of a heart attack.

Most important fact about this drug

Aspirin should not be used during the last 3 months of pregnancy unless specifically prescribed by a doctor. It may cause problems in the unborn child or complications during delivery.

How should you take this medication?

You should take aspirin as directed by your doctor or follow the directions on the package.

Do not take more than the recommended dose.

Do not use aspirin if it has a strong, vinegar-like odor.

Do not chew or crush sustained-release brands, such as Bayer time-release aspirin, or enteric-coated preparations, such as Ecotrin.

Take with a full glass of water to reduce the risk of lodging aspirin in the throat.

What side effects may occur?

Side effects cannot be anticipated. If any develop or change in intensity, inform

your doctor as soon as possible. Only your doctor can determine if it is safe for you to continue using aspirin.

■ *Side effects may include:*
Heartburn
Nausea and/or vomiting
Possible involvement in formation of
stomach ulcers and bleeding
Small amounts of blood in stool
Stomach pain
Stomach upset

Why should this drug not be prescribed?

Do not take aspirin if you are allergic to it, if you have asthma, ulcers or ulcer symptoms, or if you are taking a medication that affects the clotting of your blood, unless specifically told to do so by your doctor.

Special warnings about this medication

Aspirin should not be given to children or teenagers for flu symptoms or chicken-pox. Aspirin has been associated with the development of Reye's syndrome, a disorder that involves abnormal brain function.

If you have a continuous or high fever, or a severe or persistent sore throat, especially with a high fever, vomiting and nausea, consult your doctor. It could indicate a more serious illness.

For conditions affecting children under 12 years old that require aspirin, consult your doctor.

If pain persists for more than 10 days or if redness appears at site of inflammation, consult your doctor.

If you experience ringing in the ears or hearing loss, consult your doctor before taking more aspirin.

Keep this medication out of the reach of children.

Possible food and drug interactions when taking this medication

If aspirin is taken with certain other drugs, the effects of either could be increased, decreased, or altered. It is especially important to check with your doctor before combining aspirin with the following:

Anti-gout medications such as Zyloprim
Arthritis medications such as Motrin and
Indocin
Blood thinners such as Coumadin and
Panwarfin
Diabetes medications such as DiaBeta and
Micronase

Special information if you are pregnant or breastfeeding

The use of aspirin during pregnancy should be discussed with your doctor. Aspirin should not be used during the last 3 months of pregnancy unless specifically indicated by your doctor. It may cause problems in the fetus and complications during delivery. Aspirin may appear in breast milk and could affect a nursing infant. Ask your doctor whether it is safe to take aspirin while you are breastfeeding.

Recommended dosage

ADULTS

Treatment of Minor Pain and Fever
The usual dose is 1 or 2 tablets every 3 to 4 hours up to 6 times a day.

Prevention of Stroke
The usual dose is 1 tablet 4 times daily or 2 tablets 2 times a day.

Prevention of Heart Attack
The usual dose is 1 tablet daily. Your physician may suggest that you take a larger dose, however.

CHILDREN
Consult your doctor.

Overdosage
Any medication used in excess can have serious consequences. If you suspect symptoms of an aspirin overdose, seek medical treatment or contact a poison control center immediately.

Brand name:

ASPIRIN FREE ANACIN

See Tylenol, page 661.

Generic name:

ASPIRIN WITH CODEINE PHOSPHATE

See Empirin with Codeine, page 232.

Generic name:

ASTEMIZOLE

See Hismanal, page 279.

Brand name:

ATARAX

Generic name: Hydroxyzine hydrochloride

Why is this drug prescribed?
Atarax is an antihistamine used to relieve the symptoms of common anxiety and tension and, in combination with other medications, to treat anxiety that results from physical illness. It also relieves itching from allergic reactions and can be used as a sedative before and after general anesthesia. Antihistamines work by decreasing the effects of histamine, a chemical released in the body that narrows air passages in the lungs and contributes to inflammation. Antihistamines reduce itching and swelling and dry up secretions from the nose, eyes, and throat.

Most important fact about this drug
The effectiveness of Atarax for long-term use (more than 4 months) in the treatment of anxiety has not been established. Your doctor should re-evaluate its effects periodically.

How should you take this medication?
Take this medication exactly as prescribed by your doctor.

What side effects may occur?
Side effects cannot be anticipated. If any develop or change in intensity, inform your doctor as soon as possible. Only your doctor can determine if it is safe for you to continue taking Atarax.

Drowsiness, the most common side effect of Atarax, is usually temporary and may disappear in a few days or when dosage is reduced. Less common or rare side effects include dry mouth, involuntary motor activity, tremor, and convulsions. These usually occur with higher than recommended doses of Atarax.

Why should this drug not be prescribed?
Atarax should not be taken in early pregnancy or if you are sensitive to or have ever had an allergic reaction to it. Make sure your doctor is aware of any drug reactions you have experienced.

Special warnings about this medication
Atarax increases the effects of drugs that depress the activity of the central nervous system. If you are taking narcotics, non-narcotic analgesics, or barbiturates in combination with Atarax, their dosage should be reduced.

This medication can cause drowsiness. Driving or operating dangerous machinery or participating in any hazardous activity that requires full mental alertness is not recommended until you know how you react to Atarax.

Possible food and drug interactions when taking this medication

Atarax may increase the effects of alcohol. Avoid alcohol while taking this medication.

If Atarax is taken with certain other drugs, the effects of either could be increased, decreased, or altered. It is especially important to check with your doctor before combining Atarax with the following:

Barbiturates such as Seconal, Phenobarbital
Narcotics such as Demerol, Percocet
Non-narcotic analgesics

Special information
if you are pregnant or breastfeeding

Although the effects of Atarax during pregnancy have not been adequately studied in humans, birth defects have appeared in animal studies with this medication. If you are pregnant or plan to become pregnant, inform your doctor immediately. Atarax may appear in breast milk and could affect a nursing infant. If this medication is essential to your health, your doctor may advise you to discontinue breastfeeding until your treatment is finished.

Recommended dosage

NOTE: When treatment begins with injections, it can be continued in tablet form.

All dosages should be adjusted according to the patient's response to the drug.

For Relief of Symptoms of Anxiety and Tension From Either Mental or Physical Disorders

ADULTS

The usual dose is 50 to 100 milligrams 4 times per day.

CHILDREN UNDER AGE 6

A total dose of 50 milligrams daily, divided into smaller doses.

CHILDREN OVER AGE 6

A total dose of 50 to 100 milligrams daily, divided into smaller doses.

For Itching Due to Allergic Conditions Such as Chronic Urticaria (an Allergic Reaction Causing Skin Eruptions) and Other Allergic Skin Conditions

ADULTS

The usual dose is 25 milligrams 3 or 4 times a day.

CHILDREN UNDER AGE 6

A total dose of 50 milligrams daily, divided into smaller doses.

CHILDREN OVER AGE 6

A total dose of 50 to 100 milligrams daily, divided into smaller doses.

As a Sedative Used Before and After General Anesthesia

ADULTS

The usual dose is 50 to 100 milligrams.

CHILDREN

The usual dose is 0.6 milligram per 2.2 pounds of body weight.

Atarax tablets come in 10-, 25-, 50-, and 100-milligram strengths. Atarax syrup supplies 10 milligrams per teaspoonful.

Overdosage

Any medication taken in excess can cause

symptoms of overdose. If you suspect an overdose, seek medical attention immediately.

The most common symptoms of Atarax overdose are excessive calm and a possible drop in blood pressure.

Generic name:

ATENOLOL

See Tenormin, page 616.

Generic name:

ATENOLOL/CHLORTHALIDONE

See Tenoretic, page 614.

Brand name:

ATIVAN

Generic name: Lorazepam

Why is this drug prescribed?

Ativan is used in the treatment of anxiety disorders and for short-term (up to 4 months) relief of the symptoms of anxiety. It belongs to a class of drugs known as benzodiazepines.

Most important fact about this drug

Tolerance and dependence can develop with the use of Ativan. You may experience withdrawal symptoms if you stop using it abruptly. Only your doctor should advise you to discontinue or change your dose.

How should you take this drug?

Take this medication exactly as prescribed by your doctor. If you forget to take a dose, take it as soon as you remember. If it is almost time for your next dose, skip the one you missed and go back to your regular schedule. Never take two doses at the same time.

What side effects may occur?

Side effects cannot be anticipated. If any develop or change in intensity, inform your doctor as soon as possible. Only your doctor can determine if it is safe for you to continue taking Ativan.

- *More common side effects may include:*
  Dizziness
  Unsteadiness
  Weakness

- *Less common or rare side effects may include:*
  Agitation, change in appetite, depression, eye function disorders, headache, memory impairment, mental disorientation, nausea, sleep disturbance, stomach and intestinal disorders

- *Side effects due to rapid decrease or abrupt withdrawal from Ativan:*
  Abdominal and muscle cramps, convulsions, depressed mood, inability to fall or stay asleep, sweating, tremors, vomiting

Why should this drug not be prescribed?

If you are sensitive to or have ever had an allergic reaction to Ativan or similar drugs, you should not take this medication.

Unless you are directed to do so by your doctor, do not take this medication if you have acute narrow-angle glaucoma.

Anxiety or tension related to everyday stress usually does not require treatment with Ativan. Discuss your symptoms thoroughly with your doctor.

Special warnings about this medication

Ativan may cause you to become drowsy or less alert; therefore, driving or operating dangerous machinery or participating in any hazardous activity that requires full mental alertness is not recommended.

This drug should not be used to treat psychosis.

If you are severely depressed or have suffered from severe depression, consult with your doctor before taking this medication.

If you have decreased kidney or liver function, use of this drug should be discussed with your doctor.

If you are elderly or if you have been using Ativan for a prolonged period of time, you should be frequently monitored by your doctor.

Possible food and drug interactions when taking this medication

Ativan may intensify the effects of alcohol. Avoid alcohol while taking this medication.

If Ativan is taken with certain other drugs, the effects of either could be increased, decreased, or altered. It is especially important to check with your doctor before combining Ativan with barbiturates (Phenobarbital, Seconal, Amytal) or any sedative-type medication.

Special information if you are pregnant or breastfeeding

Do not take Ativan if you are pregnant or planning to become pregnant. There is an increased risk of birth defects. It is not known whether Ativan appears in breast milk. If this medication is essential to your health, your doctor may advise you to discontinue breastfeeding until your treatment is finished.

Recommended dosage

ADULTS

The usual recommended dosage is a total of 2 to 6 milligrams per day divided into smaller doses. The largest dose should be taken at bedtime. The daily dose may vary from 1 to 10 milligrams per day.

Anxiety:
The usual starting dose is a total of 2 to 3 milligrams per day given in 2 or 3 small doses.

For insomnia due to anxiety, a single daily dose of 2 to 4 milligrams may be given, usually at bedtime.

CHILDREN

The safety and effectiveness of Ativan have not been established in children under 12 years of age.

ELDERLY

The usual starting dosage should not exceed a total of 1 to 2 milligrams per day in divided doses to avoid oversedation and unsteadiness. This dose can be adjusted by your doctor as needed.

When higher dosage is indicated, the evening dose should be increased first.

Overdosage

Any medication taken in excess can cause symptoms of overdose. If you suspect an overdose, seek medical attention immediately.

The symptoms of Ativan overdose may include:
Coma
Confusion
Low blood pressure
Sleepiness

Brand name:

ATRETOL

See Tegretol, page 608.

Brand name:

ATROFEN

See Lioresal, page 326.

Brand name:

ATROVENT

Generic name: Ipratropium bromide

Why is this drug prescribed?
Atrovent is a bronchodilator prescribed for the maintenance treatment of bronchial spasms (wheezing) associated with chronic obstructive pulmonary disease, including chronic bronchitis and emphysema. A bronchodilator improves the passage of air into the lungs.

Most important fact about this drug
This medication is not for use in acute attacks of bronchial spasm when a rapid response is required.

How should you take this medication?
Atrovent is not intended for occasional use. In order to obtain maximum effectiveness, this medication must be used consistently throughout your course of treatment, as prescribed by your doctor.

What side effects may occur?
Side effects cannot be anticipated. If any develop or change in intensity, inform your doctor as soon as possible. Only your doctor can determine if it is safe for you to continue taking Atrovent.

■ *More common side effects may include:*
Blurred vision, cough, dizziness, dry mouth or irritation from aerosol, headache, nausea, nervousness, rapid, strong heartbeat, rash, stomach upset

■ *Less common or rare side effects may include:*
Constipation, coordination difficulty, difficulty in urinating, drowsiness, fatigue, flushing, hives, hoarseness, inability to fall or stay asleep, increased heart rate, itching, low blood pressure, loss of hair, mouth sores, sharp eye pain, tingling sensation, tremors.

Why should this drug not be prescribed?
If you are sensitive to or have ever had an allergic reaction to Atrovent or similar drugs, you should not take this medication. Make sure that your doctor is aware of any drug reactions that you have experienced.

Special warnings about this medication
Unless you are directed to do so by your doctor, do not take this medication if you have narrow angle-glaucoma, an enlarged prostate or obstruction in the neck of the bladder.

Temporary blurring of vision may occur if you accidentally spray the aerosol in your eyes.

Possible food and drug interactions when taking this medication
No drug interactions have been reported.

Special information if you are pregnant or breastfeeding
The effects of Atrovent during pregnancy have not been adequately studied. If you are pregnant or plan to become pregnant, inform your doctor immediately. It is not known whether Atrovent may appear in breast milk. If this drug is essential to your health, your doctor may advise you to stop nursing your baby until your treatment is finished.

Recommended dosage
ADULTS

The usual starting dose is 2 inhalations, 4 times per day. Additional inhalations may be taken; however, the total should not exceed 12 in 24 hours.

CHILDREN

Safety and effectiveness have not been established in children below 12 years of age.

Atrovent comes in a metered-dose inhaler with enough medication for 200 inhalations.

Overdosage

Any drug taken in excess can cause symptoms of overdose. If you suspect an overdose, seek medical attention immediately. There is no information on specific symptoms of Atrovent overdose.

Brand name:

AUGMENTIN

Generic ingredients: Amoxicillin, Clavulanate potassium

Why is this drug prescribed?

Augmentin is used in the treatment of lower respiratory, middle ear, sinus, skin, and urinary tract infections that are caused by specific bacteria. These bacteria produce a chemical enzyme called beta lactamase that makes some infections particularly difficult to treat.

Most important fact about this drug

If you have a history of allergic reactions to medicines or other substances you should discuss this thoroughly with your doctor.

How should you take this medication?

Augmentin may be taken with or without food.

Shake oral (liquid) suspension well before using. Store under refrigeration and discard after 10 days.

What side effects may occur?

Side effects cannot be anticipated. If any develop or change in intensity, inform your doctor as soon as possible. Only your doctor can determine if it is safe for you to continue taking Augmentin.

- *More common side effects may include:*
  Diarrhea/loose stools
  Itching or burning of the vagina
  Nausea or vomiting
  Skin rashes and hives

- *Less common side effects may include:*
  Abdominal discomfort, anemia, arthritis, black "hairy" tongue, blood disorders, fever, gas, headache, indigestion, inflammation of the stomach and/or large intestine, itching, joint pain, muscle pain, skin inflammation, skin peeling, sores and inflammation in the mouth and on the tongue and gums.

- *Rare side effects may include:*
  Agitation, anxiety, behavioral changes, change in liver function, confusion, dizziness, hyperactivity, insomnia.

Why should this drug not be prescribed?

If you are sensitive to or have ever had an allergic reaction to any penicillin medication or if you have an infectious disease such as mononucleosis, do not take this drug.

Augmentin and other penicillin-like medicines are generally safe; however, anyone with liver, kidney or blood disorders is at increased risk when using this drug. Alternative choices may be available to your doctor.

If you have diabetes and test your urine for the presence of sugar, you should ask your doctor or pharmacist if this medication will interfere with the type of test you use.

Special warnings about this medication

Allergic reactions to this medication can be serious and possibly fatal. Let your doctor know about previous allergic reactions to medicines, food, or other substances before using Augmentin. If you experience a reaction, report it to your doctor immediately and seek medical treatment.

Possible food and drug interactions when taking this medication

Augmentin may react with the antigout medication Benemid, resulting in changes in blood levels. A reaction with another antigout drug, Zyloprim, may cause rashes. Notify your doctor if you are taking these drugs.

Do not take Augmentin when using Antabuse (disulfiram).

Special information if you are pregnant or breastfeeding

The effects of Augmentin during pregnancy have not been adequately studied. Because there may be potential risk to the fetus, doctors usually recommend Augmentin to pregnant women only when the benefits of therapy outweigh any potential risk to the fetus. Augmentin appears in breast milk and could affect a nursing infant. If Augmentin is essential to your health, your doctor may advise you to stop nursing your baby until your treatment with this drug is finished.

Recommended dosage

ADULTS

The usual adult dose is one 250-milligram tablet every 8 hours. For more severe infections and infections of the respiratory tract, the dose should be one 500-milligram tablet every 8 hours. It is essential that you take this medicine according to your doctor's directions.

CHILDREN

The usual total daily dosage is 20 milligrams per 2.2 pounds of body weight per day, divided into 4 doses and taken every 8 hours. For middle ear infections, sinus infections, and lower respiratory infections, the dose should be 40 milligrams per 2.2 pounds per day, divided into doses every 8 hours. Severe infections should be treated with the higher recommended dose. Children weighing 88 pounds or more should be dosed according to the adult recommendations.

Overdosage

Augmentin is generally safe; however, large amounts may cause overdose symptoms, including exaggerated side effects listed above. Suspected overdoses of Augmentin must be treated immediately; contact your physician or an emergency room.

Brand name:

AURALGAN

Generic ingredients: Antipyrine, Benzocaine Glycerin
Other brand name: Auroto Otic

Why is this drug prescribed?

Auralgan is prescribed to relieve pressure, reduce inflammation and congestion, and lessen the pain and discomfort of severe middle ear infections. This drug may be used in combination with an antibiotic for killing the infecting organism.

Auralgan is also used to remove excessive or impacted earwax.

Most important fact about this drug

Discard this product 6 months after the dropper is first placed in the drug solution.

How should you use this medication?

Use this medication exactly as prescribed by your doctor.

Do not rinse the medication dropper after using; replace it in the bottle after each use. Hold the dropper assembly by the screw cap and, without squeezing the rubber bulb, insert the dropper into the drug container and screw down tightly.

What side effects may occur?

Side effects cannot be anticipated. If any develop or change in intensity, inform your doctor as soon as possible. For Auralgan, no specific side effects have been reported.

Why should this drug not be prescribed?

If you are sensitive to or allergic to any of the ingredients contained in Auralgan or similar drugs, you should not take this medication. Make sure that your doctor is aware of any drug reactions that you have experienced.

Unless directed to do so by your doctor, do not use this medication if you have a punctured eardrum.

Special warnings about this medication

Notify your doctor if irritation occurs or if you develop an allergic reaction to this medication.

Possible food and drug interactions when taking this medication

No food or drug interactions have been reported.

Special information if you are pregnant or breastfeeding

The effects of Auralgan during pregnancy have not been adequately studied. If you are pregnant or plan to become pregnant, notify your doctor immediately. It is not known whether Auralgan appears in breast milk. If this medication is essential to your health,

your doctor may advise you to discontinue breastfeeding until your treatment is finished.

Recommended dosage

ADULTS AND CHILDREN

Acute Otitis Media (Severe Middle Ear Infection)
Apply the medication drop by drop into the ear, permitting the solution to run along the wall of the ear canal until it is filled. Avoid touching the ear with the dropper. Then moisten a piece of cotton dressing material, such as gauze, with Auralgan and insert it into the opening of the ear. Repeat every 1 to 2 hours until pain and congestion are relieved.

Removal of Earwax
Before: Apply Auralgan drop by drop into the ear 3 times daily for 2 or 3 days to help detach and remove earwax from the wall of the ear canal.

After: Auralgan is useful for drying out the canal or relieving discomfort.

Before and after the removal of earwax, cotton dressing material such as gauze should be moistened with Auralgan and inserted into the opening of the ear following use of the medication.

Overdosage

No information on overdosage with Auralgan is available.

Generic name:

AURANOFIN

See Ridaura, page 542.

Brand name:

AUROTO OTIC

See Auralgan, page 48.

Brand name:

AVENTYL

See Pamelor, page 450.

Brand name:

AXID

Generic name: Nizatidine

Why is this drug prescribed?

Axid is prescribed for the treatment of active duodenal ulcers. It is also used for maintenance therapy, at a reduced dosage, after a duodenal ulcer has healed.
Axid belongs to a class of drugs known as histamine H2 blockers.

Most important fact about this drug

Although Axid can be used for up to 8 weeks, most ulcers are healed within 4 weeks of therapy.

How should you take this medication?

Take this medication exactly as prescribed by your doctor.

What side effects may occur?

Side effects cannot be anticipated. If any develop or change in intensity, inform your doctor as soon as possible. Only your doctor can determine if it is safe for you to continue taking Axid.

■ More common side effects may include:
Hives
Rash
Sleepiness
Sweating

■ Less common or rare side effects may include:
Allergic reactions, bleeding and bruising, blood disorders, breast development in males, decreased sexual drive, fever, hepatitis (inflammation of the liver), impotence, nausea, rapid heartbeat, reversible mental confusion, wheezing, yellow eyes and skin

Why should this drug not be prescribed?

If you are sensitive to or have ever had an allergic reaction to Axid or similar drugs you should not take this medication. Make sure that your doctor is aware of any drug reactions that you have experienced.

Special warnings about this medication

A stomach malignancy could be present, even if your symptoms have been relieved by Axid.

If you have moderate or severe kidney disease, your dosage should be reduced.

Possible food and drug interactions when taking this medication

If Axid is taken with certain other drugs, the effects of either could be increased, decreased, or altered. It is especially important to check with your doctor before combining Axid with aspirin, especially when taken in high doses.

Special information if you are pregnant or breastfeeding

The effects of Axid during pregnancy have not been adequately studied. If you are pregnant or plan to become pregnant, inform your doctor immediately. Axid appears in breast milk and could affect a nursing infant. If this medication is essential to your health, your doctor may advise you to discontinue breastfeeding until your treatment with this medication is finished.

Recommended dosage

ADULTS

Active Duodenal Ulcer
The usual dose is 300 milligrams once a day at bedtime. An alternate dosage regimen is 150 milligrams twice a day.

Maintenance of a Healed Duodenal Ulcer
The usual dose is 150 milligrams once a day at bedtime.

People with moderate to severe kidney disease should receive a reduced dose.

CHILDREN

The safety and effectiveness of Axid have not been established in children.

ELDERLY

Dosage should be determined by the particular needs of the elderly patient.

Overdosage

Any medication taken in excess can cause symptoms of overdose. If you suspect an overdose, seek medical attention immediately.

No specific information on Axid overdose is available.

Generic name:

AZATADINE MALEATE AND PSEUDOEPHEDRINE SULFATE

See Trinalin, page 656.

Generic name:

AZITHROMYCIN

See Zithromax, page 698.

Brand name:

AZULFIDINE

Generic name: Sulfasalazine

Why is this drug prescribed?

Azulfidine, an anti-inflammatory medicine, is prescribed for the treatment of mild to moderate ulcerative colitis (long-term, progressive bowel disease) and as an added treatment in severe ulcerative colitis. This medication is also prescribed to decrease severe attacks of ulcerative colitis.

Azulfidine EN-tabs are prescribed for patients who cannot take the regular Azulfidine tablet because of symptoms of stomach and intestinal irritation such as nausea and vomiting; for patients taking the first few doses of the drug; or for patients in whom a reduction in dosage does not lessen the stomach or intestinal side effects.

Ulcerative colitis is chronic inflammation and ulceration of the lining of large bowel and rectum. The main symptom is bloody diarrhea; the feces may also contain pus and mucus.

Most important fact about this drug

Although ulcerative colitis rarely disappears completely, the risk of recurrence can be substantially reduced by the continued use of this drug.

Azulfidine belongs to a class of drugs known as sulfonamides. Serious and sometime fatal allergic reactions have been reported with this class of drugs. Make sure your doctor is aware of any allergies you have to sulfa drugs.

How should you take this medication?

Take this medication in evenly divided doses, as determined by your doctor, preferably with food or milk to avoid stomach upset.

It is important that you drink plenty of fluids while taking this medication to avoid kidney stones.

Skin and urine may become yellow-orange in color while taking Azulfidine.

In addition, prolonged exposure to the sun should be avoided.

What side effects may occur?

Side effects cannot be anticipated. If any develop or change in intensity, inform your doctor as soon as possible. Only your doctor can determine if it is safe for you to continue taking Azulfidine.

■ *More common side effects may include:*
Diarrhea
Headache
Lack or loss of appetite
Nausea
Stomach distress
Vomiting

■ *Less common side effects may include:*
Bluish discoloration of the skin, fever, hives, itching, skin rash

■ *Rare side effects may include:*
Abdominal pain, blood in the urine, bloody diarrhea, convulsions, dizziness, drowsiness, hallucinations, hearing loss, inability to fall or stay asleep, itchy skin eruptions, joint pain, lack of muscle coordination, loss of hair, mental depression, red, slightly raised rash, ringing in the ears, sensitivity to light, skin discoloration, skin disorders, urine discoloration

Why should this drug not be prescribed?

If you are sensitive to or have ever had an allergic reaction to sulfasalazine, its breakdown products in the body, salicylates (aspirin), or other sulfa drugs, you should not take this medication. Make sure that your

doctor is aware of any drug reactions that you have experienced.

Unless you are directed to do so by your doctor, do not take Azulfidine if you have an intestinal or urinary obstruction or if you have porphyria (an inherited disorder distinguished by a disturbance of the metabolism of the substance that gives color to the skin and iris of the eyes).

Special warnings about this medication

Patients with kidney or liver damage or patients who have any blood disease should be checked very carefully by their doctor before taking Azulfidine. Deaths have been reported in these patients from allergic reactions, blood diseases, kidney or liver damage, changes in nerve and muscle impulses, and fibrosing alveolitis (inflammation of the lungs due to a thickening or scarring of tissue). Signs such as sore throat, fever, abnormal paleness of the skin, bruising, or jaundice (yellowing of the skin) may be an indication of a serious blood disorder. Frequent blood counts and urine tests should be performed by the doctor.

Azulfidine should be given with caution to patients with severe allergy or bronchial asthma.

If Azulfidine EN-tabs are passed undisintegrated, stop taking the drug and notify your doctor immediately. (You may lack the intestinal enzymes necessary to dissolve this medication.)

Possible food and drug interactions when taking this medication

If Azulfidine is taken with certain other drugs, the effects of either could be increased, decreased, or altered. It is especially important to check with your doctor before combining Azulfidine with the following:

Digoxin (Lanoxin)
Folic acid (a B-complex vitamin)

Special information
if you are pregnant or breastfeeding

The effects of Azulfidine during pregnancy have not been adequately studied. If you are pregnant or plan to become pregnant, inform your doctor immediately.
Azulfidine is secreted in breast milk and could affect a nursing infant. If this medication is essential to your health, your doctor may advise you to discontinue breastfeeding until your treatment is finished.

Recommended dosage

Your doctor will carefully individualize your dosage and monitor your response periodically.

ADULTS

The usual initial recommended dose is 3 to 4 grams daily divided into smaller doses (intervals between nighttime doses should not exceed 8 hours). In some cases the initial dosage is 1 to 2 grams daily to lessen side effects.

Maintenance Therapy
The usual maintenance dose is 2 grams daily.

CHILDREN 2 AND OLDER

The usual initial recommended dose is 40 to 60 milligrams per 2.2 pounds of body weight in each 24-hour period, divided into 3 to 6 doses.

Maintenance Therapy
The usual maintenance dose is 30 milligrams per 2.2 pounds of body weight in each 24-hour period, divided into 4 doses.

Overdosage

Symptoms of Azulfidine overdose may include:
Convulsions
Drowsiness
Nausea
Stomach and abdominal pain
Vomiting

If you suspect symptoms of an Azulfidine overdose, seek emergency medical attention immediately.

Generic name:

BACLOFEN

See Lioresal, page 326.

Brand name:

BACTRIM

Generic ingredients: Trimethoprim, Sulfamethoxazole
Other brand names: Cotrim, Septra

Why is this drug prescribed?

Bactrim, an antibacterial combination drug, is prescribed for the treatment of certain urinary tract infections, severe middle ear infections in children, long-lasting or frequently recurring bronchitis in adults that has increased in seriousness, inflammation of the intestine due to a severe bacterial infection, pneumonia in patients who have a suppressed immune system (Pneumocystis carinii pneumonia) and for travelers' diarrhea in adults.

Most important fact about this drug

Sulfamethoxazole, an ingredient in Bactrim, is one of a group of drugs called sulfonamides, which prevent the growth of bacteria in the body. However, fatalities have occurred with use of sulfonamides due to severe reactions, including Stevens-Johnson syndrome (severe eruptions around the mouth, anus, or eyes), progressive disintegration of the outer layer of the skin, sudden and severe liver damage, a severe blood disorder (agranulocytosis), and a lack of red and white blood cells because of a bone marrow disorder.

Notify your doctor at the first sign of an adverse reaction such as skin rash, sore throat, fever, joint pain, cough, shortness of breath, abnormal skin paleness, reddish or purplish skin spots, or yellowing of the skin or whites of the eyes.

Frequent blood counts by a doctor are recommended for patients taking sulfonamide drugs.

How should you take this medication?
Take Bactrim exactly as prescribed by your doctor.

It is important that you drink plenty of fluids while taking this medication in order to prevent sediment in the urine and the formation of stones.

What side effects may occur?
Side effects cannot be anticipated. If any develop or change in intensity, inform your doctor as soon as possible. Only your doctor can determine if it is safe for you to continue taking Bactrim.

■ *More common side effects may include:*
Hives
Lack or loss of appetite
Nausea
Skin rash
Vomiting

■ *Less common side effects may include:*
Abdominal pain, anemia, chills, convulsions, depression, diarrhea, fatigue, fever, hallucinations, headache, hepatitis, inability to fall or stay asleep, inability to urinate, inflammation of heart muscle, inflammation of the mouth and/or tongue, itching, joint pain, kidney failure, lack of feeling or concern, lack of muscle coordination, muscle pain, nervousness, red, raised rash, redness and swelling of the tongue, ringing in the ears, scaling of dead skin due to inflammation, sensitivity to light, severe skin welts or swelling, skin eruptions, skin peeling, vertigo, weakness, yellowing of eyes and skin

Why should this drug not be prescribed?
If you are sensitive to or have ever had an allergic reaction to trimethoprim, sulfamethoxazole or drugs of this type, you should not take this medication. Make sure that your doctor is aware of any drug reactions that you have experienced.

Unless you are directed to do so by your doctor, do not take this medication if you have been diagnosed as having megaloblastic anemia, which is a blood disorder due to a deficiency of folic acid.

This drug should not be prescribed for infants less than 2 months of age.

Bactrim is not recommended for preventative or prolonged use in middle ear infections and should not be used in the treatment of streptococcal pharyngitis (inflammation or infection of the pharynx due to streptococcus bacteria.)

Special warnings about this medication
If you have impaired kidney or liver function, have a folic acid deficiency, are a chronic alcoholic, are taking anticonvulsants, have been diagnosed as having malabsorption syndrome (abnormal intestinal absorption), are in a state of poor nutrition, or have severe allergies or bronchial asthma, caution should be exercised when taking Bactrim. Consult with your doctor.

If you are an AIDS (acquired immunodeficiency syndrome) patient and are being treated for pneumocystis carinii pneumonia, you will experience more side effects than will a patient without AIDS.

Your urine and kidney function should be monitored by your doctor during treatment with Bactrim, especially if your kidneys are not functioning properly.

Possible food and drug interactions when taking this medication

If Bactrim is taken with certain other drugs, the effects of either could be increased, decreased, or altered. It is especially important to check with your doctor before combining Bactrim with the following:

Anticonvulsants such as phenytoin (Dilantin)
Diuretics (in the elderly)
Methotrexate
Warfarin (Coumadin)

Special information
If you are pregnant or breastfeeding

The effects of Bactrim during pregnancy have not been adequately studied. If you are pregnant or plan to become pregnant, notify your doctor immediately. The drug should not be taken at term. Bactrim does appear in breast milk and could affect a nursing infant. It should not be taken while breast-feeding.

Recommended dosage

ADULTS

Urinary Tract Infections and Intestinal Inflammation
The usual adult dosage in the treatment of urinary tract infection is 1 Bactrim DS (double strength) tablet, 2 Bactrim tablets, or 4 teaspoonfuls (20 milliliters) of Bactrim Suspension every 12 hours for 10 to 14 days. The dosage for inflammation of the intestine is the same but is taken for 5 days.

Worsening of Chronic Bronchitis
The usual recommended dosage is 1 Bactrim DS (double strength) tablet, 2 Bactrim tablets, or 4 teaspoonfuls (20 milliliters) of Bactrim Suspension every 12 hours for 14 days.

Pneumocystis Carinii Pneumonia
The recommended dosage is 20 milligrams of trimethoprim and 100 milligrams of sulfamethoxazole per 2.2 pounds of body weight per 24 hours divided into equal doses every 6 hours for 14 days.

Travelers' Diarrhea
The usual recommended dosage is 1 Bactrim DS (double strength) tablet, 2 Bactrim tablets, or 4 teaspoonfuls (20 milliliters) of Bactrim Suspension every 12 hours for 5 days.

CHILDREN

Urinary Tract Infections or Middle Ear Infections
The recommended dose for children 2 months of age or older, given every 12 hours for 10 days, is determined by weight. The following table is a guideline for this dosage:

22 pounds, 1 teaspoonful (5 milliliters)
44 pounds, 2 teaspoonfuls (10 milliliters)
  1 tablet
66 pounds, 3 teaspoonfuls (15 milliliters)
  1½ tablets
88 pounds, 4 teaspoonfuls (20 milliliters)
  2 tablets or 1 DS tablet

Intestinal Inflammation
The recommended dose is identical to the dosage recommended for urinary tract and middle ear infections; however, it should be taken for 5 days.

Pneumocystis Carinii Pneumonia
The recommended dose, taken every 6 hours for 14 days, is determined by weight. The following table is a guideline for this dosage:

18 pounds, 1 teaspoonful (5 milliliters)
35 pounds, 2 teaspoonfuls (10 milliliters)
  1 tablet
53 pounds, 3 teaspoonfuls (15 milliliters)
  1½ tablets
70 pounds, 4 teaspoonfuls (20 milliliters)
  2 tablets or 1 DS tablet

The safety of repeated use of Bactrim in children under 2 years of age has not been established.

ELDERLY

There may be an increased risk of severe side effects when Bactrim is taken by elderly patients, especially in patients who have impaired kidney and/or liver function or in patients who are taking other medication. Consult with your doctor before taking Bactrim.

Bactrim DS (double strength) tablets contain 160 milligrams of trimethoprim and 800 milligrams of sulfamethoxazole.

Bactrim tablets contain 80 milligrams of trimethoprim and 400 milligrams of sulfamethoxazole.

Overdosage
Symptoms of an overdose of Bactrim include:
Blood or sediment in the urine, colic, confusion, dizziness, drowsiness, fever, headache, lack or loss of appetite, mental depression, nausea, unconsciousness, vomiting, yellowed eyes and skin

If you suspect an overdose, seek emergency medical attention immediately.

Brand name:

BACTROBAN

Generic name: Mupirocin

Why is this drug prescribed?
Bactroban is prescribed for the topical treatment of bacterial infections such as impetigo.

Most important fact about this drug
If the use of Bactroban does not clear your skin infection within 3 to 5 days, or if the infection becomes worse, notify your doctor.

How should you use this medication?
This drug is for external use only.

If you forget to apply a dose, apply it as soon as you remember. If it is almost time for the next dose, skip the one you missed and go back to your regular schedule.

What side effects may occur?
Side effects cannot be anticipated. If any develop or change in intensity, inform your doctor as soon as possible. Only your doctor can determine if it is safe for you to continue taking Bactroban.

■ *More common side effects may include:*
Burning
Pain
Stinging

■ *Less common side effects may include:*
Itching

■ *Rare side effects may include:*
Abnormal redness, dry skin, inflammation of the skin, nausea, oozing, skin rash, swelling, tenderness

Why should this drug not be prescribed?
If you are sensitive to or have ever had an allergic reaction to Bactroban or similar drugs, you should not use this medication. Make sure that your doctor is aware of any drug reactions that you have experienced.

Special warnings about this medication
Continued or prolonged use of Bactroban may result in a growth of bacteria that do not respond to this medication and can cause a secondary infection.

This drug is not intended for use in the eyes.

Possible food and drug interactions when taking this medication
There are no known drug interactions.

Special information
if you are pregnant or breastfeeding

The effects of Bactroban during pregnancy have not been adequately studied. If you are pregnant or plan to become pregnant, inform your doctor immediately.
Bactroban may appear in breast milk. Your doctor may advise you to discontinue breastfeeding until your treatment with this medication is finished.

Recommended dosage

A small amount of this medication should be applied to the affected area 3 times a day. The treated area may then be covered with gauze if desired.

Overdosage

There is no information available on overdosage.

Generic name:

BECLOMETHASONE DIPROPIONATE

Brand names: Beclovent Inhalation Aerosal, Beconase AQ Nasal Spray, Beconase Inhalation Aerosol, Vancenase AQ Nasal Spray, Vancenase Nasal Inhaler, Vanceril Inhaler

Why is this drug prescribed?

Beclomethasone is a corticosteroid. Beclovent and Vanceril are prescribed for the treatment of recurring symptoms of bronchial asthma.

Beconase and Vancenase are used for the symptomatic relief of hay fever and for the prevention of the recurrence of nasal polyps following surgical removal.

Most important fact about this drug

Beclomethasone is not a bronchodilator medication and should not be used for relief of asthma when bronchodilators and other non-steroid drugs can be used. It is not useful when rapid relief of symptoms is needed but helps to control symptoms when taken routinely.

It may be 1 to 2 weeks before full relief is obtained with beclomethasone nasal spray. The dosage of beclomethasone nasal products should not be increased and they are not immediately effective. Patients' instructions are provided with products.

How should you take this medication?

Beclomethasone is prescribed in an oral inhalant or a nasal spray form. Use this medication only as preventive therapy exactly as prescribed by your doctor. Many patients will require additional drugs to fully control asthma symptoms, but this drug may allow other drugs to be used in smaller doses.

Shake the aerosol canister well before using. Do not use or store canister near heat or open flame. Do not puncture.

You may wish to rinse your mouth after inhalation.

If you are also using a bronchodilator inhalant, it should be used before the beclomethasone inhalant is used to promote the best effects from the latter drug. Use of the two inhalers should be separated by several minutes.

What side effects may occur?

Side effects cannot be anticipated. If any develop or change in intensity, inform your doctor as soon as possible. Only your doctor can determine if it is safe for you to continue taking this medication.

■ *Side effects may include:*
Dry mouth
Fluid retention
Hives

Hoarseness
Skin rash
Wheezing

■ *When using a nasal spray, other possible side effects are:*
Headache, light-headedness, nasal burning, nasal irritation, nausea, nose and throat infections, nosebleed, runny nose, sneezing, stuffy nose, tearing eyes.

Why should this drug not be prescribed?
Beclomethasone should not be prescribed if your asthma can be controlled with bronchodilators and other non-steroid medications.

Beclomethasone should not be prescribed if you require only occasional treatment for asthma.

Beclomethasone should not be prescribed for the treatment of non-asthmatic bronchitis.

If you are sensitive to or have ever had an allergic reaction to beclomethasone or similar drugs, you should not take this medication. Make sure that your doctor is aware of any drug reactions that you have experienced.

Special warnings about this medication
When corticosteroid drugs are taken by mouth they substitute for and decrease the body's normal ability to make its own steroid chemicals as well as its ability to respond to stress.

There is a risk of causing a serious condition called "adrenal insufficiency" when patients are changed from steroid tablets taken by mouth to aerosol beclomethasone dipropionate. Although the aerosol may provide adequate control of asthma during the changeover period, it does not provide the normal amount of steroid the body needs during acute stress situations. If you are being transferred from steroid tablets to beclomethasone and you experience a period of stress or a severe asthma attack, you may require additional treatment with steroid tablets.

Transfer of patients from steroid tablet therapy to beclomethasone dipropionate aerosol may uncover allergic conditions that were previously suppressed by the steroid tablet therapy, such as runny nose, conjunctivitis, and eczema. If you are on high (immuno-suppressant) doses, avoid being exposed to chickenpox or measles; these diseases can be serious or fatal in children and in adults who have never had them.

Recommended dosage
ADULTS

Beclomethasone Oral Inhalant
The usual recommended dose for adults and children 12 years of age and over is 2 inhalations given 2 to 4 times a day. Four inhalations given twice daily have been shown to be effective in some patients. If you have severe asthma, your doctor may advise you to start with 12 to 16 inhalations a day. Daily intake should not exceed 20 inhalations.

Beclomethasone Nasal Spray
The usual dosage is 1 or 2 inhalations in each nostril 2 to 4 times a day for adults and children 12 years of age and over.

CHILDREN

Beclomethasone Oral Inhalant
Children 6 to 12 years of age: The usual recommended dose is 1 or 2 inhalations given 3 or 4 times a day. Four inhalations given twice daily have been effective for some patients. Daily intake should not exceed 10 inhalations.

Beclomethasone Nasal Spray
Children 6 to 12 years of age: The usual dosage is 1 inhalation in each nostril 3 times daily. Aerosol is *not* recommended for children below 6 years of age.

Beclomethasone should not be given to children under the age of 6 unless advised by your doctor.

Overdosage
Any medication taken in excess can have serious consequences. If you suspect an overdose, seek medical attention immediately.

Brand name:

BECLOVENT

See Beclomethasone Dipropionate, page 57.

Brand name:

BECONASE

See Beclomethasone Dipropionate, page 57.

Brand name:

BEEPEN VK

See Penicillin V, page 462.

Brand name:

BENADRYL

Generic name: Diphenhydramine hydrochloride

Why is this drug prescribed?
Benadryl is an antihistamine with drying and sedative effects. It relieves red, inflamed eyes caused by food allergies and the itching, swelling, and redness from hives and other rashes that are caused by mild allergic reactions. It also relieves the sneezing, coughing, runny or stuffy nose, and red, teary, itching eyes caused by seasonal allergies (hay fever) and the common cold. Antihistamines work by decreasing the effects of histamine, a chemical released in the body that narrows air passages in the lungs and contributes to inflammation. Antihistamines reduce itching and swelling and dry up secretions from the nose, eyes, and throat.

Benadryl is also used to treat allergic reactions to blood transfusions, to prevent and treat motion sickness, and, with other drugs, to treat anaphylactic shock (severe allergic reaction) and Parkinsonism, a nerve disorder characterized by tremors, stooped posture, shuffling walk, muscle weakness, drooling, and emotional instability.

Most important fact about this drug
Antihistamines may produce excitability in children. In the elderly they may cause dizziness, drowsiness, or low blood pressure.

How should you take this medication?
Benadryl should be taken exactly as prescribed by your doctor or follow instructions on the label.

What side effects may occur?
Side effects cannot be anticipated. If any develop or change in intensity, inform your doctor as soon as possible. Only your doctor can determine if it is safe for you to continue taking Benadryl.

■ *More common side effects may include:*
Disturbed coordination
Dizziness
Drowsiness
Increased chest congestion
Sleepiness
Stomach upset

■ *Less common or rare side effects may include:*
Anaphylactic shock (extreme allergic reaction), blurred vision, chills,

confusion, constipation, convulsions, diarrhea, difficulty sleeping, double vision, drug rash, dry mouth, nose, throat, early menstruation, excessive perspiration, extreme tiredness, frequent or difficult urination, headache, hives, increased sensitivity to sunlight, irregular heartbeat, irritability, loss of appetite, low blood pressure, nausea, nervousness, pounding heartbeat, rapid heartbeat, restlessness, ringing in the ears, stuffy nose, tightness of chest and wheezing, tingling or pins and needles, tremor, unreal sense of well-being, urinary retention, vertigo, vomiting

Why should this drug not be prescribed?

Benadryl should not be used in newborn or premature infants, or if you are breastfeeding your infant.

Do not take this medication if you are sensitive to or have ever had an allergic reaction to diphenhydramine hydrochloride or other antihistamines with a similar chemical composition.

Special warnings about this medication

Antihistamines in general should be used very cautiously if you have narrow-angle glaucoma, narrowing of the stomach or intestine because of peptic ulcer or other stomach problems, symptoms of an enlarged prostate or difficulty urinating. Antihistamines can make children less alert and, in young children, may cause excitability. Antihistamines may produce hallucinations, convulsions, or death in children, especially if too much is taken. Elderly people (60 years or older) are more likely to experience dizziness, extreme calm, and low blood pressure.

Benadryl should be used cautiously if you have a history of asthma or other chronic lung disease, increased eye pressure, an over-active thyroid, high blood pressure, or heart disease.

This medication can cause drowsiness. Driving or operating dangerous machinery or participating in any hazardous activity that requires full mental alertness is not recommended until you know how you react to Benadryl.

Antidepressants known as MAO inhibitors will intensify the drying effects of Benadryl and should not be taken at the same time.

Possible food and drug interactions when taking this medication

Benadryl may increase the effects of alcohol and alcohol may increase the sedative effects of Benadryl. Do not drink alcohol while taking this medication.

If Benadryl is taken with certain other drugs, the effects of either could be increased, decreased, or altered. It is especially important to check with your doctor before combining Benadryl with the following:

Antidepressant drugs known as MAO inhibitors, such as Marplan, and Nardil
Sedatives/hypnotics such as Nembutal and Seconal
Tranquilizers such as Xanax and Valium

Special information if you are pregnant or breastfeeding

The effects of Benadryl during pregnancy have not been adequately studied. If you are pregnant or plan to become pregnant, inform your doctor immediately. Benadryl should be used during pregnancy only if clearly needed. Antihistamine therapy is not advised for nursing mothers. If this medication is essential to your health, your doctor may advise you to discontinue breastfeeding until your treatment with Benadryl is finished.

Recommended dosage

ADULTS

The usual recommended dose is 25 to 50 milligrams 3 or 4 times daily. The sleep-aid dosage is 50 milligrams at bedtime.

Motion Sickness

For prevention of motion sickness, the first dose should be given 30 minutes before exposure to motion and similar doses should be given before meals and at bedtime for the duration of exposure.

CHILDREN (OVER 20 POUNDS)

The usual dose is 12.5 to 25 milligrams, 3 to 4 times daily. The maximum daily dosage should not exceed 300 milligrams.

This medication should not be used as a sleep aid for children under age 12. Your physician will determine the best use of the drug in response to its effects on the child.

Overdosage

Any medication taken in excess can have serious consequences. If you suspect an overdose, seek medical attention immediately. Antihistamine overdose has caused hallucinations, convulsions, and death in children.

Symptoms of Benadryl overdose may include:
Central nervous system depression or
    stimulation, especially in children.
Dry mouth
Fixed, dilated pupils
Flushing
Stomach symptoms

Generic name:

BENAZEPRIL HYDROCHLORIDE

See Lotensin, page 342.

Brand name:

BENTYL

Generic name: Dicyclomine hydrochloride

Why is this drug prescribed?

Bentyl, available in capsules, tablets, and syrup, is prescribed for the treatment of functional bowel/irritable bowel syndrome (abdominal pain, accompanied by diarrhea and constipation, which does not seem to be disease-related but is associated with stress).

Most important fact about this drug

Heat prostration (fever and heat stroke due to decreased sweating) can occur with use of this drug in hot weather. If symptoms occur, notify your doctor immediately.

How should you take this medication?

Take this medication exactly as prescribed by your doctor.

What side effects may occur?

Side effects cannot be anticipated. If any develop or change in intensity, inform your doctor as soon as possible. Only your doctor can determine if it is safe for you to continue taking Bentyl.

■ *Common side effects may include:*
    Blurred vision
    Dizziness
    Drowsiness
    Dry mouth
    Light-headedness
    Nausea
    Nervousness
    Weakness

Not all of the following side effects have been reported with dicyclomine hydrochloride, but they have been reported for similar drugs with antispasmodic action; contact your doctor if they occur.

Abdominal pain, agitation, bloated feeling, coma, confusion or excitement, constipation, decreased anxiety, decreased sweating, difficulty in carrying out voluntary movements, difficulty in urinating, disorientation, double vision, enlargement of the pupil of the eye, exaggerated feeling of well-being, eye paralysis, fainting, fatigue, hallucinations, headache, hives, impotence, inability to fall or stay asleep, inability to urinate, itching, labored, difficult breathing, lack of coordination, lack or loss of appetite, memory loss, short-term, nasal stuffiness or congestion, numbness, pounding heartbeat, rapid heartbeat, rash, sluggishness, sneezing, speech disturbance, suffocation, suppression of breast milk, taste loss, temporary cessation of breathing, throat congestion, tingling, vomiting

Why should this drug not be prescribed?

If you are sensitive to or have ever had an allergic reaction to Bentyl, you should not take this medication. Make sure that your doctor is aware of any drug reactions that you have experienced.

Unless you are directed to do so by your doctor, do not take this drug if you have an obstructive disease of the urinary tract, obstructive disease of the stomach or intestines, severe ulcerative colitis (inflammatory disease of the large intestine and rectum), reflux esophagitis (inflammation of the esophagus usually caused by the backflow of acid stomach contents), glaucoma, or myasthenia gravis (disease characterized by long-lasting fatigue and muscle weakness). The drug also should not be taken following hemorrhage severe enough to affect cardiovascular status.

This drug should not be prescribed for infants less than 6 months of age.

Special warnings about this medication

Bentyl may produce drowsiness or blurred vision. Therefore, driving a car or operating dangerous machinery or participating in any hazardous activity that requires full mental alertness is not recommended.

Diarrhea may be an early symptom of a partial intestinal blockage, especially in patients who have had an ileostomy or colostomy. If this occurs, notify your doctor immediately.

This medication should be used with caution in patients with autonomic neuropathy (abnormal condition of the peripheral nerves, which maintain many of the body's involuntary functions); liver or kidney disease; hyperthyroidism; high blood pressure; coronary heart disease; congestive heart failure; rapid, irregular heartbeat (use of this medication may increase the heartrate); hiatal hernia (protrusion of part of the stomach through the diaphragm); or known or suspected enlargement of the prostate gland.

Possible food and drug interactions when taking this medication

If Bentyl is taken with certain other drugs, the effects of either could be increased, decreased, or altered. It is especially important to check with your doctor before combining Bentyl with the following:

Amatadine (Symmetrel—used to treat Parkinson's disease)

Antacids

Antiglaucoma drugs such as Betoptic

Antihistamines

Benzodiazepines (tranquilizers such as Valium and Xanax)

Digoxin (Lanoxin—used to treat congestive heart failure)

MAO inhibitors (antidepressants such as Nardil)

Metoclopramide (Reglan, a gastrointestinal stimulant)

Narcotic analgesics (pain relievers such as Demerol)

Nitrates and nitrites

Phenothiazines (anti-psychotic drugs such as Thorazine)

Quinidine (Quinidex—prescribed for abnormal heartbeats)

Sympathomimetic drugs such as Proventil and Ventolin

Tricyclic antidepressant drugs such as Elavil and Tofranil

Special Information
If you are pregnant or breastfeeding

The effects of Bentyl during pregnancy have not been adequately studied. If you are pregnant or plan to become pregnant, notify your doctor. Bentyl does appear in breast milk and could affect a nursing infant. If this medication is essential to your health, your doctor may advise you to discontinue breastfeeding until your treatment is finished.

Recommended dosage

ADULTS

The only oral dose clearly shown to be effective is 160 milligrams per day divided into 4 equal doses. Since this dose is associated with a significant incidence of side effects, your doctor may recommend a starting dose of 80 milligrams per day divided into 4 equal doses. Depending upon your response during the first week of treatment, your doctor may increase your dose to 160 milligrams per day unless side effects appear.

If this drug is not effective within 2 weeks or side effects require doses below 80 milligrams per day, your doctor may discontinue it.

CHILDREN

Safety and effectiveness have not been established in children.

Overdosage

Symptoms of a Bentyl overdose include:
Blurred vision, central nervous system (brain and spinal cord) stimulation, difficulty in swallowing, dilated pupils, dizziness, dryness of the mouth, headache, hot, dry skin, nausea, nerve blockage causing weakness and possible paralysis, vomiting

If you suspect an overdose, seek medical attention immediately.

Brand name:

BENZAC W

See Desquam-E, page 181.

Brand name:

BENZAGEL

See Desquam-E, page 181.

Brand name:

BENZASHAVE

See Desquam-E, page 181.

Brand name:

BENZAMYCIN

Generic ingredients: Erythromycin, Benzoyl peroxide

Why is this drug prescribed?

A combination of the antibiotic Erythromycin and the antibacterial agent benzoyl peroxide, Benzamycin is effective in stopping the bacteria that cause acne and in reducing acne infection. It is used when over-the-counter preparations containing lower doses of benzoyl peroxide are not effective.

Most important fact about this drug

If excessive irritation or dryness occurs, discontinue the use of Benzamycin and notify your doctor.

How should you use this medication?

Use Benzamycin 2 times per day, once in the morning and once in the evening, or as directed by your doctor. Apply to the affected areas after thoroughly washing and rinsing with warm water. Gently pat dry.

This medication should be stored in your refrigerator and discarded after 3 months.

What side effects may occur?

Very few side effects have been reported with the use of Benzamycin. However, those reported include:

Abnormal redness of the skin
Dryness
Itching

If any develop or change in intensity, inform your doctor as soon as possible. Only your doctor can determine if it is safe for you to continue taking Benzamycin.

Why should this drug not be prescribed?

If you are sensitive to or have ever had an allergic reaction to erythromycin or benzoyl peroxide, you should not take this medication. Make sure that your doctor is aware of any drug reactions that you have experienced.

Special warnings about this medication

Benzamycin Topical Gel is for external use only. Avoid contact with your eyes and mucous membranes.

Benzamycin may bleach hair or colored fabric. Avoid contact with scalp and clothes.

Possible food and drug interactions when taking this medication

If Benzamycin is taken with other acne medications, the effects of either could be increased, decreased, or altered. It is especially important to check with your doctor before combining Benzamycin with other medications, especially Cleocin-T.

Special information
if you are pregnant or breastfeeding

The effects of Benzamycin during pregnancy have not been adequately studied. If you are pregnant or plan to become pregnant inform your doctor immediately. It is not known whether Benzamycin appears in breast milk. If this medication is essential to your health, your doctor may advise you to discontinue breastfeeding your baby until your treatment with this medication is finished.

Recommended dosage

ADULTS

Apply to affected areas twice daily, once in the morning and once in the evening.

CHILDREN

The safety and effectiveness of Benzamycin have not been established in children under 12 years of age.

Overdosage

Any medication used in excess can cause symptoms of overdose. If you suspect an overdose, seek medical attention.

Generic name:

BENZONATATE

See Tessalon, page 621.

Generic name:

BENZOYL PEROXIDE

See Desquam E, page 181.

Generic name:

BENZTROPINE MESYLATE

See Cogentin, page 122.

Generic name:

BEPRIDIL HYDROCHLORIDE

See Vascor, page 669.

Brand name:

BETAGAN

Generic name: Levobunolol hydrochloride

Why is this drug prescribed?

Betagan eyedrops are given to treat chronic open-angle glaucoma (increased pressure inside the eye). This medication is a beta blocker. It works by lowering pressure within the eyeball.

Most important fact about this drug

Although Betagan eyedrops are applied to the eye, the medication is absorbed and may have effects in other parts of the body. If you have diabetes, asthma, or other respiratory diseases, or decreased heart function, make sure the doctor is aware of the problem.

How should you use this medication?

Use Betagan eyedrops exactly as prescribed by your doctor. Some patients also need to use eye drops that constrict their pupils.

What side effects may occur?

Side effects from Betagan cannot be anticipated. If any develop, or change in intensity, inform your doctor. Only your doctor can determine whether it is safe to continue taking this medication. You may feel a momentary burning and stinging when you place the drops in your eyes. More rarely, an eye inflammation may develop.

Beta blockers may cause muscle weakness; weakened muscles around the eyes may cause double vision or drooping eyelids.

Other potential side effects include:

Burning and tingling (pins and needles), chest pain, clumsiness (temporary), depression, diarrhea, dizziness, headache, hives, iris irritation, itching, inflammation of the cornea, heart palpitations, low blood pressure, nasal congestion, nausea, rash, shortness of breath, stroke, vision problems, weakness, wheezing

Why should this drug not be prescribed?

Do not use Betagan if you have ever had an allergic reaction or are sensitive to it.

Betagan should not be prescribed if you have any of the following conditions:
Asthma
Cardiogenic shock
Diabetes
Heart block (second- or third-degree)
Heart failure
Severe chronic obstructive lung disease
Slow heartbeat (sinus bradycardia)

Special warnings about this medication

Betagan contains a sulfite preservative. In a few people, sulfites can cause an allergic reaction, which may be life-threatening. If you suffer from asthma, you are at increased risk for sulfite allergy.

Betagan may be absorbed into your bloodstream. If too much of the drug is absorbed, this may worsen asthma or other lung diseases or lead to heart failure, which sometimes happens with oral beta-blocker medications.

Beta blockers may increase the risks of anesthesia. If you are facing elective surgery, your doctor may want you to taper off Betagan prior to your operation.

Use Betagan cautiously if you have diminished lung function.

Since beta blockers may mask some signs and symptoms of low blood sugar (hypoglycemia), you should use Betagan very carefully if you have low blood sugar or if you have diabetes, and are taking insulin or an oral antidiabetic medication.

If your body tends to produce too much thyroid hormone, you should taper off Betagan very gradually rather than stopping the drug all at once. Abrupt withdrawal of any beta blocker may provoke a rush of thyroid hormone ("thyroid storm").

Possible food and drug interactions when taking this medication

If Betagan is taken with certain other drugs, the effects of either could be increased, decreased, or altered. It is especially important to check with your doctor before combining Betagan with the following:

Beta block, oral form (Inderal, Tenormin, Sectral, and others)
Epinephrine (Epifrin)
Reserpine (Serpasil and others)

Special information
if you are pregnant or breastfeeding

If you are pregnant or plan to become pregnant, notify your doctor immediately. Betagan eye drops should be used during pregnancy only if the benefit justifies the potential risk to the unborn child.

Since other beta blocker eye medications are known to appear in breast milk, Betagan eye drops should be used with caution if you are breastfeeding.

Recommended dosage

ADULTS

The recommended starting dose is 1 or 2 drops of Betagan 0.5% in the affected eye(s) once a day.

The typical dose with Betagan 0.25% is 1 or 2 drops twice daily.

In more severe or uncontrolled glaucoma, your doctor may use Betagan 0.5%, administered 2 times a day.

Overdosage

Overuse of Betagan eyedrops may produce symptoms of beta-blocker overdosage—slowed heartbeat, low blood pressure, breathing difficulty, and/or heart failure. Any medication taken in excess can have serious consequences. If you suspect an overdose of Betagan, seek medical attention immediately.

Generic name:

BETAMETHASONE DIPROPIONATE

See Diprolene, page 203.

Brand name:

BETAPEN-VK

See Penicillin V, page 462.

Generic name:

BETAXOLOL HYDROCHLORIDE (OPHTHALMIC)

See Betoptic, page 66.

Brand name:

BETOPTIC

Generic name: Betaxolol hydrochloride

Why is this drug prescribed?

Betoptic Ophthalmic Solution and Betoptic S Ophthalmic Suspension contain an ophthalmic medication that lowers internal eye pressure and is used to treat glaucoma (high pressure of the fluid in the eye).

Most important fact about this drug

Although Betoptic, a type of drug called a beta blocker, is applied directly to the eye, it may be absorbed into the bloodstream. Because it may have effects in other parts of the body, Betoptic should be used cautiously in patients with diabetes, asthma or other respiratory diseases, or decreased heart function.

How should you use this medication?

Use this medication exactly as prescribed by your doctor. You may need to take other medications at the same time.

Betoptic S Suspension should be shaken well before each dose is administered.

What side effects may occur?

Side effects cannot be anticipated. If any develop or change in intensity, inform your doctor as soon as possible. Only your doctor can determine if it is safe for you to continue using Betoptic.

■ *More common side effects may include:*
Temporary eye discomfort

■ *Less common or rare side effects may include:*
Allergic reactions, asthma, blurred vision, change in pupil sizes, crusty lashes, decreased corneal sensitivity, dead skin, depression, difficulty breathing, difficulty sleeping or drowsiness, dizziness, dry eyes, eye pain, fluid retention, hair loss, headache, hives, inflammation of the cornea, inflammation of the tongue, intolerance to light, itching, peeling skin, pupils of different sizes, red eyes and skin, shortness of breath, slow heartbeat, tearing, thickening chest secretions, vertigo, vision problems, wheezing

Why should this drug not be prescribed?

Do not use Betoptic if you are sensitive or have ever had an allergic reaction to it.

Special warnings about this medication

Before you use Betoptic tell your doctor if you have any of the following:
Asthma
Diabetes
Heart disease
Severe obstructive lung disease
Thyroid disease

Your doctor may advise you to gradually stop using Betoptic before general anesthesia.

The effectiveness of this drug for glaucoma may be reduced after long-term use.

Possible food and drug interactions while using this medication

If Betoptic is used with certain other drugs, the effects of either could be increased, decreased, or altered. It is especially important to check with your doctor before combining Betoptic with the following:

Drugs that alter mood, such as tranquilizers or sedatives
Epinephrine (Epipen)
Oral beta blockers such as Inderal and Tenormin
Reserpine (Serpasil)

Special Information
if you are pregnant or breastfeeding

The effects of Betoptic during pregnancy have not been adequately studied. If you are pregnant or plan to become pregnant, inform your doctor immediately. Betoptic may appear in breast milk and could affect a nursing infant. If this medication is essential to your health, your doctor may advise you to stop breastfeeding until your treatment with Betoptic is finished.

Recommended dosage

ADULTS

Betoptic
The usual recommended dose is 1 drop of Betoptic in the affected eye(s) twice daily.

Betoptic S
The usual recommended dose is 1 to 2 drops of Betoptic S in the affected eye(s) twice daily.

Overdosage

Any medication used in excess can have serious consequences. If you suspect an overdose of Betoptic, seek medical attention immediately.

Brand name:

BIAXIN

Generic name: Clarithromycin

Why is this drug prescribed?

Biaxin, a new antibiotic chemically related to erythromycin, is given to treat certain bacterial infections of the respiratory tract, including:

Pharyngitis ("strep throat")
Tonsillitis (inflammation of tonsils due to infection)
Sinusitis (inflammation of sinuses due to infection)
Pneumonia

It is also given to treat infections of the skin.

Most important fact about this drug

Like other antibiotics, Biaxin may cause a potentially life-threatening form of diarrhea called pseudomembranous colitis. Mild diarrhea, a fairly common Biaxin side effect, may disappear as your body gets used to the drug. However, if Biaxin gives you prolonged or severe diarrhea, stop taking the drug and call your doctor immediately.

How should you take this medication?

Take Biaxin exactly as prescribed by your doctor. You may take the medication with or without food.

Continue taking Biaxin for the full course of treatment.

What side effects may occur?

Side effects cannot be anticipated. If any side effects develop or change in intensity, tell your doctor immediately. Only your doctor can determine whether it is safe to continue taking Biaxin.

- *More common side effects may include:*
  An altered sense of taste
  Diarrhea
  Nausea

- *Other potential side effects may include:*
  Headache, indigestion, stomach pain, stomach upset

Why should this drug not be prescribed?

Do not take Biaxin if you have ever had an allergic reaction or are sensitive to it or to erythromycin or another macrolide antibiotic such as TaO and Zithromax.

Possible food and drug interactions when taking this medication

If Biaxin is taken with certain other drugs, the effects of either could be increased, decreased, or altered. It is especially important to check with your doctor before combining Biaxin with the following:

Carbamazepine (Tegretol)
Theophylline (Slo-Phyllin, Theo-Dur, and others)

Biaxin is chemically related to erythromycin. It is possible that other interactions reported with erythromycin could also occur with Biaxin.

Special information
if you are pregnant or breastfeeding

If you are pregnant or plan to become pregnant, notify your doctor immediately. Since Biaxin may have the potential to produce birth defects, it should be taken during pregnancy only if the benefits outweigh the potential risk to the unborn child.

Caution is advised when using Biaxin while breastfeeding. Like its chemical cousin erythromycin, Biaxin may make its way into breast milk.

Recommended dosage

ADULTS

Your doctor will carefully tailor your individual dosage of Biaxin depending upon the type of infection and bacteria.

The usual dose varies from 250 to 500 milligrams every 12 hours for 7 to 14 days.

CHILDREN

Biaxin is not recommended for children under 12 years of age.

Overdosage

Although no specific information is available, any medication taken in excess can have serious consequences. If you suspect an overdose of Biaxin, seek medical attention immediately.

Brand name:

BLEPH-10

See Sodium Sulamyd, page 583.

Brand name:

BRETHAIRE

See Brethine, page 69.

Brand name:

BRETHINE

Generic name: *Terbutaline sulfate*
Other brand names: *Bricanyl, Brethaire*

Why is this drug prescribed?

Brethine is a bronchodilator, (a medication which opens the bronchial tubes) prescribed for the prevention and relief of bronchial spasms in asthma. This medication is also used for the relief of bronchial spasm associated with bronchitis and emphysema.

Most important fact about this drug

If you experience an immediate allergic reaction and a worsening of a bronchial spasm, notify your doctor immediately.

How should you take this medication?

Take this drug exactly as prescribed by your doctor.

The action of Brethine may last up to 6 hours. Do not use more frequently than recommended.

What side effects may occur?

Side effects cannot be anticipated. If any develop or change in intensity, inform your doctor as soon as possible. Only your doctor can determine if it is safe for you to continue taking Brethine.

■ *More common side effects may include:*
Chest discomfort, difficulty in breathing, dizziness, drowsiness, flushed feeling, headache, increased heart rate, nausea, nervousness, pain at injection site, rapid, strong heartbeat, sweating, tremors, vomiting, weakness

■ *Less common side effects may include:*
Anxiety, dry mouth, muscle cramps.

■ *Rare side effects may include:*
Dry throat, inflammation of blood vessels due to allergic reaction, liver disorder, throat irritation, unusual taste

Why should this drug not be prescribed?

If you are sensitive to or have ever had an allergic reaction to Brethine or similar drugs, you should not take this medication. Make sure that your doctor is aware of any drug reactions that you have experienced.

Special warnings about this medication

When taking Brethine, you should not use other inhaled medications called sympathomimetics before checking with your doctor. Only your doctor can determine what is a sufficient amount of time between inhaled medication doses.

Consult with your doctor before using this medication if you have diabetes, high blood pressure, hyperthyroidism or a history of seizures.

Unless you are directed to do so by your doctor, do not take this medication if you have heart disease accompanied by an irregular heart rate.

Possible food and drug interactions when taking this medication

If Brethine is taken with certain other drugs, the effects of either could be increased, decreased, or altered. It is especially important to check with your doctor before combining Brethine with the following:

Antidepressant drugs known as MAO
  inhibitors (Nardil, Parnate)
Beta blockers (Tenormin)
Other bronchodilators
Tricyclic antidepressants (Elavil)

Special information
if you are pregnant or breastfeeding

The effects of Brethine during pregnancy have not been adequately studied. If you are pregnant or plan to become pregnant, inform your doctor immediately. It is not known whether Brethine appears in breast milk. If this drug is essential to your health, your doctor may advise you to stop nursing your baby until your treatment is finished.

Recommended dosage

For Brethine:

ADULTS

Tablets

The usual oral dose is 5 milligrams taken at approximately 6-hour intervals, 3 times per day during waking hours. If side effects are excessive, your doctor may reduce your dose to 2.5 milligrams, 3 times per day.

Do not take more than 15 milligrams in a 24-hour period.

CHILDREN

This medication is not recommended for use in children below 12 years of age.

For children 12 to 15 years of age, the usual dose is 2.5 milligrams, 3 times per day.

A total of 7.5 milligrams should not be exceeded in a 24-hour period.

For Brethaire:

The usual dosage for adults and children 12 years and older is 2 inhalations separated by a 60 second interval, repeated every 4 to 6 hours.

Overdosage

Any drug taken or used in excess can cause symptoms of an overdose. Signs of a Brethine overdose are the same as side effects. If you suspect an overdose, seek medical attention immediately.

Brand name:

BRICANYL

See Brethine, page 69.

Generic name:

BROMOCRIPTINE MESYLATE

See Parlodel, page 455.

Brand names:

BRONKOMETER/ BRONKOSOL

Generic name: Isoetharine mesylate

Why is this drug prescribed?

Bronkometer, a pocket nebulizer for administering a fine spray, and Bronkosol, a solution used for oral inhalation, are prescribed as bronchodilators to treat bronchial asthma and reversible narrowing of the airways into the lungs that may occur in association with bronchitis and emphysema.

Most important fact about this drug

Excessive use of this drug may cause it to become ineffective. If your condition is unresponsive to treatment with Bronkometer or Bronkosol, notify your doctor immediately, as he may wish to discontinue this drug and prescribe an alternate treatment.

How should you take this medication?

Use this medication exactly as prescribed by your doctor.

What side effects may occur?

Although Bronkometer and Bronkosol are relatively free of side effects, too frequent use may cause the following:

Anxiety, changes in blood pressure, dizziness, excitement, headache, inability to fall or stay asleep, nausea, pounding heartbeat, rapid heart rate, restlessness, tension, tremors, weakness

Why should this drug not be prescribed?

If you are sensitive to or have ever had an allergic reaction to isoetharine, or any other ingredients in these medications, you should not take them. Make sure that your doctor is aware of any drug reactions that you have experienced.

Special warnings about this medication

Bronkosol contains acetone sodium bisulfite, which may cause allergic-type reactions, including life-threatening or less severe asthmatic episodes, in certain patients. If you have an allergic-type reaction, notify your doctor immediately.

If you have hyperthyroidism (overactivity of the thyroid gland), high blood pressure, severe heart disease, cardiac asthma, limited heart function, or a sensitivity to sympathomimetic amines (compounds that stimulate the sympathetic nervous system, dilating for example, the airways in the lungs), consult with your doctor before taking this medication. Your dosage will be adjusted accordingly.

Possible food and drug interactions when taking this medication

If Bronkometer/Bronkosol is taken with certain other drugs, the effects of either could be increased, decreased, or altered. It is especially important to check with your doctor before combining Bronkometer/ Bronkosol with epinephrine or other compounds that stimulate the sympathetic nervous system

These drugs are direct heart stimulants and may cause an excessively rapid heart rate. However, Bronkometer and Bronkosol may be alternated with these drugs as prescribed by your doctor.

Special information if you are pregnant or breastfeeding

If you are pregnant, plan to become pregnant or are breastfeeding, inform your doctor before using Bronkometer or Bronkosol.

Recommended dosage

Bronkometer

ADULTS

The average adult dose is 1 or 2 inhalations. Occasionally, more may be required. It is important, however, to wait 1 full minute after the first 1 or 2 inhalations in order to be certain whether another is necessary. In most cases, inhalations need not be repeated more often than every 4 hours, although more frequent administration may be necessary in severe cases. The Bronkometer Inhaler System is for oral inhalation only.

Bronkosol

Bronkosol can be used with a hand nebulizer for administering a fine spray, or, in the hospital, by oxygen aerosolization (inhalation), or intermittent positive pressure breathing (IPPB).

The usual adult dose using a hand nebulizer is 4 inhalations of undiluted solution. Your doctor will determine when and how often you should repeat the dose.

Overdosage

Any medication taken in excess can have serious consequences. If you suspect an overdose, seek emergency medical treatment immediately.

Brand name:

BRONKOSOL

See Bronkometer, page 71.

Generic Name:

BUMETANIDE

See Bumex, page 72.

Brand name:

BUMEX

Generic name: Bumetanide

Why is this drug prescribed?

Bumex is used to lower the amount of water in your body by increasing the output of urine. It is prescribed in the treatment of edema, or fluid retention, associated with congestive heart failure, liver or kidney disease.

It is classified as a "loop diuretic" because of its point of action within the kidneys.

Most important fact about this drug

Bumex is a powerful drug. If taken in excessive amounts, it can severely decrease the levels of water and minerals, especially potassium, your body needs to function. Therefore, your doctor should monitor your dose carefully.

How should you take this medication?

Bumex can increase the frequency of urination and may cause loss of sleep if taken at night. Therefore, if you are taking a single dose of Bumex daily, it should be taken in the morning. If you take more than one dose a day, take the last dose no later than 6:00 PM.

If you miss a dose of Bumex, take it as soon as you remember. However, if it is almost time for your next dose, skip the missed dose and go back to your regular schedule. Never take two doses at the same time.

What side effects may occur?

Side effects cannot be anticipated. If any develop or change in intensity, inform

your doctor as soon as possible. Only your doctor can determine if it is safe for you to continue taking Bumex.

■ *More common side effects may include:*
Dizziness
Headache
Low blood pressure
Muscle cramps
Nausea

■ *Signs of too much potassium loss are:*
Dry mouth
Irregular heartbeat
Muscle cramps or pains
Unusual tiredness or weakness

■ *Less common or rare side effects may include:*
Abdominal pain, black stools, chest pain, dehydration, diarrhea, dry mouth, ear discomfort, fatigue, hearing loss, itching, joint pain, kidney failure, muscle and bone pain, nipple tenderness, premature ejaculation and difficulty maintaining erection, skin rash or hives, sweating, upset stomach, vertigo, vomiting, weakness

Why should this drug not be prescribed?
Bumex should not be used if you are unable to urinate or if you are dehydrated.

If you are sensitive to or have ever had an allergic reaction to Bumex or similar drugs, you should not take this medication. Make sure that your doctor is aware of any drug reactions that you have experienced.

Special warnings about this medication
If you are allergic to sulfur-containing drugs such as sulfonamides (anti-bacterial drugs), check with your doctor before taking Bumex.

Bumex can cause a decrease in blood platelets. Regular monitoring of your blood status by your doctor is recommended.

Bumex can cause a loss of potassium from the body. Your doctor may recommend

foods or fluids high in potassium or may want you to take a potassium supplement to help prevent this. Follow your doctor's recommendation carefully.

While taking this medication you may feel dizzy or lightheaded or actually faint when getting up from a lying or sitting position. If getting up slowly does not help or if this problem continues, notify your doctor.

If you have kidney disease or any known problems with your pancreas, notify your doctor before taking this medication.

Bumex may cause you to become drowsy or less alert when you begin taking it. If it has this effect on you, driving or operating dangerous machinery or participating in any hazardous activity that requires full mental alertness is not recommended.

Possible food and drug interactions when taking this medication
Check with your doctor before drinking alcohol while taking Bumex. The combination may cause a serious drop in blood pressure.

Drugs that are potentially harmful to the kidneys should be avoided while taking Bumex because there is no experience with the combination of these drugs.

If Bumex is taken with certain other drugs, the effects of either could be increased, decreased, or altered. It is especially important to check with your doctor before combining Bumex with the following:

High blood pressure medication
Indomethacin and other nonsteroidal
    anti-inflammatory drugs
Probenecid (Benemid)

The combination of Bumex and certain antibiotics or cisplatin may increase the risk of hearing loss.

Because Bumex can lower potassium levels, the combination of Bumex and digitalis or digoxin may increase the risk of changes in heartbeat.

The combination of Bumex and lithium may increase the levels of lithium in the body, causing it to become poisonous.

Special information
If you are pregnant or breastfeeding

The effects of Bumex during pregnancy have not been adequately studied. If you are pregnant or plan to become pregnant, inform your doctor immediately. It is not known if this medication appears in breast milk. Your doctor may advise you to discontinue breastfeeding your baby until your treatment with Bumex is finished.

Recommended dosage

Bumex is available in 0.5, 1, and 2 milligram tablets.

ADULTS

The usual total daily dose is 0.5 to 2.0 milligrams a day. For most people, this is given as a single dose. However, if the initial dose is not adequate, a second or third dose may be given at 4 to 5 hour intervals, up to a maximum daily dose of 10 milligrams.

An alternate dose schedule recommended for the control of edema is Bumex given on alternate days or for 3 to 4 days with rest periods of 1 to 2 days in between.

If you have liver failure, your dose should be kept to a minimum and increased very carefully.

CHILDREN

The safety and effectiveness of Bumex have not been established in children below the age of 18.

Overdosage

An overdose of Bumex can lead to severe dehydration, reduction of blood volume and circulatory collapse.

The signs of an overdose include:
Cramps
Dizziness
Lethargy
Loss or lack of appetite
Mental confusion
Vomiting
Weakness

If you suspect an overdose, get medical attention immediately.

Generic name:

BUPROPION HYDROCHLORIDE

See Wellbutrin, page 685.

Brand name:

BUSPAR

Generic name: Buspirone hydrochloride

Why is this drug prescribed?

BuSpar is used in the treatment of anxiety disorders and for short-term relief of the symptoms of anxiety.

Most important fact about this drug

BuSpar should not be used with antidepressant drugs known as monoamine oxidase inhibitors. Brands include Nardil and Parnate.

How should you take this medication?

Take BuSpar exactly as prescribed by your doctor. You may not feel the full effects of this drug for 1 to 2 weeks after starting the medication.

If you forget to take a dose of BuSpar, take it as soon as you remember. If it is almost time for your next dose, skip the one you missed and go back to your regular schedule. Never take two doses at the same time.

What side effects may occur?
Side effects cannot be anticipated. If any develop or change in intensity, inform your doctor as soon as possible. Only your doctor can determine if it is safe for you to continue taking BuSpar.

■ *More common side effects may include:*
Chest pain, dizziness, dream disturbances, headache, light-headedness, nasal congestion, nausea, nervousness, ringing in the ears, sore throat, unusual excitement

■ *Less common or rare side effects may include:*
Altered taste or smell, conjunctivitis, change in appetite, change in sexual function, chest congestion, dry skin, easy bruising, exaggerated feeling of well-being, eye pain, fearfulness, fever, fluid retention, flushing, frequent or painful urination, gas, hair loss, hallucinations, heart attack or failure, high blood pressure, itching, joint pain, light intolerance, loss of interest, loss of strength or fainting, low blood pressure, menstrual irregularity, muscle pain, spasms or cramps, muscle weakness, numbness, tingling, pain or weakness in hands or feet, rectal bleeding, red, itching eyes, restlessness, seizures, shortness of breath, slow heartbeat, slurred speech, stroke, stupor, uncontrolled body movements, urinary incontinence

Why should this drug not be prescribed?
If you are sensitive to or have ever had an allergic reaction to BuSpar or similar drugs, you should not take this medication. Make sure that your doctor is aware of any drug reactions that you have experienced.

Anxiety or tension related to everyday stress usually does not require treatment with BuSpar. Discuss your symptoms thoroughly with your doctor.

The use of BuSpar is not recommended if you have severe kidney or liver damage.

BuSpar should not be used to treat psychosis.

Special warnings about this medication
The effects of BuSpar on the central nervous system are unpredictable. Therefore, driving or operating dangerous machinery or participating in any hazardous activity that requires full mental alertness is not recommended.

Possible food and drug interactions when taking this medication
Although BuSpar does not intensify the affects of alcohol, it is best to avoid alcohol while taking this medication.

If BuSpar is taken with certain other drugs, the effects of either could be increased, decreased, or altered. It is especially important to check with your doctor before combining BuSpar with the following:

Haloperidol (Haldol)
MAO inhibitors (antidepressant drugs such as Nardil)
Trazodone (Desyrel)

Special information if you are pregnant or breastfeeding
The effects of BuSpar during pregnancy have not been adequately studied. If you are pregnant or plan to become pregnant, inform your doctor immediately. It is not known whether BuSpar appears in breast milk. If this medication is essential to your health, your doctor may advise you to discontinue breastfeeding until your treatment is finished.

Recommended dosage

ADULT

The recommended starting dose is a total of 15 milligrams per day divided in smaller doses, usually 5 milligrams 3 times a day. Every 2 to 3 days, the dosage may be increased by your doctor by 5 milligrams per day as needed. The daily dose should not exceed 60 milligrams per day.

CHILDREN

The safety and effectiveness of BuSpar have not been established in children under 18 years of age.

ELDERLY

The use of BuSpar in elderly patients has not been thoroughly established. However, no unusual age-related effects have been identified. The usual dose is 15 milligrams per day in divided doses.

Overdosage

Any medication taken in excess can cause symptoms of overdose. If you suspect an overdose, seek medical attention immediately.

The symptoms of BuSpar overdose may include:
Drowsiness
Nausea or vomiting
Severe stomach upset
Unusually small pupils

Generic name:

BUSPIRONE HYDROCHLORIDE

See BuSpar, page 74.

Generic name:

BUTALBITAL, ACETAMINOPHEN, AND CAFFEINE

See Fioricet, page 253.

Generic name:

BUTALBITAL, ASPIRIN, AND CAFFEINE

See Fiorinal, page 255.

Generic name:

BUTALBITAL, CODEINE, ASPIRIN, AND CAFFEINE

See Fiorinal with Codeine, page 257.

Brand name:

BUTAZOLIDIN

Generic name: Phenylbutazone

Why is this drug prescribed?

Butazolidin, a nonsteroidal anti-inflammatory drug, is used to relieve the inflammation, swelling, stiffness and joint pain associated with ankylosing spondylitis, (arthritis of the spine), acute gouty arthritis, active rheumatoid arthritis, and acute attacks of degenerative joint disease of the hips and knees.

Most important fact about this drug

This medication can cause agranulocytosis (decreased white blood cells) and aplastic anemia. Butazolidin should be used only after other nonsteroidal anti-inflammatory drugs have been tried and have failed, and you have discussed the risks and benefits of using this drug with your doctor. If there is no significant improvement in your symptoms after 1 week, the drug should be discontinued.

How should you take this medication?

Your doctor may ask you to take Butazolidin with meals or milk to avoid stomach upset.

Take this medication exactly as prescribed by your doctor.

If you are using Butazolidin for arthritis, it should be taken regularly. If you forget to take a dose, take it as soon as you remember. If it is almost time for your next dose, skip the one you missed and go back to your regular schedule. Never take two doses at the same time.

What side effects may occur?
Side effects cannot be anticipated. If any develop or change in intensity, inform your doctor as soon as possible. Only your doctor can determine if it is safe for you to continue taking Butazolidin.

■ *More common side effects may include:*
Abdominal discomfort
Heartburn
Indigestion
Nausea
Rash
Stomach upset
Swelling due to fluid retention
Water retention

■ *Less common or rare side effects may include:*
Agitation, aplastic anemia (decrease in red and white cells or platelets), bone marrow depression, changes in blood sugar, changes in kidney function, confusion, congestive heart failure, constipation, decrease in white cells, diarrhea, distended abdomen with gas, drowsiness, fever, headache, hearing loss, hepatitis, high blood pressure, inability to urinate, inflammation of mouth and tongue, inflammation of the esophagus, inflammation of the pericardium (sac that surrounds the heart), inflammation of the stomach, intestinal bleeding, itching, joint pain, kidney failure, kidney stones, lupus erythematosus (a form of arthritis), numbness, peptic ulcer, ringing in ears, salivary gland enlargement, shock, skin eruptions, sluggishness, Stevens-Johnson

syndrome (skin peeling), tremors, vomiting, weakness, worsening of inflammatory bowel disease or Crohn's disease, yellow eyes and skin.

If you develop fever, sore throat, or sores in your mouth, stomach upset and pain, symptoms of anemia, unusual bleeding or bruising, black or tarry stool, skin rashes, or significant weight gain or swelling due to fluid retention, stop taking Butazolidin immediately and contact your doctor at once.

Why should this drug not be prescribed?
If you are sensitive to or have ever had an allergic reaction to Butazolidin, aspirin, or similar drugs, of if you have had asthma attacks caused by aspirin or drugs of this type, you should not take this medication.

Special warnings about this medication
Butazolidin can cause agranulocytosis (decrease in white blood cells) and aplastic anemia (reduced red blood cell production due to bone marrow deficiencies). Your doctor should take a careful history and do a complete physical and laboratory work-up before you start this medication, and your blood should be taken periodically for continual monitoring.

Women, the elderly, and people using Butazolidin for long-term therapy are at greater risk for developing aplastic anemia or agranulocytosis.

Make sure your doctor explains the symptoms you should look for if serious side effects are developing.

Peptic ulcers and bleeding can occur without warning.

This drug should be used with caution if you have kidney or liver disease. It can cause liver inflammation in some people.

Do not take aspirin or any other anti-inflammatory medications while taking Butazolidin, unless your doctor tells you to do so.

If you are taking blood thinning medication, this drug should be used with caution. The combination may prolong bleeding time.

This medication may cause vision problems. If you experience any changes in your vision, inform your doctor.

Use with caution if you have heart disease or high blood pressure. This drug can increase water retention.

Butazolidin can cause some people to become drowsy or less alert. If it has this effect on you, driving or operating dangerous machinery or participating in any hazardous activity that requires full mental alertness is not recommended.

Possible food and drug interactions when taking this medication

If Butazolidin is taken with certain other drugs, the effects of either could be increased, decreased, or altered. It is especially important to check with your doctor before combining Butazolidin with the following:

Aspirin
Barbiturates such as Seconal, Phenobarbital, Amytal
Blood thinners such as Coumadin
Digitoxin
Insulin
Lithium
Methotrexate
Other anti-inflammatory agents
Phenytoin (Dilantin)
Rifampin
Sulfonylureas such as Diabenese, Tolazamide, Tolbutamide

Special information if you are pregnant or breastfeeding

The effects of Butazolidin during pregnancy have not been adequately studied. If you are pregnant or plan to become pregnant inform your doctor immediately. Butazolidin appears in breast milk and could affect a nursing infant. If this medication is essential to your health, your doctor may advise you to discontinue breastfeeding until your treatment is finished.

Recommended dosage

ADULTS

This medication should be used at the lowest possible dose that provides quick relief of severe symptoms.

Rheumatoid Arthritis, Ankylosing Spondylitis, Acute Degenerative Joint Disease
The starting dosage is 300 to 600 milligrams daily divided into 3 or 4 smaller doses. If there is no significant improvement in symptoms after 1 week, use of the drug should be stopped. If your symptoms improve after 1 week, your doctor should decrease your dosage to the minimal amount needed to maintain relief. If used long term, total dosage should not exceed 400 milligrams daily.

Acute Gout (Gouty Arthritis)
The starting dose is 400 milligrams, followed by doses of 100 milligrams every 4 hours. Inflammation usually subsides within 4 days, and treatment should not last longer than 1 week.

CHILDREN

The safety and effectiveness of Butazolidin have not been established in children under 14 years of age. However, your doctor may decide that the benefits outweigh the potential risks.

ELDERLY

This drug should not be used long term in elderly patients unless no alternative exists because of increased risk of side effects.

The elderly should stop therapy on or as soon as possible after the seventh day because of risk of severe or fatal reactions.

Overdosage

Any medication taken in excess can cause symptoms of overdose. If you suspect an overdose, seek medical attention immediately.

The symptoms of Butazolidin overdose may include:

Mild overdose
Abdominal pain
Drowsiness
Nausea

Severe overdose (early onset)
Agitation, bluish color of skin, coma, convulsions (more common in children), diarrhea, dizziness, hallucinations, high or low blood pressure, hyperventilation (too frequent breathing), nausea, psychosis, respiratory failure, restlessness, upper abdominal pain, very high fever, vomiting, vomiting blood

Severe overdose (late onset, 2 to 7 days)
Abnormal blood conditions, abnormal laboratory test results, acute kidney failure, blood in urine, changes in heart function, decrease in amount of urine, heart failure, swelling due to fluid retention, yellow eyes and skin

Generic name:

BUTOCONAZOLE NITRATE

See Femstat, page 252.

Brand name:

CAFERGOT

Generic ingredients: Ergotamine tartrate, Caffeine

Why is this drug prescribed?

Cafergot is prescribed for the relief or prevention of vascular headaches, for example, migraine, migraine variants, or cluster headaches.

Most important fact about this drug

It is extremely important that you do not exceed your recommended dosage, especially when Cafergot is used over long periods. There have been reports of psychological dependence in patients who have abused this drug over long periods of time. Discontinuance of the drug may produce withdrawal symptoms such as sudden, severe headaches.

The excessive use of Cafergot can also lead to ergot poisoning resulting in symptoms such as headache, pain in the legs when walking, muscle pain, numbness, coldness, and abnormal paleness of the fingers and toes. If this condition is not treated, it can lead to gangrene (tissue death due to decreased blood supply).

How should you take this medication?

Take this medication exactly as prescribed by your doctor, remaining within the limits of your recommended dosage. Start taking the drug at first sign of an attack.

What side effects may occur?

Side effects cannot be anticipated. If any develop or change in intensity, inform your doctor as soon as possible. Only your doctor can determine if it is safe for you to continue taking Cafergot.

■ *More common side effects may include:*
Itching

Nausea
Rapid heart rate
Slow heartbeat
Vomiting

■ *Complications caused by constriction of the
blood vessels can be serious. They
include:*
Chest pain
Muscle pains
Pins and needles sensation
Weakness

Although these symptoms occur most
commonly with long-term therapy at
relatively high doses, they have been reported
with short-term or normal doses.

Why should this drug not be prescribed?

If you are sensitive to or have ever had an
allergic reaction to ergotamine tartrate,
caffeine, or similar drugs, you should not take
this medication. Make sure that your
doctor is aware of any drug reactions that
you have experienced.

Unless you are directed to do so by your
doctor, do not take this medication if you
have coronary heart disease, peripheral
vascular disease (circulatory problems),
high blood pressure, impaired liver or kidney
function, or an infection, or if you are
pregnant.

Special warnings about this medication

If you experience excessive nausea and
vomiting during attacks making it
impossible for you to retain oral medication,
your doctor will probably tell you to use
rectal suppositories.

Possible food and drug interactions
when taking this medication

If Cafergot is taken with certain other drugs,
the effects of either could be increased,
decreased, or altered. It is especially important

to check with your doctor before combining
Cafergot with vasopressors such as Epipen.

Special information
if you are pregnant or breastfeeding

Do not take Cafergot if you are pregnant. If
you are pregnant, plan to become
pregnant, or are breastfeeding your baby,
consult your doctor before taking
Cafergot.

Recommended dosage

Dosage should start at the first sign of an
attack.

ADULTS

Orally
The total dose for any single attack should
not exceed 6 tablets.

Rectally
The maximum dose for an individual attack
is 2 suppositories.

The total weekly dosage should not exceed
10 tablets or 5 suppositories.

A preventive short-term dose may be given
at bedtime to certain patients, but only
as prescribed by a doctor.

Overdosage

If you suspect an overdose, seek emergency
medical treatment immediately.

Symptoms of Cafergot overdose include:
Coma, convulsions, diminished or absent
pulses, drowsiness, high or low blood
pressure, numbness, shock, stupor, tingling,
pain, and bluish discoloration of the
limbs, unresponsiveness, vomiting

Brand name:

CALAN

Generic name: Verapamil hydrochloride
Other Brand names: Calan SR, Isoptin,
Isoptin SR, Verelan

Why is this drug prescribed?

Verapamil, a type of medication called a calcium channel blocker, is prescribed for the treatment of various types of angina (chest pain, often accompanied by a feeling of choking, usually caused by lack of oxygen to the heart due to clogged arteries). It is also used for irregular heartbeat, and high blood pressure. The sustained release formula (SR) is used for the treatment of high blood pressure. Calcium channel blockers ease the heart's workload by slowing down the passage of nerve impulses through it, and hence the contractions of the heart muscle. This improves blood flow through the heart and throughout the body, reduces blood pressure, corrects irregular heartbeat, and helps prevent angina pain.

Verapamil is also being prescribed to prevent migraine headache and asthma and to treat manic depression.

Most important fact about this drug

Verapamil can reduce or eliminate angina pain caused by exertion or exercise. But be sure to discuss with your doctor how much exertion is safe for you.

How should you take this medication?

Calan, Isoptin and Verelan tablets can be taken with or without food. Calan SR and Isoptin SR should be taken with food.

Calan SR, Isoptin SR, and Verelan must be swallowed whole and should not be crushed or chewed.

Take this medication exactly as prescribed by your doctor, even if you are feeling well.

Try not to miss any doses. If the drug is not taken regularly, your condition can get worse.

If you forget to take a dose, take it as soon as you remember. If it is almost time for your next dose, skip the one you missed and go back to your regular schedule. Never take two doses at the same time.

Check with your doctor before you stop taking this drug; a slow reduction in the dose may be required.

What side effects may occur?

Side effects cannot be anticipated. If any develop or change in intensity, inform your doctor as soon as possible. Only your doctor can determine if it is safe for you to continue taking verapamil.

■ *More common side effects may include:*
Congestive heart failure, constipation, dizziness, fatigue, fluid retention, headache, low blood pressure, nausea, rash, shortness of breath, slow heartbeat

■ *Less common or rare side effects may include:*
Angina, blurred vision, breast development in males, bruising, chest pain, confusion, diarrhea, difficulty sleeping, drowsiness, dry mouth, excessive milk secretion, fainting, fever and rash, flushing, hair loss, heart attack, hives, impotence, increased urination, joint pain, limping, loss of balance, muscle cramps, pounding heartbeat, rash, shakiness, skin peeling, sleepiness, spotty menstruation, sweating, tingling or pins and needles, upset stomach

Why should this drug not be prescribed?

If you have low blood pressure or certain types of heart disease, including ventricular dysfunction, conduction disorder, sick sinus syndrome unless you have a pacemaker, or flutter or fibrillation, you should not take verapamil.

If you are sensitive to or have ever had an allergic reaction to Calan or any other brands of verapamil, or other drugs of this type, do not take this medication.

Special warnings about this medication

Verapamil may cause your blood pressure to become too low. If you experience dizziness or lightheadedness, notify your doctor.

Congestive heart failure and fluid in the lungs have occurred in people taking verapamil with other heart drugs known as beta-blockers. Make sure your doctor is aware of all medications you are taking.

If you have a certain heart condition, liver disease, kidney disease, or Duchenne dystrophy (the most common type of muscular dystrophy), verapamil should be used with caution.

Possible food and drug interactions when taking this medication

If verapamil is taken with certain other drugs, the effects of either could be increased, decreased, or altered. It is especially important to check with your doctor before combining verapamil with the following:

ACE inhibitors such as Capoten, Vasotec
Beta blockers such as Lopressor, Tenormin, Inderal
Carbamazepine (Tegretol)
Cimetidine (Tagamet)
Cyclosporine (Sandimmune)
Digitalis (Lanoxin)
Disopyramide (Norpace)
Diuretics such as Lasix, HydroDIURIL
Flecainide (Tambocor)
Inhalation anesthetics
Lithium (Eskalith)
Neuromuscular blocking agents
Nitrates such as Transderm Nitro, Isordil
Phenobarbital
Quinidine (Quinidex)
Rifampin (Rifadin)

Theophylline (Theo-Dur)
Vasodilators such as Loniten
Other high blood pressure drugs such as Minipress

Special information if you are pregnant or breastfeeding

The effects of verapamil during pregnancy have not been adequately studied. If you are pregnant or plan to become pregnant, inform your doctor immediately. The drug appears in breast milk and could affect a nursing infant. If this medication is essential to your health, your doctor may advise you to discontinue breastfeeding until your treatment is finished.

Recommended dosage

FOR CALAN AND ISOPTIN

Dosages of this medication must be adjusted to meet the individual patient's needs. In general, dosages of this medication should not exceed 480 milligrams per day. Your doctor will closely monitor your response to this drug, usually within 8 hours of the first dose.

ANGINA

Adults
The usual initial dose is 80 to 120 milligrams, 3 times per day. Lower doses of 40 milligrams 3 times a day may be used for patients who have a stronger response to this medication, such as elderly patients or those with decreased liver function. The dosage may be increased by your doctor either daily or weekly until the desired response is seen.

Elderly
A lower dose of 40 milligrams may be used for an elderly patient.

ARRHYTHMIAS
(CONTROL OF HEART RHYTHMS)

Adults

The usual dose in patients also on digitalis ranges from a total of 240 to 320 milligrams per day divided into 3 or 4 doses.

In patients not on digitalis, doses range from a total of 240 to 480 milligrams per day divided into 3 or 4 doses.

Maximum effects of this drug should be seen in the first 48 hours of use.

HIGH BLOOD PRESSURE

Adults

Effects of this drug on blood pressure should be seen within the first week of use. Any adjustment of this medication to a higher dose will be based on its effectiveness as determined by your doctor.

The usual dose of this drug, when used alone for high blood pressure, is 80 milligrams, 3 times per day. Total daily doses of 360 milligrams and 480 milligrams may be used. Smaller doses of 40 milligrams 3 times per day may be used in smaller patients.

Children

The safety and effectiveness of this drug in children has not been established.

Elderly

A starting dose of 40 milligrams, 3 times per day may be used.

FOR CALAN SR, ISOPTIN SR, AND VERELAN

Dosages for high blood pressure should be adjusted to meet each individual patient's needs.

Adults

The usual starting dose of Calan SR and Isoptin SR is 180 milligrams taken in the morning. For Verelan, it is 240 milligrams. Lower starting doses of 120 milligrams may be used in smaller patients. Your doctor will monitor your response to this drug and may adjust it each week. In addition, your doctor may increase the dose and add evening doses to the morning dose, based on the effectiveness of the drug.

You should see results from the drug within a week.

Children

The safety and effectiveness of this drug in children under age 18 have not been established.

Elderly

A lower starting dose of 120 milligrams may be used in elderly patients and then adjusted according to the patient's response.

Overdosage

Any medication taken in excess can have serious consequences. If you suspect an overdose, seek medical attention immediately.

There is no specific information available on verapamil overdose; however, a person suspected of overdose should be under observation for at least 48 hours. Fainting and low blood pressure may occur.

Brand name:

CALAN SR

See Calan, page 81.

Brand name:

CALCIMAR

Generic name: Calcitonin-salmon

Why is this drug prescribed?
Calcimar is a synthetic form of calcitonin, a naturally occurring hormone produced by the thyroid gland. Calcimar reduces the rate of calcium loss from bones. Since less calcium passes from the bones to the blood, Calcimar also helps control blood calcium levels. Calcimar is used to treat:

Paget's disease (abnormal bone growth leading to deformities).

Hypercalcemia (abnormally high calcium blood levels).

Postmenopausal bone loss (bone loss occurring after menopause).

Most important fact about this drug
Calcimar has been reported to cause serious allergic reactions (such as shock, difficulty breathing, wheezing, and swelling of the throat or tongue) in a few people.

How should you take this medication?
Calcimar is taken by injection, given by either a doctor or the patient. If you are injecting Calcimar yourself, it is important to follow your doctor's instructions carefully so that you inject Calcimar correctly.

Calcimar should be stored in the refrigerator.

Do not use Calcimar solution if it has changed color or has particles floating in it.

If you are taking Calcimar for postmenopausal bone loss, you should be sure your diet provides enough calcium and vitamin D. Foods that are good sources of calcium include dairy products (such as milk and cheese) and fish. Good sources of vitamin D include fish (such as salmon, sardines, and tuna), liver, and dairy products. Sunlight is another indirect source of vitamin D.

What side effects may occur?
Side effects cannot be anticipated. If any develop or change in intensity, inform your doctor as soon as possible. Only your doctor can determine if it is safe for you to continue taking Calcimar.

■ *More common side effects may include:*
   Inflamed skin where Calcimar
      has been injected
   Nausea
   Vomiting

■ *Less common side effects may include:*
   Flushed face, flushed hands, skin rashes

Why should this drug not be prescribed?
You should not be using Calcimar if you are allergic to it.

Special warnings about this medication
Calcimar may cause an abnormally low blood level of calcium, resulting in muscle cramps, spasms, and twitches in the face, feet, and hands.

Before taking Calcimar for the first time, you should consider having a skin test to determine whether you are allergic to the drug.

People who take Calcimar on a long-term basis should have periodic urine and blood tests to determine the ongoing effects of Calcimar.

Possible food and drug interactions when taking this medication
There are no interactions listed for this drug.

Special information if you are pregnant or breastfeeding
Pregnant women should use Calcimar only if the potential benefits clearly outweigh

any potential risks to the unborn child. Women are usually advised not to take Calcimar while breastfeeding an infant.

Recommended dosage

ADULTS

Paget's Disease
The suggested beginning dose is 100 international units, or 0.5 milliliters, per day, taken by injection. Bone pain may lessen during the first few months of treatment. Other conditions may require a longer treatment time.

Some people may find it is enough to take 0.25 milliliter daily or every other day.

It is important to let your doctor know how you respond to this drug; some people may develop an antibody to Calcimar, and it may become less effective.

Hypercalcemia (Abnormally High Blood Calcium Levels)
The suggested beginning dose is 4 international units for every kilogram (approximately 2.2 pounds) of body weight, taken by injection every 12 hours.

If needed, this dosage may be increased to 8 international units for every kilogram of body weight, by injection, every 12 hours.

The maximum dose of this drug is 8 international units for every kilogram of body weight, by injection, every 6 hours.

Postmenopausal Bone Loss (Bone Loss Occurring After Menopause)
The suggested dose is 100 international units daily, taken by injection. You should also take supplemental vitamin D (400 units per day) and calcium (such as 1.5 grams of calcium carbonate daily).

Overdosage

Any medication taken in excess can have serious consequences. If you suspect an overdose, seek medical help immediately.

Symptoms of Calcitonin overdose may include:
Nausea
Vomiting

Generic name:

CALCITONIN-SALMON

See Calcimar, page 84.

Generic name:

CALCITRIOL

See Rocaltrol, page 550.

Brand name:

CAPOTEN

Generic name: Captopril

Why is this drug prescribed?

Capoten is used in the treatment of high blood pressure and congestive heart failure. When prescribed for high blood pressure, it is effective used alone or combined with diuretics. If it is prescribed for congestive heart failure, it is generally used in combination with digitalis and diuretics. Capoten is in a family of drugs known as "ACE inhibitors." It works by preventing a chemical in your blood called angiotensin I from converting into a more potent form that increases salt and water retention in your body. Capoten also enhances blood flow throughout your blood vessels.

Most important fact about this drug

Since blood pressure declines gradually, it may take several weeks for the full effect of Capoten to occur.

Do not use potassium-containing preparations or salt-substitutes while taking Capoten.

How should you take this medication?

Capoten should be taken 1 hour before meals.

Take this medication exactly as prescribed by your doctor.

Stopping Capoten suddenly could cause your blood pressure to increase.

If you forget to take a dose, take it as soon as you remember. If it is almost time for your next dose, skip the one you missed and go back to your regular schedule. Never take two doses at the same time.

What side effects may occur?

Side effects cannot be anticipated. If any develop or change in intensity, inform your doctor as soon as possible. Only your doctor can determine if it is safe for you to continue taking Capoten.

- *More common side effects may include:* Abdominal pain, constipation, cough, diarrhea, dizziness, dry mouth, fatigue, hair loss, headache, inability to sleep, labored breathing, loss of appetite, loss of taste, nausea, peptic ulcer, rash, itching, stomach irritation, tingling or pins and needles, vomiting

- *Less common or rare side effects may include:* Anemia, blurred vision, breast development in males, cardiac arrest, changes in heart rhythm, chest pain, confusion, depression, difficulty swallowing, fever and chills, flushing, hepatitis, impotence, indigestion, inflammation of the nose, inflammation of the tongue, lack of coordination, muscle pain and/or weakness, nervousness, pallor, palpitations or other heart effects, skin inflammation, skin peeling, sleepiness, sore throat, sudden loss of strength or fainting, swelling of face, lips, tongue or throat, arms and legs, weakness, yellow eyes and skin

If you develop chest pain, swelling of your face around your lips, tongue or throat, or of your arms and legs, difficulty swallowing, sore throat, or fever and chills, you should contact your doctor immediately. You may need emergency treatment.

Why should this drug not be prescribed?

If you are sensitive to or have ever had an allergic reaction to Capoten or similar drugs, you should not take this medication. Make sure that your doctor is aware of any drug reactions that you have experienced.

Special warnings about this medication

If you are taking Capoten, a complete assessment of your kidney function should be done; kidney function should continue to be monitored.

If you are taking Capoten for your heart, be careful not to increase physical activity too quickly. Check with your doctor as to how much exercise is safe for you.

If you are taking high doses of diuretics and Capoten, you may develop excessively low blood pressure.

Capoten may cause you to become drowsy or less alert, especially if you are also taking a diuretic at the same time. If it has this effect on you, driving or operating dangerous machinery or participating in any hazardous activity that requires full mental alertness is not recommended.

Dehydration may cause a drop in blood pressure. If you experience symptoms such as excessive perspiration, vomiting and/or diarrhea, notify your doctor immediately.

Possible food and drug interactions when taking this medication

If Capoten is taken with certain other drugs, the effects of either could be increased, decreased, or altered. It is especially important to check with your doctor before combining Capoten with the following:

Adrenergic neuron blocking agents
Aspirin
Digoxin (Lanoxin)
Diuretics
Ganglionic blocking agents
Indomethacin
Lithium
Nitroglycerin
Potassium preparations
Potassium-sparing diuretics such as Lasix, Bumex, Edecrin

If you take Capoten with food, the absorption of the drug will be reduced by 30 percent to 40 percent.

Special information
if you are pregnant or breastfeeding

Capoten can cause birth defects, prematurity and death to the fetus and newborn. If you are pregnant or plan to become pregnant, make sure your doctor knows you are taking this medication. Capoten appears in breast milk and could affect a nursing infant. If this medication is essential to your health, your doctor may advise you to discontinue breastfeeding until your treatment is finished.

Recommended dosage

ADULTS

The usual starting dose is 25 milligrams taken 2 or 3 times a day. If you have any problems with your kidneys or suffer from other major health problems, your starting dose may be lower. Depending on how your blood pressure responds, your doctor may increase your dose later, up to a total of 150

milligrams a day. The maximum recommended daily dose is 450 milligrams.

Heart failure
For most patients, the usual dose is 25 milligrams 3 times a day. A daily dosage of 450 milligrams should not be exceeded.

CHILDREN

The safety and effectiveness of Capoten in children have not been established.

Capoten should be used in children only if other measures for controlling blood pressure have not been effective.

ELDERLY

Dosage should be determined by the particular needs of the elderly patient.

Overdosage

Any medication taken in excess can cause symptoms of overdose. If you suspect an overdose, seek medical attention immediately.

A sudden drop in blood pressure is the primary effect of a Capoten overdose.

Brand name:

CAPOZIDE

Generic ingredients: Captopril, Hydrochlorothiazide

Why is this drug prescribed?

Capozide is used in the treatment of high blood pressure. It combines an ACE inhibitor with a thiazide diuretic. Captopril, the ACE inhibitor, works by preventing a chemical in your blood called angiotensin I from converting into a more potent form that increases salt and water retention in your body. Captopril also enhances blood flow throughout your blood vessels. Hydrochlorothiazide, the diuretic, helps your body produce and eliminate more urine, which helps in lowering blood pressure.

Most important fact about this drug

Since blood pressure declines gradually, it may take several weeks for the full effect of Capozide to occur. Even if you are feeling well, you must continue to take this medication. It is needed to keep your blood pressure under control.

How should you take this medication?

Capozide should be taken 1 hour before meals.

Take this medication exactly as prescribed by your doctor. Stopping Capozide suddenly could cause your blood pressure to increase.

If you forget to take a dose, take it as soon as you remember. If it is almost time for your next dose, skip the one you missed and go back to your regular schedule. Never take two doses at the same time.

What side effects may occur?

Side effects can't be anticipated. If any develop or change in intensity, inform your doctor as soon as possible. Only your doctor can determine if it is safe for you to continue taking Capozide.

■ *More common side effects may include:*
Chest pain, constipation, cough, diarrhea, dizziness, fatigue, hair loss, headache, inability to sleep, itching, labored breathing, loss of appetite, loss of taste, low blood pressure, low potassium levels leading to symptoms such as dry mouth, excessive thirst, weak or irregular heartbeat, muscle pain or cramps, nausea, peptic ulcer, rapid heartbeat, rash, stomach irritation, tingling or pins and needles, vomiting

■ *Less common or rare side effects may include:*
Abdominal pain, anemia, blurred vision, breast development in males, bronchitis, bronchospasm, changes in heart rhythm, confusion, constipation, dry mouth, flushing, heart attack, hepatitis, indigestion, impotence, inflammation of nose, inflammation of pancreas, inflammation of tongue, lack of coordination, loss of appetite, loss of strength or fainting, low blood pressure on rising, muscle pain and/or weakness, nervousness, pallor, rapid heartbeat, restlessness, sensitivity to light, skin inflammation and/or peeling, sleepiness, weakness, yellow eyes and skin

Why should this drug not be prescribed?

If you are sensitive to or have ever had an allergic reaction to captopril or hydrocholorothiazide or similar drugs, or if you are sensitive to other sulfonamide-derived drugs, you should not take this medication.

If you have a history of angioedema (swelling of face, extremities and throat) or inability to urinate, you should not take this medication.

Special warnings about this medication

If you develop swelling of your face around your lips, tongue or throat or of your arms and legs or difficulty swallowing, you should contact your doctor immediately. You may need emergency treatment.

If you develop a sore throat or fever you should contact your doctor immediately. It could indicate a more serious illness.

If you are taking Capozide, a complete assessment of your kidney function should be done; kidney function should continue to be monitored.

If you have liver disease or a disease of the connective tissue (lupus erythematosus), Capozide should be used with caution.

If you have severe congestive heart failure, you should be carefully watched for low blood pressure. You should not increase physical activity too quickly.

Excessive sweating, dehydration, severe diarrhea, or vomiting could deplete your fluids and cause your blood pressure to become too low. Be careful when exercising and in hot weather.

Capozide causes some people to become drowsy or less alert. If it has this effect on you, driving or operating dangerous machinery or participating in any hazardous activity that requires full mental alertness is not recommended.

Possible food and drug interactions when taking this medication

Capozide may intensify the effects of alcohol. Do not drink alcohol while taking this medication.

If Capozide is taken with certain other drugs, the effects of either could be increased, decreased, or altered. It is especially important to check with your doctor before combining Capozide with the following:

Anesthetics (used in surgery)
Antigout drugs such as Zyloprim
Barbituates such as Phenobarbital, Seconal
Calcium salts
Cardiac glycosides such as Lanoxin
Cholestyramine (Questran Light)
Colestipol (Colestid Granules)
Corticosteroids such as Prednisone
Diazoxide (Proglycen)
Insulin
Lithium
MAO inhibitors (antidepressants such as Nardil)
Methenamine (Mandelamine)
Narcotics such as Percocet
Nitroglycerin or other nitrates
Nondepolarizing muscle relaxants (used in surgery)

Nonsteroidal anti-inflammatory drugs such as Naprosyn
Norepinephrine (Levophed)
Oral antidiabetic drugs such as Micronase
Oral blood thinners
Other antihypertensives
Potassium-sparing diuretics such as Moduretic
Potassium supplements
Probenecid (Benemid)
Salt substitutes containing potassium
Sulfinpyrazone (Anturane)

Special information if you are pregnant or breastfeeding

Capozide can cause birth defects, prematurity and death to the fetus and newborn. If you are pregnant or plan to become pregnant and are taking Capozide, contact your doctor immediately to discuss the potential hazard to your unborn child. Capozide appears in breast milk and could affect a nursing infant. If this medication is essential to your health, your doctor may advise you to discontinue breastfeeding until your treatment is finished.

Recommended dosage

ADULTS

Dosages of this drug are always individualized, and your doctor will determine what combination works best for you. This medication can and may be used in conjunction with other medications such as beta-blockers. Dosages are also adjusted for patients with decreased kidney function.

This medication should be taken 1 hour before meals.

Initial dose is one 25 milligram/15 milligram tablet, one time a day. If this is not effective, your doctor may adjust the dosage every 6 weeks to 50 milligram/15 milligram, 25 milligram/25 milligram, or 50 milligram/25 milligram tablets 1 time a day. The daily dose should not exceed 150 milligrams captopril and 50 milligrams hydrochlorothiazide.

CHILDREN

The safety and effectiveness of Capozide in children have not been established. Capozide should be used in children only if other measures for controlling blood pressure have not been effective.

ELDERLY

Dosage should be determined by the particular needs of the elderly patient.

Overdosage

Any medication taken in excess can cause symptoms of overdose. If you suspect an overdose, seek medical attention immediately.

The symptoms of Capozide overdose may include:
Coma
Hypermotility
Lethargy
Low blood pressure
Sluggishness
Stomach and intestinal irritation

Generic name:

CAPTOPRIL

See Capoten, page 85.

Generic name:

CAPTOPRIL WITH HYDROCHLOROTHIAZIDE

See Capozide, page 87.

Brand name:

CARAFATE

Generic name: Sucralfate

Why is this drug prescribed?

Carafate is an antiulcer medication prescribed for the short-term treatment (up to 8 weeks) of active duodenal ulcer, and as maintenance therapy, at a reduced dosage, after a duodenal ulcer has healed.

Most important fact about this drug

Duodenal ulcer is a recurring illness. While Carafate can cure an acute ulcer, it cannot prevent other ulcers from occurring or lessen their severity.

How should you take this medication?

Carafate works best when taken on an empty stomach. If you take an antacid to relieve pain, make sure it is not within one-half hour before or after you take Carafate.

Take this drug exactly as prescribed by your doctor.

What side effects may occur?

Side effects cannot be anticipated. If any develop or change in intensity, inform your doctor as soon as possible. Only your doctor can determine if it is safe for you to continue taking Carafate.

■ *More common side effects may include:*
Constipation

■ *Less common or rare side effects may include:*
Back pain, diarrhea, dizziness, dry mouth, gas, headache, indigestion, itching, nausea, possible allergic reactions, including hives and respiratory difficulty, rash, sleepiness, stomach upset, vertigo, vomiting

Why should this drug not be prescribed?

There are no prohibitions against the use of this drug.

Special warnings about this medication

If you have kidney failure or are on dialysis, this drug should be used with caution. Use of Carafate while taking aluminum containing antacids may increase the possibility of aluminum toxicity in patients with kidney failure.

Possible food and drug interactions when taking this medication

If Carafate is taken with certain other drugs, the effects of either could be increased, decreased, or altered. It is especially important to check with your doctor before combining Carafate with the following:

Cimetidine (Tagamet)
Ciprofloxacin (Cipro)
Digoxin (Lanoxin)
Norfloxacin (Noroxin)
Phenytoin (Dilantin)
Ranitidine (Zantac)
Tetracycline
Theophylline

Special information
if you are pregnant or breastfeeding

The effects of Carafate during pregnancy have not been adequately studied. If you are pregnant or plan to become pregnant, inform your doctor immediately. Carafate may appear in breast milk and could affect a nursing infant. If this medication is essential to your health, your doctor may advise you to discontinue breastfeeding until your treatment with this medication is finished.

Recommended dosage

ADULTS

Active Duodenal Ulcer:
The usual dose is 1 gram (1 tablet) 4 times a day on an empty stomach. While your ulcer may heal during the first 2 weeks of therapy, Carafate should be continued for 4 to 8 weeks.

Maintenance Therapy:
The usual dose is 1 gram (1 tablet) 2 times a day.

CHILDREN

The safety and effectiveness of Carafate in children have not been established.

ELDERLY

Dosage should be determined by the particular needs of the elderly patient.

Overdosage

Any medication taken in excess can cause symptoms of overdose. The risk of overdose with Carafate is low. However, if you suspect an overdose, seek medical attention immediately.

There are no specific symptoms available.

Generic name:

CARBAMAZEPINE

See Tegretol, page 608.

Brand name:

CARDENE

Generic name: Nicardipine hydrochloride

Why is this drug prescribed?

Cardene, a type of medication called a calcium channel blocker, is prescribed for the treatment of chronic stable angina (chest pain usually caused by lack of oxygen to the heart resulting from clogged arteries, brought on by exertion) and high blood pressure. When used to treat angina, Cardene is effective alone or in combination with beta-blocking medications such as Tenormin or Inderal. If it is used to treat high blood pressure, Cardene is effective alone or in combination with other high blood pressure medications. Calcium channel blockers ease the workload of the heart by slowing down the muscle contractions of the heart and the passage of nerve impulses through the heart. This improves blood flow through the heart and throughout the body, reducing blood pressure.

Most important fact about this drug

Cardene can reduce or eliminate chest (angina) pain caused by exertion or exercise. Be sure to discuss with your doctor how much exercise or exertion is safe for you to do.

How should you take this medication?

Take this medication exactly as prescribed by your doctor, even if your symptoms have disappeared.

Try not to miss any doses. If Cardene is not taken regularly, your condition may worsen.

What side effects may occur?

Side effects cannot be anticipated. If any develop or change in intensity, inform your doctor as soon as possible. Only your doctor can determine if it is safe for you to continue taking Cardene.

■ *More common side effects may include:*
Dizziness
Flushing
Headache
Increased chest (angina) pain
Indigestion
Nausea
Pounding or rapid heartbeat
Sleepiness
Swelling of feet
Weakness

■ *Less common side effects may include:*
Abnormal dreams, constipation, difficulty sleeping, drowsiness, dry mouth, excessive nighttime urination, fainting, fluid retention, muscle pain, nervousness, rash, shortness of breath, tingling or pins

and needles, tremors, vomiting, vague feeling of bodily discomfort.

■ *Rare side effects may include:*
Allergic reactions, anxiety, blurred vision, confusion, dizziness when standing, depression, hot flashes, increased movements, infection, inflammation of the nose, inflammation of the sinuses, impotence, joint pain, low blood pressure, more frequent urination, ringing in ears, sore throat, unusual chest pain, vertigo, vision changes

Why should this drug not be prescribed?

If you have advanced aortic stenosis (a narrowing of the aortic valve that causes obstruction of blood flow from the heart to the body), you should not take this medication.

If you are sensitive to or have ever had an allergic reaction to Cardene, you should not take this medication. Make sure your doctor is aware of any drug reactions you may have experienced.

Special warnings about this medication

If you experience increased chest pain when you start taking Cardene or when your dosage is increased, contact your doctor immediately.

This medication should be carefully monitored if you have congestive heart failure, especially if you are also taking a beta-blocking medication such as Tenormin or Inderal.

Cardene can cause your blood pressure to become too low, making you feel lightheaded or faint. Your doctor should check your blood pressure when you start taking Cardene and continue to monitor it while your dosage is being adjusted.

If you have liver disease or decreased liver function, this drug should be used with caution.

Possible food and drug interactions when taking this medication

If Cardene is taken with certain other drugs, the effects of either could be increased, decreased, or altered. It is especially important to check with your doctor before combining Cardene with the following:

Cimetidine (Tagamet)
Cyclosporine (Sandimmune)
Digoxin (Lanoxin)
Fentanyl (Innovar) anesthesia

Special information if you are pregnant or breastfeeding

The effects of Cardene during pregnancy have not been adequately studied. If you are pregnant or plan to become pregnant, inform your doctor immediately. Cardene may appear in breast milk and could affect a nursing infant. If this medication is essential to your health, your doctor may advise you to discontinue breastfeeding until your treatment with Cardene is finished.

Recommended dosage

ADULTS

Angina
Dosages should be adjusted to individual patient needs, usually beginning with 20 milligrams, 3 times a day. The usual regular dose is 20 to 40 milligrams, 3 times a day. Your physician may monitor your condition for at least 3 days before adjusting your dose.

High Blood Pressure
Dosages should be adjusted to individual patient needs, usually beginning with 20 milligrams 3 times a day. The usual dose is 20 to 40 milligrams 3 times a day.

Your doctor may monitor your response to this medication for a few hours after the first dose.

Your physician may also monitor your condition for at least 3 days before adjusting your dose.

Patients with reduced kidney function will be carefully supervised and may be given a starting dose of 20 milligrams 3 times a day.

Patients with reduced liver function will be monitored carefully and may be given a starting dose of 20 milligrams 2 times a day.

Patients with congestive heart failure will also be carefully monitored, and their starting dose will be slowly administered.

CHILDREN

The safety and effectiveness of this drug in children under age 18 have not been established.

ELDERLY

This drug should be used with caution in elderly patients.

Overdosage

The symptoms of overdose may include:
Confusion
Drowsiness
Severe low blood pressure
Slow heartbeat
Slurred speech

If you suspect symptoms of a Cardene overdose, seek medical attention immediately.

Brand name:

CARDIZEM

Generic name: Diltiazem hydrochloride

Why is this drug prescribed?

Cardizem, a calcium channel blocker, is used in the treatment of angina pectoris (chest pain usually caused by lack of oxygen to the heart due to clogged arteries) and chronic stable angina (caused by exertion). Cardizem SR and Cardizem CD (controlled released forms of diltiazem) are used for the control of high blood pressure. Cardizem dilates blood vessels and slows the heart to reduce blood pressure and the pain of angina.

Most important fact about this drug

Cardizem usually reduces or even stops chest pain from exercise. Be careful not to over-do because you feel well. Check with your doctor as to how much exercise is safe for you.

How should you take this medication?

Cardizem should be taken before meals and at bedtime.

Take this medication exactly as prescribed by your doctor, even if your symptoms have disappeared.

If you forget to take a dose, take it as soon as you remember. If it's almost time for your next dose, skip the missed dose and go back to your regular schedule. Never take two doses at the same time.

What side effects may occur?

Side effects cannot be anticipated. If any develop or change in intensity, inform your doctor as soon as possible. Only your doctor can determine if it is safe for you to continue taking Cardizem.

■ *More common side effects may include:*
Abnormally slow heartbeat (more common with Cardizem SR)
Dizziness
Fluid retention
Flushing (more common with Cardizem SR)
Headache
Nausea
Rash
Weakness

■ *Less common or rare side effects may include:*
Abnormal dreams, amnesia, blood disorders, congestive heart failure, constipation, depression, diarrhea, difficulty sleeping, drowsiness, dry mouth, excessive urination at night, eye irritation, fainting, hair loss, hallucinations, heart attack, hives, impotence, indigestion, irregular heartbeat, itching, joint pain, labored breathing, loss of appetite, low blood pressure, muscle cramps, nasal congestion, nervousness, nosebleed, personality change, rapid heartbeat, reddish or purplish spots on skin, ringing in ears, sexual difficulties, skin sensitivity to sunlight, taste alteration, thirst, tingling or pins and needles, tremor, unusual gait, vision changes, vomiting, weight increase

Why should this drug not be prescribed?

If you suffer from sick sinus syndrome (a form of irregular heartbeat) or have second or third degree heart block (a conduction disorder), you should not take this drug unless you have a ventricular pacemaker.

Don't take Cardizem if you have low blood pressure or an allergy to the drug.

This drug should not be given to people with lung congestion, or those having a heart attack.

Special warnings about this medication

If you suffer from sick sinus syndrome, be

aware that Cardizem can cause an abnormally slow heart rate.

If you have congestive heart failure, this drug should be used with caution.

If you suffer from kidney or liver disease, you should use Cardizem with caution.

This medication may cause your heart rate to become too slow. You should check your pulse regularly.

Possible food and drug interactions when taking this medication

If Cardizem is taken with certain other drugs, the effects of either could be increased, decreased, or altered. It is especially important to check with your doctor before combining Cardizem with the following:

Anesthetics
Beta-blockers (heart and blood pressure drugs such as Tenormin and Inderal)
Cimetidine (Tagemet)
Digoxin (Lanoxin)
Ranitidine (Zantac)

Special information if you are pregnant or breastfeeding

The effects of Cardizem during pregnancy have not been adequately studied. If you are pregnant or plan to become pregnant, inform your doctor immediately. Cardizem appears in breast milk and could affect a nursing infant. If this medication is essential to your health, your doctor may advise you to discontinue breastfeeding until your treatment with this medication is finished.

Recommended dosage

ADULT

Dosage levels must be determined by each patient's needs. However, the average daily dosage is between 180 milligrams and 360 milligrams, divided into 3 or 4 smaller doses.

The recommended dosage for Cardizem SR is 60 to 120 milligrams 2 times a day. Cardizem CD is a once-a-day form of this drug.

CHILDREN

Safety and effectiveness in children have not been established.

Overdosage

Any medication taken in excess can cause overdose. If you suspect an overdose seek medical attention immediately.

The symptoms of Cardizem overdose may include:
Heart block (conduction disorder)
Heart failure
Very low blood pressure
Very slow heartbeat

Brand name:

CARDURA

Generic name: Doxazosin mesylate

Why is this drug prescribed?

Cardura is used in the treatment of high blood pressure. It is effective when used alone or in combination with diuretics or beta-blocking medications. Doctors also prescribe Cardura to treat symptoms of benign prostatic hyperplasia (BPH), an abnormal enlargement of the prostate gland.

Most important fact about this drug

If you have high blood pressure, you must take Cardura regularly for it to be effective. Even if you are feeling well, you must continue to take Cardura to control your blood pressure.

How should you take this medication?

This medication can be taken with or without food.

Cardura should be taken exactly as prescribed by your doctor, even if your symptoms have disappeared.

Try not to miss any doses. If this medication is not taken regularly, your condition may worsen.

What side effects may occur?

Side effects cannot be anticipated. If any develop or change in intensity, inform your doctor as soon as possible. Only your doctor can determine if it is safe for you to continue taking Cardura.

■ *More common side effects may include:*
Dizziness
Drowsiness
Fatigue
Headache

■ *Less common side effects may include:*
Arthritis, constipation, depression, difficulty sleeping, eye pain, flushing, gas, inability to hold urine, indigestion, inflammation of conjunctiva (pink eye), itching, joint pain, lack of muscle coordination, low blood pressure, motion disorders, muscle cramps, muscle pain, muscle weakness, nausea, nervousness, nosebleeds, rash, ringing in ears, shortness of breath, tingling or pins and needles, weakness.

■ *Rare side effects may include:*
Abnormal thinking, abnormal vision, agitation, altered sense of smell, amnesia, back pain, breast pain, changeable emotions, changes in taste, chest pain, confusion, coughing, decreased sense of touch, diarrhea, dizziness when standing up, dry mouth, dry skin, earache, excessive urination, fainting, fecal incontinence, fever, fluid retention, flu-like symptoms, gout, hair loss, heart attack, hot flushes, inability to concentrate, inability to tolerate light, increased appetite, increased

sweating, increased thirst, infection, inflammation of the nose, stomach or intestines, infection, loss of appetite, loss of sense of personal identity, migraine headache, morbid dreams, nausea, nervousness, pain, pallor, rapid pounding heartbeat, sexual problems, sinus inflammation, slight or partial paralysis, sore throat, tremors, twitching, vertigo, weight gain, weight loss, wheezing

Why should this drug not be prescribed?

Cardura should not be taken if you are sensitive to or have ever had an allergic reaction to Cardura or such drugs as Minipren or Hytrin. Make sure that your doctor is aware of any drug reactions that you may have experienced.

Special warnings about this medication

Cardura can cause low blood pressure, especially when you first start taking the medication and when dosage is increased. This can cause you to become faint, dizzy, or light-headed, particularly when first standing up. You should avoid driving or any hazardous tasks where injury could occur for 24 hours after taking the first dose, after your dose has been increased or if Cardura has been stopped and then restarted.

If you have liver disease or are taking other medications that alter liver function, this drug should be used with caution.

Cardura may cause lowered blood counts. Your doctor should monitor your blood count while you are taking this medication.

This medication may cause you to become drowsy or sleepy. Driving or operating dangerous machinery or participating in any hazardous activity that requires full mental alertness is not recommended.

Possible food and drug interactions when taking this medication

No significant interactions have been reported.

Special information
If you are pregnant or breastfeeding

The effects of Cardura during pregnancy have not been adequately studied. If you are pregnant or plan to become pregnant, inform your doctor immediately. Cardura may appear in breast milk and could affect a nursing infant. If this medication is essential to your health, your doctor may advise you to discontinue breastfeeding until your treatment with this medication is finished.

Recommended dosage

ADULTS

All doses should be adjusted to each individual patient's needs.

The usual starting dose is 1 milligram taken 1 time per day. To minimize the potential for dizziness or fainting associated with Cardura, which may occur between 2 and 6 hours after a dose, your doctor will monitor your pressure during this period and afterwards to check the effectiveness of this medication.

After the effects of the starting dose are measured, your doctor may increase the dose to 2 milligrams per day and then, if necessary, to 4 milligrams, 8 milligrams, or 16 milligrams. As the dose increases, the potential for side effects such as dizziness, vertigo, lightheadedness, and fainting also increase.

CHILDREN

The safety and effectiveness of this drug in children have not been established.

ELDERLY

This drug should be used with caution in elderly patients.

Overdosage

Any medication taken in excess can cause symptoms of overdose. If you suspect a Cardura overdose, seek medical attention immediately.

Although no specific information is available, low blood pressure is the most likely symptom.

Generic name:

CARISOPRODOL

See Soma, page 585.

Generic name:

CARTEOLOL HYDROCHLORIDE

See Cartrol, page 97.

Brand name:

CARTROL

Generic name: Carteolol hydrochloride

Why is this drug prescribed?

Cartrol, a type of medication known as a beta blocker, is used in the treatment of high blood pressure. It is effective when used alone or when combined with other high blood pressure medications, particularly with a thiazide-type diuretic. Beta-blockers decrease the force and rate of heart contractions.

Most important fact about this drug

You must take Cartrol regularly for it to be effective. Even if you are feeling well, you need the drug to keep your blood pressure down.

How should you take this medication?

Cartrol can be taken with or without food.

Take this medication exactly as prescribed by your doctor, even if your symptoms have disappeared.

Try not to miss any doses. If this medication is not taken regularly, your condition may worsen.

If you forget to take a dose, take it as soon as you remember. If it's within 8 hours of your next scheduled dose, skip the one you missed and go back to your regular schedule. Never take two doses at the same time.

What side effects may occur?

Side effects cannot be anticipated. If any develop or change in intensity, inform your doctor as soon as possible. Only your doctor can determine if it is safe for you to continue taking Cartrol.

■ *More common side effects may include:*
Abdominal pain, back pain, chest pain, diarrhea, joint pain, leg pain, muscle cramps, nasal congestion, nausea, rash, sore throat, swelling due to fluid retention in arms and legs, tingling or pins and needles, tiredness, trouble sleeping, weakness

■ *Rare side effects may include:*
Angina pectoris (heart pain), blurred vision, bronchospasm, change in heart rhythm, cold symptoms, conjunctivitis, constipation, cough, depression, dizziness, excessive sweating, fever, flu-like symptoms, gas, gout, heart block, heart failure, hepatitis, impotence, neck and shoulder pain, nervousness, ringing in ears, stomach upset, strange dreams, urinary infection, wheezing, yellow eyes and skin

Certain other side effects have been reported for drugs similar to Cartrol. Check with your doctor if you suspect a problem.

Why should this drug not be prescribed?

If you have bronchial asthma, severely slow heartbeat, inadequate blood supply to the circulatory system (cardiogenic shock), heart block (a conduction disorder), or congestive heart failure, you should not take this medication.

Special warnings about this medication

If you have a history of severe congestive heart failure, Cartrol should be used with caution.

Cartrol should not be stopped suddenly. This can cause increased chest pain and heart attack. Dosage should be gradually reduced.

If you suffer from thyroid disease or glaucoma, this drug should be used with caution.

If you suffer from asthma, seasonal allergies or other bronchial conditions, coronary artery disease, or kidney disease, this medication should be used with caution.

This medication may mask the symptoms of low blood sugar or alter blood sugar levels. If you are diabetic, discuss this with your doctor.

Notify your doctor or dentist that you are taking Cartrol if you have a medical emergency, and before you have surgery or dental treatment.

Possible food and drug interactions while taking this medication

If Cartrol is taken with certain other drugs, the effects of either could be increased, decreased, or altered. It is especially important to check with your doctor before combining Cartrol with the following:

Antidiabetic drugs such as Micronase and Diabeta
Catecholamine-depleting drugs such as reserpine (found in several other blood pressure medications)
Digitalis
General anesthetics
Insulin

Non-steroidal anti-inflammatory drugs such as Motrin and Naprosyn

Oral calcium antagonists such as Cardizem, Procardia, and Calan

Special Information
if you are pregnant or breastfeeding

The effects of Cartrol during pregnancy have not been adequately studied. If you are pregnant or plan to become pregnant, inform your doctor immediately. Cartrol may appear in breast milk and could affect a nursing infant. If this medication is essential to your health, your doctor may advise you to discontinue breastfeeding until your treatment with this medication is finished.

Recommended dosage

ADULTS

Dosages of Cartrol are always individualized.

The usual starting dose is 2.5 milligrams 1 time a day, alone or with a diuretic. Doses may be gradually increased to 5 milligrams or 10 milligrams 1 time a day. Doses over 10 milligrams per day do not provide additional benefit and may actually reduce the effectiveness of this drug.

Patients with kidney disorders must be carefully monitored, and dosages will be adjusted to the individual patient depending on his or her level of kidney function. The maintenance dose is 2.5 or 5 milligrams 1 time a day.

CHILDREN

The safety and effectiveness of Cartrol have not been established in children.

ELDERLY

Dosage should be determined by the particular needs of the elderly patient.

Overdosage

Any medication taken in excess can have serious consequences. If you suspect an overdose, seek medical attention immediately.

There is no specific information available on Cartrol overdose; however, overdose symptoms with other beta blockers include:

Bronchospasm
Extremely slow heartbeat
Heart block
Low blood pressure
Severe congestive heart failure

Brand name:

CATAPRES

Generic name: Clonidine hydrochloride

Why is this drug prescribed?

Catapres is a medication used in the treatment of high blood pressure. It is effective when used alone or with other high blood pressure medications. Doctors also prescribe Catapres for alcohol, nicotine, or benzodiazepine (Valium) withdrawal; migraine headaches; smoking cessation programs; Tourette's syndrome; opiates/methadone detoxification; premenstrual tension; and diabetic diarrhea.

Most important fact about this drug

Catapres should not be stopped suddenly. Headache, nervousness, agitation, and rapid rise in blood pressure can occur. Severe reactions such as brain dysfunction and death have also been reported. Your doctor should therefore gradually reduce your dosage over several days to avoid withdrawal symptoms.

How should you take this medication?

Take this medication exactly as prescribed by your doctor, even if you are feeling well.

Try not to miss any doses. If Catapres is not taken regularly, your condition may worsen.

What side effects may occur?

Side effects cannot be anticipated. If any develop or change in intensity, inform your doctor as soon as possible. Only your doctor can determine if it is safe for you to continue taking Catapres.

■ *More common side effects may include:*
Constipation
Dizziness
Drowsiness
Dry mouth
Sedation (calm)
Skin reactions (Catapres-TTS)

■ *Less common side effects may include:*
Agitation, breast development in males, changes in heartbeat, changes in liver function, changes in taste, decreased sexual activity, difficulty sleeping, difficulty urinating, dizziness on standing up, excessive nighttime urination, fatigue, fluid retention, hair loss, headache, hives, impotence, itching, joint pain, leg cramps, loss of appetite, loss of sexual drive, mental depression, muscle pain, nausea, nervousness, rash, retention of urine, sluggishness, vague bodily discomfort, vomiting, weakness, weight gain

■ *Rare side effects may include:*
Anxiety, behavior changes, blurred vision, burning eyes, changes in heartbeat, congestive heart failure, delirium, dry eyes, dry nasal passages, fever, greater sensitivity to alcohol, hallucinations, hepatitis, inflammation of the parotid glands, pallor, restlessness, vivid dreams or nightmares.

Why should this drug not be prescribed?

Do not take this medication if you have ever had an allergic reaction to Catapres or to any of the components of the adhesive layer of the transdermal patch.

Special warnings about this medication

If your doctor has switched you to oral Catapres (tablet) because you had an allergic reaction, such as a rash or hives, to the transdermal skin patch, be aware that you may have a similar reaction to the Catapres tablet.

If you have severe heart or kidney disease, are recovering from a heart attack, or have a disease of the blood vessels of the brain, this drug should be used with caution.

Do not stop taking Catapres suddenly without talking to your doctor first. Severe side effects can occur. Dosage should be reduced gradually.

If you are taking Catapres and a beta blocker, (e.g., Inderal or Tenormin) and your doctor wants to stop your medication, the beta blocker should be stopped several days before the gradual withdrawal of Catapres.

Catapres may cause you to become drowsy or less alert; therefore, driving or operating dangerous machinery or participating in any hazardous activity that requires full mental alertness is not recommended.

Possible food and drug interactions when taking this medication

Catapres may increase the effects of alcohol. Do not drink alcohol while taking this medication.

If Catapres is taken with certain other drugs, the effects of either could be increased, decreased, or altered. It is especially important to check with your doctor before combining Catapres with the following:

Amitriptyline (Elavil)
Barbiturates (Nembutal, Seconal)
Sedatives
Tricyclic antidepressants (Elavil, Tofranil)

Special information
if you are pregnant or breastfeeding

The effects of Catapres during pregnancy
have not been adequately studied. If you
are pregnant or plan to become pregnant,
inform your doctor immediately.
Catapres appears in breast milk and could
affect a nursing infant. If this medication
is essential to your health, your doctor may
advise you to discontinue breastfeeding
until your treatment with this medication
is finished.

Recommended dosage

ADULTS

Dosages should be adjusted to each
individual patient's needs.

The usual starting dose is 0.1 milligram, 2
times per day (usually in the morning
and at bedtime).

The regular dose of Catapres is determined
by increasing the starting dose by 0.1
milligram per day until the desired response
is achieved. A larger portion of the
increased dose can be taken at bedtime to
reduce potential drowsiness and dry
mouth side effects that may appear when
you begin taking this drug.

The most common effective dosages range
from 0.2 milligram to 0.6 milligram per
day divided into smaller doses. The
maximum effective dose is 2.4 milligrams
per day; however, this dose is not usually
prescribed.

Patients with reduced kidney function should
be carefully monitored when taking this drug.

Transdermal Patch
The patch should be used to meet each
individual patient's needs. The patch
comes in different strengths, and your doctor
will determine which is best for you,
based on your own blood pressure response.

Patients who are using another high blood
pressure medication should not stop
taking it abruptly when they begin using the
patch, because the medication in the
patch may take a few days to work. The
original medication should be
discontinued slowly as the patch begins to
work.

The Catapres-TTS patch should be put on
a hairless, clean area of the upper arm
or body. Normally, a new one will be
applied every 7 days to a new area of
the skin. If the patch becomes loose, use
some adhesive tape or an adhesive
bandage to keep it in place.

CHILDREN

The safety and effectiveness of Catapres
in children and of Catapres-TTS in children
under 12 have not been established.

ELDERLY

Dosages are generally as above; however, the
dose for an elderly patient may be lower
than the regular starting dose initially and
adjusted until the desired effect is
reached.

Overdosage

*The symptoms of Catapres overdose may
include:*
Changes in heart function, constriction of
pupils of the eye, high blood pressure,
irritability, low blood pressure, reduced rate
of breathing, seizures, sleepiness, slow
heartbeat, slowed reflexes, sluggishness,
temporary stoppage in breathing,
vomiting, weakness

If you suspect symptoms of a Catapres overdose, seek medical attention immediately.

Brand name:

CECLOR

Generic name: Cefaclor

Why is this drug prescribed?
Ceclor, a cephalosporin antibiotic, is used in the treatment of ear, nose, throat, respiratory tract, urinary tract and skin infections caused by specific bacteria, including staph, strep, and E. coli. Uses include treatment of sore or strep throat, pneumonia, and tonsillitis.

Most important fact about this drug
Do not take this drug if you are allergic to cephalsporin antibiotics or penicillin. There is a possibility that you could be allergic to both medications. Allergic reactions to this medication can be serious and possibly fatal. If you experience a reaction, report it to your doctor immediately and seek medical treatment.

How should you take this medication?
Take this medication exactly as prescribed by your doctor. It is important that you finish taking all of this medication to obtain the maximum benefit.

This medication works fastest when taken on an empty stomach. However, your doctor may ask you to take this drug with food to avoid stomach upset.

What side effects may occur?
Side effects cannot be anticipated. If any develop or change in intensity, inform your doctor as soon as possible. Only your doctor can determine if it is safe for you to continue taking Ceclor.

■ *More common side effects may include:*
Diarrhea (loose stools)
Hives
Itching

■ *Less common or rare side effects may include:*
Blood disorders (an increase in certain types of white blood cells), hepatitis and jaundice, nausea, skin rashes accompanied by joint pain, vaginal inflammation, vomiting.

Other problems have been reported in patients taking Ceclor, though it's not known whether the drug was the cause. Check with your doctor if you suspect a side effect.

Why should this drug not be prescribed?
If you are sensitive to or have ever had an allergic reaction to Ceclor or similar drugs, you should not take this medication. Make sure that your doctor is aware of any drug reactions that you have experienced.

Unless you are directed to do so by your doctor, do not take this medication if you have a history of gastrointestinal problems, particularly colitis. You may be at increased risk for side effects.

Special warnings about this medication
Ceclor may cause a false positive result with some urine sugar tests for diabetics. Your doctor can advise you of any adjustments you might need to make in your medication or diet.

Possible food and drug interactions when taking this medication
No significant interactions have been reported.

Special information if you are pregnant or breastfeeding
The effects of Ceclor during pregnancy have not been adequately studied. If you are pregnant or plan to become pregnant, this

drug should be used only when prescribed by your doctor. Ceclor appears in breast milk and could affect a nursing infant. If this medication is essential to your health, your doctor may advise you to stop nursing your baby until your treatment with Ceclor is finished.

Recommended dosage

ADULTS

The usual adult dose is 250 milligrams every 8 hours. For more severe infections (such as pneumonia), doses may be increased as determined by your doctor.

CHILDREN

The usual daily dosage is 20 milligrams per 2.2 pounds of body weight per day in divided doses every 8 hours. In more serious infections, such as middle ear infection, the usual dose is 40 milligrams per 2.2 pounds of body weight per day in divided doses. The total daily dose should not exceed 1 gram.

Overdosage

Large amounts of Ceclor may cause overdose symptoms, including:
Diarrhea
Nausea
Stomach upset
Vomiting

If other symptoms are present, they may be related to an allergic reaction or other underlying disease. In any case, you should contact your doctor or an emergency room immediately.

Generic name:

CEFACLOR

See Ceclor, page 102.

Generic name:

CEFADROXIL MONOHYDRATE

See Duricef, page 218.

Generic name:

CEFIXIME

See Suprax, page 591.

Brand name:

CEFTIN

Generic name: Cefuroxime axetil

Why is this drug prescribed?

Ceftin, a cephalosporin antibiotic, is prescribed for mild to moderately severe bacterial infections of the throat, lungs, ears, skin, and urinary tract, and for gonorrhea.

Most important fact about this drug

If you have shown a sensitivity to penicillin or other cephalosporin, notify your doctor before taking this medication. Severe reactions have been reported in penicillin-sensitive patients. If an allergic reaction to Ceftin occurs, discontinue taking the drug and notify your doctor.

How should you take this medication?

Ceftin can be taken on a full or empty stomach. However, this drug enters the bloodstream and works faster when taken after meals.

Take this medication exactly as prescribed by your doctor. It is important that you finish taking all of this medication to obtain the maximum benefit.

If you forget to take a dose, take it as soon as you remember. If it is almost time for your next dose, take the missed dose and your next dose 5 to 6 hours later before going back to the regular schedule.

What side effects may occur?

Side effects cannot be anticipated. If any develop or change in intensity, inform your doctor as soon as possible. Only your doctor can determine if it is safe for you to continue taking Ceftin.

■ *More common side effects may include:*
Colitis
Diarrhea
Nausea
Skin rashes, redness or itching
Vomiting

■ *Less common or rare side effects may include:*
Dizziness, headache, seizures, vaginal inflammation, yeast infection

Why should this drug not be prescribed?

Ceftin should not be prescribed if you have a known allergy to penicillin, cephalosporins or other drugs.

Special warnings about this medication

Colitis has been reported with the use of Ceftin; therefore, if you develop diarrhea while taking this medication, notify your doctor.

Continued or prolonged use of Ceftin may result in an overgrowth of bacteria that does not respond to this medication and can cause a secondary infection. You should take this drug only when it is prescribed by your doctor, even if you have symptoms like those of a previous infection.

Possible food and drug interactions when taking this medication

It is important to consult with your doctor before taking this drug with probenecid (gout medication).

If diarrhea occurs while taking Ceftin, consult with your doctor before taking an anti-diarrhea medication, as certain drugs, such as Lomotil or Parepectolin, may cause your diarrhea to become worse.

This medication may cause a false test result indicating sugar in your urine.

Special information if you are pregnant or breastfeeding

The effects of Ceftin during pregnancy have not been adequately studied. If you are pregnant or plan to become pregnant, inform your doctor immediately. Ceftin appears in breast milk and could affect a nursing infant. If this medication is essential to your health, your doctor may advise you to discontinue breastfeeding until your treatment with this medication is finished.

Recommended dosage

ADULTS

The usual dose for adults and children over 12 years of age is 250 milligrams, 2 times a day. For more severe infections the dose may be increased to 500 milligrams, 2 times a day. The usual dose for urinary tract infection is 125 milligrams, 2 times a day. Dose may be increased to 250 milligrams 2 times a day for severe infection.

The usual dosage for gonorrhea is a single dose of 1 gram.

CHILDREN

Ceftin for children is available only in tablet form. If your child cannot swallow the tablet whole, the tablet may be crushed and mixed with food such as applesauce or ice cream. However, the crushed tablet has a strong, bitter taste. If your child cannot swallow the tablet or won't take the medication due to the taste, check with your doctor so that an alternative therapy can be considered.

The usual dose for children up to 12 years of age is 125 milligrams, 2 times a day.

For children with middle ear infections, the usual dosage is 125 milligrams, 2 times a day, for children under 2 years of age and 250 milligrams, 2 times a day, for children 2 years of age and older.

ELDERLY

No adjustment of the usual adult dose is necessary.

Overdosage

Any medication taken in excess can have serious consequences. Overdosage with cephalosporin antibiotics can cause cerebral irritation leading to convulsions. If you suspect an overdose, seek medical attention immediately.

Generic name:

CEFUROXIME AXETIL

See Ceftin, page 103.

Brand name:

CENTRAX

Generic name: Prazepam

Why is this drug prescribed?

Centrax is used in the treatment of anxiety disorders and for short-term relief of the symptoms of anxiety. It belongs to a class of drugs known as benzodiazepines.

Most important fact about this drug

Tolerance and dependence can occur with the use of Centrax. You may experience withdrawal symptoms if you stop using this drug abruptly. Discontinue or change your dose only in consultation with your doctor.

How should you take this medication?

Take this medication exactly as prescribed by your doctor. If you forget to take a dose, take it as soon as you remember. If it is almost time for your next dose, skip the one you missed and go back to your regular schedule. Never take two doses at the same time.

What side effects may occur?

Side effects cannot be anticipated. If any develop or change in intensity, inform your doctor as soon as possible. Only your doctor can determine if it is safe for you to continue taking Centrax.

■ *More common side effects may include:*
Dizziness
Drowsiness
Fatigue
Lack of muscular coordination
Light-headedness
Weakness

■ *Less common or rare side effects may include:*
Blurred vision, confusion, dry mouth, excessive sweating, fainting, genital and urinary tract disorders, headache, itching, joint pain, palpitations, skin rashes, slurred speech, stomach and intestinal disorders, swelling of feet, tremors, vivid dreams

Why should this drug not be prescribed?

If you are sensitive to or have ever had an allergic reaction to Centrax or similar drugs, you should not take this medication.

Unless you are directed to do so by your doctor, do not take this medication if you have acute narrow-angle glaucoma.

Centrax should not be prescribed if you are being treated for mental disorders more serious than anxiety.

Anxiety or tension related to everyday stress usually does not require treatment with Centrax. Discuss your symptoms thoroughly with your doctor.

Special warnings about this medication

Centrax may cause you to become drowsy or less alert; therefore, driving or operating dangerous machinery or participating in any hazardous activity that requires full mental alertness is not recommended.

If you are severely depressed or have suffered from severe depression, consult with your doctor before taking this medication.

Possible food and drug interactions when taking this medication

Like alcohol, Centrax is a central nervous system depressant. Do not drink alcohol while taking this medication.

If Centrax is taken with certain other drugs, the effects of either could be increased, decreased, or altered. It is especially important to check with your doctor before combining Centrax with antidepressants and central nervous system depressants, including the following:

Barbiturates (Phenobartital)
MAO inhibitors (certain drugs used for depression)
Narcotics (morphine and codeine-containing pain medication)
Phenothiazines (Thorazine, Phenergan)

Special information
if you are pregnant or breastfeeding

Do not take Centrax if you are pregnant or planning to become pregnant. There may be an increased risk of birth defects. This drug may appear in breast milk and could affect a nursing infant. If this medication is essential to your health, your doctor may advise you to discontinue breastfeeding until

your treatment with this medication is finished.

Recommended dosage

ADULTS

The usual dosage is a total of 30 milligrams per day divided into small doses. This dose should be adjusted gradually to between 20 and 60 milligrams per day according to individual need.

Centrax can also be given as a single dose taken at bedtime. The recommended starting dose is 20 milligrams. To maximize the antianxiety effect with a minimum of daytime drowsiness, the dose can be adjusted up to 40 milligrams.

CHILDREN

Safety and effectiveness have not been established in children under 18 years of age.

ELDERLY

In elderly the usual daily dose is 10 to 15 milligrams in divided doses.

Overdosage

Any medication taken in excess can cause symptoms of overdose. If you suspect an overdose seek medical attention immediately.

Generic name:

CEPHALEXIN

See Keflex, page 305.

Generic name:

CEPHALEXIN HYDROCHLORIDE

See Keftab, page 306.

Generic name:

CEPHRADINE

See Velosef, page 676.

Generic name:

CHLORDIAZEPOXIDE

See Librium, page 320.

Generic name:

CHLORDIAZEPOXIDE WITH AMITRIPTYLINE

See Limbitrol, page 324.

Generic name:

CHLORDIAZEPOXIDE WITH CLIDINIUM

See Librax, page 319.

Generic name:

CHLORHEXIDINE GLUCONATE

See Peridex, page 469.

Generic name:

CHLOROTHIAZIDE

See Diuril, page 206.

Generic name:

CHLORPROMAZINE

See Thorazine, page 625.

Generic name:

CHLORPROPAMIDE

See Diabinese, page 187.

Generic name:

CHLORTHALIDONE

See Hygroton, page 284.

Generic name:

CHLORZOXAZONE

See Parafon Forte DSC, page 454.

Brand name:

CHOLEDYL

Generic name: Oxtriphylline

Why is this drug prescribed?

Choledyl relieves and/or prevents symptoms of asthma and wheezing associated with chronic bronchitis and emphysema. Choledyl relaxes the muscles in the bronchial airways of the lungs, allowing easier breathing. Choledyl is obtained from the drug theophylline and is categorized as a xanthine derivative.

Most important fact about this drug

It is essential that you take this drug only at the prescribed dosage, and only at the times your doctor has indicated.

How should you take this medication?

Tablets should be swallowed whole. They should not be crushed, chewed, or dissolved.

Avoid consuming large amounts of caffeine-containing beverages such as coffee and tea.

Your individual dosage is determined by your response to Choledyl. Your doctor will perform blood level tests regularly to avoid over- and under-dosage. Do not change your dose without consulting your doctor.

What side effects may occur?

Side effects cannot be anticipated. If any develop or change in intensity, inform your doctor as soon as possible. Only your doctor can determine if it is safe for you to continue taking Choledyl.

■ *Side effects may include:*
Circulatory failure, convulsions, diarrhea, difficulty sleeping, flushing, hair loss, headaches, hyperexcitability, increased sugar in blood, irregular heartbeat, irritability, low blood pressure, muscle twitching, nausea, possible increase in urine production, pounding heartbeat, rapid breathing, rapid heartbeat, rash, restlessness, stomach pain, vomiting, vomiting blood

Why should this drug not be prescribed?

Choledyl should be avoided if you have an active peptic ulcer or a seizure disorder for which you do not take medication, or if you are sensitive to or have ever had an allergic reaction to any of its components.

Special warnings about this medication

This medication should be used cautiously by people who have liver disease or heart failure, a continuous high fever, or are over 55 years old (especially men and those who have chronic lung disease). Use caution also, when treating babies under 1 year old.

Your doctor should check your blood regularly while you are using Choledyl, to avoid toxicity. Irregular heartbeats, convulsions, or even death can be the first sign of toxicity, and can occur without any previous warning.

Even at nontoxic levels, Choledyl may cause your heartbeat to become irregular or worsen an already irregular heartbeat.

This medication should not be taken with other xanthine medications such as Theo-Dur.

Choledyl should be used with care if you have a history of peptic ulcer or high blood pressure.

Possible food and drug interactions when taking this medication

If Choledyl is taken with certain other drugs, the effects of either could be increased, decreased, or altered. It is especially important to check with your doctor before combining Choledyl with the following:

Other drugs that open air passages in the lungs (Proventil, Ventolin)
Allopurinol (Zyloprim)
Cimetidine (Tagamet)
Erythromycin, troleandomycin such as E.E.S., Erythrocin, Tao Capsules
Lithium carbonate (Lithobid)
Oral contraceptives
Phenytoin (Dilantin)
Rifampin (Rifadin, Rimactane)

Special information if you are pregnant or breastfeeding

The effects of Choledyl during pregnancy have not been adequately studied; and it should be used only if clearly needed. If you are pregnant or plan to become pregnant, inform your doctor immediately. Choledyl appears in breast milk and can cause irritability and other side effects in nursing infants. If this medication is essential to your health, your doctor may advise you to stop breastfeeding until your treatment with Choledyl is finished.

Recommended dosage

Choledyl tablets should not be chewed, crushed, or dissolved. Your dosage should be individualized to meet your requirements based on reduction of symptoms and improvement of your breathing and lung function. Your doctor will conduct appropriate lab tests to ensure that you are receiving proper concentrations of this medication.

Older adults and those with congestive heart failure and/or liver disease may have unusually low dosage requirements and thus may experience toxic effects at high dosages. Ideal dosages should be based on body weight.

Immediate-release dosage forms are usually given every 6 hours. This is particularly true in children, but dosing intervals up to 8 hours may be satisfactory in adults, since they eliminate the drug at a slower rate.

Some children and adults who need higher-than-average doses may benefit from using sustained-release forms of this medication (Choledyl SA).

Most recommended doses are only guidelines, since tolerance and effectiveness of this drug varies widely from individual to individual.

DOSAGE FOR NON-SUSTAINED RELEASE FORM (TABLETS AND ELIXIR)

Adults
The usual dose for adult smokers is 7.8 milligrams per 2.2 pounds of body weight to begin and then 4.7 milligrams per 2.2 pounds every 6 hours.

For healthy nonsmoking adults, the usual dose is 7.8 milligrams per 2.2 pounds of body weight to begin and then 4.7 milligrams per 2.2 pounds every 8 hours.

For older patients and those with lung and heart problems, the usual dose is 7.8 milligrams per 2.2 pounds to start and then

1.6 to 3.1 milligrams per 2.2 pounds every 8 to 12 hours.

The usual dose for adults on long-term therapy is a total of 25 milligrams per 2.2 pounds of body weight every 24 hours, divided into smaller doses taken at 6 or 8 hour intervals. Your doctor will increase this dose at 3-day intervals until your response is satisfactory.

Children
The usual dose for children aged 1 to 9 years is 7.8 milligrams per 2.2 pounds of body weight to begin and then 6.2 milligrams per 2.2 pounds every 6 hours.

Children aged 9 to 16 years take 7.8 milligrams per 2.2 pounds to begin and then 4.7 milligrams per 2.2 pounds every 6 hours.

Overdosage
It is possible for theophylline toxicity (poisoning) to occur without previous warning at normally prescribed doses of this medication. Convulsions and death may occur. Never take more than the specific doses your doctor has prescribed. If you suspect an overdose, seek medical treatment immediately. Symptoms of Choledyl overdose include:

Coma
Seizure

Generic name:

CHOLESTYRAMINE RESIN

See Questran, page 528.

Generic name:

CHOLINE MAGNESIUM TRISALICYLATE

See Trilisate, page 654.

Brand name:

CHRONULAC SYRUP

Generic name: Lactulose
Other brand name: Duphalac

Why is this drug prescribed?
Chronulac treats constipation. In people who are chronically constipated, Chronulac increases the number and frequency of bowel movements.

Most important fact about this drug
It may take 24 to 48 hours to produce a normal bowel movement.

How should you take this medication?
Take this medication exactly as prescribed by your doctor.

If you find the taste of Chronulac unpleasant, it can be taken with water, fruit juice, or milk.

Chronulac should be stored at room temperature. Under normal conditions, the liquid may darken in color, which is normal.

What side effects may occur?
Side effects cannot be anticipated. If any develop or change in intensity, inform your doctor as soon as possible. Only your doctor can determine if it is safe for you to continue taking Chronulac.

■ *Side effects may include:*
  Diarrhea
  Gas
  Intestinal cramps
  Nausea
  Potassium and fluid loss
  Vomiting

Why should this drug not be prescribed?
Chronulac contains galactose, a simple sugar. If you are on a low-galactose diet, do not take this medication.

Special warnings about this medication
This medication should be used with caution if you have diabetes.

If unusual diarrhea occurs, contact your doctor.

Possible food and drug interactions when taking this medication
If Chronulac is taken with certain other drugs, the effects of either could be increased, decreased, or altered. It is especially important to check with your doctor before combining Chronulac with non-absorbable antacids such as Maalox and Mylanta.

Special information if you are pregnant or breastfeeding
The effects of Chronulac during pregnancy have not been adequately studied. If you are pregnant or plan to become pregnant, inform your doctor immediately. Chronulac may appear in breast milk and could affect a nursing infant. If this medication is essential to your health, your doctor may advise you to stop breastfeeding until your treatment is finished.

Recommended dosage
The usual dose is 1 to 2 tablespoonfuls (15 to 30 milliliters) daily. The dose may be increased to 60 milliliters a day, if necessary. It may take 24 to 48 hours to produce a normal bowel movement.

Overdosage
Any medication taken in excess can have serious consequences. If you suspect an overdose, seek medical treatment immediately.

Symptoms of Chronulac overdose may include:
Abdominal cramps
Diarrhea

Generic name:

CIBALITH-S

See Lithobid, page 328.

Generic name:

CICLOPIROX OLAMINE

See Loprox, page 339.

Generic name:

CIMETIDINE

See Tagamet, page 600.

Brand name:

CIPRO

Generic name: Ciprofloxacin hydrochloride

Why is this drug prescribed?
Cipro, an anti-infective drug, is used in the treatment of lower respiratory infections, skin infections, bone and joint infections, urinary tract infections, and infectious diarrhea.

Because Cipro is effective only for certain types of bacterial infections, before beginning treatment your doctor may perform tests to identify the specific organisms causing your infection.

Most important fact about this drug
Serious and occasionally fatal allergic reactions, some following the first dose, have been reported in patients receiving Cipro. Some reactions were accompanied by collapse of the circulatory system, loss of consciousness, tingling, swelling of the face and throat, shortness of breath, itching, and hives.

Although such reactions are relatively rare, be sure to notify your doctor immediately at the first sign of a skin rash or any other allergic reaction.

How should you take this medication?
Cipro may be taken with or without meals but is best tolerated when taken 2 hours after a meal.

Drink plenty of fluids while taking this medication.

What side effects may occur?
Side effects cannot be anticipated. If any develop or change in intensity, inform your doctor as soon as possible. Only your doctor can determine if it is safe for you to continue taking Cipro.

■ *More common side effects may include:*
Abdominal pain/discomfort
Diarrhea
Headache
Nausea
Rash
Restlessness
Vomiting

■ *Less common side effects may include:*
Abnormal dread or fear, achiness, bad taste, bleeding in the stomach and/or intestines, blood clots in the lungs, blurred vision, bronchial spasm, change in color perception, chest pain, chills, confusion, constipation, convulsions, coughing up blood, decreased vision, depression, difficulty in swallowing, dizziness, double vision, drowsiness, eye pain, fainting, fever, fluid retention in the lungs, flushing, gas, gout flareup, hallucinations, hearing loss, heart attack, hiccups, high blood pressure, hives, inability to fall or stay asleep, inability to urinate, indigestion, intestinal inflammation, irregular heartbeat, irritability, itching, joint or back pain, joint stiffness, kidney failure, lack of muscle

coordination, lack or loss of appetite, large volumes of urine, lightheadedness, loss of sense of identity, mouth sores, neck pain, nightmares, nosebleed, overbrightness of lights, pounding heartbeat, ringing in the ears, seizures, sensitivity to light, shortness of breath, skin peeling, redness, sluggishness, swelling of the face, neck, lips, eyes, or hands, swelling of the throat, tender, red bumps on skin, tingling sensation, tremors, unusual darkening of the skin, vaginal inflammation, vague feeling of illness, weakness, yellowed eyes and skin

Why should this drug not be prescribed?

If you are sensitive to or have ever had an allergic reaction to Cipro or certain other drugs of this type, you should not take this medication. Make sure that your doctor is aware of any drug reactions that you have experienced.

Special warnings about this medication

Cipro may cause you to become dizzy or lightheaded; therefore, driving a car, operating dangerous machinery, or participating in any hazardous activity that requires full mental alertness is not recommended.

Continued or prolonged use of this drug may result in a growth of bacteria that do not respond to this medication and can cause a secondary infection. Therefore, it is important that your doctor monitor your condition on a regular basis.

Convulsions have been reported in patients receiving Cipro. If you experience a seizure or convulsion, notify your doctor immediately.

This medication may stimulate the central nervous system which may lead to tremors, restlessness, lightheadedness, confusion, and hallucinations. If these reactions occur, consult with your doctor at once.

If you have a known or suspected central nervous system disorder such as epilepsy or hardening of the arteries in the brain, consult with your doctor before taking Cipro.

You may become more sensitive to light while taking this drug. Try to stay out of the sun as much as possible.

Blood tests and tests for urine and kidney function should be performed by your doctor during prolonged treatment with Cipro.

Possible food and drug interactions when taking this medication

If Cipro is taken with certain other drugs, the effects of either could be increased, decreased, or altered. It is especially important to check with your doctor before combining Cipro with the following:

Cyclosporine (Sandimmune)
Probenecid (Benemid), an antigout medication
Sucralfate (Carafate), a stomach ulcer medication
Theophylline (Theo-Dur), a bronchodilator used to treat asthma, bronchitis, and emphysema)
Warfarin (Coumadin), a blood thinner

Serious and fatal reactions have occurred when Cipro is taken in combination with theophylline (Theo-Dur). These reactions have included cardiac arrest, seizures, status epilepticus (continuous attacks of epilepsy with no periods of consciousness), and respiratory failure.

Products containing iron, multivitamins containing zinc, or antacids containing magnesium, aluminum, or calcium, when taken in combination with Cipro, may interfere with absorption of this medication.

Cipro may increase the effects of caffeine.

Special information
if you are pregnant or breastfeeding

The effects of Cipro during pregnancy have not been adequately studied. If you are pregnant or plan to become pregnant, notify your doctor immediately. Cipro does appear in breast milk and could affect a nursing infant. If this medication is essential to your health, your doctor may advise you to discontinue breastfeeding your baby until your treatment is finished.

Recommended dosage

ADULTS

The length of treatment with Cipro depends upon the severity of infection. Generally, Cipro should be continued for at least 2 days after the signs and symptoms of infection have disappeared. The usual length of time is 7 to 14 days; however, for severe and complicated infections, treatment may be prolonged.

Bone and joint infections may require treatment for 4 to 6 weeks or longer.

Infectious diarrhea may be treated for 5 to 7 days.

Urinary Tract Infections
The usual adult dosage is 250 milligrams taken every 12 hours. Complicated infections, as determined by your doctor, may require 500 milligrams taken every 12 hours.

Lower Respiratory Tract, Skin, Bone, and Joint Infections
The usual recommended dosage is 500 milligrams taken every 12 hours. Complicated infections, as determined by your doctor, may require a dosage of 750 milligrams taken every 12 hours.

Infectious Diarrhea
The recommended dosage is 500 milligrams taken every 12 hours.

CHILDREN

Safety and effectiveness have not been established in children and adolescents less than 18 years of age.

Overdosage

Any medication taken in excess can have serious consequences. If you suspect an overdose, seek medical attention immediately.

Generic name:

CIPROFLOXACIN HYDROCHLORIDE

See Cipro, page 111.

Generic name:

CLARITHROMYCIN

See Biaxin, page 68.

Generic name:

CLEMASTINE FUMARATE

See Tavist, page 606.

Brand name:

CLEOCIN T

Generic name: Clindamycin phosphate

Why is this drug prescribed?
Cleocin T is an antibiotic used to treat acne.

Most important fact about this drug
Clindamycin has been known to cause severe colitis, which can be fatal. Symptoms, which can occur after a few days, weeks or months after beginning treatment with this drug, include severe diarrhea, severe abdominal cramps and the possibility of the passage of blood.

How should you take this medication?

Use this medication exactly as prescribed by your doctor. Excessive use of Cleocin T can cause your skin to become too dry or irritated.

What side effects may occur?

Side effects cannot be anticipated. If any develop or change in intensity, inform your doctor as soon as possible. Only your doctor can determine if it is safe for you to continue taking Cleocin T.

■ *More common side effects may include:*
Skin dryness

■ *Less common or rare side effects may include:*
Abdominal pain, bloody diarrhea, colitis, diarrhea, inflammation of hair follicles, oily skin, peeling, burning or abnormal redness of skin, skin inflammation and irritation, stomach and intestinal disturbances

Why should this drug not be prescribed?

If you are sensitive to or have ever had an allergic reaction to Cleocin T or similar drugs, you should not use this medication. Make sure that your doctor is aware of any drug reactions that you have experienced.

Unless you are directed to do so by your doctor, do not take this medication if you have a history of intestinal inflammation, ulcerative colitis or antibiotic-associated colitis.

Special warnings about this medication

Cleocin T contains an alcohol base, which can cause burning and irritation of the eyes. It also has an unpleasant taste. Caution should be exercised when applying this medication so as not to get it in the eyes, nose, mouth or other mucous membrane. In the event of accidental contact, rinse the affected area with cool water.

Use with caution if you have hay fever, asthma, or eczema.

Possible food and drug interactions when taking this medication

If diarrhea occurs while taking Cleocin T, check with your doctor before taking an antidiarrhea medication, as certain drugs may cause your diarrhea to become worse.

The diarrhea should not be treated with the commonly used drugs that slow movement through the intestinal tract, such as Lomotil or products containing paregoric.

Special information if you are pregnant or breastfeeding

The effects of Cleocin T during pregnancy have not been adequately studied. If you are pregnant or plan to become pregnant, inform your doctor immediately. Cleocin T may appear in breast milk and could affect a nursing infant. If this medication is essential to your health, your doctor may advise you to discontinue breastfeeding your baby until your treatment with this medication is finished.

Recommended dosage

ADULTS

Apply a thin film of gel, solution or lotion to the affected area 2 times a day.

Lotion: Shake well immediately before using.

CHILDREN

The safety and effectiveness of Cleocin T have not been established in children under 12 years of age.

Overdosage

Any medication taken in excess can have serious consequences. If you suspect an overdose, seek medical attention immediately.

Generic name:

CLINDAMYCIN PHOSPHATE

See Cleocin T, page 113.

Brand name:

CLINDEX

See Librax, page 319.

Brand name:

CLINORIL

Generic name: Sulindac

Why is this drug prescribed?

Clinoril, a nonsteroidal anti-inflammatory drug, is used to relieve the inflammation, swelling, stiffness and joint pain associated with rheumatoid arthritis, osteoarthritis (the most common form of arthritis), and ankylosing spondylitis (stiffness and progressive arthritis of the spine.) It is also used to treat bursitis, tendinitis, acute gouty arthritis, and other types of pain.

The safety and effectiveness of this medication in the treatment of people with rheumatoid arthritis who are incapacitated, almost or completely bedridden, in wheelchairs, or unable to care for themselves, have not been established.

Most important fact about this drug

You should have frequent check-ups with your doctor if you take Clinoril regularly. Ulcers or internal bleeding can occur without warning.

How should you take this medication?

Take this medication exactly as prescribed by your doctor.

If you are using Clinoril for arthritis, it should be taken regularly.

If you forget to take a dose, take it as soon as you remember. If it is almost time for your next dose, skip the one you missed and go back to your regular schedule. Never take two doses at the same time.

What side effects may occur?

Side effects cannot be anticipated. If any develop or change in intensity, inform your doctor as soon as possible. Only your doctor can determine if it is safe for you to continue taking Clinoril.

■ *More common side effects may include:*
Abdominal pain, constipation, diarrhea, dizziness, gas, headache, indigestion, itching, loss of appetite, nausea, nervousness, rash, ringing in ears, stomach cramps, swelling due to fluid retention, vomiting

■ *Less common or rare side effects may include:*
Abdominal bleeding, abdominal inflammation, anemia, appetite change, bloody diarrhea, blurred vision, change in color of urine, chest pain, colitis, congestive heart failure, depression, fever, hair loss, hearing loss, hepatitis, high blood pressure, inability to sleep, inflammation of lips and tongue, kidney failure, liver failure, loss of sense of taste, low blood pressure, muscle and joint pain, nosebleed, painful urination, pancreatitis, peptic ulcer, sensitivity to light, shortness of breath, skin eruptions, sleepiness, Stevens-Johnson syndrome, vaginal bleeding, weakness, yellow eyes and skin

Why should this drug not be prescribed?

If you are sensitive to or have ever had an allergic reaction to Clinoril, aspirin, or similar drugs, or if you have had asthma attacks caused by aspirin or other drugs of this type, you should not take this medication. Make sure that your doctor is aware of any drug reactions that you have experienced.

Special warnings about this medication

Peptic ulcers and bleeding can occur without warning.

This drug should be used with caution if you have kidney or liver disease; it can cause liver inflammation in some people.

Do not take aspirin or any other anti-inflammatory medications while taking Clinoril, unless your doctor tells you to do so.

Clinoril can cause vision problems. If you experience a change in your vision, inform your doctor.

If you have heart disease or high blood pressure, this drug can increase water retention. Use with caution.

If you develop pancreatitis (inflammation of the pancreas), Clinoril should be stopped immediately and not restarted.

Clinoril may cause you to become drowsy or less alert. If this happens, driving or operating dangerous machinery or participating in any hazardous activity that requires full mental alertness is not recommended.

Possible food and drug interactions when taking this medication

If Clinoril is taken with certain other drugs, the effects of either could be increased, decreased, or altered. It is especially important to check with your doctor before combining Clinoril with the following:

Anti-gout medication (Benemid)
Blood thinners such as Coumadin, Panwarfin
Aspirin

Cyclosporine (Sandimmune)
Diflunisal (Dolobid)
Dimethyl sulfoxide (DMSO)
Lithium
Loop diuretics such as Lasix
Methotrexate
Oral diabetes medications

Special information if you are pregnant or breastfeeding

The effects of Clinoril during pregnancy have not been adequately studied; drugs of this class are known to cause birth defects. If you are pregnant or plan to become pregnant, inform your doctor immediately. Clinoril may appear in breast milk and could affect a nursing infant. If this medication is essential to your health, your doctor may advise you to discontinue breastfeeding until your treatment with Clinoril is finished.

Recommended dosage

ADULTS

Osteoarthritis, Rheumatoid Arthritis, Ankylosing Spondylitis
Starting dosage is 150 milligrams 2 times a day. Take with food. Doses should not exceed 400 milligrams per day.

Acute Gouty Arthritis or Arthritic Shoulder and Joint Condition
400 milligrams daily taken in doses of 200 milligrams 2 times a day.
For acute painful shoulder, therapy lasting 7 to 14 days is usually adequate.
For acute gouty arthritis, therapy lasting 7 days is usually adequate.

The lowest dose that proves beneficial should be used.

CHILDREN

The safety and effectiveness of Clinoril have not been established in children.

ELDERLY

Dosage should be determined by the particular needs of the elderly patient.

Overdosage

Any medication taken in excess can cause symptoms of overdose. If you suspect an overdose, seek medical attention immediately.

The symptoms of Clinoril overdose may include:
Coma
Low blood pressure
Reduced output of urine
Stupor

Generic name:

CLOBETASOL PROPIONATE

See Temovate, page 611.

Brand name:

CLOMID

See Clomiphene Citrate, page 117.

Generic name:

CLOMIPHENE CITRATE

Brand names: Clomid, Serophene

Why is this drug prescribed?

Clomiphene is prescribed for the treatment of ovulatory failure in patients who wish to become pregnant and whose husbands are fertile and potent.

Most important fact about this drug

Properly timed sexual intercourse is very important for good results.

Clomiphene may cause visual disturbances, blurred vision, dizziness and light-headedness. You should use caution while driving or performing tasks requiring mental alertness under conditions of variable lighting.

The likelihood of conception diminishes with each succeeding course of treatment. Your doctor will determine the need for continuing therapy after the first course. Three courses constitute adequate therapy.

Clomiphene treatment increases the possibility and potential hazards of multiple pregnancies (twins, etc.).

How should you take this medication?

Take this medication exactly as prescribed by your doctor.

What side effects may occur?

Side effects occur infrequently and generally do not interfere with treatment at the recommended dosage of clomiphene. They tend to occur more frequently at higher doses and during long-term treatment.

■ *More common side effects include:*
Abdominal discomfort
Enlargement of the ovaries
Flushes

■ *Less common side effects include:*
Abnormal uterine bleeding, breast tenderness, depression, dizziness, fatigue, hair loss, headache, hives, inability to fall or stay asleep, increased urination, inflammation of the skin, lightheadedness, nausea, nervousness, ovarian cysts, visual disturbances, vomiting, weight gain

Why should this drug not be prescribed?

If you are pregnant or think you are, do not take this drug.

Unless directed to do so by your doctor, do not use this medication if you have an uncontrolled thyroid or adrenal disorder, an abnormality of the brain such as a pituitary tumor, liver disease or a history of liver problems, abnormal uterine bleeding of undetermined origin, ovarian cysts, or enlargement of the ovaries not caused by polycystic ovarian syndrome (hormonal disorder causing lack of ovulation).

Special warnings about this medication

Patients should be carefully evaluated for normal liver function and normal estrogen levels before they are considered for treatment with clomiphene.

It is recommended that the patient be examined for pregnancy, ovarian enlargement, or cyst formation prior to treatment with this drug and between each treatment cycle. A complete pelvic examination should be performed prior to treatment and should be repeated before each course of this medication.

Birth defects have been reported following treatment to induce ovulation with clomiphene, although no direct effects of the drug on the human fetus have been established.

Because blurring and/or other visual symptoms may occur occasionally with clomiphene treatment, driving a car or operating dangerous machinery, especially under conditions of variable lighting, is not recommended.

If you experience visual disturbance symptoms, notify your doctor immediately. Visual disturbance symptoms may include blurring, spots or flashes, double vision, intolerance to light, decreased visual sharpness, loss of peripheral vision, and distortion of space. He may recommend a complete evaluation by an eye specialist.

Ovarian hyperstimulation syndrome, (or OHSS, enlargement of the ovary) has occurred in patients receiving treatment with clomiphene. OHSS may progress rapidly and become serious. The early warning signs are severe pelvic pain, nausea, vomiting, and weight gain. Symptoms include abdominal pain, abdominal enlargement, nausea, vomiting, diarrhea, weight gain, shortness of breath, and less urine production. If you experience any of these warning signs or symptoms, notify your doctor immediately.

To lessen the risks associated with abnormal ovarian enlargement during treatment with clomiphene, the lowest effective dose should be prescribed. Patients with polycystic ovarian syndrome may be unusually sensitive to certain hormones and may respond abnormally to usual doses of this drug. If you experience pelvic pain, notify your doctor. He may discontinue your use of clomiphene until the ovaries return to pretreatment size.

Because the safety of long-term treatment with clomiphene has not been established, more than 3 courses of therapy are not recommended.

Possible food and drug interactions when taking this medication

No food or drug interactions have been reported while taking clomiphene.

Special information if you are pregnant or breastfeeding

If you become pregnant, notify your doctor immediately. You should not be taking this drug while you are pregnant.

Recommended dosage

The recommended dosage for the first course of treatment is 50 milligrams (1 tablet) daily for 5 days. If ovulation does not appear to have occurred, your doctor may prescribe additional courses of treatment, However, treatment beyond 3 courses is not recommended.

Overdosage

Taking any medication in excess can have serious consequences. If you suspect an overdose, contact your doctor immediately.

Generic name:

CLOMIPRAMINE HYDROCHLORIDE

See Anafranil, page 25.

Generic name:

CLONAZEPAM

See Klonopin, page 308.

Generic name:

CLONIDINE HYDROCHLORIDE

See Catapres, page 99.

Generic name:

CLORAZEPATE DIPOTASSIUM

See Tranxene, page 644.

Generic name:

CLOTRIMAZOLE

See Lotrimin, page 344.

Generic name:

CLOTRIMAZOLE WITH BETAMETHASONE DIPROPIONATE

See Lotrisone, page 345.

Generic name:

CLOZAPINE

See Clozaril, page 119.

Brand name:

CLOZARIL

Generic name: Clozapine

Why is this drug prescribed?

Clozaril, an antipsychotic medication recently approved for use in the U.S., is given to help people with severe schizophrenia who have failed to respond to standard treatments. Like other antipsychotic medications, Clozaril is not a cure, but it can help some mentally ill people behave more rationally and lead more normal lives.

Most important fact about this drug

Even though it does not produce some of the disturbing side effects of other antipsychotic medications, Clozaril may cause agranulocytosis, a potentially lethal disorder of the white blood cells. Because of the risk of agranulocytosis, anyone who takes Clozaril is required to have a blood test once a week. The drug is carefully controlled so that patients must get their weekly blood test before receiving the following week's supply of medication. A patient whose blood test results are abnormal will be taken off Clozaril. Usually this causes the blood cell counts to return to normal.

Clozaril can cause seizures, so it is advisable to avoid driving and other potentially hazardous activities when on Clozaril therapy.

How should you take this medication?

Take Clozaril exactly as directed by your doctor. Because of the significant risk of serious side effects associated with this drug, your doctor will periodically reassess the need for continued Clozaril therapy.

Clozaril is distributed *only* through the Clozaril Patient Management System, which ensures weekly white blood cell testing, patient monitoring, and pharmacy services prior to delivery of the next week's supply of Clozaril.

Clozaril may be taken with or without food.

What side effects may occur?
Side effects cannot be anticipated. If any develop or change in intensity, inform your doctor as soon as possible. Only your doctor can determine if it is safe for you to continue taking Clozaril.

The most feared side effect is agranulocytosis, a dangerous drop in the number of a certain kind of white blood cells. If not caught in time, agranulocytosis can lead to fever, weakness, and even death. That is why all people who take Clozaril must have a blood test every week. About 1% develop agranulocytosis and must stop taking the drug.

Seizures are another potential side effect, occurring in some 5% of people who take Clozaril. The higher the dosage, the greater the risk of seizures.

- *More common side effects may include:*
  Constipation, dizziness, drowsiness, dry mouth, fainting, fever, low blood pressure, nausea, rapid heartbeat and other heart conditions, salivation, sedation, sweating, tremors, vertigo, vision problems, vomiting

- *Less common side effects may include:*
  Abnormal stools, appetite increase, backache, bitter taste, bloodshot eyes, breast pain or discomfort, bruise, chills, confusion, coughing, dry throat, ear disorders, ejaculation problems, fainting, hallucinations, headache, hives, hot flashes, impotence, increase or decrease in libido, involuntary movement of the eyes, irritability, itching, joint pain, lethargy, lightheadedness (especially when rising quickly from a seated or lying position), loss of speech, muscle pain, nervous stomach, nosebleed, numbness, pneumonia-like symptoms, poor coordination, pounding heartbeat, rash, rectal bleeding, restlessness, runny nose, shakiness, skin inflammation, sleeplessness, sneezing, sore throat, stomach pain, stuttering, twitching, vaginal itch, a vague feeling of being sick, weakness, wheezing.

Why should this drug not be prescribed?
Clozaril is considered a somewhat risky medication because of its potential to cause agranulocytosis and seizures. It should be given only to people whose mental illness is serious, and who have not been helped by more traditional antipsychotic medications such as Haldol or Mellaril.

You should not take Clozaril if:
- You have ever had a disease or disorder of the bone marrow;
- You ever developed an abnormal white blood cell count while taking Clozaril;
- You are currently taking some other drug, such as Tegretol, with the potential to cause a decrease in white blood cell count.

Special warnings about this medication
Clozaril can cause drowsiness, especially at the start of treatment. For this reason, and also because of the potential for seizures, you should not drive, swim, climb, or operate dangerous machinery while you are taking this medication, at least in the early stages of treatment.

Even though you will have weekly blood tests while taking Clozaril, you should stay alert for early symptoms of agranulocytosis: weakness, lethargy, fever, sore throat, malaise, a flu-like feeling, or ulcers of the mucous membranes. If any such symptoms develop, tell your doctor immediately.

While taking Clozaril, do not drink or use drugs of any kind, including over-the-counter medicines, without first checking with your doctor.

If you take Clozaril, you must be monitored especially closely if you have either narrow-angle glaucoma or an enlarged prostate; Clozaril could make these conditions worse.

If you have kidney, liver, or heart disease; low blood pressure; or a history of seizures or prostate problems, you should discuss these with your doctor before taking Clozaril.

Possible food and drug interactions when taking this medication

If Clozaril is taken with certain other drugs, the effects of either could be increased, decreased, or altered. It is especially important to check with your doctor before combining Clozaril with the following:

Blood pressure medication such as Aldomet
Digoxin (Lanoxin)
Drugs that affect the central nervous system such as Valium, Xanax, and Seconal
Drugs that contain atropine such as Donnatal and Levsin
Drugs that suppress bone-marrow activity such as Tegretol
Warfarin (Coumadin and Panwarfin)

Special information
if you are pregnant or breastfeeding

If you are pregnant or plan to become pregnant, inform your doctor immediately. Clozaril treatment should be continued during pregnancy only if absolutely necessary. You should not breastfeed if you are taking Clozaril, since the drug might find its way into breast milk.

Recommended dosage

ADULTS

Your doctor will carefully individualize your dosage and monitor your response weekly.

The usual recommended initial dose is 25 milligrams 1 or 2 times daily. The dosage may be increased in increments of 25 to 50 milligrams a day to achieve a daily dose of 300 to 450 milligrams by the end of 2 weeks. The maximum dose will not exceed 900 milligrams.

Your doctor will determine long-term dosage depending upon your own response and results of the weekly blood test.

CHILDREN

Safety and efficacy have not been established for children up to 16 years of age.

Overdosage

Any medication taken in excess can have serious consequences. If you suspect an overdose, seek medical attention immediately.

Symptoms of overdose with Clozaril may include:
Coma
Delirium
Drowsiness
Excess salivation
Low blood pressure, faintness
Rapid heartbeat
Seizures
Shallow breathing

Brand name:

COGENTIN

Generic name: Benztropine mesylate

Why is this drug prescribed?

Cogentin, an antispasmodic medication, is given to help treat "parkinsonism": the muscle rigidity, tremors, and spasms that occur in Parkinson's disease and that sometimes develop as unwanted side effects of antipsychotic drugs.

Cogentin is used as adjunctive therapy. For example, people with Parkinson's disease may be given Cogentin as an adjunct to levodopa (Dopar, Larodopa) or to a levodopa/carbidopa combination (Sinemet). People with psychotic disorders may be given Cogentin as an adjunct if their antipsychotic medication (Thorazine, Stelazine, Navane, Haldol, others) causes muscle rigidity and tremors.

Most important fact about this drug

Unlike some of the other antiparkinsonian medications, Cogentin has a sedative effect. It is thus particularly suitable as a bedtime medication because it lasts through the night. Taken at night, it may help a person regain enough muscle control to move and roll over during sleep and to arise unaided in the morning.

How should you take this medication?

Take Cogentin exactly as prescribed by your doctor.

Cogentin causes dry mouth. Sucking on sugarless hard candy, sipping water, or maintaining good dental hygiene can relieve the dry mouth that may result from taking Cogentin.

Cogentin can reduce the ability to sweat, an important function by which overheating is prevented. Avoid excess sun or exercise that may cause excessive sweating.

What side effects may occur?

Side effects cannot be anticipated. If any develop or change in intensity, inform your doctor as soon as possible. Only your doctor can determine if it is safe for you to continue taking Cogentin.

■ Side effects may include:
Bowel blockage, confusion, constipation, depression, dilated pupils, disorientation, dizziness and blurry vision, dry mouth, fever, hallucinations, heat stroke, impaired memory, listlessness, nausea, nervousness, numbness in fingers, rapid heartbeat, rash, urinary retention or pain with urination, vomiting, worsening of existing psychosis

Why should this drug not be prescribed?

Do not take Cogentin if you are sensitive to it or if you have ever had an allergic reaction to it or to any similar antispasmodic medication.

Do not take Cogentin if you have angle-closure glaucoma.

Some people who take antipsychotic medications develop tardive dyskinesia, a syndrome of involuntary movements of the mouth, jaw, arms, and legs. Cogentin should not be given to treat tardive dyskinesia; it will not help, and it may make the condition worse.

Cogentin should not be given to children under the age of 3; it should be used with caution in older children.

Special warnings about this medication

Do not drive or operate dangerous machinery while taking Cogentin, since the drug may impair your mental or physical abilities.

Be sure to tell your doctor if you have ever had tachycardia (excessively rapid heartbeats) or if you have an enlarged prostate; you will require especially close monitoring while taking Cogentin in these cases.

Tell your doctor if Cogentin produces weakness in particular muscle groups. For example, if you have been suffering from neck rigidity and Cogentin suddenly causes your neck to relax so much that it feels weak, you may be taking more Cogentin than you need.

Possible food and drug interactions when taking this medication

When taken simultaneously with an antipsychotic medication (Thorazine, Stelazine, Haldol, others) or a tricyclic antidepressant medication (Elavil, Norpramine, Tofranil, others), Cogentin has occasionally caused bowel blockage or heat stroke that proved dangerous or even fatal. If you are taking Cogentin concurrently with an antipsychotic or with a tricyclic antidepressant, tell your doctor immediately if you begin to have any stomach or bowel complaint, fever, or heat intolerance.

Cogentin has a drying effect on the mouth and other moist tissues. If you take it along with another drug that also has a drying effect, you are at risk for anhidrosis (inability to sweat), heat stroke and even death from hyperthermia (high fever). Chronic illness, alcoholism, central nervous system disease, or heavy manual labor can increase this risk. In hot weather, your doctor may lower your dosage of Cogentin.

Special information if you are pregnant or breastfeeding

If you are pregnant or plan to become pregnant, inform your doctor immediately. No information is available about the safety of taking Cogentin during pregnancy or while you are breastfeeding.

Recommended dosage

Your doctor will individualize the dose of Cogentin, taking into consideration the condition being treated, the presence of other diseases, and any physical disorder.

In general, the recommended usual dose given by mouth is 1 to 2 milligrams a day, but it can range from 0.5 to 6 milligrams a day.

Overdosage

Any medication taken in excess can have serious consequences. If you suspect symptoms of an overdose of Cogentin, seek medical attention immediately. Symptoms of overdose may include any of those listed in the "side effects section" (see above) or any of the following:

Blurred vision, confusion, coma, convulsions, delirium, difficulty swallowing or breathing, dilated pupils, dizziness, dry mouth, flushed, dry skin, glaucoma, hallucinations, headache, inability to sweat, listlessness, muscle weakness, nausea, nervousness, numb fingers, painful urination, palpitations, rapid heartbeat, rash, shock, uncoordinated movements, vomiting

Brand name:

COLACE

Generic name: Docusate sodium

Why is this drug prescribed?

Colace is prescribed to help keep stools soft for easy, natural passage. This medication is useful for constipation due to hard stools, for painful anal and rectal conditions, for cardiac and other conditions in which maximum ease of passage is desirable to avoid difficulty and pain, and when it is not advisable to use peristaltic stimulants (agents that force waste toward the anus by producing wavelike contractions of digestive tract muscles).

Most important fact about this drug
Colace is a stool softener—not a laxative—and therefore is not habit-forming.

How should you take this medication?
To conceal the drug's bitter taste, Colace liquid may be taken in half a glass of milk or fruit juice or in infant formula. The proper dosage of this medication may also be added to a retention or flushing enema.

What side effects may occur?
Side effects are unlikely. The main ones reported are bitter taste, throat irritation and nausea (mainly associated with use of the syrup and liquid). Rash has occurred.

Why should this drug not be prescribed?
There are no known reasons this drug should not be prescribed.

Possible food and drug interactions when taking this medication
No food or drug interactions have been reported while taking Colace.

Special information
if you are pregnant or breastfeeding
If you are pregnant, plan to become pregnant, or are breastfeeding your baby, notify your doctor before using this medication.

Recommended dosage
Dosage should be adjusted by your doctor according to your needs.

Higher doses are recommended at the start of treatment with Colace. The effect on stools is usually seen 1 to 3 days after the first dose.

ADULTS AND OLDER CHILDREN

The suggested daily dosage is 50 to 200 milligrams.

In enemas, add 50 to 100 milligrams of Colace or 5 to 10 milliliters of Colace liquid to a retention or flushing enema, as prescribed by your doctor.

CHILDREN

The suggested daily dosage for children 6 to 12 years of age is 40 to 120 milligrams; for children 3 to 6 years of age, it is 20 to 60 milligrams; for children under 3 years of age, it is 10 to 40 milligrams.

Overdosage
Overdose is unlikely with the normal use of Colace.

Brand name:

COLBENEMID

Generic ingredients: Probenecid, Colchicine
Other brand name: Col-Probenecid

Why is this drug prescribed?
ColBENEMID is prescribed for the treatment of long-term gouty arthritis (a disease that produces pain and swelling of the joints accompanied by fever and chills) when complicated by frequent, recurrent severe attacks of gout.

Most important fact about this drug
Therapy with ColBENEMID should not be started until an acute gout attack (symptoms that come on suddenly) has subsided. However, if an acute attack occurs during therapy, your doctor may ask you to use additional colchicine or take other appropriate measures to control the attack. You should not alter the dose of ColBENEMID.

How should you take this medication?
Take this medication exactly as prescribed by your doctor.

Drink plenty of fluids to prevent blood in the urine, renal colic (sharp lower back pain produced by the passage of kidney stones), rib or backbone pain, and uric acid stones (crystallized product of metabolized protein found in the blood and excreted in the urine), which are sometimes caused by ColBENEMID. Sufficient sodium bicarbonate (antacid) or potassium citrate (a supplement) should also be taken to make the urine less acid.

What side effects may occur?
Side effects cannot be anticipated. If any develop or change in intensity, inform your doctor as soon as possible. Only your doctor can determine if it is safe for you to continue taking ColBENEMID.

■ *Side effects may include:*
Abdominal pain, anaphalactic shock (an allergic reaction including shortness of breath, increased heart rate, tingling in throat, and collapse), anemia, backbone or rib pain, blood in the urine, diarrhea, dizziness, fever, flushing, hair loss, headache, hives, lack or loss of appetite, liver damage, localized swelling or itching, muscular weakness, nausea, nerve inflammation, reddish or purplish spots, sharp back pain traveling to groin, sore gums, uric acid kidney stones, urinary frequency, vomiting

Why should this drug not be prescribed?
If you are sensitive or have ever had an allergic reaction to probenecid (anti-gout medication), colchicine (gout pain reliever), or similar drugs, you should not take this medication. Be sure that your doctor is aware of any drug reactions that you have experienced.

Unless you are directed to do so by your doctor, do not take this medication if you have any abnormal condition of the blood or uric acid kidney stones. Also, ColBENECID should not be started until a severe attack of gout has subsided.

Special warnings about this medication
Treatment with ColBENEMID may aggravate gout. If this occurs, your doctor may increase your dosage of colchicine or prescribe another treatment.

Do not use salicylates (aspirin) while taking ColBENEMID for pain relief; use acetaminophen (Tylenol, Anacin-3, for example).

Severe allergic reactions have occurred rarely with the use of this medication. Most of these reactions have occurred within several hours after restarting treatment following previous usage of the drug. Notify your doctor if you experience an allergic reaction.

This medication should be used with caution in patients with a history of peptic (stomach) ulcer.

If you have decreased kidney function, your doctor may prescribe an increased dosage of this medication.

Possible food and drug interactions when taking this medication
If ColBENEMID is taken with certain other drugs, the effects of either could be increased, decreased, or altered. It is especially important to check with your doctor before combining ColBENEMID with the following:

Indomethacin (Indocin), an anti-inflammatory
Ketamine, a non-barbiturate general anesthetic
Ketoprofen (Orudis), an anti-inflammatory
Lorazepam (Ativan), a tranquilizer
Meclofenamate (Meclomen), an anti-inflammatory
Methotrexate, a cancer drug
Naproxen (Naprosyn), an anti-inflammatory
Penicillin (ampicillin), an antibiotic
Rifampin (Rifadin), an anti-bacterial
Salicylates (aspirin)

Sulfonamides (anti-bacterial drugs)
Sulfonylureas such as Orinase, an oral
  diabetes medication
Sulindac (Clinoril), an anti-inflammatory
Theophylline, a bronchodilator
Thiopental, a general anesthetic

Special Information
If you are pregnant or breastfeeding
ColBENEMID may cause birth defects. If you
are pregnant, plan to become pregnant,
or are breastfeeding your baby, inform your
doctor immediately.

Recommended dosage
ADULTS

The recommended dosage is 1 tablet daily
for 1 week, followed by 1 tablet twice a
day thereafter.

If you have decreased kidney function, a daily
dosage of 2 tablets may be adequate.
However, if necessary, your doctor may
increase your daily dosage by 1 tablet
every 4 weeks if symptoms of gouty arthritis
are not controlled. Usually, no more than
4 tablets per day is recommended.

When severe attacks have been absent for 6
months or more, the daily dosage may
be decreased by 1 tablet every 6 months.
Laboratory blood tests may be required
to determine uric acid levels in the urine
before your doctor lowers the dosage.

Overdosage
Any medication taken in excess can have
serious consequences. Overdosage with
colchicine may result in severe, even fatal,
reactions.

If you suspect symptoms of a ColBENEMID
overdose, seek emergency medical
treatment immediately.

*Symptoms of a ColBENEMID overdose may
include:*

Bacterial infection, blood in stools, blood in
urine, bone marrow failure (decreased
formation of red and white blood cells),
coma, difficulty breathing, epilepsy, fluid
in the lungs, heart damage, kidney damage,
low blood pressure, muscle weakness,
severe diarrhea, stomach pain

Brand name:

COLESTID

Generic Name: Colestipol hydrochloride

Why is this drug prescribed?
Colestid, in conjunction with diet, is used to
help lower high levels of cholesterol in
the blood.

Most important fact about this drug
Accidentally inhaling Colestid may cause
serious effects. To avoid this NEVER take
it in its dry form. Colestid should always be
mixed with water or other liquids BEFORE
you take it.

How should you take this medication?
Colestid should be mixed with liquids such
as:

Carbonated beverages (may cause stomach
  or intestinal discomfort)
Flavored drinks
Milk
Orange juice
Pineapple juice
Tomato juice
Water

Colestid may also be mixed with:

Milk used on breakfast cereals
Pulpy fruit (such as crushed peaches, pears,
  or pineapple) or into fruit cocktail
Soups with a high liquid content (such as
  chicken noodle or tomato)

To take Colestid with beverages:

1. Measure at least 3 ounces of liquid into a glass.
2. Add the prescribed dose of Colestid to the liquid.
3. Stir until Colestid is completely mixed (it will not dissolve. and then drink the mixture.
4. Pour a small amount of the beverage into the glass, swish it around, and drink it. This will help make sure you have taken all the medication.

What side effects may occur?

Side effects cannot be anticipated. If any develop or change in intensity, inform your doctor as soon as possible. Only your doctor can determine if it is safe for you to continue taking Colestid.

■ *Most common side effects:*
Constipation
Worsening of hemorrhoids

■ *Less common side effects may include:*
Abdominal discomfort, abdominal pain, anxiety, arthritis, belching, diarrhea, distended abdomen, dizziness, drowsiness, fatigue, gas, headache, hives, loss of appetite, muscle and joint pain, nausea, shortness of breath, skin inflammation, vertigo, vomiting, weakness

Why should this drug not be prescribed?

You should not be using Colestid if you are allergic to it or any of its components.

Special warnings about this medication

Before starting treatment with Colestid, you should:

■ Be tested (and treated) for diseases that may contribute to increased blood cholesterol, such as hypothyroidism, diabetes, nephrotic syndrome (a kidney disease), dysproteinemia (a blood disease), and obstructive liver disease.

■ Be on a diet plan (approved by your doctor) that stresses low-cholesterol foods and weight loss (if necessary).

Because certain medications may increase cholesterol, you should tell your doctor all of the medications you use.

Colestid may prevent the absorption of vitamins such as A, D, and K.

Long-term use of Colestid may be connected to increased bleeding from a lack of vitamin K. Taking vitamin K1 will help relieve this condition and prevent it in the future.

Your cholesterol and triglyceride levels should be tested while you are taking Colestid.

Colestid may cause or worsen constipation. Dosages should be adjusted by your doctor. You may need to increase your intake of fiber and fluid. A stool softener also may be needed occasionally. People with coronary artery disease should be especially careful to avoid constipation. Hemorrhoids may be worsened by constipation related to Colestid.

Although there have been no reports that Colestid suppresses the thyroid gland, it is theoretically possible. This may be especially true for people who have low thyroid levels.

Possible food and drug interactions when taking this medication

Colestid may delay the absorption of other drugs. The time period between taking Colestid and taking other medications should be as long as possible. Other drugs should be taken at least 1 hour before or 4 hours after taking Colestid.

If Colestid is taken with certain other drugs, the effects of either could be increased, decreased, or altered. It is especially important to check with your doctor before combining Colestid with the following:

Chlorothiazide (Diuril)
Digitalis (Lanoxin)
Furosemide (Lasix)
Gemfibrozil (Lopid)
Penicillin G, including brands such as Pentids
Propranolol (Inderal)
Tetracycline drugs such as Sumycin
Vitamins such as A, D, and K

Special information
if you are pregnant or breastfeeding
Pregnant women and women who are breastfeeding should use Colestid only when the possible gains outweigh the possible risks to the mother and child.

Recommended dosage
ADULTS

The recommended beginning dose is from 5 to 10 grams per day.

Later, dosage can range from 5 to 30 grams per day, divided into smaller, equal doses or taken in a single dose once a day. Doses may be increased if necessary.

Overdosage
Overdoses of Colestid have not been reported. If an overdose occurred, the most likely harmful effect would be obstruction of the stomach and/or intestines. If you suspect an overdose, seek medical help immediately.

Generic name:

COLESTIPOL HYDROCHLORIDE

See Colestid, page 126.

Generic name:

COLISTIN SULFATE

See Coly-Mycin S Oral, page 128.

Generic name:

COLISTIN SULFATE, NEOMYCIN, AND HYDROCORTISONE

See Coly-Mycin S Otic, page 129.

Brand name:

COL-PROBENECID

See ColBENEMID, page 124.

Brand name:

COLY-MYCIN S ORAL

Generic name: Colistin sulfate

Why is this drug prescribed?
Coly-Mycin S Oral is used to treat diarrhea and inflammation of the stomach and intestines in infants and children. Apparently, Coly-Mycin S Oral works because of its effectiveness against bacterial infections of the intestine.

Most important fact about this drug
Do not use Coly-Mycin S Oral in amounts exceeding the recommended dose, since this may result in kidney damage. In addition, prolonged use may result in overgrowth of other forms of bacteria.

How should you take this medication?
Store Coly-Mycin S Oral in the refrigerator. Do not freeze. Shake well before using. Discard unused portion after 2 weeks.

What side effects may occur?
Side effects cannot be anticipated. If any develop or change in intensity, contact your doctor as soon as possible. Only your doctor can determine if it is safe for your child to continue taking Coly-Mycin S Oral.

No side effects have been reported when dosages within the recommended range are used.

Why should this drug not be prescribed?

Your child should not take this drug if he or she is sensitive to it or has had an allergic reaction to it.

Special warnings about this medication

If your child has azotemia (a condition marked by excessive amounts of nitrogen compounds in the blood caused by severe kidney impairment), or if your child takes dosages that exceed the recommended amount, there is a risk of kidney damage.

Prolonged use of Coly-Mycin S Oral may result in the overgrowth of other forms of bacteria.

Before beginning treatment with Coly-Mycin S Oral, kidney function should be tested; your doctor may need to do a blood test.

Possible food and drug interactions when taking this medication

No interactions have been reported.

Recommended dosage

CHILDREN

The usual dose of Coly-Mycin S Oral powder is 2.3 to 6.8 milligrams per pound of body weight per day of the Coly-Mycin S Oral powder, divided into 3 doses. For example, a 10-pound infant would usually require a total daily dose of 23 to 68 milligrams of Coly-Mycin S Oral powder (approximately one-third to 1 teaspoon of Coly-Mycin S Oral solution) 3 times a day. A 50-pound child would require a total daily dose of 115 to 340 milligrams of Coly-Mycin S Oral powder (approximately 1.5 to 4.5 teaspoons of solution) 3 times a day.

Overdosage

Although no specific information is available, any medication taken in excess can have serious consequences. If you suspect symptoms of an overdose of Coly-Mycin S Oral, seek medical attention immediately.

Brand name:

COLY-MYCIN S OTIC

Generic ingredients: Colistin sulfate, Neomycin sulfate, Hydrocortisone acetate, Thonzonium bromide

Why is this drug prescribed?

Coly-Mycin S Otic is a liquid solution used to treat ear infections. Colistin sulfate and neomycin sulfate are antibiotics used to treat the bacterial infection itself, while hydrocortisone acetate is a corticosteroid that helps reduce the inflammation, swelling, itching, and other skin reactions associated with an ear infection; thonzonium bromide facilitates the drug's effects.

Most important fact about this drug

As with other antibiotics, long-term treatment may encourage other infections. Therefore, if your ear infection does not improve within a week, your physician may want to change your medication.

How should you use this medication?

Shake well before using.

The external ear canal should be thoroughly cleaned and dried with a sterile cotton swab (applicator). The patient should lie with the infected ear facing up. Pull the earlobe down and back (for children) or up and back (for adults) to straighten the ear canal. Drop the solution into the ear. The patient should lie in this position for 5 minutes to aid in penetration of the drops into the ear. If necessary, this procedure should be repeated for the other ear. If you prefer, a sterile cotton wick or plug may be inserted into the ear canal and then soaked with the Coly-Mycin S Otic solution. This cotton wick should be moistened every 4 hours with more solution and replaced at least once every 24 hours. Avoid touching the dropper to the ear or other surfaces.

What side effects may occur?

No specific side effects are listed; however, neomycin (an ingredient in Coly-Mycin S Otic) may be associated with an increased risk of allergic skin reaction.

Why should this drug not be prescribed?

You should not take this drug if you have had an allergic reaction to any of the ingredients, or if you suffer from herpes simplex, vaccinia (cowpox), or varicella (chickenpox).

Special warnings about this medication

Treatment should not continue for more than 10 days.

If you warm Coly-Mycin S Otic before applying, do not heat the solution to above body temperature, since this will lessen its potency. Warm the drops by holding the bottle in your hand for a few minutes.

If an allergic reaction occurs, you should stop using Coly-Mycin S Otic immediately. Your doctor may also recommend that future treatment with kanamycin, paromomycin, streptomycin, and possibly gentamicin be avoided, since you may also be allergic to these medications.

Use Coly-Mycin S Otic with care if you suffer from a perforated eardrum or chronic otitis media (inflammation of the middle ear).

Possible food and drug interactions when using this medication

No interactions have been reported.

Special information
If you are pregnant or breastfeeding

The effects of Coly-Mycin S Otic during pregnancy have not been adequately studied. If you are pregnant or plan to become pregnant, inform your doctor immediately. Coly-Mycin S Otic may appear in breast milk and could affect a nursing infant. If this medication is essential to your health, your doctor may advise you to stop breastfeeding until your treatment is finished.

Recommended dosage

ADULTS

The usual dose is 5 drops (when using the supplied measured dropper) or 4 drops (when using the dropper-bottle container) in the affected ear, 3 or 4 times daily.

INFANTS AND CHILDREN

The usual dose is 4 drops (when using the supplied measured dropper) or 3 drops (when using the dropper-bottle container) in the affected ear.

Please see the "How should you use this medication" section above for more information on applying Coly-Mycin S Otic.

Overdosage

Although no specific information is available, any medication taken in excess can have serious consequences. If you suspect an overdose, seek medical treatment immediately.

Brand name:

COLYTE

Generic ingredients: Polyethylene glycol, Sodium chloride, Potassium chloride, Sodium bicarbonate, Sodium sulfate

Why is this drug prescribed?

Colyte is used to clean the bowel before an examination of the upper part of the rectum (colonoscopy) or a barium enema X-ray.

Most important fact about this drug
Colyte makes the stool watery, which cleans the bowel.

How should you take this medication?
If you are using the powdered form, dissolve Colyte in a container with enough water to produce the volume indicated in the directions. Mix well before drinking.

If you are using the jug (4-liter), add tap water to the fill line. Replace the cap, close tightly, and shake until all the ingredients are dissolved. You should not add anything else—flavorings, for example—to the solution.

Do not eat for at least 2 hours before drinking Colyte. For best results, avoid eating for 3 to 4 hours prior to administration.

You can drink clear liquids before the examination.

You should drink 8 ounces of Colyte every 10 minutes. Rapid drinking is better than drinking small amounts continuously.

The first bowel movement should occur in about 1 hour. Continue to drink Colyte until the watery stool is clear. This usually requires drinking 3 to 4 quarts.

Once Colyte has been mixed with water, it should be stored in the refrigerator and used within 48 hours. Throw out the unused portion.

What side effects may occur?
Side effects cannot be anticipated. If any occur or change in intensity, inform your doctor as soon as possible. Only your doctor can determine if it is safe for you to continue using Colyte.

■ *More common side effects may include:*
Abdominal fullness
Bloating
Nausea

■ *Less common side effects may include:*
Abdominal cramps, anal irritation, vomiting

■ *Rare side effects may include:*
Hives, runny nose, skin inflammation

Why should this drug not be prescribed?
Colyte should not be taken if you have a stomach or intestinal blockage, an inflammation of the colon (colitis) or an enlarged colon, a perforated bowel, or problems with gastric retention.

Special warnings about this medication
This drug should be used cautiously if you have chronic bowel disease (ulcerative colitis) or an impaired gag reflex, or if you are prone to vomiting.

Possible food and drug interactions when taking this medication
Any oral medication taken after you have started drinking Colyte may be flushed out of your system before it can be absorbed.

Special information if you are pregnant or breastfeeding
The effects of Colyte during pregnancy have not been adequately studied. If you are pregnant or plan to become pregnant, inform your doctor immediately. It should be used only if clearly needed.

Recommended dosage
The recommended adult dose is 240 milliliters (8 fluid ounces) every 10 minutes. Cleansing is complete when the bowels run clear. This usually requires drinking 3 to 4 liters (3 to 4 quarts) of liquid.

Overdosage
Although there is no specific information available, any medication taken in excess

can have serious consequences. If you suspect an overdose seek medical attention.

Brand name:

COMPAZINE

Generic name: Prochlorperazine

Why is this drug prescribed?

Compazine is used to control severe nausea and vomiting. It is also used to treat symptoms of psychotic disorders such as schizophrenia. Although Compazine is also prescribed for anxiety, it is not the first choice of most doctors. Other drugs that do not share Compazine's potential risks, such as Valium, are usually prescribed first.

Most important fact about this drug

Compazine may cause tardive dyskinesia—involuntary muscle spasms and twitches in the face and body. This condition may be permanent. It appears to be most common among the elderly, especially women. Ask your doctor for information about this possible risk.

How should you take this medication?

Never take more Compazine than prescribed. It can increase the risk of serious side effects.

What side effects may occur?

Side effects cannot be anticipated. If any develop or change in intensity, inform your doctor as soon as possible. Only your doctor can determine if it is safe for you to continue taking Compazine.

■ *Side effects may include:*
Abnormal muscle rigidity, abnormal secretion of milk, abnormal sugar in urine, abnormalities of posture and movement, agitation, anemia, appetite changes, asthma, blurred vision, breast development in males, chewing movements, constipation, convulsions, difficulty swallowing, discolored skin tone, dizziness, drooling, drowsiness, dry mouth, ejaculation problems, exaggerated reflexes, fever, fluid retention, fluid retention in the brain, fragmented movements, head arched backward, headache, heart attack, heels bent back on legs, high or low blood sugar, hives, impotence, inability to urinate, increased appetite, increased psychotic symptoms, increased weight, infection, insomnia, intestinal obstruction, involuntary movements of arms, hands, legs, and feet, involuntary movements of face, tongue, and jaw, irregular movements, jerky movements, jitteriness, light sensitivity, low blood pressure (sometimes fatal), mask-like face, menstrual irregularities, narrowed or dilated pupils, nasal congestion, nausea, pain in the shoulder and neck area, painful muscle spasm, parkinsonism-like symptoms, persistent, painful erections, pill-rolling motion, protruding tongue, puckering of the mouth, puffing of the cheeks, rigid arms, feet, head, and muscles, rotation of eyeballs or state of fixed gaze, shock, shuffling gait, skin itching, peeling, rash, inflammation, sore throat, mouth, and gums, spasms in back, feet and ankles, jaw, and neck, swelling and itching skin, swelling in throat, tremors, yellowed eyes and skin

Why should this drug not be prescribed?

You should not be given Compazine if you are in a coma, if you are taking large amounts of central nervous system depressants (such as alcohol, barbiturates, or narcotics), or if you have Reye's syndrome (a brain disease affecting children and adolescents).

Children under 2 years of age or weighing less than 20 pounds should not be given Compazine; and it should not be used in pediatric surgery.

Special warnings about this medication

If you suddenly stop taking Compazine, you may experience a change in appetite, dizziness, nausea, vomiting, and tremors. Follow your doctor's instructions closely when discontinuing this drug.

Compazine may obscure the signs and symptoms of brain tumors and intestinal obstruction.

You should use Compazine cautiously if you have: a brain tumor, intestinal blockage, heart disease, glaucoma, or an abnormal bone marrow or blood condition, such as leukemia, or if you are exposed to extreme heat or pesticides. Be particularly cautious if you are hypersensitive to other drugs of this type.

This drug may impair your ability to drive a car or operate potentially dangerous machinery. Do not participate in any activities that require full alertness if you are unsure about your ability.

Compazine may cause false-positive pregnancy tests and a false-positive test result for phenylketonuria (a birth defect involving damage to the central nervous system).

Possible food and drug interactions when taking this medication

If Compazine is taken with certain other drugs, the effects of either could be increased, decreased, or altered. It is especially important to check with your doctor before combining Compazine with the following:

Anticonvulsants such as Dilantin and Tegretol
Anticoagulants such as Coumadin
Guanethidine (Ismelin)
Propranolol (Inderal)
Thiazide diuretics such as Dyazide

Extreme drowsiness and other potentially serious effects can result if Compazine is combined with alcohol, narcotics, painkillers, and other central nervous system depressants.

Drugs such as Compazine should not be used with the diagnostic product Amipaque or with epinephrine (Epipen).

Special information if you are pregnant or breastfeeding

Compazine is not usually recommended for pregnant women. However, it may be prescribed for nausea and vomiting so severe that the potential benefits of the drug outweigh the potential risks. Compazine appears in breast milk and may affect a nursing infant. If this drug is essential to your health, your doctor may recommend that you stop breastfeeding until your treatment is finished.

Recommended dosage

ADULTS

To Control Severe Nausea and Vomiting
Tablets: The usual dosage is one 5-milligram or 10-milligram tablet 3 or 4 times a day.

'Spansule' Capsules: The usual starting dose is one 15-milligram capsule on getting out of bed or one 10-milligram capsule every 12 hours.

The usual rectal dosage (suppository) is 25 milligrams, taken 2 times a day.

For Non-psychotic Anxiety
Tablets: The usual dose is 5 milligrams, taken 3 or 4 times a day.

'Spansule' capsule: The usual starting dose is one 15-milligram capsule on getting up or one 10-milligram capsule every 12 hours.

Treatment should not continue for longer than 12 weeks, and daily doses should not exceed 20 milligrams.

Relatively Mild Psychotic Disorders
The usual dose is 5 or 10 milligrams, taken 3 or 4 times daily.

Moderate to Severe Psychotic Disorders
Dosages usually start at 10 milligrams, taken 3 or 4 times a day. If needed, dosage may be gradually increased; 50 to 75 milligrams daily has been helpful for some people.

More Severe Psychotic Disorders
Dosages may range from 100 to 150 milligrams per day.

CHILDREN

The lowest effective dose of Compazine should be used, since children may be sensitive to this drug. If a child becomes restless or excited after taking Compazine, do not give the child another dose.

Use Compazine cautiously in children who are seriously ill (with diseases such as chicken pox or measles) or who are dehydrated.

Children under 2 years of age or weighing less than 20 pounds should not be given Compazine.

For Severe Nausea and Vomiting
An oral or rectal dose of Compazine is usually not needed for more than 1 day.

Children 20 to 29 Pounds
The usual dose is 2½ milligrams 1 or 2 times daily. Total daily amount should not exceed 7.5 milligrams.

Children 30 to 39 Pounds
The usual dose is 2½ milligrams 2 or 3 times daily. Total daily amount should not exceed 10 milligrams.

Children 40 to 85 Pounds
The usual dose is 2½ milligrams 3 times daily, or 5 milligrams 2 times daily.

Total daily amount should not exceed 15 milligrams.

For Psychotic Disorders

Children 2 to 5 Years Old
The starting oral or rectal dose is 2½ milligrams 2 or 3 times daily. Do not exceed 10 milligrams the first day and 20 milligrams thereafter.

Children 6 to 12 Years Old
The starting oral or rectal dose is 2½ milligrams 2 or 3 times daily. Do not exceed 10 milligrams the first day and 25 milligrams thereafter.

ELDERLY

In general, elderly people take lower dosages of Compazine. Because elderly people may develop low blood pressure while taking Compazine, they should be closely monitored. Elderly people (especially elderly women) may be more susceptible to tardive dyskinesia—a possibly permanent condition. Tardive dyskinesia causes involuntary muscle spasms and twitches in the face and body. Elderly people should consult their doctor for information about these potential risks.

Overdosage
Any medication taken in excess can have serious consequences. An overdose of Compazine can be fatal. If you suspect an overdose, seek medical help immediately.

Symptoms of Compazine overdose may include:
Agitation
Coma
Convulsions
Dry mouth
Extreme sleepiness
Fever
Intestinal blockage
Irregular heart rate
Restlessness

Category:

CONTRACEPTIVES

See Oral Contraceptives, page 437.

Brand name:

CORGARD

Generic name: Nadolol

Why is this drug prescribed?

Corgard is used in the treatment of angina pectoris (chest pain, usually caused by lack of oxygen to the heart due to clogged arteries) and high blood pressure.

When prescribed for high blood pressure, it is effective when used alone or in combination with other high blood pressure medications. Corgard is a type of drug known as a beta blocker. It decreases the force and rate of heart contractions.

Most important fact about this drug

If you have high blood pressure, you must take Corgard regularly for it to be effective. Even if you are feeling well, you need this medication to keep your blood pressure down.

How should you take this medication?

Corgard can be taken with or without food.

Take this medication exactly as prescribed by your doctor, even if your symptoms have disappeared.

Try not to miss any doses. Corgard is taken once a day. If it is not taken regularly, your condition may worsen.

If you forget to take a dose, take it as soon as you remember. If it's within 8 hours of your next scheduled dose, skip the one you missed and go back to your regular schedule. Never take two doses at the same time.

What side effects may occur?

Side effects cannot be anticipated. If any develop or change in intensity, inform your doctor as soon as possible. Only your doctor can determine if it is safe for you to continue taking Corgard.

■ *More common side effects may include:*
Change in behavior
Changes in heartbeat
Dizziness or lightheadedness
Mild drowsiness
Slow heartbeat
Weakness or tiredness

■ *Less common or rare side effects may include:*
Abdominal discomfort, asthma-like symptoms, bloating, confusion, constipation, cough, decreased sex drive, diarrhea, dry eyes, dry mouth, dry skin, facial swelling, gas, headache, heart failure, impotence, indigestion, itching, loss of appetite, low blood pressure, nasal stuffiness, nausea, rash, ringing in ears, slurred speech, vision changes, vomiting, weight gain

Why should this drug not be prescribed?

If you have a slow heartbeat, bronchial asthma, heart block, cardiogenic shock or active heart failure you should not take this medication.

Special warnings about this medication

If you have a history of congestive heart failure, Corgard should be used with caution. Corgard should not be stopped suddenly. It can cause increased chest pain and heart attack. Dosage should be gradually reduced.

If you suffer from asthma, chronic bronchitis, emphysema, seasonal allergies or other bronchial conditions or kidney or liver disease, this medication should be used with caution.

Ask your doctor if you should check your pulse while taking Corgard. It can cause your heartbeat to become too slow.

This medication may mask the symptoms of low blood sugar or alter blood sugar levels. If you are diabetic, discuss this with your doctor.

This medication may cause you to become drowsy or less alert; therefore, driving or operating dangerous machinery or participating in any hazardous activity that requires full mental alertness is not recommended until you know how you respond to this medication.

Notify your doctor or dentist that you are taking Corgard if you have a medical emergency or before you have surgery or dental treatment.

Possible food and drug interactions when taking this medication

If Corgard is taken with certain other drugs, the effects of either could be increased, decreased, or altered. It is especially important to check with your doctor before combining Corgard with the following:

Antidiabetic drugs, including Insulin and oral
   drugs like Micronase
Catecholamine-depleting drugs such as
   reserpine
General anesthetics

Special Information
If you are pregnant or breastfeeding

The effects of Corgard during pregnancy have not been adequately studied. If you are pregnant or plan to become pregnant, inform your doctor immediately. Corgard appears in breast milk and could affect a nursing infant. If this medication is essential to your health, your doctor may advise you to discontinue breastfeeding until your treatment with this medication is finished.

Recommended dosage

ADULTS

Dosage must be individualized.

Angina Pectoris
The usual starting dose is 40 milligrams once daily. The usual maintenance dose is 40 or 80 milligrams, once a day. Doses up to 160 or 240 milligrams, once a day may be needed.

High Blood Pressure
The usual starting initial dose is 40 milligrams once daily.

The usual maintenance dose is 40 or 80 milligrams, once a day. Doses up to 240 or 320 milligrams once a day may be needed.

Dosage for kidney patients must be adjusted.

CHILDREN

The safety and effectiveness of Corgard have not been established in children.

ELDERLY

Dosage should be determined by the particular needs of the elderly patient.

Overdosage

Any medication taken in excess can cause symptoms of overdose. If you suspect an overdose, seek medical attention immediately.

The symptoms of Corgard overdose may include:
Difficulty in breathing
Heart failure
Low blood pressure
Slow heartbeat

Brand name:

CORTISPORIN OPHTHALMIC SUSPENSION

Generic ingredients: Polymyxin B sulfate, Neomycin sulfate, Hydrocortisone

Why is this drug prescribed?

Cortisporin Ophthalmic Suspension is a combination of the cortisone-like drug, hydrocortisone, and two antibiotics. It is prescribed to treat superficial bacterial infections of the eye and to provide relief from inflammatory conditions such as irritation, swelling, redness, and general eye discomfort.

Most important fact about this drug

Prolonged use of this medication may result in glaucoma, with potential damage to the optic nerve and visual problems. Prolonged use also may suppress your immune response and thus increase the hazard of secondary eye infections. Your doctor may measure your eye pressure periodically if you are using this product for 10 days or longer.

How should you use this medication?

Cortisporin should be used as prescribed by your doctor.

It should be shaken well before using.

Keep this medicine from freezing.

What side effects may occur?

Side effects cannot be anticipated. If any develop or change in intensity, inform your doctor as soon as possible. Only your doctor can determine if it is safe for you to continue using Cortisporin.

■ *Side effects may include:*
  Cataract formation (results in blurred vision); delayed wound healing; increased eye pressure with possible development of glaucoma and, infrequently, optic nerve damage; irritation when drops are instilled; localized allergic reactions (itching, swelling, redness); other infections, particularly fungal infections of the cornea, and bacterial eye infection

Why should this drug not be prescribed?

Cortisporin should not be used if you have certain viral or fungal diseases of the eye, including inflammation of the cornea caused by herpes simplex, chickenpox or cow pox, or if you are sensitive to or have ever had an allergic reaction to any of its ingredients.

Special warnings about this medication

Steroids such as hydrocortisone may hide the existence of an infection or worsen an existing one. If you are using this medication for more than 10 days, your doctor should routinely check your eye pressure.

Neomycin, one of the ingredients in Cortisporin, may cause an allergic reaction, usually itching, redness and swelling, or failure to heal. These symptoms subside quickly once the medication is stopped. You are more likely to be sensitive to neomycin if you are sensitive to the following antibiotics: kanamycin, paromomycin, streptomycin and possibly gentamicin.

This medication should be used with extreme caution if you have herpes simplex.

If you develop a sensitivity to Cortisporin, avoid other topical medications that contain neomycin.

Persistent fungus infections have occurred with long-term Cortisporin use.

Possible food and drug interactions when taking this medication

No interactions have been reported.

Special information
if you are pregnant or breastfeeding

Although the effects of Cortisporin during pregnancy have not been adequately studied, steroids should be used during pregnancy only if the benefits outweigh the dangers to the fetus. If you are pregnant or plan to become pregnant, inform your doctor immediately. Hydrocortisone, when taken orally, appears in breast milk. Since medication may be absorbed into the bloodstream when it is applied to the eye, your doctor may advise you to stop breastfeeding until your treatment with Cortisporin is finished.

Recommended dosage

ADULTS

The usual recommended dose is 1 or 2 drops in the affected eye every 3 or 4 hours, depending on the severity of the condition. Cortisporin may be used more often if necessary.

Overdosage

Any medication used in excess can have serious consequences. If you suspect an overdose, seek medical treatment immediately.

Brand name:

CORZIDE

Generic ingredients: Nadolol, Bendroflumethiazide

Why is this drug prescribed?

Corzide is a combination drug used in the treatment of high blood pressure. It combines a beta blocker and a thiazide diuretic. Nadolol, the beta blocker, decreases the force and rate of heart contractions. Bendroflumethiazide, the diuretic, helps your body produce and eliminate more urine, which helps in lowering blood pressure.

Most important fact about this drug

Since blood pressure lowers gradually, it may take several weeks for the full effect of Corzide to occur. Even if you are feeling well, you must continue to take this medication.

How should you take this medication?

Corzide may be taken with or without food.

Take this medication exactly as prescribed by your doctor, even if your symptoms have disappeared.

Try not to miss any doses. Corzide is taken once a day. If this medication is not taken regularly, your condition may worsen.

If you forget to take a dose, take it as soon as you remember. If it's within 8 hours of your next scheduled dose, skip the one you missed and go back to your regular schedule. Never take two doses at the same time.

What side effects may occur?

Side effects cannot be anticipated. If any develop or change in intensity, inform your doctor as soon as possible. Only your doctor can determine if it is safe for you to continue taking Corzide.

■ *More common side effects may include:*
Asthma-like symptoms
Changes in heart rhythm
Cold hands and feet
Dizziness
Fatigue
Low blood pressure
Low potassium (dry mouth, excessive thirst, weak or irregular heartbeat, muscle pain or cramps)
Slow heartbeat

■ *Less common or rare side effects may include:*
Abdominal discomfort, anemia, bloating, blurred vision, change in behavior,

changes in liver function, constipation, cough, decrease in white blood cells, diarrhea, dry mouth, eyes or skin, facial swelling, gas, headache, heart block, heart failure, hepatitis, impotence, indigestion, inflammation of the pancreas, itching, jaundice, loss of appetite, lowered sex drive, muscle spasm, nasal stuffiness, nausea, rash, ringing in ears, sedation, sensitivity to light, slurred speech, sweating, tingling or pins and needles, vertigo, vomiting, weakness, weight gain, wheezing

Why should this drug not be prescribed?

If you have bronchial asthma, slow heartbeat, heart block (conduction disorder), inadequate blood supply to the circulatory system (cardiogenic shock), active congestive heart failure, inability to urinate, or if you are sensitive to or have ever had an allergic reaction to Corzide, its ingredients, or similar drugs, you should not take this medication.

Special warnings about this medication

If you have a history of congestive heart failure, Corzide should be used with caution.

Corzide should not be stopped suddenly. This can cause increased chest pain and heart attack. Dosage should be gradually reduced.

If you suffer from asthma, seasonal allergies, emphysema or other bronchial conditions, or kidney or liver disease, this medication should be used with caution.

Ask your doctor if you should check your pulse while taking Corzide. It can cause your heartbeat to become too slow.

Corzide may mask the symptoms of low blood sugar or alter blood sugar levels. If you are diabetic, discuss this with your doctor.

This medication can cause you to become drowsy or less alert; therefore, activity that requires full mental alertness is not recommended until you know how you respond to this medication.

Notify your doctor or dentist that you are taking Corzide if you have a medical emergency, or before you have surgery or dental treatment.

Possible food and drug interactions when taking this medication

Corzide may intensify the effects of alcohol. Do not drink alcohol while taking this medication.

If Corzide is taken with any other drug, the effects of either could be increased, decreased, or altered. It is especially important to check with your doctor before combining Corzide with the following:

Amphotericin B
Antidepressant drugs known as MAO
    inhibitors such as Nardil
Antidiabetic drugs, including insulin and oral
    drugs such as Micronase
Antigout drugs, such as Benemid
Barbiturates
Blood thinners such as Coumadin and
    Panwarfin
Calcium salt
Cardiac glycosides
Catecholamine-depleting drugs, such as
    reserpine
Cholestyramine (Questran)
Colestipol (Colestid)
Corticosteroids such as Prednisone
Diazoxide
General anesthetics
Lithium
Methenamine (Mandelamine)
Narcotics such as Percocet
Nondepolarizing muscle relaxants
Nonsteroidal anti-inflammatory drugs such
    as Motrin

Other antihypertensives
Sulfinpyrazone

Special information
if you are pregnant or breastfeeding
The effects of Corzide during pregnancy have
not been adequately studied. If you are
pregnant or plan to become pregnant, inform
your doctor immediately. Corzide appears
in breast milk and could affect a nursing
infant. If this medication is essential to
your health, your doctor may advise you to
discontinue breastfeeding until your
treatment with Corzide is finished.

Recommended dosage
ADULTS

Dosages of this drug are always
individualized.

This drug may be taken with or without
meals.

Usual dose is 1 Corzide 40/5 milligram tablet
per day or 1 Corzide 80/5 milligram
tablet per day if the desired effect is not
reached. Your doctor can and may
gradually add another high blood pressure
medication to this drug gradually.

Dosages will also be adjusted in patients with
decreased kidney function.

CHILDREN

The safety and effectiveness of Corzide have
not been established in children.

ELDERLY

Dosage should be determined by the
particular needs of the elderly patient.

Overdosage
Any medication taken in excess can cause
symptoms of overdose. If you suspect an
overdose, seek medical attention immediately.

*The symptoms of Corzide overdose may
include:*
Abdominal irritation
Central nervous system depression
Coma
Extremely slow heartbeat
Heart failure
Lethargy
Low blood pressure
Wheezing

Brand name:

COTRIM

See Bactrim, page 53.

Brand name:

COUMADIN

Generic name: Warfarin sodium

Why is this drug prescribed?
Coumadin is an anticoagulant (blood thinner).
It is prescribed to:

Prevent and/or treat a blood clot that has
formed within a blood vessel;

Prevent blood clots from reaching the lungs;

Aid in the prevention of blood clots that may
form in blood vessels anywhere in the
body after a heart attack.

Most important fact about this drug
The most serious risks associated with
Coumadin treatment are hemorrhage (severe
bleeding resulting in the loss of a large
amount of blood) in any tissue or organ and,
less frequently, the destruction of skin
tissue cells (necrosis). The risk of hemorrhage
usually depends on the dosage and length
of treatment with this drug.

Hemorrhage and necrosis have been reported to result in death or permanent disability. Severe necrosis can lead to the removal of damaged tissue or amputation of a limb. Necrosis appears to be associated with blood clots located in the area of tissue damage and usually occurs within a few days of starting Coumadin treatment.

How should you take this medication?

The objective of treatment with a blood thinner is to control the blood-clotting process without causing severe bleeding, so that a clot does not form and cut off the blood supply necessary for normal bodily function. Therefore, it is very important that you take this medication exactly as prescribed by your doctor and that your doctor monitor your condition on a regular basis.

Effective treatment with minimal complications depends upon the cooperation of patients and their communication with the doctor.

Do not take or discontinue any other medication unless directed to do so by your doctor. Avoid alcohol, salicylates such as aspirin, large amounts of green leafy vegetables, or drastic changes in your diet.

You should carry an identification card that indicates you are taking Coumadin.

Do not change from one brand of this drug to another without consulting your doctor or pharmacist.

Coumadin may cause a red-orange discoloration of urine.

What side effects may occur?

Side effects cannot be anticipated. If any develop or change in intensity, inform your doctor as soon as possible. Only your doctor can determine if it is safe for you to continue taking Coumadin.

■ *More common side effects may include:*
Hemorrhage: Signs and symptoms of severe bleeding resulting in the loss of large amounts of blood depend upon the location and extent of bleeding.

Symptoms include: Chest, abdomen, joint or other pain, destruction of skin tissue and other tissue, difficult breathing or swallowing, headache, paralysis, shortness of breath, unexplained shock, unexplained swelling

■ *Less common side effects may include:*
Abdominal and other cramping, allergic reactions, diarrhea, fever, hives, loss of hair, nausea, purple toes, severe or long-lasting inflammation of the skin

Why should this drug not be prescribed?

This drug should not be prescribed for any condition where the danger of hemorrhage may be greater than the potential benefits of treatment. Unless directed to do so by your doctor, do not take this medication if you are being treated for one of the following conditions:

A tendency to hemorrhage
An abnormal blood condition
Balloon-like swelling of a blood vessel in the brain or heart
Bleeding tendencies associated with ulceration or bleeding of the stomach, intestines, or the genital or urinary system
Eclampsia (a rare and serious pregnancy disorder producing life-threatening convulsions)
Excessive bleeding of brain blood vessels
Inflammation, due to bacterial infection, of the membrane that lines the inside of the heart
Inflammation of the sac that surrounds the heart or an escape fluid from the heart sac

Malignant hypertension (extremely elevated blood pressure that damages the inner linings of blood vessels, the heart, spleen, kidneys and brain)

Preeclampsia (an abnormal pregnancy condition that can lead to eclampsia)

Pregnancy

Recent or contemplated traumatic surgery resulting in large, open surfaces

Recent or future surgery of the central nervous system or eye

Spinal cord puncture or other diagnostic or therapeutic procedures that cause bleeding

Threatened abortion (symptoms such as vaginal bleeding during pregnancy that signal a spontaneous loss of the baby)

Unsupervised senility, alcoholism, or psychosis (severe mental disorder that causes a person to lose contact with reality) are conditions that would hamper a patient's ability to follow or comply with a prescribed dosage regimen, making use of this drug inadvisable.

Special warnings about this medication

Treatment with blood thinners may increase the risk that fatty plaque will break away from the wall of an artery and lodge at another point, causing the blockage of a blood vessel.

There is an increased risk of developing blood clots if you have one of the following conditions:

An infectious disease or intestinal disorder

A history of recurrent blood clot disorders in a patient or his or her family

Inflammation of a blood vessel

Moderate to severe high blood pressure

Moderate to severe kidney or liver dysfunction

Polycythemia vera (blood disorder)

Severe allergic disorders

Severe diabetes

Surgery resulting in large exposed raw surfaces

Trauma that may result in internal bleeding

Patients with congestive heart failure may become more sensitive to Coumadin, requiring more frequent laboratory monitoring by the doctor.

If you are taking Coumadin, your doctor should periodically check the time it takes for you blood to start the clotting process (prothrombin time). Numerous factors such as travel and changes in diet, environment, physical state, and medication may alter your response to treatment with an anticoagulant. Prothrombin time should also be monitored after your release from the hospital and whenever other medications are started, discontinued, or taken haphazardly.

If you are elderly or in a weakened state while taking Coumadin, it is recommended that your doctor monitor you on a regular basis.

Notify your doctor if any illness, such as diarrhea, infection, or fever develops; if any unusual symptoms, such as pain, swelling, or discomfort, appear, or if prolonged bleeding from cuts, increased menstrual flow, vaginal bleeding, nosebleeds, bleeding of gums from brushing, unusual bleeding or bruising, red or dark brown urine, or red or tarry black stool occurs.

Possible food and drug interactions when taking this medication

Alcohol may increase or decrease the time it takes your blood to begin the clotting process. The use of alcohol is not recommended.

Consult your doctor before making any change in your medications. The drug listed below are of particular concern.

Drugs used to dissolve blood clots:
Streptokinase (Streptase)
Urokinase (Abbokinase)

The following drugs may increase the time it takes for your blood to begin the clotting process when taken alone or in combination with Coumadin:

Allopurinol (Zyloprim)
Aminosalicylic acid
Amiodarone hydrochloride (Cordarone)
Anabolic steroids (Anadrol-50)
Anesthetics, inhalation (Ethrane)
Antibiotics
Bromelains (Bromase)
Chenodiol (bile salt that reduces cholesterol secretion)
Chloral hydrate (Noctec)
Chlorpropamide (Diabinese)
Chymotrypsin (pancreatic enzymes)
Cimetidine (Tagamet)
Clofibrate (Atromid-S)
Dextran
Dextrothyroxine
Diazoxide (Proglycem)
Diflunisal (Dolobid)
Disulfiram (Antabuse)
Diuretics (Hydromox, Diulo)
Ethacrynic acid (Edecrin)
Fenoprofen (Nalfon)
Fluoroquinolone antibiotics (Cipro)
Glucagon (used to treat low blood sugar)
Ibuprofen (Motrin)
Indomethacin (Indocin)
Influenza virus vaccine (Flu-Imune)
Lovastatin (Mevacor)
Mefenamic acid (Ponstel)
Methyldopa (Aldomet)
Methylphenidate (Ritalin)
Metronidazole (Flagyl)
Miconazole (Monistat)
MAO inhibitors (Nardil)
Nalidixic acid (NegGram)
Naproxen (Naprosyn)
Narcotics (Percocet, Demerol)
Pentoxifylline (Trental)
Phenobarbital

Phenylbutazone (Butazolidin)
Phenytoin (Dilantin)
Propafenone (Rythmol)
Pyrazolones (Butazolidin)
Quinidine (Quinidex)
Quinine (Quinamm)
Ranitidine (Zantac)
Salicylates (Aspirin)
Sulfinpyrazone (Anturane)
Sulfonamides
Sulindac (Clinoril)
Tamoxifen (Nolvadex)
Thyroid drugs (Synthroid)
Tolbutamide (Orinase)
Trimethoprim/sulfamethoxazole (Bactrim)

The following drugs may decrease the time it takes for your blood to begin the clotting process if taken alone or in combination with Coumadin:

Adrenocortical steroids (Prednisone)
Aminoglutethimide (Cytadren)
Antacids
Antihistamines (Benadryl)
Barbiturates (Phenobarbital)
Carbamazepine (Tegretol)
Chloral hydrate (Noctec)
Chlordiazepoxide (Librium)
Cholestyramine (Questran)
Diuretics (Hydromox, Diulo)
Ethchlorvynol (Placidyl)
Glutethimide (Doriden)
Griseofulvin (Gris-PEG)
Haloperidol (Haldol)
Meprobamate (Miltown)
Nafcillin (Unipen)
Oral contraceptives
Paraldehyde (used as a hypnotic and sedative)
Primidone (Mysoline)
Ranitidine (Zantac)
Rifampin (Rifadin)
Sucralfate (Carafate)
Trazodone (Desyrel)
Vitamin C

Special information
if you are pregnant or breastfeeding
Coumadin should not be taken by women who are or may become pregnant since the drug passes through the placental barrier and may cause fatal hemorrhage in the fetus. There have also been reports of birth malformations in children born to mothers who have been treated with Coumadin during pregnancy. If you become pregnant while taking this drug, discuss the possible risks with your doctor. Coumadin may appear in breast milk and could affect a nursing infant. If this medication is essential to your health, discuss breastfeeding with your doctor.

Recommended dosage

ADULTS

The administration and dosage of Coumadin must be individualized for each patient by a doctor according to the patient's sensitivity to the drug.

A common starting dosage for adults is 10 milligrams per day for 2 to 4 days. Individualized daily dosage adjustments are based on the results of tests that determine the amount of time it takes for the blood clotting process to begin.

A maintenance dose of 2 to 10 milligrams per day is satisfactory for most patients. The duration of treatment should be individualized.

CHILDREN

Safety and effectiveness have not been established in children below the age of 18.

Overdosage
Signs and symptoms of Coumadin overdose reflect abnormal bleeding. They include:
Blood in stools or urine
Excessive menstrual bleeding
Black stools
Reddish or purplish spots on skin
Excessive bruising
Excessive bleeding from superficial injuries

If you suspect an overdose, seek emergency medical treatment immediately.

Generic name:

CROMOLYN SODIUM

Brand names: Intal Capsules (for inhalation), Intal Solution (for nebulizer), Intal Aerosol Spray, Nasalcrom Nasal Solution, Opticrom Ophthalmic Solution

Why is this drug prescribed?
Cromolyn sodium is an antiasthmatic/ antiallergic medication. Different forms of the drug are used either to treat bronchial asthma, to prevent asthma attacks, or to prevent and treat seasonal and chronic allergies.

The drug works by preventing "mast cells" from releasing certain substances that can cause allergic reactions or too much bronchial activity. It also helps prevent bronchial constriction caused by exercise, aspirin, cold air, and certain environmental pollutants, such as toluene and sulfur dioxide.

Most important fact about this drug
Cromolyn sodium should be taken only as directed by your doctor. When taken for severe bronchial asthma, it can be 4 weeks before you feel its maximum benefit. Some people, however, will receive relief of symptoms sooner. Do not discontinue the inhalation capsules or nasal solution abruptly without the advice of your doctor.

How should you take this medication?
These capsules should not be swallowed.

Each cromolyn sodium capsule should be inhaled using the Spinhaler turbo-inhaler.

One capsule is usually inhaled 4 times daily at regular intervals. Although cromolyn sodium is tasteless, it may leave a slightly bitter taste after inhalation. Capsules should be stored at room temperature and the Spinhaler replaced every 6 months.

Cromolyn sodium nebulizer solution should be inhaled using a power-operated nebulizer equipped with an appropriate face mask. Hand operated nebulizers are not suitable. It is important that the solution be inhaled at regular intervals, usually 4 times per day.

Cromolyn sodium aerosol spray can be used for either chronic asthma or to prevent an asthma attack. For chronic asthma, it must be inhaled at regular intervals, as directed by your doctor, usually 2 sprays inhaled 4 times daily. To prevent an asthma attack caused by exercise, cold air, etc., the usual dose of 2 inhalation sprays should be taken between 10 and 60 minutes before exercising or exposure to cold or pollutants.

The nasal solution Nasalcrom should be used with a metered nasal spray device, which should be replaced every 6 months. The nasal passages should be cleared before administering the spray. The nasal solution is used for nasal congestion due to seasonal (for example, pollen) or chronic allergies. For seasonal allergies, treatment is more effective if started before the start of the allergy season. Treatment should then continue throughout the season. For year-round allergies, treatment may be required for up to 4 weeks before results occur. The additional use of other allergy medications, such as antihistamines or decongestants, may also be necessary during initial treatment.

Opticrom eyedrops should not be used while wearing soft contact lenses. Lenses may be worn a few hours after the drug has been stopped. The eyedrops are used for allergic disorders of the eye and are taken at regular intervals, usually 1 to 2 drops in each eye, 4 to 6 times per day. Your eyes may initially sting or burn when the eyedrops are used. Relief from allergy symptoms may occur within a few days, but treatment may be necessary for up to 6 weeks. The drops should be stored below 30°C (86°F) and protected from direct sunlight. The eyedrop bottle should be discarded 4 weeks after it is opened.

What side effects may occur?

Side effects cannot be anticipated. If any develop or change in intensity, inform your doctor as soon as possible. Only your doctor can determine if it is safe for you to continue taking cromolyn sodium.

■ *More common side effects may include:*
Fleeting cough
Mild wheezing

■ *Less common or rare side effects may include:*
Angioedema (chest pain, swelling of face around lips, tongue and throat, arms and legs, sore throat, fever, chills, difficulty swallowing), bad taste in mouth, coughing and wheezing, dizziness, ear problems, headache, hives, joint swelling and pain, nasal congestion, nasal itching or burning, nausea, nose bleed, painful urination or frequent urination, sneezing, rash, teary eyes, tightness in throat

Why should this drug not be prescribed?

If you are sensitive to or have ever had an allergic reaction to cromolyn sodium, lactose, or similar drugs of this type, you should not take this medication. Make sure that your doctor is aware of any drug reactions that you have experienced.

Special warnings about this medication

Asthma symptoms may recur if the recommended dosage of cromolyn sodium is reduced or discontinued. Cromolyn sodium has no role in the treatment of an acute asthmatic attack once it has begun; if it is persistent, it may cause a condition called status asthmaticus. Obtain medical help immediately if you experience a severe attack.

Possible food and drug interactions when taking this medication

If you are taking other prescription or non-prescription drugs, this should be discussed with your doctor to determine if these drugs would interact with cromolyn sodium.

Special information if you are pregnant or breastfeeding

The effects of cromolyn sodium during pregnancy have not been adequately studied. If you are pregnant or plan to become pregnant, inform your doctor immediately. It is not known if cromolyn sodium passes into breast milk. However, as with all medication, a nursing woman should use this drug only after careful consultation with her doctor.

Recommended dosage

INTAL CAPSULES FOR INHALATION
INTAL SOLUTION FOR NEBULIZER

Adults

For management of bronchial asthma, the usual dosage is 20 milligrams (1 capsule or ampule) inhaled 4 times daily at regular intervals, using the Spinhaler turbo-inhaler or power-operated nebulizer. If you have chronic asthma, this drug's effectiveness depends on your taking it regularly, as directed, and only after an attack has been controlled and you can inhale adequately.

For the prevention of an acute attack following exercise or exposure to cold, dry air, environmental agents, etc., the usual dose is 1 capsule or ampule inhaled shortly (no more than 1 hour) before exposure to the irritant. Inhalation may be repeated as needed for continued protection during prolonged exposure.

Children

For children 5 years old and over for the capsules, and 2 years old and over for the solution, the usual starting dose is 1 capsule or ampule (20 milligrams) inhaled 4 times a day at regular intervals.

INTAL AEROSOL SPRAY

Adults and Children 5 Years Old and Over

For the management of bronchial asthma, the usual starting dose is 2 metered sprays taken at regular intervals, 4 times daily. This is the maximum dose that should be taken, and lower dosages may be effective in younger patients. This drug should be used only after an asthma attack has been controlled and you can inhale adequately.

For the prevention of an acute asthma attack, the usual dose is inhalation of two metered sprays shortly before exposure to the irritant.

NASALCROM NASAL SOLUTION

Adults and Children 6 Years Old and Over

For the prevention and treatment of allergies caused by exposure to certain irritants, the usual dosage is 1 spray in each nostril 3 to 6 times per day at regular intervals, using the metered spray device.

OPTICROM EYEDROPS

Adults and Children

For the treatment of allergic eye disorders, the usual dosage is 1 to 2 drops instilled in each eye 4 to 6 times per day at regular intervals. Treatment for up to 6 weeks is sometimes required.

Overdosage

Any medication taken in excess can have serious consequences. If you suspect an overdose, seek medical attention immediately.

Symptoms of cromolyn sodium overdose may include:
Difficulty breathing
Heart failure
Low blood pressure
Slow heartbeat

Brand name:

CUTIVATE

Generic name: Fluticasone propionate

Why Is this drug prescribed?

Cutivate cream and ointment are prescribed for the relief of the inflammatory and itchy symptoms of skin disorders known to be responsive to corticosteroid treatment.

Most important fact about this drug

Absorption of this drug through the skin can affect the whole body as opposed to just the surface being treated.

The drug has produced dysfunction of the thyroid, pituitary, and adrenal glands, symptoms of Cushing's syndrome (weight gain, reddening of the face and neck, growth of excess facial hair, high blood pressure, and mental disturbances) hyperglycemia (excess glucose in the blood), and glucosuria (urinary excretion of glucose).

The use of a large amount of this medication over large surface areas and the application of airtight dressings or bandages may cause this absorption. Your doctor should monitor your condition and periodically check the endocrine system, which controls your thyroid, pituitary, and adrenal gland function, if you are receiving a large dose of any potent steroid preparation applied to a large area of your skin.

How should you use this medication?

Use this medication exactly as prescribed by your doctor. It is for external use only. Avoid contact with the eyes.

What side effects may occur?

Side effects cannot be anticipated. If any develop or change in intensity, inform your doctor as soon as possible. Only your doctor can determine if it is safe for you to continue taking Cutivate.

■ *More common side effects may include:*
Burning
Dryness
Itching
Numbness of fingers

■ *Less common side effects may include:*
Infection, inflammation of hair follicles, inflammation of the skin around the mouth, irritation, prickly heat, skin eruptions resembling acne, stretch marks

Less common side effects occur more frequently with the use of airtight bandages.

Why should this drug not be prescribed?

If you are sensitive to or have ever had an allergic reaction to fluticasone propionate or other drugs of this type, you should not use this medication. Make sure that your doctor is aware of any drug reactions that you have experienced.

Special warnings about this medication

Do not use this drug for any disorder other than the one for which it was prescribed.

The treated skin area should not be bandaged, covered, or wrapped unless you have been directed to do so by your doctor.

The use of tight-fitting diapers or plastic pants is not recommended for a child being treated in the diaper area. These garments may act as airtight dressings or bandages.

If an irritation or allergic reaction develops while using Cutivate, notify your doctor.

Possible food and drug interactions when taking this medication

No interactions with food or other drugs have been reported.

Special information if you are pregnant or breastfeeding

The effects of Cutivate during pregnancy have not been adequately studied. If you are pregnant or plan to become pregnant, inform your doctor immediately. It is not known whether this medication appears in breast milk. If this drug is essential to your health, your doctor may advise you to discontinue breastfeeding until your treatment is finished.

Recommended dosage

ADULTS

Apply a thin film of Cutivate cream or ointment to the affected skin areas 2 times a day. Rub in gently.

Your doctor may recommend airtight bandages or dressings if the medication is being used for psoriasis (a skin disorder characterized by patches of red, dry, scale-covered skin) or other stubborn skin conditions.

CHILDREN

Safety and effectiveness of this drug have not been established in children and infants.

Overdosage

A severe overdosage is unlikely with the use of Cutivate; however, long-term or prolonged use can produce various side effects.

Generic name:

CYCLOBENZAPRINE HYDROCHLORIDE

See Flexeril, page 261.

Brand name:

CYCLOCORT

Generic name: Amcinonide

Why is this drug prescribed?

Cyclocort is prescribed for the relief of the inflammatory and itchy symptoms of skin disorders that are responsive to corticosteroid treatment.

Most important fact about this drug

Absorption of this drug through the skin can affect the whole body as opposed to only the area being treated. It has produced reduced thyroid, pituitary, and adrenal gland function, symptoms of Cushing's syndrome (weight gain, reddening of the face and neck, growth of excess facial hair, high blood pressure, and mental disturbances), hyperglycemia (excess glucose in the blood), and glucosuria (urinary excretion of glucose) in some patients.

The use of this medication over large surface areas, prolonged use, and application of airtight dressings or bandages may cause this absorption. Your doctor should monitor your condition and periodically check the endocrine system, which controls your thyroid, pituitary, and adrenal gland function, if you are receiving a large dose of any potent steroid preparation applied to a large area of your skin.

How should you use this medication?

Use this medication exactly as prescribed by your doctor. It is for external use only. Avoid contact with the eyes.

What side effects may occur?

Side effects cannot be anticipated. If any develop or change in intensity, inform your doctor as soon as possible. Only your doctor can determine if it is safe for you to continue taking Cyclocort.

- *More common side effects may include:*
  Burning
  Itching
  Soreness
  Stinging

- *Less common or rare side effects may include:*
  Dryness, excessive growth of hair, infection, inflammation of hair follicles, inflammation of the skin around the mouth, irritation, prickly heat, skin eruptions resembling acne, softening of the skin, stretch marks

Why should this drug not be prescribed?

If you are sensitive to or have ever had an allergic reaction to amcinonide or other drugs of this type, you should not take this medication. Make sure that your doctor is aware of any drug reactions that you have experienced.

Special warnings about this medication

Do not use this drug for any disorder other than the one for which it was prescribed.

The use of tight-fitting diapers or plastic pants is not recommended for a child being treated in the diaper area. These garments may act as airtight dressings or bandages.

The treated skin area should not be bandaged, covered, or wrapped unless you have been directed to do so by your doctor.

If an irritation or allergic reaction develops while you are using Cyclocort, notify your doctor.

Possible food and drug interactions when taking this medication

No interactions with food or other drugs have been reported.

Special information if you are pregnant or breastfeeding

The effects of Cyclocort during pregnancy have not been adequately studied. If you are pregnant or plan to become pregnant, inform your doctor immediately. It is not known whether this medication appears in breast milk. If this drug is essential to your health, your doctor may advise you to discontinue breastfeeding until your treatment is finished.

Recommended dosage

ADULTS

A thin film of Cyclocort is usually applied to the affected area 2 or 3 times a day, depending on the severity of the condition.

The lotion may be applied topically to the specified areas, particularly hairy areas, 2 times per day. The lotion should be rubbed into the affected area completely, and the area should not be washed and should be protected from clothing or rubbing until the lotion has dried.

Your doctor may recommend airtight bandages or dressings if you are being treated for psoriasis (a skin disorder characterized by patches of red, dry, scale-covered skin) or other stubborn skin conditions. If an infection develops, stop bandaging the area.

CHILDREN

Topical use of Cyclocort on children should be limited to the smallest amount that is effective. Long-term treatment may interfere with the growth and development of children.

Overdosage

A severe overdosage is unlikely with the use of Cyclocort; however, long-term or prolonged use can produce various side effects.

Generic name:

CYCLOPHOSPHAMIDE

See Cytoxan, page 154.

Generic name:

CYCLOSPORINE

See Sandimmune, page 563.

Brand name:

CYLERT

Generic name: Pemoline

Why is this drug prescribed?

Cylert is used to help treat children who have attention deficit disorder with hyperactivity. However, this condition does not always require drug treatment. Drugs such as Cylert should be taken as part of a comprehensive treatment plan offering psychological and educational support to help the child become more stable.

Children who have attention deficit disorder with hyperactivity may show signs of:

Emotional mood swings
Hyperactivity
Impulsive actions
Moderate to severe distractibility
Short attention span

Most important fact about this drug

Because long-term use of drugs such as Cylert may affect a child's growth, children who take this drug for extended periods should be carefully monitored.

How should you take this medication?

Cylert should be taken once a day, in the morning.

What side effects may occur?

Side effects cannot be anticipated. If any develop or change in intensity, inform your doctor as soon as possible. Only your doctor can determine if it is safe for your child to continue taking Cylert.

■ *More common side effects may include:*
Insomnia

■ *Other side effects may include:*
Dizziness, drowsiness, hallucinations, headache, increased irritability, involuntary fragmented movements of the face, eyes, lips, tongue, arms, and legs, liver problems, loss of appetite, mild depression, nausea, seizures, skin rash, stomachache, suppressed growth (in children), uncontrolled vocal outbursts (such as grunts, shouts, and obscene language), weight loss, yellowing of skin or eyes

■ *Rare side effects may include:*
A rare form of anemia with symptoms such as bleeding gums, bruising, chest pain, fatigue, headache, nosebleeds, and pallor

Why should this drug not be prescribed?

You should not be using Cylert if you are allergic to it or if you have liver problems.

Special warnings about this medication

Cylert may cause dizziness. Warn your child to be cautious while climbing stairs or participating in activities that require mental alertness.

Although there have been no reports that Cylert is physically addictive, it is chemically similar to a class of drugs that are potentially addictive. Therefore, anyone who has a history of drug or alcohol abuse should use Cylert cautiously.

Long-term, excessive use of Cylert has caused temporary psychotic symptoms in some adults.

Although no cause-and-effect relationship has ever been established, there have been rare reports of death related to liver problems in some people taking Cylert.

Children who take this drug on a long-term basis should be carefully monitored because there have been reports that drugs such as Cylert can stunt growth.

You should use Cylert cautiously if you have kidney problems.

Psychotic children who take Cylert may experience increasingly disordered thoughts and behavioral disturbances.

Possible food and drug interactions when taking this medication

If Cylert is taken with certain other drugs, the effects of either could be increased, decreased, or altered. It is especially important to check with your doctor before combining Cylert with the following:

Antiepileptic medications such as Tegretol. Other central nervous system drugs, such as Ritalin

Special Information
If you are pregnant or breastfeeding

Pregnant women should use Cylert only if it is clearly necessary. Women who breastfeed should use this drug cautiously because it might appear in breast milk and affect the baby.

Recommended dosage

The recommended beginning dose is 37.5 milligrams daily. Dosages may be gradually increased if needed. Most patients take doses ranging from 56.25 to 75 milligrams a day. The maximum recommended daily dose of Cylert is 112.5 milligrams. Significant improvement is gradual and may not be apparent until the third or fourth week of treatment with Cylert.

Your doctor may occasionally stop treatment with Cylert to see whether behavioral problems return and whether further treatment with Cylert is necessary.

Overdosage

Any medication taken in excess can have serious consequences. If you suspect an overdose, seek medical help immediately.

Symptoms of Cylert overdose may include: Agitation, coma, confusion, convulsions, delirium, dilated pupils, euphoria, extremely high temperature, flushing, hallucinations, headache, high blood pressure, increased heart rate, increased reflex reactions, muscle twitches, sweating, tremors, vomiting

Generic name:

CYPROHEPTADINE HYDROCHLORIDE

See Periactin, page 467.

Brand name:

CYTOTEC

Generic name: Misoprostol

Why is this drug prescribed?

Cytotec, a synthetic prostaglandin (hormone-like substance), reduces the production of stomach acid and protects the stomach lining. People who take nonsteroidal anti-inflammatory drugs (NSAIDS) may be given Cytotec tablets to help prevent stomach ulcers.

Aspirin and other NSAIDS such as Motrin, Naprosyn, Ponstel, and others, which are widely used to control the pain and inflammation of arthritis, are generally hard on the stomach. If you must take an NSAID for a prolonged period of time, and if you are elderly or have ever had a stomach ulcer, your doctor may want you to take Cytotec for as long as you take the NSAID.

Most important fact about this drug

You must not become pregnant while using Cytotec. This drug causes uterine contractions that could lead to miscarriage. If miscarriage does occur, there is a risk that it might be incomplete. This could lead to bleeding, hospitalization, surgery, infertility, or even death. It is vitally important to use reliable contraception while taking Cytotec.

How should you take this medication?

Take Cytotec exactly as prescribed by your doctor. A typical dosage is four 200-microgram tablets per day, to be taken with food. If you cannot tolerate this dosage, your doctor may have you take four 100-microgram tablets per day. Take the final dosage at bedtime.

Never give Cytotec to any other person: the dosage might be wrong, and if the other person is pregnant, the drug might harm the unborn baby.

What side effects may occur?

Cytotec may cause abdominal cramps, diarrhea, and/or nausea, especially during the first few weeks of treatment. These symptoms may disappear as your body gets used to the drug. Taking Cytotec with food can help minimize these problems. If you have prolonged difficulty (more than 8 days), or if you have severe diarrhea, cramping and/or nausea, call your doctor.

■ *Other side effects may include:*
Abnormal taste, abnormal vision, aches, allergic reactions, anxiety, blood disorders, blood in urine, breast pain, breathing difficulty, bronchitis, changes in appetite, chest pain, constipation, deafness, depression, dizziness, drowsiness, earache, excessive sweating, fainting, fatigue, fever, fluid retention, gas, gastrointestinal bleeding, inflammation/infection, gout, headache, heavy menstrual bleeding, high blood pressure, impotence, inflammation of the eyelids and gums, irregular heart rate, loss of hair, loss of sexual desire, low blood pressure, menstrual pain, modified menstrual cycle, nervous system disturbances, nose bleeding, pain, pallor, phlebitis, pneumonia, rash, rectal disorders, rigors (alternating chills, fever and a feeling of heat and perspiration), ringing in ears, speech impairment, spotting (light bleeding between menstrual periods), thirst, upper respiratory tract infection, upset stomach, urinary tract infection, urination difficulty (painful or large volumes), uterine cramps, vomiting, weakness, weight changes

Cytotec may cause uterine bleeding even if you have gone through menopause. However, postmenopausal bleeding could be a sign of some other gynecological problem. If you experience any such bleeding while taking Cytotec, notify your doctor at once.

Why should this drug not be prescribed?

Do not take Cytotec if you are sensitive or have ever had an allergic reaction to it or to another prostaglandin medication.

Do not take Cytotec if you are pregnant or might become pregnant while taking it.

Special warnings about this medication

Since Cytotec may cause diarrhea, you should use this drug very cautiously if you have inflammatory bowel disease or any other condition in which dehydration would be particularly dangerous.

To reduce the risk of diarrhea, take Cytotec with food and avoid taking it with a magnesium-containing antacid, such as Di-Gel, Gelusil, Maalox, Mylanta, and others. Have frequent medical checkups.

Possible food and drug interactions when taking this medication

If Cytotec is taken with certain other drugs, the effects of either could be increased, decreased, or altered. It is especially important to check with your doctor before combining Cytotec with anti-arthritis medication containing phenylbutazone, such as Butazolidin or Butazolidin Alka.

Special information if you are pregnant or breastfeeding

If you are pregnant or plan to become pregnant, inform your doctor immediately. Because Cytotec can cause miscarriage, it should not be taken during pregnancy. If you are a woman of childbearing age, you should not take Cytotec unless you have thoroughly discussed the risks with your doctor and believe you are able to take effective contraceptive measures.

You will need to pass a pregnancy test at about 2 weeks before starting to take

Cytotec. To be sure you are not pregnant at the start of Cytotec treatment, your doctor will have you take your first dose on the second or third day of your menstrual period.

Even the most scrupulous contraceptive measures sometimes fail. If you believe you may have become pregnant while taking Cytotec, stop taking the drug and contact your doctor immediately.

Recommended dosage

ADULTS

The recommended oral dose of Cytotec for the prevention of NSAID-induced stomach ulcers is 200 micrograms 4 times daily with food. The last dose of the day should be at bedtime.

If this dose cannot be tolerated, a dose of 100 micrograms can be used.

Cytotec should be taken for the duration of NSAID therapy as prescribed by your doctor.

For Patients with Kidney Impairment
Adjustment of the dosing schedule in patients with impaired kidney function is not routinely needed, but dosage can be reduced if the 200-microgram dose is not tolerated.

Overdosage

Any medication taken in excess can have serious consequences. If you suspect symptoms of an overdose of Cytotec, seek medical attention immediately.

Symptoms of Cytotec overdose may include:
Abdominal pain
Breathing difficulty
Convulsions
Diarrhea
Fever
Heart palpitations
Low blood pressure

Sedation (extreme drowsiness)
Slowed heartbeat
Stomach or intestinal discomfort
Tremors

Brand name:

CYTOXAN

Generic name: Cyclophosphamide

Why is this drug prescribed?

Cytoxan, an anticancer drug, works by interfering with the growth of malignant cells. It may be used alone but is often given with other anticancer medications.

Cytoxan is used in the treatment of the following types of cancer:

Breast cancer
Leukemias (cancers affecting the white
    blood cells)
Malignant lymphomas (Hodgkin's disease or
    cancer of the lymph nodes)
Multiple myeloma (a malignant condition or
    cancer of the plasma cells)
Advanced mycosis fungoides (cancer of the
    skin and lymph nodes)
Neuroblastoma (a malignant tumor of
    the adrenal gland or sympathetic
    nervous system)
Ovarian cancer (adenocarcinoma)
Retinoblastoma (a malignant tumor of the
    retina)

In addition, Cytoxan may sometimes be given to children who have "minimal change" nephrotic syndrome (kidney damage resulting in loss of protein in the urine) and who have not responded well to treatment with adrenal corticosteroids.

Most important fact about this drug

Cytoxan may cause bladder damage, probably from toxic by-products of the drug that are excreted in the urine. Potential problems include bladder infection with bleeding and fibrosis of the bladder.

While you are being treated with Cytoxan, drink 3 or 4 liters of fluid a day to help prevent bladder problems. Forcing fluids will dilute your urine and make you urinate frequently, thus minimizing the Cytoxan by-products' contact with your bladder.

How should you take this medication?

Take Cytoxan exactly as prescribed by your doctor. You will undergo frequent blood tests, and the doctor will adjust your dosage depending on the evolution of your white blood cell count; a dosage reduction is necessary if the count drops below a certain level. You will also have frequent urine tests to check for blood in the urine, a sign of bladder damage.

Take Cytoxan on an empty stomach. If stomach upset is severe, take with food.

If you are unable to swallow the tablet form, you may be given an oral solution made from the injectable form of Cytoxan and Aromatic Elixir. This solution should be stored in the refrigerator and used within 14 days.

What side effects may occur?

Side effects cannot be anticipated. If any develop or change in intensity, inform your doctor immediately. Only your doctor can determine if it is safe for you to continue using Cytoxan.

One possible Cytoxan side effect is the development of a secondary cancer, typically of the bladder, lymph nodes, or bone marrow. A secondary cancer may occur up to several years after the drug is given.

Noncancerous bladder problems may occur during Cytoxan therapy (see "Most important fact about this drug" section, above).

■ *More common side effects may include:*
Loss of appetite
Nausea and vomiting

■ *Less common side effects may include:*
Abdominal pain, darkening of skin and
fingernails, decreased sperm count,
diarrhea, impaired wound healing, mouth
sores, new tumor growth, prolonged
impairment of fertility or temporary sterility
in men, rash, temporary failure to
menstruate, temporary hair loss

Why should this drug not be prescribed?

Do not take this medication if you have ever
had an allergic reaction to it. Also, tell
your doctor if you have ever had an allergic
reaction to another alkylating anticancer
drug such as Alkeran, CeeNU, Emcyt,
Leukeran, Myleran, or Zanosar.

In adults, Cytoxan should not be given for
"minimal change" nephrotic syndrome or
any other kidney disease.

Also, Cytoxan should not be given to anyone
who is unable to produce normal blood
cells due to severely depressed bone marrow
function.

Special warnings about this medication

You are at increased risk for toxic side effects
from Cytoxan if you have any of the
following conditions:

Blood disorder (low white blood cell or
    platelet count)
Bone marrow tumors
Kidney disorder
Liver disorder
Past anticancer therapy
Past X-ray therapy

Possible food and drug interactions when taking this medication

If Cytoxan is taken with certain other drugs,
the effects of either could be increased,

decreased, or altered. It is especially important
to check with your doctor before
combining Cytoxan with the following:

Adriamycin (another anticancer drug)
Anectine (used in anesthesia)
Phenobarbital

If you take adrenal steroid hormones because
you have had your adrenal glands
removed, you are at increased risk for toxic
effects from Cytoxan; your dosage of both
steroids and Cytoxan may need to be
modified.

Special information if you are pregnant or breastfeeding

If you are pregnant or plan to become
pregnant, inform your doctor immediately.
When taken during pregnancy, Cytoxan
can cause defects in the unborn baby. Women
taking Cytoxan should use effective
contraception.

Cytoxan does find its way into breast milk.
A new mother will need to choose
between taking this drug and nursing her
baby.

Recommended dosage

ADULTS AND CHILDREN

Malignant Diseases
Your doctor will tailor your dosage according
to your condition and other drugs taken with
Cytoxan.

The recommended oral dosage range is 1 to
5 milligrams per 2.2 pounds of body
weight per day.

"Minimal Change" Nephrotic Syndrome
The recommended oral dosage is 2.5 to 3
milligrams per 2.2 pounds of body weight
per day for a period of 60 to 90 days.

Overdosage

Any medication taken in excess can have serious consequences. If you suspect an overdose, seek medical attention immediately.

Brand name:

DDAVP

Generic name: Desmopressin acetate

Why is this drug prescribed?

DDAVP is an antidiuretic hormone given to prevent or control the frequent urination and loss of water associated with diabetes insipidus (a rare condition characterized by very large quantities of diluted urine and excessive thirst). It is also used to treat frequent passage of urine and increased thirst in patients with certain brain injuries, and to help stop some types of childhood bedwetting.

DDAVP is available as a nasal spray in a pump bottle, or as nose drops to be instilled using a soft plastic tube. An injectable form of DDAVP is also available.

Most important fact about this drug

DDAVP is not effective for the treatment of nephrogenic diabetes insipidus, a form of the disorder caused by malfunctioning kidneys. This condition may be present from birth or may develop as a result of a kidney disease called pyelonephritis.

How should you use this medication?

Use DDAVP exactly as prescribed. The spray and drops are for nasal use only; never swallow the medication.

Your doctor may increase or decrease your dosage, depending on how you respond to DDAVP. Your response will be judged by how long you are able to sleep without having to get up to urinate and how much urine your kidneys produce.

Keep your DDAVP nasal spray or nose drops in the refrigerator. If you travel, you may store the medication at controlled room temperature (72 degrees Fahrenheit) for up to three weeks.

The DDAVP nasal spray pump bottle accurately delivers exactly 50 doses of the medication. After the fiftieth dose, the amount of medication that comes out with each spray will no longer be a full dose. When this happens, throw the bottle away even if it is not completely empty.

Since the DDAVP spray bottle delivers only a standard-sized dose, infants or children who need less medication should be given the nose drops instead of the spray.

If scars or swelling inside the nose make it difficult to absorb DDAVP efficiently, your doctor may consider giving you an injectable form of the drug.

What side effects may occur?

Too high a dosage of DDAVP may produce headache or nausea, which will probably disappear when the dosage is reduced. Some people have complained of nosebleed, sore throat, cough, or a cold or other upper respiratory infections after taking DDAVP.

Other potential side effects include:
Abdominal cramps (mild), chills, conjunctivitis (inflamed eyelids), depression, disruption in the output of tears, dizziness, flushing, nasal congestion, nostril pain, rash, runny or stuffy nose, swelling around the eyes, upset stomach, weakness

Why should this drug not be prescribed?

Do not use DDAVP if you are sensitive to it or have ever had an allergic reaction to it.

Special warnings about this medication

Patients who have central cranial diabetes insipidus, especially elderly and very young patients, should limit their fluid intake. Otherwise, water intoxication and too little sodium in the blood could lead to seizures.

If you have cystic fibrosis or any other condition that causes a mineral imbalance (low level of sodium in the blood), you should use DDAVP with extreme caution: This medication could place you at greater risk of seizures.

Because DDAVP may cause a rise in blood pressure, use this medication cautiously if you have high blood pressure and/or coronary artery disease.

Possible food and drug interactions when taking this medication

If DDAVP is taken with certain other drugs, the effects of either could be increased, decreased, or altered. It is especially important to check with your doctor before combining DDAVP with epinephrine (adrenaline) or any other drug used to increased blood pressure.

Special information if you are pregnant or breastfeeding

If you are pregnant or plan to become pregnant, inform your doctor immediately. Although DDAVP is not known to cause birth defects, it should be used with caution. DDAVP should be taken during pregnancy only if clearly needed.

DDAVP apparently does not appear in breast milk. However, check with your doctor before using the drug while breastfeeding.

Recommended dosage

Your doctor will carefully tailor your dosage to meet your individual needs.

PRIMARY NOCTURNAL ENURESIS (BEDWETTING)

Children 6 Years of Age and Older
The usual recommended dose taken through

the nose is 20 micrograms or 0.2 milliliters at bedtime. Dosage requirements range from 10 to 40 micrograms. It is recommended that one-half the dose be taken in each nostril.

CENTRAL CRANIAL DIABETES INSIPIDUS

Adults
The usual recommended dosage range for adults is 0.1 to 0.4 milliliter daily, either as a single dose or in divided doses.

Children
The usual dosage range for children aged 3 months to 12 years is 0.05 to 0.3 milliliter daily, either as a single dose or divided into 2 doses. About one-quarter to one-third of cases can be controlled by a single daily dose of DDAVP administered by nose spray.

Overdosage

An overdose of DDAVP may cause headache or nausea. Lowering the dosage should correct any problems.

Any medication taken in excess can have serious consequences. If you suspect an overdose of DDAVP, seek medical attention.

Brand name:

DALMANE

Generic name: Flurazepam hydrochloride

Why is this drug prescribed?

Dalmane is used for the relief of insomnia, difficulty falling asleep, waking up frequently at night or waking up early in the morning. It belongs to a class of drugs known as benzodiazepines.

Most important fact about this drug

Tolerance and dependence can occur with the use of Dalmane. You may experience withdrawal symptoms if you stop using this drug abruptly. Discontinue or change your dose only in consultation with your doctor.

How should you take this medication?

Take this medication exactly as prescribed by your doctor.

What side effects may occur?

Side effects cannot be anticipated. If any develop or change in intensity, inform your doctor as soon as possible. Only your doctor can determine if it is safe for you to continue taking Dalmane.

■ *More common side effects may include:*
Dizziness
Drowsiness
Falling
Lack of muscular coordination
Light-headedness
Staggering

■ *Less common or rare side effects may include:*
Apprehension, bitter taste, blood disorder, blurred vision, body and joint pain, burning eyes, chest pains, confusion, constipation, depression, diarrhea, difficulty in focusing, dry mouth, exaggerated feeling of well-being, excessive salivation, excitement, faintness, flushes, genital and urinary tract disorders, hallucinations, headache, heartburn, hyperactivity, irritability, itching, loss of appetite, low blood pressure, nausea and vomiting, nervousness, palpitation, restlessness, shortness of breath, skin rash, slurred speech, stimulation, stomach upset and abdominal pain, sweating, talkativeness, weakness

■ *Side effects due to rapid decrease or abrupt withdrawal from Dalmane:*
Abdominal and muscle cramps
Convulsions
Depressed mood
Inability to fall asleep or stay asleep
Sweating

Tremors
Vomiting

Why should this drug not be prescribed?

If you are sensitive to or have had an allergic reaction to Dalmane or similar drugs, you should not take this medication. Make sure that your doctor is aware of any drug reactions that you have experienced.

Special warnings about this medication

Dalmane will cause you to become drowsy or less alert; therefore, driving or operating dangerous machinery or participating in any hazardous activity that requires full mental alertness is not recommended.

If you are severely depressed or have suffered from severe depression, consult with your doctor before taking this medication.

If you have decreased kidney or liver function or chronic respiratory or lung disease, use of this drug should be discussed with your doctor.

Possible food and drug interactions when taking this medication

Alcohol intensifies the effects of Dalmane. Do not drink alcohol while taking this medication.

If Dalmane is taken with certain other drugs, the effects of either could be increased, decreased, or altered. It is especially important to check with your doctor before combining Dalmane with an antihistamine, sleep-inducing medication or any drug that affects the central nervous system such as tranquilizers.

Special information if you are pregnant or breastfeeding

Do not take Dalmane if you are pregnant or planning to become pregnant. There is an increased risk of birth defects. This drug may appear in breast milk and could affect a nursing infant. If this medication is essential to your health, your doctor may advise you to discontinue breastfeeding until your treatment with Dalmane is finished.

Recommended dosage

ADULTS

The usual recommended dose is 30 milligrams at bedtime; however 15 milligrams may be all that is necessary. Your dose should be individualized to your needs by your doctor.

CHILDREN

Safety and effectiveness of Dalmane have not been established in children under 15 years of age.

ELDERLY

Dosage should be limited to the smallest effective amount to avoid over-sedation, dizziness, confusion or lack of muscle coordination. The usual recommended initial dose is 15 milligrams.

Overdosage

Any medication taken in excess can cause symptoms of overdose. If you suspect an overdose, seek medical attention immediately.

The symptoms of Dalmane overdose may include:
Coma
Confusion
Low blood pressure
Sleepiness

Brand name:

DANTRIUM

Generic name: Dantrolene sodium

Why is this drug prescribed?

Dantrium, a muscle relaxant, is given to relieve muscle spasm caused by conditions such as cerebral palsy, multiple sclerosis, spinal cord injury, or stroke.

In addition, Dantrium is used to prevent or manage malignant hyperthermia, a life-threatening rapid rise in body temperature that sometimes develops as an adverse reaction to anesthesia.

Most important fact about this drug

Dantrium has the potential of causing serious or even fatal liver damage, including hepatitis and jaundice. Women and people of either sex who are past the age of 35 seem to be at increased risk for Dantrium-related liver damage as do those taking other medications at the same time.

Before you take Dantrium, your doctor will perform blood tests to evaluate your liver function; these tests should be repeated at regular intervals while you are taking Dantrium.

How should you take this medication?

Dantrium is available in capsule and injectable form. Take Dantrium capsules exactly as prescribed by your doctor.

Dantrium may cause dizziness, light-headedness, and drowsiness. You should use caution when driving or performing tasks that require alertness.

Avoid alcoholic beverages and other drugs that can cause drowsiness.

Dantrium can make skin more sensitive to sunlight. Avoid prolonged exposure.

Dantrium may cause feelings of suffocation; exercise caution while eating to avoid choking. This danger is greatest on the day of administration of the injectable form.

You may notice a decrease in the strength of your grip and weakness in your leg muscles, especially when walking down stairs, after receiving the injectable form of Dantrium.

What side effects may occur?

Side effects cannot be anticipated. If any develop or change in intensity, inform your doctor as soon as possible. Only your doctor can determine if it is safe for you to continue taking Dantrium.

■ *More common side effects may include:*
Diarrhea
Dizziness
Drowsiness
Fatigue
Malaise
Weakness

■ *Less common side effects may include:*
Abdominal cramps, acne-like rash, chills, confusion, constipation, depression, difficulty swallowing, fever, hives, itching, light-headedness, loss of appetite, nervousness, rapid heart rate, speech disturbances, stomach irritation with bleeding, stomach upset, swelling, unusual hair growth, urinary frequency and other urinary problems, visual disturbances

Diarrhea may abate if the dosage is reduced. If not, Dantrium treatment should be stopped temporarily. If the diarrhea starts again as soon as Dantrium is given, treatment with Dantrium should be stopped permanently.

Why should this drug not be prescribed?

Do not take this medication if you are sensitive to it or have ever had an allergic reaction to it.

You should not take Dantrium if you have active liver disease, such as hepatitis or cirrhosis.

If you use the spasms of your leg or trunk muscles to help you to sit upright, stand,

or walk, Dantrium may be unsuitable for you; by relaxing these muscles, the medication could actually increase your disability.

Special warnings about this medication

If you have heart disease or obstructive lung disease, or if you have ever had liver disease, you should be monitored very closely while taking Dantrium.

Do not drive, climb, or operate dangerous machinery while taking Dantrium, since the sedative effect could impair your judgment or coordination.

Because of the risk of liver damage, your doctor will stop Dantrium therapy after 45 days if the drug has not helped you by that time.

Possible food and drug interactions when taking this medication

While taking Dantrium, check with your doctor before taking tranquilizers of any kind.

In women over the age of 35, the risk of liver damage from Dantrium is increased if estrogen (e.g., Premarin) is taken simultaneously.

While taking Dantrium, it is advisable to avoid taking the heart medication verapamil (Calan, Isoptin); in some people this combination of drugs may cause heart problems.

Special information if you are pregnant or breastfeeding

If you are pregnant or plan to become pregnant, inform your doctor immediately. No information is available about the safety of Dantrium during pregnancy. The drug should not be taken by women who are breastfeeding.

Recommended dosage

CHRONIC SPASTICITY

Adults
Your doctor will tailor your dose depending on the severity of your condition.

The usual initial dose is 25 milligrams once daily. Your doctor may increase the total daily dose by 25 milligrams every 4 to 7 days until optimal results are obtained or until a dosage of 100 milligrams 4 times a day is reached.

Children
The usual starting dose is 0.5 milligram per 2.2 pounds of body weight 2 times daily; this is increased to 0.5 milligram per 2.2 pounds 3 or 4 times daily and then by increments of 0.5 milligram per 2.2 pounds up to as high as 3.0 milligrams per 2.2 pounds 2, 3, or 4 times daily, if necessary.

Doses higher than 100 milligrams 4 times daily should not be used in children.

MALIGNANT HYPERTHERMIA

Dosages for maligant hyperthermia are closely monitored by your doctor, usually in the hospital.

Overdosage

Although no specific information is available on Dantrium overdosage, any medication taken in excess can have serious consequences. If you suspect an overdose, seek emergency medical attention immediately.

Generic name:

DANTROLENE SODIUM

See Dantrium, page 159.

Brand name:

DARVOCET-N

Generic ingredients: Propoxyphene napsylate, Acetaminophen
Other brand names: Darvon-N (contains propoxyphene napsylate only)

Why is this drug prescribed?

Darvocet-N is a mild narcotic pain reliever prescribed for the relief of mild to moderate pain, with or without fever.

Darvon-N is prescribed for the relief of mild to moderate pain.

Most important fact about this drug

Tolerance and dependence can occur with the use of propoxyphene when it is taken in higher than recommended doses over long periods of time.

How should you take this medication?

Take Darvocet-N and Darvon-N exactly as prescribed by your doctor. Do not increase the amount you take without your doctor's approval. If you miss a dose of this medication, do not double your dosage. Do not take this drug for any reason other than its proper indications.

Do not give these drugs to others who may have similar symptoms.

What side effects may occur?

Side effects cannot be anticipated. If any develop or change in intensity, inform your doctor as soon as possible. Only your doctor can determine if it is safe for you to continue taking propoxyphene.

■ *More common side effects may include:*
Drowsiness
Dizziness
Nausea
Sedation
Vomiting

If these side effects occur, it may help if you lie down after taking the medication.

■ *Less common side effects may include:* Abdominal pain, constipation, feelings of elation or discomfort, hallucinations, headache, lightheadedness, minor visual disturbances, skin rashes, weakness

Why should this drug not be prescribed?

If you are sensitive to or have ever had an allergic reaction to propoxyphene, acetaminophen (Tylenol), or drugs of this type, you should not take this medication. Make sure that your doctor is aware of any drug reactions that you have experienced.

Unless you are directed to do so by your doctor, do not take this medication if you are severely depressed or have ever suffered from severe depression.

Special warnings about this medication

Propoxyphene may cause you to become drowsy or less alert; therefore, driving or operating dangerous machinery or participating in any hazardous activity that requires full mental alertness is not recommended until you know your response to this drug.

If you have a kidney or liver disorder, consult with your doctor before taking propoxyphene.

Possible food and drug interactions when taking this medication

Propoxyphene is a central nervous system depressant and intensifies the effects of alcohol. Heavy use of alcohol with this drug may cause overdose symptoms. Therefore, use of alcohol should be avoided with this medication.

If propoxyphene is taken with certain other drugs, the effects of either could be increased, decreased, or altered. It is especially important to check with your doctor before combining propoxyphene with the following:

Anticonvulsants such as Tegretol
Antidepressant drugs such as Elavil
Antihistamines such as Benadryl
Muscle relaxants such as Flexeril
Sleep aids such as Halcion
Tranquilizers such as Xanax, Valium
Warfarin-like drugs such as Coumadin

The use of these drugs with propoxyphene increases their sedative or calming effects and may lead to overdose symptoms, including death.

Severe neurologic disorders, including coma, have occurred with the use of propoxyphene in combination with anticonvulsant drugs (e.g., Tegretol).

Special information if you are pregnant or breastfeeding

Do not take propoxyphene if you are pregnant or planning to become pregnant unless you are directed to do so by your doctor. Temporary drug dependence may occur in newborns when the mother has taken this drug consistently in the weeks before delivery. Propoxyphene does appear in breast milk. However, no adverse effects have been found in nursing infants.

Recommended dosage

ADULTS

The usual dose of Darvocet-N 50 is 2 tablets given every 4 hours for pain as needed. The usual dose of Darvocet-N 100 is 1 tablet given every 4 hours for pain as needed.

Your doctor may prescribe reduced total daily dosage if you have kidney or liver impairment.

The maximum recommended dose of Darvon-N is 6 tablets per day or 60 milliliters of Darvon-N suspension per day.

CHILDREN

The safety and effectiveness of propoxyphene have not been established in children.

ELDERLY

Your doctor will prescribe a dose individualized to suit your needs.

Overdosage

Symptoms of an overdose of Darvon-N, alone or in combination with other drugs, may include weakness, difficulty breathing, confusion, anxiety, and more severe drowsiness and dizziness. Extreme overdosage may lead to unconsciousness and death.

Symptoms of an overdose of Darvocet-N may include changes in heart rhythm, coma, convulsions, dilated pupils, low blood pressure, lowered heart function, stoppage in breathing, stupor.

If you suspect symptoms of a Darvocet-N or Darvon-N overdose, seek medical attention immediately.

Brand name:

DARVON

Generic name: Propoxyphene hydrochloride
Other brand name: Darvon Compound-65
(Compound-65 also contains aspirin and caffeine)

Why is this drug prescribed?

Propoxyphene is a mild narcotic prescribed for the relief of mild to moderate pain. Darvon Compound-65 is prescribed for the relief of mild to moderate pain, either when pain is present alone or when it is accompanied by fever.

Most important fact about this drug

Tolerance and dependence can occur with the use of propoxyphene when taken in higher than recommended doses over long periods of time.

How should you take this medication?

Take propoxyphene exactly as prescribed by your doctor. Do not increase the amount you take without your doctor's approval. If you miss a dose of this medication, do not double your dosage. Do not take these drugs for any reason other than their proper indications. Do not give these drugs to others who may have similar symptoms.

What side effects may occur?

Side effects cannot be anticipated. If any develop or change in intensity, inform your doctor as soon as possible. Only your doctor can determine if it is safe for you to continue taking propoxyphene.

■ *More common side effects may include:*
Dizziness
Drowsiness
Nausea
Sedation
Vomiting

If these side effects occur, it may help if you lie down after taking the medication.

■ *Less common or rare side effects may include:*
Abdominal pain, constipation, feelings of elation or discomfort, hallucinations, headache, lightheadedness, minor visual disturbances, skin rashes, weakness

Why should this drug not be prescribed?

If you are sensitive to or have ever had an allergic reaction to propoxyphene, aspirin, caffeine, or drugs of this type, you should not take this medication. Make sure that your doctor is aware of any drug reactions that you have experienced.

Unless you are directed to do so by your doctor, do not take this medication if you are severely depressed or have ever suffered from severe depression.

Because there is a possible association between aspirin and Reye's syndrome, Darvon Compound-65 should not be given to children and teenagers who have chickenpox or flu unless prescribed by a doctor.

Special warnings about this medication

Propoxyphene may cause you to become drowsy or less alert; therefore, driving or operating dangerous machinery or participating in any hazardous activity that requires full mental alertness is not recommended until you know your response to this drug.

Darvon Compound-65 contains aspirin and caffeine. If you have an ulcer, consult with your doctor before taking Darvon Compound-65. Aspirin may irritate the stomach lining and may cause bleeding.

If you have a kidney or liver disorder, consult with your doctor before taking propoxyphene.

Aspirin may cause asthma attacks. If you have had an asthma attack while taking aspirin, consult with your doctor before taking Darvon Compound-65.

Possible food and drug interactions when taking this medication

Propoxyphene is a central nervous system depressant and intensifies the effects of alcohol. Heavy use of alcohol with this drug may cause overdose symptoms. Therefore, limit your use of alcohol with this medication.

If propoxyphene is taken with certain other drugs, the effects of either could be increased, decreased, or altered. It is especially important to check with your doctor before combining propoxyphene with the following:

Anticonvulsants such as Tegretol
Antidepressant drugs such as Elavil
Antihistamines such as Benadryl
Muscle relaxants such as Flexeril
Sleep aids
Tranquilizers such as Xanax, Valium
Warfarin-like drugs such as Coumadin

The use of these drugs with propoxyphene increases their sedative or calming effects and may lead to overdose symptoms, including death.

The use of anticoagulants (blood thinners) in combination with propoxyphene may cause bleeding. If you are taking an anticoagulant, consult with your doctor before taking this drug.

The use of aspirin in combination with uricosuric (antigout) drugs may alter the effects of the antigout medication in the body. Consult with your doctor before taking Darvon Compound-65.

Severe neurologic disorders, including coma, have occurred with the use of propoxyphene in combination with anticonvulsant drugs (e.g., Tegretol).

Special information if you are pregnant or breastfeeding

Do not take propoxyphene if you are pregnant or planning to become pregnant, unless you are directed to do so by your doctor. Temporary drug dependence may occur in newborns when the mother has taken this drug consistently in the weeks before delivery. The use of Darvon Compound-65 (which contains aspirin) during pregnancy may cause problems in the unborn child or complications during delivery. Propoxyphene does appear in breast milk. However, no adverse effects have been found in nursing infants.

Recommended dosage

ADULTS

The usual dose of Darvon is 1 capsule (65 milligrams) taken every 4 hours as needed for pain.

The usual dose of Darvon Compound-65 is 1 capsule (65 milligrams propoxyphene hydrochloride, 389 milligrams aspirin, and 32.4 milligrams caffeine) taken every 4 hours as needed for pain.

The maximum propoxyphene hydrochloride dose is 390 milligrams for 1 day.

Your doctor may prescribe a reduced total daily dosage if you have kidney or liver impairment.

CHILDREN

The safety and effectiveness of propoxyphene have not been established in children.

ELDERLY

Your doctor will prescribe a dose individualized to suit your needs.

Overdosage

Symptoms of an overdose of Darvon, alone or in combination with other drugs, may include weakness, difficulty breathing, confusion, anxiety, and more severe drowsiness and dizziness. Extreme overdosage may lead to unconsciousness and death.

Symptoms of an overdose of Darvon Compound-65 may include:
Coma
Convulsions

Decreased heart function
Dilated pupils
Low blood pressure
Stupor
Temporary stoppage in breathing

Brand name:

DECADRON TABLETS

Generic name: Dexamethasone

Why is this drug prescribed?

Decadron, a corticosteriod drug, is used to reduce inflammation and relieve symptoms in a variety of disorders, including rheumatoid arthritis and severe cases of asthma. It may be given to people to treat primary or secondary adrenal cortex insufficiency (lack of sufficient adrenal hormone). It is also given to help treat the following disorders:

Severe allergic conditions such as
    drug-induced allergies
Blood disorders such as leukemia and various
    anemias
Certain cancers (along with other drugs)
Skin diseases such as severe psoriasis
Collagen (connective tissue) diseases such as
    systemic lupus erythematosus
Digestive tract disease such as ulcerative
    colitis
High serum levels of calcium associated with
    cancer
Fluid retention due to nephrotic syndrome
    (a condition in which damage to the
    kidneys causes loss of protein in the
    urine)
Eye diseases of various kinds
Lung diseases (tuberculosis)

Most important fact about this drug

Decadron decreases your resistance to infection and may mask some of the signs and symptoms of a new infection, making it difficult to diagnose.

You should not be vaccinated or immunized while taking Decadron, especially in high doses. Decadron may prevent your body from producing the proper antibodies to build up immunity.

How should you take this medication?

Decadron should be taken exactly as prescribed by your doctor.

If you are taking large doses, your doctor may advise you to take Decadron with meals and to take antacids between meals, to prevent a peptic ulcer from developing.

Decadron should not be stopped suddenly without checking with your doctor. If you have been using this medication for long-term treatment, it should be reduced gradually.

The lowest possible dose should always be used, and as symptoms subside, dosage should be reduced gradually.

What side effects may occur?

Side effects cannot be anticipated. If any develop or change in intensity, inform your doctor as soon as possible. Only your doctor can determine if it is safe for you to continue taking Decadron.

■ *Side effects may include:*
Abdominal distention, allergic reactions, blood clots, bone fractures and degeneration, bruises, cataracts, congestive heart failure, convulsions, cushingoid symptoms (moon face, weight gain, high blood pressure, emotional disturbances, growth of facial hair in women), emotional disturbances, excessive hairiness, fluid and salt retention, general feeling of illness, glaucoma, headache, hiccups, high blood pressure, hives, increased appetite, increased eye pressure, increased pressure in head, increased sweating, increases in amounts of insulin or hypoglycemic medications needed in

diabetes, inflammation of the esophagus, inflammation of the pancreas, irregular menstruation, loss of muscle mass, low potassium levels in blood leading to symptoms such as dry mouth, excessive thirst, weak or irregular heartbeat, and muscle pain or cramps, menstruation, muscle weakness and disease, nausea, osteoporosis, peptic ulcer, perforated small and large bowel, poor healing of wounds, protruding eyeballs, ruptured tendons, suppression of growth in children, thin, fragile skin, tiny red or purplish spots on the skin, vertigo, weight gain

Why should this drug not be prescribed?

Decadron should not be used if you have a fungal infection, or if you are sensitive or allergic to any of its ingredients.

Special warnings about this medication

Decadron can alter the way your body responds to unusual stress. If you are injured, need surgery, or develop an acute illness, inform your doctor. Your dosage may need to be increased.

Decadron may reactivate a dormant case of tuberculosis. If you have inactive tuberculosis and must take Decadron for an extended period, your doctor will prescribe anti-TB medication as well.

When you stop taking Decadron after long-term therapy, you may develop withdrawal symptoms such as fever, muscle or joint pain, and a feeling of illness.

Long-term use of Decadron may cause cataracts, glaucoma, and eye infections.

Decadron should be used cautiously if you have an underactive thyroid, cirrhosis, or herpes simplex of the eye, or if you have recently had a heart attack.

Aspirin should be used cautiously with Decadron if you have a blood-clotting disorder.

Decadron should also be given with caution if you have any of the following conditions:

Diverticulitis or other inflammatory condition of the intestine
High blood pressure
Certain kidney disease
Active or dormant peptic ulcer
Myasthenia gravis (a muscle disorder)
Osteoporosis (brittle bones)
Ulcerative colitis with impending danger of infection

Steroids may alter male fertility.

This medication can aggravate existing emotional problems or cause emotional disturbances. Symptoms range from euphoria (an exaggerated sense of well-being) and difficulty sleeping to mood swings and psychotic episodes. If you experience any changes in mood, contact your doctor.

Possible food and drug interactions when taking this medication

If Decadron is taken with certain other drugs, the effects of either could be increased, decreased, or altered. It is especially important to check with your doctor before combining Decadron with the following:

Blood-thinning medications such as Coumadin and Panwarfin
Ephedrine
Indomethacin (Indocin)
Phenobarbital
Phenytoin (Dilantin)
Potassium-depleting diuretics such as HydroDIURIL
Rifampin (Rifadin, Rimactane)

Special information if you are pregnant or breastfeeding

The effects of Decadron during pregnancy have not been adequately studied. If you are pregnant or plan to become pregnant, inform your doctor immediately. Infants born to mothers who have taken substantial doses of corticosteroids during pregnancy should be carefully watched for adrenal problems. Corticosteroids appear in breast milk and can suppress growth in infants. If Decadron is essential to your health, your doctor may advise you to stop breastfeeding until your treatment with Decadron is finished.

Recommended dosage

ADULTS

Your doctor will tailor your individual dose to the condition being treated. Initial doses range from 0.75 milligram to 9 milligrams a day.

After the drug produces a satisfactory response, your doctor will gradually lower the dose to the minimum effective level.

Overdosage

Reports of overdose with this medication are rare. However, if you suspect an overdose, seek medical treatment immediately.

Brand name:

DECADRON TURBINAIRE AND RESPIHALER

Generic name: Dexamethasone sodium phosphate

Why is this drug prescribed?

Decadron is a synthetic adrenocortical steroid (a hormone created in the laboratory). Decadron Turbinaire is used to treat nasal problems caused by allergy, inflammation, and polyps. Decadron Respihaler treats bronchial asthma and similar bronchial conditions that have not improved with other therapies.

Most important fact about this drug

You should not be vaccinated or immunized while taking Decadron, especially in high doses. Decadron may prevent your body from producing the proper antibodies to build up immunity.

How should you take this medication?

Decadron should be taken exactly as prescribed by your doctor.

Decadron should be stored at room temperature. Since the contents are under pressure, make sure the container is not broken, stored in extreme heat, or burned.

What side effects may occur?

Side effects cannot be anticipated. If any develop or change in intensity, inform your doctor as soon as possible. Only your doctor can determine whether it is safe to continue using Decadron.

■ *More common side effects of Decadron Turbinaire may include:*
Headache
Nasal dryness
Nasal irritation

■ *Less common side effects of Decadron Turbinaire may include:*
Bronchial asthma, hives, lightheadedness, loss of smell, nausea, nosebleeds, perforated nasal septum (dividing wall of the nose), rebound nasal congestion, throat discomfort

■ *Side effects of Decadron Resphilaler may include:*
Coughing
Fungal infections in the throat
Hoarseness
Throat irritation

■ *Side effects that may occur when Decadron is absorbed into the bloodstream:*

Abdominal distension, abnormal skin redness, allergic skin reactions, blood clots, cataracts, congestive heart failure, convulsions, development of Cushing's syndrome (moon face, emotional disturbances, high blood pressure, weight gain, and growth of facial and body hair in women), diabetes, dizziness, emotional disturbances, eroding of femoral and humeral heads, fractures of the long bones, fractures of the vertebra, fragile skin, glaucoma, headache, hiccups, high blood pressure, hives, increased appetite, increased eye pressure, increased pressure in head, increased sweating, loss of muscle mass, menstrual irregularities, muscle diseases caused by steroid use, muscle weakness, nausea, osteoporosis, peptic ulcer with possible perforation and bleeding, perforated small or large bowel, poor wound healing, potassium loss, protruding eyeballs, reddish or purplish spots on the skin, ruptured tendons, salt and fluid retention, vague feeling of weakness, weight gain

Why should this drug not be prescribed?

Do not use Decadron if you have a fungal infection or if you have ever had an allergic reaction or are sensitive to any of its ingredients. Decadron Turbinaire should not be used if you have tuberculosis, a nasal condition caused by a virus or a fungus, or herpes simplex infection of the eye. Decadron Respihaler should not be used if sputum cultures show that you have a yeast infection (*Candida albicans*).

Special warnings about this medication

Decadron Respihaler should not be used for occasional or isolated attacks of asthma or for severe asthmatic attacks. However, it should be used if you have not had adequate results from other non-steroid therapies, or if you are taking corticosteroids orally and your doctor wants to reduce the amount of steroids in your bloodstream.

Decadron can alter the way your body responds to unusual stress. If you are injured, need surgery, or develop an acute illness, tell your doctor. Your dosage may need to be increased.

If you develop a fungus infection of the larynx or pharynx while using the Decadron Respihaler, stop using the respihaler and start taking prescribed medication to treat the fungus infection.

Corticosteroids such as Decadron may mask the symptoms of infection and make you more susceptible to infections.

Using Decadron for a long time may cause cataracts, glaucoma, and eye infections.

Large doses of Decadron may raise blood pressure, increase salt and water retention, and increase potassium loss. If this happens, your doctor may tell you to restrict salt in your diet or suggest you take a potassium supplement.

Decadron should be used with extreme caution if you have dormant tuberculosis or test positive for tuberculosis. Decadron may reactivate the disease.

When you stop taking Decadron after long-term therapy, you may develop withdrawal symptoms such as fever, muscle or joint pain, and weakness.

Decadron should be used with care if you have an underactive thyroid or cirrhosis.

The lowest possible dose should be used to control your condition, and reduction of Decadron should be gradual.

Decadron may aggravate existing emotional problems or cause emotional disturbances. Symptoms range from euphoria (an exaggerated sense of well-being) and difficulty sleeping to mood swings, personality changes, severe depression, and psychotic episodes. If you experience any changes in mood, call your doctor.

Aspirin should be used cautiously with Decadron if you have a clotting disorder.

Decadron should be used with care if you have ulcerative colitis, diverticulitis (an inflammation of the digestive tract), peptic ulcer, kidney disease, high blood pressure, osteoporosis, myasthenia gravis (muscle weakness, especially in the face and neck), or if you have recently had a heart attack.

Long-term therapy with Decadron may affect the growth and development of children 6 years and older and should be carefully checked by your doctor. This medication is not recommended for children under 6 years of age.

Steroids may alter male fertility.

Possible food and drug interactions when taking this medication

If Decadron is taken with certain other drugs, the effects of either could be increased, decreased, or altered. It is especially important to check with your doctor before combining Decadron with the following:

Blood thinners such as Coumadin
Ephedrine
Phenytoin (Dilantin)
Phenobarbital
Potassium-depleting diuretics such as Dyazide and Esidrix
Rifampin (Rifadin, Rimactane)

Special information if you are pregnant or breastfeeding

The effects of Decadron during pregnancy have not been adequately studied. If you are pregnant or plan to become pregnant, inform your doctor immediately. Infants born to mothers who have taken substantial doses of corticosteroids during pregnancy should be carefully watched for adrenal problems. Corticosteroids appear in breast milk and could affect infant growth or cause other damaging effects. Decadron is not recommended for nursing mothers. If Decadron is essential to your health, your doctor may advise you to stop breastfeeding until your treatment with Decadron is finished.

Recommended dosage

TURBINAIRE

Adults
The usual initial dosage is 2 sprays in each nostril, 2 or 3 times a day.

Children (6 to 12 years of age)
The usual initial dosage is 1 or 2 sprays in each nostril 2 times a day, depending on age.

Dosage should be gradually reduced when improvement occurs. The maximum daily dosage for adults is 12 sprays and for children, 8 sprays. Therapy should be stopped as soon as possible. If symptoms return, your doctor may start the medication again.

RESPIHALER

Adults
The recommended initial dose is 3 inhalations, 3 or 4 times a day.

Children
The recommended initial dose is 2 inhalations, 3 or 4 times a day.

Dosage should be gradually reduced when improvement occurs. The maximum daily dosage for adults is 3 inhalations per dose, 12 inhalations per day; and for children, 2 inhalations per dose, 8 inhalations per day. If you are taking corticosteroids orally, your dosage should be reduced or stopped before reduction of Respihaler dosage is begun.

Overdosage

There have been rare reports of toxicity (poisoning) and death following steroid overdose. If you suspect Decadron overdose, seek medical treatment immediately.

Brand name:

DECONAMINE

Generic ingredients: Chlorpheniramine maleate, d-Pseudoephedrine hydrochloride

Why is this drug prescribed?

Deconamine is an antihistamine and decongestant used for the temporary relief of persistent runny nose, sneezing, and nasal congestion caused by upper respiratory infections (the common cold), sinus inflammation, or hay fever. It is also used to help clear nasal passages and shrink swollen membranes; and to drain the sinuses and relieve sinus pressure. Antihistamines work by decreasing the effects of histamine, a chemical released in the body that narrows air passages in the lungs and contributes to inflammation. Antihistamines reduce itching and swelling and dry up secretions from the nose, eyes, and throat.

Most important fact about this drug

Deconamine may cause you to become drowsy or less alert. Driving or operating dangerous machinery or participating in any hazardous activity that requires full mental alertness is not recommended until you know how you react to Deconamine.

How should you take this medication?

Deconamine should be taken exactly as prescribed by your doctor.

What side effects may occur?

Side effects cannot be anticipated. If any develop or change in intensity, inform your doctor as soon as possible. Only your doctor can determine if it is safe for you to continue taking Deconamine.

The most common side effect is mild to moderate drowsiness.

■ *Less common or rare side effects may include:*
Anaphylactic shock (extreme allergic reaction), anemia, anxiety, blood disorders, blurred vision, breathing difficulty, central nervous system (CNS) depression or stimulation, chills, confusion, constipation, convulsions, diarrhea, difficulty sleeping, disturbed coordination, dizziness, double vision, drug rash, dry mouth, nose, and throat, early menstruation, excessive perspiration, excitation, fatigue, extreme calm (sedation), fear, frequent or difficult urination, hallucination, headache, hives, hysteria, increased chest congestion, irregular heartbeat, irritability, lightheadedness, loss of appetite, low blood pressure, nausea, nerve inflammation, nervousness, painful urination, pallor, pounding heartbeat, rapid heartbeat, restlessness, ringing in ears, sensitivity to light, stomach upset, stuffy nose, tightness of chest, tingling in arms and legs, tremor, unwarranted sense of well-being, urinary retention, vertigo, vomiting, weakness, wheezing

Why should this drug not be prescribed?
Deconamine should not be used if you have severe high blood pressure or severe heart disease, are taking an antidepressant drug known as an MAO inhibitor (Parnate), or are sensitive to or have ever had an allergic reaction to antihistamines or any of the ingredients in this medication.

Special warnings about this medication
Deconamine should be used with extreme caution if you have narrow-angle glaucoma, narrowing peptic ulcer or certain gastric obstructions, symptoms of an enlarged prostate, or difficulty urinating.

Also use caution if you have bronchial asthma, emphysema, chronic lung disease, high blood pressure, heart disease, diabetes, increased eye pressure, or an overactive thyroid.

Deconamine may cause excitability, especially in children.

Nervousness, dizziness, or sleeplessness may occur at higher doses.

Pseudoephedrine, one of the ingredients in Deconamine, may produce central nervous system (brain and spinal cord) stimulation, which can result in convulsions, or cardiovascular collapse with low blood pressure.

Possible food and drug interactions when taking this medication
Alcohol increases the sedative effect of Deconamine. Avoid it while taking this medication.

If Deconamine is taken with certain other drugs, the effects of either may be increased, decreased, or altered. It is especially important to check with your doctor before combining Deconamine with the following:

Antidepressant drugs known as MAO inhibitors such as Marplan, Nardil
Mecamylamine (Inversine)
Methyldopa (Aldomet)
Reserpine (Serpasil)
Sedatives/hypnotics such as Nembutal, Seconal
Tranquilizers such as Xanax, Valium
Veratrum alkaloids

Special information if you are pregnant or breastfeeding
The effects of Deconamine during pregnancy have not been adequately studied. If you are pregnant or plan to become pregnant, notify your doctor immediately. Deconamine may appear in breast milk and could affect a nursing infant. If this medication is essential to your health, your doctor may advise you

to discontinue breastfeeding until your treatment with Deconamine is finished.

Recommended Dosage

DECONAMINE TABLETS

Adults And Children Over 12 Years
The usual dosage is 1 tablet 3 or 4 times daily.

Children Under 12 Years
Deconamine Syrup is recommended.

DECONAMINE SYRUP

Adults And Children Over 12 Years
The usual dose is 1 to 2 teaspoonfuls (5 to 10 milliliters) 3 or 4 times daily.

Children 6 To 12 Years
The usual dose is ½ to 1 teaspoonful (2.5 to 5 milliliters) 3 or 4 times daily, not to exceed 4 teaspoonfuls in 24 hours.

Children 2 To 6 Years
The usual dose is ½ teaspoonful (2.5 milliliters) 3 or 4 times daily, not to exceed 2 teaspoonfuls in 24 hours.

Children Under 2 years
Take as directed by the physician.

DECONAMINE SR CAPSULES

Adults And Children Over 12 Years
The usual dose is 1 capsule every 12 hours.

Children Under 12 Years
Deconamine Syrup is recommended.

Overdosage

Any medication taken in excess can have serious consequences. If you suspect an overdose, seek medical attention immediately.

The symptoms of Deconamine overdose include central nervous system (CNS) stimulation and changes in heart function.

Brand name:

DELTASONE

Generic name: Prednisone
Other brand name: Orasone

Why is this drug prescribed?

Deltasone, a corticosteroid drug, is used to reduce inflammation and alleviate symptoms in a variety of disorders, including rheumatoid arthritis and severe cases of asthma. It may be given to treat primary or secondary adrenal cortex insufficiency (lack of sufficient adrenal hormone in the body). It is used in treating all of the following:

Allergic conditions (severe)
Blood disorders
Certain cancers (along with other drugs)
Collagen diseases, including systemic lupus
 erythematosus (a disease of the
 connective tissue)
Eye diseases of various kinds
Flare-ups of multiple sclerosis
Fluid retention due to "nephrotic syndrome"
 (a condition in which damage to the
 kidneys causes protein to be lost in
 the urine)
Lung diseases, including tuberculosis
Prevention of organ rejection
Rheumatoid arthritis and related disorders
Skin diseases
Trichinosis with complications
Ulcerative colitis or enteritis (severe flare-ups)

Most important fact about this drug

Unfortunately, Deltasone decreases your resistance to infection; thus it is possible for you to get a new infection while taking this medication. Deltasone may also mask some of the signs and symptoms of a new infection, which makes it difficult for a doctor to know what the problem is.

How should you take this medication?

Take Deltasone exactly as prescribed by your doctor. You should always be given the *lowest* possible effective dosage.

If you need long-term Deltasone treatment, your doctor may prescribe alternate-day therapy, in which you take the medication only every other morning. The "resting day" gives your adrenal glands a chance to produce some hormone naturally so they will not lose the ability.

If you have been taking Deltasone for a period of time, you will probably need an increased dosage of the medication before, during, and after any stressful situation. Always consult your doctor if you are anticipating stress and think you may need a temporary dosage increase.

When stopping Deltasone treatment, tapering off is better than quitting abruptly. Your doctor will probably have you decrease the dosage very gradually over a period of days or weeks.

You should take Deltasone with food to avoid stomach upset.

If you are on alternate-day therapy or have been prescribed a single daily dose, take it in the morning with breakfast (around 8 AM). If you have been prescribed several doses per day, take them at evenly spaced intervals around the clock.

Patients on long-term Deltasone therapy should wear or carry identification.

What side effects may occur?

Side effects cannot be anticipated. If any develop or change in intensity, inform your doctor as soon as possible. Only your doctor can determine if it is safe for you to continue taking Deltasone.

Deltasone may cause euphoria, mood changes, personality changes, severe depression, insomnia, or even psychotic behavior. It may worsen any existing emotional instability.

At high dosage, Deltasone may cause fluid retention and high blood pressure. If this happens, you may need a low-salt diet and a potassium supplement.

With prolonged Deltasone treatment, eye problems may develop (e.g., a viral or fungal eye infection, cataracts, or glaucoma).

If you take Deltasone over the long term, the buildup of adrenal hormones in your body may cause Cushing's syndrome, marked by weight gain, a "moon-faced" appearance, thin, fragile skin, muscle weakness, brittle bones, purplish stripe marks on the skin, and other symptoms. Females are more likely than males to develop Cushing's syndrome. Alternate-day therapy may help prevent its development.

■ *Other potential side effects from Deltasone include:*
   Bone fractures, bulging eyes, convulsions, distended abdomen, face redness, glaucoma, headache, hives; other allergic-type reactions, increased pressure inside eyes or skull, inflamed esophagus, irregular menstrual periods, muscle weakness or disease, osteoporosis, pancreatitis, peptic ulcer, poor healing of wounds, stunted growth (in children), sweating, thin, fragile skin, vertigo

Why should this drug not be prescribed?

Do not take Deltasone if you have ever had an allergic reaction to it.

You should not be treated with Deltasone if you have a systemic fungus infection, such as candidiasis or cryptococcosis.

Special warnings about this medication

Do not get a smallpox vaccination or any other immunization while you are taking Deltasone. The vaccination might not "take," and might do harm to the nervous system.

Deltasone may reactivate a dormant case of tuberculosis. If you have inactive TB and must take Deltasone for an extended time, you should be given anti-TB medication as well.

If you have an underactive thyroid gland or cirrhosis of the liver, your doctor will probably need to prescribe Deltasone for you at a lower-than-average dosage.

If you have an eye infection caused by the herpes simplex virus, Deltasone should be used with great caution; there is a potential danger than the cornea will become perforated.

Deltasone should also be given with caution if you have any of the following conditions:

Diverticulitis or other disorder of the intestine
High blood pressure
Kidney disorder
Myasthenia gravis (a muscle-weakness disorder)
Osteoporosis (brittle bones)
Peptic ulcer
Ulcerative colitis with danger of infection

Long-term treatment with Deltasone may stunt growth. If this medication is given to a child, the youngster's growth should be monitored carefully.

Diseases such as chickenpox or measles can be very serious or even fatal in children and adults who are taking this drug. Avoid being exposed to these diseases.

Possible food and drug interactions when taking this medication

Deltasone may decrease your carbohydrate tolerance or activate a latent case of diabetes. If you are already taking insulin or oral medication for diabetes, make sure your doctor knows this; you may need an increased dosage while you are being treated with Deltasone.

If you have a blood-clotting disorder caused by a vitamin K deficiency (hypoprothrombinemia) and are taking Deltasone, check with your doctor before you use aspirin.

You may be at risk of convulsions if you take the immunosuppressant drug cyclosporine (Sandimmune) while being treated with Deltasone.

Special information if you are pregnant or breastfeeding

If you are pregnant or plan to become pregnant, inform your doctor immediately. Deltasone should be taken during pregnancy only if clearly needed and only if the benefit outweighs the potential risks to your unborn child.

Recommended dosage

Dosage is determined by the condition being treated and your response to the drug. Typical starting doses can range from 5 milligrams to 60 milligrams a day. Once you respond to the drug, your doctor will lower the dose gradually to the minimum effective amount. For treatment of acute attacks of multiple sclerosis, doses of as much as 200 milligrams per day may be given for a week.

Overdosage

Long-term high doses of Deltasone may produce Cushing's syndrome (see "side effects" section). Although no specific information is available regarding short-term overdosage, any medication taken in excess can have serious consequences. If you suspect an overdose of Deltasone, seek medical attention immediately.

Brand name:

DEMEROL

Generic name: Meperidine hydrochloride

Why is this drug prescribed?
Demerol, a narcotic analgesic, is prescribed for the relief of moderate to severe pain.

Most important fact about this drug
Do not take Demerol if you are currently taking antidepressant drugs known as MAO (monoamine oxidase) inhibitors (Parnate, Nardil) or have used them in the previous 2 weeks. These drugs taken in combination with one another have caused unpredictable, severe, and occasionally fatal reactions. If a narcotic is needed, your doctor should perform a sensitivity test in which repeated, small doses of morphine are administered over the course of several hours while your condition and vital signs are carefully observed.

How should you take this medication?
Take Demerol exactly as prescribed by your doctor. Do not increase the amount or length of time you take this drug without your doctor's approval.

If you are taking Demerol in syrup form, each dose of the syrup should be taken in ½ glass of water.

What side effects may occur?
Side effects cannot be anticipated. If any develop or change in intensity, inform your doctor as soon as possible. Only your doctor can determine if it is safe for you to continue taking Demerol.

■ *More common side effects may include:*
Dizziness
Light-headedness
Nausea
Sedation
Sweating
Vomiting

If any of these side effects occur, it may help if you lie down after taking the medication.

■ *Less common or rare side effects may include:*
Agitation, constipation, difficulty in urinating or inability to urinate, disorientation, dry mouth, fainting, fast heartbeat, feeling of elation, flushing of the face, hallucinations, headache, hives, impairment of mental and physical performance, itching, low blood pressure, mental and physical sluggishness, mental clouding, palpitations, rashes, restlessness, severe convulsions, slow heartbeat, tremors, troubled and slowed breathing, uncoordinated muscle movements, visual disturbances, weakness

Why should this drug not be prescribed?
If you are sensitive to or have ever had an allergic reaction to Demerol or other narcotic painkillers, you should not use this medication. Make sure that your doctor is aware of any drug reactions that you have experienced.

Do not take Demerol with monoamine oxidase inhibitors such as Nardil and Parnate.

Special warnings about this medication
Demerol may impair the mental and/or physical abilities required for the performance of potentially hazardous tasks such as driving a car or operating machinery.

Tolerance and mental and physical dependence can occur with the use of Demerol when it is taken repeatedly. If you have a history of drug dependence, consult with your doctor before taking this drug.

Demerol should be used with caution if you have a severe liver or kidney disorder, hypothyroidism (underactive thyroid gland), Addison's disease (adrenal gland failure), an enlarged prostate, a urethral stricture (narrowing of the urethra), a head injury, an acute abdominal condition, an irregular heartbeat, or a history of convulsions.

This drug should also be used with caution in patients having a severe asthma attack, patients with frequently recurring lung disease, patients who are unable to inhale or exhale an extra volume of air when needed, or patients who have any preexisting breathing difficulties.

Because Demerol may cause unusually slow or troubled breathing and may increase the pressure from fluid surrounding the brain and spinal cord, this drug should be used in patients with head injury only if it is determined absolutely necessary by the doctor.

Demerol may cause orthostatic hypotension (a drop in blood pressure upon rising from a horizontal position).

Possible food and drug interactions when taking this medication
Demerol is a central nervous system depressant and intensifies the effects of alcohol. Do not drink alcohol while taking this medication.

If Demerol is taken with certain other drugs, the effects of either could be increased, decreased, or altered. It is especially important to check with your doctor before combining Demerol with the following:

Antihistamines such as Benadryl
General anesthetics
MAO inhibitors such as Nardil, Parnate
Other central nervous system depressants
Other narcotic analgesics such as Percocet, Tylenol with codeine
Phenothiazines such as Thorazine
Sedative/hypnotics such as Valium, Halcion
Tranquilizers such as Xanax
Tricyclic antidepressants such as Elavil, Tofranil

If such combined drug therapy is being considered, the dose of one or both medications should be reduced to avoid difficulty in breathing, low blood pressure, sedation, or coma.

**Special information
if you are pregnant or breastfeeding**
Do not take Demerol if you are pregnant or planning to become pregnant unless you are directed to do so by your doctor. Demerol appears in breast milk and could affect a nursing infant. If this medication is essential to your health, your doctor may advise you to discontinue breastfeeding your baby until your treatment is finished.

Recommended dosage

ADULTS

The usual dosage of Demerol is 50 milligrams to 150 milligrams every 3 or 4 hours, to be determined by your doctor according to your response and the severity of the pain.

CHILDREN

The usual dosage is 0.5 milligram to 0.8 milligram per pound of body weight, taken every 3 or 4 hours, as determined by your doctor.

ELDERLY

Your doctor may reduce the dosage.

Overdosage
Symptoms of an overdose of Demerol include:
Bluish discoloration of the skin
Cold and clammy skin
Coma
Extreme sleepiness progressing to a state of unresponsiveness
Limp, weak muscles
Low blood pressure
Slow heartbeat
Troubled or slowed breathing

In severe overdosage, the patient may stop breathing, and circulatory collapse, heart attack, and death may occur.

If you suspect an overdose, seek emergency medical treatment immediately.

Brand name:

DEMULEN

See Oral Contraceptives, page 437.

Brand name:

DEPAKENE

Generic name: Valproic acid

Why is this drug prescribed?

Depakene is an anticonvulsant medication used to treat seizures.

Most important fact about this drug

Fatalities from liver failure have occurred in patients taking Depakene. The risk of liver failure is most pronounced in children under the age of 2 years, especially if they are taking other anticonvulsants, have congenital metabolic disorders, have severe seizure disorders with mental retardation, and/or suffer from organic brain disease. When Depakene is administered to these children, it should be the only anticonvulsant prescribed and should be used with extreme caution. The risk of fatal liver disease decreases considerably with age. However, all patients should watch for signs of liver failure (including loss of control of seizures, weakness, lethargy, loss of appetite, facial swelling, and vomiting), and your doctor will probably carry out periodic liver function tests.

How should you take this medication?

If it irritates the stomach or intestines, take Depakene with food.

To avoid irritating the mouth and throat, Depakene capsules should be swallowed whole, not chewed.

What side effects may occur?

Side effects cannot be anticipated. If any develop or change in intensity, inform your doctor as soon as possible. Only your doctor can determine if it is safe for you to continue taking Depakene.

■ *More common side effects may include:*
Indigestion
Nausea
Vomiting

■ *Less common or rare side effects may include:*
Abdominal cramps, aggression, anemia, bleeding, blood disorders, breast enlargement, breast milk not associated with pregnancy or nursing, bruising, changes in behavior, coma, constipation, depression, diarrhea, difficulty in speaking, dizziness, double vision, drowsiness, emotional upset, hair loss, headache, involuntary eye movements, involuntary jerking or tremors, irregular menstrual periods, itching, lack of coordination, liver disease, loss of or increased appetite, pancreatic inflammation, rash, sedation, sensitivity to light, skin lesions, spots before the eyes, swelling of the arms and legs due to fluid retention, swollen glands, weakness, weight loss or gain

Why should this drug not be prescribed?

You should not take this drug if you have liver disease or liver dysfunction, or if you have had an allergic reaction to it.

Special warnings about this medication

Liver failure has occurred in patients taking Depakene (see "Most important fact about this drug" above). Depakene should be discontinued immediately if a liver problem occurs or is suspected. Be especially cautious if you have ever had liver disease or if you are taking other anticonvulsants or have a congenital metabolic disorder.

Because of the potential for side effects involving blood disorders, your doctor will probably test your blood before Depakene therapy and at regular intervals during use. Bruising, hemorrhaging, or clotting disorders usually mean the dosage should be reduced or the drug should be stopped altogether.

Since Depakene may cause drowsiness, you should not drive a car, operate heavy machinery, or engage in hazardous activity until you know how you react to the drug.

Possible food and drug interactions when taking this medication

If Depakene is taken with certain other drugs, the effects of either could be increased, decreased, or altered. It is especially important to check with your doctor before combining Depakene with the following:

Aspirin
Carbamazepine (Tegretol)
Clonazepam (Klonopin)
Dicumarol
Ethosuximide (Zarontin)
Oral contraceptives
Phenobarbital and other barbiturates
Phenytoin (Dilantin)
Primidone (Mysoline)
Warfarin blood thinners (Coumadin)

Extreme drowsiness and other serious effects may occur if Depakene is taken with alcohol or other depressants such as Halcion, Restoril, or Xanax.

Special information if you are pregnant or breastfeeding

If taken during pregnancy, Depakene may harm the fetus. The drug is not recommended

for pregnant women unless the benefits of therapy clearly outweigh the risks. In fact, women of childbearing potential should take Depakene only if it has been shown to be essential in the control of seizures. Since Depakene appears in breast milk, nursing mothers should use it only with caution.

Recommended dosage

The usual starting dose is 15 milligrams per 2.2 pounds of body weight per day. Your doctor may increase the dose at weekly intervals by 5 to 10 milligrams per 2.2 pounds per day until seizures are controlled or side effects become too severe. The daily dose should not exceed 60 milligrams per 2.2 pounds per day.

Overdosage

Any medication taken in excess can have serious consequences. Severe overdosage of Depakene can cause coma. If you suspect an overdose, seek medical help immediately.

Brand name:

DEPAKOTE

Generic name: Divalproex sodium (Valproic acid)

Why is this drug prescribed?

Depakote, an epilepsy medication, is used in the treatment of certain types of seizures. It can be used alone, or with other seizure-prevention medication to treat simple and complex absence seizures, and multiple seizures, including absence seizures.

Most important fact about this drug

Depakote can cause serious liver damage, especially during the first six months of therapy. Liver function tests should be done by your doctor before Depakote is prescribed and repeated frequently once you start taking the medication. Your doctor needs to know as soon as possible if this drug is having an adverse effect on your liver so therapy can be stopped or changed.

How should you take this medication?

The tablet should be swallowed whole (don't chew or crush it), with water. It has a special coating to avoid upsetting your stomach.

If you are taking the sprinkle capsule, it can be swallowed whole or sprinkled on a teaspoon of soft food such as applesauce or pudding. Swallow it immediately, without chewing. The sprinkle capsules are large enough to be opened easily.

Depakote can be taken with meals or snacks to avoid upset stomach.

This medication must be taken exactly as your doctor prescribes.

If you take Depakote once a day and forget to take it, take your dose as soon as you remember. If you don't remember until the next day, skip the missed dose and return to your regular schedule. Never take two doses at the same time.

If you take Depakote twice a day or more and forget to take your dose, take your dose if it's within six hours of the missed dose, and take the rest of the doses at equal intervals during the day. Never take two doses at the same time.

What side effects may occur?

Side effects cannot be anticipated. If any develop or change in intensity, inform your doctor as soon as possible. Because Depakote is often used with other anti-seizure drugs, it may not be possible to determine whether a side effect is due to Depakote alone. Only your doctor can determine if it is safe for you to continue taking Depakote.

■ *More common side effects may include:*
Change in menstrual periods
Drowsiness
Indigestion
Nausea
Temporary hair loss
Vomiting
Weight gain

■ *Less common or rare side effects may include:*
Abdominal cramps, anemia, behavior problems, blood disorders, constipation, depression, diarrhea, dizziness, double vision, emotional upset, fluid retention, headache, involuntary rapid movement of eyeball, itching, lack of muscular coordination, loss of appetite, seeing "spots before your eyes", sensitivity to light, skin rash, speech difficulties, tremor, unusual bleeding and bruising, weakness

Why should this drug not be prescribed?

You should not take this medication if you have liver disease or severe liver dysfunction.

If you are sensitive to or have ever had an allergic reaction to Depakote or similar drugs, you should not take this medication.

Special warnings about this medication

This medication can severely impair the liver.

Notify your doctor or dentist that you are taking Depakote if you have a medical emergency or before you have surgery or dental treatment.

Depakote causes some people to become drowsy or less alert. Driving or operating dangerous machinery or participating in any hazardous activity that requires full mental alertness is not recommended until you are certain the drug does not have this effect on you.

Possible food and drug interactions when taking this medication

Depakote depresses activity of the central nervous system, and may increase the effects of alcohol. Do not drink alcohol while taking this medication.

If Depakote is taken with certain other drugs, the effects of either could be increased, decreased, or altered. It is especially important to check with your doctor before combining Depakote with the following:

Anticoagulants (blood thinners such as Coumadin)
Aspirin
Barbiturates such as phenobarbital
Oral contraceptives
Other seizure medications, including Carbamazepin (Tegretol), Clonazepam (Klonopin), Ethosuximide (Zarontin), and Phenytoin (Dilantin)

Special information if you are pregnant or breastfeeding

Depakote may produce birth defects during the first three months of pregnancy. If you are pregnant or plan to become pregnant, inform your doctor immediately. Depakote appears in breast milk and could affect a nursing infant. If Depakote is essential to your health, your doctor may advise you to discontinue breastfeeding until your treatment with this medication is finished.

Recommended dosage

ADULTS AND CHILDREN

Dosage is determined by your body weight. The usual recommended initial dose is 15 milligrams per 2.2 pounds per day, increased at 1 week intervals by 5 to 10 milligrams per 2.2 pounds per day until your doctor feels that the desired effect has been reached. The maximum recommended daily dosage is 60 milligrams per 2.2 pounds. If your total dosage is more than 250 milligrams per day, it should be divided into smaller individual doses.
The best dosage may be determined with the aid of a blood test.

Overdosage

Any medication taken in excess can cause symptoms of overdose. If you suspect an overdose, seek medical attention immediately.

The symptom of Depakote overdose is deep coma.

Generic name:

DESIPRAMINE HYDROCHLORIDE

See Norpramin, page 435.

Generic name:

DESMOPRESSIN ACETATE

See DDAVP, page 156.

Generic name:

DESONIDE

See Tridesilon, page 650.

Brand name:

DESOWEN

See Tridesilon, page 650.

Generic name:

DESOXIMETASONE

See Topicort, page 642.

Brand name:

DESQUAM-E

Generic name: Benzoyl peroxide
Other brand names: Benzac W, Benzagel,
BenzaShave, Theroxide

Why is this drug prescribed?

Desquam-E Gel is a topical acne medication used to treat various types of acne. It can be used alone or with other drugs, including antibiotics and products that contain retinoic acid or sulfur and salicylic acid.

Most important fact about this drug

Significant clearing of the skin should occur after 2 to 3 weeks of treatment with Desquam-E. If used with sunscreens containing PABA (para-amino benzoic acid), it may cause temporary skin discoloration.

How should you use this medication?

The affected area should be cleansed before the medication is applied. Desquam-E should then be gently rubbed in.

What side effects may occur?

Side effects cannot be anticipated. If any develop or change in intensity, notify your doctor as soon as possible. Only your doctor can determine whether it is safe for you to continue using Desquam-E.

■ *Side effects may include:*
Allergic reaction (itching, rash) in area where the medication was applied
Excessive drying (red and peeling skin and possible swelling)

Why should this drug not be prescribed?

Do not use Desquam-E if you are sensitive or allergic to benzoyl peroxide.

Special warnings about this medication

Desquam-E is for external use only.
Avoid contact with your eyes, nose, or throat.

If you are sensitive to medications derived from benzoic acid (certain topical anesthetics) or to cinnamon, you may also be sensitive to Desquam-E.

If Desquam-E comes in contact with hair or colored fabric, it may bleach the color.

Possible food and drug interactions when taking this medication

If Desquam-E is used with sunscreens containing PABA (para-amino benzoic acid), it may cause temporary skin discoloration.

Special information
if you are pregnant or breastfeeding

The effects of Desquam-E during pregnancy have not been adequately studied. It should be used only if clearly needed. If you are pregnant or plan to become pregnant, inform your doctor immediately. This medication may appear in breast milk and could affect a nursing infant. If this medication is essential to your health, your doctor may advise you to stop breastfeeding until your treatment with Desquam-E is finished.

Recommended dosage

ADULTS AND CHILDREN 12 YEARS
AND OVER

Desquam-E Emollient Gel should be gently rubbed into all affected areas once or twice a day. If you are fair-skinned or live in an excessively dry climate, you should probably start with one application a day. Desquam-E can continue to be used for as long as your doctor thinks it is necessary.

Overdosage

Although no specific information is available on Desquam-E overdosage, any medication taken in excess can have serious consequences. If you suspect an overdose, seek medical attention immediately.

Brand name:

DESYREL

Generic name: Trazodone hydrochloride

Why is this drug prescribed?
Desyrel is prescribed for the treatment of depression with or without anxiety.

Most important fact about this drug
Desyrel has been associated with the occurrence of priapism, a persistent painful erection of the penis. Male patients who experience prolonged or inappropriate erections should discontinue this drug and consult with their doctor.

How should you take this medication?
Desyrel should be taken shortly after a meal or light snack. The risk of dizziness or lightheadedness may increase if you take the drug under fasting conditions. Take Desyrel exactly as prescribed by your doctor.

What side effects may occur?
Side effects cannot be anticipated. If any develop or change in intensity, inform your doctor as soon as possible. Only your doctor can determine if it is safe for you to continue taking Desyrel.

■ More common side effects may include:
Abdominal or stomach disorder, aches or pains in muscles and bones, allergic skin reaction, anger or hostility, bad taste in mouth, blurred vision, brief loss of consciousness, confusion, constipation, decreased appetite, decreased concentration, decreased sex drive, diarrhea, disorientation, dizziness or light-headedness, drowsiness, dry mouth, excitement, fatigue, fluid retention and swelling, fullness or heaviness in the head, headache, high or low blood pressure, impaired memory, inability to fall or stay asleep, nasal or sinus congestion, nausea or vomiting, nervousness, nightmares or vivid dreams, rapid heartbeat, red, tired, itchy eyes, ringing in the ears, shortness of breath, sudden loss of strength or fainting, sweating or clammy skin, tingling sensation, tremors, uncoordinated movements, weight gain or loss

■ Less common or rare side effects may include:
Agitation, allergic reactions, anemia, blood in the urine, breast enlargement or filling, chest pain, delayed urine flow, double vision, early menstruation, ejaculation abnormalities, excess salivation, gas, grand mal seizures, hair loss, hallucinations or delusions, heart attack, impaired speech, impotence, increased appetite, increased sex drive, increased urinary frequency, jaundice, lack of muscle coordination, liver disorders, mild degree of mania or elevated mood, milk production, missed menstrual periods, muscle twitches, numbness, prolonged erections, rash and itching, restlessness, slow heartbeat, swelling due to fluid retention, temporary interruption of normal breathing, weakness

Why should this drug not be prescribed?
If you are sensitive to or have ever had an allergic reaction to Desyrel or similar drugs, you should not take this medication. Make sure that your doctor is aware of any drug reactions that you have experienced.

Special warnings about this medication
Desyrel may cause you to become drowsy or less alert and may affect your judgment. Therefore, driving or operating dangerous machinery or participating in any hazardous activity that requires full mental alertness is not recommended.

Notify your doctor or dentist that you are taking this drug if you have a medical emergency, and before you have surgery or dental treatment. Stop using the drug if you are going to have elective surgery.

Possible food and drug interactions when taking this medication

Desyrel may intensify the effects of alcohol. Do not drink alcohol while taking this medication.

If Desyrel is taken with certain other drugs, the effects of either could be increased, decreased, or altered. It is especially important to check with your doctor before combining Desyrel with the following:

Antidepressant drugs known as MAO
    inhibitors, including Nardil and
    Parnate
Barbiturates such as Seconal
Digoxin (Lanoxin)
Drugs for high blood pressure
Other antidepressants such as Prozac or
    Norpramim
Phenytoin (Dilantin)

Special information
if you are pregnant or breastfeeding

The effects of Desyrel during pregnancy have not been adequately studied. If you are pregnant or planning to become pregnant, inform your doctor immediately. This medication may appear in breast milk. If treatment with this drug is essential to your health, your doctor may advise you to discontinue breastfeeding your baby until your treatment is finished.

Recommended dosage

ADULTS

The usual starting dosage is a total of 150 milligrams per day, divided into 2 or more smaller doses. Your doctor may increase your dose by 50 milligrams per day every 3 or 4 days. Total dosage should not exceed 400 milligrams per day in divided

doses. Once an adequate response has been achieved, your doctor may gradually reduce your dose. Because this medication makes you drowsy, your doctor may tell you to take the largest dose at bedtime.

CHILDREN

The safety and effectiveness of Desyrel have not been established in children below 18 years of age.

ELDERLY

Your dose should be determined by your doctor.

Overdosage

Any medication taken in excess can cause overdose. Death from overdose has occurred when Desyrel has been taken in combination with other drugs.

Symptoms of an overdose may include:
Breathing failure
Drowsiness
Irregular heartbeat
Prolonged, painful erection
Seizures
Vomiting

If you suspect an overdose, seek medical attention immediately.

Generic name:

DEXAMETHASONE

See Decadron Tablets, page 165.

Generic name:

DEXAMETHASONE SODIUM PHOSPHATE

See Decadron Turbinaire and Respihaler, page 167.

Generic name:

DEXCHLORPHENIRAMINE MALEATE

See Polaramine, page 489.

Brand name:

DEXEDRINE

Generic name: Dextroamphetamine sulfate

Why is this drug prescribed?

Dexedrine, a stimulant drug available in liquid, tablet, or sustained-release capsule form, is prescribed to help treat the following conditions:

1. Narcolepsy (recurrent "sleep attacks")
2. Attention-deficit disorder with hyperactivity. (The total treatment program should include social, psychological, and educational guidance along with Dexedrine.)
3. Short-term treatment of obesity (along with a behavioral modification program).

Most important fact about this drug

Because it is a stimulant, this drug has high abuse potential. The stimulant effect may give way to a letdown period of depression and fatigue. Although the letdown can be relieved by taking another dose, this soon becomes a vicious circle.

If you habitually take Dexedrine in doses higher than recommended, you may eventually become dependent on the drug and suffer from withdrawal symptoms when it is unavailable.

How should you take this medication?

Take Dexedrine exactly as prescribed by your doctor. If it is prescribed in liquid or tablet form, you may need up to 3 doses a day. The sustained-release capsules permit once-a-day dosing.

Do not take Dexedrine late in the day, since this could cause insomnia. If you experience insomnia or an unwanted loss of appetite while taking this drug, notify your doctor; you may need a lower dosage.

It is likely that your doctor will periodically take you off Dexedrine to determine whether you still need it.

Do not chew or crush the sustained release form, Dexedrine Spansules.

Do not increase the dosage, except on your doctor's advice.

Dexedrine may mask extreme fatigue and cause dizziness, impairing your ability to perform tasks requiring alertness or drive an automobile.

Do not use Dexedrine to improve mental alertness or stay awake. Do not share it with others.

What side effects may occur?

Side effects cannot be anticipated. If any develop or change in intensity, inform your doctor as soon as possible. Only your doctor can determine if it is safe for you to continue taking Dexedrine.

■ *More common side effects may include:* Excessive restlessness or overstimulation (a common Dexedrine side effect that may aggravate any existing tendency toward tics).

■ *Other side effects may include:* Constipation, diarrhea, dizziness, dry mouth, euphoria, headache, heart palpitations, high blood pressure, hives, rapid heartbeat, sleeplessness, stomach and intestinal disturbances, tremors, uncontrollable twitching or jerking, unpleasant taste in the mouth

Unless you are being treated for obesity, you may find appetite suppression and weight loss to be unwanted side effects.

Dexedrine may cause impotence or affect sexual desire.

■ *Effects of chronic heavy abuse of Dexedrine may include:*
Hyperactivity, insomnia, irritability, personality changes, schizophrenia-like thoughts and behavior, severe skin disease

Why should this drug not be prescribed?
Do not take Dexedrine if you are sensitive or have ever had an allergic reaction to it. Also, do not take Dexedrine if you have a history of alcohol or drug abuse.

Do not take Dexedrine for at least 14 days after taking a monoamine oxidase inhibitor (MAO inhibitor) type of antidepressant such as Marplan, Nardil, or Parnate. Dexedrine and MAO inhibitor antidepressants may interact to cause a sharp, potentially life-threatening rise in blood pressure.

Dexedrine should not be prescribed for you if you suffer from any of the following conditions:

Agitation
Cardiovascular disease
Glaucoma
Hardening of the arteries
High blood pressure
Overactive thyroid gland

Special warnings about this medication
In the treatment of obesity, only a short course of Dexedrine should be prescribed. When the drug's appetite-suppressing effect no longer seems to work, it is time to stop taking Dexedrine—not take more of it. Increasing the dosage will lead to drug dependence.

Be aware that one of the inactive ingredients in Dexedrine is a yellow food coloring called tartrazine (Yellow No. 5). In a few people, particularly those who are allergic to aspirin, tartrazine can cause a severe allergic reaction.

Dexedrine may impair judgment or coordination. Do not drive or operate dangerous machinery until you know how you react to the medication.

There is some concern that Dexedrine may stunt a child's growth. For the sake of safety, any child who takes Dexedrine should have his or her growth monitored.

Possible food and drug interactions when taking this medication
If Dexedrine is taken with certain foods or drugs, the effects of either could be increased, decreased, or altered. It is especially important to check with your doctor before combining Dexedrine with the following:

■ Substances that *dampen* the effects of Dexedrine:
Ammonium chloride
Chlorpromazine (Thorazine)
Fruit juices
Glutamic acid hydrochloride
Guanethidine
Haloperidol (Haldol)
Lithium carbonate (Lithobid)
Methenamine
Reserpine (Serpasil)
Sodium acid phosphate
Vitamin C (as ascorbic acid)

■ Substances that *boost* the effects of Dexedrine:
Baking soda
Darvon
Diamox
Diuretics (Diuril)

MAO-inhibitor antidepressants such as
Marplan, Nardil, and Parnate

■ Substances that *have decreased effect* when
taken with Dexedrine:
Adrenergic blockers such as Dibenzyline
and Regitine
Antihistamines
Blood pressure medications
Ethosuximide (Zarontin)
Veratrum alkaloids

■ Substances that *have increased effect* when
taken with Dexedrine:
Demerol
Dilantin
Levophed
Phenobarbital
Tricyclic antidepressants such as Elavil and
Tofranil

Special Information
if you are pregnant or breastfeeding
If you are pregnant or plan to become
pregnant, inform your doctor immediately.
Animal studies suggest that Dexedrine might
cause birth defects. Babies born to women
taking Dexedrine may be premature or have
low birth weight. They may also be
unhappy, agitated, or apathetic due to
withdrawal symptoms. Since Dexedrine
finds its way into breast milk, it should not
be taken by a nursing mother.

Recommended dosage
Regardless of what the drug is to be used
for, amphetamines such as Dexedrine
should be taken at the lowest effective dosage,
and dosage should be individually
adjusted.

NARCOLEPSY

Adults
The usual dose is 5 to 60 milligrams per day,
divided into smaller, equal doses,
depending on individual patient response.

Children
Narcolepsy seldom occurs in children under
12 years of age; however, when it does,
Dexedrine may be used.

The suggested initial dose for patients aged
6 to 12 is 5 milligrams per day. Your
doctor may increase the daily dose in
increments of 5 milligrams at weekly
intervals until it becomes effective.

Patients 12 years of age and older will be
started with 10 milligrams daily. The daily
dosage may be raised in increments of 10
milligrams at weekly intervals until
effective. If side effects such as insomnia or
anorexia appear, the dosage will probably
be reduced.

"Spansule" capsules may be used for once-a-
day dosage wherever appropriate. With
tablets or elixir, take the first dose on
awakening; additional doses (1 or 2) are
taken at intervals of 4 to 6 hours.

ATTENTION DEFICIT DISORDER WITH
HYPERACTIVITY

This drug is not recommended for children
under 3 years of age.

Children from 3 to 5 Years of Age
The usual starting dose is 2.5 milligrams daily,
in tablet or elixir form. The daily dosage
may be raised in increments of 2.5 milligrams
at weekly intervals until an effective dose
is reached.

Children 6 Years of Age and Older
The usual starting dose is 5 milligrams once
or twice daily. The daily dosage may be
raised in increments of 5 milligrams at weekly
intervals until response is satisfactory.
Only in rare cases does the dose exceed a
total of 40 milligrams per day.

"Spansule" capsules may be used for once-a-
day dosage wherever appropriate.

With tablets or elixir, the first dose should be taken on awakening; additional doses (1 or 2) are taken at intervals of 4 to 6 hours. Your doctor may interrupt the schedule occasionally to determine if there is a recurrence of behavioral symptoms sufficient to require continued therapy.

OBESITY

The usual dosage is one 10- or 15-milligram "Spansule" capsule daily, taken in the morning, or up to 30 milligrams daily as tablets or elixir, divided into doses of 5 to 10 milligrams taken 30 to 60 minutes before meals.

Dexedrine is not recommended for this use in children under 12 years of age.

Overdosage
If you suspect an overdose of Dexedrine, seek medical attention immediately.

Symptoms of an acute Dexedrine overdose may include:
Abdominal cramps, assaultiveness, coma, confusion, convulsions, diarrhea, fever, hallucinations, heightened reflexes, high or low blood pressure, irregular heartbeat, nausea, panic, rapid breathing, restlessness, tremor, vomiting

Generic name:

DEXTROAMPHETAMINE SULFATE

See Dexedrine, page 184.

Brand name:

DIABETA

See Micronase, page 377.

Brand name:

DIABINESE

Generic name: Chlorpropamide

Why is this drug prescribed?
Diabinese is an oral antidiabetic medication used to treat Type II (non-insulin-dependent) diabetes. Diabetes occurs when the body fails to produce enough insulin or is unable to use it properly. Insulin is believed to work by helping sugar penetrate the cell wall so it can be used by the cell.

There are actually two forms of diabetes: Type I insulin-dependent and Type II non-insulin-dependent. Type I usually requires insulin injection for life, while Type II diabetes can usually be treated by dietary changes and/or oral antidiabetic medications such as Diabinese. Apparently, Diabinese controls diabetes by stimulating the pancreas to secrete more insulin. Occasionally, Type II diabetics must take insulin injections on a temporary basis, especially during stressful periods or times of illness.

Most important fact about this drug
Drugs such as Diabinese may possibly lead to more heart problems than diet treatment alone, or treatment with diet and insulin. If you have heart problems, you may want to discuss this with your doctor.

Patients taking Diabinese must remember that this medication is an aid to, and not a substitute for, good diet and exercise. Failure to follow a sound diet and exercise plan may lead to serious and potentially fatal complications, such as hypoglycemia (described below). Patients should also remember that Diabinese is *not* an oral form of insulin, and is not a substitute for injected insulin.

How should you take this medication?

Ordinarily, your doctor will ask you to take a single daily dose of Diabinese each morning with breakfast. However, if a single dose upsets your stomach, he or she may ask you take Diabinese in smaller doses throughout the day.

To prevent low blood sugar levels (hypoglycemia):

- You should understand the symptoms of hypoglycemia

- Know how exercise affects your blood sugar levels

- Maintain an adequate diet

- Keep a source of quick-acting sugar with you all the time

Avoid alcohol. If you drink alcohol, it may cause breathlessness and facial flushing.

What side effects may occur?

Side effects cannot be anticipated. If any develop or change in intensity, inform your doctor as soon as possible. Only your doctor can determine if it is safe for you to continue taking Diabinese.

Side effects from Diabinese are rare and seldom require discontinuation of the medication.

- *More common side effects include:*
  Diarrhea
  Hunger
  Itching
  Loss of appetite
  Nausea
  Stomach upset
  Vomiting

- *Less common or rare side effects may include:*
  Anemia and other blood disorders, cholestatic jaundice (caused by obstructed bile flow), hives, proctocolitis (inflammation of the rectum and/or colon), sensitivity to light

Diabinese, like all oral antidiabetics, can result in hypoglycemia (low blood sugar). The risk of hypoglycemia can be increased by missed meals, alcohol, other medications, and excessive exercise. To avoid hypoglycemia, closely follow the dietary and exercise regimen suggested by your physician.

- *Symptoms of mild hypoglycemia may include:*
  Cold sweat, fast heartbeat, fatigue, headache, nausea, nervousness

- *Symptoms of more severe hypoglycemia may include:*
  Coma, pale skin, shallow breathing

Contact your doctor immediately if these symptoms of severe low blood sugar occur.

Why should this drug not be prescribed?

You should not take Diabinese if you have ever had an allergic reaction to it.

Diabinese should not be taken if you are suffering from diabetic ketoacidosis (a life-threatening medical emergency caused by insufficient insulin and marked by excessive thirst, nausea, fatigue, pain below the breastbone, and a fruity breath).

Special warnings about this medication

If you are taking Diabinese, you should check your blood and urine periodically for the presence of abnormal sugar (glucose) levels.

Remember that it is important that you closely follow the diet and exercise regimen established by your doctor.

Even patients with well-controlled diabetes may find that stress, illness, surgery, or fever results in a loss of control over their diabetes. In these cases, the patient's physician may recommend that Diabinese be discontinued temporarily and injected insulin administered.

In addition, the effectiveness of any oral antidiabetic, including Diabinese, may decrease with time. This may occur either because of a diminished responsiveness to the medication or a worsening of the diabetes.

Possible food and drug interactions when taking this medication

When you take Diabinese with certain other drugs, the effects of either could be increased, decreased, or altered. It is important that you consult with your doctor before taking Diabinese with the following:

Adrenal corticosteroids such as Deltasone
Anabolic steroids
Aspirin in large doses
Barbiturates (Seconal)
Beta blockers such as Inderal and Tenormin
Calcium channel blockers such as Cardizem and Procardia
Chloramphenicol (Chloromycetin)
Coumarin (Coumadin)
Diuretics chlorothiazide, hydrochlorothiazide
Epinephrine (Epipen)
Estrogens such as Premarin
Isoniazid (Laniazid)
MAO inhibitors (antidepressants such as Nardil and Parnate)

Nicotinic acid (Nicobid, Nicolar)
Nonsteroidal anti-inflammatory agents such as Advil, Motrin, Naprosyn, Nuprin
Oral miconazole
Oral contraceptives
Phenothiazines
Phenylbutazone (Butazolidin)
Phenytoin (Dilantin)
Probenecid (Benemid, ColBENEMID)
Sulforamides such as Bactrim
Thyroid medication such as Synthroid and Proloid

Alcohol should be avoided since excessive alcohol consumption can cause low blood sugar and other reactions.

Special information
if you are pregnant or breastfeeding

The effects of Diabinese during pregnancy have not been adequately established. If you are pregnant or plan to become pregnant you should inform your doctor immediately. Since studies suggest the importance of maintaining normal blood sugar (glucose) levels during pregnancy, your physician may prescribe injected insulin.

To minimize the risk of low blood sugar (hypoglycemia) in newborn babies, Diabinese, if prescribed during pregnancy, should be discontinued at least 1 month before the expected delivery date.

Since Diabinese appears in breast milk, it is not recommended for nursing mothers. If diet alone does not control glucose levels, then insulin should be considered.

Recommended Dosage

Dosage levels must be determined by each patient's needs.

ADULTS

Usually an initial daily dose of 250 milligrams is recommended for stable, middle-aged, non-insulin-dependent patients. After 5 to 7 days, this dosage may be adjusted in increments of 50 to 125 milligrams every 3 to 5 days to achieve optimum benefits. Patients with mild diabetes may respond well to daily doses of 100 milligrams or less of Diabinese, while patients with severe diabetes may require 500 milligrams daily. Maintenance doses above 750 milligrams are not recommended.

ELDERLY

Elderly, malnourished, or debilitated patients, and patients with impaired kidney and liver function usually receive an initial dose of 100 to 125 milligrams.

CHILDREN

Safety and effectiveness have not been established.

Overdosage

An overdose of Diabinese can cause low blood sugar (see "What side effects may occur?" for symptoms).

Eating sugar or a sugar-based product will often correct the condition. If you suspect an overdose, seek medical attention immediately.

Brand name:

DIAMOX

Generic name: Acetazolamide

Why is this drug prescribed?

Diamox controls fluid secretion. It is used in the treatment of glaucoma, epilepsy (petit mal and unlocalized seizures), congestive heart failure and drug-induced fluid retention. It is also used to prevent or relieve the symptoms of acute mountain sickness in climbers attempting a rapid climb and those who feel sick during a gradual climb. It is called a carbonic anhydrase inhibitor. By slowing down or stopping the action of the enzyme carbonic anhydrase, Diamox lowers pressure in the eye and also acts as a mild diuretic.

Most important fact about this drug

This drug is considered to be a sulfa drug because of its chemical properties. Severe reactions have been reported with sulfa drugs. If you develop a rash, bruises, sore throat or fever contact your doctor immediately.

How should you take this medication?

Diuretics can cause your body to lose too much potassium. Ask your doctor for the warning signs of too much potassium loss. Also ask whether you should eat specific foods that are rich in potassium, or take a potassium supplement to avoid this problem.

Take this medication exactly as prescribed by your doctor.

If you forget to take a dose, take it as soon as you remember. If it is almost time for your next dose, skip the one you missed and go back to your regular schedule. Never take two doses at the same time.

What side effects may occur?

Side effects cannot be anticipated. If any develop or change in intensity, inform your doctor as soon as possible. Only your doctor can determine if it is safe for you to continue taking Diamox.

■ *More common side effects may include:*
Change in taste
Diarrhea
Increase in amount or frequency of
  urination
Loss of appetite

Low potassium (leading to symptoms like dry mouth, excessive thirst, weak or irregular heartbeat, muscle pain or cramps)
Nausea
Ringing in the ears
Tingling or pins and needles in hands or feet
Vomiting

■ *Less common or rare side effects may include:*
Black or bloody stools, blood in urine, confusion, convulsions, drowsiness, fever, high sugar levels in urine, hives, hypersensitivity reaction, liver dysfunction, rash, sensitivity to light, skin peeling, vision changes, weakness or loss of muscle tone

Why should this drug not be prescribed?
Do not take this medication if your sodium or potassium levels are low, or if you have kidney or liver disease or dysfunction, including cirrhosis or Addison's disease.

Diamox should not be used as a long-term treatment for chronic noncongestive angle-closure glaucoma, a disorder of the eyes.

Special warnings about this medication
Aspirin should be used with extreme caution if you are taking Diamox.

If you have emphysema or other breathing disorders, this drug should be used with caution.

Possible food and drug interactions when taking this medication
If Diamox is taken with certain other drugs, the effects of either could be increased, decreased, or altered. It is especially important to check with your doctor before combining Diamox with the following:

Amphetamines
Aspirin and other over-the-counter medications
Lithium
Methenamine (Urex)
Oral hypoglycemic agents such as Micronase
Quinidine

Special information
if you are pregnant or breastfeeding
The effects of Diamox during pregnancy have not been adequately studied. If you are pregnant or plan to become pregnant, inform your doctor immediately. Diamox may appear in breast milk and could affect a nursing infant. If this medication is essential to your health, your doctor may advise you to discontinue breastfeeding until your treatment with Diamox is finished.

Recommended dosage

ADULTS

This medication is available in both oral and injectable form. Dosages are for the oral form only.

Glaucoma
This medication is used as an addition to regular glaucoma treatment. Dosages for open-angle glaucoma range from 250 milligrams to 1 gram per 24 hours in two or more smaller doses. Your doctor should supervise your dosage and watch the effect of this medication carefully if you are using it for glaucoma. It should be individualized for each patient's needs. In secondary glaucoma and before surgery in acute congestive (closed-angle) glaucoma, the usual dosage is 250 milligrams every 4 hours or, in some cases, 250 milligrams twice a day. The injectable form of this drug is occasionally used in acute cases.

The usual dosage of Diamox Sequels (sustained-release capsules) is 1 capsule 2 times a day, usually morning and evening. Dosage may be increased to 1 gram.

Dosage should be adjusted carefully, and your physician should monitor you continuously.

Epilepsy
The daily dosage is 8 to 30 milligrams per 2.2 pounds in 2 or more doses. Typical dosage may range from 375 to 1,000 milligrams per day. Dosage is adjusted to the individual patient's needs; Diamox can be used with other anticonvulsant medication.

Congestive Heart Failure
The usual starting dosage to reduce fluid retention in congestive heart failure patients is 250 milligrams to 375 milligrams per day or 5 milligrams per 2.2 pounds of body weight, taken in the morning. Diamox is usually given on alternate days for this problem, but individual patient needs determine the dose.

Edema Due to Medication
The usual dose is 250 to 375 daily for 1 to 2 days, alternating with a day of rest. Individual patient needs determine the dose.

Acute Mountain Sickness
The usual dose is 500 milligrams to 1,000 milligrams in 2 or more doses, using either tablets or sustained-release capsules. Doses of this medication are often begun prior to attempting to reach high altitudes. Higher dose levels are determined by individual patient needs.

CHILDREN

The safety and effectiveness of Diamox in children have not been established. However, doses of 8 milligrams to 30 milligrams per 2.2 pounds have been used in children with various forms of epilepsy. Individual patient needs determine the proper dose.

ELDERLY

Dosage should be determined by the particular needs of the elderly patient.

Diamox tablets come in strengths of 125 and 250 milligrams. Diamox Sequels (sustained-release capsules) contain 500 milligrams of acetazolamide.

Overdosage
Any medication taken in excess can cause symptoms of overdose. If you suspect an overdose, seek medical attention immediately.

There is no specific information available about signs of Diamox overdose, but chemical imbalances, high acid levels in the bloodstream, and central nervous system effects might be expected.

Generic name:

DIAZEPAM

See Valium, page 667.

Generic name:

DICLOFENAC SODIUM

See Voltaren, page 682.

Generic name:

DICLOXACILLIN SODIUM

See Dynapen, page 223.

Generic name:

DICYCLOMINE HYDROCHLORIDE

See Bentyl, page 61.

Generic name:

DIETHYLPROPION HYDROCHLORIDE

See Tenuate, page 618.

Generic name:

DIETHYLSTILBESTROL (DES)

Why is this drug prescribed?

Diethylstilbestrol (DES), a synthetic estrogen (female hormone) available in regular or sustained-release tablets, is often given as part of the treatment for some inoperable kinds of breast cancer and prostate cancer.

Most important fact about this drug

DES must not be taken during pregnancy. In the past it was sometimes given in early pregnancy to try to prevent miscarriage. Now we know that if the unborn child is female (a so-called DES daughter), she may grow up to develop cancer or other tissue abnormalities of the cervix or vagina. DES may also cause malformation of the fetal heart or limbs.

How should you take this medication?

Take DES exactly as prescribed by your doctor. If you are being treated for inoperable prostate cancer, your initial dosage of DES may later be reduced.

What side effects may occur?

Side effects cannot be anticipated. If any develop or change in intensity, inform your doctor as soon as possible. Only your doctor can determine if it is safe for you to continue taking DES.

- *Serious potential side effects of DES include:*
  Blood clots (thrombosis, heart attack, stroke)
  Blood sugar problems
  Endometrial cancer
  Gallbladder disease
  High blood pressure
  Liver tumor

- *Additional side effects you may experience include:*
  Abnormal uterine bleeding, fluid retention, jaundice

DES can produce many of the same side effects as oral contraceptives. Grouped by physical category, these include:

- Bladder irritation, breakthrough bleeding, cervical changes, menstrual changes, painful or missed periods, premenstrual syndrome, vaginal yeast infection:
- Breast tenderness, breast enlargement, or secretion from the breasts;
- Abdominal cramps, bloating, jaundice, nausea, vomiting;
- Abnormal body hair growth, rash and skin eruptions, scalp hair loss, skin pigmentation;
- Intolerance to contact lenses;
- Depression, dizziness, headache, involuntary movements, migraine;
- Swelling due to fluid retention, weight gain or loss, changed sex drive.

Why should this drug not be prescribed?

Do not take this medication if you are sensitive to it or have ever had an allergic reaction to it.

You should have a complete physical before starting treatment with DES, and should not be given the drug if you have any of the following:

Abnormal, undiagnosed genital bleeding
Breast cancer (except in certain cases)
Estrogen-dependent tumor of any kind
History of a blood clot due to estrogen
Pregnancy
Thrombophlebitis (Inflammation of part of a vein)

Special warnings about this medication

DES should never be used as a "morning-after pill" for birth control.

DES increases the risk of cancer of the endometrium (lining of the uterus). If you are taking DES and you notice any unusual bleeding from the vagina, notify your doctor immediately.

There is some suspicion that DES may also be capable of triggering other kinds of cancer. If breast cancer runs in your family, or if you have ever had breast nodules, breast fibrocystic disease, or an abnormal mammogram, make sure you tell this to your doctor before you take DES.

If you are diabetic, you should monitor your blood or urine glucose level carefully, since DES decreases glucose tolerance

DES causes fluid retention, and this may aggravate certain conditions, such as epilepsy, migraine, and heart or kidney disease.

Possible food and drug interactions when taking this medication

If DES is taken with certain other drugs, the effects of either could be increased, decreased, or altered. It is especially important to check with your doctor before combining DES with the following:

Warfarin (Coumadin)
Vitamin C

Special information if you are pregnant or breastfeeding

As noted, DES must not be taken during pregnancy because of the high risk of harm to the fetus. If you are pregnant and are taking DES, contact your doctor immediately to discuss the option of terminating the pregnancy. No specific information is available about DES and breastfeeding. In general, a nursing mother should not take drugs. It may be necessary to choose between taking DES and breastfeeding your baby.

Recommended dosage

ADULTS

Inoperable Progressing Prostate Cancer
The usual starting dose is 1 to 3 milligrams daily, more in advanced cases. The dosage may later be reduced to an average of 1 milligram daily.

Inoperable Progressing Breast Cancer in Specific Groups of Men and Postmenopausal Women
The usual dose is 15 milligrams daily.

Overdosage

An acute overdose of DES may cause abdominal cramps, loss of appetite, diarrhea, nausea, and vomiting. After a large dose, vaginal bleeding may occur.

Chronic overdosage with DES may cause facial skin darkening ("mask of pregnancy"), fluid retention and swelling, headache, leg cramps, male breast development, sun sensitivity, and vertigo.

Any medication taken in excess can have serious consequences. If you suspect an overdose of DES, seek medical attention immediately.

Generic name:

DIFLORASONE DIACETATE

See Psorcon, page 525.

Generic name:

DIFLUNISAL

See Dolobid, page 208.

Generic name:

DIGOXIN

See Lanoxin, page 310.

Brand name:

DILANTIN

Generic name: Phenytoin sodium

Why is this drug prescribed?
Dilantin is an antiepileptic drug, prescribed to control grand mal seizures (a type of seizure in which the patient experiences a sudden loss of consciousness immediately followed by generalized convulsions) and temporal lobe seizures (a type of seizure caused by disease in the cortex of the temporal lobe of the brain affecting smell, taste, sight, hearing, memory, and movement).

Dilantin may also be used to prevent and treat seizures occurring during and after neurosurgery (surgery of the brain and spinal cord).

Most important fact about this drug
If you have been taking Dilantin regularly, do not stop abruptly. Abrupt withdrawal of Dilantin may precipitate prolonged or repeated epileptic seizures without any recovery of consciousness between attacks. Status epilepticus is a medical emergency that may be fatal if not treated promptly.

How should you take this medication?
Take Dilantin exactly as prescribed by your doctor. It is important that you strictly follow the prescribed dosage regimen and tell your doctor about any condition that makes it impossible for you to take Dilantin orally as prescribed.

One dose a day: if you miss a dose, take the missed dose as soon as you remember. However, if you do not remember the missed dose until the next day, skip it and go back to your regular dosing schedule. Do not take double doses.

More than one dose a day: take the missed dose as soon as possible. However, if it is within 4 hours of your next dose, skip the missed dose and go back to your regular schedule. Do not take double doses.

If you are given Dilantin Oral Suspension, shake well before using. Use the specially marked measuring spoon, a plastic syringe, or a medicine measuring cup to measure each dose accurately.

Swallow Dilantin Kapseals whole.

Dilantin Infatabs can be either chewed thoroughly and then swallowed, or swallowed whole.

Dilantin Infatabs are not to be used for once-a-day dosing.

Do not change from one brand of Dilantin to another without consulting your doctor. Different products may not work the same way.

Depending on the type of seizure disorder, your doctor may give you another drug with Dilantin.

Dilantin may interact with many prescription and nonprescription drugs. Consult your doctor or pharmacist before taking other drugs.

What side effects may occur?
Side effects cannot be anticipated. If any develop or change in intensity, inform your doctor as soon as possible. Only your doctor can determine whether it is safe for you to continue taking Dilantin.

■ *More common side effects may include:*
Decreased coordination

Involuntary eyeball movement
Mental confusion
Slurred speech
Unsteady movement

■ *Other side effects may include:*
Abnormal hair growth, abnormal muscle
tone, blood disorders, brief episodes
of nervousness, constipation, dizziness,
enlargement of lips, headache, inability
to fall asleep or stay asleep, motor twitching,
nausea, overgrowth of gum tissue,
Peyronie's disease (a disorder of the penis
that causes the penis to bend on an
angle during erection, often making
intercourse painful or difficult), rapid
and spastic involuntary movement, skin
rash, tremors, vomiting

Why should this drug not be prescribed?
If you have ever had an allergic reaction or
are sensitive to phenytoin or to similar
anticonvulsants used to treat epilepsy, do not
take Dilantin. Make sure your doctor is
aware of any drug reactions that you have
experienced.

Dilantin is not indicated for seizures due to
hypoglycemia (low blood sugar) and is
not effective for petit mal seizures (epilepsy
characterized by brief moments of
unconsciousness occasionally accompanied by
muscle spasms or twitching).

Special warnings about this medication
Tell your doctor if you develop a skin rash.
If the rash is scale-like, characterized by
reddish or purplish spots (bruises), or consists
of fluid-filled blisters, your doctor may
recommend that you stop using this drug and
prescribe an alternative treatment.

There is a possible relationship between the
use of Dilantin and the development of
certain diseases of the lymph system, including
Hodgkin's disease (cancer of lymph
tissue). These diseases may occur with or
without symptoms, which include fever,
rash, joint pain, and swollen lymph glands.

Use Dilantin cautiously if you have porphyria
(an inherited disorder that affects the
chemical and physical bodily process of
substances that give color to the skin).

Because the liver is the main site of Dilantin
conversion, patients with impaired liver
function, elderly patients, or people who are
seriously ill may show early signs of drug
poisoning.

Practicing good dental hygiene minimizes the
development of gingival hyperplasia
(excessive formation of the gums over the
teeth) and its complications.

Avoid drinking alcoholic beverages while
taking Dilantin.

Possible food and drug interactions when taking this medication
If Dilantin is taken with certain other drugs,
the effects of either could be increased,
decreased, or altered. It is especially important
to check with your doctor before
combining Dilantin with the following:

Alcohol
Amiodarone antiarrhythmic (Cordarone)
Antacids containing calcium
Anticoagulants such as the blood thinner
    Coumadin
Carbamazepine (Tegretol, an anticonvulsant)
Chloramphenicol (Chloromycetin)
Chlordiazepoxide (Librium)
Cortiscosteroids (hormone steroid drugs such
    as prednisone)
Diazepam (Valium)
Digitoxin (Crystodigin)
Disulfiram (Antabuse)
Doxycycline (Vibramycin)
Estrogens such as Premarin
Ethosuximide (Zarontin)
Furosemide (Lasix)

H2-antagonists such as Tagamet and Zantac
Halothane (inhaled anesthetic)
Isoniazid (tuberculosis drug)
Methylphenidate (Ritalin, a central nervous system stimulant)
Molindone hydrochloride (Moban, an antipsychotic)
Oral contraceptives such as Ortho-Novum
Phenobarbital
Phenothiazines such as tranquilizers, antiemetics, and antihistamines
Phenylbutazone (Butazolidin, a non-steroid anti-inflammatory)
Quinidine (Quinidex, a drug used to treat heart arrhythmias)
Reserpine (Rau-Sed)
Rifampin (Rifadin)
Salicylates (anti-inflammatory, fever-reducing aspirin)
Sodium valproate (anticonvulsant)
Succinimides (class of anticonvulsants)
Sucralfate (Carafate, a peptic ulcer drug)
Sulfonamides (antibacterial drugs)
Theophylline (bronchodilator used to treat asthma, bronchitis)
Tolbutamide (antidiabetic)
Trazodone (Desyrel, an antidepressant)
Valproic acid (Depakene, an anticonvulsant)

Tricyclic antidepressants may cause seizures in susceptible people, making a dosage adjustment of Dilantin necessary.

Hyperglycemia (high blood sugar) may occur in patients taking Dilantin. People with diabetes may experience increased serum glucose levels due to Dilantin.

Abnormal softening of the bones may occur in patients taking Dilantin because of Dilantin's interference with vitamin D metabolism.

Special Information
If you are pregnant or breastfeeding

If you are pregnant or plan to become pregnant, inform your doctor immediately.

Because of the possibility of birth defects with antiepileptic drug such as Dilantin, your doctor will determine whether to discontinue the drug. Do not stop taking Dilantin on your own. Breastfeeding is not recommended during treatment with Dilantin.

Recommended dosage

The Dilantin dosage should be individualized to provide maximum benefit. Your doctor will monitor your blood levels closely while you are taking Dilantin or when switching you from one drug to another.

ADULTS

Standard Daily Dosage
Patients who have not had any previous treatment may start by taking one 100-milligram Dilantin (Extended Phenytoin Sodium Capsule) 3 times daily, with the dosage then adjusted according to individual requirements.

The satisfactory maintenance dosage for most adults is 1 capsule 3 to 4 times a day.
The dosage may be increased up to 2 capsules 3 times a day, if necessary.

Once-A-Day Dosage
Only Extended Phenytoin Sodium Capsules are recommended for once-a-day use.

In adults, if seizure control is established with divided doses of three 100-milligram Dilantin capsules daily, once-a-day dosage with 300 milligrams of Extended Phenytoin Sodium Capsules may be started.

CHILDREN

The initial dosage is 5 milligrams per 2.2 pounds of body weight per day in 2 or 3 equally divided doses, with the subsequent dosage individualized to a maximum daily dosage of 300 milligrams. The recommended daily maintenance dosage is usually 4 to 8 milligrams per 2.2 pounds. Children over

6 years of age may require the minimum adult dose (300 milligrams per day).

Overdosage
Any medication taken in excess can have serious consequences. If you suspect an overdose of Dilantin, seek medical attention immediately.

Symptoms of Dilantin overdose may include:
Difficulty in pronouncing words correctly
Involuntary eyeball movement
Lack of muscle coordination
Nausea
Sluggishness
Slurred speech
Tremors
Vomiting

Brand name:

DILAUDID

Generic name: Hydromorphone hydrochloride

Why is this drug prescribed?
Dilaudid, a narcotic analgesic, is prescribed for the relief of moderate to severe pain such as that due to:

Bilary colic (pain caused by an obstruction in the gallbladder or bile duct)
Burns
Cancer
Heart attack
Injury (soft tissue and bone)
Renal colic (sharp lower back and groin pain usually caused by the passage of a stone through the ureter)
Surgery

Most important fact about this drug
High dose tolerance leading to mental and physical dependence can occur with the use of Dilaudid when it is taken repeatedly. Physical dependence (need for continual doses

to prevent withdrawal symptoms) can occur after only a few days of narcotic use, although it usually takes several weeks.

How should you take this medication?
Take Dilaudid exactly as prescribed by your doctor. Never increase the amount you take without your doctor's approval.

What side effects may occur?
Side effects cannot be anticipated. If any develop or change in intensity, inform your doctor as soon as possible. Only your doctor can determine if it is safe for you to continue taking Dilaudid.

■ *Side effects may include:*
Anxiety, constipation, dizziness, drowsiness, fear, impairment of mental and physical performance, inability to urinate, mental clouding, mood changes, nausea, restlessness, sedation, sluggishness, troubled and slowed breathing, vomiting

Why should this drug not be prescribed?
If you are sensitive to or have ever had an allergic reaction to Dilaudid or narcotic pain killers you should not take this medication. Make sure that your doctor is aware of any drug reactions that you have experienced.

Unless told to do so by your doctor, do not take this drug if you have unusual pressure on the skull due to a head injury or if you experience troubled or slow breathing due to a lung obstruction or lung disease such as emphysema or status asthmaticus (a prolonged asthma attack that does not respond to standard treatment).

Special warnings about this medication
Dilaudid may impair the mental and/or physical abilities required for the performance of potentially hazardous tasks such as driving a car or operating machinery.

Dilaudid should be used with caution if you are in a weakened condition or if you have a severe liver or kidney disorder, hypothyroidism (underactive thyroid gland), Addison's disease (adrenal gland failure), an enlarged prostate, a urethral stricture (narrowing of the urethra), or a head injury.

Dilaudid suppresses the cough reflex; therefore, caution should be exercised when Dilaudid is used for pain after an operation or in patients with a lung disease.

High doses of Dilaudid may produce labored or slowed breathing. This drug also affects centers that control breathing rhythm and may produce irregular and periodic breathing.

Narcotics such as Dilaudid may mask or hide the symptoms of sudden or severe abdominal conditions, making diagnosis and treatment difficult.

Possible food and drug interactions when taking this medication

Dilaudid is a central nervous system depressant and intensifies the effects of alcohol. Do not drink alcohol while taking this medication.

If Dilaudid is taken with certain other drugs, the effects of either could be increased, decreased, or altered. It is especially important to check with your doctor before combining Dilaudid with the following:

Antiemetics (drugs that prevent or lessen
  nausea and vomiting)
Antihistamines such as Benadryl
General anesthetics
Other central nervous system depressants
  such as Nembutal, Restoril
Other narcotic analgesics such as Demerol,
  Percocet
Phenothiazines such as Thorazine
Sedative/hypnotics such as Valium, Halcion
Tranquilizers such as Xanax
Tricyclic antidepressants such as Elavil,
  Tofranil

When such combined drug therapy is being considered, the dose of one or both medications should be reduced.

Special information
if you are pregnant or breastfeeding

Do not take Dilaudid if you are pregnant or plan to become pregnant unless you are directed to do so by your doctor. Drug dependence occurs in newborns when the mother has taken narcotic drugs regularly during pregnancy. Withdrawal signs include irritability and excessive crying, tremors, overactive reflexes, increased breathing rate, increased stools, sneezing, yawning, vomiting, and fever. Dilaudid may appear in breast milk and could affect a nursing infant. If this medication is essential to your health, your doctor may advise you to discontinue breastfeeding your baby until your treatment is finished.

Recommended dosage

ADULTS

Oral

The usual recommended dose of Dilaudid is 2 milligrams every 4 to 6 hours as determined by your doctor. Severity of pain, your individual response, and your size are used to determine your exact dosage. More severe pain may require 4 milligrams or more every 4 to 6 hours.

Rectal

Dilaudid suppositories (3 milligrams) may provide relief for a longer period of time. The usual adult dose is 1 suppository inserted rectally every 6 to 8 hours or as directed by your doctor.

CHILDREN

The safety and effectiveness of Dilaudid have not been established in children.

ELDERLY

Elderly patients should be very careful when using Dilaudid. Your doctor will prescribe a dose individualized to suit your needs.

Overdosage

Symptoms of an overdose of Dilaudid include: Bluish tinge to skin, cold and clammy skin, coma, extreme sleepiness progressing to a state of unresponsiveness, labored or slowed breathing, limp, weak muscles, low blood pressure, slow heart rate

In severe overdosage, the patient may stop breathing, and shock, heart attack, and death may occur.

If you suspect an overdose, seek emergency medical treatment immediately.

Generic name:

DILTIAZEM HYDROCHLORIDE

See Cardizem, page 94.

Brand name:

DIMETANE-DC

Generic ingredients: Brompheniramine maleate, Phenylpropanolamine hydrochloride, Codeine phosphate

Why is this drug prescribed?

Dimetane-DC Cough Syrup (Dimetane-DC) is an antihistamine/decongestant/cough suppressant combination that relieves coughs, nasal congestion, and upper respiratory symptoms caused by allergies and the common cold. Brompheniramine, the antihistamine, reduces itching and dries up secretions from the nose, eyes, and throat. Phenylpropanolamine, the decongestant, clears nasal stuffiness and makes breathing easier. Codeine calms a cough.

Most important fact about this drug

Dimetane-DC may cause you to become drowsy or less alert. Alcohol will intensify this effect. Driving or operating dangerous machinery or participating in any hazardous activity that requires full mental alertness is not recommended until you know how you react to Dimetane-DC.

How should you take this medication?

Take this medication exactly as prescribed by your doctor.

Do not exceed the directed dosage.

What side effects may occur?

Side effects cannot be anticipated. If any side effects develop or change in intensity, tell your doctor as soon as possible. Only your doctor can determine whether it is safe to continue taking Dimetane-DC.

■ *More common side effects may include:* Dizziness/lightheadedness Drowsiness Dry mouth, nose, and throat

■ *Less common or rare side effects may include:* Constipation, convulsions, diarrhea, difficulty sleeping, difficulty urinating, disturbed coordination, drug rash, false sense of well-being, headache, high blood pressure, hives, increased sensitivity to sunlight, irregular heartbeat, irritability, itching, loss of appetite, nausea, nervousness/restlessness, shortness of breath, stomach upset, tightness in chest, tremor, vision changes, vomiting, weakness, wheezing

Why should this drug not be prescribed?

This medication should not be used for newborn or premature infants or by nursing mothers.

Dimetane-DC should be avoided if you have severe high blood pressure or heart disease, including a history of heart attack or stroke; if you are taking antidepressant drugs known as MAO inhibitors (Nardil and others); if you have asthma or other breathing disorders; or if you have ever had an allergic reaction or are sensitive to any of its ingredients.

Special warnings about this medication

Dimetane-DC should be used cautiously if you have a history of bronchial asthma, narrow angle glaucoma, stomach or bladder obstruction, diabetes, or thyroid disease.

Codeine can cause drug dependence and tolerance with continued use and should be carefully monitored by your doctor.

Antihistamine overdosage can cause hallucinations and convulsions, especially in infants and small children.

Possible food and drug interactions when taking this medication

Dimetane-DC may increase the effects of alcohol. Do not drink alcohol while taking this medication.

If Dimetane-DC is taken with certain other drugs, the effects of either drug could be increased, decreased, or altered. It is especially important to check with your doctor before combining Dimetane-DC with the following:

Sedatives/hypnotics such as Phenobarbital, Halcion, and Seconal
Tranquilizers such as Xanax and Valium
Medications for anxiety such as Librium and Valium
MAO inhibitor drugs such as Nardil and Marplan
Medications for high blood pressure such as Aldomet

Special information
if you are pregnant or breastfeeding

If you are pregnant or plan to become pregnant, inform your doctor immediately. No information is available about the safety of Dimetane-DC during pregnancy.

Dimetane-DC should not be taken if you are breastfeeding. If Dimetane-DC is essential to your health, your doctor may advise you to stop breastfeeding until your treatment is finished.

Recommended dosage

ADULTS AND CHILDREN
12 YEARS AND OVER

The recommended dosage is 2 teaspoonfuls every 4 hours.

CHILDREN 6 TO UNDER 12 YEARS OLD

The usual dosage is 1 teaspoonful every 4 hours.

CHILDREN 2 TO UNDER 6 YEARS OLD

The dosage is ½ teaspoonful every 4 hours.

CHILDREN 6 MONTHS TO UNDER 2 YEARS OLD

Dosage will be determined by your doctor.

Do not take more than 6 doses in 24 hours.

Overdosage

Any medication taken in excess can cause overdose. Antihistamines may cause convulsions and death, especially in infants and small children. If you suspect an overdose, seek medical treatment immediately.

Symptoms of Dimetane-DC overdose may include:
Anxiety, breathing difficulty, convulsions, disorientation, excitation or stimulation, extreme sleepiness leading to loss of consciousness, fever, hallucinations, irregular heartbeat, rapid heartbeat

Brand name:

DIPENTUM

Generic name: Olsalazine sodium

Why is this drug prescribed?
Dipentum is an anti-inflammatory drug used by people who are allergic to sulfasalazine (Azulfidine) to maintain long-term freedom from symptoms of ulcerative colitis (chronic inflammation and ulceration of the large intestine and rectum).

Most important fact about this drug
People with a history of kidney disease should have urine and blood tests to check kidney function while taking Dipentum.

How should you take this medication?
Take Dipentum in evenly divided doses with food.

What side effects may occur?
Side effects cannot be anticipated. If any develop or change in intensity, inform your doctor as soon as possible. Only your doctor can determine if it is safe for you to continue taking Dipentum.

Diarrhea is the most common side effect.

■ Other side effects may include:
Abdominal pain/cramping, bloating, depression, difficulty breathing, dizziness, drowsiness, fatigue, feeling of tiredness, headache, heartburn, increased blood in stool, indigestion, inflamed mucous lining in mouth, insomnia, joint pain, lightheadedness, loss of appetite, nausea, rectal bleeding, skin itching, skin rash, sluggishness, upper respiratory infection, vertigo, vomiting

Cases of rare forms of hepatitis (symptoms may include aching muscles, chills, fever, headache, joint pain, loss of appetite, vomiting, and yellowish skin) have been reported in some people taking Dipentum.

Why should this drug not be prescribed?
You should not be using Dipentum if you are allergic to salicylates such as aspirin.

Special warnings about this medication
If diarrhea occurs, contact your doctor.

If you have a history of kidney disease, remember that your kidney function should be monitored while taking Dipentum.

Possible food and drug interactions when taking this medication
No drug interactions are known.

Special information if you are pregnant or breastfeeding
Pregnant women should use Dipentum only if the possible gains warrant the possible risks to the unborn child. Women who breastfeed an infant should use Dipentum cautiously, because it is not known whether this drug appears in breast milk and what effect it might have on a nursing infant.

Recommended dosage

ADULTS

The usual dose is a total of 1 gram per day, divided into 2 equal doses.

CHILDREN

Safety and effectiveness have not been established in children.

Overdosage
There have been no reports of Dipentum overdose. However, should you suspect an overdose, seek medical help immediately.

Generic name:

DIPHENHYDRAMINE HYDROCHLORIDE

See Benadryl, page 59.

Generic name:

DIPHENOXYLATE WITH ATROPINE SULFATE

See Lomotil, page 333.

Generic name:

DIPIVEFRIN HYDROCHLORIDE

See Propine, page 513.

Brand name:

DIPROLENE

Generic name: Betamethasone dipropionate

Why is this drug prescribed?

Diprolene, a synthetic cortisone-like steroid available in cream, lotion, or ointment form, is used to treat certain itchy rashes and other inflammatory skin conditions.

Most important fact about this drug

When you use Diprolene, you inevitably absorb some of the steroid through the skin and into the bloodstream. To keep absorption to a minimum, leave the skin exposed to the air or, at most, covered loosely by clothing after applying Diprolene. If you use an airtight bandage, too much of the steroid will get into your blood, possibly leading to undesirable effects.

How should you use this medication?

Apply Diprolene in a thin film, exactly as prescribed by your doctor. A typical regimen is one or two applications per day.

Be careful not to use the medication for longer than prescribed. If you do, you may disrupt your body's ability to make its own adrenal-corticoid hormones. You may safely use Diprolene AF Cream or Diprolene Ointment, the milder forms of the

medication, for up to three consecutive weeks. Diprolene Cream and Diprolene Lotion, which are stronger, should be used for no more than two consecutive weeks.

Once you have applied Diprolene, never cover the skin with an airtight bandage or other tight dressing.

For a fungal or bacterial skin infection, you will need antifungal or antibacterial medication in addition to Diprolene. If improvement is not prompt, you should stop using Diprolene until the infection is visibly clearing.

What side effects may occur?

Side effects cannot be anticipated. A possible side effect of Diprolene is stinging or burning of the skin where the medication is applied.

■ *Other side effects on the skin may include:* Acne-like eruptions, atrophy, "broken" capillaries (fine reddish lines), cracking or tightening, dryness, infected hair follicles, irritation, itching, prickly heat, rash, redness, sensitivity

Using too much Diprolene, or using Diprolene for too long, may produce side effects elsewhere in the body: see the "Overdosage" section below.

Why should this drug not be prescribed?

Do not use Diprolene if you are sensitive to it or have ever had an allergic reaction to it.

Special warnings about this medication

Diprolene is for external use only. Avoid getting it into your eyes.

Do not use Diprolene to treat any condition other than the one for which it was prescribed.

Possible food and drug interactions when using this medication

No interactions have been reported.

Special information
if you are pregnant or breastfeeding

It is not known whether Diprolene, when applied to skin, causes any problem during pregnancy or while breastfeeding. Nevertheless, let your doctor know if you are planning to become pregnant.

Recommended dosage

ADULTS

Diprolene products are not to be used with airtight dressings.

Cream or ointment
Apply a thin film to the affected skin areas once or twice daily. Treatment should be limited to 45 grams per week.

Diprolene Cream is more potent than the ointment or AF cream. Limit treatment with the cream to 14 days.

Lotion
Apply a few drops of Diprolene Lotion to the affected area once or twice daily and massage lightly until the lotion disappears.

Treatment must be limited to 14 days, and amounts greater than 50 milliliters per week should not be used.

CHILDREN

Use of Diprolene Cream Ointment, and AF Cream is not recommended for children under 12 years of age.

Overdosage

With copious or prolonged use of Diprolene, hormone absorbed into the bloodstream may cause high blood sugar, sugar in the urine, and Cushing's syndrome.

Symptoms of Cushing's syndrome may include:
Acne, depression, high blood pressure, humped upper back, insomnia, moonfaced appearance, muscle weakness, obese trunk,

paranoia, stretch marks, susceptibility to bruising, fractures, and infections, retardation of linear growth, delayed weight gain, wasted limbs

Cushing's syndrome may also trigger the development of diabetes mellitus.

Left uncorrected, Cushing's syndrome may become serious. If you suspect your use of Diprolene has led to Cushing's syndrome, seek medical attention immediately.

Generic name:

DIPYRIDAMOLE

See Persantine, page 472.

Brand name:

DISALCID

Generic name: Salsalate

Why is this drug prescribed?

Disalcid, a nonsteroidal anti-inflammatory drug, is used to relieve the symptoms of rheumatoid arthritis, osteoarthritis (the most common form of arthritis), and other rheumatic disorders.

Most important fact about this drug

Medicines containing salicylate or aspirin may be associated with the development of Reye's syndrome, a disorder that causes abnormal brain and liver function. It occurs mostly in children who have taken aspirin or other medication containing salicylate to relieve symptoms of the flu or chickenpox. Disalcid contains a salicylate and is not recommended if you have flu symptoms or chickenpox.

How should you take this medication?

Disalcid should be taken exactly as prescribed by your doctor.

Food may slow the absorption of Disalcid. However, your doctor may ask you to take Disalcid with food in order to avoid stomach upset.

What side effects may occur?

Side effects cannot be anticipated. If any develop or change in intensity, inform your doctor as soon as possible. Only your doctor can determine if it is safe for you to continue taking Disalcid.

■ *Side effects may include:*
Hearing impairment
Nausea
Rash
Ringing in the ears
Vertigo

Why should this drug not be prescribed?

Disalcid should not be taken if you are sensitive to or have ever had an allergic reaction to salsalate.

Special warnings about this medication

Disalcid should be used with extreme caution if you have chronic kidney disease or a peptic ulcer.

Salicylates occasionally cause asthma in people who are sensitive to aspirin. Although Disalcid contains a salicylate, it is less likely than aspirin to cause this reaction.

Possible food and drug interactions when taking this medication

If Disalcid is taken with certain other drugs, the effects of either could be increased, decreased, or altered. It is especially important to check with your doctor before combining Disalcid with the following:

ACE inhibitors (blood pressure drugs such as Capoten and Vasotec)
Acetazolamide (Diamox)
Aspirin and other drugs containing salicylates such as Bufferin and Empirin

Blood-thinning medications (Coumadin, Panwarfin)
Corticosteroids such as Deltasone and Decadron
Medications for gout such as Zyloprim and Benemid
Methotrexate (Rheumatrex)
Naproxen (Anaprox, Naprosyn)
Oral diabetics such as Glucotrol and Tolinase
Penicillin
Phenytoin (Dilantin)
Sulfinpyrazone (Anturane)
Thiopental (barbiturate used for anesthesia)
Thyroid hormone (Synthroid)

Special information
if you are pregnant or breastfeeding

The effects of Disalcid during pregnancy have not been adequately studied. If you are pregnant or plan to become pregnant, inform your doctor immediately. Disalcid may appear in breast milk and could affect a nursing infant. If this medication is essential to your health, your doctor may advise you to stop breastfeeding until your treatment with Disalcid is finished.

Recommended dosage

You may not feel the full benefit of this medication for 3 to 4 days.

ADULTS

The usual dosage is 3,000 milligrams daily, divided into smaller doses as follows:

(1) 2 doses of two 750-milligram tablets; (2) 2 doses of three 500-milligram tablets/capsules; or (3) 3 doses of two 500-milligram tablets/capsules.

CHILDREN

Dosage recommendations and indications for Disalcid use in children have not been established.

ELDERLY

Some elderly patients may require a lower dosage to achieve desired blood levels and to avoid the more common side effects.

Overdosage

Any medication taken in excess can have serious consequences. Deaths have occurred from salicylate overdose. If you suspect an overdose, seek medical treatment immediately.

Symptoms of Disalcid overdose may include: Confusion, dehydration, diarrhea, drowsiness, headache, high body temperature, hyperventilation, ringing in the ears, sweating, vertigo, vomiting

Generic name:

DISOPYRAMIDE PHOSPHATE

See Norpace, page 433.

Brand name:

DIULO

See Zaroxolyn, page 694.

Brand name:

DIURIL

Generic name: Chlorothiazide

Why is this drug prescribed?

Diuril is used in the treatment of high blood pressure and other conditions that require the elimination of excess fluid (water) from the body. These conditions include congestive heart failure, cirrhosis of the liver, corticosteroid and estrogen therapy, and kidney disease. When used for high blood pressure, Diuril can be used alone or with other high blood pressure medications. Diuril contains a form of thiazide, a diuretic that prompts your body to produce and eliminate more urine, which helps lower blood pressure.

Most important fact about this drug

If you have high blood pressure, you must take Diuril regularly for it to be effective. Even if you are feeling well, you must continue to take this medication. It's needed to keep your blood pressure under control.

Diuretics can cause your body to lose too much potassium. Ask your doctor for the warning signs of potassium depletion. Also ask whether you should eat specific foods that are rich in potassium or take a potassium supplement to avoid this problem.

How should you take this medication?

Take Diuril exactly as prescribed by your doctor. Stopping Diuril suddenly could cause your condition to worsen.

If you forget to take a dose, take it as soon as you remember. If it is almost time for your next dose, skip the one you missed and go back to your regular schedule. Never take two doses at the same time.

What side effects may occur?

Side effects cannot be anticipated. If any develop or change in intensity, inform your doctor as soon as possible. Only your doctor can determine if it is safe for you to continue taking Diuril.

■ *More common side effects may include:*
Diarrhea
Dizziness on standing up
Headache
Light-headedness
Loss of appetite
Low blood pressure

Low potassium (leading to symptoms like
   dry mouth, excessive thirst, weak
   or irregular heartbeat, muscle pain or
   cramps)
Stomach upset
Weakness

■ *Less common or rare side effects may
   include:*
Abdominal cramps, anemia, changes in
blood sugar, constipation, difficulty
breathing, dizziness, fever, fluid in lungs,
high levels of sugar in urine, hives,
hypersensitivity reactions, inflammation of
the pancreas, inflammation of the
salivary glands, lung inflammation, muscle
spasms, nausea, rash, reddish or
purplish spots on skin, restlessness,
sensitivity to light, Stevens-Johnson
syndrome, stomach irritation, tingling or
pins and needles, vertigo, vision
changes, vomiting, yellow eyes and skin

Why should this drug not be prescribed?
If you are unable to urinate, you should not
take this medication. If you are sensitive
to or have ever had an allergic reaction to
Diuril or similar drugs, or if you are
sensitive to other sulfonamide-derived drugs,
you should not take this medication.

Special warnings about this medication
If you are taking Diuril, a complete
assessment of your kidney function should
be done; kidney function should continue
to be monitored. Use with caution if you
have severe kidney disease.

If you have liver disease, diabetes, gout, or
collagen vascular disease (lupus
erythematosus), Diuril should be used with
caution.

If you have bronchial asthma or a history
of allergies you may be at greater risk
for an allergic reaction to this medication.

Dehydration, excessive sweating, severe
diarrhea or vomiting could deplete your
body's fluids and cause your blood pressure
to become too low. Be careful when
exercising and in hot weather.

Notify your doctor or dentist that you are
taking Diuril if you have a medical
emergency, and before you have surgery or
dental treatment.

Possible food and drug interactions when taking this medication
Diuril may increase the effects of alcohol. Do
not drink alcohol while taking this
medication.

If Diuril is taken with certain other drugs,
the effects of either may be increased,
decreased, or altered. It is especially important
to check with your doctor before
combining Diuril with the following:

Barbiturates such as phenobarbital
Corticosteroids such as Prednisone,
   ACTH
Drugs to treat diabetes such as Insulin,
   Micronase
Lithium
Narcotics such as Percocet
Nonsteroidal anti-inflammatory drugs such
   as Naprosyn
Norepinephrine (Levophed)
Other drugs for high blood pressure
Skeletal muscle relaxants such as tubocurarine

Special information if you are pregnant or breastfeeding
The effects of Diuril during pregnancy have
not been adequately studied. If you are
pregnant or plan to become pregnant, inform
your doctor immediately. Diuril appears
in breast milk and could affect a nursing
infant. If this medication is essential to
your health, your doctor may advise you to
discontinue breastfeeding until your
treatment is finished.

Recommended dosage

ADULTS

Diuril comes in tablets, an oral suspension, and an intravenous preparation, reserved for emergencies. Dosages below are for the oral preparations.

Diuresis
The usual dose is 0.5 gram to 1 gram 1 or 2 times per day. Your doctor may have you take this medication on alternate days or on some other on-off schedule.

High Blood Pressure
The starting dose is 0.5 gram to 1 gram per day, taken as one dose or two or more smaller doses. Dosages will be adjusted to the individual patient's need.

CHILDREN

Dosages for children should be adjusted according to weight, generally 10 milligrams per pound of body weight daily in 2 doses.

Under 6 months
Dosage may be up to 15 milligrams per pound of body weight per day in 2 doses.

Under 2 years
The usual dosage is 125 milligrams to 375 milligrams per day in 2 doses. The liquid form of this drug may be used in children under 2 years of age at ½ to 1½ teaspoons (2.5 to 7.5 milliliters) per day.

2 to 12 years
375 milligrams to 1 gram daily in 2 doses. The liquid form of this medication may be used in children 2 to 12 years at 1½ to 4 teaspoons (7.5 milliliters to 20 milliliters) per day.

ELDERLY

Dosage should be determined by the particular needs of the elderly patient.

Overdosage

Any medication taken in excess can cause symptoms of overdose. If you suspect an overdose, seek medical attention immediately.

Signs of Diuril overdose may include:
Dehydration and symptoms of low potassium (dry mouth, excessive thirst, weak or irregular heartbeat, muscle pain or cramps)
Electrolyte depletion

Generic name:

DIVALPROEX SODIUM

See Depakote, page 178.

Generic name:

DOCUSATE SODIUM

See Colace, page 123.

Brand name:

DOLOBID

Generic name: Diflunisal

Why is this drug prescribed?

Dolobid, a nonsteroidal anti-inflammatory drug, is used to treat mild to moderate pain and relieve the inflammation, swelling, stiffness and joint pain associated with rheumatoid arthritis and osteoarthritis (the most common form of arthritis).

Most important fact about this drug

You should have frequent check-ups with your doctor if you take Dolobid regularly. Ulcers or internal bleeding can occur without warning.

How should you take this medication?

Dolobid should be taken with food or an antacid, and with a full glass of water or milk. Never take it on an empty stomach.

Tablets should be swallowed whole, not chewed or crushed.

Take this medication exactly as prescribed by your doctor.

If you are using Dolobid for arthritis, it should be taken regularly.

If you forget to take a dose, take it as soon as you remember. If it is almost time for your next dose, skip the one you missed and go back to your regular schedule. Never take two doses at the same time.

What side effects may occur?

Side effects cannot be anticipated. If any develop or change in intensity, inform your doctor as soon as possible. Only your doctor can determine if it is safe for you to continue taking Dolobid.

■ *More common side effects may include:*
Abdominal pain, constipation, diarrhea, dizziness, fatigue, gas, headache, inability to sleep, indigestion, nausea, rash, ringing in ears, sleepiness, vomiting

■ *Less common or rare side effects may include:*
Abdominal bleeding, anemia, blurred vision, confusion, depression, disorientation, dry mouth and nose, fluid retention, hepatitis, hives, inflammation of lips and tongue, itching, kidney failure, lightheadedness, loss of appetite, nervousness, painful urination, peptic ulcer, pins and needles, protein or blood in urine, rash, sensitivity to light, skin eruptions, Stevens-Johnson syndrome, vertigo, weakness, yellow eyes and skin

Why should this drug not be prescribed?

If you are sensitive to or have had an allergic reaction to Dolobid, aspirin, or similar drugs, or if you have had asthma attacks caused by aspirin or other drugs of this type, you should not take this medication. Make sure that your doctor is aware of any drug reactions that you have experienced.

Special warnings about this medication

Peptic ulcers and bleeding can occur without warning.

This drug should be used with caution if you have kidney or liver disease; and it can cause liver inflammation in some people.

Do not take aspirin or any other anti-inflammatory medications while taking Dolobid, unless your doctor tells you to do so.

Dolobid can cause vision problems. If you experience any changes in your vision, inform your doctor.

Dolobid may prolong bleeding time. If you are taking blood-thinning medication, this drug should be taken with caution.

If you have heart disease or high blood pressure, this drug can increase water retention. Use with caution.

Dolobid may cause you to become drowsy or less alert; therefore, driving or operating dangerous machinery or participating in any hazardous activity that requires full mental alertness is not recommended.

Possible food and drug interactions when taking this medication

If Dolobid is taken with certain other drugs, the effects of either could be increased, decreased, or altered. It is especially important to check with your doctor before combining Dolobid with the following:

Acetaminophen
Antacids
Aspirin
Cyclosporine (Sandimmune)
Methotrexate
Naproxen (Naprosyn)
Oral anticoagulants (Blood thinners)
The arthritis medication Sulindac (Clinoril)
The diuretic hydrochlorothiazide

Special information
If you are pregnant or breastfeeding
The effects of Dolobid during pregnancy have not been adequately studied. If you are pregnant or plan to become pregnant inform your doctor immediately. Dolobid appears in breast milk and could affect a nursing infant. If this medication is essential to your health, your doctor may advise you to discontinue breastfeeding until your treatment with Dolobid is finished.

Recommended dosage
ADULTS

Mild to Moderate Pain
Starting dose is 1,000 milligrams, followed by 500 milligrams every 8 to 12 hours, depending on the patient. Your physician may adjust your dosage according to age, weight and severity of symptoms.

Osteoarthritis and Rheumatoid Arthritis
500 to 1,000 milligrams per day in 2 doses of 250 milligrams or 500 milligrams.

The lowest dose that proves beneficial should be used.

Maximum maintenance dosage is 1,500 milligrams per day.

CHILDREN
Safety and effectiveness of Dolobid have not been established in children under 12 years of age. However, your doctor may decide that the benefits of this medication may outweigh the potential risks.

ELDERLY
Dosage should be determined by the particular needs of the elderly patient.

Overdosage
Any medication taken in excess can cause symptoms of overdose. If you suspect an overdose, seek medical attention immediately.

The symptoms of Dolobid overdose may include:
Abnormally rapid heartbeat, coma, diarrhea, disorientation, drowsiness, hyperventilation, nausea, ringing in the ears, stupor, sweating, vomiting

Brand name:

DONNAGEL-PG

Generic ingredients: Powdered opium, Kaolin, Pectin, Hyoscyamine sulfate, Atropine sulfate, Scopolamine hydrobromide

Why is this drug prescribed?
Donnagel-PG is used to treat diarrhea.

Most important fact about this drug
The opium in Donnagel-PG may be habit-forming.

This medication should not be used for more than 2 days, or if you have a high fever, unless specifically indicated by your doctor.

How should you take this medication?
Take this medication exactly as prescribed by your doctor.

Do not take more than the recommended dosage.

Do not take Donnagel-PG for diarrhea associated with antibiotic-caused inflammation of the colon or diarrhea caused by bacteria.

Shake well before using.

What side effects may occur?
Side effects cannot be anticipated. If any appear or change in intensity, inform your doctor as soon as possible. Only your doctor can determine if it is safe for you to continue taking Donnagel-PG.

- *Side effects (more common at high dosages) may include:*
  Blurred vision
  Difficult urination
  Dry mouth
  Flushing and dryness of the skin

Why should this drug not be prescribed?
Donnagel-PG should not be used if you have glaucoma, advanced kidney or liver disease, or are sensitive to or allergic to any of its ingredients.

Special warnings about this medication
Remember, diarrhea may signal a serious problem. Donnagel-PG should not be taken for more than 2 days, or if you have a fever, unless your doctor has specifically told you to do so.

Unless directed to do so by your doctor, do not use Donnagel-PG if you have glaucoma or excessive eye pressure or are elderly (undiagnosed glaucoma or excessive pressure could exist). Do not give the drug to children under 6 years of age without first consulting your doctor.

If you develop blurred vision, a rapid pulse, or dizziness, stop taking the medication.

If your mouth becomes dry, your dosage may need to be reduced.

If eye pain develops, stop taking the medication and see your doctor immediately. This could indicate undiagnosed glaucoma.

Donnagel-PG should be used with care if you have a bladder obstruction or an enlarged prostate.

Possible food and drug interactions when taking this medication
No interactions are listed.

Special information
if you are pregnant or breastfeeding
The effects of Donnagel-PG during pregnancy have not been adequately studied. If you are pregnant or plan to become pregnant, inform your doctor immediately. Donnagel-PG may appear in breast milk and could affect a nursing infant. If this medication is essential to your health, your doctor may advise you to stop breastfeeding until your treatment with Donnagel-PG is finished.

Recommended dosage
ADULTS AND CHILDREN OVER 12 YEARS

The usual dose is 2 tablespoons (1 fluid ounce) initially, then 1 tablespoon every 3 hours.

CHILDREN 6 TO 12 YEARS OLD

The usual dose is 2 teaspoonfuls initially, then 1 or 2 teaspoonfuls every 3 hours.

CHILDREN UNDER 6 YEARS OLD

Your physician will determine the dosage according to your child's body weight. It should not be more than 4 doses in 24 hours.

Overdosage

Any medication taken in excess can have serious consequences. No specific symptoms of overdosage have been reported, but if you suspect an overdose seek medical treatment immediately.

Brand name:

DONNATAL

Generic ingredients: Phenobarbital, Hyoscyamine sulfate, Atropine sulfate, Scopolamine hydrobromide

Why is this drug prescribed?

Donnatal is a mild antispasmodic medication used with other drugs for relief of cramps and pain associated with various stomach, intestinal and bowel disorders, including irritable bowel syndrome, acute colitis and duodenal ulcer. One of its ingredients, phenobarbital, is a mild sedative.

(Note: The FDA classifies Donnatal as being "possibly" effective for these disorders. Some medical experts question the effectiveness of this drug in all cases.)

Most important fact about this drug

Phenobarbital, one of the ingredients of Donnatal, can be habit-forming. If you have a history of drug dependence or are addiction-prone, do not take Donnatal.

How should you take this medication?

Donnatal should be taken one-half hour to 1 hour before meals.

Take this medication exactly as prescribed by your doctor.

If you forget to take a dose, take it as soon as you remember. If it is almost time for your next dose, skip the one you missed and go back to your regular schedule. Never take two doses at the same time.

What side effects may occur?

Side effects cannot be anticipated. If any develop or change in intensity, inform your doctor as soon as possible. Only your doctor can determine if it is safe for you to continue taking Donnatal.

■ *More common side effects may include:*
Blurred vision
Constipation
Decreased sweating
Drowsiness
Dry mouth

■ *Less common or rare side effects may include:*
Agitation, allergic reaction, bloated feeling, difficulty sleeping, difficulty urinating, dilation of the pupil of the eye, dizziness, excitement, headache, impotence, loss of taste, muscular and bone pain, nausea, nervousness, pounding heartbeat, rapid heartbeat, skin rash or hives, suppression of lactation, vomiting, weakness

Why should this drug not be prescribed?

Do not take Donnatal if you suffer from glaucoma, diseases that block the urinary tract or gastrointestinal tracts, or myasthenia gravis, a condition in which the muscles become progressively paralyzed. Also, Donnatal should not be used by people with intestinal atony, unstable cardiovascular status, ulcerative colitis, or hiatal hernia.

If you are sensitive to or have ever had an allergic reaction to Donnatal, its ingredients, or similar drugs, you should not take this medication. Make sure your doctor is aware of any drug reactions that you have experienced.

Special warnings about this medication

If you suffer from high blood pressure, over-active thyroid (hyperthyroidism), abnormal heartbeat or heart, kidney, or liver disease, you should use Donnatal with caution.

Donnatal can decrease sweating. If you are exercising or are subjected to high temperatures, be careful of heat prostration.

If you have a gastric ulcer or have an ileostomy or colostomy, this medication should be used with caution.

Donnatal may cause you to become drowsy or less alert. Driving or operating dangerous machinery or participating in any hazardous activity that requires full mental alertness is not recommended.

Possible food and drug interactions when taking this medication

Donnatal may intensify the effects of alcohol. Check with your doctor before using alcohol with this medication.

If Donnatal is taken with certain other drugs, the effects of either could be increased, decreased, or altered. It is especially important to check with your doctor before combining Donnatal with the following:

Adrenal corticosteroids
Anticoagulants (Blood-thinning medication) such as Coumadin
Antidepressants such as Elavil
Antihistamines such as Benadryl
Barbiturates such as Seconal
Digitalis (Lanoxin)
Narcotics such as Percocet
Tranquilizers such as Valium

Special information if you are pregnant or breastfeeding

The effects of Donnatal during pregnancy have not been adequately studied. If you are pregnant or plan to become pregnant, this drug should be used only when prescribed by your doctor. It is not known whether Donnatal appears in breast milk. If this medication is essential to your health, your doctor may advise you to discontinue breastfeeding until your treatment is finished.

Recommended dosage

ADULTS

All dosages should be adjusted to individual patient needs.

Tablets or Capsules
The usual dosage is 1 or 2 tablets or capsules, 3 or 4 times a day.

Liquid
The usual dosage is 1 or 2 teaspoonfuls, 3 or 4 times a day.

Donnatal Extentabs
The usual dosage is 1 tablet every 12 hours. Your doctor may tell you to take 1 tablet every 8 hours, if necessary.

CHILDREN

Dosage is determined by body weight and can be given every 4 to 6 hours. Follow your doctor's instructions carefully when giving this medication to a child.

Overdosage

Any medication taken in excess can cause symptoms of overdose. If you suspect an overdose, seek medical attention immediately.

The symptoms of Donnatal overdose may include:
Blurred vision
Central nervous system stimulation
Difficulty swallowing
Dilated pupils
Dizziness
Dry mouth
Headache
Hot and dry skin
Nausea
Vomiting

Brand name:

DORAL

Generic name: Quazepam

Why is this drug prescribed?

Doral, a sleeping medication available in tablet form, is taken as short-term treatment for insomnia. Symptoms of insomnia may include difficulty falling asleep, frequent awakenings throughout the night, or very early morning awakening.

Most important fact about this drug

Doral is a chemical cousin of Valium and is potentially addictive. Over time, your body will get used to the prescribed dosage of Doral, and you will no longer derive any benefit from it. That is the point at which to stop taking this medication. If you were to increase the dosage against medical advice, the drug would again work as a sleeping pill—but only until your body adjusted to the higher dosage. That, in a nutshell, is the vicious circle that can lead to addiction. If you use Doral only as prescribed, however, you will not become addicted to it.

How should you take this medication?

Take Doral exactly as prescribed by your doctor—one dose per day, at bedtime. Keep in touch with your doctor; if you respond very well, it may be possible to cut your dosage in half after the first few nights. The older or more run-down you are, the more desirable it is to try for this early dosage reduction.

If you have been taking Doral regularly for 6 weeks or so, you may experience withdrawal symptoms if you stop "cold turkey," or even if you reduce the dosage without specific instructions on how to do it. Always follow your doctor's advice for tapering off gradually from Doral.

Alcohol should be avoided during treatment with Doral.

Until you know how this medicine affects you, do not drive a car or operate potentially dangerous machinery.

What side effects may occur?

Side effects cannot be anticipated. If any develop or change in intensity, inform your doctor as soon as possible. Only your doctor can determine if it is safe for you to continue taking Doral.

■ *More common side effects may include:*
Dizziness
Drowsiness
Dry mouth
Fatigue
Headache
Indigestion

■ *Less common side effects may include:*
Abdominal pain, abnormal taste, abnormal thinking, changes in sex drive, confusion, constipation, diarrhea, impotence, incontinence, irregular menstrual periods, irritability, itching, jaundice, muscle spasms, nervousness, nightmares, rash, slurred or otherwise abnormal speech, urinary retention, vague feeling of being sick, vision problems, weakness

Some people who have taken Doral nightly for several weeks begin to experience increased wakefulness in the final third of the night and anxiety the following day.

In rare instances, Doral produces agitation, sleep disturbances, hallucinations, or stimulation—exactly the opposite of the desired effect. If this should happen to you, stop taking Doral immediately.

Why should this drug not be prescribed?

Do not take Doral if you are sensitive to it, or if you have ever had an allergic or if you have ever had an allergic reaction to it or to another Valium-type medication.

You should not take Doral if you know or suspect that you have sleep apnea (short periods of arrested breathing that occur during sleep).

Special warnings about this medication

Because Doral may decrease your daytime alertness, do not drive, climb, or operate dangerous machinery until you find out how the drug affects you. In some cases, Doral's sedative effect may last for several days after the last dose.

If you are suffering from depression, Doral may make your depression worse.

If you have a history of alcohol or drug abuse, you are at special risk for addiction to Doral.

Never increase the dosage of Doral on your own. Tell your doctor right away if the medication no longer seems to be working.

Possible food and drug interactions when taking this medication

If Doral is taken with certain other drugs, the effects of either could be increased, decreased, or altered. It is especially important to check with your doctor before combining Doral with the following:

Antiseizure medications such as Dilantin and Tegretol
Antihistamines such as Benadryl
Mood-altering medications such as Thorazine and Clozaril
Other central nervous system depressants such as Xanax and Valium

Do not drink alcohol while taking Doral.

Special information if you are pregnant or breastfeeding

Because Doral may cause fetal malformations, it should not be taken during pregnancy. If you do take Doral while pregnant, inform your doctor immediately. If you want to have a baby, tell your doctor; plan to discontinue taking Doral before getting pregnant.

Babies whose mothers are taking Doral at the time of birth may experience withdrawal symptoms from the drug. Such babies may be "floppy" (flaccid) instead of having normal muscle tone.

Since Doral does pass into breast milk, you should not take this medication if you are nursing a baby.

Recommended dosage

ADULTS

The recommended initial dose is 15 milligrams daily. Your doctor may later reduce this dosage to 7.5 milligrams.

CHILDREN

Safety and efficacy of Doral in children under 18 years old have not been established.

ELDERLY AND DEBILITATED PATIENTS

Your doctor will tailor your dose to your specific needs.

Overdosage

Any medication taken in excess can have serious consequences. If you suspect an overdose of Doral, seek medical attention immediately.

Symptoms of an overdose of Doral may include:
Coma
Confusion
Somnolence

Brand name:

DORYX

Generic name: Doxycycline hyclate
Other brand names: Vibramycin, Vibra-Tabs

Why is this drug prescribed?
Doxycycline is a broad-spectrum tetracycline antibiotic used against a wide variety of bacterial infections, including, Rocky Mountain spotted fever and other fevers caused by ticks, fleas, and lice; urinary tract infections; trachoma (chronic infections of the eye); and some gonococcal infections in adults. It is also used with other medications to treat severe acne and amoebic dysentery (diarrhea caused by severe parasitic infection of the intestines).

Occasionally doctors prescribe doxycycline to treat Lyme disease. This is not yet an officially approved use for this drug.

Most important fact about this drug
Children under 8 years old and women in the last half of pregnancy should not take this medication. It may cause developing teeth to become permanently discolored (yellow-gray-brown).

How should you take this medication?
Take doxycycline with a full glass of water or other liquid to avoid irritating your throat or stomach. Doxycycline can be taken with or without food. However, if the medicine does upset your stomach, you may wish to take it with a glass of milk or after you have eaten.

Take this medication exactly as prescribed by your doctor, even if your symptoms have disappeared.

Doxycycline capsules must be swallowed whole.

If you are taking an oral suspension form of doxycycline such as Vibramycin Oral Suspension, store in the refrigerator. Do not freeze. Shake well before using.

What side effects may occur?
Side effects cannot be anticipated. If any develop or change in intensity, inform your doctor as soon as possible. Only your doctor can determine if it is safe for you to continue taking doxycycline.

■ *More common side effects may include:*
Angioedema (chest pain; swelling of face, around lips, tongue and throat, arms and legs; sore throat, fever, and chills; difficulty swallowing), bulging foreheads in infants, diarrhea, difficulty swallowing, discolored teeth in infants and children (more common during long-term use of tetracycline), inflammation of the tongue, loss of appetite, nausea, rash, rectal or genital itching, severe allergic reaction (hives, itching, and swelling), skin sensitivity to light, vomiting

■ *Less common or rare side effects may include:*
Aggravation of lupus erythematosus (disease of the connective tissue), skin inflammation and peeling, throat inflammation and ulcerations

Why should this drug not be prescribed?
If you are sensitive to or have ever had an allergic reaction to doxycycline or drugs of this type, you should not take this medication. Make sure your doctor is aware of any drug reactions that you have experienced.

Special warnings about this medication
As with other antibiotics, treatment with doxycycline may result in a growth of bacteria that do not respond to this medication and can cause a secondary infection.

You may become more sensitive to sunlight while taking doxycycline. Be careful if you are going out in the sun or using a sunlamp.

Birth control pills that contain estrogen may not be as effective while you are taking tetracycline drugs. Ask your doctor or pharmacist if you should use another form of birth control while taking doxycycline.

Possible food and drug interactions when taking this medication

If doxycycline is taken with certain other drugs, the effects of either could be increased, decreased, or altered. It is especially important to check with your doctor before combining doxycycline with the following:

Antacids containing aluminum, calcium, or magnesium, or iron-containing preparations (Maalox, Mylanta, and others)
Blood-thinning medications such as Coumadin and Panwarfin
Penicillin (V-Cillin K, Pen VK, others)
Sodium bicarbonate

Special information
if you are pregnant or breastfeeding

Doxycycline should not be used during pregnancy. Tetracycline can damage developing teeth during the last half of pregnancy. If you are pregnant or plan to become pregnant, inform your doctor immediately. Tetracyclines such as doxycycline appear in breast milk and can affect a nursing infant. If this medication is essential to your health, your doctor may advise you to discontinue breastfeeding until your treatment is finished.

Recommended dosage

ADULTS

The usual dose of oral doxycycline is 200 milligrams on the first day of treatment (100 milligrams every 12 hours) followed by a maintenance dose of 100 milligrams per day. The maintenance dose may be taken as a single dose or as 50 milligrams every 12 hours.

Your doctor may prescribe 100 milligrams every 12 hours for severe infections such as chronic urinary tract infection.

For Uncomplicated Gonorrhoea (Except Anorectal Infections in Men)
The usual dose is 100 milligrams by mouth, twice a day for 7 days. An alternate, single-day treatment is 300 milligrams, followed in 1 hour by a second 300 milligram dose.

For Primary and Secondary Syphilis
The usual dose is 300 milligrams a day, divided into smaller, equal doses for at least 10 days.

CHILDREN

For children above 8 years of age, the recommended dosage schedule for those weighing 100 pounds or less is 2 milligrams per pound of body weight, divided into 2 doses, on the first day of treatment, followed by 1 milligram per pound of body weight given as a single daily dose or divided into 2 doses on subsequent days.

For more severe infections, up to 2 milligrams per pound of body weight may be used.

For children over 100 pounds, the usual adult dose should be used.

Overdosage

Any medication taken in excess can have serious consequences. If you suspect an overdose, seek medical treatment immediately.

Generic name:

DOXAZOSIN MESYLATE

See Cardura, page 95.

Generic name:

DOXEPIN HYDROCHLORIDE

See Sinequan, page 581.

Generic name:

DOXYCYCLINE HYCLATE

See Doryx, page 216.

Brand name:

DUPHALAC

See Chronulac Syrup, page 110.

Brand name:

DURICEF

Generic name: Cefadroxil monohydrate
Other brand name: Ultracef

Why is this drug prescribed?

Duricef, a cephalosporin antibiotic, is used in the treatment of nose, throat, urinary tract and skin infections that are caused by specific bacteria, including staph, strep, and E. coli.

Most important fact about this drug

Do not take this drug if you are allergic to cephalosporin antibiotics or penicillin. There is a possibility that you could be allergic to both medications. Allergic reactions to this medication can be serious and possibly fatal. If you experience a reaction, report it to your doctor immediately and seek medical treatment.

How should you take this medication?

Take this medication exactly as prescribed by your doctor. It is important that you finish taking all of this medication to obtain the maximum benefit.

What side effects may occur?

Side effects cannot be anticipated. If any develop or change in intensity, inform your doctor as soon as possible. Only your doctor can determine if it is safe for you to continue taking Duricef.

■ *More common side effects may include:*
Diarrhea

■ *Less common or rare side effects may include:*
Colitis, nausea, redness and swelling of skin, skin rash and itching, vaginal inflammation, vomiting

Why should this drug not be prescribed?

If you are sensitive to or have ever had an allergic reaction to a cephalasporin antibiotic, you should not take Duricef.

Special warnings about this medication

If you have allergies, particularly to drugs, or often develop diarrhea when taking other antibiotics, you should tell your doctor before Duricef is prescribed.

Use with caution if you have a history of gastrointestinal disease, particularly colitis.

Continued or prolonged use of Duricef may result in a growth of bacteria that do not respond to this medication and can cause a secondary infection.

Possible food and drug interactions when taking this medication

No significant interactions have been reported.

Special information
if you are pregnant or breastfeeding

The effects of Duricef during pregnancy have not been adequately studied. If you are pregnant or plan to become pregnant, inform your doctor immediately. Duricef may appear in breast milk and could affect a nursing infant. If this medication is essential to your health, your doctor may advise you to stop nursing your baby until your treatment time with Duricef is finished.

Recommended dosage

ADULTS

Urinary Tract Infections
The usual dosage for uncomplicated infections is a total of 1 to 2 grams per day in a single dose or 2 smaller doses. For all other urinary tract infections, the usual dosage is a total of 2 grams per day taken in 2 doses.

Skin and Skin Structure Infections
The usual dose is a total of 1 gram per day in a single dose or 2 smaller doses.

Throat Infections — Strep Throat and Tonsillitis:
The usual dosage is a total of 1 gram per day in a single or 2 smaller doses for 10 days.

CHILDREN

For urinary tract and skin infections, the usual dose is 30 milligrams per 2.2 pounds of body weight per day, divided and taken every 12 hours. For throat infections, the recommended dose per day is 30 milligrams per 2.2 pounds of body weight in single or 2 smaller doses. In the treatment of strep throat, the dose should be taken for at least 10 days.

ELDERLY

If you are elderly or have kidney disease, your dose may be reduced by your doctor.

Overdosage

Duricef is generally safe. However, large amounts may cause overdose symptoms, including seizures or the side effects listed above. Suspected overdoses of Duricef must be treated immediately, and you should contact your physician or an emergency room.

Brand name:

DYAZIDE

Generic ingredients: Hydrochlorothiazide, Triamterene

Why is this drug prescribed?

Dyazide is a diuretic used in the treatment of high blood pressure and other conditions that require the elimination of excess water from the body. When used for high blood pressure, Dyazide can be taken alone or with other high blood pressure medications. Diuretics help your body produce and eliminate more urine, which helps lower blood pressure. Triamterene, one of the ingredients, helps to minimize the potassium loss that can be caused by the other component, hydrochlorothiazide.

Most important fact about this drug

Your doctor may not prescribe Dyazide if you have certain kidney problems, are unable to urinate, or have pre-existing problems with high potassium levels in your body.

Your doctor will check your potassium level frequently.

How should you take this medication?

Dyazide should be taken early in the day.

To avoid stomach upset, Dyazide may be taken with food.

Avoid prolonged exposure to sunlight.

Avoid potassium-containing salt substitutes.

What side effects may occur?

Side effects cannot be anticipated. If any occur or change in intensity, inform your doctor as soon as possible. Only your doctor can determine if it is safe for you to continue taking Dyazide.

■ *Side effects may include:*
Abdominal pain, anemia, blurred vision, breathing difficulty, change in potassium level causing symptoms such as dry mouth, excessive thirst, weak or irregular heartbeat, muscle pain, and cramps, constipation, diabetes, diarrhea, dizzinesss, dizziness when standing up, dry mouth, fatigue, fluid in lungs, headache, hives, impotence, irregular heartbeat, kidney failure, kidney stones, muscle cramps, nausea, rash, sensitivity to light, strong allergic reaction (localized hives, itching, and swelling or in severe cases, shock), tingling or pins and needles, vertigo, vision changes, vomiting, weakness, worsening of lupus, yellow eyes and skin

Why should this drug not be prescribed?

If you are unable to urinate or have any serious kidney disease, if you have high potassium levels in your blood, or if you are taking other drugs that prevent loss of potassium, you should not take Dyazide. Potassium-containing salt substitutes should not be used, and potassium supplements should be used only when specifically indicated by your doctor.

If you are sensitive to or have ever had an allergic reaction to triamterene, hydrochlorothiazide, or similar drugs, or if you are sensitive to other sulfa drugs, you should not take this medication.

Special warnings about this medication

If you are taking Dyazide and have kidney disease, a complete assessment of your kidney function should be done; kidney function should continue to be monitored.

Dyazide should be used with caution if you are taking a type of blood pressure medication called an ACE inhibitor, such as Vasotec or Capoten.

If you have liver disease, diabetes, cirrhosis of the liver, heart failure, or kidney stones, this medication should be used with care.

If you suffer from a salt deficiency, be careful to avoid becoming dehydrated when exercising and in hot weather.

Possible food and drug interactions when taking this medication

If Dyazide is taken with certain other drugs, the effects of either could be increased, decreased, or altered. It is especially important to check with your doctor before combining Dyazide with the following:

ACE inhibitors (Capoten, Vasotec, others)
ACTH
Amphotericin B
Blood-thinning medications such as Coumadin and Panwarfin
Corticosteroids such as Deltasone
Drugs for hypoglycemia such as Diabinese
Gout medications such as Zyloprim
Laxatives
Lithium (Eskalith)
Low-salt milk
Methenamine
Nonsteroidal anti-inflammatory drugs such as Voltaren and Dolobid
Norepinephrine (Levophed)
Other drugs that minimize potassium loss or contain potassium
Other high blood pressure medications (Minipress, Vasotec, others)
Salt substitutes containing potassium
Sodium polystyrene sulfonate
Tubocurarine

Special information
if you are pregnant or breastfeeding

The effects of Dyazide during pregnancy have not been adequately studied. If you are pregnant or plan to become pregnant, inform your doctor immediately. Dyazide appears in breast milk and could affect a nursing infant. If this medication is essential to your health, your doctor may advise you to discontinue breastfeeding until your treatment is finished.

Recommended dosage

ADULTS

The usual dose of Dyazide is 1 or 2 capsules once daily, with appropriate monitoring of blood potassium levels by your doctor.

CHILDREN

Safety and effectiveness in children have not been established.

Overdosage

Any medication taken in excess can have serious consequences. If you suspect an overdose, seek medical treatment immediately.

Symptoms of Dyazide overdose may include:
Fever
Flushed face
Nausea
Production of large amounts
    of pale urine
Vomiting
Weakness
Weariness

Brand name:

DYNACIRC

Generic name: Isradipine

Why is this drug prescribed?

DynaCirc, a type of medication called a calcium channel blocker, is prescribed for the treatment of high blood pressure. It is effective when used alone or with a thiazide-type diuretic. Calcium channel blockers ease the workload of the heart by slowing down the muscle contractions of the heart and the passage of nerve impulses through the heart. This improves blood flow through the heart and throughout the body and reduces blood pressure.

Most important fact about this drug

If you have high blood pressure, you must take DynaCirc regularly for it to be effective. Even if you are feeling well, you must continue to take DynaCirc to control your blood pressure.

How should you take this medication?

Take this medication exactly as prescribed by your doctor, even if your symptoms have disappeared.

Try not to miss any doses. If DynaCirc is not taken regularly, your condition may worsen.

What side effects may occur?

Side effects cannot be anticipated. If any develop or change in intensity, inform your doctor as soon as possible. Only your doctor can determine if it is safe for you to continue taking DynaCirc.

■ *More common side effects may include:*
    Chest pain
    Dizziness
    Fatigue
    Fluid retention
    Flushing
    Headache
    Pounding heartbeat

■ *Less common side effects may include:*
    Diarrhea, increased urinary frequency, nausea, rapid heartbeat, rash, shortness of breath, stomach upset, unusually frequent urination, vomiting, weakness

■ *Rare side effects may include:*
Constipation, cough, decreased sex drive, depression, difficulty sleeping, drowsiness, dry mouth, excessive nighttime urination, excessive sweating, fainting, changes in heartbeat, heart attack, heart failure, hives, impotence, itching, leg and foot cramps, low blood pressure, nervousness, numbness, severe dizziness, sluggishness, stroke, throat discomfort, tingling or pins and needles, vision changes

Why should this drug not be prescribed?

If you are sensitive to or have ever had an allergic reaction to DynaCirc or similar drugs of this type, you should not take this medication. Tell your doctor about any drug reactions you have experienced.

Special warnings about this medication

DynaCirc can cause your blood pressure to become too low. If you feel lightheaded or faint, contact your doctor.

This medication should be carefully monitored if you have congestive heart failure, especially if you are also taking a beta-blocking medication—(e.g., Tenormin, Inderal)

Possible food and drug interactions when taking this medication

If DynaCirc is taken with certain other drugs, the effects of either could be increased, decreased, or altered. It is especially important to check with your doctor before combining DynaCirc with the following:

Beta blockers (Tenormin, Lopressor)
Fentanyl, an anesthetic
Propranolol (Inderal)

Special information if you are pregnant or breastfeeding

The effects of DynaCirc during pregnancy have not been adequately studied. If you are pregnant or plan to become pregnant, consult your doctor immediately. DynaCirc may appear in breast milk and could affect a nursing infant. If this medication is essential to your health, your doctor may advise you to discontinue breastfeeding until your treatment with DynaCirc is finished.

Recommended dosage

ADULTS

All dosages should be adjusted to meet the individual patient's needs.

The usual starting dose is 2.5 milligrams, 2 times a day, either alone or in combination with a thiazide diuretic drug. DynaCirc may lower blood pressure 2 to 3 hours after taking the first dose, but the full effect of the drug may not take place for 2 to 4 weeks.

After a 2- to 4-week trial, your doctor may increase the dosage by 5 milligrams per day every 2 to 4 weeks until a maximum dose of 20 milligrams per day is reached. Side effects may increase or become more common after a 10-milligram dose.

Patients with kidney or liver disease should still begin treatment with a 2.5-milligram dose 2 times per day; however, they should be closely monitored, since their conditions may change the effects of this drug.

ELDERLY

This drug's effects may be stronger in elderly patients, who should be closely monitored. The usual starting dose should still be 2.5 milligrams 2 times per day.

Overdosage

Although no specific information is available, the symptoms of overdose with other calcium channel blockers include drowsiness, severe low blood pressure and slow heartbeat.

If you suspect symptoms of a DynaCirc overdose, seek medical attention immediately.

Brand name:

DYNAPEN

Generic name: Dicloxacillin sodium

Why is this drug prescribed?

Dynapen is a penicillin-like antibiotic that treats certain bacterial infections caused by staph (staphylococci).

Most important fact about this drug

Dynapen should not be taken if you have had an allergic reaction to any form of penicillin. Make sure your doctor is aware of any allergic reactions you have experienced.

How should you take this medication?

Dynapen should be taken exactly as prescribed by your doctor. It is important to take the entire amount prescribed, even if fever or other symptoms have disappeared.

Unless your doctor has told you otherwise, Dynapen should be taken 1 hour before meals or 2 hours after eating.

Dynapen Suspension should be stored in the refrigerator. Do not freeze. Shake well before using. Discard after 14 days. If you store the liquid form of Dynapen at room temperature, it should be discarded after 7 days.

Do not take any additional medications, including nonprescription drugs such as antacids, laxatives or vitamins, without your doctor's approval.

If you have previously experienced an allergic reaction to penicillin, you should wear a medical identification tag or bracelet.

What side effects may occur?

Side effects cannot be anticipated. If any develop or change in intensity, inform your doctor as soon as possible. Only your doctor can determine if it is safe for you to continue taking Dynapen.

■ Side effects may include:
Allergic reactions, delayed, allergic reactions, immediate, black or hairy tongue, diarrhea, feeling of being sick, fever, hives, itching, low blood pressure, nausea, serum sickness-like symptoms (joint and muscle pain with fever and hives), stomach pain, vomiting, wheezing

Why should this drug not be prescribed?

Do not take Dynapen if you have ever had an allergic reaction to any penicillin medication.

Special warnings about this medication

Your doctor should take a complete drug and allergy history before prescribing Dynapen. Serious and, rarely, fatal allergic reactions have occurred with penicillin use. If you develop any allergic symptoms, contact your doctor immediately.

If you experience shortness of breath, wheezing, skin rash, mouth irritation, black tongue, sore throat, nausea, vomiting, diarrhea, fever, swollen joints or unusual bruising or bleeding, stop taking Dynapen and contact your doctor immediately.

Possible food and drug interactions when taking this medication

If Dynapen is taken with certain other drugs, the effects of either could be increased, decreased, or altered. It is especially important to check with your doctor before combining Dynapen with the following:

Probenecid (Benemid)
Tetracycline drugs such as Achromycin V

Special information
if you are pregnant or breastfeeding
The effects of Dynapen during pregnancy have not been adequately studied. If you are pregnant or plan to become pregnant, inform your doctor immediately. Penicillin appears in breast milk and may affect a nursing infant.

If this medication is essential to your health, your doctor may advise you to stop breastfeeding until your treatment with Dynapen is finished.

Recommended dosage

ADULTS

Mild to Moderate Infections
The usual dose is 125 milligrams every 6 hours.

Severe Infections
The usual dose is 250 milligrams every 6 hours.

CHILDREN

Mild to Moderate Infections
The usual dose is 12.5 milligrams per 2.2 pounds of body weight per day divided into equal doses and taken every 6 hours.

Severe Infections
The usual dose is 25 milligrams per 2.2 pounds per day divided into equal doses and taken every 6 hours.

Overdosage
Any medication used in excess can have serious consequences. If you suspect a Dynapen overdose, seek medical attention immediately.

Brand name:

E-MYCIN

See Erythromycin, Oral, page 239.

Brand name:

E.E.S.

See Erythromycin, Oral, page 239.

Brand name:

ERYC

See Erythromycin, Oral, page 239.

Generic name:

ECHOTHIOPHATE IODIDE

See Phospholine Iodide, page 481.

Generic name:

ECONAZOLE NITRATE

See Spectazole, page 586.

Brand name:

ECOTRIN

See Aspirin, page 40.

Brand name:

EFUDEX

Generic name: Fluorouracil

Why is this drug prescribed?
Efudex is an antineoplastic (drug used to control or kill cancer cells) prescribed for the

treatment of solar keratoses (a small red or flesh-colored wartlike growth caused by overexposure to the sun). Such growths may develop into skin cancer.

When conventional methods are impractical, as in the case of difficult treatment sites, Efudex is also useful in the treatment of superficial basal cell carcinomas or slow-growing malignant tumors of the face usually found at the edge of the nostrils, eyelids, or lips.

Most important fact about this drug

If an airtight dressing is used to cover the skin being treated, there may be inflammatory reactions in the normal skin around the treated area. If covering the treated area is necessary, use a porous gauze dressing to avoid skin reactions.

How should you take this medication?

Use this medication exactly as prescribed by your doctor.

Efudex should be applied with care near the eyes, nose, and mouth.

Wash hands immediately after applying.

What side effects may occur?

Side effects cannot be anticipated. If any develop or change in intensity, inform your doctor as soon as possible. Only your doctor can determine if it is safe for you to continue using Efudex.

■ *More common side effects may include:*
Burning
Discoloration of the skin
Itching
Pain

■ *Less common side effects may include:*
Allergic skin inflammation, hair loss, pus, scaling, scarring, sensitivity to light, soreness, swelling, tearing, tenderness

Why should this drug not be prescribed?

If you are sensitive to or have ever had an allergic reaction to Efudex or similar drugs, you should not take this medication. Make sure that your doctor is aware of any drug reactions that you have experienced.

Special warnings about this medication

Prolonged exposure to ultraviolet rays should be avoided while under treatment with Efudex.

Remember to wash your hands immediately after applying.

Skin reaction to this drug may be unsightly during treatment and, in some cases, for several weeks after treatment has ended.

Solar keratoses that do not respond to this drug should be biopsied (removal of small amount of tissue to be examined under a microscope) to confirm the skin disease.

Your doctor will perform follow-up biopsies if you are being treated for superficial basal cell carcinoma.

Possible food and drug interactions when taking this medication

There are no reported food or drug interactions

Special information if you are pregnant or breastfeeding

The effects of Efudex during pregnancy have not been adequately studied. If you are pregnant, plan to become pregnant, or are breastfeeding your baby, consult your doctor immediately.

Recommended dosage

When Efudex is applied to affected skin, the skin becomes abnormally red, blisters form, and the surface skin wears away. A lesion or sore forms at the affected site, and the diseased or cancerous skin cells die before a new layer of skin forms.

ADULTS

Actinic or Solar Keratosis
Apply cream or solution 2 times a day in an amount sufficient to cover the affected area. Medication should be continued until the inflammatory response reaches the stage where the skin wears away, a sore or lesion forms, and the skin cells die, at which time use of the medication should stop. The usual length of treatment is from 2 to 4 weeks. Complete healing of the affected area may not be evident for 1 to 2 months after ending the treatment.

Superficial Basal Cell Carcinomas
Only the 5% strength of this medication is recommended. Apply cream or solution 2 times a day in an amount sufficient to cover the affected area. Treatment should be continued for at least 3 to 6 weeks but may be needed for as long as 10 to 12 weeks before the lesions are gone.

Your doctor will want to monitor your condition to make sure it has been cured.

Overdosage
Although no specific information is available on Efudex overdosage, any medication used in excess can have serious consequences. If you suspect an overdosage, seek medical attention immediately.

Brand name:

ELAVIL

*Generic name: Amitriptyline hydrochloride
Other brand name: Endep*

Why is this drug prescribed?
Elavil is prescribed for the relief of symptoms of mental depression. Some evidence exists

for the use of Elavil in certain other medical conditions, but only your doctor can make this decision. Elavil is one of a group of drugs called tricyclic antidepressants.

Most important fact about this drug
You may experience adverse side effects if you stop using this drug abruptly. Only your doctor should advise you to discontinue or change your dose.

How should you take this medication?
Elavil should be taken exactly as prescribed by your doctor. It may need to be taken for several weeks before you feel better. However, some side effects, such as mild drowsiness, may appear early in therapy and disappear after a few days.

If you forget to take a dose of this medication, take it as soon as you remember. However, if it is almost time for your next dose, skip the missed dose. Never take two doses at the same time.

If you miss a bedtime dose taken once daily, do not take that dose in the morning. It may cause side effects while you are awake.

What side effects may occur?
Side effects cannot be anticipated. If any develop or change in intensity, inform your doctor as soon as possible. Only your doctor can determine if it is safe for you to continue taking Elavil.

■ *Side effects may include:*
Abnormal movements, anxiety, black tongue, blurred vision, breast development in males, breast enlargement, coma, confusion, constipation, delusions, diarrhea, difficult or frequent urination, difficulty in speech, dilation of pupils, disorientation, disturbed concentration, dizziness on getting up, dizziness or lightheadedness, drowsiness, dry mouth, excessive or spontaneous flow of milk, excitement,

fainting, fatigue, fluid retention, hair loss, hallucinations, headache, heart attack, hepatitis, high fever, high or low blood sugar, hives, impotence, inability to sleep, increased or decreased sex drive, increased perspiration, increased pressure within the eye, inflammation of the mouth, intestinal obstruction, irregular heartbeat, lack or loss of coordination, loss of appetite, nausea, numbness, rapid and/or pounding heartbeat, rash, red or purple spots on skin, restlessness, ringing in the ears, sensitivity to light, stomach upset, strange taste, stroke, swelling due to fluid retention in the face and tongue, swelling of testicles, tingling, pins and needles, tremors, urinary retention, vomiting, weakness, weight gain or loss

■ *Side effects due to rapid decrease or abrupt withdrawal from Elavil include:*
Headache
Nausea
Vague feeling of bodily discomfort

■ *Side effects due to gradual dosage reduction may include:*
Dream and sleep disturbances
Irritability
Restlessness

These do not indicate an addiction to the drug.

Why should this drug not be prescribed?

If you are sensitive to or have ever had an allergic reaction to Elavil or similar drugs, you should not take this medication. Make sure that your doctor is aware of any drug reactions that you have experienced.

Elavil should not be taken if you are taking other antidepressants known as MAO inhibitors (Nardil, Parnate).

Unless you are directed to do so by your doctor, do not take this medication if you are recovering from a heart attack.

Special warnings about this medication

Elavil may cause you to become drowsy or less alert; therefore, driving or operating dangerous machinery or participating in any hazardous activity that requires full mental alertness is not recommended.

While taking this medication, you may feel dizzy or lightheaded or actually faint when getting up from a lying or sitting position. If getting up slowly doesn't help or if this problem continues, notify your doctor.

Elavil should be used with caution if you have a history of seizures, urinary retention, glaucoma or other chronic eye conditions or a heart or circulatory system disorder, or if you are receiving thyroid medication. You should discuss all of your medical problems with your doctor before taking this medication.

Some side effects of Elavil may last from 3 to 7 days after you stop taking it. Your doctor may want you to continue taking this medication after you no longer feel depressed to prevent these symptoms from returning. Your continued need for this drug should be determined by your doctor.

Possible food and drug interactions when taking this medication

Elavil may intensify the effects of alcohol. Do not drink alcohol while taking this medication.

If Elavil is taken with certain other drugs, the effects of either could be increased, decreased, or altered. It is especially important that you consult with your doctor before taking this drug in combination with the following:

Allergy medicine
Anticholinergics such as Bentyl
Antihistamines
Barbiturates such as Phenobarbital

Cimetidine (Tagamet)
Cold medicine
Contraceptives
Disulfiram (Antabuse)
Estrogens
Ethchlorvynol (Placidyl)
Fluoxetine (Prozac)
Guanethidine (Ismelin)
Histamine blockers such as cimetidine
     (Tagamet)
Muscle relaxants
Neuroleptics such as Thorazine
Other central nervous system depressants
Pain killers
Parkinsonism drugs such as Cogentin
Sedatives
Seizure medication
Sleep medicine
Sympathomimetics (Ventolin, Proventil)
Thyroid hormones
Tranquilizers

Special information
if you are pregnant or breastfeeding

The effects of Elavil during pregnancy have
not been adequately studied. If you are
pregnant or planning to become pregnant,
inform your doctor immediately. This
medication appears in breast milk. If Elavil
is essential to your health, your doctor
may advise you to discontinue breastfeeding
until your treatment is finished.

Recommended dosage

ADULTS

The usual starting dosage is 75 milligrams
per day divided into 2 or more smaller
doses. This dose may be increased gradually,
by your doctor, to 150 milligrams per
day. The total daily dose should not exceed
300 milligrams.

An alternative starting dose of 50 milligrams
to 100 milligrams at bedtime may be
recommended by your doctor. This bedtime
dose may be increased by 25 or 50

milligrams up to a total of 150 milligrams
per day as determined by your doctor.

Your doctor may prescribe a maintenance dose
of Elavil to be taken once daily, usually
at bedtime.

Your doctor may want to perform a blood
test to help in deciding the best dose for
you.

CHILDREN

Use of Elavil is not recommended for children
under 12 years of age.

The usual dose for adolescents 12 years of
age and over is 10 milligrams, 3 times a
day, with 20 milligrams taken at bedtime.

ELDERLY

The usual dose is 10 milligrams taken 3 times
a day, with 20 milligrams taken at
bedtime.

Elavil Tablets come in strengths of 10, 25,
50, 75, 100 and 150 milligrams.

Elavil Injection is supplied in 10-milliliter vials.

Overdosage

Deaths by deliberate or accidental overdose
have occurred with Elavil.

Symptoms of Elavil overdose may include:
Abnormally low blood pressure
Congestive heart failure
Convulsions
Dilated pupils
Drowsiness
Rapid or irregular heartbeat
Reduction of body temperature
Unresponsiveness or coma

*Other symptoms that are contrary to the effect
of this medication are:*
Agitation
Excessive movement and redness

Extremely high body temperature
Rigid muscles
Vomiting

If you suspect an overdose, seek medical attention immediately.

Brand name:

ELDEPRYL

Generic name: Selegiline hydrochloride

Why is this drug prescribed?
Eldepryl is prescribed along with levodopa/caridopa (Sinemet) for patients with Parkinson's disease. It is used when the response to levodopa/caridopa is deteriorating. There is no evidence that Eldepryl works without the simultaneous use of levodopa (Larodopa) or levodopa/caridopa (Sinemet).

Parkinson's disease, which causes muscle rigidity and difficulty with walking and talking, involves the progressive degeneration of a particular type of nerve cell. Early on, Larodopa or Sinemet alone may alleviate the symptoms of the disease. In time, however, these medications work less well; their effectiveness seems to switch on and off at random, and the patient may begin to experience side effects such as involuntary movements and "freezing" in mid-motion.

Eldepryl may be prescribed at this stage of the disease to help restore the effectiveness of Larodopa or Sinemet. A patient who begins to take Eldepryl may need a reduced dosage of the other medication.

Most important fact about this drug
Eldepryl is chemically related to MAO inhibitor antidepressants, such as Marplan, Nardil, and Parnate. With these particular antidepressants, patients who take them must avoid tyramine-rich foods such as aged cheeses and meats, yogurt, and fermented beverages, or run the risk of a life-threatening rise in blood pressure. Fortunately, however, patients taking Eldepryl have no dietary restrictions of this type, as long as they take the medication at the correct dosage.

How should you take this medication?
Take Eldepryl exactly as prescribed by your doctor. It is important not to exceed the recommended daily dosage. Taking too much Eldepryl could cause a dangerous rise in blood pressure.

What side effects may occur?
Side effects cannot be anticipated. If any develop or change in intensity, inform your doctor as soon as possible. Only your doctor can determine if it is safe for you to continue taking Eldepryl.

■ *Side effects may include:*
Abdominal pain, aches, agitation, anemia, angina (chest pain upon exertion), anxiety, back pain, blurred vision, body ache, chills, confusion, decreased penis sensation, delusions, depression, diarrhea, dizziness, drowsiness, dry mouth, eyelid spasm, facial grimace, fainting, falling down, freezing, general feeling of illness, hair loss, hallucinations, headache, heart palpitations, heart rhythm abnormalities, inability to carry out purposeful movements, increased sweating, increased tremor, Insomnia, irritability, leg pain, lethargy, lightheadedness upon standing up, loss of balance, lower back pain, muscle cramps, nausea, poor appetite, rash, restlessness (desire to keep moving), ringing in the ear, shortness of breath, slowed body movements, stiff neck, tension, transient "high", urinary problems, vivid dreams or nightmares, vomiting, weakness, weight loss

Why should this drug not be prescribed?

Do not take Eldepryl if you are sensitive or have ever had an allergic reaction to it.

Special warnings about this medication

Never take Eldepryl at a higher dosage than prescribed; doing so could put you at risk for a dangerous rise in blood pressure.

If dizziness or light-headedness occurs when rising from a sitting or lying position, rising more slowly may help.

Possible food and drug interactions when taking this medication

If Eldepryl is taken with certain other drugs, the effects of either could be increased, decreased, or altered. It is especially important to check with your doctor before combining Eldepryl with the following:

Fluoxetine (Prozac)
Meperidine (Demerol)
Other narcotic drugs such as Percocet and
  Tylenol with Codeine

If you have taken Prozac, you should wait at least 5 weeks after the last dose before starting to take Eldepryl.

If you anticipate taking Prozac, do not take the first dose until at least 14 days after your last dose of Eldepryl.

Eldepryl may worsen side effects caused by your usual dosage of levodopa.

Special information if you are pregnant or breastfeeding

If you are pregnant or plan to become pregnant, inform your doctor immediately. Although Eldepryl is not known to cause specific birth defects, it should not be taken during pregnancy unless it is clearly needed.

It is not known whether Eldepryl finds its way into breast milk. As a general rule, a nursing mother should not take any drug unless it is clearly necessary.

Recommended dosage

ADULTS

The recommended dose of Eldepryl is 10 milligrams per day divided into 2 smaller doses of 5 milligrams each, taken at breakfast and lunch. There is no evidence that additional benefit will be obtained from higher doses.

Higher doses should ordinarily be avoided because of the increased risk of side effects.

CHILDREN

The use of Eldepryl in children has not been evaluated.

Overdosage

Although no specific information is available about Eldepryl overdosage, it is assumed, because of chemical similarities, that the symptoms would resemble those of overdose with an MAO inhibitor antidepressant.

Symptoms of MAO *inhibitor overdose may include:*
Agitation, chest pain, clammy skin, coma, convulsions, dizziness, drowsiness, extremely high fever, faintness, fast, irregular pulse, irritability, hallucinations, headache (severe), high blood pressure, hyperactivity, lockjaw, low blood pressure (severe), shallow breathing, sweating

It is important to note that after an acute overdose, symptoms may not appear for up to 12 hours and may not reach their full force for 24 hours or more. If you suspect an Eldepryl overdose, seek medical attention immediately. Hospitalization is recommended, with continuous observation and monitoring for at least 2 days.

Brand name:

ELOCON

Generic name: Mometasone furoate

Why is this drug prescribed?

Elocon is a cortisone-like steroid available in cream, ointment, or lotion form. It is used to treat certain itchy rashes and other inflammatory skin conditions.

Most important fact about this drug

When you use Elocon cream, ointment, or lotion, some of the medication passes through the skin and into the bloodstream. After you apply Elocon you should leave the skin exposed to the air or, at most, covered loosely by clothing. Using an airtight bandage would permit more of the medication to be absorbed into your blood; this could produce various side effects.

How should you use this medication?

Use Elocon exactly as prescribed by your doctor. Apply a thin film of the cream or ointment or a few drops of the lotion to the affected skin once a day. Massage it in until it disappears. Avoid getting it into your eyes.

For the most effective and economical use of Elocon lotion, hold the tip of the bottle very close to (but not touching) the affected skin and squeeze the bottle gently.

Once you have applied Elocon, never cover the skin with an airtight bandage, a tight diaper, plastic pants or any other airtight dressing. This could encourage excessive absorption of the medication into your bloodstream.

Be careful not to use Elocon for a longer time than prescribed. If you do, you may disrupt your ability to make your own natural adrenal corticoid hormones (hormones secreted by the outer layer of the adrenal gland).

What side effects may occur?

Side effects cannot be anticipated. If any develop or change in intensity, notify your doctor as soon as possible. Only your doctor can determine if it is safe for you to continue using Elocon.

■ *Side effects may include:*
Acne-like pimples, allergic skin rash, boils, burning, damaged skin, dryness, excessive hairiness, infected hair follicles, infection of the skin, irritation, itching, light colored patches on skin, prickly heat, rash around the mouth, skin thinning and atrophy, softening of the skin, stretch marks, tingling or stinging

Why should this drug not be prescribed?

Do not use Elocon if you are sensitive or have ever had an allergic reaction to it or any other corticosteroid medication.

Special warnings about this medication

Elocon is for external use only. Avoid getting it into your eyes. Do not use it to treat anything other than the condition for which it was prescribed.

Possible food and drug interactions when using this medication

No interactions have been noted.

Special information if you are pregnant or breastfeeding

If you are pregnant or plan to become pregnant, inform your doctor immediately. Elocon should not be used during pregnancy unless the benefit outweighs the potential risk to the unborn child.

You should not use Elocon while breastfeeding, since absorbed hormone could make its way into the breast milk and perhaps harm the nursing baby. If you are a new mother, you should contact your doctor, who will help you decide between breastfeeding and taking Elocon.

Recommended dosage

ADULTS

Apply a thin film of Elocon Cream or Ointment to the affected skin areas once daily. Do not use airtight dressings.

Apply a few drops of Elocon Lotion to the affected areas once daily and massage lightly until it disappears. For the most effective and economical use, hold the nozzle of the bottle very close to (but not touching) the affected areas and gently squeeze the bottle.

CHILDREN

Use should be limited to the least amount necessary. Use of steroids over a long period of time may interfere with growth and development.

Overdosage

With extensive or long-term use of Elocon, hormone absorbed into the bloodstream may cause Cushing's syndrome.

Symptoms of Cushing's syndrome may include:

Acne, depression, excessive hair growth, high blood pressure, humped upper back, insomnia, moonfaced appearance, obese trunk, paranoia, stretch marks, wasted limbs, stunted growth (in children), susceptibility to bruising, fractures and infections

Cushing's syndrome may also trigger diabetes mellitus.

If it is left uncorrected, Cushing's syndrome may become serious. If you suspect your long-term use of Elocon has led to Cushing's syndrome, seek medical attention immediately.

Brand name:

EMPIRIN

See Aspirin, page 40.

Brand name:

EMPIRIN WITH CODEINE

Generic ingredients: Aspirin, Codeine phosphate

Why is this drug prescribed?

Empirin with Codeine is a narcotic anti-inflammatory medication. It relieves mild, moderate, and severe pain.

Most important fact about this drug

Codeine can be habit-forming when taken over a long period of time or in high doses. Do not take more of the drug, or use it for a longer period of time than your doctor has indicated.

How should you take this medication?

Empirin with Codeine should be taken exactly as prescribed by your doctor.

It should be taken with food or a full glass of milk or water to lessen stomach upset.

What side effects may occur?

Side effects cannot be anticipated. If any develop or change in intensity, inform your doctor as soon as possible. Only your doctor can determine if it is safe for you to continue using Empirin with Codeine.

■ *More common side effects may include:*
  Constipation
  Decreased breathing
  Dizziness
  Drowsiness
  Light-headedness
  Nausea
  Vomiting

■ *Less common side effects may include:*
Aggravation of peptic ulcer, anaphylactic shock, asthma, bruising or bleeding, exaggerated feeling of depression, exaggerated sense of well-being, excessive bleeding following injury or surgery, mild to severe allergic reactions (anaphylactic shock, asthma), itching, ringing in ears, rashes, skin rashes, stomach pain, upset stomach or heartburn

Why should this drug not be prescribed?

Empirin with Codeine should not be used if you: are sensitive or allergic to aspirin or codeine, experience severe bleeding, have blood clotting disorder or severe vitamin K deficiency, are taking blood-thinning medications, have a peptic ulcer or other serious gastrointestinal lesions, or have liver damage. Children or teenagers with symptoms of chickenpox or the flu should not take Empirin with Codeine because of the danger of contracting Reye's Syndrome.

Special warnings about this medication

Aspirin can cause severe allergic reactions including anaphylactic shock (shortness of breath, violent cough, difficulty breathing, bluish skin color caused by lack of oxygen, fever, rash or hives, irregular pulse, convulsions or collapse).

Aspirin can cause bleeding if you have a peptic ulcer or other gastrointestinal lesions or a bleeding disorder. It may also prolong bleeding time after an injury or surgery. It can also hide symptoms of serious abdominal conditions.

Codeine should be used cautiously if you have a head injury or other brain lesions. It can depress breathing, cause drowsiness, and increase pressure in your head.

Empirin with Codeine should be used cautiously if you are elderly or debilitated or have severe kidney or liver disease, gallstones or gallbladder disease, a breathing disorder, an irregular heartbeat, inflammatory disorders of the gastrointestinal tract, an underactive thyroid, Addison's disease (a disorder of the adrenal glands), an enlarged prostate or narrowing of the urethra, blood-clotting disorders, head injuries, or an acute abdominal condition.

Empirin with Codeine is not recommended for long-term use unless specifically indicated by your doctor.

Aspirin should be used with care if you have a history of allergies. Sensitivity reactions are relatively common in people with asthma and nasal polyps.

Empirin with Codeine may make you drowsy or less alert. Be careful driving, operating machinery, or using appliances that require full mental alertness until you know how you react to this medication.

Alcohol and other depressants should be avoided while using this medication.

Remember, this medication can be habit-forming and should be taken exactly as prescribed by your doctor. Do not take more of the medication, or use it more often, than your doctor has indicated.

Possible food and drug interactions when taking this medication

The effects of alcohol may be increased if taken with Empirin with Codeine. Avoid using alcohol while taking this medication.

If Empirin with Codeine is taken with certain other drugs, the effects of either could be increased, decreased, or altered. It is especially important to check with your doctor before combining Empirin with Codeine with the following:

Blood thinners such as Coumadin and
Panwarfin

Corticosteroids such as Medrol and
Meticorten

Furosemide (Lasix)

General anesthetics

Insulin

MAO inhibitors such as antidepressants
Marplan and Nardil

Methotrexate

Mercaptopurine

Nonsteroidal anti-inflammatory drugs such
as Advil, Motrin, and Indocin

Oral diabetes medications such as Diabinese,
Tolinase

Other narcotic analgesics such as Percodan and
Tylox

Penicillin

Probenecid (Benemid and others)

Sedative-hypnotics such as phenobarbital and
Nembutal

Sulfa drugs such as Azo Gantrisin and Septra

Sulfinpyrazone (Anturane)

Tranquilizers such as Xanax and Valium

Vitamin C

Special information
If you are pregnant or breastfeeding

The effects of Empirin with Codeine during
pregnancy have not been adequately
studied. If you are pregnant or plan to
become pregnant, inform your doctor
immediately. Aspirin and codeine appear in
small amounts in breast milk and may
affect a nursing infant. If this medication is
essential to your health, your doctor may
advise you to stop breastfeeding until your
treatment with this medication is finished.

Recommended dosage

Dosage is determined by the severity of your
pain and your response to this
medication. Your doctor may prescribe more
than the usual recommended dose if your
pain is severe or you have become tolerant
to the pain relief of codeine.

The usual adult dose for Empirin with
Codeine No. 2 and No. 3 is 1 or 2
tablets every 4 hours as needed. The usual
adult dose for Empirin with Codeine No.
4 is 1 tablet every 4 hours as required.

Overdosage

Any medication taken in excess can have
serious consequences. Empirin with
Codeine can cause severe breathing difficulties
if too much is taken. If you suspect an
overdose of Empirin with Codeine, seek
medical treatment immediately.

*Symptoms of Empirin with Codeine overdose
may include:*
Bluish skin color due to lack of oxygen,
circulatory collapse, clammy skin, coma,
constricted pupils, delirium, delusions,
dizziness, double vision, excitability,
garbled speech, hallucinations, muscle
unresponsiveness, shortness of breath, skin
eruptions, slow and shallow breathing, stupor

*Symptoms of Empirin with Codeine overdose
in children may include:*
Confusion, convulsions, dehydration, difficulty
hearing, dim vision, dizziness, drowsiness,
extremely high body temperature, headache,
nausea, rapid breathing, ringing in ears,
sweating, thirst, vomiting

Generic name:

ENALAPRIL MALEATE

See Vasotec, page 674.

Generic name:

ENALAPRIL MALEATE WITH
HYDROCHLOROTHIAZIDE

See Vaseretic, page 671.

Brand name:

ENDEP

See Elavil, page 226.

Brand name:

ENDURON

Generic name: Methyclothiazide

Why is this drug prescribed?

Enduron is used in the treatment of high blood pressure and other conditions that require the elimination of excess fluid (water) from the body. These conditions include congestive heart failure, cirrhosis of the liver, corticosteroid and estrogen therapy, and kidney disease. When used for high blood pressure, Enduron can be used alone or with other high blood pressure medications. Enduron contains a form of thiazide, a diuretic that prompts your body to produce and eliminate more urine, which helps lower blood pressure.

Most important fact about this drug

If you have high blood pressure, you must take Enduron regularly for it to be effective. Even if you are feeling well, you must continue to take this medication. It is needed to keep your blood pressure under control.

Diuretics can cause your body to lose too much potassium. Ask your doctor for the warning signs of potassium depletion. Also ask whether you should eat specific foods that are rich in potassium or take a potassium supplement to avoid this problem.

How should you take this medication?

Take Enduron exactly as prescribed by your doctor. If you forget to take a dose, take it as soon as you remember. If it is almost time for your next dose, skip the one you missed and go back to your regular schedule. Never take two doses at the same time.

What side effects may occur?

Side effects cannot be anticipated. If any develop or change in intensity, inform your doctor as soon as possible. Only your doctor can determine if it is safe for you to continue taking Enduron.

■ *Side effects may include:*
Anemia, blood disorders, constipation, cramping, diarrhea, difficulty breathing, dizziness, dizziness upon standing up, fever, fluid in lungs, headache, high blood sugar, high levels of sugar in urine, hives, hypersensitivity reactions, inflammation of the pancreas, inflammation of the salivary glands, loss of appetite, lung inflammation, muscle spasms, nausea, rash, reddish or purplish spots on the skin, restlessness, sensitivity to light, Stevens-Johnson syndrome (skin peeling), stomach irritation, symptoms of low potassium levels, such as dry mouth, excessive thirst, weak or irregular heartbeat, muscle pain or cramps, tingling or pins and needles, upset stomach, vertigo, vision changes, vomiting, weakness, yellow eyes and skin

Why should this drug not be prescribed?

If you are unable to urinate, you should not take this medication.

If you are sensitive to or have ever had an allergic reaction to Enduron or similar drugs, or if you are sensitive to other sulfonamide-derived drugs, you should not take this medication.

Special warnings about this medication

If you are taking Enduron, a complete assessment of your kidney function should be done; kidney function should continue to be monitored.

If you have liver disease, diabetes, gout, or collagen vascular disease (lupus erythematosus), Enduron should be used with caution.

If you have bronchial asthma or a history of allergies, you may be at greater risk for an allergic reaction to this medication.

Dehydration, excessive sweating, severe diarrhea or vomiting could deplete your body's fluids and cause your blood pressure to become too low. Be careful when exercising and in hot weather.

Notify your doctor or dentist that you are taking Enduron if you have a medical emergency, and before you have surgery or dental treatment.

Possible food and drug interactions when taking this medication

Enduron may intensify the effects of alcohol. Do not drink alcohol while taking this medication.

If Enduron is taken with certain other drugs, the effects of either could be increased, decreased, or altered. It is especially important to check with your doctor before taking Enduron with the following:

Barbiturates such as phenobarbital
Corticosteroids such as prednisone and ACTH
Digitalis (Lanoxin)
Insulin
Lithium (Eskalith, Lithobid)
Narcotics such as Percocet
Norepinephrine (Levophed)
Other high blood pressure medications
Tubocurarine

Special information
if you are pregnant or breastfeeding

The effects of Enduron during pregnancy have not been adequately studied. If you are pregnant or plan to become pregnant, inform your doctor immediately. Enduron appears in breast milk and could affect a nursing infant. If this medication is essential to your health, your doctor may advise you to discontinue breastfeeding until your treatment is finished.

Recommended dosage

ADULTS

Doses of this drug should be individualized to each patient and given at the lowest dose that allows the maximum effect.

Edema
The usual dose is 2.5 milligrams to a maximum of 10 milligrams 1 time a day.

High Blood Pressure
The usual dose is 2.5 milligrams to 5 milligrams 1 time per day. If results are not satisfactory in 8 to 12 weeks, another diuretic will be added rather than increasing the dose.

This medication is often used in combination with other antihypertensive drugs (such as deserpidine [Harmonyl]). However, your doctor will determine whether or not this is appropriate.

Enduron is supplied in 2.5- and 5-milligram tablets.

Overdosage

Any medication taken in excess can cause symptoms of overdose. If you suspect an overdose, seek medical attention immediately.

The symptoms of Enduron overdose may include:
Confusion
Muscular weakness

Stomach and intestinal disturbances
Weakness

Brand name:

ENTEX LA

*Generic ingredients: Guaifenesin,
Phenylpropanolamine hydrochloride
Other brand name: Nolex LA*

Why is this drug prescribed?
Entex LA is used to treat the symptoms of bronchitis, the common cold, sinusitis, nasal congestion, and throat infections.

Entex LA is a combination of two medications, phenylpropanolamine (a decongestant) and guaifenesin (an expectorant), specially formulated to deliver prolonged therapeutic benefit. Phenylpropanolamine helps reduce congestion in the nasal passages, while guaifenesin breaks up mucus in the lower respiratory tract, making it easier to expectorate.

Most important fact about this drug
People who have severe high blood pressure, who are sensitive to phenylpropanolamine in a sympathomimetic drug (such as Dristan Decongestant), or who take antidepressant medications known as MAO inhibitors (such as Nardil) should not take Entex LA.

How should you take this medication?
Entex LA tablets may be broken in half to make them easier to swallow but must not be chewed or crushed.

What side effects may occur?
Side effects cannot be anticipated. If any develop or change in intensity, inform your doctor as soon as possible. Only your doctor can determine if it is safe for you to continue taking Entex LA.

■ *Side effects may include:*
Difficulty urinating (in patients with a prostate condition)
Headache
Inability to sleep or difficulty sleeping
Irritated stomach
Nausea
Nervousness
Restlessness

Why should this drug not be prescribed?
You should not use Entex LA if you have severe high blood pressure, are sensitive to sympathomimetic drugs (such as Dristan Decongestant), or take antidepressant medications known as MAO inhibitors (such as Nardil).

Special warnings about this medication
Entex LA should be used cautiously by people with the following conditions:

Diabetes
Glaucoma or other eye problems
Heart disease
High blood pressure
Hyperthyroidism (excessive thyroid gland activity)
Prostate condition

Possible food and drug interactions when taking this medication
Entex LA should not be used by people who take antidepressant medications known as MAO inhibitors (such as Nardil).

Special information
if you are pregnant or breastfeeding
The effects of Entex LA during pregnancy have not been adequately studied. If you are pregnant or plan to become pregnant, notify your doctor immediately. Entex LA appears in breast milk and could affect a nursing infant. If this medication is essential to your health, your doctor may advise you to discontinue breastfeeding until treatment with this drug is finished.

Recommended dosage

ADULTS AND CHILDREN 12 YEARS AND OLDER

The usual dosage is 1 tablet 2 times a day (every 12 hours).

CHILDREN 6 TO 12 YEARS OLD

The usual dosage is one-half tablet 2 times a day (every 12 hours).

Tablets may be broken in half to make them easier to swallow but must not be chewed or crushed.

CHILDREN UNDER 6 YEARS OLD

Entex LA is not recommended for this age group.

The safety and effectiveness of Entex LA have not been established in children.

ELDERLY

The elderly should take Entex LA with caution.

Older adults may experience convulsions, difficulty breathing, and hallucinations.

Overdosage

Any medication taken in excess can cause symptoms of overdose. If you suspect symptoms of an Entex LA overdose, seek medical help immediately.

Symptoms of Entex LA overdose may include:
High blood pressure
Perspiration
Sleepiness

Brand name:

EPITOL

See Tegretol, page 608.

Brand name:

EQUANIL

See Miltown, page 382.

Generic name:

ERGOLOID MESYLATES

See Hydergine, page 280.

Generic name:

ERGOTAMINE TARTRATE WITH CAFFEINE

See Cafergot, page 79.

Brand name:

ERY-TAB

See Erythromycin, Oral, page 239.

Brand name:

ERYCETTE

See Erythromycin, Topical, page 242.

Brand name:

ERYTHROCIN

See Erythromycin, Oral, page 239.

Generic name:

ERYTHROMYCIN ETHYLSUCCINATE WITH SULFISOXAZOLE ACETYL

See Pediazole, page 460.

Generic name:

ERYTHROMYCIN WITH BENZOYL PEROXIDE

See Benzamycin, page 63.

Generic name:

ERYTHROMYCIN, ORAL

Brand names: E.E.S., E-Mycin, ERYC, Ery-tab, Erythrocin, Ilosone, PCE

Why is this drug prescribed?

Erythromycin is an antibiotic used to treat many kinds of infections, including:

Chlamydia
Diphtheria
Ear infections
Gonorrhea
Intestinal infections
Legionnaire's disease
Prevention of recurrent rheumatic fever and bacterial endocarditis in people who are allergic to penicillin or who have congenital or rheumatic heart disease
Rheumatic fever
Skin infections
Syphilis
Upper and lower respiratory tract infections
Urinary tract infections
Whooping cough

Most important fact about this drug

Erythromycin, like any other antibiotic, works best when there is a constant amount of drug in the blood. To help keep the drug amount constant, it is important not to miss any doses. Also, it is advisable to take the doses at evenly spaced times around the clock.

How should you take this medication?

Take erythromycin exactly as prescribed by your doctor.

Most people can take erythromycin with or without meals. However, food may decrease the effectiveness of erythromycin in some people.

Your doctor may advise you to take erythromycin 30 minutes to 2 hours before meals.

Chewable forms of erythromycin should be crushed or chewed before being swallowed.

Delayed-release or enteric-coated forms of erythromycin in capsules or tablets should be swallowed whole. Do not crush or break. If you are not sure about the form of erythromycin you are taking, ask your pharmacist.

The liquid form of erythromycin should be kept in the refrigerator. Do not freeze.

What side effects may occur?

Side effects cannot be anticipated. If any develop or change in intensity, inform your doctor as soon as possible. Only your doctor can determine whether it is safe to continue taking this medication.

More common side effects may include:
Abdominal pain
Diarrhea
Loss of appetite
Nausea
Vomiting

Less common side effects may include:
Hives, skin eruptions, yellow eyes and skin

Rare side effects may include:
Chest pain, confusion, dizziness, hallucinations, hearing loss (reversible), inflammation of the large intestine, palpitations, rapid heartbeat, seizures, severe allergic reaction, vertigo

Why should this drug not be prescribed?

You should not use erythromycin if you have ever had an allergic reaction or are sensitive to it. Erythromycin should not be used with Seldane or Hismanal.

Special warnings about this medication

If you have ever had liver disease, consult with your doctor before taking erythromycin.

If new infections (called superinfections) occur, talk to your doctor. You may need to be treated with a different antibiotic.

Possible food and drug interactions when taking this medication

If erythromycin is taken with certain other drugs, the effects of either could be increased, decreased, or altered. It is especially important to check with your doctor before combining erythromycin with the following:

Carbamazepine (Tegretol)
Cyclosporine (Sandimmune)
Digoxin (Lanoxin)
Ergotamine (Cafergot)
Hexobarbital
Lovastatin (Mevacor)
Other antibiotics
Blood thinning drugs such as Coumadin
Phenytoin (Dilantin)
Terfenadine (Seldane)
Theophylline (Theo-Dur)
Triazolam (Halcion)

Special information
if you are pregnant or breastfeeding

If you are pregnant or plan to become pregnant, inform your doctor immediately. Erythromycin appears in breast milk and could affect a nursing infant. If this medication is essential to your health, your doctor may advise you to discontinue breastfeeding until your treatment is finished.

Recommended dosage

Dosage instructions are determined by the type (and severity) of infection being treated and may vary slightly for different brands of erythromycin. The following are recommended dosages for PCE, one of the most commonly prescribed brand.

ADULTS

Streptococcal Infections
The usual dose is 250 milligrams every 6 hours, 333 milligrams every 8 hours, or 500 milligrams every 12 hours. Depending on the severity of the infection, the dose may be increased to a total of 4 grams a day. However, when the daily dosage is larger than 1 gram, twice-a-day doses are not recommended, and the drug should be taken more often in smaller doses.

To treat streptococcal infections of the upper respiratory tract (tonsillitis or strep throat), erythromycin should be taken for 10 days. The usual dosage in long-term prevention to prevent recurring attacks of rheumatic fever is 250 milligrams twice daily.

Gonorrhea
The usual dosage is 3 grams in a single oral dose.

To Prevent Bacterial Endocarditis (Inflammation and Infection of the Heart Lining and Valves) in Patients Who Are Allergic to Penicillin
The oral regimen is 1 gram of erythromycin taken one-half to 2 hours before dental surgery or surgical procedures of the upper respiratory tract, followed by 500 milligrams every 6 hours for 8 doses.

Urinary Tract Infections Due to Chlamydia Trachomatis *During Pregnancy*
Although the optimal dose and duration of therapy have not been established, the suggested treatment is 500 milligrams of

erythromycin by mouth 4 times a day or 666 milligrams orally every 8 hours on an empty stomach for at least 7 days. For women who cannot tolerate this regimen, a decreased dose of 500 milligrams orally every 12 hours, 333 milligrams orally every 8 hours, or 250 milligrams by mouth 4 times a day should be used for at least 14 days.

For Patients with Uncomplicated Urinary, Reproductive Tract, or Rectal Infections Caused by Chlamydia Trachomatis *When Tetracycline Cannot Be Taken*
The usual dosage is 500 milligrams of erythromycin by mouth 4 times a day or 333 milligrams orally every 8 hours for at least 7 days.

For Patients with Nongonococcal Urethral Infections When Tetracycline Cannot Be Taken
The usual dosage is 500 milligrams of erythromycin by mouth 4 times a day or 666 milligrams orally every 8 hours for at least 7 days.

Syphilis
The usual dosage is 30 to 40 grams divided into smaller doses over a period of 10 to 15 days.

Intestinal Infections
The usual dosage is 500 milligrams every 12 hours, 333 milligrams every 8 hours, or 250 milligrams every 6 hours for 10 to 14 days.

Legionnaires' Disease
Although the optimal dosage has not been established, doses utilized in reported clinical data were 1 to 4 grams daily, divided into smaller doses.

CHILDREN

Age, weight, and severity of the infection determine the correct dosage.

The usual dosage is from 30 to 50 milligrams daily for each 2.2 pounds of body weight, divided into equal doses.

For more severe infections, this dosage may be doubled, but it should not exceed 4 grams per day.

Children weighing over 44 pounds should follow the recommended adult dose schedule.

The dosage for children weighing under 44 pounds is determined by their weight.

Conjunctivitis (Pinkeye) in the Newborn Caused by Chlamydia Trachomatis *(a Sexually Transmitted Infection Passed on by the Mother)*
The usual dosage of oral erythromycin suspension is 50 milligrams for each 2.2 pounds of body weight daily, divided into 4 doses, for at least 2 weeks.

Pneumonia in Infants Caused by Chlamydia Trachomatis
Although the most effective length of treatment has not been established, the recommended therapy is oral erythromycin suspension, 50 milligrams for each 2.2 pounds of body weight daily, divided into 4 doses, for at least 3 weeks.

Whooping Cough
Although the optimal dosage and duration have not been established, clinical studies utilized 40 to 50 milligrams for each 2.2 pounds of body weight daily, divided into smaller doses for 5 to 14 days.

ELDERLY

Erythromycin should be used with caution in elderly patients.

Overdosage
Any medication taken in excess can have serious consequences. If you suspect an overdose, seek medical help immediately.

*Symptoms of erythromycin overdose
may include:*
Diarrhea
Nausea
Stomach cramps
Vomiting

Generic name:

ERYTHROMYCIN, TOPICAL

Brand names: A/T/S, Erycette, T-Stat

Why is this drug prescribed?
Erythromycin topical (applied directly to the
skin) is used for the treatment of acne.

Most important fact about this drug
These brands of erythromycin are for external
use only and should not be used in or
around the eyes, nose or mouth.

How should you use this medication?
Erythromycin topical should be used exactly
as prescribed by your doctor.

Thoroughly wash the affected area with soap
and water and pat dry before applying
medication.

Rub or lightly spread the medication over the
affected area. A/T/S Topical Gel should
not be rubbed in.

What side effects may occur?
Side effects cannot be anticipated. If any
develop or change in intensity, inform
your doctor as soon as possible. Only your
doctor can determine if it is safe for you
to continue using erythromycin topical.

■ *Side effects may include:*
Burning sensation
Dryness
Hives
Irritation of the eyes
Itching

Oiliness
Peeling
Scaling
Tenderness
Unusual redness of the skin

Why should this drug not be prescribed?
Erythromycin topical should not be used if
you are sensitive to or have ever had an
allergic reaction to any of the ingredients.

Special warnings about this medication
The use of antibiotics can stimulate the
growth of other bacteria that are resistant
to the antibiotic you are taking. If new
infections (called superinfections) occur,
talk to your doctor. You may need to be
treated with a different antibiotic drug.

The use of other topical acne medications in
combination with erythromycin topical
may cause irritation, especially with the use
of peeling, scaling, or abrasive medications.

The safety and effectiveness of A/T/S has not
been established in children.

Possible food and drug interactions
when using this medication
If erythromycin topical is used with certain
other drugs, the effects of either could be
increased, decreased, or altered. It is especially
important to check with your doctor
before combining erythromycin topical with
the following:

Other topical acne medications

Special information
if you are pregnant or breastfeeding
The effects of erythromycin topical during
pregnancy have not been adequately
studied. If you are pregnant or plan to
become pregnant, inform your doctor
immediately. Erythromycin topical may appear
in breast milk and could affect a nursing
infant. If this medication is essential to your

health, your doctor may advise you to stop breastfeeding until your treatment with erythromycin topical is finished.

Recommended dosage

A/T/S TOPICAL SOLUTION

Apply the solution to the affected area(s) 2 times a day, in the morning and at night. Moisten the applicator or a pad with A/T/S, then rub over the affected area(s). Make sure the area(s) is (are) thoroughly washed with soap and water and patted dry before applying medication. If there is no improvement after 6 to 8 weeks, consult your doctor.

A/T/S/ TOPICAL GEL

Apply a thin film of gel to the affected area(s). Spread the medication lightly. Do not rub it in. Make sure the area(s) is (are) thoroughly washed with soap and water and patted dry before applying medication. Thoroughly wash your hands after application of the medication. If there has been no improvement after 6 to 8 weeks, talk to your doctor.

ERYCETTE TOPICAL SOLUTION

Rub the pledget over the affected area(s) 2 times a day. Make sure the area(s) is (are) thoroughly washed with soap and water and patted dry before applying medication. Additional pledgets can be used, if needed. Each pledget should be used just once and then thrown away.

T-STAT TOPICAL SOLUTION

The solution or pads should be applied over the affected area(s) 2 times a day. Make sure the area(s) is (are) thoroughly washed with soap and water and patted dry before applying medication. Additional pads can be used, if needed. T-Stat should be applied with the applicator top or disposable pads. If you use the pads or your fingertips, wash your hands after application.

Reducing the frequency of applications may reduce peeling and drying.

Overdosage

Although overdosage is unlikely, any medication used in excess can have serious consequences. If you suspect an overdose, seek medical treatment immediately.

Brand name:

ESGIC

See *Fioricet, page 253.*

Brand name:

ESIDRIX

See *HydroDIURIL, page 281.*

Generic name:

ESTAZOLAM

See *ProSom, page 516.*

Generic name:

ESTROGENS, CONJUGATED

See *Premarin, page 498.*

Brand name:

ETHMOZINE

Generic name: Moricizine hydrochloride

Why is this drug prescribed?

Ethmozine is prescribed for the treatment of certain life-threatening heartbeat irregularities.

Most important fact about this drug

Because Ethmozine may actually cause or worsen heartbeat irregularities (arrhythmias) in some patients, treatment with this drug is usually started in the hospital.

How should you take this medication?

Take Ethmozine exactly as prescribed by your doctor, even if you feel better.

An imbalance of minerals in your body fluids could have a negative effect on the way the drug works; any such imbalance should be identified and corrected before you begin treatment with Ethmozine.

What side effects may occur?

Side effects cannot be anticipated. If any develop or change in intensity, inform your doctor as soon as possible. Only your doctor can determine if it is safe for you to continue taking Ethmozine.

The most dangerous side effect, which occurs in approximately 4% of patients treated with Ethmozine, is a new heartbeat irregularity; if such an irregularity develops, the drug must be stopped.

■ *More common side effects may include:*
Breathing difficulties
Dizziness
Fatigue
Headache
Nausea
Pounding heartbeat

■ *Less common side effects may include:*
Abdominal pain, abnormal walking, agitation, anxiety, blurred vision, chest pain, clumsiness, confusion, decreased sex drive, depression, diarrhea, double vision, dry mouth, eye pain, fainting, fever, hives, impotence, indigestion, itching, loss of memory, muscle pain, nervousness, numbness, rash, ringing in the ears, sore throat, speech disorder, stomach upset,

sweating, swelling of the lips and tongue, tingling, tremors, urinary problems, visual problems, vomiting, weakness

Why should this drug not be prescribed?

Do not take Ethmozine if you are sensitive to it or have ever had an allergic reaction to it.

In addition, you should not be treated with Ethmozine if you have any of the following heart (or heart-related) conditions:

Cardiogenic shock
Heart block, bifascicular block unless you have a pacemaker
Second- or third-degree atrioventricular block (AV block)

Special warnings about this medication

Because of its potential to cause new heartbeat abnormalities, Ethmozine is reserved for the treatment of life-threatening heartbeat irregularities originating in the ventricle (lower half of the heart).

Extreme caution is advised if you have a heart condition called "sick sinus syndrome," since Ethmozine could make this condition worse.

You will need a lower-than-average dosage of Ethmozine and close monitoring if you have liver or kidney function problems. If you develop signs of a liver problem while being treated with Ethmozine, your doctor may stop the drug.

While taking Ethmozine, you will need especially close monitoring if you have congestive heart failure, or if you have a pacemaker.

Possible food and drug interactions when taking this medication

If Ethmozine is taken with certain other drugs, the effects of either could be increased, decreased, or altered. It is especially important to check with your doctor before combining Ethmozine with the following:

Cimetidine (Tagamet)
Theophylline (Theo-Dur and other brands)

Special information if you are pregnant or breastfeeding

If you are pregnant or plan to become pregnant, inform your doctor immediately. Although there is no evidence to date of any specific birth defects caused by Ethmozine, this drug should be used during pregnancy only if clearly needed. Ethmozine does make its way into breast milk, and has the potential to harm a nursing infant. Thus, you may need to choose between taking Ethmozine and breastfeeding your baby.

Recommended dosage

ADULTS

Your doctor will individualize your dose according to your heart condition and any other disorders you may have, such as liver and kidney problems.

The usual recommended dosage ranges from 600 milligrams to 900 milligrams daily, given every 8 hours in 3 equally divided doses.

CHILDREN

Safety and effectiveness have not been established in children under the age of 18.

Overdosage

An overdose of Ethmozine may produce very serious consequences.

Symptoms of Ethmozine overdose may include any of the following:
Arrested breathing
Coma
Fainting

Heartbeat abnormalities
Heart attack
Lethargy
Low blood pressure
Vomiting
Worsening of congestive heart failure

If you suspect an overdose of Ethmozine, seek medical attention immediately.

Generic name:

ETODOLAC

See Lodine, page 331.

Brand name:

EULEXIN

Generic name: Flutamide

Why is this drug prescribed?

Eulexin is used along with another drug, Lupron, to treat prostate cancer. Eulexin belongs to a class of drugs known as antiandrogens. It blocks the effect of the male hormone testosterone. Giving Eulexin with Lupron, which decreases the body's testosterone levels, is one way of treating prostate cancer.

Most important fact about this drug

Taking Eulexin and Lupron together is essential in this form of treatment. You should not interrupt their doses or stop taking either of these medications without consulting your doctor.

How should you take this medication?

Take Eulexin exactly as prescribed by your doctor. Do not use more or less Eulexin, and do not use Eulexin more often than instructed by your doctor.

What side effects may occur?

Side effects cannot be anticipated. If any develop or change in intensity, inform your doctor immediately. Only your doctor can determine if it is safe for you to continue taking Eulexin. Eulexin is always given with another antiandrogen drug. When a side effect develops, it is difficult to know which drug is responsible.

■ *Side effects may include:*

Anemia, anxiety, breast tissue swelling and tenderness, confusion, decreased sexual ability, depression, diarrhea, drowsiness, fluid retention, high blood pressure, hot flashes, impotence, jaundice and liver damage, loss of appetite, loss of sex drive, lung disorder, nausea, nervousness, rash, sun sensitivity (rashes, blisters upon exposure to sun), upset stomach, urine discoloration (amber or yellow-green), vomiting

Why should this drug not be prescribed?

Do not take Eulexin if you have ever had an allergic reaction or are sensitive to it, or to any of the colorings or other inactive ingredients in the capsules.

Special warnings about this medication

Eulexin may cause liver damage in some people. You should have liver function tests (specific blood tests) before you start treatment with Eulexin, and at regular intervals thereafter. If a liver problem does develop, you may need to take less Eulexin or to stop taking the drug altogether. Report any signs or symptoms that might suggest liver damage to your doctor right away. Warning signs include dark urine, itching, flu-like symptoms, jaundice (a yellowing of the skin and eyes), persistent appetite loss, and persistent tenderness on the right side of the upper abdomen.

Possible food and drug interactions when taking this medication

If you are already taking the anticoagulant drug warfarin (Coumadin, Panwarfin), you will need to be monitored especially closely after treatment with Eulexin begins. Your doctor may need to lower your dosage of warfarin.

Recommended dosage

The recommended Eulexin dosage is 2 capsules 3 times a day at 8-hour intervals for a total daily dosage of 750 milligrams.

Overdosage

Although no specific information is available, any medication taken in excess can have serious consequences. If you suspect an overdose of Eulexin, seek medical attention immediately.

Brand name:

EUTHROID

Generic name: Liotrix

Why is this drug prescribed?

Euthroid is a synthetic thyroid hormone replacement drug. It is used to treat an underactive thyroid in children and adults.

Most important fact about this drug

Although Euthroid will speed up your metabolism, it is not effective as a weight-loss drug and should not be taken for that purpose. Too much Euthroid may cause life-threatening side effects, especially if you take it with appetite suppressants.

How should you take this medication?

Take Euthroid exactly as prescribed by your doctor. There is no "typical" dosage; the amount you need will depend on how much thyroid hormone your body produces on its own. Take no more or less than the prescribed amount. Take your dose at the same time every day for consistent effect.

In most cases, thyroid replacement medication is taken for the rest of your life.

Euthroid can be taken with food or on an empty stomach.

What side effects may occur?
When Euthroid is given at the correct dosage, side effects are rare. However, an excessive dosage or a too-rapid increase in dosage may lead to overstimulation of the thyroid gland. Symptoms of overstimulation may include:

Changes in appetite
Diarrhea
Fever
Headache
Increased heart rate
Irritability
Nausea
Nervousness
Sleeplessness
Sweating
Weight loss

Why should this drug not be prescribed?
You should not take Euthroid if you have ever had an allergic reaction to it; if your thyroid gland is making too much thyroid hormone; or if your adrenal glands are not making enough corticosteroid hormones.

Special warnings about this medication
Euthroid should be used cautiously if you have heart disease, diabetes, or an adrenal gland insufficiency, or if you are elderly.

If you are diabetic or are taking a blood-thinning medication, the dosage may have to be adjusted.

Euthroid may cause partial hair loss in children during the first few months of treatment. The hair loss is usually temporary.

Euthroid contains Yellow No. 5 dye, which may cause an allergic reaction.

Possible food and drug interactions when taking this medication
If Euthroid is taken with certain other drugs, the effects of either could be increased, decreased, or altered. It is especially important to check with your doctor before combining Euthroid with the following:

Blood-thinning medications such as Coumadin
Cholestyramine (Questran)
Diabetes medications such as insulin, Diabinese, and Glucotrol
Estrogen (Premarin)
Oral contraceptives

Special information if you are pregnant or breastfeeding
Thyroid hormones are safe for use during pregnancy. Minimal amounts of thyroid hormone appear in breast milk. Although no serious adverse reactions have been reported in nursing infants, this medication should be used cautiously if you are breastfeeding. Ask your doctor whether you should breastfeed while taking Euthroid.

Recommended dosage
Your doctor will tailor the dosage to meet your individual requirements, taking into consideration the status of your thyroid gland and any other medical conditions you may have.

Overdosage
Any medication taken in excess can have serious consequences. Too much thyroid medication produces the symptoms of an overactive thyroid. If you suspect an overdose, seek medical treatment immediately.

Symptoms of Euthroid overdose may include:
Change in bowel habits
Diarrhea
Excessive sweating
Heart palpitations
Heat intolerance
Increased pulse rate
Nervousness

Brand name:

FML S.O.P.

Generic name: Fluorometholone

Why is this drug prescribed?
FML S.O.P. is a steroid (cortisone-like) eye ointment that is used to treat irritation and inflammation of the eyelid and eyeball.

Most important fact about this drug
FML S.O.P. should be used with extreme caution to treat an inflammation of the cornea due to various viral or fungal infections. Frequent monitoring of your condition by your doctor is recommended.

Wearing contact lenses while using steroid eye ointments may increase your chances of developing an eye infection.

How should you use this medication?
Use this ointment exactly as prescribed by your doctor. Do not discontinue treatment until advised to do so.

What side effects may occur?
There are no reported side effects of FML S.O.P. However, if you suspect any are developing, notify your doctor as soon as possible. Only your doctor can determine whether it is safe to continue using FML S.O.P.

Why should this drug not be prescribed?
If you have ever had an allergic reaction or are sensitive to fluorometholone or similar drugs (anti-inflammatories, steroids), do not use this ointment. Tell your doctor about any drug reactions you have experienced.

Do not use this ointment if you have a severe eye inflammation due to various viral or fungal infections of the eye unless your doctor tells you to do so.

Special warnings about this medication
Prolonged use of FML S.O.P. ointment may result in glaucoma (elevated pressure in the eye causing optic nerve damage and loss of vision) cataract formation (eye disorder causing the lens of the eye to become less transparent, or the development of eye infection from fungi or viruses.

The use of topical corticosteroids such as FML S.O.P. has been known to cause punctures when used in the presence of diseases that cause thinning of the cornea or sclera (tough, opaque covering at the back of the eyeball).

The use of a corticosteroid medication could hide the presence of a pus-producing eye infection or cause the infection to become worse.

Internal pressure of the eye should be checked frequently by your doctor.

Possible food and drug interactions when taking this medication
No interactions with food or other drugs have been reported.

Special information
if you are pregnant or breastfeeding
If you are pregnant or plan to become pregnant, tell your doctor immediately. No information is available about the safety of FML S.O.P. during pregnancy.

FML S.O.P. may appear in breast milk and could affect a nursing infant. If using FML S.O.P. is essential to your health, your doctor may advise you to stop breastfeeding until your treatment is finished.

Recommended dosage
ADULTS

Apply a small amount of ointment (one-half inch ribbon) between the lower eyelid and eyeball 1 to 3 times a day. During the first 24 to 48 hours, the dosage may be increased to 1 application every 4 hours.

CHILDREN

The safety and effectiveness of FML S.O.P. have not been established in children under 2 years of age.

Overdosage

Overdosage with FML S.O.P. will not ordinarily cause severe problems. If FML S.O.P. is accidentally ingested, drink fluids to dilute the medication.

Generic name:

FAMOTIDINE

See Pepcid, page 464.

Brand name:

FASTIN

Generic name: Phentermine hydrochloride

Why is this drug prescribed?

Fastin, an appetite suppressant, is prescribed for short-term use (a few weeks) as part of an overall diet plan for the reduction of weight. Fastin should be used along with a behavior modification program.

Most important fact about this drug

Loss of effectiveness (tolerance) of Fastin and other related drugs may develop within a few weeks. You should discontinue the use of the medication rather than increase the dosage when it becomes less effective.

Appetite suppressants such as Fastin are no substitute for a proper diet.

How should you take this medication?

Take this medication exactly as prescribed by your doctor.

Fastin may be habit-forming and can be addicting.

You should not share Fastin with others.

Avoid alcoholic beverages while taking this medication.

What side effects may occur?

Side effects cannot be anticipated. If any develop or change in intensity, inform your doctor as soon as possible. Only your doctor can determine if it is safe for you to continue taking Fastin.

■ *Side effects may include:*
Abdominal discomfort, blood pressure elevation, changes in sex drive, constipation, diarrhea, dizziness, dryness of the mouth, feelings of discomfort, feelings of elation, headache, hives, impotence, inability to fall or stay asleep, increased heart rate, nausea, overstimulation, palpitations (pounding sensation of the heart), restlessness, tremors, unpleasant taste, vomiting

Why should this drug not be prescribed?

If you are sensitive or have ever had an allergic reaction to phentermine hydrochloride or compounds that have a similar effect, you should not take this medication. Make sure that your doctor is aware of any drug reactions that you have experienced.

Unless directed to do so by your doctor, do not take this drug if you have hardening of the arteries, symptoms of heart or blood vessel disease, an overactive thyroid, glaucoma or moderate to severe high blood pressure, or you are in an agitated state, have a history of drug abuse or are taking or have taken an MAO inhibitor (anti-depressant drugs such as Nardil and Parnate) within the last 14 days.

Special warnings about this medication

Fastin may impair your ability to engage in potentially hazardous activities. Therefore, you should take extreme care while driving a car or operating machinery.

Psychological dependence has occurred while taking this drug. Consult with your doctor if you rely on this drug to maintain a state of well-being.

The abrupt withdrawal of this medication following prolonged usage of high doses may result in extreme fatigue, mental depression, and sleep disturbances.

Signs of long-term poisoning with this class of drugs include severe skin disorders, a pronounced inability to fall or stay asleep, irritability, hyperactivity, and personality changes. The most severe symptom is psychosis, a major mental disorder in which the person becomes detached from reality.

Possible food and drug interactions when taking this medication

The use of alcohol in combination with Fastin may result in an unfavorable drug reaction.

If Fastin is taken with certain other drugs, the effects of either could be increased, decreased, or altered. It is especially important that you check with your doctor before combining Fastin with the following:

Antidiabetic drugs such as insulin
Antihypertensive drugs such as guanethidine
MAO inhibitors (antidepressants such as
  Nardil)

Special information
if you are pregnant or breastfeeding

The effects of Fastin during pregnancy have not been adequately studied. If you are pregnant, plan to become pregnant or are breastfeeding, notify your doctor immediately.

Recommended dosage

ADULTS

The recommended dosage is 1 capsule approximately 2 hours after breakfast for appetite control. Late evening medication should be avoided because of the possibility of insomnia (inability to fall asleep). Taking 1 capsule daily has been found to be adequate for suppression of the appetite for 12 to 14 hours.

CHILDREN

This drug is not recommended for use in children under 12 years of age.

Overdosage

Any medication taken in excess can have serious consequences.

If you suspect Fastin overdose, seek emergency medical treatment immediately.

Symptoms of Fastin overdose may include: Abdominal cramps, assaultiveness, confusion, diarrhea, failure of the blood to circulate through the system, hallucinations, high or low blood pressure, irregular heartbeat, nausea, panic states, rapid breathing, restlessness, tremors, vomiting

In cases of fatal poisoning, convulsions and coma usually precede death.

Fatigue and depression may follow the stimulant effects of Fastin.

Brand name:

FELDENE

Generic name: Piroxicam

Why is this drug prescribed?

Feldene, a nonsteroidal anti-inflammatory drug, is used to relieve the inflammation, swelling, stiffness and joint pain associated with rheumatoid arthritis and osteoarthritis (the most common form of arthritis). It is also used in the treatment of other types of pain.

Most important fact about this drug
You should have frequent check-ups with your doctor if you take Feldene regularly. Ulcers or internal bleeding can occur without warning.

How should you take this medication?
Feldene should be taken with food or an antacid, and with a full glass of water. Never take it on an empty stomach.

Take this medication exactly as prescribed by your doctor.

If you are using Feldene for arthritis, it should be taken regularly.

If you forget to take a dose, take it as soon as you remember. If it is almost time for your next dose, skip the one you missed and go back to your regular schedule. Never take two doses at the same time.

What side effects may occur?
Side effects cannot be anticipated. If any develop or change in intensity, inform your doctor as soon as possible. Only your doctor can determine if it is safe for you to continue taking Feldene.

- *More common side effects may include:* Abdominal pain or discomfort, anemia, constipation, diarrhea, dizziness, fluid retention, gas, headache, heartburn, indigestion, inflammation of inside of mouth, itching, loss of appetite, nausea, rash, ringing in ears, sleepiness, stomach upset, vertigo

- *Less common or rare side effects may include:* Abdominal bleeding, black, bloody stools,

blurred vision, bruising, congestive heart failure (worsening of), depression, dry mouth, eye irritations, fever, hepatitis, high blood pressure, hives, inability to sleep, labored breathing, low or high blood sugar, nervousness, nosebleed, skin eruptions, Stevens-Johnson syndrome (itchy rash), sweating, swollen eyes, vomiting, vomiting blood, weight loss or gain, worsening of angina, yellow eyes and skin

Why should this drug not be prescribed?
If you are sensitive to or have ever had an allergic reaction to Feldene, aspirin, or similar drugs, or if you have had asthma attacks caused by aspirin or other drugs of this type, you should not take this medication. Make sure that your doctor is aware of any drug reactions that you have experienced.

Special warnings about this medication
Peptic ulcers and bleeding can occur without warning.

This drug should be used with caution if you have kidney or liver disease, and it can cause liver inflammation in some people.

Do not take aspirin or any other anti-inflammatory medications while taking Feldene, unless your doctor tells you to do so.

If you have heart disease or high blood pressure, this drug can increase water retention. Use with caution.

Feldene may cause you to become drowsy or less alert; therefore, driving or operating dangerous machinery or participating in any hazardous activity that requires full mental alertness is not recommended.

Possible food and drug interactions when taking this medication
If Feldene is taken with certain other drugs, the effects of either could be increased,

decreased, or altered. It is especially important to check with your doctor before combining Feldene with the following:

Anticoagulants (blood thinners)
Lithium

Special information
if you are pregnant or breastfeeding

The effects of Feldene during pregnancy have not been adequately studied. If you are pregnant or plan to become pregnant, inform your doctor immediately. Feldene appears in breast milk and could affect a nursing infant. If this medication is essential to your health, your doctor may advise you to discontinue breastfeeding until your treatment with this medication is finished.

Recommended dosage

ADULTS

Rheumatoid Arthritis and Osteoarthritis:
The usual dose is 20 milligrams a day in one dose. It is possible to divide this dose. Feldene's full effects will not be achieved for 7 to 12 days, although some relief of symptoms will occur soon after you take the medication.

The lowest dose that proves beneficial should be used.

CHILDREN

The safety and effectiveness of Feldene have not been established in children.

ELDERLY

Dosage should be determined by the particular needs of the elderly patient.

Overdosage

Any medication taken in excess can cause symptoms of overdose. If you suspect an overdose, seek medical attention immediately.

No specific symptoms are documented.

Generic name:

FELODIPINE

See Plendil, page 487.

Brand name:

FEMSTAT

Generic name: Butoconazole nitrate

Why is this drug prescribed?

Femstat Vaginal Cream is prescribed for the treatment of yeast-like fungal infections of the vulva and vagina.

Most important fact about this drug

To obtain maximum benefit, it is important that you continue to use Femstat Vaginal Cream during menstruation and that you finish using all of the medication, even if your symptoms have disappeared.

How should you use this medication?

Use this medication exactly as prescribed by your doctor.

What side effects may occur?

Side effects cannot be anticipated. If any develop or change in intensity, inform your doctor as soon as possible. Only your doctor can determine if it is safe for you to continue using Femstat.

■ *Side effects may include:*
Itching of the fingers
Soreness
Swelling
Vaginal discharge
Vulvar itching
Vulvar or vaginal burning

Why should this drug not be prescribed?

If you are sensitive to or have ever had an allergic reaction to butoconazole nitrate or any other ingredients in Femstat Cream, you should not use this medication. Make sure that your doctor is aware of any drug reactions that you have experienced.

Special warnings about this medication
If symptoms persist, or if irritation or sensitization (an allergic reaction) develops while using this medication, notify your doctor.

Possible food and drug interactions when taking this medication
No interactions with other drugs have been reported.

Special information if you are pregnant or breastfeeding
The effects of Femstat Cream during the first trimester (first three months) of pregnancy have not been adequately studied. However, women using this cream for 3 to 6 days during the second or third trimester of pregnancy have experienced no adverse effects or complications, nor have their infants. It is not known whether this drug appears in breast milk. If Femstat is essential to your health, your doctor may advise you to discontinue breastfeeding your baby until your treatment is finished.

Recommended dosage

ADULTS

Non-pregnant Patients
The recommended dose is 1 applicatorful of cream inserted vaginally at bedtime for 3 days. Your doctor may extend your treatment for an additional 3 days if necessary.

Pregnant Patients (2nd and 3rd trimesters only)
The recommended dose is 1 applicatorful of cream inserted vaginally at bedtime for 6 days.

CHILDREN

Safety and effectiveness have not been established in children.

Overdosage
No overdosage has been reported.

Generic name:

FENOPROFEN CALCIUM

See Nalfon, page 398.

Generic name:

FINASTERIDE

See Proscar, page 515.

Brand name:

FIORICET

Generic ingredients: Butalbital, Acetaminophen, Caffeine
Other brand name: Esgic

Why is this drug prescribed?
Fioricet, a strong, non-narcotic pain reliever and muscle relaxant, is prescribed for the relief of tension headache symptoms caused by muscle contractions in the head, neck, and shoulder area. It combines a non-narcotic, sedative barbiturate (butalbital), a non-aspirin pain reliever (acetaminophen), and caffeine.

Most important fact about this drug
Mental and physical dependence can occur with the use of barbiturates such as butalbital when these drugs are taken in higher than recommended doses over long periods of time.

How should you take this medication?
Take Fioricet exactly as prescribed by your doctor. Do not increase the amount you take without your doctor's approval.

What side effects may occur?

Side effects cannot be anticipated. If any develop or change in intensity, inform your doctor as soon as possible. Only your doctor can determine if it is safe for you to continue taking Fioricet.

■ *More common side effects may include:*
Dizziness
Drowsiness

If these side effects occur, it may help if you lie down after taking the medication.

■ *Less common or rare side effects may include:*
Depression, gas, light-headedness, mental confusion, nausea, vomiting

Why should this drug not be prescribed?

If you are sensitive to or have ever had an allergic reaction to barbiturates, acetaminophen, caffeine, or other drugs of this type, you should not take this medication. Make sure that your doctor is aware of any drug reactions that you have experienced.

Unless you are directed to do so by your doctor, do not take this medication if you have porphyria (an inherited metabolic disorder affecting the liver or bone marrow).

Special warnings about this medication

Fioricet may cause you to become drowsy or less alert; therefore, driving or operating dangerous machinery or participating in any hazardous activity that requires full mental alertness is not recommended until you know your response to this drug.

If you are being treated for severe depression or have a history of severe depression or drug abuse, consult with your doctor before taking Fioricet.

Possible food and drug interactions when taking this medication

Butalbital is a central nervous system (brain and spinal cord) depressant and intensifies the effects of alcohol. Use of alcohol with this drug may also cause overdose symptoms. Therefore, use of alcohol should be avoided.

If Fioricet is taken with certain other drugs, the effects of either could be increased, decreased, or altered. It is especially important to check with your doctor before combining Fioricet with the following:

Antihistamines such as Benadryl
Antipsychotics such as Haldol, Thorazine
Drugs to treat depression such as Elavil
Muscle relaxants such as Flexeril
Narcotic pain relievers such as Darvon
Sleep aids such as Halcion
Tranquilizers such as Xanax, Valium

Fioricet may decrease the effect of anticoagulants (blood thinners). If you are taking an anticoagulant, consult with your doctor before taking this drug.

Special information
if you are pregnant or breastfeeding

The effects of Fioricet during pregnancy have not been adequately studied. If you are pregnant or plan to become pregnant, inform your doctor immediately. Butalbital does appear in breast milk. If this medication is essential to your health, your doctor may advise you to discontinue breastfeeding your baby until your treatment is finished.

Recommended dosage

ADULTS

The usual dose of Fioricet is 1 or 2 tablets taken every 4 hours as needed. Do not exceed a total dose of 6 tablets per day.

CHILDREN

The safety and effectiveness of Fioricet have not been established in children under 12 years of age.

ELDERLY

This drug may cause excitement, depression, and confusion in elderly patients.
Therefore, your doctor will prescribe a dose individualized to suit your needs.

Overdosage

Symptoms of Fioricet overdose are mainly attributed to its barbiturate component. These symptoms may include:
Coma
Confusion
Drowsiness
Low blood pressure
Shock
Slow or troubled breathing

Overdose due to the acetaminophen component of Fioricet may cause kidney and liver damage or coma due to low blood sugar. Death due to liver failure has also been reported.

Symptoms of liver damage include:
Excess perspiration
Feeling of bodily discomfort
Nausea
Vomiting

If you suspect an overdose, seek emergency medical treatment immediately.

Brand name:

FIORINAL

Generic ingredients: Butalbital, Aspirin, Caffeine
Other brand name: Isollyl

Why is this drug prescribed?

Fiorinal, a strong, non-narcotic pain reliever and muscle relaxant, is prescribed for the relief of tension headache pain symptoms caused by stress or muscle contraction in the head, neck, and shoulder area. It combines a non-narcotic, sedative barbiturate (butalbital) with a pain reliever (aspirin) and a stimulant (caffeine).

Most important fact about this drug

Mental and physical dependence can occur with the use of barbiturates such as butalbital when taken in higher than recommended doses over long periods of time.

How should you take this medication?

Take Fiorinal exactly as prescribed by your doctor. Do not increase the amount you take without your doctor's approval.

What side effects may occur?

Side effects cannot be anticipated. If any develop or change in intensity, inform your doctor as soon as possible. Only your doctor can determine if it is safe for you to continue taking Fiorinal.

■ *More common side effects may include:*
Dizziness
Drowsiness

■ *Less common or rare side effects may include:*
Gas, light-headedness, nausea, vomiting

Why should this drug not be prescribed?

If you are sensitive to or have ever had an allergic reaction to barbiturates (central nervous system depressants), aspirin, caffeine, or drugs of this type, you should not take this medication. Make sure that your doctor is aware of any drug reactions that you have experienced.

Unless you are directed to do so by your doctor, do not take this medication if you have porphyria (an inherited metabolic disorder affecting the liver or bone marrow).

Because there is a possible association between aspirin and Reye's syndrome, Fiorinal should not be given to children and teenagers who have chickenpox or flu unless prescribed by a doctor.

Special warnings about this medication

Fiorinal may cause you to become drowsy or less alert, therefore, driving or operating dangerous machinery or participating in any hazardous activity that requires full mental alertness is not recommended until you know your response to this drug.

Fiorinal contains aspirin. If you have a stomach (peptic) ulcer or a disorder affecting the blood clotting process, consult your doctor before taking Fiorinal. Aspirin may irritate the stomach lining and may cause bleeding.

If you have chronic (long-lasting or frequently recurring) tension headaches and your prescribed dose of Fiorinal does not relieve the pain, consult with your doctor. Taking more of this drug than your doctor has prescribed may cause dependence and symptoms of overdose.

Possible food and drug interactions when taking this medication

Butalbital is a central nervous system (brain and spinal cord) depressant and intensifies the effects of alcohol. Use of alcohol with this drug may also cause overdose symptoms. Therefore, use of alcohol should be avoided.

If butalbital is taken with certain other drugs, the effects of either could be increased, decreased, or altered. It is especially important to check with your doctor before combining butalbital with other central nervous system depressants including sedatives and tranquilizers such as Halcion and Xanax.

The use of anticoagulants (blood thinners) in combination with Fiorinal may cause bleeding. If you are taking an anticoagulant, consult with your doctor before taking this drug.

Special information if you are pregnant or breastfeeding

The effects of Fiorinal during pregnancy have not been adequately studied. If you are pregnant or plan to become pregnant, inform your doctor immediately. Butalbital and aspirin appear in breast milk. If this medication is essential to your health, your doctor may advise you to discontinue breastfeeding until your treatment with this medication is finished.

Recommended dosage

ADULTS

The usual dose of Fiorinal is 1 or 2 tablets or capsules taken every 4 hours. Do not exceed a total dose of 6 tablets or capsules per day.

CHILDREN

The safety and effectiveness of butalbital have not been established in children under 12 years of age.

Overdosage

Any medication taken in excess can have serious consequences. If you suspect an overdose, seek medical attention immediately.

Symptoms of an overdose of Fiorinal are mainly attributed to its barbiturate component. These symptoms may include:
Coma
Confusion
Drowsiness
Low blood pressure
Shock
Slow or troubled breathing

Symptoms attributed to the aspirin component of Fiorinal may include:
Abdominal pain
Deep, rapid breathing
Delirium
High fever
Rapid heartbeat
Restlessness
Ringing in the ears
Seizures
Vomiting

Brand name:

FIORINAL WITH CODEINE

Generic ingredients: Butalbital, Codeine phosphate, Aspirin, Caffeine

Why is this drug prescribed?

Fiorinal with Codeine, a strong narcotic pain reliever and muscle relaxant, is prescribed for the relief of tension headache pain caused by stress and muscle contraction in the head, neck, and shoulder area. It combines a sedative-barbiturate (butalbital), a narcotic pain reliever and cough suppressant (codeine), a non-narcotic pain and fever reliever (aspirin), and a stimulant (caffeine).

Most important fact about this drug

Mental and physical dependence can occur with the use of barbiturates, such as butalbital, and narcotics, such as codeine, when these drugs are taken in higher than recommended doses over long periods of time.

How should you take this medication?

Take Fiorinal with Codeine exactly as prescribed by your doctor. Do not increase the amount you take without your doctor's approval.

What side effects may occur?

Side effects cannot be anticipated. If any develop or change in intensity, inform your doctor as soon as possible. Only your doctor can determine if it is safe for you to continue taking Fiorinal with Codeine.

- *More common side effects may include:*
  Abdominal pain
  Dizziness
  Drowsiness
  Intoxicated feeling
  Nausea

- *Less common side effects may include:*
  Agitation, difficulty swallowing, dry mouth, earache, excessive sweating, fainting, fatigue, fever, headache, heartburn, heavy eyelids, high energy, hot spells, increased heart rate, increased urination, itching, leg pain, muscle fatigue, nasal stuffiness, numbness, ringing in the ears, shaky feeling, sluggishness, tingling, vomiting

- *Rare side effects may include:*
  Anxiety, chest pain, constipation, constriction of pupils, decreased sex drive, depression, diarrhea, disorientation, fainting, fluid retention, flushing, hallucinations, hiccups, hives, hyperactivity, inability to fall or stay asleep, increased or decreased appetite, increased sexual activity, inflammation of stomach and intestine, inflammation of the esophagus, mouth burning, nervousness, nosebleed, palpitations, salivation, sedation, skin rash and welts, slurred speech, twitching, unconsciousness, urinary difficulty, vertigo, weakness

- *Side effects of this drug's components may include:*
  Anemia, hepatitis, high blood sugar, internal bleeding, irritability, kidney damage, peptic ulcer, stomach upset, tremors

Why should this drug not be prescribed?

If you are sensitive to or have ever had an allergic reaction to butalbital, codeine, aspirin, caffeine, or drugs of this type, you should not take this medication. Make sure that your doctor is aware of any drug reactions that you have experienced.

Unless you are directed to do so by your doctor, do not take this medication if you are being treated for a blood disease, severe vitamin K deficiency, severe liver damage, nasal polyps (growths or nodules), asthma due to aspirin or other nonsteroidal anti-inflammatory drugs such as Motrin, swelling due to fluid retention, peptic ulcer, or porphyria (an inherited metabolic disorder affecting the liver and bone marrow).

Because there is a possible association between aspirin and Reye's syndrome, Fiorinal with Codeine should not be given to children and teenagers who have chickenpox or flu unless prescribed by a doctor.

Special warnings about this medication

Fiorinal with Codeine may cause you to become drowsy or less alert; therefore, driving or operating dangerous machinery or participating in any hazardous activity that requires full mental alertness is not recommended.

Codeine may cause unusually slow or troubled breathing and may increase the pressure caused by fluid surrounding the brain and spinal cord in patients with head injury. Therefore, Fiorinal with Codeine should be used with caution only as prescribed by your doctor.

If you have chronic (long-lasting or frequently recurring) tension headaches and your prescribed dose of Fiorinal with Codeine does not relieve the pain, consult with your doctor. Taking more of this drug than your doctor has prescribed may cause dependence and symptoms of overdose.

If you have a history of drug dependence, consult with your doctor before taking Fiorinal with Codeine.

If you are being treated for a kidney, liver, or blood clotting disorder, consult with your doctor before taking Fiorinal with Codeine.

Possible food and drug interactions when taking this medication

Fiorinal with Codeine is a central nervous system (affecting the brain and spinal cord) depressant and intensifies the effects of alcohol. Use of alcohol with this drug may also cause overdose symptoms. Therefore, use of alcohol should be avoided.

If butalbital is taken with certain other drugs, the effects of either could be increased, decreased, or altered. It is especially important to check with your doctor before combining Fiorinal with Codeine with the following:

Anticoagulants (blood thinners)
Antidepressant drugs such as Elavil, Sinequan
Antidiabetic drugs such as Micronase
Antigout medications such as Zyloprim
Antihistamines such as Benadryl
Central nervous system depressants such as
    Nembutal, Restoril
Corticosteroids such as prednisone
General anesthetics
MAO inhibitors (drugs used for severe
    depression, such as Nardil)
Methotrexate (antimetabolite—cancer drug)
Nonsteroidal anti-inflammatory drugs such
    as Motrin, Indocin
Other narcotic analgesics such as Darvon,
    Vicodin
Sedative/hypnotics such as Nembutal,
    phenobarbital
6-Mercaptopurine (antimetabolite—cancer
    drug)
Tranquilizers such as Librium, Xanax, Valium

The use of anticoagulants (blood thinners) in combination with Fiorinal with Codeine may cause bleeding. If you are taking an anticoagulant, consult with your doctor before taking this drug.

Special information
If you are pregnant or breastfeeding
The effects of Fiorinal with Codeine during pregnancy have not been adequately studied. If you are pregnant or plan to become pregnant, inform your doctor immediately. Butalbital, aspirin, caffeine, and codeine appear in breast milk. If this medication is essential to your health, your doctor may advise you to discontinue breastfeeding until your treatment with this medication is finished.

Recommended dosage

ADULTS

The usual dose of Fiorinal with Codeine is 1 or 2 capsules taken every 4 hours. Do not exceed a total dose of 6 capsules per day.

CHILDREN

The safety and effectiveness of butalbital have not been established in children under 12 years of age.

ELDERLY

Your doctor will prescribe a dose individualized to suit your needs.

Overdosage
Symptoms of an overdose of Fiorinal with Codeine are mainly attributed to its barbiturate and codeine ingredients.

Symptoms attributed to the barbiturate ingredient of Fiorinal with Codeine may include:
Coma
Confusion
Dizziness
Drowsiness

Low blood pressure
Shock
Slow or troubled breathing

Symptoms attributed to the codeine ingredient of Fiorinal with Codeine may include:
Convulsions
Loss of consciousness
Pinpoint pupils
Troubled and slowed breathing

Symptoms attributed to the aspirin ingredient of Fiorinal with Codeine may include:
Abdominal pain
Deep, rapid breathing
Delirium
High fever
Restlessness
Ringing in the ears
Seizures
Vomiting

If you suspect symptoms of a Fiorinal with Codeine overdose, seek emergency medical treatment immediately.

Brand name:

FLAGYL

Generic name: Metronidazole
Other brand name: Metryl

Why is this drug prescribed?
Flagyl is an antibacterial drug that effectively treats certain vaginal and urinary tract infections in men and women; amebic dysentery; and infections of the abdomen, liver, skin, bones and joints, brain, lungs (including pneumonia), and heart caused by bacterial organisms that are susceptible to metronidazole.

Most important fact about this drug
Do not drink alcoholic beverages while taking Flagyl. Alcohol can cause abdominal cramps, nausea, vomiting, headaches, and

flushing. When you have stopped taking Flagyl, wait another 24 hours (one day) before consuming any alcohol.

How should you take this medication?

Flagyl can be taken with or without food.

If you are being treated for trichomoniasis (vaginal infection that is often sexually transmitted), the male partner should use a condom for the duration of treatment.

What side effects may occur?

Side effects cannot be anticipated. If any develop or change in intensity, tell your doctor immediately. Only your doctor can determine whether it is safe to continue taking Flagyl.

Two serious side effects that have occurred with Flagyl are seizures and numbness or tingling in the arms, legs, hands, and feet. If you experience either of these symptoms, stop taking the medication and call your doctor immediately.

■ *More common side effects may include:*
Abdominal cramps
Constipation
Diarrhea
Headache
Loss of appetite
Nausea
Upset stomach
Vomiting

■ *Less common side effects may include:*
Blood disorders, confusion, dark urine, decreased libido, depression, difficulty sleeping, dizziness, dry mouth (or vagina or vulva), fever, flushing, furry tongue, hives, inability to hold urine, increased production of pale urine, irritability, lack of muscle coordination, metallic taste, occasional joint pain, painful or difficult urination, pelvic pressure, rash, stuffy nose, vertigo, weakness, yeast infection (candida) in vagina

Why should this drug not be prescribed?

Flagyl should not be used during the first 3 months of pregnancy to treat vaginal infections. Do not take Flagyl if you have ever had an allergic reaction or are sensitive to metronidazole or similar drugs.

Special warnings about this medication

If you experience seizures or numbness or tingling in your arms, legs, hands, or feet, stop taking Flagyl and call your doctor immediately.

Flagyl should be used cautiously if you have severe liver disease.

Active or undiagnosed yeast infections may appear or worsen when you take Flagyl.

Possible food and drug interactions when taking this medication

Alcohol consumption can cause cramps, nausea, vomiting, headaches, and flushing. Do not drink alcohol while taking Flagyl and avoid drinking any alcohol for another 24 hours after your last dose of Flagyl.

If Flagyl is taken with certain other drugs, the effects of either could be increased, decreased, or altered. It is especially important to check with your doctor before combining Flagyl with any of the following:

Blood thinners such as Coumadin and
    Panwarfin
Cimetidine (Tagamet)
Disulfiram (Antabuse)
Lithium (Lithobid, Cibalith-S Syrup)
Phenobarbital
Phenytoin (Dilantin)

Special information if you are pregnant or breastfeeding

This medication should only be used if it is clearly needed.

No information is available about the safety of Flagyl during pregnancy.

If you are pregnant or plan to become pregnant, tell your doctor immediately.

Flagyl appears in breast milk and could affect a nursing infant. If Flagyl is essential to your health, your doctor may advise you to stop breastfeeding until your treatment is finished.

Recommended dosage

ADULT

Trichomoniasis
One-day treatment: 2 grams of Flagyl, given either as a single dose or in 2 divided doses (1 gram each) in the same day.

Seven-day course of treatment: 250 milligrams 3 times daily for 7 consecutive days. The dosage regimen should be individualized for male and female patients.

Acute Intestinal Amebiasis (Acute Amebic Dysentery)
750 milligrams taken orally 3 times daily for 5 to 10 days.

Amebic Liver Abscess
500 milligrams or 750 milligrams taken orally 3 times daily for 5 to 10 days.

Anaerobic Bacterial Infections
The usual adult oral dosage is 7.5 milligrams per 2.2 pounds of body weight every 6 hours.

CHILDREN

Amebiasis
35 to 50 milligrams for each 2.2 pounds of body weight per day, divided into 3 doses, taken orally, for 10 days.

ELDERLY

The actions of metronidazole may be altered in elderly patients, and it may be necessary to have your blood levels monitored and the dosage adjusted.

Overdosage

Any medication taken in excess can have serious consequences. Flagyl has been used for suicide attempts; accidental overdoses have also occurred. If you suspect an overdose, seek medical treatment immediately.

Symptom of Flagyl overdose may include:
Lack of muscle coordination
Nausea
Vomiting

Generic name:

FLAVOXATE HYDROCHLORIDE

See Urispas, page 666.

Generic name:

FLECAINIDE ACETATE

See Tambocor, page 604.

Brand name:

FLEXERIL

Generic name: Cyclobenzaprine hydrochloride

Why is this drug prescribed?

Flexeril is a skeletal muscle relaxant prescribed to relieve muscle spasms resulting from injuries such as sprains, strains, or pulls. Combined with rest and physical therapy, cyclobenzaprine provides relief of muscular stiffness and pain.

Flexeril should be used only for short periods (no more than 3 weeks). Since the type of injury that cyclobenzaprine treats (such as a sprained ankle) should improve in a few weeks, there is no reason to use it for a longer period.

Most important fact about this drug

Flexeril may cause you to become drowsy or less alert; therefore, driving or operating dangerous machinery or participating in any hazardous activity that requires full mental alertness is not recommended.

How should you take this medication?
Flexeril may be taken with or without food.

If you forget to take a dose, take it as soon as you remember. If it is almost time for your next dose, skip the missed dose and resume your regular schedule.

What side effects may occur?
Side effects cannot be anticipated. If any develop or change in intensity, inform your doctor as soon as possible. Only your doctor can determine if it is safe for you to continue taking Flexeril.

■ *More common side effects may include:*
Dizziness
Drowsiness
Dry mouth

■ *Less common or rare side effects may include:*
Abnormal heartbeats, abnormal sensations, abnormal thoughts or dreams, agitation, anxiety, bloated feeling, blurred vision, confusion, constipation, convulsions, decreased appetite, depressed mood, diarrhea, difficulty falling or staying asleep, difficulty speaking, disorientation, double vision, excitement, fainting, fatigue, fluid retention, gas, hallucinations, headache, heartburn, hepatitis, hives, increased heart rate, indigestion, inflammation of the stomach, itching, lack of coordination, liver diseases, loss of sense of taste, low blood pressure, muscle twitching, nausea, nervousness, palpitations, rash, ringing in the ears, stomach and intestinal pain, sweating, swelling of the tongue or face, thirst, tingling in hands or feet, tremors, unpleasant taste in the mouth, urinating more or less than usual, vague feeling of bodily discomfort, vertigo, vomiting, weakness, yellow eyes and skin

Why should this drug not be prescribed?
You should not take this drug if you are taking antidepressant drugs known as MAO inhibitors (such as Nardil or Parnate) or have taken an MAO inhibitor within the last 2 weeks, if you have ever had an allergic reaction to Flexeril, or if you have hyperthyroidism, (excessive thyroid gland activity).

In addition, you should not take Flexeril if you have recently had a heart attack or if you have congestive heart failure, heart block or conduction disturbances, and irregular heartbeats.

This drug should not be used for long-term treatment of more severe muscular injuries.

Special warnings about this medication
You should use Flexeril with caution if you have a history of urinary retention problems or glaucoma or if you are taking anticholinergic (antispasmodic) medications (such as Donnatal or Bentyl).

Possible food and drug interactions when taking this medication
Serious, potentially fatal reactions may occur if Flexeril is taken with antidepressant drugs known as MAO inhibitors (such as Nardil, Parnate) or if 2 weeks have not passed since the last MAO inhibitor was taken. You should closely follow your doctor's advice regarding discontinuation of MAO inhibitors before taking Flexeril.

If Flexeril is taken with certain other drugs, the effects of either could be increased, decreased, or altered. It is especially important to check with your doctor before combining Flexeril with the following:

Alcohol

Barbiturates (such as phenobarbital)

Guanethidine (Esimil, Ismelin) and other high blood pressure drugs

Other depressants (such as Halcion and Xanax)

Special information if you are pregnant or breastfeeding

The effects of Flexeril during pregnancy have not been adequately studied. If you are pregnant or plan to become pregnant, inform your doctor immediately. It is not known if Flexeril appears in breast milk. However, cyclobenzaprine is related to tricyclic antidepressants, and some of those drugs do appear in breast milk. If this medication is essential to your health, your doctor may advise you to discontinue breast feeding your baby until your treatment is finished.

Recommended dosage

ADULTS

The usual dose is 10 milligrams 3 times a day. Daily dosage should not exceed 60 milligrams.

Your doctor may prescribe a dose individualized to suit your needs.

CHILDREN

Safety and effectiveness of cyclobenzaprine have not been established for children under the age of 15.

Overdosage

Any medication taken in excess can cause symptoms of overdose. Severe overdosage of Flexeril can cause death. If you suspect symptoms of a Flexeril overdose, seek medical attention immediately.

Symptoms of Flexeril overdose may include: Agitation, coma, confusion, congestive heart failure, convulsions, dilated pupils, disturbed concentration, drowsiness, hallucinations, high or low temperatures, increased heartbeats, irregular heart rhythms, muscle stiffness, overactive reflexes, severe low blood pressure, stupor, vomiting

Brand name:

FLOXIN

Generic name: Ofloxacin

Why is this drug prescribed?

Floxin is an antibiotic. It has been used effectively to treat lower respiratory tract infections, including chronic bronchitis and pneumonia, sexually transmitted diseases (except syphilis), urinary tract infections, and skin infections.

Most important fact about this drug

Floxin kills many types of bacteria. It is used to treat infections in many locations of the body. The safety of Floxin in children or adolescents under 18 years old, or in pregnant or nursing women, has not been established.

How should you take this medication?

Floxin may make you feel dizzy or lightheaded. Be careful driving, operating machinery, or doing any activity that requires full mental alertness until you know how you react to this medication.

It is important that you tell your doctor if you have a history of seizures or other central nervous system disorders.

Floxin should be taken on an empty stomach.

It is important to drink plenty of fluids while taking Floxin.

Mineral supplements, vitamins with iron or minerals, or antacids containing calcium, aluminum or magnesium should not be taken 2 hours before or 2 hours after taking Floxin.

You should take Floxin exactly as directed by your doctor.

Complete the full course of therapy for best results and to decrease the risk of a relapse of the infection.

What side effects may occur?

Side effects cannot be anticipated. If any develop or change in intensity, inform your doctor as soon as possible. Only your doctor can determine if it is safe for you to continue taking Floxin.

■ *More common side effects may include:*
Diarrhea
Difficulty sleeping
Dizziness
Headache
Nausea

■ *Less common or rare side effects may include:*
Anxiety, body pain, burning, irritation, pain, itching or rash of the female genitals, changes in thinking and perception, chest pain, chills, confusion, continual runny nose, constipation, cough, decreased appetite, depression, disturbed dreams or sleep disorders, dry mouth, excessive perspiration, exhaustion, fainting, false sense of well-being, fatigue, fever, fluid retention, gas, hallucinations, hearing loss, high blood pressure, increased urination, inflammation of the colon, intolerance to light, involuntary eyeball movement, itching, joint pain, low blood pressure when standing up, menstrual changes, muscle pain, nervousness, painful or difficult swallowing, painful or difficult urination, possible aggravation of myasthenia gravis, pounding heartbeat, rash, ringing in the ears, severe allergic reaction, skin flaking, sleepiness, Stevens-Johnson syndrome (skin peeling), stomach pain and cramps, taste distortion, thirst, tingling or pins and needles, upset stomach, vaginal discharge, vaginal infection, vague feeling of weakness, vertigo, visual disturbances, vomiting, weakness, weight loss

Why should this drug not be prescribed?

Floxin should not be taken if you are sensitive to or have ever had an allergic reaction to ofloxacin or to quinolone medications.

Special warnings about this medication

The safety of this medication in children or adolescents under 18 years old or pregnant or nursing women has not been established.

Floxin, used in high doses for short periods of time, may hide or delay the symptoms of syphilis, but is not effective in treating syphilis. If you are taking Floxin for gonorrhea, your doctor should test you for syphilis and then perform a follow-up test after 3 months of treatment.

Serious and sometimes fatal allergic reactions have occurred in patients being treated with ofloxacin, some after only one dose. If you develop any allergic symptoms (rash, fever, itching, hives, swelling of the face or throat, difficulty breathing, tingling), stop taking the medication and contact your doctor immediately.

Convulsions, increased pressure in the head, psychosis, tremors, restlessness, lightheadedness, confusion, and hallucinations have been reported with drugs of this type. If you experience any of these symptoms, contact your doctor immediately.

Floxin should be used with care if you have kidney disease, a brain disorder, epilepsy, or are prone to seizures.

Because increased sensitivity to sunlight can occur with Floxin, exposure to excessive sunlight should be avoided.

Possible food and drug interactions when taking this medication

If Floxin is taken with certain other drugs, the effects of either could be increased, decreased, or altered. It is especially important to check with your doctor before combining Floxin with the following:

Antacids
Blood thinners such as Coumadin
Calcium supplements
Iron supplements
Multivitamins containing zinc
Theophylline-containing drugs, such as Theo-
    Dur and others

Special information if you are pregnant or breastfeeding

The effects of Floxin during pregnancy have not been adequately studied; however, abnormalities, decreased fetal weight, and deaths have occurred in animals. If you are pregnant or plan to become pregnant, inform your doctor immediately. This medication should not be used during pregnancy unless your doctor has determined that the benefit outweighs the risk to the unborn baby. Floxin appears in breast milk and could affect a nursing infant. If this medication is essential to your health, your doctor may advise you to stop breastfeeding until your treatment with Floxin is finished.

Recommended dosage

The usual daily dose of Floxin is 200 milligrams to 400 milligrams orally every 12 hours as described below:

LOWER RESPIRATORY TRACT INFECTIONS

Exacerbation of Chronic Bronchitis
The usual dose is 400 milligrams every 12 hours for 10 days, for a total daily dose of 800 milligrams.

Pneumonia
The usual dose is 400 milligrams every 12 hours for 10 days, for a total daily dose of 800 milligrams.

SEXUALLY TRANSMITTED DISEASES

Gonorrhea
The usual dose is 400 milligrams in a single dose, for a total dose of 400 milligrams.

Cervicitis/Urethritis Due to C. Trachomatis and/or N. Gonorrhoeae
The usual dose is 300 milligrams every 12 hours for 7 days, for a total daily dose of 600 milligrams.

MILD TO MODERATE SKIN AND SKIN STRUCTURE INFECTIONS

The usual dose is 400 milligrams every 12 hours for 10 days, for a total daily dose of 800 milligrams.

URINARY TRACT INFECTIONS

Cystitis Due to E. Coli or K. Pneumoniae
The usual dose is 200 milligrams every 12 hours for 3 days, for a total daily dose of 400 milligrams.

Cystitis Due to Other Organisms
The usual dose is 200 milligrams every 12 hours for 7 days, for a total daily dose of 400 milligrams.

Complicated Urinary Tract Infections
The usual dose is 200 milligrams every 12 hours for 10 days, for a total daily dose of 400 milligrams.

Prostatitis
The usual dose is 300 milligrams every 12 hours for 6 weeks, for a total daily dose of 600 milligrams.

Dosages should be reduced in patients with impaired kidney function.

Overdosage

Although no specific information is available, any medication taken in excess can have serious consequences. If you suspect an overdose, seek medical treatment immediately.

Generic name:

FLUNISOLIDE

See AeroBid, page 9.

Generic name:

FLUOCINONIDE

See Lidex, page 322.

Generic name:

FLUOROMETHOLONE

See FML, page 248.

Generic name:

FLUOROURACIL

See Efudex, page 224.

Generic name:

FLUOXETINE HYDROCHLORIDE

See Prozac, page 523.

Generic name:

FLUPHENAZINE HYDROCHLORIDE

See Prolixin, page 510.

Generic name:

FLURAZEPAM HYDROCHLORIDE

See Dalmane, page 157.

Generic name:

FLURBIPROFEN

See Ansaid, page 31.

Generic name:

FLUTAMIDE

See Eulexin, page 245.

Generic name:

FLUTICASONE PROPIONATE

See Cutivate, page 147.

Generic name:

FOSINOPRIL SODIUM

See Monopril, page 391.

Brand name:

FULVICIN P/G

See Gris-PEG, page 273.

Generic name:

FUROSEMIDE

See Lasix, page 314.

Brand name:

GANTRISIN

Generic name: Sulfisoxazole

Why is this drug prescribed?

Gantrisin is prescribed for the treatment of severe, long-lasting, or recurring urinary tract infections not caused by an obstruction or foreign body. These include pyelonephritis (bacterial kidney inflammation), pyelitis (inflammation of the part of the kidney that drains urine into the ureter), and cystitis (inflammation of the bladder). This drug is an antibacterial sulfonamide that halts the growth and spread of certain bacteria.

This drug is also used to treat bacterial meningitis, and is prescribed as a preventive measure for people who have been exposed to meningitis.

Some middle ear infections are treated with Gantrisin in combination with penicillin or erythromycin.

Toxoplasmosis (parasitic disease transmitted by infected cats, their feces or litter boxes, and undercooked meat) can be treated with Gantrisin in combination with pyrimethamine (Daraprim). Malaria that does not respond to the drug chloroquine (Aralen) can be treated with Gantrisin in combination with other drug treatment.

Gantrisin is also used in the treatment of bacterial infections such as trachoma and inclusion inflammation conjunctivitis (eye infections), nocardiosis (bacterial disease affecting the lungs, skin, and brain), and chancroid (venereal disease causing enlargement and ulceration of lymph nodes in the groin).

Most important fact about this drug

Fatalities have occurred with the use of sulfonamides because of severe reactions, including sudden and severe liver damage, agranulocytosis (a severe blood disorder), and aplastic anemia (a lack of red and white blood cells because of a bone marrow disorder).

Notify your doctor at the first sign of an adverse reaction such as skin rash, sore throat, fever, joint pain, cough, shortness of breath, abnormal skin paleness, reddish or purplish skin spots or yellowing of the skin or whites of the eyes.

Patients taking sulfonamides should have frequent blood counts.

How should you take this medication?

Take Gantrisin exactly as prescribed by your doctor.

It is important that you drink plenty of fluids while taking this medication in order to prevent crystals in the urine and the formation of stones.

What side effects may occur?

Side effects cannot be anticipated. If any develop or change in intensity, inform your doctor as soon as possible. Only your doctor can determine if it is safe for you to continue taking Gantrisin.

■ Side effects may include:
Abdominal pain, allergic reactions, chills, convulsions, depression, diarrhea, fatigue, fever, hallucinations, headache, hives, inability to fall or stay asleep, inability to urinate, inflammation of heart muscle, inflammation of the eye, inflammation of the mouth, itching, joint pain, lack of feeling or concern, lack of muscle coordination, lack or loss of appetite, muscle pain, nausea, red, raised rash, reddish or purplish skin spots, redness and inflammation of the tongue, ringing in the ears, scaling of dead skin due to inflammation, scant urine output, sensitivity

to light, severe skin welts or swelling, skin eruptions, skin rash, swelling due to fluid retention, vertigo, vomiting, weakness

Why should this drug not be prescribed?

If you are sensitive to or have ever had an allergic reaction to Gantrisin or sulfa drugs, you should not take this medication. Make sure that your doctor is aware of any drug reactions that you have experienced.

This drug should not be prescribed for infants less than 2 months of age. You should not take Gantrisin if you are pregnant or planning to become pregnant, or if you are nursing a baby.

Special warnings about this medication

If you have impaired kidney or liver function, or if you have severe allergies or bronchial asthma, caution should be exercised when taking Gantrisin. Consult with your doctor.

An analysis of your urine and kidney function should be performed by your doctor during treatment with Gantrisin, especially for patients with impaired kidney function.

Possible food and drug interactions when taking this medication

If Gantrisin is taken with certain other drugs, the effects of either could be increased, decreased, or altered. It is especially important to check with your doctor before combining this drug with the following:

Methotrexate, an anticancer drug
Sulfonylureas, drugs that reduce blood sugar, such as Micronase
Warfarin (Coumadin, a blood thinner)

Special information if you are pregnant or breastfeeding

If you are pregnant or planning to become pregnant, or if you are breastfeeding, you should not take Gantrisin.

Recommended dosage

ADULTS

The recommended starting dose is 2 to 4 grams. A maintenance dose of 4 to 8 grams per day, divided into 4 to 6 doses, is recommended.

CHILDREN

This medication should not be prescribed for infants under 2 months of age except in the treatment of congenital toxoplasmosis (a parasitic infection contracted by pregnant women and passed along to the fetus).

The usual maintenance dose for children 2 months of age or older is 150 milligrams per 2.2 pounds of body weight divided into 4 to 6 doses taken over 24 hours.

The usual starting dose is one-half of the regular maintenance dose, or 75 milligrams per 2.2 pounds of body weight divided into 4 to 6 doses taken over 24 hours. Doses should not exceed 6 grams over 24 hours.

Overdosage

Any medication taken in excess can have serious consequences. If you suspect an overdose, seek emergency medical treatment immediately.

Symptoms of an overdose of Gantrisin include:
Blood or sediment in the urine
Dizziness
Drowsiness
Fever
Headache
Lack or loss of appetite
Nausea
Unconsciousness
Vomiting
Yellowing of skin and whites of eyes

Brand name:

GARAMYCIN OPHTHALMIC

Generic name: Gentamicin sulfate
Other brand name: Gentacidin

Why is this drug prescribed?

Garamycin ophthalmic, an antibiotic, is prescribed for the topical treatment of eye infections such as conjunctivitis (pink eye), keratitis (inflammation of the cornea), blepharitis (inflammation of the eyelids), corneal ulcers, acute meibomianitis (inflammation of the glands on the eyelids), and dacryocystitis (inflammation of the tear sac). It is available in solution and ointment form.

Most important fact about this drug

Garamycin Ophthalmic Solution should never be applied to the front part (anterior chamber) of the eye or under the upper eyelid.

How should you use this medication?

Use this medication exactly as prescribed by your doctor.

What side effects may occur?

Occasional eye irritation may occur with the use of Garamycin Ophthalmic Solution.

Occasional burning or stinging in the eye may occur with the use of Garamycin Ophthalmic Ointment.

Why should this drug not be prescribed?

If you are sensitive to or have ever had an allergic reaction to Gentamicin or certain other drugs of this type (e.g. aminoglycosides), you should not take this medication. Make sure that your doctor is aware of any drug reactions that you have experienced.

Special warnings about this medication

Continued or prolonged use of this drug may result in a growth of bacteria or fungi that do not respond to this medication and can cause a secondary infection. Should this occur, notify your doctor.

Ophthalmic ointments may slow corneal healing.

Recommended dosage

ADULTS AND CHILDREN

Garamycin Ophthalmic Solution
Put 1 or 2 drops into the affected eye every 4 hours. For severe infections, your doctor may increase your dosage up to a maximum of 2 drops once every hour.

Garamycin Ophthalmic Ointment
Apply a small amount to the affected eye 2 or 3 times a day.

Generic name:

GEMFIBROZIL

See Lopid, page 335.

Brand name:

GENTACIDIN

See Garamycin Opthalmic, page 269.

Generic name:

GENTAMICIN SULFATE

See Garamycin Opthalmic, page 269.

Brand name:

GENUINE BAYER

See Aspirin, page 40.

Generic name:

GLIPIZIDE

See Glucotrol, page 270.

Brand name:

GLUCOTROL

Generic name: Glipizide

Why is this drug prescribed?

Glucotrol is an oral antidiabetic medication used to treat Type II (non-insulin-dependent) diabetes. In diabetics the body either does not make enough insulin or the insulin that is produced no longer works properly.

There are actually two forms of diabetes: Type I insulin-dependent and Type II non-insulin-dependent. Type I usually requires insulin injection for life, while Type II diabetes can usually be treated by dietary changes and/or oral antidiabetic medications such as Glucotrol. Apparently, Glucotrol controls diabetes by stimulating the pancreas to secrete more insulin. Occasionally, Type II diabetics must take insulin injections on a temporary basis, especially during stressful periods or times of illness.

Most important fact about this drug

Patients taking Glucotrol must remember that this medication is not a substitute for a good diet and exercise plan. It merely enhances treatment of the condition. Failure to follow a sound diet and exercise plan may lead to serious and potentially fatal complications, such as low blood sugar levels (known as hypoglycemia). Patients should also remember that Glucotrol is *not* an oral form of insulin and should not be substituted for injected insulin.

How should you take this medication?

In general, to achieve the best control over blood sugar levels, Glucotrol should be taken 30 minutes before a meal. However, the exact dosing schedule as well as the dosage amount must be determined by your physician.

What side effects may occur?

Side effects from Glucotrol are rare and seldom require discontinuation of the medication.

■ *More common side effects may include:*
Constipation, diarrhea, dizziness, drowsiness, headache, hives, itching, low blood sugar, nausea, sensitivity to light, skin rash and eruptions, stomach pain

■ *Less common or rare side effects may include:*
Anemia and other blood disorders, yellow eyes and skin

Glucotrol, like all oral antidiabetic drugs, can cause low blood sugar. This risk is increased by missed meals, alcohol, other medications, and/or excessive exercise. To avoid low blood sugar, you should closely follow the dietary and exercise regimen suggested by your physician.

■ *Symptoms of mild low blood sugar may include:*
Blurred vision
Cold sweats
Dizziness
Fast heartbeat
Fatigue
Headache
Hunger
Light-headedness
Nausea
Nervousness

■ *Symptoms of more severe low blood sugar may include:*
Coma
Disorientation
Pale skin
Seizures
Shallow breathing

Ask your doctor what steps you should take if you experience mild hypoglycemia. If symptoms of severe low blood sugar occur, contact your doctor immediately. Severe hypoglycemia should be considered a medical emergency, and prompt medical attention is essential.

Why should this drug not be prescribed?
You should not take Glucotrol if you have had an allergic reaction to it previously.

Glucotrol should not be taken if you are suffering from diabetic ketoacidosis (a life-threatening medical emergency caused by insufficient insulin and marked by excessive thirst, nausea, fatigue, pain below the breastbone, and a fruity breath).

Special warnings about this medication
Oral antidiabetic medication has been associated with an increased risk of death from cardiovascular conditions. One study of another oral antidiabetic medication called tolbutamide (Orinase) in non-insulin-dependents found that patients receiving tolbutamide had a cardiovascular mortality rate 2.5 times greater than subjects treated with diet alone—although no significant increase in overall mortality was found. Although this study concerned tolbutamide, a general warning involving the increased risk of severe heart disease has been applied to all oral antidiabetics.

If you are taking Glucotrol, you should check your blood and urine periodically for the presence of abnormal sugar (glucose) levels.

Even patients with well-controlled diabetes may find that stress, illness, surgery, or fever results in a lack of control over their diabetes. In these cases, the patient's physician may recommend that Glucotrol be discontinued temporarily and injected insulin administered.

In addition, the effectiveness of any oral antidiabetic, including Glucotrol, may decrease with time. This may occur because of either a diminished responsiveness to the medication or a worsening of the diabetes.

Possible food and drug interactions when taking this medication
It is essential that you closely follow your physician's dietary guidelines and that you inform your physician of any medication, either prescription or non-prescription, that you are taking. Specific medications that affect Glucotrol include:

Anabolic steroids such as Androl-50
Aspirin
Chloramphenicol (Chloromycetin)
Corticosteroids such as prednisone
Coumarin (Coumadin)
Estrogens such as Premarin
Heart and blood pressue medications called beta blockers such as Tenormin, Lopressor
Heart medications called calcium channel blockers such as Cardizem, Procardia XL
Isoniazid
MAO Inhibitors (antidepressant drugs such as Nardil
Miconazole (Monistat)
Nicotinic acid (Nicobid)
Nonsteroidal anti-inflammatory drugs such as Motrin
Oral contraceptives
Phenothiazine drugs such as Mellaril
Phenylbutazone (Butazolidin)
Phenytoin (Dilantin)
Probenecid (Benemid)

Sulfonamide drugs such as Bactrium
Thiazide diuretics such as Diuril, HydroDiuril
Thyroid medications such as Synthroid,
  Proloid

Alcohol must be used carefully, since excessive
alcohol consumption can cause low blood
sugar.

Special information
if you are pregnant or breastfeeding

The effects of Glucotrol during pregnancy
have not been adequately studied.
Therefore, if you are pregnant, or planning
to become pregnant, you should take
Glucotrol only on the advice of your
physician. Since studies suggest the
importance of maintaining normal blood sugar
(glucose) levels during pregnancy, your
physician may prescribe injected insulin during
pregnancy. To minimize the risk of low
blood sugar in newborn babies, Glucotrol,
if prescribed during pregnancy, should be
discontinued at least one month before the
expected delivery date. Although it is not
known if Glucotrol crosses into breast milk,
other oral antidiabetics do appear in
human milk. Because of the potential for
hypoglycemia in nursing infants, a decision
must be made to either discontinue Glucotrol
or stop nursing. If Glucotrol is discontinued
and if diet alone does not control glucose
levels, then insulin injection should be
considered.

Recommended dosage

Dosage levels must be determined by each
patient's needs.

ADULTS

The usual recommended starting dose is 5
milligrams taken before breakfast. Depending
upon blood glucose response, this initial
dose may be increased in increments of
2.5 to 5 milligrams. The maximum
recommended daily dose is 40 milligrams;

total daily dosages above 15 milligrams
are usually divided into 2 equal doses that
are taken before meals.

CHILDREN

The safety and effectiveness of this drug in
children have not been established.

ELDERLY

Elderly patients or patients with liver disease
usually receive a starting dose of 2.5
milligrams. To lessen the risk of hypoglycemia,
the usual dose in these patients should
be determined cautiously.

Overdosage

An overdose of Glucotrol can cause low
blood sugar. These symptoms include:
Cold sweat
Fatigue
Headache
Nausea
Nervousness
Rapid heartbeat

*Symptoms of more severe low blood sugar
include:*
Coma
Disorientation
Pale skin
Seizures
Shallow breathing

Contact your doctor immediately if these
symptoms of severe low blood sugar
occur.

Eating sugar or a sugar-based product will
often correct the condition. If you suspect
an overdose, seek medical attention
immediately.

Generic name:

GLYBURIDE

See Micronase, page 377.

Brand name:

GRIS-PEG

Generic name: Griseofulvin
Other brand names: Grisactin, Fulvicin P/G

Why is this drug prescribed?
Gris-PEG is prescribed for the treatment of the following ringworm infections:

Athlete's foot
Barber's itch (inflammation of the facial hair follicles)
Ringworm of the body
Ringworm of the groin and thigh
Ringworm of the nails
Ringworm of the scalp

Because Gris-PEG is effective for only certain types of fungal infections, before treatment your doctor may perform tests to identify the type of fungus responsible for the infection.

Most important fact about this drug
If you are being treated with Gris-PEG for an extended period of time, your doctor should perform regular tests, including periodic monitoring of kidney function, liver function, and blood cell production.

How should you take this medication?
Take this medication exactly as prescribed by your doctor.

It is important that you finish taking all of this medication, even if you are feeling better, in order to remove any traces of the infecting organism. Cure is confirmed by laboratory tests.

To minimize stomach irritation, take Gris-PEG at meal times or with food or milk.

Observe good hygiene during treatment to help control infection and prevent reinfection.

What side effects may occur?
Side effects cannot be anticipated. If any develop or change in intensity, inform your doctor as soon as possible. Only your doctor can determine if it is safe for you to continue taking Gris-PEG.

■ *More common side effects may include:*
Hives
Skin rashes

■ *Less common side effects may include:*
Confusion, diarrhea, dizziness, fatigue, headache, impairment of performance of routine activities, inability to fall or stay asleep, nausea, oral thrush (mouth inflammation), upper abdominal pain, vomiting

■ *Rare side effects may include:*
Swelling and itching of areas of skin, tingling sensation in hands and feet

Why should this drug not be prescribed?
If you are sensitive to or have ever had an allergic reaction to Gris-PEG or other drugs of this type, you should not take this medication. Make sure that your doctor is aware of any drug reactions that you have experienced.

Unless you are directed to do so by your doctor, do not take this medication if you have liver damage or porphyria (inherited metabolic disorder of the liver or bone marrow). Do not take Gris-PEG while pregnant.

Special warnings about this medication
Gris-PEG is derived from a species of penicillin; although penicillin-sensitive patients have been treated without difficulty, notify your doctor if you are sensitive or allergic to penicillin.

Because sensitivity to light is occasionally associated with the use of Gris-PEG, avoid exposure to intense natural or artificial sunlight.

Notify your doctor if you develop lupus erythematosus (a form of arthritis) or lupus-like signs and symptoms (arthritis, red butterfly rash over the nose and cheeks, tiredness, weakness, sensitivity to sunlight, skin lesions) while taking this drug.

This drug should not be used for minor or trivial infections that will respond to topical medications alone.

The safety and effectiveness of Gris-PEG have not been established for the prevention of fungal infections.

Possible food and drug interactions when taking this medication

Gris-PEG may intensify the effects of alcohol. Do not drink alcohol while taking this medication.

If Gris-PEG is taken with certain other drugs, the effects of either could be increased, decreased, or altered. It is especially important to check with your doctor before combining Gris-PEG with the following:

Warfarin-type anticoagulants (blood thinners such as Coumadin)
Barbiturates (antianxiety drugs, anticonvulsants, and sedatives such as phenobarbital)
Oral contraceptives such as Ortho-Novum

Special information
If you are pregnant or breastfeeding

Gris-PEG should not be used by pregnant patients. If you become pregnant while taking this drug, notify your doctor immediately. There is a potential hazard to the fetus.

If you are breastfeeding your infant, consult with your doctor before taking Gris-PEG.

Recommended dosage

The recommended treatment periods for various ringworm infections are:
Ringworm of the scalp—4 to 6 weeks
Ringworm of the body—2 to 4 weeks
Athlete's foot—4 to 8 weeks

The recommended treatment period, depending on the rate of growth, for ringworm of the fingernails is at least 4 months and for ringworm of the toenails at least 6 months.

ADULTS

Ringworm of the Body, Groin and Thigh, Scalp
The recommended daily dosage is 375 milligrams taken as a single dose or divided into smaller doses, as determined by your doctor.

Athlete's Foot, Ringworm of the Nails
The recommended daily dosage is 750 milligrams divided into smaller doses, as determined by your doctor.

CHILDREN

A single daily dose is effective in children with ringworm of the scalp. The recommended dosage is 3.3 milligrams per pound of body weight per day. The following dosage schedule is suggested:

35 to 60 pounds:
   125 to 187.5 milligrams daily
Over 60 pounds:
   187.5 to 375 milligrams daily

A recommended dosage has not been established in children 2 years of age and under.

Overdosage

Any medication taken in excess can have dangerous consequences. If you suspect an overdose, seek emergency medical treatment immediately.

Brand name:

GRISACTIN

See *Gris-PEG, page 273.*

Generic name:

GRISEOFULVIN

See *Gris-PEG, page 273.*

Generic name:

GUANABENZ ACETATE

See *Wytensin, page 687.*

Generic name:

GUANFACINE HYDROCHLORIDE

See *Tenex, page 612.*

Brand name:

HABITROL

See *Nicotine Patches, page 416.*

Brand name:

HALCION

Generic name: Triazolam

Why is this drug prescribed?

Halcion is used for short-term treatment of insomnia. It is a member of the benzodiazepine class of drugs, many of which are used as tranquilizers. Exactly how benzodiazepines work has not been established; however, many researchers believe that they achieve their calming effect by altering the levels of certain neurotransmitters (chemical messengers), in the brain.

Most important fact about this drug

Because of Halcion's sedative effects, you should not operate heavy machinery, drive an automobile, engage in hazardous tasks, or consume alcohol or other mental depressants while you are taking the drug.

Do not use Halcion for more than 7 to 10 days without first consulting your doctor.

Do not increase the prescribed dose except on the advice of your doctor.

If you develop unusual and disturbing thoughts or behavior during treatment with Halcion, you should discuss them with your doctor immediately.

How should you take this medication?

To help avoid stomach upset, Halcion may be taken with food.

What side effects may occur?

Side effects cannot be anticipated. If any develop or change in intensity, inform your doctor as soon as possible. Only your doctor can determine if it is safe for you to continue taking Halcion.

■ *More common side effects may include:*
Coordination problems
Dizziness
Drowsiness
Headache
Light-headedness
Nausea/vomiting
Nervousness

■ *Less common or rare side effects may include:*
Aggressiveness, agitation, behavior problems, burning tongue, changes in sexual drive, chest pain, confusion, congestion,

constipation, cramps/pain, delusions, depression, diarrhea, disorientation, dreaming abnormalities, dry mouth, exaggerated sense of well-being, excitement, fainting, falling, fatigue, hallucinations, impaired urination, inappropriate behavior, incontinence, inflammation of the tongue and mouth, irritability, itching, loss of appetite, loss of sense of reality, memory impairment, memory loss (e.g. traveler's amnesia), menstrual irregularities, morning "hangover" effects, muscle spasms in the shoulders or neck, nightmares, rapid heart rate, restlessness, ringing in the ears, skin inflammation, sleep disturbances including insomnia, sleepwalking, slurred or difficult speech, stiff, awkward movements, taste changes, tingling or pins and needles, tiredness, visual disturbances, weakness, worsening of depression including suicidal thinking, yellowing of the skin and white of the eyes

Why should this drug not be prescribed?

You should not take this drug if you are pregnant or if you have had an allergic reaction to it or to other benzodiazepines.

Special warnings about this medication

It is important to take Halcion exactly as prescribed, since benzodiazepine abuse has been associated with drug dependence and addiction. Patients with a history of alcoholism, drug abuse, or personality disorders should use Halcion with caution.

Abrupt discontinuation of Halcion should be avoided, since it has been associated with withdrawal symptoms (convulsions, cramps, tremor, vomiting, sweating, feeling ill, perceptual problems, and insomnia). A gradual dosage tapering schedule is usually recommended for patients taking more than the lowest dose of Halcion for longer

than a few weeks. The usual treatment period is 7 to 10 days.

"Traveler's amnesia" has been reported by patients who took Halcion to induce sleep while traveling. To avoid this condition, you should take Halcion only when a full night of sleep is possible.

Tell your doctor if you are pregnant, think you may be pregnant, or are planning to become pregnant, or if you are breast-feeding, before taking Halcion.

You may suffer increased anxiety during the daytime while taking Halcion.

After discontinuing the drug, you may experience a "rebound insomnia" for the first 2 nights—that is, insomnia may be worse than before you took the sleeping pill.

You should be aware that anterograde amnesia (forgetting events after an injury) has been associated with benzodiazepines—some reports suggest a higher rate with Halcion than with other benzodiazepines.

You should be cautious about using this drug if you have liver or kidney problems, lung problems, or a tendency to temporarily stop breathing while you are asleep.

Possible food and drug interactions when taking this medication

If Halcion is taken with certain other drugs, the effects of either could be increased, decreased, or altered. It is especially important to check with your doctor before combining Halcion with the following:

Cimetidine (Tagamet)
Erythromycin (PCE, E-Mycin)
Monoamine Oxidase Inhibitors (antidepressant drugs such as Nardil and Parnate)

In addition, excessive drowsiness and other potentially dangerous side effects may occur if Halcion is combined with alcohol or other central nervous system depressants such as barbiturates (Seconal), antihistamines (Benadryl), other psychotropic drugs (Thorazine, Valium), and anticonvulsants (Dilantin, Tegretol).

Special information if you are pregnant or breastfeeding

Since benzodiazepines have been associated with fetal damage, you should not take Halcion if you are pregnant, think you may be pregnant, or are planning to become pregnant, or if you are breastfeeding.

Recommended dosage

ADULTS

The usual dose is 0.25 milligram before bedtime. The dose should never be more than 0.5 milligram.

CHILDREN

Safety and efficacy for children under the age of 18 have not been established.

ELDERLY

To decrease the possibility of oversedation, dizziness, or impaired coordination, the usual starting dose is 0.125 milligram. This may be increased to 0.25 milligram if necessary.

In general, the lowest effective dose for all patients should be used.

Overdosage

Any medication taken in excess can have serious consequences. Severe overdosage of Halcion can be fatal. If you suspect an overdose, seek medical help immediately.

Symptoms of Halcion overdose may include:
Apnea (temporary cessation of breathing)
Coma
Confusion
Excessive sleepiness

Problems in coordination
Seizures
Shallow or difficult breathing
Slurred speech

Brand name:

HALDOL

Generic name: Haloperidol

Why is this drug prescribed?

Haldol is used to reduce the symptoms of psychotic disorders such as schizophrenia, and to control tics (uncontrolled muscle contractions of face, arms, or shoulders) and the unintended utterances that mark Gilles de la Tourette's syndrome. It is also used in short-term treatment of children with severe behavior problems, including hyperactivity and combativeness.

Most important fact about this drug

Haldol may cause tardive dyskinesia—a condition characterized by involuntary muscle spasms and twitches in the face and body. This condition can be permanent, and appears to be most common among the elderly, especially women. Ask your doctor for information about this possible risk.

How should you take this medication?

Haldol may be taken with food or after eating. If taking Haldol in a liquid concentrate form, you will need to dilute it with milk or water.

You should not take Haldol with coffee, tea, or other caffeinated beverages, or with alcohol.

Haldol causes dry mouth. Sucking on sugarless hard candy or ice chips may help alleviate the problem.

What side effects may occur?

Side effects cannot be anticipated. If any side effects develop or change in intensity, inform your doctor as soon as possible. Only your doctor can determine if it is safe for you to continue taking this medication.

■ *Side effects may include:*
Abnormal secretion of milk, agitation, anemia, anxiety, appetite changes, blurred vision, breast pain, breast development in males, cataracts, catatonic state, chewing movements, confusion, constipation, coughing, deeper breathing, dehydration, depression, diarrhea, dizziness, drowsiness, dry mouth, exaggerated feeling of well-being, exaggerated reflexes, excessive salivation, fever, hair loss, hallucinations, headache, heat stroke, high or low blood sugar, impotence, increased libido, indigestion, involuntary movements, irregular blood pressure, pulse, and heartbeat, irregular menstrual periods, lack of muscular coordination, muscle spasms, nausea, Parkinson-like symptoms, persistent abnormal erections, physical rigidity and stupor, protruding tongue, puckering of mouth, puffing of checks, rapid heartbeat, restlessness, rigid arms, feet, head, and muscles, rotation of eyeballs, seizures, sensitivity to light, skin rash, eruptions, sleeplessness, sluggishness, sweating, swelling of breasts, twitching in the body, neck, shoulders and face, urinary retention, vertigo, visual problems, vomiting, wheezing or asthma-like symptoms, yellowing of skin and whites of eyes

Why should this drug not be prescribed?
Haldol should not be given to comatose individuals. Do not take Haldol with central nervous system depressants such as alcohol, barbiturates, or narcotics. Avoid Haldol if you have Parkinson's disease or are hypersensitive to the drug.

Special warnings about this medication
You should use Haldol cautiously if you have ever had breast cancer, a severe cardiovascular disorder, chest pain, glaucoma, seizures, or an allergy to medication of this type.

Temporary muscle spasms and twitches may occur if you suddenly stop taking Haldol. Follow your doctor's instructions closely when discontinuing the drug.

This drug may impair your ability to drive a car or operate potentially dangerous machinery. Do not participate in any activities that require full alertness if you are unsure of your response to Haldol.

Possible food and drug interactions when taking this medication
If Haldol is taken with certain other drugs, the effects of either could be increased, decreased, or altered. It is especially important to check with your doctor before combining Haldol with the following:

Anticonvulsants such as Dilantin and
 Tegretol
Anticoagulants/blood thinners such as
 Dicumarol
Lithium (Eskalith)

Extreme drowsiness and other potentially serious effects can result if Haldol is combined with alcohol, narcotics, painkillers, sleeping medications, or other central nervous system depressants.

Drugs such as Haldol should not be used with epinephrine (EpiPen).

Special information if you are pregnant or breastfeeding
Pregnant women should use Haldol only if clearly needed. The effects of Haldol during pregnancy have not been adequately studied. If you are pregnant or plan to become pregnant, inform your doctor immediately. Haldol should not be used by women who are breastfeeding an infant.

Recommended dosage
Doses should be tailored to the individual.

ADULTS

Moderate Symptoms
The usual dosage is 1 to 6 milligrams daily. This amount should be divided into 2 or 3 smaller doses per day.

Severe Symptoms
The usual dosage is 6 to 15 milligrams daily. This amount should be divided into 2 or 3 smaller doses per day.

CHILDREN

Children younger than 3 years old should not take Haldol.

For children between the ages of 3 and 12, weighing approximately 33 to 88 pounds, doses should start at 0.5 milligram per day.

If needed, dosages may be increased.

For Psychotic Disorders
The daily dose may range from 0.05 milligram to 0.15 milligram for every 2.2 pounds of body weight.

For Non-Psychotic Behavior Disorders and Tourette's Disorder
The daily dose may range from 0.05 milligram to 0.075 milligram for every 2.2 pounds of body weight.

ELDERLY

In general, elderly people take dosages of Haldol in the lower ranges. Elderly people (especially elderly women) may be more susceptible to tardive dyskinesia—a possibly irreversible condition marked by involuntary muscle spasms and twitches in the face and body. Elderly people should consult their doctor for information about these potential risks.

Doses may range from 1 to 6 milligrams daily.

Overdosage
Any medication taken in excess can have serious consequences. An overdosage of Haldol can be fatal. If you suspect an overdose, seek medical help immediately.

Symptoms of Haldol overdose may include: Catatonic state, coma, decreased breathing, low blood pressure, rigid muscles, sedation, tremor, weakness

Generic name:

HALOPERIDOL

See Haldol, page 277.

Brand name:

HISMANAL

Generic name: Astemizole

Why is this drug prescribed?
Hismanal is an antihistamine prescribed to reduce allergy symptoms. Two conditions that astemizole is useful for are hay fever and hives.

Most important fact about this drug
Take this drug only as needed. Do not attempt to hurry its onset or increase its effect with larger doses than your doctor has prescribed.

How should you take this medication?
Astemizole should be taken on an empty stomach—for example, 1 hour before you eat or 2 hours after eating. Taking the drug with food may make it less effective.

Store your medication in a cool, dry place away from heat or direct sunlight and keep it away from children.

What side effects may occur?

Side effects cannot be anticipated. If any develop or change in intensity, inform your doctor as soon as possible. Only your doctor can determine if it is safe for you to continue taking Hismanal.

■ *More common side effects may include:* Diarrhea, dizziness, drowsiness, dry mouth, fatigue, headache, increase in appetite, inflammation of the eyelids, joint pain, nausea, nervousness, sore throat, stomach and intestinal pain, weight gain

■ *Less common side effects may include:* Asthma-like symptoms, depression, fluid retention, itching, muscle pain, nosebleeds, palpitations, sensitivity to light, skin rash

■ *Rare side effects may include:* Convulsions

Why should this drug not be prescribed?

You should not be taking this medication if you have a known allergy to Hismanal.

Special warnings about this medication

If you are being treated for a lower respiratory tract disease such as asthma or for liver or kidney disease, consult with your doctor before taking Hismanal.

Possible food and drug interactions when taking this medication

Taking this drug with food can decrease its effectiveness. Hismanal should not be taken with erythromycin or the antifungal drug Nizoral.

Special information if you are pregnant or breastfeeding

The effects of Hismanal during pregnancy have not been adequately studied. Therefore, this medication should be prescribed only when the benefits of therapy outweigh any potential risk to the fetus. It is not known whether Hismanal appears in breast milk. If this medication is essential to your health, your doctor may advise you to stop nursing your baby until your treatment with this drug is finished.

Recommended dosage

ADULTS

The usual dose for adults and children 12 years and over is 10 milligrams (1 tablet) once daily.

CHILDREN

Safety and effectiveness in children under 12 have not been established.

Overdosage

Hismanal is generally safe; however, large amounts may cause overdose symptoms, including serious irregular heartbeat. If you suspect an overdose, get medical help immediately.

Brand name:

HUMULIN

See Insulin, page 297.

Brand name:

HYDERGINE

Generic name: Ergoloid mesylates

Why is this drug prescribed?

Hydergine helps relieve the signs and symptoms of the decline in mental capacity (decline in cognitive and interpersonal skills, motivation, self-care, and mood) thought to be related to aging or some form of dementia (such as Alzheimer's or senility) in people over age 60.

Most important fact about this drug

Hydergine should not be used for the treatment of acute or chronic mental disorders.

How should you take this medication?

Take Hydergine exactly as prescribed by your doctor.

Allow the sublingual tablets to dissolve completely under the tongue. Do not crush or chew sublingual tablets.

What side effects may occur?

Side effects cannot be anticipated. If any develop or change in intensity, notify your doctor as soon as possible. Only your doctor can determine whether it is safe to continue taking Hydergine.

■ *Side effects may include:*
Irritation below the tongue with the sublingual dose
Stomach upset
Temporary nausea

Why should this drug not be prescribed?

Do not use hydergine preparations if you have ever had an allergic reaction or are sensitive to ergoloid mesylates, or if you have a mental disorder.

Special warnings about this medication

Since the symptoms treated with Hydergine are of unknown origin and may change or evolve into a specific disease, your doctor will make a specific diagnosis before prescribing Hydergine and then watch closely for any changes in your condition.

Possible food and drug interactions when taking this medication

No interactions have been reported.

Special information if you are pregnant or breastfeeding

Hydergine is not intended for use by women of childbearing age.

Recommended dosage

ADULTS

The usual dose of Hydergine is 1 milligram, 3 times a day. The relief of symptoms usually occurs gradually and may take 3 to 4 weeks.

Overdosage

Any medication taken in excess can have serious consequences. If you suspect an overdose, seek medical attention immediately.

Brand name:

HydroDIURIL

Generic name: Hydrochlorothiazide
Other brand name: Esidrix

Why is this drug prescribed?

HydroDIURIL is used in the treatment of high blood pressure and other conditions that require the elimination of excess fluid (water) from the body. These conditions include congestive heart failure, cirrhosis of the liver, corticosteroid and estrogen therapy, and kidney disorders. When used for high blood pressure, HydroDIURIL can be used alone or with other high blood pressure medications. HydroDIURIL contains a form of thiazide, a diuretic that prompts your body to produce and eliminate more urine, which helps lower blood pressure.

Most important fact about this drug:

If you have high blood pressure, you must take HydroDIURIL regularly for it to be effective. Even if you are feeling well, continue to take it. You need the medication to keep your blood pressure under control.

Diuretics can cause your body to lose too much potassium. Ask your doctor for the warning signs of potassium depletion. Also, ask whether you should eat specific foods that are rich in potassium or take a potassium supplement to avoid this problem.

How should you take this medication?
Take HydroDIURIL exactly as prescribed by your doctor.

What side effects may occur?
Side effects cannot be anticipated. If any develop or change in intensity, inform your doctor as soon as possible. Only your doctor can determine if it is safe for you to continue taking HydroDIURIL.

■ *Side effects may include:*
Abdominal cramping
Diarrhea
Dizziness upon standing up
Headache
Loss of appetite
Low blood pressure
Low potassium leading to symptoms such as dry mouth, excessive thirst, weak or irregular heartbeat, muscle pain or cramps
Stomach irritation
Stomach upset
Weakness

■ *Less common or rare side effects may include:*
Anemia, blood disorders, changes in blood sugar, constipation, difficulty breathing, dizziness, fever, fluid in the lung, high levels of sugar in the urine, hives, hypersensitivity reactions, inflammation of the lung, inflammation of the pancreas, inflammation of the salivary glands, kidney failure, muscle spasms, nausea, rash, reddish or purplish spots on the skin, restlessness, sensitivity to light, Stevens-Johnson syndrome (skin peeling), tingling or pins and needles, vertigo, vision changes, vomiting, yellow eyes and skin

Why should this drug not be prescribed?
If you are unable to urinate, you should not take this medication.

If you are sensitive to or have ever had an allergic reaction to HydroDIURIL or similar drugs, or if you are sensitive to other sulfonamide-derived drugs, you should not take this medication.

Special warnings about this medication
If you are taking HydroDIURIL, your kidney function should be given a complete assessment, and should continue to be monitored.

If you have liver disease, diabetes, gout, or collagen vascular disease (lupus erythematosus), HydroDIURIL should be used with caution.

If you have bronchial asthma or a history of allergies, you may be at greater risk for an allergic reaction to this medication.

Dehydration, excessive sweating, severe diarrhea or vomiting could deplete your body's fluids and cause your blood pressure to become too low. Be careful when exercising and in hot weather.

Possible food and drug interactions when taking this medication
HydroDIURIL may increase the effects of alcohol. Do not drink alcohol while taking this medication.

If HydroDIURIL is taken with certain other drugs, the effects of either could be increased, decreased, or altered. It is especially important to check with your doctor before combining HydroDIURIL with the following:

Barbiturates such as phenobarbital
Corticosteroids such as prednisone and ACTH

Drugs to treat diabetes such as insulin or
  Micronase
Lithium
Narcotics such as Percocet
Nonsteroidal anti-inflammatory drugs such
  as Naprosyn
Norepinephrine (Levophed)
Other high blood pressure medications
Skeletal muscle relaxants, such as tubocurarine

Special information
if you are pregnant or breastfeeding

The effects of HydroDIURIL during pregnancy
have not been adequately studied. If you
are pregnant or plan to become pregnant,
inform your doctor immediately.
HydroDIURIL appears in breast milk and
could affect a nursing infant. If this
medication is essential to your health, your
doctor may advise you to discontinue
breastfeeding until your treatment is finished.

Recommended dosage

Dosage should be adjusted to each patient's
needs. The smallest dose that is effective
should be used.

ADULTS

Diuresis
The usual dose is 50 milligrams to 100
milligrams, 1 or 2 times per day. Your
doctor may put you on a day on, day off
schedule or some other alternate day
schedule to suit your needs.

High Blood Pressure
The usual dose is 50 milligrams to 100
milligrams a day in 1 or 2 doses. Dosages
should be adjusted when used with other high
blood pressure medications.

CHILDREN

Dosages for children should be adjusted
according to weight, generally 1 milligram
per pound of body weight in 2 doses per day.
Infants under 6 months may need 1.5
milligrams per pound per day in 2 doses.

Under 2 years
Based on the above, the dosage is 12.5
milligrams to 37.5 milligrams per day in
2 doses.

2 to 12 years
The dosage, based on body weight, is 37.5
milligrams to 100 milligrams in 2 doses.

HydroDIURIL tablets come in strengths of
25, 50 and 100 milligrams.

Overdosage

Any medication taken in excess can cause
symptoms of overdose. If you suspect an
overdose, seek medical attention immediately.

*The symptoms of HydroDIURIL overdose
may include:*
Dry mouth
Electrolyte imbalance
Excessive thirst
Muscle pain or cramps
Symptoms of low potassium such as
  dehydration
Weak or irregular heartbeat

Generic name:

HYDROCHLOROTHIAZIDE

See HydroDIURIL, page 281.

Generic name:

HYDROCODONE WITH
ACETAMINOPHEN

See Vicodin, page 678.

Generic name:

HYDROCORTISONE WITH
ACETIC ACID

See VoSoL, page 684.

Generic name:

HYDROMORPHONE HYDROCHLORIDE

See Dilaudid, page 198.

Generic name:

HYDROXYCHLOROQUINE SULFATE

See Plaquenil, page 485.

Generic name:

HYDROXYZINE HYDROCHLORIDE

See Atarax, page 42.

Brand name:

HYGROTON

Generic name: Chlorthalidone
Other brand name: Thalitone

Why is this drug prescribed?

Chlorthalidone is a diuretic (water pill) used to treat high blood pressure and fluid retention associated with congestive heart failure, cirrhosis of the liver (a disease of the liver caused by damage to its cells), corticosteroid and estrogen therapy, and kidney disease. When used for high blood pressure, chlorthalidone may be used alone or in combination with other high-blood-pressure medications. Diuretics help your body produce and eliminate more urine, which helps lower blood pressure.

Most important fact about this drug

If you have high blood pressure, you must take chlorthalidone regularly for the drug to be effective. Even if you are feeling well, you must continue to take this medication.

It is necessary to keep your blood pressure under control.

Diuretics can cause your body to lose too much potassium. Ask your doctor for the warning signs of potassium depletion. Also ask whether you should eat specific foods that are rich in potassium or take a potassium supplement to avoid this problem.

How should you take this medication?

Diuretics such as chlorthalidone increase urination; therefore chlorthalidone should be taken in the morning. Avoid overexposure to sun and do not use a sunlamp.

Chlorthalidone should be taken exactly as prescribed by your doctor.

Chlorthalidone may be taken with food.

What side effects may occur?

Side effects cannot be anticipated. If any side effects develop or change in intensity, tell your doctor immediately. Only your doctor can determine whether it is safe to continue taking chlorthalidone.

■ *Side effects may include:*
Allergic reaction, anemia, changes in blood sugar, change in potassium levels causing symptoms like dry mouth, excessive thirst, weak or irregular heartbeat, muscle pain or cramps, constipation, cramping, diarrhea, dizziness, dizziness upon standing up, flaky skin, headache, hives, impotence, inflammation of the pancreas, itching, loss of appetite, low blood pressure, muscle spasms, nausea, rash, restlessness, sensitivity to light, stomach irritation, tingling or pins and needles, vision changes, vomiting, weakness, yellow eyes and skin

Why should this drug not be prescribed?

If you are unable to urinate or if you have ever had an allergic reaction or are sensitive to chlorthalidone or other sulfa drugs, do not take chlorthalidone.

Special warnings about this medication

Chlorthalidone should be used carefully if you have kidney or liver disease.

If you have a history of bronchial asthma, you may be more likely to have an allergic reaction to chlorthalidone.

Chlorthalidone is a strong diuretic that can cause the potassium or salt levels in your blood to become too low.

Be careful in hot weather not to become dehydrated. Contact your doctor if you experience excess thirst, tiredness, restlessness, muscle pains or cramps, nausea, vomiting, or increased heart rate or pulse.

This medication may aggravate lupus erythematosus, a disease of the connective tissue.

Tell your doctor if you have ever had an allergic reaction to other diuretics; or if you have asthma, kidney or liver disease, gout, or lupus.

Possible food and drug interactions when taking this medication

Drinking alcohol may increase the chance of dizziness occurring. Do not drink alcohol while taking this medication.

If Chlorthalidone is taken with certain other drugs, the effects of either could be increased, decreased, or altered. It is especially important to check with your doctor before combining chlorthalidone with the following:

Appetite-control medicines
Cholestyramine or colestipol (Questran, Colestid)
Cortiscosteroids such as prednisone

Decongestants (medicines for asthma, colds, cough, hay fever, or sinus)
Digitalis (Lanoxin)
Insulin
Lithium (Lithobid)
Oral hypoglycemics (drugs that lower blood sugar)
Other high blood pressure medications such as Catapres and Aldomet

Special information if you are pregnant or breastfeeding

If you are pregnant or plan to become pregnant, inform your doctor immediately. Information is not available about the safety of chlorthalidone during pregnancy.

Chlorthalidone may appear in breast milk and could affect a nursing infant. If chlorthalidone is essential to your health, your doctor may advise you to stop breastfeeding until your treatment is finished.

Recommended dosage

Your doctor will tailor your individual chlorthalidone dose, starting with the lowest possible dose to obtain a satisfactory response.

ADULTS

High Blood Pressure

The usual recommended initial dose for high blood pressure is a single dose of 25 milligrams. Your doctor may increase the dose to 100 milligrams once daily.

Edema (Fluid Retention)

The usual recommended initial dose is 50 to 100 milligrams daily or 100 milligrams every other day. Some patients may require 150 to 200 milligrams at these intervals. Some patients may require up to 200 milligrams daily.

Once desired control of blood pressure or edema has been achieved, your doctor may adjust your maintenance dose, which may be lower than your initial dose.

Overdosage

Any medication taken in excess can have serious consequences. If you suspect an overdose, seek medical treatment immediately.

Symptoms of chlorthalidone overdose may include:
Confusion
Dizziness
Nausea
Weakness

Generic name:

HYOSCYAMINE SULFATE

See Levsin, page 316.

Brand name:

HYTRIN

Generic name: Terazosin hydrochloride

Why is this drug prescribed?

Hytrin, an antihypertensive medication in tablet form, is given to reduce high blood pressure. It may be used alone, or your doctor may also prescribe other blood-pressure-lowering medication, such as a diuretic or a beta blocker.

Hytrin is also prescribed for the treatment of benign prostatic hyperplasia (BPH), an abnormal enlargement of the prostate gland.

Most important fact about this drug

With the first dose or the first few doses of Hytrin, be aware that you are likely to feel dizzy or faint whenever you rise from a sitting or lying position. This effect, due to lowered blood pressure, should disappear as your body becomes used to Hytrin.

How should you take this medication?

Take Hytrin exactly as prescribed by your doctor. You may take the tablets with or without food.

The starting dose of Hytrin is always low: one 1-milligram tablet to be taken at bedtime. Your doctor will increase the dosage gradually until the amount that is best for you is determined.

What side effects may occur?

Side effects cannot be anticipated. If any develop or change in intensity, inform your doctor as soon as possible. Only your doctor can determine if it is safe for you to continue taking Hytrin.

■ *Most common side effects may include:*
Blurred vision
Dizziness
Drowsiness
Headache
Heart palpitations
Nausea
Stuffy nose
Swollen wrists and ankles
Weakness

If these symptoms persist, tell your doctor. Your dosage of Hytrin may be higher than needed.

■ *Less common side effects may include:*
Anxiety, bronchitis, conjunctivitis ("pink eye"), constipation, diarrhea, dry mouth, facial swelling, fever, flu or cold symptoms (cough, sore throat, runny nose), flushing, frequent urination, gas, gout, impotence, increased heart rate, indigestion, inflamed sinuses, insomnia, irregular heartbeat, itching, joint pain and swelling, lightheadedness, muscle aches, nervousness, nosebleed, numbness or tingling, pain in the abdomen, chest, or shoulder, rash, ringing in the ears, shortness of breath, stomach upset,

sweating, urinary incontinence, urinary tract infection, vision changes, vomiting

Why should this drug not be prescribed?

Do not take Hytrin if you are sensitive to it or have ever had an allergic reaction to it.

Special warnings about this medication

When your blood pressure falls in response to Hytrin, fainting may occur. Other less severe reactions include dizziness, heart palpitations, lightheadedness, and drowsiness. If your occupation is such that these symptoms might cause serious problems, make sure your doctor knows this from the start; your Hytrin dosage should be increased very cautiously.

Regardless of your occupation, avoid driving, climbing and other hazardous tasks at the following times:

■ After your first dose of Hytrin
■ With each new dosage increase
■ When you re-start Hytrin after any treatment interruption

Possible food and drug interactions when taking this medication

If Hytrin is combined with other blood pressure medications, your doctor may gradually adjust the dosages.

Special information if you are pregnant or breastfeeding

If you are pregnant or plan to become pregnant, notify your doctor immediately. Hytrin is not recommended during pregnancy unless the benefit outweighs the potential risk to the unborn baby.

It is not known whether Hytrin can make its way into breast milk. Caution is advised when using Hytrin during breastfeeding.

Recommended dosage

ADULTS

The usual initial dose is 1 milligram at bedtime. The dose may be slowly increased to achieve the desired blood pressure response. The usual recommended dose range is 1 milligram to 5 milligrams administered once a day; however, some patients may benefit from doses as high as 20 milligrams per day.

If Hytrin administration is discontinued for several days or longer, therapy should be reinstituted using the initial dosing regimen.

Overdosage

If you take too much Hytrin, dizziness, lightheadedness and fainting may occur within 90 minutes. A large overdose may lead to shock. If you suspect symptoms of an overdose of Hytrin, seek medical attention immediately.

Generic name:

IBUPROFEN

See Motrin, page 393.

Brand name:

ILETIN

See Insulin, page 297.

Brand name:

ILOSONE

See Erythromycin, Oral, page 239.

Generic name:

IMIPRAMINE HYDROCHLORIDE

See Tofranil, page 633.

Brand name:

IMODIUM

Generic name: Loperamide hydrochloride

Why is this drug prescribed?

Imodium is prescribed for the control and relief of symptoms of diarrhea not known to be caused by a specific organism and for diarrhea associated with long-term inflammatory bowel disease. This drug is also prescribed for reducing the volume of discharge from an ileostomy (a surgical opening of the small intestine onto the abdominal wall through which feces pass).

Most important fact about this drug

If your diarrhea does not stop after a few days or a fever develops, notify your doctor immediately.

Your doctor may use Imodium for diarrhea associated with antibiotic therapy with extreme caution.

How should you take this medication?

Take this medication exactly as prescribed by your doctor.

Do not take more than the directed dose.

Imodium may cause dryness of the mouth. You may want to use sugarless hard candy, sugarless gum, or water to relieve dryness.

Imodium may cause drowsiness and/or dizziness. You should exercise extra caution while driving or performing tasks requiring mental alertness.

What side effects may occur?

Side effects reported from the use of Imodium are difficult to distinguish from symptoms associated with diarrhea. Those reported, however, were more commonly observed during the treatment of long-lasting diarrhea.

■ *Side effects may include:*
  Abdominal pain or discomfort
  Allergic reactions, including skin rash
  Constipation
  Dizziness
  Drowsiness
  Dry mouth
  Nausea and vomiting
  Tiredness

Why should this drug not be prescribed?

If you are sensitive to or have ever had an allergic reaction to Imodium, you should not take this medication. Make sure that your doctor is aware of any drug reactions that you have experienced.

Unless you are directed to do so by your doctor, do not take Imodium if constipation must be avoided.

Special warnings about this medication

Imodium should not be used in the case of acute dysentery (an inflammation of the intestines characterized by abdominal pain, watery—sometimes bloody— stools, and fever, caused by bacteria, viruses, or parasites).

Dehydration may occur in patients who have diarrhea. It is important that you drink plenty of fluids while taking Imodium.

Imodium should be used with special caution in young children because of the diverse rate of response in this age-group.

Patients with liver dysfunction should be monitored closely by their doctor for signs of central nervous system dysfunction, such as drowsiness or convulsions.

Possible food and drug interactions when taking this medication

There are no reported food or drug interactions.

Special information if you are pregnant or breastfeeding

The effects of Imodium during pregnancy have not been adequately studied. If you are pregnant or plan to become pregnant, notify your doctor. It is not known whether Imodium appears in breast milk and could affect a nursing infant. If this medication is essential to your health, your doctor may advise you to discontinue breastfeeding until your treatment is finished.

Recommended dosage

ADULTS

Severe Diarrhea

The recommended starting dosage is 2 capsules (4 milligrams) followed by 1 capsule (2 milligrams) after each unformed stool. Daily dosage should not exceed 8 capsules (16 milligrams). Improvement should be observed within 48 hours.

Long-Lasting or Frequently Recurring Diarrhea

The recommended starting dosage is 2 capsules (4 milligrams) followed by 1 capsule (2 milligrams) after each unformed stool until diarrhea is controlled, after which the dosage of Imodium should be reduced by your doctor to meet your individual needs. When the ideal daily dosage has been established, this amount may then be given as a single dose or in divided doses. The average maintenance dosage is 2 to 4 capsules per day, not to exceed 8 capsules. If improvement is not observed after treatment with 8 capsules (16 milligrams) per day for at least 10 days, notify your doctor.

CHILDREN

Imodium is not recommended in children under 2 years of age.

Severe Diarrhea

In children 2 to 5 years of age or 40 pounds or less, the non-prescription liquid medication (Imodium A-D) should be used. For children between the ages of 6 and 12, either Imodium capsules (2 milligrams per capsule) or Imodium A-D Liquid (1 milligram per teaspoonful) may be used.

For children 2 to 12 years of age, the following schedule for capsules or liquid will usually fulfill starting dosage requirements:

2 to 5 years (28-44 pounds):
  1 milligram (1 teaspoonful of Imodium A-D liquid) taken 3 times a day (3 milligrams daily)

6 to 8 years (45-66 pounds):
  2 milligrams taken 2 times a day (4 milligrams daily)

8 to 12 years (66 pounds and over):
  2 milligrams taken 3 times a day (6 milligrams daily)

After the first day of treatment, it is recommended that subsequent Imodium doses (1 milligram per 22 pounds of body weight) be given only after a loose stool. The total daily dosage should not exceed the recommended dosages for the first day.

Long-Lasting or Frequently Recurring Diarrhea

A corrective treatment dosage has not been established for children with long-lasting or frequently recurring diarrhea.

Overdosage

Any medication taken in excess can have serious consequences. If you suspect an Imodium overdose, seek medical attention immediately.

Symptoms of an Imodium overdosage may include:
Constipation
Dizziness, drowsiness, and slowed breathing
Irritation of the stomach and intestines
Nausea and vomiting

In the event of an Imodium overdosage, the patient should be watched for at least 24 hours.

Generic name:

INDAPAMIDE

See Lozol, page 346.

Brand name:

INDERAL

Generic ingredient: Propranolol hydrochloride

Why is this drug prescribed?
Inderal, a type of medication known as a beta blocker, is used in the treatment of high blood pressure, angina pectoris (chest pain, usually caused by lack of oxygen to the heart due to clogged arteries), changes in heart rhythm, prevention of migraine headache, hereditary tremors, hypertrophic subaortic stenosis (a condition related to exertional angina), and tumors of the adrenal gland. It is also used to reduce the risk of death from recurring heart attack. When used for the treatment of high blood pressure, it is effective alone or combined with other high blood pressure medications, particularly thiazide-type diuretics. Beta blockers decrease the force and rate of heart contractions.

Most important fact about this drug
If you have high blood pressure, you must take Inderal regularly for it to be effective. Even if you are feeling well, you need the drug to keep your blood pressure down.

How should you take this medication?
Inderal works best when taken before meals.

Take this medication exactly as prescribed by your doctor, even if your symptoms have disappeared.

Try not to miss any doses. If this medication is not taken regularly, your condition may worsen.

If you forget to take a dose, take it as soon as you remember. If it's within 8 hours of your next scheduled dose, skip the one you missed and go back to your regular schedule. Never take two doses at the same time.

What side effects may occur?
Side effects cannot be anticipated. If any develop or change in intensity, inform your doctor as soon as possible. Only your doctor can determine if it is safe for you to continue taking propranolol.

■ *Side effects may include:*
Abdominal cramps, colitis, congestive heart failure, constipation, decreased sexual ability, depression, diarrhea, difficulty breathing, disorientation, dry eyes, fever with sore throat, hair loss, hallucinations, headache, light-headedness, low blood pressure, lupus erythematosus (a form of immune system disorder), nausea, rash, reddish or purplish spots on skin, short-term memory loss, slow heartbeat, tingling, prickling in hands, tiredness, trouble sleeping, upset stomach, visual changes, vivid dreams, vomiting, weakness, worsening of heart block

Why should this drug not be prescribed?

If you have inadequate blood supply to the circulatory system (cardiogenic shock), heart block (conduction disorder), a slow heartbeat, bronchial asthma, or severe congestive heart failure, you should not take this medication.

Special warnings about this medication

If you have a history of congestive heart failure, Inderal usage should be monitored by your doctor.

Inderal should not be stopped suddenly. This can cause increased chest pain and heart attack. Dosage should be gradually reduced.

If you suffer from asthma or other bronchial conditions, coronary artery disease or kidney or liver disease, this medication should be used with caution.

Ask your doctor if you should check your pulse while taking Inderal. This medication can cause your heartbeat to become too slow.

This medication may mask the symptoms of low blood sugar or alter blood sugar levels. If you are diabetic, discuss this with your doctor.

Notify your doctor or dentist that you are taking Inderal if you have a medical emergency, and before you have surgery or dental treatment.

Possible food and drug interactions while taking this medication

If Inderal is taken with certain other drugs, the effects of either could be increased, decreased, or altered. It is especially important to check with your doctor before combining Inderal with the following:

Aluminum hydroxide gel (Amphojel)
Antipyrine (Auralgan)

Calcium channel blocking drugs such as Cardizem, Procardia, and Calan
Catecholamine-depleting drugs such as reserpine (found in several other blood pressure medications)
Chlorpromazine (Thorazine)
Cimetidine (Tagamet)
Haloperidol (Haldol)
Lidocaine
Nonsteroidal anti-inflammatory drugs such as Motrin and Naprosyn
Phenobarbitone
Phenytoin (Dilantin)
Rifampin (Rifadin)
Theophylline (Bronkaid)
Thyroxine
Verapamil

Special information if you are pregnant or breastfeeding

The effects of Inderal during pregnancy have not been adequately studied. If you are pregnant or plan to become pregnant, inform your doctor immediately. Inderal appears in breast milk and could affect a nursing infant. If this medication is essential to your health, your doctor may advise you to discontinue breastfeeding until your treatment with this medication is finished.

Recommended dosage

ADULTS

All dosages for Inderal, for any problem, must be individualized.

Your doctor will determine when and how often you should take this drug, so remember to take it exactly as your doctor directs.

Hypertension
The usual starting dose is 40 milligrams 2 times a day. This dose may be in combination with a diuretic. Dosages are gradually increased to between 120

milligrams and 240 milligrams per day for maintenance. In some cases, a dose of 640 milligrams per day may be needed. Depending on the patient, maximum effect of this drug may take from a few days to several weeks. In some patients, dosing 3 times a day may work better.

Angina Pectoris
The usual daily dosage is 80 milligrams to 320 milligrams divided into 2, 3 or 4 smaller doses. When treatment is being discontinued, dosages should be reduced gradually over a period of several weeks.

Arrhythmias
The usual dose is 10 milligrams to 30 milligrams 3 or 4 times a day, before meals and at bedtime.

Myocardial Infarction
The usual daily dosage is 180 milligrams to 240 milligrams divided into smaller doses. The usual maximum dose is 240 milligrams, although your doctor may increase the dose when treating myocardial infarction with angina or high blood pressure.

Migraine
The usual starting dosage is 80 milligrams per day divided into smaller doses. Dosages can be increased gradually to between 160 milligrams and 240 milligrams per day. If this dose does not relieve your symptoms in 4 to 6 weeks, this drug should be slowly withdrawn.

Tremors
The usual starting dose is 40 milligrams, 2 times per day. Symptoms will usually be relieved with a dose of 120 milligrams per day; however, on occasion, dosages of 240 milligrams to 320 milligrams per day may be necessary.

Hypertrophic Subaortic Stenosis
The usual dose is 20 milligrams to 40 milligrams, 3 to 4 times a day, before meals and at bedtime.

Before Adrenal Gland Vascular Tumor Surgery
The usual dose is 60 milligrams a day in divided doses for 3 days before surgery in combination with an alpha-blocker drug.

Propranolol may also be prescribed for patients with inoperable tumor in doses of 30 milligrams a day given in divided doses.

CHILDREN

Propranolol must be carefully individualized for use in children and is indicated only for high blood pressure. Doses in children are calculated by body weight, and range from 2 milligrams to 4 milligrams per 2.2 pounds daily in 2 equally divided doses. The maximum dose is 16 milligrams per 2.2 pounds per day.

If treatment is stopped, this drug must be gradually reduced over a 7 to 14 day period.

ELDERLY

Dosage should be determined by the particular needs of the elderly patient.

Inderal is also available in a sustained-release formulation, called Inderal LA, for once-a-day dosing.

Overdosage
Any medication taken in excess can cause symptoms of overdose. If you suspect an overdose, seek medical attention immediately.

No specific information on Inderal overdosage is available; however, overdose symptoms with other beta blockers include extremely slow heartbeat, heart block, low blood pressure, heart conduction problems, severe congestive heart failure, seizures, and, in some cases, bronchospasm (asthmatic attack), and low blood sugar.

Brand name:

INDERIDE

Generic ingredients: Inderal (Propranolol hydrochloride), Hydrochlorothiazide

Why is this drug prescribed?

Inderide is used in the treatment of high blood pressure. It combines a beta blocker (Inderal) with a thiazide diuretic (hydrochlorothiazide). Beta-blockers decrease the force and rate of heart contractions. Diuretics help your body produce and eliminate more urine, which also helps lower blood pressure.

Most important fact about this drug

This medication should be used only if your doctor has determined that the precise amount of each ingredient in Inderide meets your specific needs.

Diuretics can cause your body to lose too much potassium. Ask your doctor about the warning signs of too much potassium loss. Also ask whether you should eat specific foods that are rich in potassium or take a potassium supplement to avoid this problem.

How should you take this medication?

Take Inderide exactly as prescribed by your doctor, even if your symptoms have disappeared.

Try not to miss any doses. If this medication is not taken regularly, your condition may worsen.

What side effects may occur?

Side effects cannot be anticipated. If any develop or change in intensity, inform your doctor as soon as possible. Only your doctor can determine if it is safe for you to continue taking Inderide.

■ *Side effects may include:*
  Allergic reactions (including fever, rash,

aching and sore throat), anemia, blood disorders, blurred vision, collagen vascular disease (lupus erythematosus, a form of immune system disorder), constipation, congestive heart failure, cramps, decreased mental clarity, depression, diarrhea, difficulty breathing, difficulty sleeping, disorientation, dizziness, dizziness when standing, dry eyes, emotional changeability, exhaustion, fatigue, hair loss, hallucinations, headache, high blood sugar, hives, increased skin sensitivity to sunlight, inflammation of the large intestine, inflammation of the pancreas, inflammation of the salivary glands, light-headedness, loss of appetite, low blood pressure, male impotence, muscle spasms, nausea, restlessness, short-term memory loss, slow heartbeat, stomach irritation, sugar in the urine, tingling or pins and needles, upset stomach, vertigo, visual disturbances, vivid dreams, vomiting, weakness, wheezing, yellow eyes and skin

Why should this drug not be prescribed?

If you have inadequate blood supply to the circulatory system (cardiogenic shock), heart block (conduction disorder), slow heartbeat, bronchial asthma, or congestive heart failure you should not take this medication.

Do not take Inderide if you are unable to urinate or if you are sensitive to or have ever had an allergic reaction to any of its ingredients or to sulfa drugs.

Special warnings about this medication

Inderide should not be stopped suddenly. This can cause increased chest pain and heart attack. Dosage should be gradually reduced.

If you suffer from asthma, seasonal allergies or other bronchial conditions, or kidney or liver disease, this medication should be used with caution.

This medication may mask the symptoms of low blood sugar or alter blood sugar levels.

If you are diabetic, discuss this with your doctor.

If you have a history of allergies or bronchial asthma, you may be more likely to have an allergic reaction to Inderide.

Inderide may interfere with the glaucoma screening test. Intraocular pressure may increase when the medication is stopped.

Notify your doctor or dentist that you are taking Inderide if you have a medical emergency and before you have surgery or dental treatment.

Possible food and drug interactions when taking this medication

If Inderide is taken with certain other drugs, the effects of either could be increased, decreased, or altered. It is especially important to check with your doctor before combining Inderide with the following:

ACTH (adrenocorticotropic hormone)
Alcohol
Aluminum hydroxide gel (Mylanta)
Antipyrine
Calcium channel blocking drugs such as
    Calan, Cardizem and Procardia XL
Chlorpromazine (Thorazine)
Cimetidine (Tagamet)
Corticosteroids such as Prednisone
Digitalis (Lanoxin)
Haloperidol (Haldol)
Insulin
Lidocaine (Xylocaine)
Nonsteroidal anti-inflammatory drugs such
    as Motrin
Norepinephrine (Levophed)
Phenobarbitone
Phenytoin (Dilantin)
Reserpine and other catecholamine-depleting
    drugs such as Serpasil
Rifampin (Rifadin)
Theophylline (Theo-Dur)

Thyroxine (Thyroid medication Synthroid)
Tubocurarine

Special information
if you are pregnant or breastfeeding

The effects of Inderide during pregnancy have not been adequately studied. If you are pregnant or plan or become pregnant, inform your doctor immediately. Inderide appears in breast milk and could affect a nursing infant. If Inderide is essential to your health, your doctor may advise you to discontinue breastfeeding until your treatment is finished.

Recommended dosage

ADULTS

Each dose of this medication must be determined according to the individual patient's response to Inderide's main ingredients, Inderal and hydrochlorothiazide.

The usual dose is one Inderide tablet, 2 times per day. (If more than 160 milligrams of propranolol are required per day, then a combination product such as Inderide should not be used because you would be getting too much of the diuretic.)

Your doctor may use this medication in combination with other high blood pressure drugs to achieve the desired effect.

CHILDREN

The safety and effectiveness of this drug in children have not been established.

ELDERLY

This drug should be used with caution in elderly patients

Overdosage

Any medication taken in excess can cause symptoms of overdose. If you suspect an overdose, seek medical attention immediately.

The symptoms of Inderide overdose may include:
Coma
Heart Failure
Increased urination
Irritation and overactivity of the stomach and
    intestines
Low blood pressure
Slow heartbeat
Sluggishness
Stupor
Wheezing

Brand name:

INDOCIN

Generic name: Indomethacin

Why is this drug prescribed?

Indocin, a nonsteroidal anti-inflammatory drug, is used to relieve the inflammation, swelling, stiffness and joint pain associated with moderate or severe rheumatoid arthritis and osteoarthritis (the most common form of arthritis), and ankylosing spondylitis (arthritis of the spine). It is also used to treat bursitis, tendinitis, (acute painful shoulder) acute gouty arthritis, and other kinds of pain.

Most important fact about this drug

You should have frequent checkups with your doctor if you take Indocin regularly. Ulcers or internal bleeding can occur without warning.

How should you take this medication?

Indocin should be taken with food or an antacid, and with a full glass of water. Never take on an empty stomach.

Take this medication exactly as prescribed by your doctor.

If you are using Indocin for arthritis, it should be taken regularly.

If you forget to take a dose, take it as soon as you remember. If it is almost time for your next one, skip the one you missed and go back to your regular schedule. Never take two doses at the same time.

If you are using the liquid or suppositories, they should be stored in the refrigerator.

What side effects may occur?

Side effects cannot be anticipated. If any develop or change in intensity inform your doctor as soon as possible. Only your doctor can determine if it is safe for you to continue taking Indocin.

■ *More common side effects may include:*
Abdominal pain, constipation, depression, diarrhea, dizziness, fatigue, headache, heartburn, indigestion, nausea, ringing in the ears, sleepiness or excessive drowsiness, stomach pain, stomach upset, vertigo, vomiting

■ *Less common or rare side effects may include:*
Anemia, anxiety, asthma, behavior disturbances, bloating, blurred vision, breast changes, changes in heartbeat, chest pain, coma, congestive heart failure, convulsions, decrease in white blood cells, fever, fluid in lungs, fluid retention, flushing, gas, hair loss, hepatitis, high or low blood pressure, hives, itching, increase in blood sugar, insomnia, kidney failure, labored breathing, light-headedness, loss of appetite, mental confusion, muscle weakness, nosebleed, peptic ulcer, problems in hearing, rash, rectal bleeding, Stevens-Johnson syndrome (skin peeling), stomach or intestinal bleeding, sweating, twitching, unusual redness of skin, vaginal bleeding, weight gain, worsening of epilepsy, yellow eyes and skin

Why should this drug not be prescribed?

If you are sensitive to or have ever had an allergic reaction to Indocin, aspirin, or similar drugs, or if you have had asthma attacks caused by aspirin or other drugs of this type, you should not take this medication. Make sure that your doctor is aware of any drug reactions that you have experienced.

Do not use Indocin suppositories if you have a history of rectal inflammation or recent rectal bleeding.

Special warnings about this medication

Indocin prolongs bleeding time. If you are taking blood-thinning medication, this drug should be taken with caution.

Your doctor should prescribe the lowest possible effective dose. The incidence of side effects increases as dosage increases.

Peptic ulcers and bleeding can occur without warning.

This drug should be used with caution if you have kidney or liver disease, and it can cause liver inflammation in some people.

Do not take aspirin or any other anti-inflammatory medications while taking Indocin, unless your doctor tells you to do so.

If you have heart disease or high blood pressure, this drug can increase water retention.

This drug can mask the symptoms of an existing infection.

Indocin may cause you to become drowsy or less alert; therefore, driving or operating dangerous machinery or participating in any hazardous activity that requires full mental alertness is not recommended.

Possible food and drug interactions when taking this medication

If Indocin is taken with certain other drugs, the effects of either could be increased, decreased or altered. It is especially important to check with your doctor before combining Indocin with the following:

Anticoagulants (blood thinners)
Aspirin
Beta-adrenergic blockers such as Tenormin, Inderal
Captopril (Capoten)
Cyclosporine (Sandimmune)
Diflunisal (Dolobid)
Digoxin (Lanoxin)
Lithium
Loop diuretics (Lasix)
Methotrexate (cancer drug)
Potassium-sparing diuretics such as Aldactone
Probenecid (Benemid, ColBENEMID)
Thiazide-type diuretics such as Diuril
Triamterene (Dyazide)

Special information
if you are pregnant or breastfeeding

The effects of Indocin during pregnancy have not been adequately studied. If you are pregnant or plan to become pregnant inform your doctor immediately. Indocin appears in breast milk and could affect a nursing infant. If this medication is essential to your health, your doctor may advise you to discontinue breastfeeding until your treatment with this medication is finished.

Recommended dosage

ADULTS

This medication is available in liquid, capsule and suppository form. The following dosages are for capsule form. If you prefer the liquid form ask your doctor to make the proper substitution. Do not try to convert the medication or dosage yourself.

Moderate to Severe Rheumatoid Arthritis, Osteoarthritis, Ankylosing Spondylitis
The usual dose is 25 milligrams 2 or 3 times a day, increasing to a total daily dose of 150 to 200 milligrams. Your doctor should monitor you carefully for side effects when you are taking this drug.

Your doctor may prescribe a single daily 75-milligram capsule of Indocin SR in place of regular Indocin.

Bursitis or Tendinitis
The usual dose is 75 to 150 milligrams daily divided into 3 to 4 small doses for 1 to 2 weeks, until symptoms disappear.

Acute Gouty Arthritis
The usual dose is 50 milligrams 3 times a day until pain is reduced to a tolerable level (usually 3 to 5 days). Your doctor will advise you when to stop taking this drug for this condition. Keep him informed of its effects on your symptoms.

CHILDREN

The safety and effectiveness of Indocin have not been established in children under 14 years of age. However, your doctor may decide that the benefits of this medication may outweigh the potential risks.

ELDERLY

Dosage should be determined by the particular needs of the elderly patient.

Overdosage

Any medication taken in excess can cause symptoms of overdose. If you suspect an overdose seek medical attention immediately.

The symptoms of Indocin overdose may include:
Convulsions
Disorientation
Dizziness
Intense headache
Lethargy
Mental confusion
Nausea, vomiting
Numbness
Tingling or pins and needles

Generic name:

INDOMETHACIN

See Indocin, page 295.

Generic name:

INSULIN

Available formulations:

Insulin, Human:
  Humulin
Insulin, Human Isophane Suspension:
  Humulin N
Insulin, Human NPH:
  Insulatard NPH Human
  Novolin N
Insulin, Human Regular:
  Novolin R
  Humulin BR & R
  Velosulin Human
Insulin, Human Regular and Human NPH mixture:
  Humulin 70/30
  Mixtard Human 70/30
  Novolin 70/30
Insulin, Human, Zinc Suspension:
  Humulin L & U
  Novolin L
Insulin, NPH:
  NPH Iletin I (also II, Beef; II, Pork)
  Insulatard NPH
  NPH Insulin
Insulin Regular and NPH mixture
  Mixtard 70/30
  Novolin 70/30

Insulin, Zinc Crystals
  NPH Iletin I
Insulin, Regular:
  Iletin I Regular (also II, Beef; II, Pork)
  Regular Insulin
  Velosulin
Insulin, Zinc Suspension:
  Iletin I, Lente
  Protamine, Zinc and Iletin
  Iletin I, Semilente
  Iletin I, Ultralente
  Lente Insulin
  Semilente Insulin
  Ultralente Insulin

Why is this drug prescribed?

Insulin is prescribed for diabetes mellitus when this condition does not improve with oral medications or by modifying your diet. Insulin is a hormone produced by the pancreas, a large gland that lies near the stomach. This hormone is necessary for the body's correct use of food, especially sugar. Insulin apparently works by helping sugar penetrate the cell wall, where it is then utilized by the cell. In people with diabetes, the body either does not make enough insulin or the insulin that is produced no longer works properly.

There are actually two forms of diabetes: Type I insulin-dependent and Type II non-insulin-dependent. Type I usually requires insulin injection for life, while Type II diabetes can usually be treated by dietary changes and/or oral antidiabetic medications (e.g., Diabinese, Glucotrol). Occasionally, Type II diabetics must take insulin injections on a temporary basis, especially during stressful periods or times of illness.

The various insulin brands above differ in several ways: for example, in the source (animal, human, or synthetic), in the time requirements for the insulin to take effect, and in the length of time the insulin remains working.

Regular insulin is manufactured from beef and pork pancreas, begins working within 30 to 60 minutes, and lasts for 6 to 8 hours. Variations of insulin have been developed to satisfy the needs of individual patients. For example, zinc suspension insulin is an intermediate-acting insulin that starts working within 1 to 1½ hours and lasts approximately 24 hours. Insulin combined with zinc and protamine is a longer-acting insulin that takes effect within 4 to 6 hours and lasts up to 36 hours. The time and course of action may vary considerably in different individuals or at different times in the same individual.

Animal-based insulin is a very safe product. However, some components may cause an allergic reaction (see below). Therefore, genetically engineered human insulin has been developed to lessen the chance of an allergic reaction. It is structurally identical to the insulin produced by your body's pancreas. However, some human insulin may be produced in a semi-synthetic process that begins with animal-based ingredients, which may cause an allergic reaction.

Most important fact about this drug

Regardless of the type of insulin your doctor has prescribed, you should follow carefully the dietary guidelines he or she has recommended. Failure to follow these guidelines or to take your insulin as prescribed may result in serious and potentially fatal complications such as hypoglycemia (lowered blood sugar levels).

How should you take this medication?

Take your insulin exactly as prescribed, being careful to follow your doctor's dietary recommendations.

Your doctor should tell you what to do if you miss an insulin injection or meal. Also, always keep a spare supply of insulin, and an extra syringe and needle on hand.

What side effects may occur?
While side effects from insulin use are rare, allergic reactions or low blood sugar (sometimes called "an insulin reaction") may pose significant health risks. Your doctor should be notified if any of the following occur.

■ *Mild allergic reactions*
Swelling, itching or redness at the injection site (usually disappears within a few days or weeks).

■ *More serious allergic reactions*
Fast pulse
Low blood pressure
Perspiration
Rash over entire body
Shortness of breath
Wheezing

Other side effects are virtually eliminated when the correct dose of insulin is matched with the proper diet and level of physical activity. Low blood sugar may develop in poorly controlled or unstable diabetes. Consuming sugar or a sugar-containing product will usually correct the condition. It can be brought about by taking too much insulin, missing or delaying meals, exercising or working more than usual, an infection or illness, a change in the body's need for insulin, drug interactions, or consuming alcohol.

■ *Symptoms of low blood sugar include:*
Blurred vision
Cold sweats
Dizziness
Fatigue
Headache
Hunger
Light-headedness
Nausea
Nervousness
Rapid heartbeat

■ *Symptoms of more severe low blood sugar include:*
Coma
Disorientation
Pale skin
Seizures
Shallow breathing

Contact your doctor immediately if any symptoms of severe low blood sugar occur. Remember too, the symptoms associated with an under supply of insulin, which can be brought on by taking too little, overeating or fever and infection.

■ *Symptoms of insufficient insulin include:*
Drowsiness
Flushing
Fruity breath
Loss of appetite
Thirst

This condition can lead to loss of consciousness or death.

Why should this drug not be prescribed?
Insulin should be used only to correct diabetic conditions.

Special warnings about this medication
Wear personal identification that states clearly that you are diabetic and, if you have been diagnosed as Type I, that you are insulin dependent. Carry a sugar-containing product (e.g. hard candy) to offset any symptoms of low blood sugar.

Do not change the type of insulin or even the model and brand of syringe or needle you use without your physician's instruction. Failure to use the proper syringe may lead to improper dosage levels of insulin. If you become ill from any cause, especially with nausea and vomiting, your insulin requirements may change. Test your urine and/or blood and let your doctor know at once.

If you are taking insulin, you should check your glucose levels with home blood and urine testing devices. If your blood tests consistently show above-normal sugar levels or your urine tests consistently show the presence of sugar, your diabetes is not properly controlled, and you should let your doctor know.

To avoid infection or contamination, use disposable needles and syringes or sterilize your reusable syringe and needle carefully.

Store insulin in a refrigerator (but not in the freezer) or in another cool, dark place. Do not expose insulin to heat or direct sunlight.

Possible food and drug interactions when taking this medication

Follow your physician's dietary guidelines as closely as you can and inform your physician of any medication, either prescription or non-prescription, that you are taking. Specific medications, depending on the amount present, that affect insulin levels or its effectiveness include:

Adrenal corticosteroids such as prednisone
Anabolic steroids
Appetite suppressants such as Tenuate
Aspirin, large doses
Beta blockers such as Tenormin, Lopressor
Diuretics such as Lasix, Dyazide, HydroDIURIL
Epinephrine (Epipen)
Estrogens such as Premarin
MAO Inhibitors such as Nardil, Eldepryl
Nicotine such as Nicoderm, Habitrol
Phenytoin (Dilantin)

Thyroid medications (Synthroid, Proloid)
Triamterene (Dyrenium)

Use alcohol carefully, since excessive alcohol consumption can cause low blood sugar. Don't drink unless your doctor has approved.

Special information
if you are pregnant or breastfeeding

Insulin is considered safe for pregnant women, but pregnancy may make managing your diabetes more difficult.

Properly controlled diabetes is essential for the health of the mother and fetus; therefore, it is extremely important that pregnant women follow closely their physician's dietary guidelines and prescribing instructions.

Since insulin does not pass into breast milk, it is safe for nursing mothers.

Recommended dosage

Your doctor will specify which insulin to use, how much, and when and how often to inject it. Proper control of your diabetes requires close and constant cooperation with your doctor. Failure to use your insulin as prescribed may result in serious and potentially fatal complications.

Some insulins should be clear and some have a cloudy precipitate. Find out what your insulin should look like and check it carefully before using.

Overdosage

An overdose of insulin can cause low blood sugar (hypoglycemia). These symptoms include:
Cold sweats
Fatigue
Headache
Nausea
Nervousness
Rapid heartbeat

Symptoms of more severe low blood sugar include:
Coma
Disorientation
Pale skin
Seizures
Shallow breathing

Contact your doctor immediately if these symptoms of severe low blood sugar occur.

Eating sugar or a sugar-based product will often correct the condition. If you suspect an overdose, seek medical attention immediately.

Brand name:

INTAL

See Cromolyn Sodium, page 144.

Generic name:

IODINATED GLYCEROL WITH DEXTROMETHORPHAN

See Tussi-Organidin, page 658.

Brand name:

IONAMIN

Generic name: Phentermine resin

Why is this drug prescribed?

Ionamin, an appetite suppressant, is prescribed for short-term use (a few weeks) as part of an overall diet plan for reduction of weight. Ionamin should be used along with a behavior modification program.

Most important fact about this drug

Loss of effectiveness (tolerance) of Ionamin and other related drugs may develop within a few weeks. You should discontinue the medicine rather than increase the dosage when it becomes less effective.

Appetite suppressants such as Ionamin are no substitute for proper dieting.

How should you take this medication?

Take this medication exactly as prescribed by your doctor.

Ionamin capsules should be swallowed whole.

Ionamin may be habit-forming and can be addicting. Therefore, you should not share Ionamin with others.

What side effects may occur?

Side effects cannot be anticipated. If any develop or change in intensity, inform your doctor as soon as possible. Only your doctor can determine if it is safe for you to continue taking Ionamin.

■ *Side effects may include:*
Abdominal discomfort, blood pressure elevation, changes in sex drive, constipation, diarrhea, dizziness, dryness of the mouth, feelings of discomfort, feelings of elation, headache, hives, impotence, inability to fall or stay asleep, increased heart rate, nausea, overstimulation, palpitations, restlessness, tremors, unpleasant taste, vomiting

Why should this drug not be prescribed?

If you are sensitive to or have ever had an allergic reaction to phentermine, sympathomimetic amines (drugs that stimulate the central nervous system and elevate blood pressure), or similar drugs (appetite-suppressing medications), you should not take Ionamin. Make sure that your doctor is aware of any drug reactions that you have experienced.

Unless directed to do so by your doctor, do not take this drug if you have hardening of the arteries, symptoms of heart and blood vessel disease, an overactive thyroid, glaucoma, moderate to severe high blood pressure, are in an agitated state, have a history of drug abuse, or are taking or have taken MAO inhibitors (antidepressants, such as Nardil) within the past 14 days.

Special warnings about this medication

Ionamin may impair your ability to drive a car or operate machinery safely.

The abrupt withdrawal of this medication following prolonged use of high doses may result in extreme fatigue, mental depression, and sleep disturbances.

Caution should be exercised taking this drug in patients with even mild high blood pressure.

Insulin requirements may be altered for patients with diabetes mellitus.

Possible food and drug interactions when taking this medication

Ionamin may intensify the effects of alcohol and produce unfavorable reactions. Therefore, the use of alcohol is not recommended while taking this medication.

If Ionamin is taken with certain other drugs, the effects of either could be increased, decreased, or altered. It is especially important to check with your doctor before combining Ionamin with the following:

Antidiabetic drugs (insulin)
Adrenergic neuron blocking drugs (drugs that lower blood pressure) such as Normodyne

Special information if you are pregnant or breastfeeding

The safe use of Ionamin during pregnancy has not been established. If you are pregnant, plan to become pregnant, or are breastfeeding, notify your doctor.

Recommended dosage

ADULTS

The recommended dosage is 1 capsule taken daily, before breakfast or 10 to 14 hours before bedtime. For individuals exhibiting greater drug responsiveness, Ionamin '15' will usually suffice. Ionamin '30' is recommended for less responsive patients.

CHILDREN

Ionamin is not recommended for children under 12 years of age.

Overdosage

Overdosage of similar drugs such as Fastin has resulted in fatal poisoning, usually ending in convulsions and coma.

If you suspect an Ionamin overdose, seek emergency treatment immediately.

Symptoms of Ionamin overdosage may include:
Abdominal cramps, assaultiveness, confusion, diarrhea, hallucinations, high or low blood pressure, irregular heartbeats, nausea, panic states, rapid breathing, restlessness, tremors, vomiting

Generic name:

IPRATROPIUM BROMIDE

See Atrovent, page 46.

Generic name:

ISOETHARINE MESYLATE

See Bronkometer, page 71.

Brand name:

ISOLLYL

See Fiorinal, page 255.

Brand name:

ISOPTIN

See Calan, page 81.

Brand name:

ISOPTIN SR

See Calan, page 81.

Brand name:

ISOPTO-CARPINE

See Pilocar, page 483.

Brand name:

ISORDIL

Generic name: Isosorbide dinitrate
Other brand name: Sorbitrate

Why is this drug prescribed?

Isosorbide dinitrate is prescribed to relieve or prevent angina pectoris (suffocating chest pain). Angina pectoris occurs when the arteries and veins become constricted and sufficient oxygen does not reach the heart. Isosorbide dinitrate dilates the blood vessels by relaxing the muscles in their walls. Oxygen flow improves as the vessels relax, and chest pain subsides.

In swallowed capsules or tablets, isosorbide dinitrate helps to *prevent* chest pain from occurring.

In chewable or sublingual (held under the tongue) tablets, isosorbide dinitrate can help relieve chest pain that has *already occurred* or may be about to begin.

Most important fact about this drug

Isosorbide dinitrate may cause severe low blood pressure (possibly marked by dizziness or fainting), especially when you are standing or if you sit up quickly. People taking diuretic medication or those who have low blood pressure should use isosorbide dinitrate with caution.

How should you take this medication?

Swallowed capsules or tablets should be taken on an empty stomach. While regular tablets may be crushed for easier use, sustained- or prolonged-release products should not be crushed or altered.

What side effects may occur?

Side effects cannot be anticipated. If any develop or change in intensity, inform your doctor as soon as possible. Only your doctor can determine if it is safe for you to continue taking isosorbide dinitrate.

Headache is the most common side effect; usually, standard headache treatments with over-the-counter pain products will relieve the pain. The headaches associated with isosorbide dinitrate usually subside within 2 weeks after treatment with the drug begins.

■ *Other common side effects may include:*
Dizziness
Low blood pressure
Weakness

■ *Less common or rare side effects may include:*
Collapse, Fainting, flushed skin, nausea, pallor, perspiration, rash, restlessness, vomiting

Why should this drug not be prescribed?

You should not take isosorbide dinitrate if you have had a previous allergic reaction to it or to other nitrates or nitrites.

Special warnings about this medication

You should use isosorbide dinitrate with caution if you have anemia, glaucoma, a previous head injury, heart attack, heart disease, low blood pressure, and/or thyroid disease.

If you stop using isosorbide dinitrate, you should follow your doctor's plan for a gradual withdrawal schedule. Abruptly stopping this medication could result in additional chest pain.

Some people may develop a tolerance to isosorbide dinitrate, which causes its effects to be reduced over time. Tell your doctor if you think isosorbide dinitrate is starting to lose its effectiveness.

Since isosorbide dinitrate can cause dizziness, you should observe caution while driving, operating machinery, or performing other tasks that demand concentration.

Possible food and drug interactions when taking this medication

If isosorbide dinitrate is taken with certain other drugs, the effects of either could be increased, decreased, or altered.

Extreme low blood pressure (marked by dizziness, fainting, numbness) may occur if isosorbide dinitrate is taken with certain other high blood pressure drugs.

Alcohol may interact with isosorbide dinitrate and produce a swift decrease in blood pressure, possibly causing dizziness and fainting.

Special information if you are pregnant or breastfeeding

Although animal studies of isosorbide dinitrate at extremely high doses (35 to 150 times the recommended human dose) have shown this drug to be harmful to animal fetuses, conclusive human studies have not been conducted. As a result, isosorbide dinitrate should be used only when the benefits of therapy clearly outweigh the potential risks to the fetus. If you are pregnant or plan to become pregnant, inform your doctor immediately. It is not known if isosorbide dinitrate appears in breast milk; therefore, nursing mothers should use isosorbide dinitrate with caution.

Recommended dosage

ADULTS

The usual *sublingual* starting dose for the *treatment* of angina pectoris is 2.5 milligrams to 5 milligrams. This initial dose should be increased gradually until the pain subsides or side effects prove bothersome.

The usual *sublingual* starting dose for the *prevention* of angina pectoris is usually 5 or 10 milligrams every 2 to 3 hours.

For preventive therapy of chronic stable angina pectoris, the usual starting dose for *swallowed, immediately released* medication is 5 to 20 milligrams. This initial dose may be increased to 10 to 40 milligrams every 6 hours.

For preventive therapy of chronic stable angina pectoris with *controlled-release* isosorbide dinitrate, the usual initial dose is 40 milligrams. This dose may be increased to doses of 40 to 80 milligrams given every 8 to 12 hours.

CHILDREN

The safety and effectiveness of isosorbide dinitrate have not been established for children.

Overdosage

Any medication taken in excess can have serious consequences. Severe overdosage of isosorbide dinitrate may result in death. If you suspect an overdose, seek medical help immediately.

Symptoms of isosorbide dinitrate overdose may include:
Bloody diarrhea, coma, confusion, convulsions, fainting, fever, flushed skin (later cold and blue), nausea, palpitations, paralysis, rapid decrease in blood pressure, rapid, then difficult and slow breathing, slow pulse, sweating, throbbing headache, vertigo, visual disturbances, vomiting

Generic name:

ISOSORBIDE DINITRATE

See Isordil, page 303.

Generic name:

ISOTRETINOIN

See Accutane, page 1.

Generic name:

ISRADIPINE

See DynaCirc, page 221.

Brand name:

JANIMINE

See Tofranil, page 633.

Brand name:

KEFLEX

Generic name: Cephalexin

Why is this drug prescribed?
This medication, a cephalosporin antibiotic, is prescribed for mild to moderately severe bacterial infections of the lungs, ears, skin, urinary tract, throat and bone.

Most important fact about this drug
If you have shown a sensitivity to penicillin, cephalosporins or any other drug, notify your doctor before taking this medication. Severe reactions have been reported in penicillin-sensitive patients.

How should you take this medication?
Keflex can be taken with or without food. However, if the medication causes stomach upset, you may wish to take it after you have eaten.

If you are taking a liquid form of Keflex, use a specially marked measuring spoon to measure each dose accurately. The liquid should be stored in a refrigerator and can be kept for up to 14 days.

It is important that you finish taking all of this medication to obtain the maximum benefit. Do not miss any doses.

If you are taking this medicine 2 times a day and you miss a dose, take the missed dose right away and your next dose 5 to 6 hours later. Then go back to your regular schedule.

If you are taking the drug 3 times a day and miss a dose, take the missed dose right away and your next dose 2 to 4 hours later. Then return to your regular schedule.

What side effects may occur?
Side effects cannot be anticipated. If any develop or change in intensity, inform your doctor as soon as possible. Only your doctor can determine if it is safe for you to continue taking Keflex.

■ *More common side effects may include:*
Mild diarrhea

■ *Less common side effects may include:*
Abdominal pain, colitis, indigestion, skin rash—itching, redness or swelling

■ *Rare side effects may include:*
Agitation, confusion, dizziness, fatigue, genital or rectal itching, hallucinations, headache, hepatitis and jaundice, joint pain and inflammation, nausea, vaginal discharge, vomiting

Why should this drug not be prescribed?

If you are sensitive to or have ever had an allergic reaction to Keflex or similar drugs, you should not take this medication. Make sure that your doctor is aware of any drug reactions that you have experienced.

Special warnings about this medication

If you have a history of stomach or intestinal disease such as colitis, check with your doctor before taking Keflex.

If your symptoms do not improve within a few days or if they get worse, notify your doctor immediately.

If you are a diabetic, it is important to note that Keflex may cause false urine sugar tests results. Notify your doctor that you are taking this medication before being tested for sugar in the urine.

Do not give this medication to other people or use it for other infections before checking with your doctor.

Possible food and drug interactions when taking this medication

If diarrhea occurs while taking Keflex, consult with your doctor before taking diarrhea medication. Common diarrhea medications such as Lomotil or Donnagel PG may make your diarrhea worse or last longer.

Special information
if you are pregnant or breastfeeding

The effects of Keflex during pregnancy have not been established. If you are pregnant or plan to become pregnant, inform your doctor immediately. Keflex appears in breast milk and could affect a nursing infant. If this medication is essential to your health, your doctor may advise you to discontinue breastfeeding until your treatment with this drug is finished.

Recommended dosage

ADULTS

The usual adult dose is 250 milligrams every 6 hours. For strep throat, skin infections and cystitis in adults and children over 15 years of age, a dose of 500 milligrams may be taken every 12 hours. Larger doses may be taken as determined by your doctor.

CHILDREN

The usual recommended daily dose is 25 to 50 milligrams for every 2.2 pounds of body weight, in divided doses. For strep throat in children over 1 year of age and for skin infections, the total daily dose may be divided and given every 12 hours.

Overdosage

Any medication taken in excess can cause overdose. If you suspect an overdose, seek medical attention immediately.

The symptoms of an overdose of Keflex may include:
Blood in the urine
Diarrhea
Nausea
Upper abdominal pain
Vomiting

Brand name:

KEFTAB

Generic name: Cephalexin hydrochloride

Why is this drug prescribed?

Keftab, a cephalosporin antibiotic, is prescribed for bacterial infections of the respiratory tract, bone, skin, genitals, and urinary system. Because Keftab is effective for only certain types of bacterial infections, before beginning treatment your doctor may perform tests to identify the organisms causing infection.

Most important fact about this drug
If you are sensitive to or have ever had an allergic reaction to penicillin, cephalosporins, or drugs of this type, notify your doctor before taking this medication. Severe, allergic reactions have been reported in penicillin-sensitive patients.

How should you take this medication?
Keftab may be taken with or without meals.

Take Keftab at even intervals around the clock as prescribed by your doctor.

To obtain maximum benefit, it is important that you finish taking all of this medication, even if you are feeling better.

What side effects may occur?
Side effects cannot be anticipated. If any develop or change in intensity, inform your doctor as soon as possible. Only your doctor can determine if it is safe for you to continue taking Keftab.

■ *More common side effects may include:* Diarrhea

■ *Less common or rare side effects may include:*
Abdominal pain, agitation, colitis (inflammation of the large intestine), confusion, dizziness, fatigue, fever, genital and rectal itching, hallucinations, headache, hepatitis, hives, indigestion, inflammation of joints, inflammation of the stomach, joint pain, nausea, rash, seizures, shock, skin peeling, skin redness, swelling due to fluid retention, vaginal discharge, vaginal inflammation, vomiting, yellowing of skin and whites of eyes

Why should this drug not be prescribed?
If you are sensitive to or have ever had an allergic reaction to the cephalosporin group of antibiotics, you should not use this medication. Make sure that your doctor is aware of any drug reactions that you have experienced.

Special warnings about this medication
If you have a history of stomach or intestinal disease, especially colitis, check with your doctor before taking Keftab.

If diarrhea occurs while taking Keftab, check with your doctor before taking a remedy. Certain diarrhea medications (Lomotil, Paregoric) may increase your diarrhea or make it last longer.

Prolonged use of Keftab may result in an overgrowth of bacteria that do not respond to the medication, causing a secondary infection. Your doctor should monitor your use of this drug on a regular basis.

If you have a kidney disorder, check with your doctor before taking Keftab. You may need a reduced dose.

If you are a diabetic, it is important to note that Keftab may cause false results in tests for urine sugar. Notify your doctor that you are taking this medication before being tested. Do not change your diet or dosage of diabetes medication without first consulting with your doctor.

Possible food and drug interactions when taking this medication
No interactions with other drugs have been reported.

Special information if you are pregnant or breastfeeding
The effects of Keftab during pregnancy have not been adequately studied. If you are pregnant or plan to become pregnant, notify

your doctor immediately. Keftab does appear in breast milk and could affect a nursing infant. If this medication is essential to your health, your doctor may advise you to discontinue breastfeeding until your treatment is finished.

Recommended dosage

ADULTS

Throat, Skin, and Urinary Tract Infections
The usual adult dosage is 500 milligrams taken every 12 hours. Cystitis (bladder infection) therapy should be continued for 7 to 14 days.

Other Infections
The usual recommended dosage is 250 milligrams taken every 6 hours. For more severe infections, larger doses may be needed, as determined by your doctor.

CHILDREN

Safety and effectiveness have not been established in children.

Overdosage

Any medication taken in excess can have serious consequences.

Symptoms of Keftab overdose may include:
Blood in the urine
Diarrhea
Nausea
Upper abdominal pain
Vomiting

If you suspect an overdose, seek emergency medical treatment immediately.

Generic name:

KETOCONAZOLE

See Nizoral, page 423.

Generic name:

KETOPROFEN

See Orudis, page 445.

Brand name:

KLONOPIN

Generic name: Clonazepam

Why is this drug prescribed?
Klonopin belongs to a class of drugs known as benzodiazepines. It is used alone or along with other medications to treat convulsive disorders such as epilepsy.

Most important fact about this drug
Tolerance and dependence can occur with use of Klonopin. You may experience withdrawal symptoms if you stop using this drug abruptly. Discontinue or change your dose only in consultation with your doctor.

How should you take this medication?
Klonopin should be taken exactly as prescribed by your doctor.

If you are taking Klonopin for epilepsy, make sure you take your doses every day at the same time. If you are taking Klonopin regularly and forget to take a dose, take it within an hour of the missed time. If it is almost time for your next dose, skip the one you missed and go back to your regular schedule. Never take two doses at the same time.

What side effects may occur?
Side effects cannot be anticipated. If any develop or change in intensity, inform your doctor as soon as possible. Only your doctor can determine if it is safe for you to continue taking Klonopin.

■ *More common side effects may include:*
  Behavior problems (especially in children)

Drowsiness
Lack of muscular coordination

■ *Less common or rare side effects may include:*
Abnormal eye movements, anemia, chest congestion, coated tongue, confusion, constipation, diarrhea, double vision, dry mouth, fecal incontinence, fever, fluid retention, "glassy-eyed" appearance, hair loss, mental depression, hallucinations, involuntary rapid movement of the eyeballs, loss of or increased appetite, loss of voice, memory loss, muscle weakness, nausea, painful or difficult urination, rapid heartbeat, runny nose, shortness of breath, skin rash, sore gums, speech difficulties, uncontrolled body movement, unusual bleeding or bruising, urinary incontinence, vertigo, weight loss or gain

■ *Side effects due to rapid decrease or abrupt withdrawal from Klonopin may include:*
Abdominal and muscle cramps
Behavior disorders
Convulsions
Hallucinations
Psychosis
Restlessness
Sleeping difficulties
Tremors

Why should this drug not be prescribed?
If you are sensitive to or have ever had an allergic reaction to Klonopin or similar drugs, you should not take this medication. Make sure that your doctor is aware of any reactions that you have experienced.

You should not take this medication if you have acute narrow angle glaucoma or severe liver disease.

Special warnings about this medication
Klonopin may cause you to become drowsy or less alert; therefore, driving or operating dangerous machinery or participating in any hazardous activity that requires full mental alertness is not recommended.

If you experience several different types of seizure disorders, this drug may increase the possibility of grand mal seizures (epilepsy). Inform your doctor if this occurs. You doctor may wish to prescribe an additional anticonvulsant drug or increase your dose.

Because of the possibility that an adverse effect on physical or mental development could become apparent only after many years, your doctor will weigh the benefits of this drug against its risks.

Possible food and drug interactions when taking this medication
Klonopin is a central nervous system depressant and its effects may be intensified by alcohol. Do not drink while taking this medication.

If Klonopin is taken with certain other drugs, the effects of either could be increased, decreased, or altered. It is especially important to check with your doctor before combining Klonopin with the following:

Antianxiety agents such as Valium
Barbiturates such as phenobarbital
Butyrophenones (Haldol)
Hypnotics such as Halcion
MAO inhibitors (a type of antidepressant)
Narcotics (morphine and codeine-containing drugs)
Other anticonvulsants
Phenothiazines such as Thorazine
Thioxanthenes (Navane)
Tricyclic antidepressants such as Elavil
Valproic acid (Depakote)

Special information
if you are pregnant or breastfeeding
The effects of Klonopin during pregnancy have not been adequately studied. If you are pregnant or plan to become pregnant, inform

your doctor immediately. Klonopin may appear in breast milk and could affect a nursing infant. If this medication is essential to your health, your doctor may advise you to discontinue breastfeeding until your treatment with this medication is finished.

Recommended dosage

ADULTS

Starting dose should not exceed 1.5 milligrams per day, divided into 3 doses. Your daily dosage may be increased by 0.5 to 1 milligram every 3 days until seizures are controlled. The maximum daily dose should not exceed 20 milligrams.

CHILDREN

Starting dose for children up to 10 years old or up to 66 pounds should be between 0.01 and 0.03 milligram per 2.2 pounds of body weight daily, not to exceed 0.05 milligram per 2.2 pounds daily. The daily dosage should be given in 2 or 3 smaller doses. This may be increased by no more than 0.25 to 0.5 milligram every 3 days until seizures are controlled. If the dose cannot be divided into 3 equal doses, the largest dose should be given at bedtime. The maximum maintenance dose is 0.1 to 0.2 milligram per 2.2 pounds daily.

Overdosage

Any medication taken in excess can cause symptoms of overdose. If you suspect an overdose, seek medical attention immediately.

The symptoms of Klonopin overdose may include:
Coma
Confusion
Sleepiness
Slowed reaction time

Brand name:

KLOR-CON

See Micro-K, page 376.

Generic name:

LABETALOL HYDROCHLORIDE

See Normodyne, page 429.

Generic name:

LACTULOSE

See Chronulac Syrup, page 110.

Brand name:

LANOXIN

Generic name: Digoxin

Why is this drug prescribed?
Lanoxin is used in the treatment of congestive heart failure, irregular heartbeat, and other heart problems. It improves the strength and efficiency of your heart, which leads to better circulation of blood and reduction of uncomfortable swelling that is common in patients with congestive heart failure. Lanoxin is in a class of drugs known as cardiac glycosides.

Most important fact about this drug
If you are taking other prescription or non-prescription drugs, this should be discussed with your doctor to determine whether these drugs would interact with Lanoxin or increase the risk of side effects.

How should you take this medication?
Lanoxin should usually be taken after your morning meal, exactly as prescribed by your doctor.

If you forget to take a dose, take it as soon as you remember, if it is within 12 hours of the missed dose. If you remember later, take Lanoxin at the next scheduled time. Never take two doses at the same time.

Your doctor may require you to check your pulse rate while taking Lanoxin. Slowing or quickening of your pulse rate could mean you are developing side effects to your prescribed dose of medication. The amount of Lanoxin needed to help most patients is very close to the amount that could cause serious problems from overdose.

What side effects may occur?

Side effects cannot be anticipated. If any develop or change in intensity, inform your doctor as soon as possible. Only your doctor can determine if it is safe for you to continue taking Lanoxin.

The amount of Lanoxin must be very carefully monitored to avoid side effects of overdose.

■ *Side effects may include:*
Apathy, blurred vision, change in heartbeat, diarrhea, dizziness, headache, loss of appetite, lower stomach pain, nausea or vomiting, psychosis, weakness, yellow vision

Why should this drug not be prescribed?

If you are sensitive to or have ever had an allergic reaction to Lanoxin or similar drugs, you should not take this medication. Make sure that your doctor is aware of any drug reactions that you have experienced.

Lanoxin should not be given to patients with ventricular fibrillation. It should not be used, alone or with other drugs, to treat obesity. It can cause irregular heartbeat and other dangerous reactions that can be fatal.

Special warnings about this medication

Notify your doctor or dentist that you are taking Lanoxin if you have a medical emergency and before you have surgery or dental treatment.

Even if you have no symptoms, do not change your dose or discontinue the use of Lanoxin before consulting with your doctor.

Possible food and drug interactions when taking this medication

If Lanoxin is taken with certain other drugs, the effects of either could be increased, decreased, or altered. It is especially important to check with your doctor before combining Lanoxin with the following:

Antacids
Antiarrhythmics (quinidine)
Antibiotics (Neomycin, Tetracycline)
Antihyperlipidemics such as Questran Light
Beta blockers such as Tenormin, Inderal
Calcium
Calcium channel blockers such as Calan SR,
    Cardizem
Certain anticancer drugs
Corticosteroids such as Decadron, Deltasone
Diphenoxylate (Lomotil)
Diuretics
Kaolin-pectin
Propantheline (Pro-Banthine)
Succinylcholine
Sulfasalazine (Azulfidine)
Sympathomimetics such as Ventolin, Proventil
Thyroid hormones such as Synthroid

Special information if you are pregnant or breastfeeding

The effects of Lanoxin during pregnancy have not been adequately studied. If you are pregnant or plan to become pregnant, inform your doctor immediately. Lanoxin appears in breast milk and could affect a nursing infant. If this medication is essential to your health, your doctor may advise you to discontinue breastfeeding.

Recommended dosage

Several factors must be considered when your doctor determines your dosage: (1) the disease being treated; (2) body weight; (3) kidney function; (4) age; and (5) other diseases you have or drugs you are taking.

ADULTS

If you are receiving Lanoxin for the first time, you may be rapidly "digitalized" (a larger first dose may be taken, followed by smaller maintenance doses), or gradually "digitalized" (maintenance doses only), depending on your doctor's recommendation. When a daily maintenance dose is prescribed, you may require a 0.125 milligram or 0.25 milligram tablet once daily. The exact dose should be determined by your doctor, based on your needs. Your doctor should monitor your kidney function closely in determining your dose and may want to periodically perform a blood test.

CHILDREN

Infants and young children usually receive divided daily doses; children over 10 need adult dosages in proportion to body weight as determined by your doctor.

Overdosage

Symptoms of Lanoxin overdose include:
Irregular heartbeat
Loss of appetite
Nausea
Vomiting

In infants and children, irregular heartbeat is the most common sign of overdose. Suspected overdoses of Lanoxin must be treated immediately, and you should contact your doctor or emergency room.

Brand name:

LARODOPA

Generic name: Levodopa

Why is this drug prescribed?

Larodopa (L-dopa) relieves the symptoms of Parkinson's disease and of Parkinsonism (a nerve disorder characterized by tremor, drooling, stooped posture, a shuffling walk, and muscle weakness) caused by carbon monoxide and manganese poisoning. Larodopa is also used in elderly people whose parkinsonism is related to hardening of the arteries in the brain.

Most important fact about this drug

Vitamin B_6 (pyridoxine hydrochloride) in oral doses of 10 to 25 milligrams, rapidly reverses the effects of Larodopa. Make sure your doctor is aware of any vitamin supplements you take and whether they contain Vitamin B_6 (pyridoxine hydrochloride).

How should you take this medication?

Larodopa should be taken exactly as prescribed by your doctor. It may take several weeks to a few months before you notice the maximum benefits from Larodopa.

Some elderly patients may experience difficulty in retention of full dentures.

Larodopa should be taken with food.

What side effects may occur?

Side effects cannot be anticipated. If any side effects develop or change in intensity, tell your doctor immediately. Only your doctor can determine whether it is safe to continue taking Larodopa.

■ *Side effects may include:*
Agitation, anemia, anxiety, bitter taste, bizarre breathing patterns, blood clots in legs, blurred

vision, burning sensation of the tongue, changes in heart rate or rhythm (slow, pounding), confusion, constant erection in men, constipation, dark sweat and/or urine, depression, sometimes with suicidal tendencies, development of duodenal ulcers, diarrhea, difficult or painful swallowing, difficulty sleeping, dilated pupils, dizziness, double vision, dry mouth, excessive salivation, exhaustion, false sense of well-being, fixation of the eyeballs upward, fluid retention, flushing, gas, hair loss, hallucinations and delusions, headache, hiccups, high blood pressure, hoarseness, Horner's syndrome (drooping upper eyelid, lack of facial sweating, constricted pupil), hot flashes, inability to hold urine, increased hand tremor, increased sweating, jaw muscle spasms, lack of muscle coordination, loss of appetite, mental changes, including paranoia and psychosis, muscle twitching and continuous blinking, nausea, nightmares, numbness, "on-off" phenomenon (sudden, unexpected complete or almost complete loss of movement coupled with tremor and muscle rigidity), rash, stimulation, stomach bleeding, teeth grinding during sleep, urinary retention, vomiting, weakness and faintness, weight gain or loss.

Why should this drug not be prescribed?
Larodopa should not be taken if you have narrow-angle glaucoma, a history of melanoma or skin lesions that could be cancerous, or if you have ever had allergic reaction or are sensitive to Larodopa. If you are taking a monoamine oxidase (MAO) inhibitor antidepressant drug, such as Marplan, Nardil or Parnate, it should be stopped two weeks before starting therapy with Larodopa.

Special warnings about this medication
Larodopa may darken sweat or urine. Medically, this is not harmful.

Larodopa should be used cautiously if you have heart or lung disease, an irregular heartbeat, bronchial asthma, or kidney, liver or glandular disease.

If you have a history of active peptic ulcer, this drug can cause abdominal hemorrhage and should be used with care.

Depression can develop with the use of Larodopa.

If you are taking Larodopa for long-term use, your doctor should evaluate your liver, heart, kidney, and blood function periodically.

If you have well-controlled chronic wide-angle glaucoma or are taking high blood pressure medications, Larodopa should be used cautiously.

Possible food and drug interactions when taking this medication
If Larodopa is taken with certain other drugs, the effects of either drug could be increased, decreased, or altered. It is especially important to check with your doctor before combining Larodopa with the following:

Antidepressants known as MAO inhibitor drugs (Nardil, Marplan, and others)
High-blood-pressure drugs such as Catapres and Aldomet
Vitamin formulations containing vitamin B_6 (pyridoxine hydrochloride)

Special information if you are pregnant or breastfeeding
If you are pregnant or plan to become pregnant, inform your doctor immediately. No information is available about the safety of Larodopa during pregnancy. Because Larodopa may appear in breast milk and could affect a nursing infant, it should not be used by nursing mothers.

Recommended dosage

ADULTS

Your doctor will tailor your individual dosage to achieve exact blood levels of Larodopa and to minimize side effects.

The usual recommended initial dose of Larodopa is 0.5 to 1 gram daily, divided into 2 or more doses with food.

Your doctor may gradually increase your dose every 3 to 7 days to achieve desired relief. The maximum daily dose should not exceed 8 grams.

ELDERLY

Elderly patients may require a lower dosage of Larodopa.

Overdosage

Any medication taken in excess can have serious consequences. If you suspect an overdose, seek medical treatment immediately.

Brand name:

LAROTID

See Amoxil, page 23.

Brand name:

LASIX

Generic name: Furosemide

Why is this drug prescribed?

Lasix is used in the treatment of high blood pressure and other conditions that require the elimination of excess fluid (water) from the body. These conditions include congestive heart failure, cirrhosis of the liver, and kidney disease. When used to treat high blood pressure, Lasix is effective alone or in combination with other high blood pressure medications. Diuretics help your body produce and eliminate more urine, which helps lower blood pressure. Lasix is classified as a "loop diuretic" because of its point of action in the kidneys.

Most important fact about this drug

Lasix is a powerful diuretic that can cause severe water loss if not carefully monitored. Your doctor should adjust your dosage so that you get the maximum benefit with the least amount of medication.

Diuretics can cause your body to lose too much potassium. Ask your doctor for the warning signs of potassium depletion. Also ask whether you should eat specific foods that are rich in potassium or take a potassium supplement to avoid this problem.

How should you take this medication?

Take this medication exactly as prescribed by your doctor.

If you forget to take a dose, take it as soon as you remember. If it is almost time for your next dose, skip the one you missed and go back to your regular schedule. Never take two doses at the same time.

What side effects may occur?

Side effects cannot be anticipated. If any develop or change in intensity, inform your doctor as soon as possible. Only your doctor can determine if it is safe for you to continue taking Lasix.

■ *Side effects may include:*
Anemia, constipation, cramping, diarrhea, dizziness, dizziness upon standing, fever, headache, high blood sugar, hives, inflammation of lymph or blood vessels, inflammation of the pancreas, itching, loss of appetite, low potassium (leading to symptoms like dry mouth, excessive thirst, weak or irregular heartbeat, muscle pain or cramps), muscle spasms, nausea, rash, reddish or purplish spots on the skin,

restlessness, ringing in the ears or hearing loss, sensitivity to light, skin inflammation, stomach or mouth irritation, vertigo, vision changes, vomiting, weakness, yellow eyes and skin

Why should this drug not be prescribed?

If you are sensitive to or have ever had an allergic reaction to Lasix or diuretics, or if you are unable to urinate, you should not take this medication.

Special warnings about this medication

If you have kidney disease, liver disease, diabetes, gout, or connective tissue disease (lupus erythematosus), Lasix should be used with caution.

If you are allergic to sulfa drugs, you may also be allergic to Lasix.

If you have high blood pressure, avoid over-the-counter medications that may increase blood pressure, including cold remedies and appetite suppressants.

Your skin may be more sensitive to the effects of sunlight.

Possible food and drug interactions when taking this medication

Lasix may increase the effects of alcohol. Do not drink alcohol while taking this medication.

If Lasix is taken with certain other drugs, the effects of either could be increased, decreased, or altered. It is especially important to consult with your doctor before taking Lasix with any of the following:

Aminoglycoside antibiotics such as Garamycin
Aspirin
Barbiturates such as phenobarbital
Ethacrynic acid (Edecrin)
Indomethacin (Indocin)
Lithium

Narcotics such as Percocet
Norepinephrine (Levophed)
Other high blood pressure medications
Succinylcholine (Anectine)
Tubocurarine

Special information if you are pregnant or breastfeeding

The effects of Lasix during pregnancy have not been adequately studied. If you are pregnant or plan to become pregnant, inform your doctor immediately. Lasix appears in breast milk and could affect a nursing infant. If this medication is essential to your health, your doctor may advise you to discontinue breastfeeding until your treatment is finished.

Recommended dosage

Dosages of this medication, which is a strong diuretic, should be adjusted to meet the individual patient's needs. It is available in both oral and injectable form. The injectable form is used only in emergency situations or in cases where patients cannot take oral medication. Dosages shown here are for the oral form only.

ADULTS

Edema
Patients are started with a single dose of 20 to 80 milligrams. If needed, the same dose can be repeated 6 to 8 hours later. Dosage may also be raised by 20 milligrams to 40 milligrams with each successive administration until the desired effect is achieved. This dosage is then taken once or twice daily thereafter. Dosages should be adjusted according to individual patient response and carefully monitored by laboratory tests. The maximum daily dose is 600 milligrams.

High Blood Pressure
The usual starting dose is 80 milligrams per day divided into 2 doses. Dosages should be adjusted, and this medication can be used with other high blood pressure medication if blood pressure is carefully monitored.

CHILDREN

The usual initial dose is 2 milligrams per 2.2 pounds of body weight. Subsequent doses may be increased by 1 to 2 milligrams per 2.2. pounds. Doses are spaced 6 to 8 hours apart. Children's doses should be adjusted to the minimum dose needed to achieve maximum effect and should not exceed 6 milligrams per 2.2 pounds.

ELDERLY

Dosage should be determined by the particular needs of the elderly patient.

Overdosage

Any medication taken in excess can cause symptoms of overdose. If you suspect an overdose, seek medical attention immediately.

The symptoms of Lasix overdose may include:
Dehydration
Low blood pressure
Muscle pain or cramps
Weak or irregular heartbeat

Brand name:

LEVLEN

See Oral Contraceptives, page 437.

Generic name:

LEVOBUNOLOL HYDROCHLORIDE

See Betagan, page 65.

Generic name:

LEVODOPA

See Larodopa, page 312.

Generic name:

LEVODOPA/CARBIDOPA

See Sinemet, page 578.

Brand name:

LEVOTHROID

See Synthroid, page 598.

Generic name:

LEVOTHYROXINE SODIUM

See Synthroid, page 598.

Brand name:

LEVOXINE

See Synthroid, page 598.

Brand name:

LEVSIN

Generic name: Hyoscyamine sulfate
Other brand name: Anaspaz

Why is this drug prescribed?

Levsin is an antispasmodic medication that comes in the form of regular tablets that are dissolved under the tongue, sustained-release capsules, liquid, drops, and as an injectable solution. Levsin is given to help treat various stomach, intestinal, and urinary tract disorders that involve cramps, colic, or other painful muscle contractions. Because Levsin has a drying effect, it may also be used to dry a runny nose or to dry excess secretions before anesthesia is administered.

In inflammation of the pancreas, Levsin may be given to help control excess secretions and reduce pain. Levsin may also be given in Parkinson's disease to help reduce the muscle rigidity and tremors, and to help control the drooling and excess sweating.

Levsin is administered as part of the preparation for certain diagnostic X-rays (e.g., of the duodenum or kidneys).

Most important fact about this drug

If you take Levsin for a stomach disorder, you may also need to take antacid medication. Antacids make Levsin more difficult for the body to absorb. To minimize this problem, take Levsin before meals and the antacids after meals.

How should you take this medication?

Take Levsin exactly as prescribed by your doctor. You may need only a single daily dose or up to four evenly spaced doses per day. Although the sublingual tablets (Levsin/SL) are designed to be dissolved under the tongue, they may also be chewed or swallowed.

What side effects may occur?

Side effects cannot be anticipated. If any side effects develop or change in intensity, tell your doctor immediately. Only your doctor can determine whether it is safe for you to continue taking Levsin.

■ *Side effects include:*
Allergic reactions, bloating, blurred vision, confusion, constipation, decreased sweating, dilated pupils, dizziness, drowsiness, dry mouth, excitement, headache, impotence, insomnia, itching, heart palpitations, loss of sense of taste, nausea, nervousness, urinary hesitancy and retention, vomiting, weakness

Why should this drug not be prescribed?

Do not take Levsin if you have ever had an allergic reaction or are sensitive to any of its ingredients. Also, you should not be given Levsin if you have any of the following:

Bowel or digestive tract obstruction or paralysis
Glaucoma
Myasthenia gravis (a disorder in which muscles become weak and tire easily)
Ulcerative colitis (severe)
Urinary obstruction

Levsin is not appropriate if you have diarrhea, especially if you have an ileostomy or a colostomy.

Special warnings about this medication

Since Levsin decreases sweating, you are vulnerable to heat stroke if you take it while you have a fever or are in a very hot environment.

Because Levsin may make you dizzy or drowsy, or blur your vision, do not drive, operate other machinery, or do any other hazardous work while taking this medication.

The injectable form of Levsin contains a sulfite, which could cause problems, including severe allergic reactions. People with asthma are more likely than others to be allergic to sulfites.

Possible food and drug interactions when taking this medication

If Levsin is taken with certain other drugs, the effects of either drug could be increased, decreased, or altered. It is especially important to check with your doctor before combining Levsin with the following:

Amantadine (Symmetrel)
Antidepressant drugs known as MAO inhibitors such as Marplan, Nardil, and Parnate
Antihistamines such as Benadryl

Haloperidol (Haldol)
Phenothiazines such as Thorazine
Tricyclic antidepressants such as Elavil and
   Tofranil

Special information
if you are pregnant or breastfeeding

If you are pregnant or plan to become
pregnant, inform your doctor immediately.
Although it is not known whether Levsin can
cause birth defects, pregnant women should
avoid all drugs except those necessary
to health.

Levsin is excreted in human milk and should
be used with caution if you are nursing
an infant.

Recommended dosage

Your doctor will tailor your dose of Levsin
according to the condition being treated
and severity of symptoms.

LEVSIN/SL AND LEVSIN TABLETS

The tablets may be swallowed or placed under
the tongue.

*Adults and Children 12 Years of Age
and Older*
The usual recommended dose is 1 to 2 tablets
every four hours. Do not take more than
12 tablets in 24 hours.

Children 2 to Under 12 Years of Age
The usual recommended dose is one-half to 1
tablet every four hours. Do not give a child
more than 6 tablets in 24 hours.

LEVSIN ELIXIR

*Adults and Children 12 Years of Age
and Older*
The recommended dosage is 1 to 2
teaspoonfuls every four hours or as
needed, but no more than 12 teaspoonfuls
in 24 hours.

Children 2 to Under 12 Years of Age
The usual dosage is one-quarter to 1 teaspoonful every 4 hours or as needed. Do
not give a child more than 6 teaspoonfuls
in 24 hours.

LEVSIN DROPS

*Adults and Children 12 Years of Age
and Older*
The recommended dosage is 1 to 2 milliliters
every 4 hours or as needed, but no more
than 12 milliliters in 24 hours.

Children 2 to Under 12 Years of Age
The usual dosage is one-quarter to 1 milliliter every 4 hours or as needed. Do not
give a child more than 6 milliliters in 24
hours.

Children Under 2 Years of Age
The dosage is based on body weight.
The doses may be repeated every 4 hours
or as needed.

WEIGHT	USUAL DOSE	DO NOT EXCEED IN 24 HOURS
2.3 kilograms (5 lbs)	3 drops	18 drops
3.4 kilograms (7.5 lbs)	4 drops	24 drops
5 kilograms (11 lbs)	5 drops	30 drops
7 kilograms (15 lbs)	6 drops	36 drops
10 kilograms (22 lbs)	8 drops	48 drops
15 kilograms (33 lbs)	11 drops	66 drops

LEVSINEX TIMECAPS

*Adults and Children 12 Years of Age and
Older*
The recommended dosage is 1 to 2
TIMECAPS every 12 hours. The dosage
may be adjusted to 1 TIMECAP every 8
hours if needed. Do not take more than
4 TIMECAPS in 24 hours.

Children 2 to Under 12 Years of Age
The usual dosage is 1 TIMECAP every 12
hours. Do not give a child more than 2
TIMECAPS in 24 hours.

Overdosage
Any medication taken in excess can have
serious consequences. If you suspect an
overdose of Levsin, seek medical attention
immediately.

Symptoms of Levsin overdose may include:
Blurred vision
Central nervous system stimulation
Dilated pupils
Dizziness
Dry mouth
Headache
Hot, dry skin
Nausea
Swallowing difficulty
Vomiting.

Brand name:

LIBRAX

*Generic ingredients: Chlordiazepoxide
hydrochloride, Clidinium bromide
Other brand name: Clindex*

Why is this drug prescribed?
Librax is a combination of a benzodiazepine
(chlordiazepoxide hydrochloride) and an
anticholingergic medication (clidinium
bromide). Librax is used, in combination
with other therapy, for the treatment of peptic
ulcer, irritable bowel syndrome, and acute
enterocolitis (inflammation of the colon and
small intestine).

Most important fact about this drug
Because of its sedative effects, you should not
operate heavy machinery, drive, engage
in hazardous tasks, or consume alcohol or
other drugs that make you drowsy while
taking Librax.

How should you take this medication?
Take this medication as directed by your
doctor. Other therapy may be prescribed
to be used at the same time.

Take Librax before meals. Avoid alcoholic
beverages.

What side effects may occur?
Many side effects cannot be anticipated. If
any develop or change in intensity, inform
your doctor as soon as possible. Only your
doctor can determine if it is safe for you
to continue taking Librax.

■ *Side effects may include:*
Blurred vision, changes in sex drive,
confusion, constipation, drowsiness, dry
mouth, fainting, jaundice, lack of
coordination, liver dysfunction, loss of
consciousness, minor menstrual irregularities,
muscle spasms, muscle stiffness, nausea,
skin eruptions, swelling due to fluid
retention, tremors, urinary difficulties

Why should this drug not be prescribed?
You should not take this drug if you have
glaucoma (elevated pressure in the eye),
prostatic hypertrophy (enlarged prostate), or
benign bladder neck obstruction. If you
are sensitive to or have ever had an allergic
reaction to Librax or any of its
ingredients, you should not take this
medication. Make sure that your doctor
is aware of any drug reactions that you have
experienced.

Special warnings about this medication
Take Librax exactly as prescribed, since
benzodiazepine abuse has been associated
with drug dependence and addiction. Patients
with a history of alcoholism, drug abuse,
or personality disorders should use Librax
with caution.

In addition, you should not stop taking Librax
suddenly, because of the risk of

withdrawal symptoms (convulsions, cramps, tremors, vomiting, sweating, feeling ill, perceptual problems, and insomnia). A gradual dosage tapering schedule is usually recommended for patients taking Librax for an extended period of time.

Elderly patients should take the lowest effective dose of Librax to reduce the possibility of side effects such as confusion, excessive drowsiness, and shaky movements.

Long-term treatment with Librax may call for periodic blood and liver function tests.

Possible food and drug interactions when taking this medication

If Librax is taken with certain other drugs, the effects of either could be increased, decreased, or altered. It is especially important to check with your doctor before combining Librax with the following:

Antidepressant drugs known as MAO
  inhibitors, such as Nardil and Parnate
Oral anticoagulants such as Coumadin
Phenothiazines such as Stelazine and
  Thorazine

In addition, you may experience excessive drowsiness and other potentially dangerous side effects if Librax is combined with alcohol or other drugs that make you drowsy.

Special information if you are pregnant or breastfeeding

Several studies have found an increased risk of birth defects if Librax is taken during the first 3 months of pregnancy. Therefore, Librax is rarely recommended for use by pregnant woman. If you are pregnant, plan to become pregnant, or are breastfeeding, inform your doctor immediately.

Recommended dosage

ADULTS

The usual dose is 1 or 2 capsules, 3 or 4 times a day before meals and at bedtime.

ELDERLY

The lowest dose that is effective should be used.

Overdosage

Any medication taken in excess can have serious consequences. Severe overdosage of Librax can be fatal. If you suspect symptoms of a Librax overdose, seek medical help immediately.

Symptoms of Librax overdose may include:
Blurred vision
Coma
Confusion
Constipation
Excessive sleepiness
Excessively dry mouth
Slow reflexes
Urinary difficulties

Brand name:

LIBRITABS

See Librium, page 320.

Brand name:

LIBRIUM

Generic name: Chlordiazepoxide
Other brand name: Libritabs

Why is this drug prescribed?

Librium is used in the treatment of anxiety disorders and for short-term relief of the symptoms of anxiety, withdrawal symptoms of acute alcoholism and anxiety and apprehension before surgery. It belongs to a class of drugs known as benzodiazepines.

Most important fact about this drug

Tolerance and dependence can occur with the use of Librium. You may experience withdrawal symptoms if you stop using this drug abruptly. Discontinue or change your dose only on advice of your doctor.

How should you take this medication?

Take this medication exactly as prescribed by your doctor.

What side effects may occur?

Side effects cannot be anticipated. If any develop or change in intensity, inform your doctor as soon as possible. Only your doctor can determine if it is safe for you to continue taking Librium.

- *More common side effects may include:*
  Confusion
  Drowsiness
  Lack of muscle coordination

- *Less common or rare side effects may include:*
  Constipation, fainting, increased or decreased sex drive, jaundice, minor menstrual irregularities, nausea, skin rash or eruptions, stiffness, swelling due to fluid retention, yellow eyes and skin

- *Side effects due to rapid decrease or abrupt withdrawal from Librium include:*
  Abdominal and muscle cramps
  Convulsions
  Return of anxiety or increase in severity of symptoms
  Sweating
  Tremors
  Vomiting

Why should this drug not be prescribed?

If you are sensitive to or have ever had an allergic reaction to Librium or similar drugs, you should not take this medication.

Anxiety or tension related to everyday stress usually does not require treatment with Librium. Discuss your symptoms thoroughly with your doctor.

Special warnings about this medication

Librium may cause you to become drowsy or less alert; therefore, driving or operating dangerous machinery or participating in any hazardous activity that requires full mental alertness is not recommended.

If you are severely depressed or have suffered from severe depression, consult with your doctor before taking this medication.

This drug may cause children to become less alert.

If you have a hyperactive, aggressive child taking Librium, inform your doctor if contrary reactions such as excitement, stimulation or acute rage occur.

Consult with your doctor before taking Librium if you are being treated for porphyria (a rare metabolic disorder) or kidney or liver disease.

Possible food and drug interactions when taking this medication

Librium is a central nervous system depressant and may intensify the effects of alcohol or have an additive effect. Do not drink alcohol while taking this medication.

If Librium is taken with certain other drugs, the effects of either could be increased, decreased, or altered. It is especially important to check with your doctor before combining Librium with the following:

Anticoagulants (blood thinners)
Antidepressant drugs known as MAO inhibitors
Barbiturates
Narcotics
Tranquilizers known as phenothiazines

Special Information
if you are pregnant or breastfeeding

Do not take Librium if you are pregnant or planning to become pregnant. There may be in increased risk of birth defects. This drug may appear in breast milk and could affect a nursing infant. If the medication is essential to your health, your doctor may advise you to discontinue breastfeeding until your treatment with the drug is finished.

Recommended dosage

ADULTS

Mild or Moderate Anxiety
The usual recommended dose is 5 or 10 milligrams, 3 or 4 times per day.

Severe Anxiety
The usual recommended dose is 20 to 25 milligrams, 3 or 4 times per day.

Apprehension and Anxiety before Surgery
On days preceding surgery, the usual recommended dose is 5 to 10 milligrams, 3 or 4 times per day.

Withdrawal Symptoms of Acute Alcoholism
The usual recommended starting oral dose is 50 to 100 milligrams per day, followed by repeated doses, up to a maximum of 300 milligrams per day to control agitation. The dose should then be reduced as much as possible.

CHILDREN

The usual recommended dose for children 6 years of age and older is 5 milligrams, 2 to 4 times per day. This dose may need to be increased to 10 milligrams, 2 or 3 times per day, in some children. The drug is not recommended for children under 6.

ELDERLY

The dosage should be limited to the smallest effective amount to avoid oversedation or impaired muscle coordination. The usual recommended dose is 5 milligrams, 2 to 4 times per day.

Overdosage

Any medication taken in excess can cause symptoms of overdose. If you suspect an overdose, seek medical attention immediately.

The symptoms of Librium overdose may include:
Coma
Confusion
Diminished reflexes
Sleepiness

Brand name:

LIDEX

Generic name: Fluocinonide

Why is this drug prescribed?

Lidex is a topical corticosteroid (one applied directly to the skin). It relieves the itching and inflammation of a wide variety of skin problems including redness and swelling.

Most important fact about this drug

Lidex is for external use only and should be used only as prescribed by your doctor.

Do not use Lidex in your eyes. If the medication gets in your eyes and causes irritation, immediately flush your eyes with a large amount of water.

How should you use this medication?

You should not bandage or cover the areas being treated with Lidex unless advised to do so by your doctor. Tell your doctor if you experience any skin reactions, especially if your doctor has advised you to use bandages.

Apply Lidex as directed by your doctor. Do not use more of the medication than suggested by your doctor.

What side effects may occur?

Side effects cannot be anticipated. If any develop or change in intensity, inform your doctor immediately. Only your doctor can determine if it is safe for you to continue using Lidex.

■ *Side effects may include:*
Acne-like eruptions, burning, dryness, excessive hair growth, infection of the skin, irritation, itching, lack of skin color, prickly heat, skin inflammation (from contact with an object such as a watch band or poison ivy), skin loss, stretch marks

Why should this drug not be prescribed?

You should not be using Lidex if you are allergic to any of the components in this preparation.

Special warnings about this medication

Do not use Lidex more often or for a longer time than your doctor ordered. If large doses of corticosteroid are applied over a large area for an extended period of time, especially when treated area is covered, this may increase the risk of absorption through the skin. The amount of drug absorbed may be enough to produce side effects. These side effects may include increased sugar in your blood and urine and Cushing's syndrome, characterized by a moon-shaped face, emotional disturbances, high blood pressure, weight gain, and growth of body hair in women.

Some factors that may increase the absorption of topical corticosteroids include:

Using bandages over the area where topical corticosteroids are applied;

Using topical corticosteroids over a large area of skin or on broken skin; or

Using topical corticosteroids for an extended period of time.

Children may absorb a proportionally greater amount of corticosteroid drugs and may be more sensitive to the effects of these drugs.

Effects experienced by children may include:
Bulges on the head
Delayed weight gain
Headache
Slow growth

Topical corticosteroids should be discontinued if irritation develops, and another treatment should be used.

Extended treatment time with any topical corticosteroid product may cause skin to waste away. This may also occur with short-term use of topical corticosteroids on the face and on areas of the body that bend.

Possible food and drug interactions when taking this medication

No interactions have been reported with Lidex.

Special information if you are pregnant or breastfeeding

Pregnant women should not use topical corticosteroids in large amounts or for long periods of time. During pregnancy, topical corticosteroids should be used only if the possible gains outweigh the possible risks to the baby.

Women who breastfeed an infant should use topical corticosteroids cautiously.

Recommended dosage

ADULTS

Lidex is applied to the affected areas in a thin film 2 to 4 times a day. If hair covers the infected area, part the hair so that topical corticosteroids can be applied directly.

CHILDREN

Children should be given the smallest effective dose of topical corticosteroids.

Children being treated with these medications in the diaper area should not wear plastic pants or tight diapers.

Overdosage

Topical corticosteroids can be absorbed in amounts large enough to have temporary effects on the adrenal, hypothalamic, and pituitary glands.

Some effects of corticosteroid drugs may include:
Abnormal sugar levels in urine
Excessive blood sugar levels
Symptoms of Cushing's syndrome

Symptoms of Cushing's syndrome may include:
Easily bruised skin
Increased blood pressure
Mood swings
Water retention
Weak muscles
Weight gain

If you suspect Lidex overdose may have occurred, seek medical help immediately.

Brand name:

LIMBITROL

Generic ingredients: Chlordiazepoxide, Amitriptyline hydrochloride

Why is this drug prescribed?

Limbitrol is a combination of an antidepressant and an antianxiety drug. It is used in the treatment of moderate to severe depression associated with moderate to severe anxiety.

Some symptoms of depression and anxiety are expected to show improvement during the first week of treatment with Limbitrol.

Most important fact about this drug

Tolerance and dependence can occur with the use of Limbitrol. You may experience withdrawal symptoms if you stop using this drug abruptly. Discontinue or change your dose only on advice of your doctor.

How should you take this medication?

Take this medication exactly as prescribed by your doctor.

What side effects may occur?

Side effects cannot be anticipated. If any develop or change in intensity, inform your doctor as soon as possible. Only your doctor can determine if it is safe for you to continue taking Limbitrol.

■ *More common side effects may include:*
Bloating
Blurred vision
Constipation
Dizziness
Drowsiness
Dry mouth

■ *Less common or rare side effects may include:*
Confusion, fatigue, impotence, lack or loss of appetite, nasal congestion, restlessness, sluggishness, unresponsiveness, tremors, vivid dreams, weakness, yellow eyes and skin

■ *Side effects from rapid decrease or abrupt withdrawal from Limbitrol include:*
Abdominal and muscle cramps, convulsions, headache, inability to fall asleep or stay asleep, nausea, restlessness, return of original symptoms or an increase in intensity, sweating, tremors, vague bodily discomfort, vomiting

The following side effects have not been reported with the use of Limbitrol. Because this drug is a combination of chlordiazepoxide and amitriptyline, the following effects associated with one or both of these drugs may possibly occur with Limbitrol.

Abnormally rapid heart rate, apprehension, black tongue, blood disorders, breast enlargement, brief loss of consciousness, delusions, diarrhea, dilation of the pupils of the eye, elevation or lowering of blood sugar levels, exaggerated sense of well-being, excessive or spontaneous flow of milk, hair loss, hallucinations, headache, heart attack, high blood pressure, inability to pass urine, increased or decreased sex drive, increased perspiration, indigestion, inflammation of the mouth, itching, irregular heartbeat, lack of muscle coordination, low blood pressure, mild degree of mania, minor menstrual irregularities, nausea, numbness, obstruction of bowels, peculiar taste, poor concentration, poor coordination, rapid or strong heartbeat, sensitivity to light, skin rash or eruptions, stroke, swelling in face and tongue, swelling of the salivary glands, swelling of the testicles, tingling, urinary frequency, vomiting, weight gain or loss

Why should this drug not be prescribed?

If you are sensitive to or have ever had an allergic reaction to benzodiazepine or tricyclic antidepressants, you should not take this medication.

Unless you are directed to do so by your doctor, do not take this medication if you are in the acute recovery phase following a heart attack.

Do not take this medication if you are being treated for angle-closure glaucoma or the inability to pass urine, unless you are directed to do so by your doctor.

If you are taking an MAO inhibitor (drug used to treat depression), consult with your doctor before taking Limbitrol. Convulsions and death have occurred when these two drugs are taken together.

Special warnings about this medication

Limbitrol may cause you to become drowsy or less alert; therefore, driving or operating dangerous machinery or participating in any hazardous activity that requires full mental alertness is not recommended.

This drug, especially when given in high doses, can cause irregular heartbeat, an increase in heart rate, heart attack or stroke. If you are being treated for a heart or circulatory disorder, consult with your doctor before taking Limbitrol.

Consult with your doctor before taking this medication if you are severely depressed or have been treated for severe depression.

Limbitrol should be discontinued several days before you have elective surgery and should be used with caution in electroconvulsive therapy. This should be discussed with your doctor.

Possible food and drug interactions when taking this medication

Limbitrol is a central nervous system depressant and may intensify the effects of alcohol. Do not drink alcohol while taking this medication.

If Limbitrol is taken with certain other drugs, the effects of either could be increased, decreased, or altered. It is especially important to check with your doctor before combining Limbitrol with the following:

Antidepressant drugs known as MAO inhibitors
Barbiturates such as phenobarbital
Cimetidine (Tagamet)
Other mood-altering drugs

The blood-pressure medication Guanethidine
Thyroid medication

Severe constipation may occur if you take
Limbitrol in combination with
anticholinergic-type drugs such as Donnatal
or Bentyl.

Special information
if you are pregnant or breastfeeding

Do not take Limbitrol if you are pregnant
or planning to become pregnant. There
is an increased risk of birth defects. This drug
may appear in breast milk and could
affect a nursing infant. If this medication is
essential to your health, your doctor may
advise you to discontinue breastfeeding until
your treatment is finished.

Recommended dosage

ADULTS

Limbitrol tablets
The usual recommended starting dosage is a
total of 3 or 4 tablets per day divided
into smaller individual doses. The larger
portion of the daily dose may be taken
at bedtime. A single bedtime dose may be
sufficient. Your dose should be
individualized to your needs by your doctor.

Limbitrol DS
The usual recommended starting dosage is a
total of 3 or 4 tablets per day divided
into smaller individual doses. This may be
increased to 6 tablets per day or decreased
to 2 tablets per day, depending on individual
need as determined by your doctor.

CHILDREN

Safety and effectiveness have not been
established in children under 12 years old.

ELDERLY

The usual dose should be limited to the
smallest effective amount, as determined

by your doctor, to avoid oversedation,
confusion and loss of muscle control.

Overdosage

Any medication taken in excess can cause
symptoms of overdose. If you suspect an
overdose, seek medical attention
immediately.

*The symptoms of Limbitrol overdose
may include:*
Abnormally fast heart rate, agitation, coma,
confusion, congestive heart failure,
convulsions, dilated pupils, drowsiness,
excessive body or limb movements, high
fever, irregular heartbeat, muscle rigidity,
reduction of body temperature, severe low
blood pressure, stupor, vomiting

Brand name:

LIORESAL

Generic name: Baclofen
Other brand name: Atrofen

Why is this drug prescribed?

Lioresal is a muscle relaxant that helps relieve
the symptoms and pain of muscle spasms
caused by multiple sclerosis (MS), particularly
from muscles that control joints, from
rhythmic expansion and contraction of
muscles (clonus), and from muscular
stiffness. Lioresal may also be of some help
to people with spinal cord injuries and
diseases.

Most important fact about this drug

Hallucinations and seizures have occurred
when Lioresal is stopped suddenly. The
dosage should be reduced gradually when the
medication is discontinued.

How should you take this medication?

Lioresal should be taken exactly as prescribed
by your doctor.

What side effects may occur?

Side effects cannot be anticipated. If any side effects develop or change in intensity, tell your doctor immediately. Only your doctor can determine whether it is safe for you to continue taking Lioresal.

■ *More common side effects may include:*
Dizziness
Exhaustion
Temporary drowsiness
Weakness

■ *Less common side effects may include::*
Confusion, constipation, difficulty sleeping, headache, increased urination, low blood pressure, nausea

■ *Rare side effects may include:*
Abdominal pain, abnormal muscle tone, especially sudden muscle spasms, bed-wetting, blood in stool, blood in urine, blurred vision, constricted (small), or dilated pupils, depression, diarrhea, double vision, dry mouth, ejaculation difficulty, epileptic seizure, excessive perspiration, excessive urination at night, excitement, fainting, false sense of well-being (euphoria), hallucinations, impotence, improper alignment of the eyes, involuntary movement of eyeball, itching, lack of muscle coordination, loss of appetite, muscle pain, painful or difficult urination, pounding heartbeat, rash, ringing in ears, shortness of breath, slurred speech, stiffness, stuffy nose, swelling of ankles, taste distortion, tingling or a feeling of "pins and needles," tremor, vomiting, weight gain

Why should this drug not be prescribed?

Do not take Lioresal if you have ever had an allergic reaction or are sensitive to baclofen.

Special warnings about this medication

Lioresal may alter the effectiveness of seizure medications. If you have epilepsy, you should be carefully monitored while taking Lioresal.

Your doctor should gradually reduce your dosage when it is time to stop taking Lioresal. Hallucinations and seizures have occurred when Lioresal is withdrawn suddenly.

Lioresal should be used cautiously if you have kidney disease or if the muscle spasms help support posture, balance, and locomotion.

Lioresal can cause you to become tired or less alert. Be careful driving or operating machinery or appliances that require full mental alertness until you know how you react to this medication.

Possible food and drug interactions when taking this medication

Lioresal may increase the effects of alcohol. Do not drink alcohol while taking this medication.

If Lioresal is taken with certain other drugs, the effects of either could be increased, decreased, or altered. It is especially important to check with your doctor before combining Lioresal with the following:

Central nervous system (brain and spinal cord) depressants such as sedatives and tranquilizers

Special information
if you are pregnant or breastfeeding

If you are pregnant or plan to become pregnant, inform your doctor immediately. No information is available about the safety of Lioresal during pregnancy.

Lioresal may appear in breast milk and could affect a nursing infant. If Lioresal is essential to your health, your doctor may advise you to stop breastfeeding until your treatment is finished.

Recommended dosage

ADULTS

Your doctor will tailor your individual dose based on the severity of your symptoms.

The recommended initial dose is 5 milligrams 3 times a day. Your doctor may increase the dose to 20 milligrams 3 times a day at 3-day intervals. The maximum daily dose should not exceed 80 milligrams (20 milligrams 4 times a day).

CHILDREN

Lioresal is not recommended for children under 12 years of age.

Overdosage

Any medication taken in excess can have serious consequences. If you suspect an overdose, seek medical treatment immediately.

Symptoms of Lioresal overdose may include:
Breathing difficulty
Coma
Drowsiness
Eye adaptation disorders
Loss of muscle tone
Seizures
Vomiting

Generic name:

LIOTRIX

See Euthroid, page 246.

Generic name:

LISINOPRIL

See Zestril, page 696.

Generic name:

LITHIUM CARBONATE

See Lithobid, page 328.

Brand name:

LITHOBID

Generic name: Lithium carbonate
Other brand name: Cibalith-S (lithium citrate)

Why is this drug prescribed?

Both Lithobid slow-release tablets and Cibalith-S syrup contain the antimanic medication lithium, which is used as an antipsychotic medication.

Lithium is given to help calm people in a hyperexcited, out-of-control state called mania. A manic episode (of manic-depressive illness) may involve some or all of the following symptoms:

Aggressiveness
Elation
Extreme tendency to "go off on a tangent"
Fast, urgent talking
Frenetic physical activity
Grandiose, unrealistic ideas
Hostility
Little need for sleep
Poor judgment

Once the mania subsides, lithium treatment may be continued over the long term, at a somewhat lower dosage, to prevent future manic episodes.

Most important fact about this drug

If the lithium dosage is too low, you will derive no benefit; if it is too high, you will experience undesirable effects. You and your doctor will need to work together to find the correct dosage. Initially, this means frequent blood tests are required to find out how much lithium is actually circulating in your bloodstream. As long as you take lithium, you will need to monitor yourself for adverse effects and promptly report any new symptoms to your doctor.

Watch for the signs of lithium toxicity, such as vomiting, unsteady walking, diarrhea, drowsiness, or weakness.

How should you take this medication?
Take Lithobid exactly as prescribed by your doctor.

Take Lithobid immediately after meals or with food or milk to avoid stomach upset.

Do not change from one brand of lithium preparation to another without consulting your doctor or pharmacist.

Even if you have been taking lithium for an extended period, you should have a blood test and a checkup at least every 2 months to make sure the dosage is still right for you. The blood sample should always be drawn just before you take your next regular dose. If you have been experiencing lithium side effects, be sure to tell your doctor.

You should drink 10 to 12 glasses of water or fluid a day. To minimize the risk of toxic side effects from lithium, eat a balanced diet that includes some salt and lots of liquids. In case of protracted sweating or diarrhea, make sure you get extra liquids and salt.

If you develop an infection that causes fever, diarrhea, or vomiting, you may need to cut back on your lithium dosage or even quit taking it temporarily. While you are ill, keep in close touch with your doctor.

Lithobid tablets are meant to be swallowed whole. Never crush or chew them; the sudden "dump" of lithium could have the effect of an overdose.

What side effects may occur?
Side effects cannot be anticipated. If any develop or change in intensity, inform your doctor as soon as possible. Only your doctor can determine if it is safe for you to continue taking Lithobid.

■ *More common side effects may include:* Diarrhea, drowsiness, fatigue, fever, frequent urination, headache, mild thirst, minor memory impairment, muscle weakness, slight hand tremor, vomiting, weight gain

■ *Less common side effects may include:* Abnormal heartbeat rhythm, ankle or wrist swelling, appetite loss, baldness, blackout spells, blurred vision, collapsed blood vessels, coma, confusion, dehydration, diarrhea, dizziness, drowsiness, drying, thinning hair, dry mouth, dry skin, excessive thirst, excessive weight gain, frequent urination, goiter, grimace or muscle distortion, hair follicle infections, hair loss, incontinence of urine or feces, involuntary eyeball movement, itching, lack of coordination, lack of sensation in skin, lethargy, low blood pressure, metallic taste, muscle irritability, nausea, overactive thyroid, physical and mental slowness, restlessness, seizures, skin numbness, skin ulcers, sleepiness, sluggishness, slurred speech, stupor, temporary blind spot in the eye, tendency to sleep, tremor, underactive thyroid, vertigo, weight loss, worsening of brain disorders, worsening of psoriasis, writhing movements

Why should this drug not be prescribed?
Do not take either Lithobid or Cibalith-S if you are sensitive to lithium or have ever had an allergic reaction to lithium.

Also, do not take either of these medications if you are debilitated or severely dehydrated, or if you have cardiovascular or kidney disease.

Special warnings about this medication

Lithium may affect your judgment or coordination. Do not drive, climb, or perform hazardous tasks until you find out how lithium affects you.

Be aware that, for any individual, there is a thin line between the dosage of lithium that works well and the dosage that starts to produce overdose effects. Stay in close touch with your doctor, and report any new symptoms immediately.

Possible food and drug interactions when taking this medication

Lithium may intensify or prolong the effects of certain drugs used in anesthesia. If you are facing surgery, make sure the surgeon and anesthesiologist know you are taking lithium.

If lithium is taken with certain other drugs, the effects of either could be increased, decreased, or altered. It is especially important to check with your doctor before combining lithium with the following:

Antipsychotic drugs such as Haldol
ACE-inhibitor blood pressure drugs such as
   Capoten or Vasotec
Anti-inflammatory drugs such as Indocin,
   Feldene, or others
Asthma drugs
Bicarbonate of soda
Diuretics such as Lasix or HydroDIURIL
Iodine-containing preparations such as
   potassium iodide

Special Information
if you are pregnant or breastfeeding

The use of lithium during pregnancy is usually not recommended because of the possibility that it might cause birth defects. If you are pregnant or plan to become pregnant, inform your doctor immediately.

Lithium is excreted in breast milk and is considered potentially harmful to a nursing infant. If this medication is essential to your health, your doctor may advise you to discontinue breastfeeding while you are taking it.

Recommended dosage

ADULTS

Lithobid
The usual dose is 900 milligrams, 2 times a day, or 600 milligrams, 3 times a day, for a total of 1,800 milligrams per day.

Cibalith-S
The usual dose is 10 milliliters or 2 teaspoons, 3 times a day.

Your doctor will individualize your dosage according to blood levels. Your blood levels will be checked at least twice a week when the drug is first prescribed and on a regular basis thereafter.

Long-term Control
Dosage will vary from one individual to another, but the following dosages will usually maintain the desired blood levels of these drugs:

Lithobid
900 milligrams to 1200 milligrams per day given in 2 or 3 divided doses.

Cibalith-S
5 milliliters or 1 teaspoon 3 or 4 times a day.

Blood levels in most cases should be checked every 2 months.

ELDERLY

Elderly patients often respond to a reduced dosage and may exhibit signs of overdose at blood levels ordinarily tolerated by younger patients.

Overdosage

Any medication taken in excess can have serious consequences. If you suspect symptoms of an overdose of lithium, seek medical attention immediately.

Initial signs of lithium overdose include blurred vision, appetite loss, vomiting, diarrhea, drowsiness and sluggishness, giddiness and staggering, trembling, lack of coordination, and slurred speech.

A more severe overdose may produce psychotic thinking, stiffened limbs, psychosis, seizures, fainting, coma, or even death.

Brand name:

LO/OVRAL

See Oral Contraceptives, page 437.

Brand name:

LODINE

Generic name: Etodolac

Why is this drug prescribed?

Lodine, a nonsteroidal anti-inflammatory drug, is used to relieve the inflammation, swelling, stiffness, and joint pain associated with acute and long-term treatment of osteoarthritis (the most common form of arthritis). It is also used to relieve other types of pain.

Most important fact about this drug

You should have frequent checkups with your doctor if you take Lodine regularly. Ulcers or internal bleeding can occur without warning.

How should you take this medication?

Your doctor may ask you to take Lodine with food or an antacid, and with a full glass of water. Never take it on an empty stomach.

Take this medication exactly as prescribed by your doctor.

If you are using Lodine for arthritis, it should be taken regularly.

What side effects may occur?

Side effects cannot be anticipated. If any develop or change in intensity, inform your doctor as soon as possible. Only your doctor can determine if it is safe for you to continue taking Lodine.

■ *More common side effects may include:*
Abdominal pain, black stools, blurred vision, chills, constipation, depression, diarrhea, dizziness, fever, gas, increased frequency of urination, indigestion, inflammation of stomach, itching, nausea, nervousness, rash, ringing in ears, painful or difficult urination, vomiting, weakness

■ *Less common or rare side effects may include:*
Abdominal bleeding, abnormal intolerance of light, anemia, asthma, congestive heart failure, dry mouth, fainting, flushing, hepatitis, high blood pressure, hives, inability to sleep, inflammation of mouth, loss of appetite, peptic ulcer, rapid heartbeat, rash, sleepiness, Stevens-Johnson syndrome (peeling skin), sweating, swelling (fluid retention), thirst, visual disturbances

Why should this drug not be prescribed?

If you are sensitive to or have ever had an allergic reaction to Lodine, aspirin, or similar drugs, or if you have had asthma attacks caused by aspirin or other drugs of this type, you should not take this medication. Make sure that your doctor is aware of any drug reactions that you have experienced.

Special warnings about this medication

Peptic ulcers and bleeding can occur without warning.

This drug should be used with caution if you have kidney or liver disease; and it can cause liver inflammation in some people.

Do not take aspirin or any other anti-inflammatory medications while taking Lodine, unless your doctor tells you to do so.

If you are taking Lodine over an extended period of time, your doctor should check your blood for anemia.

This drug can increase water retention. Use with caution if you have heart disease or high blood pressure.

Possible food and drug interactions when taking this medication

If Lodine is taken with certain other drugs, the effects of either could be increased, decreased, or altered. It is especially important to check with your doctor before combining Lodine with the following:

Aspirin
Cyclosporine (Sandimmune)
Diuretics such as HydroDIURIL
Digoxin (Lanoxin)
Lithium (Lithobid, others)
Methotrexate
Phenylbutazone (Butazolidin)

Special information
if you are pregnant or breastfeeding

The effects of Lodine during pregnancy have not been adequately studied. If you are pregnant or plan to become pregnant, inform your doctor immediately. Lodine may appear in breast milk and could affect a nursing infant. If this medication is essential to your health, your doctor may advise you to discontinue breastfeeding until your treatment with this medication is finished.

Recommended dosage

ADULTS

General Pain Relief
Take 200 to 400 milligrams every 6 to 8 hours as needed. Do not take more than 1,200 milligrams a day. For patients weighing less than 132 pounds, the maximum dose is 20 milligrams per 2.2 pounds.

Osteoarthritis
Starting dose is a total of 800 to 1,200 milligrams per day divided into smaller doses, followed by 600 to 1,200 milligrams per day in divided doses (i.e., 400 milligrams 2 or 3 times a day; 300 milligrams, 2, 3 or 4 times a day). For patients weighing less than 132 pounds the maximum dose is 20 milligrams per 2.2 pounds.

The lowest dose that proves beneficial should be used.

CHILDREN

The safety and effectiveness of Lodine have not been established in children.

Overdosage

Any medication taken in excess can cause symptoms of overdose. If you suspect an overdose, seek medical attention immediately.

The symptoms of Lodine overdose may include:
Drowsiness
Lethargy
Nausea
Stomach pain
Vomiting

Brand name:

LOESTRIN

See Oral Contraceptives, page 437.

Brand name:

LOMOTIL

Generic ingredients: Diphenoxylate hydrochloride, Atropine sulfate

Why is this drug prescribed?
Lomotil is used in the treatment of diarrhea. In severe cases, replacement of lost fluid and electrolytes may also be prescribed.

Most important fact about this drug
Lomotil is not a harmless drug, so never exceed your recommended dosage. Keep the drug out of the reach of children and leave it in a child-resistant container. Overdosage of this medication can suppress breathing and induce coma, possibly leading to permanent brain damage or death. Use this drug with care and caution.

How should you take this medication?
Lomotil can be habit-forming. Take it exactly as prescribed by your doctor.

Lomotil may cause dry mouth. Suck sugarless hard candies or chew sugarless gum if desired.

What side effects may occur?
Side effects cannot be anticipated. If any develop or change in intensity, inform your doctor as soon as possible. Only your doctor can determine if it is safe for you to continue taking Lomotil.

■ Side effects may include:
Abdominal discomfort, confusion, depression, dizziness, dry mouth, feeling of elation, general feeling of not being well, headache, hives, inflammation of the pancreas, intestinal blockage, itching, lack or loss of appetite, loss of muscle function in the lower portion of the intestine, nausea, numbness of arms and legs, restlessness, sedation/drowsiness, sluggishness, swelling due to fluid retention, swelling of the gums, vomiting

■ Lomotil contains atropine sulfate, which may cause the following side effects:
Dryness of the skin and mucous membranes, flushing, inability to urinate, rapid heartbeat, very high body temperature

Why should this drug not be prescribed?
If you are sensitive to or have ever had an allergic reaction to diphenoxylate or atropine, you should not take this medication. Make sure that your doctor is aware of any drug reactions that you have experienced.

Unless you are directed to do so by your doctor, do not take Lomotil if you have obstructive jaundice (a disease in which bile made in the liver does not reach the intestines because of a bile duct obstruction, such as gallstones) or diarrhea associated with pseudomembranous enterocolitis (inflammation of the colon and the small intestine) or enterotoxin-producing bacteria (an enterotoxin is a poisonous substance that affects the stomach and intestines).

Special warnings about this medication
Lomotil may produce drowsiness or dizziness. Therefore, driving a car, operating dangerous machinery, or participating in any hazardous activity that requires full mental alertness is not recommended.

This drug may interrupt peristalsis (contractions of the digestive tract that force food through the tubes and waste toward the anus). This can result in fluid retention in the intestine, which may increase the dehydration and electrolyte imbalance associated with diarrhea.

If you have severe ulcerative colitis, your doctor will want to monitor your condition while you are taking this drug. If your abdomen becomes distended, or enlarged, notify your doctor.

Lomotil should be used with extreme caution if you have kidney and liver disease or if your liver is not functioning normally.

Lomotil should be used with caution in children, since side effects may occur even with recommended doses, especially in patients with Down's syndrome (a congenital disorder that causes mental retardation).

Since addiction to diphenoxylate hydrochloride is possible at high doses, the recommended dosage should never be exceeded.

Possible food and drug interactions when taking this medication

Lomotil may intensify the effects of alcohol. Do not drink alcohol while taking this medication.

If Lomotil is taken with certain other drugs, the effects of either could be increased, decreased, or altered. It is especially important to check with your doctor before combining Lomotil with the following:

Barbiturates (anticonvulsants and sedatives such as phenobarbital)
MAO inhibitors (antidepressants such as Nardil)
Tranquilizers (drugs that produce calming effects such as Xanax)

Special information
If you are pregnant or breastfeeding

The effects of Lomotil during pregnancy have not been adequately studied. If you are pregnant or plan to become pregnant, notify your doctor immediately. Lomotil may appear in breast milk and could affect a nursing infant. If this medication is essential to your health, your doctor may advise you to discontinue breastfeeding until your treatment is finished.

Recommended dosage

ADULTS

The recommended starting dosage is 2 tablets 4 times a day or 10 milliliters (2 regular teaspoonfuls) of liquid 4 times per day.

Most patients will require this dosage until control has been achieved. After that, the dosage may be reduced to meet individual requirements. Control may often be obtained with as little as 5 milligrams (2 tablets or 10 milliliters of liquid) per day.

CHILDREN

Lomotil is not recommended in children under 2 years of age.

A child's nutritional status and degree of dehydration must be considered before this drug is prescribed.

In children under 13 years of age, use only Lomotil liquid and administer with the plastic dropper. The recommended starting dosage is 0.3 to 0.4 milligrams per 2.2 pounds of body weight per day, divided into 4 equal doses. The following table provides approximate starting dosage recommendations for children:

2 years (24-31 pounds)
    1.5-3.0 milligrams/4 times daily
3 years (26-35 pounds)
    2.0-3.0 milligrams/4 times daily
4 years (31-44 pounds)
    2.0-4.0 milligrams/4 times daily
5 years (35-51 pounds)
    2.5-4.5 milligrams/4 times daily
6-8 years (38-71 pounds)
    2.5-5.0 milligrams/4 times daily
9-12 years (51-121 pounds)
    3.5-5.0 milligrams/4 times daily

Your doctor may reduce the dosage as soon as symptoms are controlled. A maintenance dosage may be as low as one-quarter of the starting dose. If no response occurs within 48 hours, Lomotil is unlikely to work.

Overdosage
Symptoms of an overdose of Lomotil may include:
Coma, dryness of skin and mucous membranes, enlargement of the pupils of the eyes, extremely high body temperature, flushing, involuntary eyeball movement, lower than normal muscle tone, pinpoint pupils, rapid heartbeat, restlessness, sluggishness, suppressed breathing

Suppressed breathing may be seen as late as 30 hours after an overdose.

If you suspect an overdose, seek medical attention immediately.

Generic name:

LOPERAMIDE HYDROCHLORIDE

See Imodium, page 288.

Brand name:

LOPID

Generic name: Gemfibrozil

Why is this drug prescribed?
Lopid is prescribed, along with a special diet, for treatment of patients with very high levels of serum triglycerides (a fatty substance in the blood) who are at risk of having pancreatitis (inflammation of the pancreas) and who do not respond adequately to a strict diet.

This drug can also be prescribed to reduce the risk of coronary heart disease in patients who have failed to respond to weight loss, diet, exercise, and other triglyceride- or cholesterol-lowering drugs.

Most important fact about this drug
Lopid should be considered for use only when reasonable attempts to lower cholesterol levels through a regular routine of diet and exercise have failed. However, taking this medication does not reduce the importance of adhering to a diet and exercise program prescribed for you by your doctor.

Excess body weight and excess alcohol intake may be important risk factors leading to a condition in which there is an unusually high content of fat stored in the body. These risk factors should be reduced, if possible, before any drug therapy is attempted.

How should you take this medication?
Take this medication exactly as prescribed by your doctor.

What side effects may occur?
Side effects cannot be anticipated. If any develop or change in intensity, inform your doctor as soon as possible. Only your doctor can determine if it is safe for you to continue taking Lopid.

■ *More common side effects may include:*
Abdominal pain, acute appendicitis, constipation, diarrhea, eczema, fatigue, headache, indigestion, nausea/vomiting, rash, vertigo

■ *Less common or rare side effects may include:*
Anemia, blood disorders, blurred vision, confusion, convulsions, decreased male fertility, decreased sex drive, depression, dizziness, fainting, hives, impotence, inflammation of the colon, irregular heartbeat, itching, joint pain, laryngeal swelling, muscle disease, muscle pain, muscle weakness, painful extremities, sleepiness, synovitis, tingling sensation, weight loss, yellow eyes and skin

Why should this drug not be prescribed?

There is a possibility that Lopid may cause malignancy, gallbladder disease, abdominal pain leading to appendectomy, or other serious, possibly fatal, abdominal disorders. This drug should not be used with patients who have mildly elevated cholesterol levels, since the benefits do not outweigh the severe side effect risks.

If you are sensitive to or have ever had an allergic reaction to Lopid or similar drugs, you should not take this medication. Make sure that your doctor is aware of any drug reactions that you have experienced.

Unless you are directed to do so by your doctor, do not take this medication if you are being treated for severe kidney or liver disorders or gallbladder disease.

Special warnings about this medication

Periodic blood level tests are recommended during the first 12 months of therapy with Lopid because of blood diseases associated with the use of this medication.

Liver disorders have occurred with the use of this drug. Therefore, periodic liver function tests are recommended.

If you are being treated for any disease that contributes to increased blood cholesterol, such as an overactive thyroid, diabetes, nephrotic syndrome (kidney and blood vessel disorder), dysproteinemia (excess of protein in the blood), or obstructive liver disease, consult with your doctor before taking Lopid.

Lopid should begin to reduce cholesterol levels during the first 3 months of therapy. If adequate reduction of cholesterol is not obtained, this medication should be discontinued. Therefore, it is important that your doctor check your progress regularly.

The use of this medication may cause gallstones leading to possible gallbladder surgery. Treatment with this drug should be discontinued if gallstones are found.

The use of this drug may be associated with myositis, a muscle disease. If you have muscle pain, tenderness, or weakness, consult with your doctor. If myositis is suspected, treatment with this drug should be discontinued.

Possible food and drug interactions when taking this medication

If Lopid is taken with certain other drugs, the effects of either could be increased, decreased, or altered. It is especially important to check with your doctor before combining Lopid with the following:

Blood-thinning drugs such as Coumadin
Lovastatin (Mevacor)

Caution should be exercised when anticoagulants (blood thinners) are given in conjunction with Lopid. The dose of the anticoagulant should be reduced to prevent bleeding complications.

In patients who have had an unsatisfactory response to either Lopid or Mevacor, the potential benefit of the combination of these two drugs does not outweigh the risk of severe muscle disease, rhabdomyolysis (a severe disease of the muscles and bones), and acute kidney failure.

Special information
if you are pregnant or breastfeeding

The effects of Lopid during pregnancy have not been adequately studied. If you are pregnant or plan to become pregnant, inform your doctor immediately. Because this medication causes tumors in animals, it may have an effect on nursing infants. If Lopid is essential to your health, your doctor may advise you to discontinue breastfeeding until your treatment with Lopid is finished.

Recommended dosage

ADULTS

The recommended dose is 1,200 milligrams divided into 2 doses, given 30 minutes before the morning and evening meals.

CHILDREN

Safety and effectiveness of Lopid have not been established for use in children.

ELDERLY

This drug should be used with caution in elderly patients.

Overdosage

There have been no reported cases of overdose with Lopid. However, should you suspect symptoms of a Lopid overdose, seek medical attention immediately.

Brand name:

LOPRESSOR

Generic name: Metoprolol tartrate

Why is this drug prescribed?

Lopressor, a type of medication known as a beta blocker, is used in the treatment of high blood pressure, angina pectoris (chest pain, usually caused by lack of oxygen to the heart due to clogged arteries), and heart attack. When prescribed for high blood pressure, it is effective when used alone or in combination with other high blood pressure medications. Beta-blockers decrease the force and rate of heart contractions.

Most important fact about this drug

If you have high blood pressure, you must take Lopressor regularly for it to be effective. Even if you are feeling well, you need the medication to keep your blood pressure under control.

How should you take this medication?

Lopressor should be taken with food or immediately after you have eaten.

Take this medication exactly as prescribed by your doctor, even if your symptoms have disappeared.

Try not to miss any doses. If this medication is not taken regularly, your condition may worsen.

If you forget to take a dose, skip the one you missed and go back to your regular schedule. Never take two doses at the same time.

What side effects may occur?

Side effects cannot be anticipated. If any develop or change in intensity, inform your doctor as soon as possible. Only your doctor can determine if it is safe for you to continue taking Lopressor.

■ *More common side effects may include the following:*
Depression
Diarrhea
Dizziness
Itching
Rash
Shortness of breath
Slow heartbeat
Tiredness

■ *Less common or rare side effects may include:*
Blurred vision, cold hands and feet, confusion, congestive heart failure, constipation, difficult or labored breathing, dry eyes, dry mouth, gas, hair loss, headache, heart attack, heartburn, low blood pressure, muscle pain, nausea, nightmares, rapid heartbeat, ringing in ears, short-term memory loss, stomach pain, swelling due to fluid retention, trouble sleeping, wheezing, worsening of heart block

Why should this drug not be prescribed?

If you have a slow heartbeat, heart block (conduction disorder), low blood pressure, cardiogenic shock, or heart failure, you should not take this medication.

Special warnings about this medication

If you have a history of congestive heart failure, Lopressor should be used with caution.

Do not stop Lopressor abruptly. This can cause increased chest pain and heart attack. Dosage should be gradually reduced.

If you suffer from asthma, seasonal allergies or other bronchial conditions, or liver disease, this medication should be used with caution.

Ask your doctor if you should check your pulse while taking Lopressor. This medication can cause your heartbeat to become too slow.

This medication may mask some symptoms of low blood sugar in diabetics or alter blood sugar levels. If you are diabetic, discuss this with your doctor.

Lopressor may cause you to become drowsy or less alert; therefore, driving or operating dangerous machinery or participating in any hazardous activity that requires full mental alertness is not recommended until you know how you respond to this medication.

Notify your doctor or dentist that you are taking Lopressor if you have a medical emergency or before you have surgery or dental treatment.

Notify your doctor if you have any difficulty in breathing.

Possible food and drug interactions when taking this medication

If Lopressor is taken with certain other drugs, the effects of either could be increased, decreased, or altered. It is especially important to check with your doctor before combining Lopressor with catecholamine-depleting drugs such as reserpine.

Special information if you are pregnant or breastfeeding

The effects of Lopressor during pregnancy have not been adequately studied. If you are pregnant or plan to become pregnant, inform your doctor immediately. Lopressor appears in breast milk and could affect a nursing infant. If this medication is essential to your health, your doctor may advise you to discontinue breastfeeding until your treatment with this medication is finished.

Recommended dosage

ADULTS

Dosages of Lopressor should be individualized by your doctor. It should be taken with or immediately following meals.

Hypertension
The usual starting dosage is a total of 100 milligrams a day in 1 or 2 doses, whether taken alone or with a diuretic. Dosage may be increased gradually up to 400 milligrams a day. Generally, the effectiveness of each dosage increase will be seen within a week.

Angina Pectoris
The usual starting dosage is a total of 100 milligrams a day in 2 doses. Dosage may be increased gradually up to 400 milligrams a day. Generally, the effectiveness of each dosage increase will be seen within a week. If treatment is to be discontinued, this drug should be gradually withdrawn over a period of 1 to 2 weeks.

Heart Attack
Lopressor can be used for treatment of heart attack both in the hospital during the early phases and after a patient's condition is

stabilized. Dosages are prescribed according to the individual patient's needs.

CHILDREN

The safety and effectiveness of Lopressor have not been established in children.

Overdosage

Any medication taken in excess can cause symptoms of overdose. If you suspect an overdose, seek medical attention immediately.

The symptoms of Lopressor overdose may include:
Asthma-like symptoms
Heart failure
Low blood pressure
Slow heartbeat

Brand name:

LOPROX

Generic name: Ciclopirox olamine

Why is this drug prescribed?

Loprox antifungal medication, is prescribed for the treatment of the following skin infections due to various species of fungi:

Athlete's foot
Fungal infection of the groin (jock itch)
Fungal infection of non-hairy parts of the skin
Cutaneous candidiasis (yeastlike fungal
  infection of the skin)
Tinea versicolor—infection of the skin that
  is characterized by yellow or tan
  patches.

Loprox is available in cream and ointment forms.

Most important fact about this drug

Loprox is not for use in the eyes.

How should you use this medication?

Use this medication for the full treatment time even though your symptoms may have improved. Notify your doctor if there is no improvement after 4 weeks.

What side effects may occur?

Loprox rarely causes side effects. If any develop or change in intensity, inform your doctor as soon as possible. Only your doctor can determine if it is safe for you to continue using Loprox.

■ *Rare side effects may include:*
  Burning, itching, redness, worsening of
  infection symptoms

Why should this drug not be prescribed?

If you are sensitive to or have ever had an allergic reaction to ciclopirox olamine or similar drugs, you should not take this medication. Make sure that your doctor is aware of any drug reactions that you have experienced.

Special warnings about this medication

If the affected area of skin shows signs of increased irritation (redness, itching, burning, blistering, swelling, oozing), notify your doctor.

Avoid the use of airtight dressings or bandages.

Special information
if you are pregnant or breastfeeding

The effects of Loprox during pregnancy have not been adequately studied. If you are pregnant or plan to become pregnant, inform your doctor immediately. It is not known whether this drug appears in breast milk. If this medication is essential to your health, your doctor may advise you to discontinue breastfeeding your baby until your treatment is finished.

Recommended dosage

ADULTS

Gently massage Loprox Cream 1% or Lotion 1% into the affected and surrounding skin areas two times a day, in the morning and evening. For most infections, improvement usually occurs within the first week of treatment. Patients with tinea versicolor usually show signs of improvement after 2 weeks of treatment.

CHILDREN

Safety and effectiveness have not been established in children under 10 years of age.

Overdosage

Any medication taken in excess can have serious consequences. If you suspect an overdose, seek medical treatment immediately.

Generic name:

LORAZEPAM

See Ativan, page 44.

Brand name:

LORELCO

Generic name: Probucol

Why is this drug prescribed?

Lorelco is used, along with diet, to lower cholesterol levels in the blood of patients with primary hypercholesterolemia (a genetic defect that causes a lack of low-density lipoprotein [LDL] receptors, which remove cholesterol from the bloodstream). Lorelco lowers *total serum cholesterol,* which means that it not only reduces LDL, or "bad," cholesterol but

may reduce HDL (high-density lipoprotein), or "good," cholesterol. The risk of lowering HDL cholesterol while lowering LDL cholesterol is unknown.

Most important fact about this drug

Lorelco should be considered for use only when reasonable attempts to lower cholesterol levels through a regular routine of diet and exercise, weight reduction, and control of diabetes have failed. However, taking this medication does not reduce the importance of adhering to a diet and exercise program prescribed for you by your doctor.

Before treatment with Lorelco is prescribed, your doctor should test to make sure that your persistently high cholesterol levels are due to a lipid (fat) disorder and not a secondary condition such as hypothyroidism, poorly controlled diabetes, liver disease, or a kidney disorder.

How should you take this medication?

Take this medication exactly as prescribed by your doctor.

What side effects may occur?

Side effects cannot be anticipated. If any develop or change in intensity, inform your doctor as soon as possible. Only your doctor can determine if it is safe for you to continue taking Lorelco.

■ *Side effects when treatment with Lorelco begins may include:*
Brief loss of consciousness or fainting
Chest pain
Dizziness
Nausea
Rapid, strong heartbeat
Vomiting

■ *Side effects during treatment may include:*
Abdominal pain, blurred vision, bruising, conjunctivitis (inflammation of the eyelid), diarrhea, diminished sense of taste and

smell, dizziness, excessive nighttime urination, excessive perspiration, fainting, gas, headache, impotence, inability to fall or stay asleep, indigestion, irregular heartbeat, itching, loss of appetite, nausea, rash, ringing in the ears, stomach or intestinal bleeding, swelling due to fluid retention, tearing, tingling sensation, vomiting

Why should this drug not be prescribed?

If you are sensitive to or have ever had an allergic reaction to Lorelco or similar drugs, you should not use this medication. Make sure that your doctor is aware of any drug reactions that you have experienced.

Unless you are directed to do so by your doctor, do not take this medication if you have had recent heart damage, have progressive heart disease, have serious abnormal heart rhythm, or experience unexplained fainting spells or other conditions that your doctor considers dangerous.

Special warnings about this medication

If you are being treated for any disease that contributes to increased blood cholesterol, such as hyperthyroidism, diabetes, nephrotic syndrome (kidney and blood vessel disorder), or obstructive liver disease, consult with your doctor before taking this medication.

Lorelco should begin to reduce cholesterol levels during the first 3 to 4 months of therapy. If adequate reduction of cholesterol is not obtained, this medication should be discontinued. Therefore, it is important that your doctor check your progress regularly.

Possible food and drug interactions when taking this medication

If Lorelco is taken with certain other drugs, the effects of either could be increased, decreased, or altered. It is especially important to check with your doctor before combining Lorelco with the following:

Antiarrhythmics such as Norpace
Clofibrate (Atromid-S)
Phenothiazines (drugs for depression such as Thorazine and Compazine)
Depression medications known as tricyclic antidepressants such as Elavil

Special information if you are pregnant or breastfeeding

The effects of Lorelco during pregnancy have not been adequately studied. If you are pregnant or plan to become pregnant, inform your doctor immediately. It is recommended that women who plan to become pregnant be withdrawn from this drug and birth control procedures be used for at least six months. Lorelco may appear in breast milk and could affect a nursing infant. If this medication is essential to your health, your doctor may advise you to discontinue breastfeeding until your treatment is finished.

Recommended dosage

ADULTS

The recommended and maximum dose is 1,000 milligrams per day, divided into 2 doses of 500 milligrams each (two 250-milligram tablets or one 500-milligram tablet), taken with the morning and evening meals.

CHILDREN

The safety and effectiveness of this drug have not been established in children.

ELDERLY

This drug should be used with caution in elderly patients.

Overdosage

Any medication taken in excess can cause symptoms of overdose. If you suspect symptoms of a Lorelco overdose, seek medical attention immediately.

Brand name:

LORTAB

See Vicodin, page 678.

Brand name:

LOTENSIN

Generic name: Benazepril hydrochloride

Why is this drug prescribed?
Lotensin, an angiotensin-converting enzyme, is used in the treatment of high blood pressure. It is effective when used alone or in combination with thiazide diuretics. Lotensin is in a family of drugs called ACE inhibitors. It works by preventing a chemical in your blood called angiotensin I from converting into a more potent enzyme that increases salt and water retention in your body. Lotensin also enhances blood flow throughout your blood vessels.

Most important fact about this drug
Since blood pressure lowers gradually, it may take 1 to 2 weeks for the full effect of Lotensin to occur. Even if you are feeling well, you must continue to take the medication to control your blood pressure.

How should you take this medication?
Lotensin can be taken with or without food.

Do not use salt substitutes containing potassium.

Take Lotensin exactly as prescribed by your doctor. Suddenly stopping Lotensin could cause your blood pressure to increase.

What side effects may occur?
Side effects cannot be anticipated. If any develop or change in intensity, inform your doctor as soon as possible. Only your doctor can determine if it is safe for you to continue taking Lotensin.

■ *More common side effects may include:*
Cough
Dizziness
Fatigue
Headache
High potassium levels (dry mouth, excessive thirst, weak or irregular heartbeat, muscle pain or cramps)
Nausea

If you develop swelling of your face, around the lips, tongue, or throat; swelling of arms and legs; sore throat, fever, and chills; or difficulty swallowing, you should contact your doctor immediately. You may need emergency treatment.

■ *Less common or rare side effects may include:*
Allergic reactions, anxiety, arthritis, asthma, bronchitis, chest pain, constipation, dark tarry stool containing blood, decreased sex drive, difficulty sleeping, dizziness when standing, fainting, fluid retention, impotence, infection, inflammation of the skin, inflammation of the stomach, itching, joint pain, low blood pressure, muscle pain, nervousness, pounding heartbeat, rash, shortness of breath, sinus inflammation, sweating, swelling of arms, legs, face, tingling or pins and needles, urinary infections, vomiting, weakness

Why should this drug not be prescribed?
If you are sensitive to or have ever had an allergic reaction to Lotensin or other angiotensin-converting enzyme (ACE) inhibitors, do not take this medication.

Special warnings about this medication
Your kidney function should be assessed when you start taking Lotensin and then monitored for the first few weeks.

Lotensin can cause low blood pressure, especially if you are also taking a diuretic. You may feel lightheaded or faint, especially during the first few days of therapy. If these symptoms occur, contact your doctor. Your dosage may need to be adjusted or discontinued.

If you have congestive heart failure, this drug should be used with caution.

Do not use potassium supplements or salt substitutes containing potassium without talking to your doctor first.

If you develop a sore throat or fever, you should contact your doctor immediately. It could indicate a more serious illness.

Excessive sweating, dehydration, severe diarrhea, or vomiting could make you lose too much water, causing your blood pressure to become too low.

Possible food and drug interactions when taking this medication

If Lotensin is taken with certain other drugs, the effects of either could be increased, decreased, or altered. It is especially important to check with your doctor before combining Lotensin with the following:

Diuretics such as Dyazide, Lasix
Potassium supplements such as Slow-K
Potassium-sparing diuretics such as Moduretic
Lithium (Eskalith)

Special information
if you are pregnant or breastfeeding

Lotensin can cause birth defects, prematurity, or death to the fetus and newborn. If you are pregnant or plan to become pregnant and are taking Lotensin, contact your doctor immediately to discuss the potential hazard to your unborn child. Minimal amounts of Lotensin appear in breast milk. If this medication is essential to your health, your doctor may advise you to discontinue breastfeeding until your treatment with this medication is finished.

Recommended dosage

ADULTS

For patients not taking a diuretic drug, the usual starting dose is 10 milligrams, 1 time per day. Regular total dosages range from 20 to 40 milligrams per day taken in either a single dose or divided into 2 equal doses. The maximum dose is 80 milligrams per day. Your doctor will closely monitor the effect of this drug and adjust it according to the individual patient's needs.

For patients already taking a diuretic, the diuretic should be stopped, if possible, 2 to 3 days before taking Lotensin. This reduces the possibility of fainting or lightheadedness. If blood pressure cannot be controlled by Lotensin alone, then diuretic use should begin again. If the diuretic cannot be discontinued, the starting dosage of Lotensin should be 5 milligrams.

For patients with reduced kidney function, the dosages should be individualized according to the amount of reduced function. The usual starting dose in these instances is 5 milligrams per day, adjusted upwards to a maximum of 40 milligrams per day.

CHILDREN

The safety and effectiveness of Lotensin have not been established in children.

ELDERLY

Lotensin should be used with caution in elderly patients.

Overdosage

Although there is no specific information available, a sudden drop in blood pressure would most likely be the primary symptom of Lotensin overdose.

If you suspect symptoms of a Lotensin overdose, seek medical attention immediately.

Brand name:

LOTRIMIN

Generic name: Clotrimazole
Other brand name: Mycelex

Why is this drug prescribed?
Lotrimin is used to treat Candida (yeast infection), fungus infections in the vagina and fungus skin infections (tinea versicolor). Lotrimin works by inhibiting the growth of certain yeast and fungus organisms.

Most important fact about this drug
Lotrimin should never be used for eye infections.

How should you take this medication?
Wash your hands before and after applying Lotrimin. Gently massage Lotrimin into the affected and surrounding skin area twice a day, in the morning and at night.

What side effects may occur?
Side effects cannot be anticipated. If any develop or change in intensity, inform your doctor as soon as possible. Only your doctor can determine if it is safe for you to continue using Lotrimin.

■ Side effects may include:
  Blistering
  Burning
  Hives
  Irritated skin
  Itching
  Peeling
  Reddened skin
  Stinging
  Swelling due to fluid retention

Why should this drug not be prescribed?
You should not be using Lotrimin if you have had an allergic reaction to it.

Special warnings about this medication
Contact your doctor if you experience increased skin irritations (such as redness, itching, burning, blistering, swelling, or oozing).

Use Lotrimin for the full treatment time, even if your symptoms have improved.

If your symptoms have not improved after 4 weeks of treatment, notify your doctor.

Possible food and drug interactions when taking this medication
None have been reported.

Special information if you are pregnant or breastfeeding
Lotrimin should be used during the first trimester of pregnancy only if clearly needed. Nursing mothers should use Lotrimin cautiously and only when clearly needed.

Recommended dosage

ADULTS, ELDERLY, AND CHILDREN

Wash your hands before and after you use Lotrimin. Apply Lotrimin in the morning and evening. Use enough Lotrimin to massage into the affected area.

Symptoms usually improve during the first week of treatment with Lotrimin.

Overdosage
Although any medication used in excess can cause symptoms of overdose, serious overdose of Lotrimin that is applied to the skin is unlikely. If you suspect symptoms of a serious Lotrimin overdose, however, seek medical help immediately.

Brand name:

LOTRISONE

Generic ingredients: Clotrimazole, Betamethasone dipropionate

Why is this drug prescribed?

Lotrisone, a combination of a corticosteroid (betamethasone) and an antifungal (clotrimazole), is used to treat skin infections caused by fungus, such as athlete's foot.

Betamethasone treats symptoms (such as itching, redness, swelling, and inflammation) that result from fungus infections, while clotrimazole treats the cause of the infection by inhibiting the growth of certain yeast and fungus organisms.

Most important fact about this drug

Lotrisone contains a corticosteroid drug (betamethasone). Corticosteroid drugs can affect hormone levels. Therefore, if you are using a large dose of Lotrisone, you should be evaluated on a regular basis to be certain that your hormones are at their correct levels.

How should you use this medication?

Wash your hands before and after applying Lotrisone. Gently massage Lotrisone into the affected and surrounding skin area twice a day, in the morning and evening.

Lotrisone should be applied sparingly to the groin area, and it should not be used for longer than 2 weeks. Loose-fitting clothing should be worn.

What side effects may occur?

Side effects cannot be anticipated. If any develop or change in intensity, inform your doctor as soon as possible. Only your doctor can determine if it is safe for you to continue using Lotrisone.

■ *More common side effects may include:*
Blistering, hives, infection, irritated skin, itching, peeling, reddened skin, skin eruptions, stinging, swelling due to fluid retention, tingling sensation

■ *Less common side effects may include:*
Acne, burning, dryness, excessive hair growth, inflamed hair follicles, inflamed skin, irritated skin around mouth, loss of skin color

Why should this drug not be prescribed?

You should not use Lotrisone if you are sensitive to its ingredients, clotrimazole and betamethasone, or to other corticosteroid or imidazole medications.

Special warnings about this medication

Corticosteroid drugs (such as betamethasone) can affect the functioning of the adrenal, hypothalamic, and pituitary glands and temporarily produce sugar in the urine, excessive blood sugar levels, and a disorder called Cushing's syndrome. Symptoms of Cushing's syndrome include easily bruised skin, increased blood pressure, low level of potassium, low sex hormone levels, mood swings, water retention, weak muscles, and weight gain.

Lotrisone should never be used for eye infections.

Even if your symptoms have decreased, use Lotrisone for the full treatment time.

If you are using Lotrisone to treat jock itch (tinea cruris) or a fungal infection of the skin, called tinea corporis, and there has been no improvement after 1 week, notify your doctor.

If you are using Lotrisone to treat athlete's foot (tinea pedis), notify your doctor if there is no improvement after 2 weeks of treatment.

Lotrisone should not be used for longer than 4 weeks.

Any skin area treated with Lotrisone should not be bandaged.

Possible food and drug interactions when taking this medication

None have been reported.

Special information
if you are pregnant or breastfeeding

Pregnant women should not use corticosteroid drugs in large amounts or for prolonged periods of time. Lotrisone should be used during pregnancy only if the potential benefits justify the potential risk to the fetus. Nursing mothers should use Lotrisone with caution and only when clearly needed.

Recommended dosage

ADULTS AND CHILDREN OVER
12 YEARS OLD

If you are using a large dose of Lotrisone, you should be evaluated on a regular basis to be certain that your hormones are at their correct levels.

Wash your hands before and after using Lotrisone. Do not bandage any skin area treated with Lotrisone. Wear loose-fitting clothes while being treated with Lotrisone in the groin area.

Improvement usually occurs within 3 to 5 days.

"Jock Itch" (Tinea Cruris) or Fungal Skin Infections (Tinea Corporis)
Gently massage Lotrisone into the affected and surrounding skin areas twice a day, in the morning and the evening, for 2 weeks. Lotrisone should be applied sparingly to the groin area. Notify your doctor if there has been no improvement after 1 week of treatment.

Athlete's Foot (Tinea Pedis)
Gently massage Lotrisone into the affected and surrounding skin areas twice a day, in the morning and the evening, for 4 weeks. Notify your doctor if there has been no improvement after 2 weeks of treatment.

CHILDREN

The safety and effectiveness of Lotrisone have not been established for children under 12 years of age. Children may absorb proportionally larger amounts of topical Lotrisone and be more sensitive to its effects than are adults.

ELDERLY

Elderly patients should use Lotrisone cautiously.

Overdosage

Any medication used in excess can have serious consequences. Serious overdose of Lotrisone that is applied to the skin is unlikely. However, seek medical help immediately if you suspect symptoms of a serious Lotrisone overdose.

Generic name:

LOVASTATIN

See Mevacor, page 371.

Brand name:

LOZOL

Generic name: Indapamide

Why is this drug prescribed?

Lozol is used in the treatment of high blood pressure, either alone or in combination with other high blood pressure medications. Lozol is also used to relieve salt and fluid retention. During pregnancy, Lozol may be prescribed to relieve fluid retention caused by a specific condition or when fluid retention causes extreme discomfort that is not relieved by rest.

Most important fact about this drug
If you have high blood pressure, you must take Lozol regularly for it to be effective. Keep taking Lozol even if you are feeling well. You need the medication to keep your blood pressure under control.

Diuretics can cause your body to lose too much potassium. Ask your doctor for the warning signs of potassium depletion. Also ask whether you should eat specific foods that are rich in potassium or take a potassium supplement to avoid this problem.

How should you take this medication?
Take Lozol exactly as prescribed by your doctor. Suddenly stopping Lozol could cause your condition to worsen.

Lozol is best taken in the morning.

If you forget to take a dose, take Lozol as soon as you remember. If it is almost time for your next dose, skip the one you missed and go back to your regular schedule. Never take two doses at the same time.

What side effects may occur?
Side effects cannot be anticipated. If any side effects develop or change in intensity, tell your doctor immediately. Only your doctor can determine whether it is safe to continue taking Lozol. Most side effects are mild and temporary.

■ *More common side effects may include:*
Agitation
Anxiety
Dizziness
Headache
Irritability

Muscle cramps or spasms
Nervousness
Numbness in hands and feet
Tension
Weakness, fatigue, loss of energy or tiredness

■ *Less common or rare side effects may include:*
Abdominal pain or cramps, blurred vision, constipation, depression, diarrhea, dizziness when standing up too quickly, drowsiness, dry mouth, excessive urination at night, flushing, frequent urination, hives, impotence or reduced sex drive, inflammation of blood vessels, insomnia, irregular heartbeat, itching, light-headedness, loss of appetite, nausea, pounding heartbeat, premature heart contractions, production of large amounts of pale urine, rash, runny nose, stomach irritation, tingling in hands and feet, vertigo, vomiting, weak or irregular heartbeat, weight loss

Why should this drug not be prescribed?
Avoid using Lozol if you are unable to urinate (anuria) or if you have ever had an allergic reaction or are sensitive to indapamide or other sulfa-containing drugs.

Special warnings about this medication
Severely low salt levels and low potassium levels have occurred with Lozol use, especially in elderly women. Symptoms disappear when salt and potassium supplements are given.

Potassium and salt loss are a common occurrence with diuretics. The risk of potassium loss increases when larger doses are used, if you have cirrhosis, or if you are also using corticosteroids or ACTH. Your doctor should check your blood regularly, especially if you have an irregular heartbeat or are taking heart medications.

Lozol should be used with care if you have gout or high uric acid levels, liver disease, diabetes, or lupus erythematosus, a disease of the connective tissue.

This medication should be used with caution if you have severe kidney disease. Your kidney function should be given a complete assessment and should continue to be monitored.

In general, diuretics should not be taken if you are taking lithium, as they increase the risk of lithium poisoning.

Possible food and drug interactions when taking this medication
If Lozol is taken with certain other drugs, the effects of either could be increased, decreased, or altered. It is especially important to check with your doctor before combining Lozol with the following:

Lithium (Lithobid, Eskalith)
Norepinephrine (drug used to treat cardiac arrest and to maintain blood pressure)
Other high blood pressure medications

Special information
if you are pregnant or breastfeeding
If you are pregnant or plan to become pregnant, tell your doctor immediately. No information is available about the safety of Lozol during pregnancy.

Lozol may appear in breast milk and could affect a nursing infant. If Lozol is essential to your health, your doctor may advise you to stop breastfeeding until your treatment is finished.

Recommended dosage
ADULTS

High Blood Pressure and Fluid Buildup in Congestive Heart Failure
The usual starting dose is 2.5 milligrams as a single daily dose taken in the morning.

Your doctor may increase your dosage to 5 milligrams taken once daily to obtain satisfactory response.

In general, doses of 5 milligrams and more do not appear to provide additional effects on blood pressure or heart failure, but are associated with a greater degree of potassium loss.

Overdosage
Any medication taken in excess can have serious consequences. If you suspect an overdose, seek medical treatment immediately.

Symptoms of Lozol overdose may include:
Electrolyte imbalance (potassium or salt depletion due to too much fluid loss)
Nausea
Stomach disorders
Vomiting
Weakness

Brand name:

LUDIOMIL

Generic name: Maprotiline hydrochloride

Why is this drug prescribed?
Ludiomil is used to treat depression and anxiety associated with depression. It is also used for depression in people with manic-depressive illness. Ludiomil is classified as a tetracyclic antidepressant that apparently works by boosting the sensitivity of nerve junctions in the brain.

Most important fact about this drug

Seizures have been associated with Ludiomil, particularly when taken in amounts larger than prescribed, if taken with phenothiazines (such as Stelazine). To reduce the risk of seizures, be sure to follow your doctor's instructions for taking this medication.

How should you take this medication?

The total daily dosage of Ludiomil may be taken in a single daily dose or divided into smaller amounts.

Improvement may not be seen for 2 to 3 weeks. You should not discontinue Ludiomil therapy unless instructed by your doctor.

Ludiomil may cause sensitivity to light. Avoid prolonged exposure to the sun. Use sunscreens and wear protective clothing until you learn your tolerance.

Avoid alcoholic beverages while taking Ludiomil.

What side effects may occur?

Side effects cannot be anticipated. If any develop or change in intensity, inform your doctor as soon as possible. Only your doctor can determine if it is safe for you to continue taking this medication.

■ *More common side effects may include:*
Agitation, anxiety, blurred vision, constipation, dizziness, drowsiness, dry mouth, fatigue, headache, insomnia, nausea, nervousness, tremors, weakness

■ *Rare side effects may include:*
Abdominal cramps, allergies, bitter taste in the mouth, black tongue, bleeding sores, blocked intestine, breast development in the male, breast enlargement in the female, confusion (especially in elderly people), decreased memory, delusions, diarrhea, difficulty swallowing, difficulty urinating, dilated pupils, disorientation, excessive or spontaneous milk excretion, excessive sweating, fainting, feeling of unreality, fever, flushing, frequent urination, hair loss, hallucinations, heart attack, high blood pressure, impotence, increased or decreased libido, increased psychotic symptoms, increased salivation, inflammation of the mouth, involuntary movement, irregular heart rate, low blood pressure, low or high blood sugar, mania, nasal congestion, nightmares, numbness, overactivity, palpitations, rapid heartbeat, red, black and blue spots on skin, restlessness, ringing in the ears, seizures, sensitivity to light, skin itching, skin rash, speech disorder, stomach pain, stroke, swelling due to fluid retention, swelling of testicles, tingling, twitches, unstable movements and gait, vomiting, weight loss or gain, yellowish skin tone

Why should this drug not be prescribed?

Ludiomil should not be used if you have had a recent heart attack.

Do not use Ludiomil if you have taken one of the antidepressant drugs known as MAO inhibitors (Parnate, Nardil), within the preceding 14 days.

Ludiomil should not be used by people who have had seizures.

Do not take Ludiomil if you are known to be hypersensitive to it.

Special warnings about this medication

Use Ludiomil cautiously if you have glaucoma, heart disease, heart attacks, thyroid disease or a history of difficulty urinating.

This drug may impair your ability to drive a car or operate potentially dangerous machinery. Do not participate in any activities that require full alertness if you are unsure of your response to the drug.

Possible food and drug interactions when taking this medication

People who take MAO inhibitors such as Nardil should not take Ludiomil.

If Ludiomil is taken with certain other drugs, the effects of either could be increased, decreased, or altered. It is especially important to check with your doctor before combining Ludiomil with the following:

Anticholinergics (medicines for abdominal complaints, Bentyl)
Benzodiazepines (tranquilizers such as Valium)
Cimetidine (Tagamet)
Guanethidine (Ismelin)
Phenothiazines (anti-psychotic medications such as Stelazine)
Sympathomimetics such as Ventolin
Thyroid medications such as Synthroid

Extreme drowsiness and other potentially serious effects can result if Ludiomil is combined with alcohol, sleeping medications such as Seconal, and other central nervous system depressants.

Special information
if you are pregnant or breastfeeding

The effects of Ludiomil during pregnancy have not been adequately studied. If you are pregnant or plan to become pregnant, inform your doctor immediately. Pregnant women should use Ludiomil only if clearly needed. Ludiomil appears in breast milk and could affect a nursing infant. Women who nurse infants should use the drug cautiously and only when the potential benefits clearly outweigh the potential risks.

Recommended dosage

Dosages should start at a low level and increase gradually if needed.

ADULTS

For Mild to Moderate Depression
Dosages usually start at 75 milligrams a day, taken as a single daily dose or divided into smaller doses. If needed, this amount may gradually be increased to a maximum of 150 milligrams daily.

For Moderate to Severe Depression
For hospitalized patients, dosages as high as 225 milligrams daily may be prescribed.

CHILDREN

Safety for children under 18 years old have not been established.

ELDERLY

For Mild to Moderate Depression
Dosages usually start at 25 milligrams a day. They may range up to 50 to 75 milligrams daily if necessary.

Overdosage

Any medication taken in excess can have serious consequences. An overdose of Ludiomil can be fatal. If you suspect an overdose, seek medical help immediately.

Symptoms of Ludiomil overdose may include:
Agitation, bluish skin, convulsions, dilated pupils, drowsiness, fever, heart failure, involuntary slow, writhing movement with the hands, irregular heart rate, lack of coordination, loss of consciousness, low blood pressure, muscle rigidity, rapid heartbeat, restlessness, shock, vomiting

Brand name:

LURIDE

Generic name: Sodium fluoride

Why is this drug prescribed?

Luride is prescribed to strengthen children's teeth during the period when the teeth are still developing.

Studies have shown that people who live where the drinking water contains a certain level of fluoride have fewer cavities than others. Fluoride helps prevent cavities in three ways: by increasing the teeth's resistance to dissolving on contact with acid, by strengthening teeth, and by slowing down the growth of mouth bacteria.

Luride may be given to children who live where the water fluoride level is 0.7 parts per million or less.

Most important fact about this drug

Before Luride is prescribed, it is important for the doctor to know the fluoride content of the water your child drinks every day. Your water company, or a private laboratory, can tell you the level of fluoride in your water.

How should you take this medication?

Give your child Luride exactly as prescribed by your doctor. It is preferable to give the tablet at bedtime after the child's teeth have been brushed. The youngster may chew and swallow the tablet or simply suck on it until it dissolves. The liquid form of this medicine is to be taken by mouth. It may be dropped directly into the mouth or mixed with water or fruit juice. Always store Luride drops in the original plastic dropper bottle.

What side effects may occur?

Side effects cannot be anticipated. If any side effects develop, tell your doctor immediately. Only your doctor can determine whether it is safe for your child to continue taking Luride.

In rare cases, Luride may cause an allergic rash or some other unexpected effect.

Why should this drug not be prescribed?

Your child should not take Luride if he or she is sensitive to it or has had an allergic reaction to it in the past.

Special warnings about this medication

Do not give full-strength tablets (1 milligram) to children under the age of 3.

Possible food and drug interactions when taking this medication

Avoid giving your child Luride along with dairy products. The calcium in dairy products may interact with the fluoride to create calcium fluoride, which the body cannot absorb well.

Recommended dosage

Since this drug is used to supplement water with low fluoride content, consult your physician to determine the proper amount based on the local water content. Also check with your doctor if you move to a new area, change to bottled water, or begin using a water-filtering device. Dosages are determined by both age and the fluoride content of the water.

INFANTS AND CHILDREN

The following daily dosages are recommended for areas where the drinking water contains fluoride at less than 0.3 parts per million:

Infants to 2 Years of Age
1 quarter-strength (0.25 milligram) tablet
or 2 drops
2 to 3 Years of Age
1 half-strength (0.5 milligram) tablet or
4 drops
3 to 12 Years of Age
1 full-strength (1 milligram) tablet or 8
drops

For areas where the fluoride content of
drinking water is between 0.3 and 0.7
parts per million, the recommended daily
dosage is one-half the above dosages.

Overdosage

Any medication taken in excess can have
serious consequences. Taking too much
fluoride for a long period of time may cause
discoloration of the teeth. Notify your
doctor or dentist if you notice white, brown,
or black spots on the teeth.

Brand name:

MS CONTIN

Generic name: Morphine sulfate

Why is this drug prescribed?

MS Contin, a controlled-release tablet
containing morphine, is used to relieve
moderate to severe pain. While regular
morphine is usually given every four
hours, MS Contin is typically given every 12
hours—only twice a day. MS Contin is
intended for people who need a morphine
painkiller for more than just a few
days.

Most important fact about this drug

Like other narcotics, MS Contin is potentially
addictive. If you take MS Contin for some
time and then stop abruptly, you could
experience withdrawal symptoms. For this
reason, do not make dosage changes on your
own; always consult your doctor.

In the case of terminal illness, it is
inappropriate to worry about addiction;
adequate pain relief should continue even if
treatment eventually does cause drug
dependence.

How should you take this medication?

Take MS Contin exactly as prescribed by your
doctor—typically one tablet every 12
hours. Swallow the tablets whole. If you crush
or chew the tablets, a dangerously large
amount of morphine could enter your
bloodstream all at once.

It is illegal to share MS Contin or any other
potent narcotic painkiller with anyone
else.

Give MS Contin ample time to work before
determining that you need to take more
of this drug.

Do not drink alcoholic beverages while using
MS Contin.

What side effects may occur?

Side effects cannot be anticipated. If any side
effects develop or change in intensity, tell
your doctor immediately. Only your doctor
can determine whether it is safe to
continue taking MS Contin.

As with other narcotics, the most hazardous
potential side effect of MS Contin is
respiratory depression (dangerously slow
breathing). If you are older or debilitated,
you are particularly vulnerable to respiratory
depression; you may be at special risk
at any age if you have a lung or breathing
problem.

Other hazards from MS Contin are apnea
(short periods of arrested breathing),
decreased circulation, shock, and cardiac
arrest.

■ *More common side effects may include:*
  Constipation
  Depressed or irritable mood
  Dizziness
  Euphoria
  Light-headedness
  Nausea
  Sedation
  Sweating
  Vomiting

You may be able to lessen these side effects by lying down.

■ *Less common side effects may include:*
  Agitation, appetite loss, biliary tract spasm, chills, constipation, cramps, diarrhea, dreams, cry mouth, facial flushing, faintness, passing out, hallucinations, disorientation, headache, heart palpitations, high blood pressure, hives, insomnia, itching, larynx spasm, low blood pressure, mood changes, morbid sensations, "pinpoint" pupils, rash, rigid muscles, seizure, sexual drive or performance problems, sweating, swelling, taste alterations, tremor, uncoordinated muscle movements, urine retention or hesitancy, vision disturbances, weakness

If you stop taking MS Contin after a long period of use, you will probably experience some degree of narcotic withdrawal syndrome. Even without treatment, your withdrawal symptoms will probably disappear within a week or two. However, you could experience a second phase of withdrawal, involving aching muscles, irritability, and insomnia, which might last for 2 to 6 months.

Why should this drug not be prescribed?
Do not take MS Contin if you have ever had an allergic reaction or are sensitive to it, or if you have acute or severe bronchial asthma.

If breathing function is depressed, MS Contin should not be given unless there is resuscitation equipment nearby.

MS Contin should not be given to anyone suspected of suffering a failure of normal intestinal activity.

Special warnings about this medication
MS Contin should not be given to anyone who might have a brain injury, or the beginnings of an abdominal problem requiring surgery; the drug could mask the symptoms, making correct diagnosis difficult or impossible.

Caution is advised in giving MS Contin to people facing biliary tract surgery, since the drug could make their condition worse. MS Contin should be given with extreme caution if any of the following are present:

Addison's disease
Alcoholism
Coma
Delirium tremens ("DT's")
Drug-related psychosis
Enlarged prostate or constricted urethra
Hypothyroidism
Kidney disorder
Kyphoscoliosis
Liver disorder
Lung disorder
Swallowing difficulty

If given to an epileptic person, MS Contin could increase the likelihood of a seizure.

Since MS Contin can impair judgment and coordination, do not drive, climb, or operate hazardous equipment while taking this drug.

Possible food and drug interactions when taking this medication
If MS Contin is taken with certain other drugs, the effects of either could be

increased, decreased, or altered. It is especially important to check with your doctor before combining MS Contin with the following:

Alcohol

Certain analgesics such as Talwin, Nubain, Stadol, and Buprenex

General anesthetics

Phenothiazines such as Thorazine and Phenergan

Sedatives or hypnotic drugs such as Dalmane, Valium, Halcion, and Xanax

Skeletal muscle relaxants such as Flexeril and Valium

Tranquilizers such as Librium

Special information
if you are pregnant or breastfeeding

If you are pregnant or plan to become pregnant, inform your doctor immediately. Although there is no evidence so far that a pregnant woman's short-term use of MS Contin can harm her unborn baby, this drug should be taken during pregnancy only if the benefit to the mother justifies a possible risk to the child.

MS Contin is not recommended for use as a painkiller during childbirth. If a woman takes this drug shortly before giving birth, her baby may have trouble breathing.

Babies born to mothers who use morphine chronically may suffer from drug withdrawal symptoms. Since some of the morphine from MS Contin appears in breast milk, do not take this medication while breastfeeding. If you do nurse while using MS Contin, your baby could experience withdrawal symptoms once you stop taking this medication.

Recommended dosage

ADULTS

MS Contin tablets are swallowed whole, and are not to be broken, chewed, or crushed.

Because of the potent nature of MS Contin, your doctor will determine which dosage form will work best and how often you should take the drug based on your individual needs.

Overdosage

Any medication taken in excess can have serious consequence. If you suspect an overdose of MS Contin, seek medical attention immediately.

Symptoms of MS Contin overdose may include:

Cold, clammy skin

Flaccid muscles

Lowered blood pressure

"Pinpoint" pupils

Sleepiness leading to stupor and coma

Slowed breathing

Slow pulse rate

Brand name:

MACROBID

See Macrodantin, page 354.

Brand name:

MACRODANTIN

Generic name: Nitrofurantoin
Other brand name: Macrobid

Why is this drug prescribed?

Nitrofurantoin, an antibacterial drug, is prescribed for the treatment of urinary tract infections caused by certain strains of bacteria.

Because nitrofurantoin is effective against only certain types of bacteria, your doctor may perform appropriate tests before treatment in order to identify the organisms causing infection.

Most important fact about this drug

Respiratory (breathing) disorders have occurred in patients taking nitrofurantoin. The drug can cause inflammation of the lungs characterized by coughing, difficulty breathing and wheezing. Pulmonary fibrosis (an abnormal increase in fibrous tissue of the lungs) can develop gradually without symptoms and can cause death. An allergic reaction to this drug is also possible and may occur without warning. Symptoms include a feeling of ill health and a persistent cough. However, these reactions, occur rarely and generally in patients receiving nitrofurantoin therapy for 6 months or longer.

Sudden and severe lung reactions are characterized by fever, chills, cough, chest pain, and difficulty breathing. These acute reactions usually occur within the first week of treatment and subside when therapy with nitrofurantoin is stopped.

Close monitoring of your condition by your doctor is recommended, especially if you are receiving long-term treatment with this medication. Full recovery from a lung disorder caused by nitrofurantoin depends upon early detection and treatment.

How should you take this medication?

To improve absorption of the drug, nitrofurantoin should be taken with food.

Take this medication exactly as prescribed by your doctor.

What side effects may occur?

Side effects cannot be anticipated. If any develop or change in intensity, inform your doctor as soon as possible. Only your doctor can determine if it is safe for you to continue taking nitrofurantoin.

■ *More common side effects may include:*
Lack or loss of appetite
Nausea
Vomiting

■ *Less common or rare side effects may include:*
Abdominal pain/discomfort, chills, cough, chest pain, diarrhea, difficulty breathing, fever, hair loss, hives, inflammation of the nerves, causing symptoms of numbness, tingling, pain or muscle weakness, itchy, red skin patches, joint pain, muscle pain, peeling skin, rash, skin inflammation, skin swelling or welts, swelling due to fluid retention, yellowing of the skin and whites of the eyes

Why should this drug not be prescribed?

If you are sensitive to or have ever had an allergic reaction to nitrofurantoin or other drugs of this type, you should not take this medication. Make sure that your doctor is aware of any drug reactions that you have experienced.

Unless you are directed to do so by your doctor, do not take this medication if you have a kidney disorder such as anuria (failure of the kidneys to produce urine) or oliguria (production of a small amount of urine by the kidneys).

Nitrofurantoin should not be taken at term of pregnancy, or given to infants under 1 month of age.

Special warnings about this medication

Fatalities have been reported from hepatitis (liver disease) during treatment with nitrofurantoin. Long-lasting, active hepatitis can occur without warning; therefore, patients receiving long-term treatment with this drug should be monitored periodically by their doctor for changes in liver function.

Fatalities from peripheral neuropathy, a nervous system disorder, have been reported in patients taking nitrofurantoin.

If you have a kidney disorder, anemia, diabetes mellitus, an electrolyte imbalance, a debilitating disease, or a vitamin B deficiency, caution should be exercised when taking this medication. Consult with your doctor.

Hemolytic anemia (below-normal hemoglobin content in the blood caused by the destruction of red blood cells) has occurred in patients taking nitrofurantoin.

This drug, in certain unpredictable instances, may affect sperm production, causing a decrease in sperm count.

Continued or prolonged use of this drug may result in growth of bacteria that do not respond to it. This can cause a secondary infection, so it is important that your doctor monitor your condition on a regular basis.

Possible food and drug interactions when taking this medication

If nitrofurantoin is taken with certain other drugs, the effects of either could be increased, decreased, or altered. It is especially important to check with your doctor before combining nitrofurantoin with the following:

Magnesium trisilicate (Gaviscon), a compound of magnesium with antacid and absorbent properties used to treat peptic ulcers and digestive disorders

Uricosuric drugs (medications that increase the amount of the uric acid excreted in the urine, such as the antigout drug, Benemid)

Special information if you are pregnant or breastfeeding

The safety of nitrofurantoin during pregnancy and breastfeeding has not been established. If you are pregnant or breastfeeding or you plan to become pregnant or breastfeed, inform your doctor immediately.

Recommended dosage

Treatment with nitrofurantoin should be continued for 1 week or for at least 3 days after obtaining a urine specimen free of infection. If your infection has not cleared up, your doctor should re-evaluate your case.

ADULTS

The recommended dosage of Macrodantin is 50 to 100 milligrams taken 4 times a day. The lower dosage level is recommended for uncomplicated urinary tract infections as determined by your doctor. For long-term treatment, your doctor may reduce your dosage to 50 to 100 milligrams taken at bedtime.

The recommended dosage of Macrobid is one 100-milligram capsule every 12 hours for 7 days.

CHILDREN

This medication should not be prescribed for children under 1 month of age.

The recommended dosage of Macrodantin for infants and children over 1 month of age is 5 to 7 milligrams per 2.2 pounds of body weight, divided into 4 doses in 24 hours.

For the long-term treatment of children, the doctor may prescribe daily doses as low as 1 milligram per 2.2 pounds of body weight taken in 1 or 2 doses per day.

Overdosage

An overdose of nitrofurantoin has not resulted in any specific symptoms other than vomiting. If vomiting does not occur soon after an excessive dose, it should be induced.

If you suspect an overdose, seek emergency medical treatment immediately.

Generic name:

MAPROTILINE HYDROCHLORIDE

See Ludiomil, page 348.

Brand name:

MAXZIDE

Generic ingredients: Triamterene, Hydrochlorothiazide

Why is this drug prescribed?

Maxzide is a diuretic combination used in the treatment of high blood pressure or other conditions that require the elimination of excess fluid (water) from the body. When used for high blood pressure, Maxzide can be used alone or with other high blood pressure medications. Diuretics help your body produce and eliminate more urine, which helps lower blood pressure. Triamterene, one of the ingredients, helps to minimize potassium loss, which can be caused by the other component, hydrochlorothiazide.

Most important fact about this drug

This medication should be used only if your doctor has determined that the precise amount of each ingredient in Maxzide meets your specific needs. It cannot be exchanged with Dyazide, a combination of the same ingredients in different amounts.

How should you take this medication?

Take Maxzide exactly as prescribed by your doctor. Stopping Maxzide suddenly could cause your condition to worsen.

Avoid potassium-containing salt substitutes, potassium supplements, and potassium-enriched diets.

What side effects may occur?

Side effects cannot be anticipated. If any develop or change in intensity, inform your doctor as soon as possible. Only your doctor can determine if it is safe for you to continue taking Maxzide.

■ *Side effects may include:*
Abdominal cramps, anemia, anxiety, change in potassium levels causing symptoms like dry mouth, excessive thirst, weak or irregular heartbeat, muscle pain or cramps, change in taste, chest pain, constipation, decreased sexual performance, depression, diarrhea, difficulty breathing, difficulty sleeping, discolored urine, dizziness, dizziness on standing up, drowsiness, dry mouth, fatigue, fever, headache, hives, hypersensitivity reaction, inflammation of the pancreas, inflammation of the salivary glands, kidney stones, loss of appetite, muscle cramps, muscle weakness, nausea, rapid heartbeat, rash, reddish or purplish spots on the skin, restlessness, sensitivity to light, shortness of breath, stomach irritation, tingling or pins and needles, vertigo, vision changes, vomiting, yellow eyes and skin

Why should this drug not be prescribed?

If you are unable to urinate or have any serious kidney disease, if you have high potassium levels in your blood, or are taking other drugs that prevent loss of potassium, you should not take this medication.

If you are sensitive to or have ever had an allergic reaction to triamterene, hydrochlorothiazide, or similar drugs, or if you are sensitive to other sulfonamide-derived drugs, you should not take this medication. Make sure that your doctor is aware of any drug reactions that you may have experienced.

Potassium supplements or other diuretics that minimize potassium loss should not be used while taking Maxzide, unless specifically indicated by your doctor.

Special warnings about this medication

If you are taking Maxzide and have kidney disease, a complete assessment of your kidney function should be done; kidney function should continue to be monitored.

If you are taking an ACE-inhibitor type of blood pressure medication such as Vasotec, Maxzide should be used with extreme caution.

If you have liver disease, diabetes, gout, or collagen vascular disease (lupus erythematosus), Maxzide should be used with caution.

If you have bronchial asthma or a history of allergies, you may be at greater risk for an allergic reaction to this medication.

Dehydration, excessive sweating, severe diarrhea or vomiting could deplete your fluids and cause your blood pressure to become too low. Be careful when exercising and in hot weather.

Notify your doctor or dentist that you are taking Maxzide if you have a medical emergency, and before you have surgery.

Possible food and drug interactions when taking this medication

Maxzide may increase the effects of alcohol. Avoid alcohol while taking this medication.

If Maxzide is taken with certain other drugs, the effects of either could be increased, decreased, or altered. It is especially important

to check with your doctor before taking Maxzide with the following:

ACE inhibitors such as Vasotec
Barbiturates such as phenobarbital
Indomethacin (Indocin)
Lithium (Lithobid)
Narcotics such as Percocet
Norepinephrine (Levophed)
Other drugs that minimize loss of potassium
    such as Midamor
Other high blood pressure medications
Potassium-containing salt substitutes
Tubocurarine

Special information
if you are pregnant or breastfeeding

The effects of Maxzide during pregnancy have not been adequately studied. If you are pregnant or plan to become pregnant, inform your doctor immediately. Maxzide appears in breast milk and could affect a nursing infant. If this medication is essential to your health, your doctor may advise you to discontinue breastfeeding until your treatment with this medication is finished.

Recommended dosage

ADULTS

It is important that potassium levels be carefully monitored when you are taking either strength of this medication. Your doctor will adjust dosage based on your individual condition.

The usual dose of Maxzide-25 MG is 1 or 2 tablets a day in a single dose.

The usual dose of Maxzide is 1 tablet daily.

CHILDREN

The safety and effectiveness of Maxzide have not been established in children.

ELDERLY

Dosage should be determined by the particular needs of the elderly patient.

Each tablet of Maxzide contains 75 milligrams of triamterene and 50 milligrams of hydrochlorothiazide.

Each tablet of Maxzide-25 MG contains 37.5 milligrams of triamterene and 25 milligrams of hydrochlorothiazide.

Overdosage

Any medication taken in excess can cause symptoms of overdose. If you suspect an overdose, seek medical attention immediately.

No specific information is available on Maxzide. However, an overdose of triamterene can cause dehydration, nausea, vomiting, weakness, low blood pressure and too much potassium in the blood. An overdose of hydrochlorothiazide can cause dehydration, sluggishness—possibly leading to coma—and stomach and intestinal irritation, as well as lowered blood levels of potassium chloride and sodium.

Generic name:

MECLIZINE HYDROCHLORIDE

See Antivert, page 33.

Generic name:

MECLOFENAMATE SODIUM

See Meclomen, page 359.

Brand name:

MECLOMEN

Generic name: Meclofenamate sodium

Why is this drug prescribed?

Meclomen, a nonsteroidal anti-inflammatory analgesic, is used for the relief of mild to moderate pain. It is also used in the treatment of menstrual pain and heavy menstrual blood loss (when the cause is unknown) and to relieve the inflammation, swelling, stiffness, and joint pain associated with acute and chronic rheumatoid arthritis and osteoarthritis (the most common form of arthritis).

Most important fact about this drug

You should have frequent check-ups with your doctor if you use Meclomen regularly. Ulcers or internal bleeding can occur without warning.

How should you take this medication?

Your doctor may ask you to take Meclomen with food or an antacid to avoid stomach upset. Never take it on an empty stomach.

Take this medication exactly as prescribed by your doctor.

If you are using Meclomen for arthritis, it should be taken regularly.

If you forget to take a dose, take it as soon as you remember. If it is almost time for your next dose, skip the one you missed and go back to your regular schedule. Never take two doses at the same time.

What side effects may occur?

Side effects cannot be anticipated. If any develop or change in intensity, inform your doctor as soon as possible. Only your doctor can determine if it is safe for you to continue taking Meclomen.

■ *More common side effects may include:*
Abdominal pain, constipation, diarrhea, dizziness, gas, headache, heartburn, hives, inflammation of the mouth, itching, loss of appetite, nausea and/or vomiting, peptic ulcer, rash, ringing in ears, swelling due to fluid retention, upset stomach

■ *Less common or rare side effects may include:*
Abdominal bleeding, anemia, blurred vision

and/or vision loss, change in taste, colitis, conjunctivitis, depression, excessive urination at night, fatigue, hair loss, inability to sleep, inflammation of skin, lupus (a disease of the immune system), rapid heartbeat, scaling of skin, skin peeling, tingling or pins and needles, yellow eyes and skin

Why should this drug not be prescribed?

If you are sensitive to or have ever had an allergic reaction to Meclomen, aspirin, or similar drugs (anti-inflammatories), or if you have had asthma attacks caused by aspirin or other drugs of this type, you should not take this medication. Make sure that your doctor is aware of any drug reactions that you have experienced.

Special warnings about this medication

Peptic ulcers and bleeding can occur without warning.

This drug should be used with caution if you have kidney or liver disease.

Do not take aspirin or any other anti-inflammatory medications while taking Meclomen, unless your doctor tells you to do so.

If you are taking this medication for an extended period of time, your doctor should check your blood for anemia.

This medication should not be used for spotting or bleeding between menstrual cycles.

Meclomen may intensify the effects of alcohol. Do not drink alcohol while taking this medication.

This medication may cause vision problems. If you experience any changes in your vision, inform your doctor.

Meclomen may prolong bleeding time. If you are taking blood-thinning medication, this drug should be used with caution.

Meclomen may mask the usual signs of infection. Use with care in the presence of an existing infection.

This drug can cause water retention. It should be used with caution if you have high blood pressure or poor heart function.

Possible food and drug interactions when taking this medication

If Meclomen is taken with certain other drugs, the effects of either could be increased, decreased, or altered. It is especially important to check with your doctor before taking Meclomen with the following:

Anticoagulants (blood thinners)
Aspirin
Methotrexate
The gout medication probenecid

Special information if you are pregnant or breastfeeding

The effects of Meclomen during pregnancy have not been adequately studied. If you are pregnant or plan to become pregnant, inform your doctor immediately. Meclomen appears in breast milk and could affect a nursing infant. If this medication is essential to your health, your doctor may advise you to discontinue breastfeeding until your treatment with this medication is finished.

Recommended dosage

ADULTS

This drug can be taken with milk or at meals.

Mild to Moderate Pain
The usual dose is 50 milligrams every 4 to 6 hours. Higher doses to a maximum of 400 milligrams per day may be needed.

Excessive Menstrual Blood Loss and Pain
The usual dose is 100 milligrams 3 times a day for up to 6 days, starting at the onset of your period.

Rheumatoid Arthritis and Osteoarthritis
The usual dose is a total of 200 to 400 milligrams a day divided into 3 to 4 equal doses. Doses should be adjusted to each individual so that the smallest dose can be used. Maximum daily dose is 400 milligrams.

CHILDREN

The safety and effectiveness of Meclomen have not been established in children under 14 years of age.

ELDERLY

Dosage should be determined by the particular needs of the elderly patient.

Overdosage

Any medication taken in excess can cause symptoms of overdose. If you suspect an overdose, seek medical attention immediately.

Little information is available, but the most common symptoms are:
Agitation
Changes in kidney function
Irrational behavior
Seizures

Brand name:

MEDROL

Generic name: Methylprednisolone

Why is this drug prescribed?

Medrol, a corticosteroid drug, is used to reduce inflammation and improve symptoms in a variety of disorders, including rheumatic arthritis, acute gouty arthritis, and severe cases of asthma. Medrol may be given to people to treat primary or secondary adrenal cortex insufficiency (lack of or insufficient adrenal cortical hormone in the body). It is also given to help treat following disorders:

Severe allergic conditions (drug-induced allergic state)
Blood disorders (leukemia and various anemias)
Certain cancers (along with other drugs)
Skin diseases (severe psoriasis)
Collagen (connective tissue) diseases (systemic lupus erythematosus)
Digestive tract diseases (ulcerative colitis)
High serum levels of calcium associated with cancer
Fluid retention due to nephrotic syndrome (a condition in which damage to kidney causes loss of protein in urine)
Various eye diseases
Lung diseases (tuberculosis)

Most important fact about this drug

Medrol decreases your resistance to infection; thus it is possible to get a new infection while taking this medication. Medrol may also mask some of the signs and symptoms of new infection, which makes it difficult for a doctor to diagnose the problem.

How should you take this medication?

Medrol should be taken exactly as prescribed by your doctor. It can be taken every day or every other day, depending on the condition being treated.

Medrol should not be stopped suddenly without checking with your doctor. If you have been using Medrol for a long time, the dose should be reduced gradually.

Medrol may cause stomach upset. Take Medrol with meals or snacks.

If your doctor has prescribed a single daily dose or alternate-day doses, take this medicine in the morning with breakfast around 8 AM. If you are taking multiple doses, take Medrol at evenly spaced intervals throughout the day.

The lowest possible dose of Medrol should always be used and, as symptoms subside, the dose should be reduced gradually.

What side effects may occur?
Side effects cannot be anticipated. If any side effects develop or change in intensity, tell your doctor immediately. Only your doctor can determine whether it is safe to continue taking Medrol.

■ *Side effects may include:*
Abdominal swelling, allergic reactions, bone fractures, bruising, congestive heart failure, cataracts, convulsions, Cushingoid symptoms (moon face, weight gain, high blood pressure, emotional disturbances, growth of facial hair in women), face redness, fluid and salt retention, glaucoma, high blood pressure, increased eye pressure, increased sweating, increase in amounts of insulin or hypoglycemic medications needed, inflammation of the esophagus, inflammation of the pancreas, irregular menstruation, muscle wasting and weakness, poor healing of wounds, protruding eyes, stomach ulcer, suppression of growth in children, symptoms of diabetes, thin, fragile skin, tiny red or purplish spots on the skin, vertigo

Why should this drug not be prescribed?
Medrol should not be used if you have a fungal infection or if you are sensitive or allergic to steroids (corticosteroids)

Special warnings about this medication
The 24-milligram Medrol tablet contains FD&C Yellow No. 5 (tartrazine), which has caused allergic reactions (including asthma) in some people. Although this is rare, it is more common in people who are sensitive to aspirin.

Medrol can alter the way your body responds to unusual stress. If you are injured, need surgery, or develop an acute illness, inform your doctor. Your dosage may need to be increased.

You should not be vaccinated or immunized while taking Medrol, especially in high doses. Medrol may prevent your body from producing the proper antibodies to build up immunity and may cause nervous system problems.

Long-term use of Medrol may cause cataracts, glaucoma (increased eye pressure), and eye infections.

Large doses of Medrol may cause high blood pressure, salt and water retention, and potassium and calcium loss. It may be necessary to restrict your salt intake and take a potassium supplement.

Medrol may reactivate dormant cases of tuberculosis. If you have inactive tuberculosis and must take Medrol for an extended period of time, your doctor will prescribe anti-TB medication as well.

Medrol should be used cautiously if you have an underactive thyroid, liver cirrhosis, or herpes simplex (virus infection) of the eye.

This medication may aggravate existing emotional problems or cause new ones. You may experience euphoria (an exaggerated sense of well-being) and difficulty sleeping, mood swings, or mental problems. If you have any changes in mood, contact your doctor.

Medrol should also be given with caution if you have any of the following conditions:

Diverticulitis or other inflammatory condition of the intestine
High blood pressure
Certain kidney diseases
Active or dormant peptic ulcer

Myasthenia gravis (a muscle weakness
   disorder)
Osteoporosis (brittle bones)
Ulcerative colitis with impending danger of
   infection

Long-term use of Medrol can slow the growth
and development of infants and children.

Use aspirin cautiously with Medrol if you
have a blood-clotting disorder.

Avoid exposure to chickenpox and measles.

Possible food and drug interactions when taking this medication

If Medrol is taken with certain other drugs,
the effects of either drug could be increased,
decreased, or altered. It is especially
important to check with your doctor before
combining Medrol with the following:

Aspirin
Cyclosporine (Sandimmune)

Special information
If you are pregnant or breastfeeding

If you are pregnant or plan to become
pregnant, tell your doctor immediately.
There is no information about the safety of
Medrol during pregnancy. Babies born to
mothers who have taken doses of Medrol
(corticosteroids) during pregnancy should
be carefully watched for adrenal problems.

Medrol may appear in breast milk and could
affect a nursing infant. If Medrol is
essential to your health, your doctor may
advise you to stop breastfeeding until your
treatment with Medrol is finished.

Recommended dosage

The starting dose of Medrol tablets may vary
from 4 milligrams to 48 milligrams per
day, depending on the specific problem being
treated.

Once the doctor is satisfied with your
response, he will gradually lower the
dosage to the smallest effective amount.

Overdosage

Any medication taken in excess can have
serious consequences. If you suspect an
overdose, seek medical treatment immediately.

Symptoms of Medrol overdose may include:
Acid indigestion
Excessive sweating
Fatigue
Muscle weakness
Swelling of arms and legs
Upset stomach

Generic name:

MEDROXYPROGESTERONE ACETATE

See Provera, page 521.

Generic name:

MEFENAMIC ACID

See Ponstel, page 492.

Brand name:

MEGACE

Generic name: Megestrol acetate

Why is this drug prescribed?

Megace is a synthetic progestational drug (a
drug that has the same effect as the
female hormone progesterone) that is used
to treat cancer of the breast and uterus.
Megace is usually prescribed when a tumor
cannot be removed by surgery or tumor
has recurred after surgery, or when other
drugs or radiation therapy are ineffective.

Most important fact about this drug

Megace is not effective in preventing miscarriage. In the vast majority of women, the cause of miscarriage is a defective egg, which cannot be corrected with medication. Furthermore, several reports suggest that the use of progestational drugs in the early months of pregnancy can cause birth defects.

How should you take this medication?

Take this medication exactly as prescribed by your doctor.

Megace works best when taken on an empty stomach, but this drug can be taken with food if it upsets your stomach.

What side effects may occur?

Side effects cannot be anticipated. If any develop or change in intensity, inform your doctor as soon as possible. Only your doctor can determine if it is safe to continue taking Megace.

■ *A frequent side effect is:*
  Weight gain

■ *Less common side effects may include:*
  Breakthrough bleeding, carpal tunnel syndrome, fluid retention, hair loss, high blood pressure, increase in blood sugar, nausea, rash, shortness of breath, tumor flare, vomiting

■ *Rare side effects may include:*
  Blood clots in lung, inflammation of a vein (thrombophlebitis)

Why should this drug not be prescribed?

Megace should not be used as a diagnostic test for pregnancy.

Special warnings about this medication

Avoid becoming pregnant while taking this medication. Megace can cause damage to a fetus and should not be used during pregnancy.

Possible food and drug interactions when taking this medication

No interactions have been reported.

Special Information if you are pregnant or breastfeeding

The use of Megace during the first 4 months of pregnancy is not recommended. If you are pregnant or plan to become pregnant, notify your doctor immediately. Because there is the possibility of adverse effects on the newborn, nursing should be discontinued if Megace is required for the treatment of cancer.

Recommended Dosage

ADULTS

Breast Cancer
The usual dose is 160 milligrams per day (40 milligrams, taken 4 times a day).

Endometrial Cancer
The usual dose is 40 to 320 milligrams per day, taken in divided doses.

It takes at least 2 months of continuous treatment with Megace before its effectiveness can be evaluated.

Overdosage

Although no specific information about Megace is available, any medication taken in excess can have serious consequences. If you suspect an overdose, seek medical treatment immediately.

Generic name:

MEGESTROL ACETATE

See Megace, page 363.

Brand name:

MELLARIL

Generic names: Thioridazine hydrocholoride

Why is this drug prescribed?
Mellaril is used to reduce the symptoms of psychotic disorders, such as schizophrenia, and to treat depression and anxiety in adults. Mellaril is also used in the treatment of agitation, fears, sleep disturbances, and anxiety in elderly people, and for certain behavior problems in children.

Most important fact about this drug
Mellaril may cause tardive dyskinesia—a condition marked by involuntary muscle spasms and twitches in the face and body. This condition may be permanent, and appears to be most common among the elderly, especially women. Ask your doctor for information about this possible risk.

How should you take this medication?
If you are taking Mellaril in a liquid concentrate form, you will need to dilute it with a liquid such as distilled water, soft tap water, or juice. Mellaril tastes best if it is diluted immediately prior to using.

Do not change from one brand to another without consulting your doctor.

You should not take Mellaril with alcohol.

What side effects may occur?
Side effects cannot be anticipated. If any develop or change in intensity, inform your doctor as soon as possible. Only your doctor can determine if it is safe for you to continue taking Mellaril.

■ Side effects may include:
Abnormal lack of movement, abnormal muscle rigidity, abnormal secretion of milk, agitation, anemia, asthma, blurred vision, breast development in males, changed mental state, changes in sex drive, chewing movements, confusion (especially at night), constipation, diarrhea, difficulty urinating, discolored eyes, drowsiness, dry mouth, excitement, eye spasms, eyes in a fixed position, eyeball rotation or state of fixed gaze, fever, fluid accumulation and swelling, headache, inhibition of ejaculation, intestinal blockage, involuntary movements, irregular blood pressure, pulse and heartbeat, irregular or missed menstrual periods, jaw spasm, loss or increase of appetite, mouth puckering, muscle rigidity, narrow pupils, nasal congestion, nausea, overactivity, pain in the shoulder and neck area, painful muscle spasm, paleness, protruding tongue, psychotic reactions, puffing of cheeks, rapid heartbeat, redness of the skin, restlessness, rigid arms, feet, head, and muscles, rigidity and masklike face, sensitivity to light, skin itching, pigmentation, rash (inflammation, eruptions), sluggishness, strange dreams, sweating, swelling in the throat, swelling of breasts, swollen glands, tremors, vomiting, weight gain, yellowing of the skin and whites of eyes

Why should this drug not be prescribed?
Do not give Mellaril to a comatose person. Do not take this drug if you are taking central nervous system depressants (such as alcohol, barbiturates, or narcotics) or if you have heart disease accompanied by severe high or low blood pressure.

Special warnings about this medication
Before using Mellaril, tell your doctor if you have ever had glaucoma; heart, liver, lung, kidney, or thyroid disease; or if you are exposed to extreme heat or pesticides.

This drug may impair your ability to drive a car or operate potentially dangerous machinery. Do not participate in any activities that require full alertness if you are unsure about your ability.

Mellaril may cause false positive results in tests for pregnancy and phenylketonuria (a birth defect involving damage to the central nervous system).

Possible food and drug interactions when taking this medication

If Mellaril is taken with certain other drugs, the effects of either could be increased, decreased, or altered. It is especially important to check with your doctor before combining Mellaril with the following:

Epinephrine
Pindolol (Visken)
Propranolol (Inderal)

Extreme drowsiness and other potentially serious effects can result if Mellaril is combined with alcohol or other central nervous system depressants such as narcotics, painkillers, and sleeping medications.

Special information
If you are pregnant or breastfeeding

Pregnant women should use Mellaril only if clearly needed. If you are pregnant or plan to become pregnant, inform your doctor immediately. Mellaril may appear in breast milk and can affect a nursing infant.

Recommended dosage

Doses should be tailored to the individual. The smallest effective amount should be used.

ADULTS

For Psychotic Disorders
The initial dose ranges from 150 to 300 milligrams a day. This amount is divided into 3 equal doses. If needed, this amount may be increased to 800 milligrams a day, taken in 2 to 4 small doses. Once symptoms improve, dosages should be decreased to the minimum amount needed.

For Treatment of Depression and Anxiety
The initial dose is 75 milligrams a day. This amount is divided into 3 doses per day. Doses may range from 20 to 200 milligrams a day, divided into 2 to 4 doses.

CHILDREN

For Treatment of Behavior Problems
Mellaril should not be given to children younger than 2 years old. For children 2 to 12 years old, doses are determined by body weight. Total daily doses range from .05 milligram to 3 milligrams for every 2.2 pounds of body weight.

The usual beginning dose for children with moderate disorders is from 20 to 30 milligrams a day.

ELDERLY

In general, elderly people take dosages of Mellaril in the lower range. Elderly people (especially elderly women) may be more susceptible to tardive dyskinesia—a possibly irreversible condition marked by involuntary muscle spasms and twitches in the face and body. Elderly people should consult their doctor for information about these potential risks.

The usual starting dosage 25 milligrams 3 times a day. The total dosage ranges from 20 to 200 milligrams a day, divided into 2 to 4 doses.

For Treatment of Depression, Anxiety and Sleep Disturbances
The initial dose is 75 milligrams a day. This amount is divided into 3 doses per day. Doses may range from 20 to 200 milligrams a day, divided into 3 or 4 doses.

Overdosage

Any medication taken in excess can have serious consequences. An overdose of Mellaril can be fatal. If you suspect an overdose, seek medical help immediately.

Symptoms of Mellaril overdose may include:
Agitation
Coma
Convulsions
Dry mouth
Extreme drowsiness
Extreme low blood pressure
Fever
Intestinal blockage
Irregular heart rate
Restlessness

Generic name:

MEPERIDINE HYDROCHLORIDE

See Demerol, page 175.

Generic name:

MEPROBAMATE

See Miltown, page 382.

Generic name:

MESALAMINE

See Rowasa, page 556.

Brand name:

METAPREL

See Alupent, page 20.

Generic name:

METAPROTERENOL SULFATE

See Alupent, page 20.

Generic name:

METHAZOLAMIDE

See Neptazane, page 412.

Generic name:

METHENAMINE AND BELLADONNA ALKALOIDS

See Urised, page 664.

Brand name:

METHERGINE

Generic name: Methylergonovine maleate

Why is this drug prescribed?

Methergine, a blood-vessel constrictor, is given to prevent or control hemorrhage from the uterus following childbirth. It works by causing the uterine muscles to contract, therefore reducing the mother's blood loss. Methergine comes in tablet or injectable forms.

Most important fact about this drug

Some blood-vessel disorders and certain infections make use of Methergine dangerous. Make sure your doctor is aware of these and other medical conditions.

How should you take this medication?

Take Methergine tablets exactly as prescribed by your doctor. If you miss a dose of this medicine, do not take the missed dose at all and do not double the next one. Instead, go back to your regular schedule.

What side effects may occur?
Side effects cannot be anticipated. If any develop or change in intensity, inform your doctor as soon as possible. Only your doctor can determine if it is safe for you to continue taking Methergine.

■ *More common side effects may include:*
High blood pressure, which may cause a headache or even a seizure. In some people however, Methergine may cause low blood pressure.

Nausea and vomiting occasionally occur as side effects of Methergine.

■ *Rare side effects may include:*
Bad taste, blood in urine, chest pains (temporary), diarrhea, dizziness, edema, hallucinations, leg cramps, nasal congestion, noise in ears, palpitations, shortness of breath, sweating

Why should this drug not be prescribed?
You should not take Methergine if you are allergic to it, if you are pregnant, or if you have high blood pressure or toxemia.

Special warnings about this medication
It may be dangerous to take Methergine if you have an infection, certain blood vessel disorders, or a liver or kidney problem. Inform your doctor if you think you have any such condition.

Possible food and drug interactions when taking this medication
If Methergine is taken with certain other drugs, the effects of either may be increased, decreased or altered. It is especially important to check with your doctor before combining Methergine with the following:

Other blood-vessel constrictors such as Epipen
Other ergot-derived medications such as
  Ergotrate

Special information if you are pregnant or breastfeeding
Methergine should not be taken during pregnancy. Although no specific information is available about possible effects of Methergine on a nursing baby, the general rule is that a mother who is breastfeeding should not take any drug unless it is clearly needed.

Recommended dosage
The usual dose is 1 tablet, 0.2 milligram, 3 or 4 times daily after childbirth for a maximum of 1 week.

Overdosage
Any medication taken in excess can have serious consequences. If you suspect symptoms of a Methergine overdose, seek medical attention immediately.

Symptoms of Methergine overdose may include:
Abdominal pain, coma, convulsions, elevated blood pressure, hypothermia (drop in body temperature), lowered blood pressure, nausea, numbness, slowed breathing, tingling of the extremities, vomiting

Generic name:

METHOCARBAMOL

See Robaxin, page 549.

Generic name:

METHOTREXATE

Brand name: Rheumatrex

Why is this drug prescribed?
Methotrexate is an anticancer drug used in the treatment of lymphoma (cancer of the lymph nodes) and certain forms of leukemia. It is also given to treat some forms of

cancers of the uterus, breast, lung, head and neck, and ovary. Methotrexate is also given to treat rheumatoid arthritis when other treatments have proved ineffective, and is sometime used to treat very severe and disabling psoriasis (a skin disease characterized by thickened patches of red, inflamed skin often covered by silver scales).

Most important fact about this drug

It is important to remember that in the treatment of psoriasis and rheumatoid arthritis methotrexate is taken once a week, not once a day. Accidentally taking the recommended weekly dosage on a daily basis can lead to fatal overdosage. Be sure to read the patient instructions that come with the package.

How should you take this medication?

Before you start taking methotrexate, you should have a chest X-ray plus blood tests to determine your blood cell counts, liver enzyme levels, and the efficiency of your kidney function. While you are taking methotrexate, the blood tests should be repeated at regular intervals; if you develop a cough or chest pain, the chest X-ray should be repeated.

Take methotrexate exactly as prescribed, and promptly report to your doctor any new symptoms that may develop.

Methotrexate is given at a higher dosage for cancer than for psoriasis or rheumatoid arthritis. After high-dose methotrexate treatment, a drug called leukovorin may be given to limit the toxic effects.

What side effects may occur?

Side effects cannot be anticipated. If any develop or change in intensity, inform your doctor as soon as possible. Only your doctor can determine whether it is safe for you to continue taking methotrexate.

■ *More common side effects may include:*
Abortion, acne, blurred vision, chills and fever, decreased resistance to infection, diarrhea, dizziness, fatigue, flu-like general discomfort, hair loss, headaches, hives, infection of hair follicles, loss of appetite, mouth ulcers or sores on the lips, nausea or vomiting, rash or itching, red patches on skin, sore throat, stomach pain, sun sensitivity, vaginal discharge, weakness

■ *Rare side effects may include:*
Abnormal behavior, abnormal reflexes, back pain, chest pain, confusion, cough, diabetes, fever, irritability, loss of coordination, loss of sexual desire, muscular pain, ringing in the ears, shortness of breath, sleepiness, sweating

If you are taking methotrexate for psoriasis, you may also experience hair loss and/or sun sensitivity, and your patches of psoriasis may seem to burn.

Methotrexate can sometimes cause serious lung damage that makes it necessary to curtail the treatment. If you experience a dry cough, fever, or breathing difficulties while taking methotrexate, be sure to tell your doctor right away.

During and immediately after treatment with methotrexate, fertility may be impaired. Men may have an abnormally low sperm count; women may have menstrual irregularities.

Why should this drug not be prescribed?

Do not take this medication if you are sensitive to it or it has given you an allergic reaction.

Methotrexate treatment is not suitable for you if you suffer from psoriasis or rheumatoid arthritis and also have one of the following conditions:

Abnormal blood cell count
Alcoholic liver disease or other chronic liver
   disease
Alcoholism
Immune-system deficiency

Special warnings about this medication

Older or physically debilitated people are
particularly vulnerable to toxic effects
from methotrexate.

Methotrexate should be administered with
great caution if you have any of the
following:

Active infection
Peptic ulcer
Ulcerative colitis

Possible food and drug interactions
when taking this medication

If you are being given methotrexate for the
treatment of cancer or psoriasis, you
should not take aspirin or other nonsteroidal
painkillers such as Advil or Naprosyn;
this combination could increase the toxic
effects of methotrexate. If you are taking
methotrexate for rheumatoid arthritis, you
may be able to continue taking aspirin
or a nonsteroidal painkiller, but your doctor
should monitor you carefully.

Other drugs that may increase the toxic effects
of methotrexate include:

Cisplatin (Platinol), an anticancer drug
Phenylbutazone (Butazolidin)
Phenytoin (Dilantin), a seizure medication
Probenecid (Benemid), a gout medication
Sulfonamides such as Bactrim, Gantrisin, and
   others

The sulfa drug Bactrim may increase
methotrexate's toxic effect on the bone
marrow, where new blood cells are made.

Certain antibiotics, including tetracycline and
chloramphenicol, may reduce the
effectiveness of methotrexate. This is also true
of vitamin preparations that contain folic
acid.

Special information
if you are pregnant or breastfeeding

A woman should not start methotrexate
therapy until the doctor is sure she is not
pregnant. Because methotrexate causes birth
defects and miscarriages, it must not be
taken during pregnancy. In fact, a couple
should avoid pregnancy if either the man
or the woman is taking methotrexate. After
the end of methotrexate treatment, a man
should wait at least 3 months, and a woman
should wait for the completion of at least
one menstrual cycle, before attempting to
conceive a child.

Methotrexate should not be given to a woman
who is breastfeeding; it does pass into
breast milk and may harm a nursing baby.

Recommended dosage

Treatment with methotrexate is highly
individualized. Your doctor will carefully
tailor your dosage of methotrexate in order
to avoid serious side effects and possible
under- or over-dosing.

Overdosage

Taken in excess, methotrexate can cause
serious and even fatal damage to the liver,
kidneys, bone marrow, lungs, or other parts
of the body. Symptoms of overdosage may
include lung or breathing problems, mouth
ulcers, or diarrhea. Initially, however,
serious damage caused by methotrexate may
be apparent only in the results of blood
tests. For this reason, careful, regular
monitoring by your doctor is necessary.
If for any reason you suspect symptoms of
an overdose of methotrexate, seek medical
attention immediately.

Generic name:

METHYCLOTHIAZIDE

See Enduron, page 235.

Generic name:

METHYLDOPA

See Aldomet, page 15.

Generic name:

METHYLERGONOVINE MALEATE

See Methergine, page 367.

Generic name:

METHYLPHENIDATE HYDROCHLORIDE

See Ritalin, page 546.

Generic name:

METHYLPREDNISOLONE

See Medrol, page 361.

Generic name:

METHYLTESTOSTERONE

See Android, page 29.

Generic name:

METHYSERGIDE MALEATE

See Sansert, page 565.

Generic name:

METOCLOPRAMIDE HYDROCHLORIDE

See Reglan, page 534.

Generic name:

METOLAZONE

See Zaroxolyn, page 694.

Generic name:

METOPROLOL TARTRATE

See Lopressor, page 337.

Generic name:

METRONIDAZOLE

See Flagyl, page 259.

Brand name:

METRYL

See Flagyl, page 259.

Brand name:

MEVACOR

Generic name: Lovastatin

Why is this drug prescribed?

Mevacor is used, along with diet, to lower cholesterol levels in the blood of patients with primary hypercholesterolemia (too much cholesterol), a genetic condition that causes a lack of the low-density lipoprotein (LDL) receptors that remove cholesterol from the bloodstream. However, Mevacor is usually prescribed only when a low-fat, and low-cholesterol diet do not lower cholesterol levels enough.

Most important fact about this drug

Mevacor should be considered for use only when reasonable attempts to lower cholesterol levels through a regular routine of diet and exercise and, if necessary, weight reduction have failed. Even though you are taking this medicine, you must stick to a diet and exercise program prescribed for you by your doctor.

Studies have established that high LDL (low-density lipoprotein) cholesterol and low HDL (high-density lipoprotein) cholesterol are both risk factors for coronary heart disease. Lowering LDL cholesterol with diet and medication can decrease the rate of non-fatal heart attacks and death from heart disease.

How should you take this medication?

Take Mevacor exactly as prescribed by your doctor.

Mevacor should be taken with meals.

What side effects may occur?

Mevacor is generally well tolerated. Any side effects that have occurred have usually been mild and short-lived. If any side effects develop or change in intensity, inform your doctor as soon as possible. Only your doctor can determine if it is safe for you to continue taking Mevacor.

■ *Side effects may include:*
  Abdominal pain/cramps, altered sense of taste, blurred vision, constipation, diarrhea, dizziness, gas, headache, heartburn, indigestion, itching, muscle cramps, muscle pain, nausea, rash, weakness

Why should this drug not be prescribed?

If you are sensitive to or have ever had an allergic reaction to Mevacor, or similar (anti-cholesterol) drugs, you should not take this medication. Make sure that your doctor is aware of any drug reactions that you have experienced.

Unless you are directed to do so by your doctor, do not take this medication if you are being treated for an acute muscle disease or liver disease or are at risk of developing kidney failure because of muscle tumors.

Do not take this drug if you are pregnant or nursing.

Special warnings about this medication

If you are being treated for any disease that contributes to increased blood cholesterol, such as hypothyroidism, diabetes, nephrotic syndrome (kidney and blood vessel disorder), dysproteinemia (an excess of protein in the blood), or liver disease, consult with your doctor before taking this medication.

It is recommended that liver function tests be performed by your doctor before treatment with Mevacor begins, every 6 weeks during the first 3 months of therapy, every 8 weeks during the rest of the first year, and periodically (about 6-month intervals) thereafter.

This drug should be used with caution if you consume substantial quantities of alcohol or have a past history of liver disease.

Possible food and drug interactions when taking this medication

If Mevacor is taken with certain other drugs, the effects of either could be increased, decreased, or altered. It is especially important to check with your doctor before combining Mevacor with the following:

Blood-thinning drugs such as Coumadin Cyclosporine (Sandimmune) and other
  immunosuppressive drugs (medication
  that lowers the body's defense reaction
  to a foreign or invading substance)

Erythromycin
Gemfibrozil (Lopid)
Nicotinic acid or niacin (Nicobid)

If you are taking Mevacor in combination with nicotinic acid or with immunosuppressive drugs such as cyclosporine, your doctor should carefully monitor you for any signs and symptoms of muscle pain, tenderness, or weakness, especially with fever or general bodily discomfort, particularly during the starting months of therapy and any time your dose is increased.

Special information
if you are pregnant or breastfeeding

Mevacor should be administered to women of childbearing age only when such patients are highly unlikely to conceive. If you become pregnant while taking this drug, discontinue using it and notify your physician immediately. There may be a potential hazard to the fetus. This medication may appear in breast milk and may have an effect on nursing infants. If this medication is essential to your health, you should discontinue breastfeeding until your treatment with this medication is finished.

Recommended dosage

ADULTS

The recommended starting dose is 20 milligrams once a day, taken with the evening meal. The maximum recommended dose is 80 milligrams per day, taken as a single dose or divided into smaller doses, as determined by your doctor. Adjustments to any dose, as determined by your doctor, should be made at intervals of 4 weeks or more.

If you are taking immunosuppressive drugs in combination with Mevacor, your dose should begin with 10 milligrams and should not exceed 20 milligrams per day.

Cholesterol levels should be monitored periodically by your doctor. He may decide to reduce the dose if your cholesterol level falls below the targeted range.

In patients with reduced kidney function, dosage should be increased above 20 milligrams a day very cautiously.

CHILDREN

The safety and effectiveness of this drug have not been established in children.

ELDERLY

This drug should be used with caution in elderly patients.

Overdosage

There have been no reported cases of overdose with Mevacor. However, if you suspect an overdose, seek medical attention immediately.

Generic name:

MEXILETINE HYDROCHLORIDE

See Mexitil, page 373.

Brand name:

MEXITIL

Generic name: Mexiletine hydrochloride

Why is this drug prescribed?

Mexitil is used to treat severe irregular heartbeat (arrhythmias). Irregular heart rhythms are generally divided into two main types: heartbeats that are faster than normal (tachycardia), or heartbeats that are slower than normal (bradycardia). Arrhythmias are often caused by drugs or disease but can occur in otherwise healthy people with no history of heart disease or other illness.

Most important fact about this drug
Your doctor should carefully monitor your heartbeat to make sure Mexitil is producing the desired effect.

How should you take this medication?
Mexitil should be taken with food or an antacid.

Take this medication exactly as prescribed by your doctor.

If you are taking Mexitil, forget to take a dose, and remember within 4 hours, take it as soon as you remember. If more than 4 hours has passed, skip the missed dose and return to your regular schedule. Never take two doses at the same time.

What side effects may occur?
Side effects cannot be anticipated. If any develop or change in intensity, inform your doctor as soon as possible. Only your doctor can determine if it is safe for you to continue taking Mexitil.

■ *More common side effects may include:*
Abdominal pain/cramps, appetite changes, blurred vision, changes in sleep habits, chest pain, possibly crushing, confusion, constipation, depression, diarrhea, dizziness, dry mouth, fatigue, fever, headache, heartburn, joint pain, light-headedness, nausea, nervousness, numbness, poor coordination, pounding heartbeat, rash, ringing in ears, shortness of breath, speech difficulties, swelling due to fluid retention, tingling or pins and needles, tremors, upset stomach, vision changes, vomiting, weakness, worsening of irregular heartbeat

■ *Less common or rare side effects may include:*
Behavior changes, congestive heart failure, decreased sex drive, difficulty swallowing, difficulty urinating, excessive perspiration, fainting, hallucinations, hair loss, hepatitis, hiccups, high blood pressure, hot flashes, impotence, irregular heartbeat, loss of consciousness, low blood pressure, peptic ulcer, seizures, short-term memory loss, skin inflammation, skin peeling, sore throat, vague feeling of bodily discomfort

Why should this drug not be prescribed?
This drug should not be used if you have heart failure, heart block (a conduction disorder) without a pacemaker, or structural heart disease or if you have recently had a heart attack.

Special warnings about this medication
If you have heart block and have a pacemaker, you should be continuously monitored while taking Mexitil.

Mexitil can aggravate low blood pressure and severe congestive heart failure and should be used cautiously by people with these conditions.

You should be monitored carefully if you have liver disease or abnormal liver function as a result of congestive heart failure.

Avoid diets that change the pH (acid/alkaline content) of your urine. A significant pH change will alter the excretion of Mexitil from your body. Talk to your doctor or pharmacist about proper diet.

Blood disorders have occurred with Mexitil use. Make sure your doctor performs periodic blood tests while you are using this medication.

If you have a seizure disorder, Mexitil should be used with caution.

Possible food and drug interactions when taking this medication
If Mexitil is taken with certain other drugs, the effects of either may be increased, decreased, or altered. It is especially important

that you consult with your doctor before taking any of the following:

Antacids such as Maalox
Caffeine products such as No-Doz
Cimetidine (Tagamet)
Other antiarrhythmic drugs such as Norpace and Quinidex
Phenobarbital
Phenytoin (Dilantin)
Rifampin (Rifadin)
Theophylline products such as Theo-Dur

Special Information
if you are pregnant or breastfeeding

The effects of Mexitil during pregnancy have not been adequately studied. If you are pregnant or plan to become pregnant, inform your doctor immediately. Mexitil appears in breast milk and could affect a nursing infant. If this medication is essential to your health, your doctor may advise you to discontinue breastfeeding until your treatment is finished.

Recommended dosage

Treatment is usually begun in the hospital.

ADULTS

The dosage of Mexitil must be adjusted to each individual patient's needs on the basis of response and tolerance to effects of the drug that are related to the dose.

The usual starting dose is 200 milligrams every 8 hours when quick control of an arrhythmia is not necessary. A minimum of 2 to 3 days between dose adjustments is recommended. Dosage may be adjusted up or down in 50- or 100-milligram increments.

Satisfactory control can be achieved in most patients with 200 to 300 milligrams taken every 8 hours with food or antacids.

If satisfactory response has not been achieved at 300 milligrams every 8 hours, a dose of 400 milligrams every 8 hours may be used.

Total daily dose should not exceed 1,200 milligrams.

When it is essential to immediately control a ventricular arrhythmia (irregular beats in the heart's two main chambers), an initial dose of 400 milligrams of Mexitil may be given, followed by a 200-milligram dose in 8 hours. Effects of this drug are usually seen within 30 minutes to 2 hours.

Your doctor will closely monitor the effects of this drug to make sure the desired effect is achieved and your dose is adjusted properly.

In general, patients with reduced kidney function will require the usual doses of Mexitil, but patients with severe liver disease may require lower doses and must be monitored closely.

Some patients who tolerate this drug well may be transferred to a 12-hour dosage schedule that will make it easier and more convenient to take Mexitil. If adequate effects are achieved on a Mexitil dose of 300 milligrams or less every 8 hours, your doctor may decide to divide the daily total into 2 doses given every 12 hours.

CHILDREN

The safety and efficacy of this drug have not been established in children.

ELDERLY

The use of this drug by an elderly patient should be carefully monitored, and dosages should be adjusted according to the individual patient's needs.

Overdosage

Any medication taken in excess can have serious consequences. There have been deaths reported with Mexitil overdose. If you suspect an overdose, seek medical attention immediately.

The symptoms of Mexitil overdose may include:
Low blood pressure
Nausea
Seizures
Slow heartbeat
Tingling or pins and needles

Generic name:

MICONAZOLE NITRATE

See Monistat, page 390.

Brand name:

MICRO-K

Generic name: Potassium chloride
Other brand names: Klor-Con, Slow-K

Why is this drug prescribed?
Micro-K is used to treat or prevent low potassium levels in people who may face potassium loss caused by digitalis (Lanoxin) and non-potassium-sparing diuretics (such as Diuril and Dyazide) and certain diseases.

Potassium plays an essential role in the proper functioning of a wide range of systems in the body, including the kidneys, muscles, and nerves. As a result, a potassium deficiency may have a wide range of effects, including dry mouth, thirst, reduced urination, weakness, fatigue, drowsiness, low blood pressure, restlessness, muscle cramps, abnormal heart rate, nausea, and vomiting.

Micro-K, Klor-Con, and Slow-K are slow-release potassium formulations.

Most important fact about this drug
There have been reports of intestinal and gastric ulcers and bleeding associated with use of slow-release potassium chloride medications. Micro-K should be used only by people who cannot take potassium chloride in liquid or effervescent forms.

Do not change from one brand of potassium chloride to another without consulting your doctor or pharmacist.

How should you take this medication?
Micro-K should be taken with meals and with water or some other liquid.

Tell your doctor if you have difficulty swallowing Micro-K. You may sprinkle the contents of the capsule onto a spoonful of soft food. Tablets should not be crushed, chewed, or sucked.

What side effects may occur?
Side effects cannot be anticipated. If any develop or change in intensity, inform your doctor as soon as possible. Only your doctor can determine if it is safe for you to continue taking Micro-K.

■ *Side effects may include:*
Diarrhea
Nausea
Stomach pain or discomfort
Stomach and intestinal ulcers and bleeding, blockage, or perforation
Vomiting

Why should this drug not be prescribed?
You should not be using Micro-K in a solid form if you are taking any drug or have any condition that could stop or slow Micro-K as it goes through the gastrointestinal tract.

If you have high potassium levels, you should not use Micro-K.

Special warnings about this medication
Before taking Micro-K, tell your doctor if you have ever had acute dehydration, heat cramps, adrenal insufficiency, diabetes, heart disease, kidney disease, liver disease, ulcers, or severe burns.

Possible food and drug interactions when taking this medication

If Micro-K is taken with certain other drugs, the effects of either could be increased, decreased, or altered. It is important to check with your doctor before combining Micro-K with the following:

ACE inhibitors such as Vasotec and Capoten
Anticholinergic drugs such as Bentyl
Digitalis (Lanoxin)
Potassium-sparing diuretics such as Midamor and Aldactone

Also tell your doctor if you use salt substitutes.

Special information
if you are pregnant or breastfeeding

Micro-K is generally considered safe for pregnant women or women who breastfeed their babies.

Recommended dosage

Dosages must be adjusted for each individual. Following are typical dosages of Micro-K.

ADULTS

To Treat Low Potassium Levels

Micro-K, Klor-Con 8, Slow-K
The usual dosage is 5 to 12 tablets or capsules per day.

Micro-K 10, Klor-Con 10
4 to 10 tablets or capsules per day.

To Prevent Low Potassium Levels

Micro-K, Klor-Con 8, Slow-K
The usual dosage is 2 or 3 tablets or capsules per day.

Micro-K 10, Klor-Con 10
2 tablets or capsules per day.

If you are taking more than 2 tablets or capsules per day, your total daily dose should be divided into smaller doses.

CHILDREN

It has not been determined if Micro-K is safe for children.

ELDERLY

Elderly patients should use Micro-K cautiously.

Overdosage

Any medication taken in excess can have serious consequences. Overdoses of Micro-K may result in potentially fatal levels of potassium. Overdose symptoms may not be noticeable in their early stages. Therefore, if you have any reason to suspect an overdose, seek medical help immediately.

Symptoms of potassium overdose may include:
Blood in stools
Cardiac arrest
Irregular heartbeat
Muscle paralysis
Muscle weakness

Brand name:

MICRONASE

Generic name: Glyburide
Other brand name: Diabeta

Why is this drug prescribed?

Micronase is an oral antidiabetic medication used to treat Type II (non-insulin-dependent) diabetes. Diabetes occurs when the body either does not make enough insulin or when the insulin that is produced no longer works properly. Insulin works by helping sugar get inside the cell, where it is then used for energy.

There are two forms of diabetes: Type I (insulin-dependent) and Type II (non-insulin-dependent). Type I diabetes usually requires insulin injection for life, while Type II diabetes can usually be treated by dietary changes, exercise and/or oral antidiabetic medications such as Micronase. This medication controls diabetes by stimulating the pancreas to secrete more insulin and by helping insulin to work better. Occasionally, Type II diabetics must take insulin injections, sometimes only temporarily during stressful periods or times of illness or, if an oral antidiabetic medication fails to control blood sugars on a long-term basis.

Most important fact about this drug

Micronase-type drugs may possibly lead to more heart problems than diet treatment alone or treatment with diet and insulin. If you have heart problems, you may want to discuss this with your doctor.

Always consider Micronase an addition to, not a substitute for, diet therapy. The safest and most desirable way to control Type II diabetes is to keep your weight and blood sugar down through diet and exercise. Micronase or another antidiabetic drug should be considered only if a diet and exercise program fail to correct your high blood sugar.

How should you take this medication?

In general, Micronase should be taken with breakfast or the first main meal of the day.

To help prevent low blood sugar levels (hypoglycemia), you should:

Understand the symptoms of hypoglycemia.
Know how exercise affects your blood sugar levels.
Maintain an adequate diet.
Keep a source of quick-acting sugar product with you at all times.

What side effects may occur?

Side effects cannot be anticipated. If any develop or change in intensity, inform your doctor as soon as possible. Only your doctor can determine if it is safe for you to continue taking Micronase.

Many side effects from Micronase are rare and seldom require discontinuation of the medication.

■ *More common side effects may include:*
Bloating
Heartburn
Nausea

■ *Less common or rare side effects may include:*
Anemia and other blood disorders, blurred vision, changes in taste, headache, hepatic porphyria (a condition frequently characterized by sensitivity to light, stomach pain and nerve damage, caused by excessive levels of porphyrin in the liver), hepatitis, hives, itching, skin rash, skin eruptions

Micronase, like all oral antidiabetics, may cause hypoglycemia (low blood sugar). The risk of hypoglycemia can be increased by missed meals, alcohol, other medications, fever, trauma, infection, surgery, or excessive exercise. To avoid hypoglycemia, you should closely follow the dietary and exercise plan suggested by your physician.

Symptoms of mild hypoglycemia may include:
Cold sweat
Drowsiness
Fast heartbeat
Headache
Nausea
Nervousness

Symptoms of more severe hypoglycemia may include:
Coma
Pale skin
Seizures
Shallow breathing

Contact your doctor immediately if these symptoms of severe low blood sugar occur.

Ask your doctor what you should do if you experience mild hypoglycemia. If hypoglycemia becomes severe, breathing may become shallow, the skin may become pale, and seizures or coma may result. Severe hypoglycemia should be considered a medical emergency, and prompt medical attention is essential.

Why should this drug not be prescribed?
You should not take Micronase if you have had an allergic reaction to it.

Micronase should not be taken if you are suffering from diabetic ketoacidosis (a life-threatening medical emergency caused by insufficient insulin and marked by excessive thirst, nausea, fatigue, pain below the breastbone, and fruity breath).

In addition, Micronase should not be used as the sole therapy in treating Type I (insulin-dependent) diabetics.

Special warnings about this medication
If you are taking Micronase, you should check your blood or urine periodically for abnormal sugar (glucose) levels.

It is important that you closely follow the diet and exercise plan recommended by your doctor.

Even patients with well-controlled diabetes may find that stress, illness, surgery, or fever result in a loss of control over their diabetes. In these cases, the patient's physician may recommend that Micronase be discontinued temporarily and injected insulin administered.

In addition, the effectiveness of any oral antidiabetic, including Micronase, may decrease with time. This may occur either because of a diminished responsiveness to the medication or a worsening of the diabetes.

Like other antidiabetic drugs, Micronase may produce severe low blood sugar if the dosage is wrong. While taking Micronase, you are particularly susceptible to episodes of low blood sugar if: you suffer from a kidney or liver problem; you have a lack of adrenal or pituitary hormone; or you are elderly, run-down, malnourished, hungry, exercising heavily, drinking alcohol, or using more than one glucose-lowering drug.

Possible food and drug interactions when taking this medication
If Micronase is taken with certain other drugs, the effects of either could be increased, decreased, or altered. It is especially important to check with your doctor before combining Micronase with the following:

Adrenal corticosteroids such as prednisone
Anabolic steroids such as testosterone or
    danazol
Beta blockers such as Inderal or Tenormin
Calcium channel blockers such as Cardizem,
    Procardia
Chloramphenicol (Chloromycetin)
Coumarins such as Coumadin
Estrogens such as Premarin
Furosemide (Lasix)
Isoniazids such as Laniazid, Rifamate, or
    Tubizid
MAO inhibitors such as Nardil or Parnate
Nicotinic acid (Niacin, Nicobid)
Nicolar
Nonsteroidal anti-inflammatory agents such
    as Advil, aspirin, Butazolidin, Motrin,
    Naprosyn, or Nuprin
Miconazole
Oral contraceptives
Phenytoin (Dilantin)
Phenothiazines such as Stelazine or Mellaril

Probenecid (Benemid, ColBENEMID)
Sulfonamides such as Sulfocetamide
Sympathomimetics such as Proventil or
　　Ventolin
Thiazide diurctics such as Diuril or
　　HydroDIURIL
Thyroid medication such as Synthroid or
　　Proloid

Alcohol must be used carefully, since excessive
alcohol consumption can cause low blood
sugar, and may produce such symptoms as
headaches, nausea, chest pains, low blood
pressure, blurred vision, dizziness and
confusion.

Special information
if you are pregnant or breastfeeding

The effects of Micronase during pregnancy
have not been adequately studied in
humans. This drug should be used during
pregnancy only if the benefit outweighs
the potential risk to the unborn baby. Since
studies suggest the importance of
maintaining normal blood sugar (glucose)
levels during pregnancy, your physician
may prescribe injected insulin during
pregnancy.

While it is not known if Micronase enters
breast milk, other similar medications do.
Therefore, patients should discuss with their
doctors whether to discontinue the
medication or to stop breastfeeding. If the
medication is discontinued, and if diet
alone does not control glucose levels, then
insulin injection should be considered.

Recommended dosage

Dosage levels must be determined based on
each patient's needs.

ADULTS

Usually an initial daily dose of 2.5 to 5
milligrams is recommended. Maintenance
therapy usually ranges from 1.25 to 20

milligrams daily. Daily doses greater than
20 milligrams are not recommended. In most
cases once-a-day dosing is recommended;
however, patients taking more than 10
milligrams a day may respond better to
twice-a-day dosing.

CHILDREN

The safety and effectiveness of Micronase have
not been established in children.

ELDERLY

Elderly, malnourished or debilitated patients,
or patients with impaired kidney and liver
function, usually receive lower initial and
maintenance doses to minimize the risk of
low blood sugar (hypoglycemia).

Overdosage

An overdose of Micronase can cause low
blood sugar (hypoglycemia.)

Symptoms of mild hypoglycemia may include:
Cold sweat
Drowsiness
Fast heartbeat
Headache
Nausea
Nervousness

*Symptoms of more severe hypoglycemia
include:*
Coma
Pale skin
Seizure
Shallow breathing

Contact your doctor immediately if these
symptoms of severe low blood sugar
occur. Eating sugar or a sugar-based product
will often correct mild hypoglycemia. If
you suspect symptoms of a Micronase
overdose, seek medical attention
immediately.

Brand name:

MIDRIN

Generic ingredients: Isometheptene mucate, Dichloralphenazone, Acetaminophen

Why is this drug prescribed?
Midrin is prescribed for the treatment of headaches, including vascular (e.g., migraine) and tension headaches.

Most important fact about this drug
Midrin is only used after the headache starts. It is not used to prevent headaches.

How should you take this medication?
You should start taking Midrin at the first sign of a migraine attack.

Do not take more than the maximum dose of Midrin.

Take this medication exactly as prescribed by your doctor.

What side effects may occur?
Side effects cannot be anticipated. If any side effects develop or change in intensity, tell your doctor immediately. Only your doctor can determine whether it is safe to continue taking Midrin.

■ *Side effects may include:*
Short periods of dizziness
Skin rash

Why should this drug not be prescribed?
Unless directed to do so by your doctor, do not take Midrin if you have glaucoma and/or severe kidney disease, high blood pressure, organic heart disease (physical defect of the heart), liver disease, or if you are currently taking antidepressant drugs known as MAO inhibitors, such as Nardil.

Special warnings about this medication
Exercise caution when taking Midrin if you have high blood pressure or any abnormal condition of the blood vessels outside of the heart, or after recent cardiovascular attacks (heart attack or blood vessel disorders).

Possible food and drug interactions when taking this medication
If you are taking antidepressants known as MAO inhibitors, for example, Nardil, check with your doctor before taking Midrin.

Acetaminophen, one of the ingredients contained in Midrin, is also present in many nonprescription pain relievers such as Tylenol. Taking these pain relievers with Midrin could lead to an overdose of acetaminophen and possible liver damage. Consult your doctor before taking any nonprescription pain medication while you are taking Midrin.

Special information if you are pregnant or breastfeeding
If you are pregnant, plan to become pregnant, or are breastfeeding your baby, check with your doctor before taking Midrin.

Recommended dosage

ADULTS

Relief of Migraine Headache
The usual dosage is 2 capsules at once, followed by 1 capsule every hour until headache is relieved, up to 5 capsules within a 12-hour period.

Relief of Tension Headache
The usual dosage is 1 or 2 capsules every 4 hours up to a maximum of 8 capsules a day.

Overdosage
Any medication taken in excess can have serious consequences. If you suspect a Midrin overdose, seek emergency medical treatment immediately.

Brand name:

MILTOWN

Generic name: Meprobamate
Other brand name: Equanil

Why is this drug prescribed?

Miltown is a tranquilizer used in the treatment of anxiety disorders and for short-term relief of the symptoms of anxiety.

Most important fact about this drug

Tolerance and dependence can occur with the use of Miltown. You may experience withdrawal symptoms if you stop using this drug abruptly. Discontinue this drug or change your dose only on your doctor's advice.

If you develop a skin rash, sore throat, fever, or shortness of breath, contact your doctor immediately. You may be having an allergic reaction to the drug.

How should you take this medication?

Take Miltown exactly as prescribed by your doctor. If you forget to take a dose, take it as soon as you remember. If it is almost time for your next dose, skip the one you missed and go back to your regular schedule. Never take two doses at the same time.

What side effects may occur?

Side effects cannot be anticipated. If any develop or change in intensity, inform your doctor as soon as possible. Only your doctor can determine if it is safe for you to continue taking Miltown.

■ *More common side effects may include:*
Diarrhea, dizziness, drowsiness, fainting, feeling of well-being, headache, inappropriate excitement, itchy rash, loss of muscle coordination, nausea, rapid or irregular heartbeat, skin eruptions, slurred speech, swelling due to fluid retention, tingling sensation, vertigo, vision problems, vomiting, weakness

■ *Less common or rare side effects may include:*
Breathing difficulty, chills, high fever, inflammation of mouth, redness and swelling of skin, Stevens-Johnson syndrome (peeling skin)

■ *Side effects due to rapid decrease in dose or abrupt withdrawal from Miltown:*
Anxiety
Confusion
Convulsions
Hallucinations
Inability to fall or stay asleep
Lack or loss of appetite
Lack or loss of muscle control
Muscle twitching
Tremors
Vomiting

Withdrawal symptoms usually become apparent within 12 to 48 hours after discontinuation of this medication.

Why should this drug not be prescribed?

If you are sensitive to or have ever had an allergic reaction to Miltown or similar drugs such as carisoprodol (Soma), you should not take this medication.

Anxiety or tension related to everyday stress usually does not require treatment with Miltown. Discuss your symptoms thoroughly with your doctor.

Special warnings about this medication

Miltown may cause you to become drowsy or less alert; therefore, driving or operating dangerous machinery or participating in any hazardous activity that requires full mental alertness is not recommended.

Long-term use of this drug should be evaluated by your doctor periodically for its usefulness.

If you have liver or kidney disorders, check with your doctor before using this medication.

If you have epilepsy, use of this drug may bring on seizures. Consult with your doctor before taking it.

Possible food and drug interactions when taking this medication

Miltown is a central nervous system depressant and may intensify the effects of alcohol. Do not drink alcohol while taking this medication.

If Miltown is taken with certain other drugs, the effects of either could be increased, decreased, or altered. It is especially important to check with your doctor before combining Miltown with mood-altering drugs and other central nervous system depressants such as the following:

Antidepressant drugs known as MAO
   inhibitors (Nardil, others)
Barbiturates such as Seconal or phenobarbital
Major tranquilizers known as phenothiazines
Narcotics such as Percocet or Demerol

Special information
if you are pregnant or breastfeeding

Do not take Miltown if you are pregnant or planning to become pregnant. There is an increased risk of birth defects. Miltown appears in breast milk and could affect a nursing infant. If this medication is essential to your health, your doctor may advise you to discontinue breastfeeding until your treatment is finished.

Recommended dosage

ADULTS

Miltown 200 and 400
The usual dosage is 1,200 milligrams to 1,600 milligrams per day divided into 3 or 4 doses. A daily dose above 2,400 milligrams is not recommended.

Miltown 600
The usual dose is 1 tablet, 2 times a day. A daily dose above 2,400 milligrams is not recommended.

CHILDREN

Miltown 200 and 400
The usual dose for children 6 to 12 years of age is 200 to 600 milligrams per day divided into 2 or 3 doses.

Miltown 200 and 400 are not recommended for use in children under age 6.

Miltown 600 is not recommended for use in children.

ELDERLY

The usual dose should be limited to the smallest effective amount as determined by your doctor to avoid oversedation.

Overdosage

Any medication taken in excess can cause symptoms of overdose. If you suspect an overdose, seek medical attention immediately.

The symptoms of Miltown overdose may include:
Coma
Drowsiness
Lack or loss of muscle control
Shock
Sluggishness and unresponsiveness

Brand name:

MINIPRESS

Generic name: Prazosin hydrochloride

Why is this drug prescribed?

Minipress is used to treat high blood pressure. It is effective when used alone or when used with other high blood pressure medications such as diuretics or beta-blocking medications (drugs that ease heart contractions), such as Tenormin.

Minipress is also prescribed for the treatment of benign prostatic hyperplasia (BPH), an abnormal enlargement of the prostate gland.

Most important fact about this drug

If you have high blood pressure, you must take Minipress regularly for it to be effective. Even if you are feeling well, you must continue to take Minipress. If you stop, your high blood pressure will return.

How should you take this medication?

Minipress can be taken with or without food.

This medication should be taken exactly as prescribed by your doctor even if your symptoms have disappeared.

Try not to miss any doses. If this medication is not taken regularly, your blood pressure will increase.

If you forget to take a dose, take it as soon as you remember. If it is almost time for your next dose, skip the one you missed and go back to your regular schedule. Never take two doses at the same time.

What side effects may occur?

Side effects cannot be anticipated. If any develop or change in intensity, inform your doctor as soon as possible. Only your doctor can determine if it is safe for you to continue taking Minipress.

■ *More common side effects may include:*
Dizziness
Drowsiness
Headache
Lack of energy
Nausea
Palpitations (pounding heartbeat)
Weakness

■ *Less common side effects may include:*
Blurred vision, constipation, depression, diarrhea, dizziness on standing up, dry mouth, fainting, fluid retention, frequent urination, nasal congestion, nervousness, nosebleeds, rash, red eyes, shortness of breath, vertigo, vomiting

■ *Rare side effects may include:*
Abdominal discomfort/pain, excessive perspiration, fever, hair loss, hallucinations, impotence, inability to hold urine, inflammation of the pancreas, itching, itchy, purple spots on wrists, forearms, thighs, joint pain, persistent, painful erection, rapid heartbeat, ringing in ears, tingling or pins and needles

Why should this drug not be prescribed?

There are no known reasons to avoid this drug.

Special warnings about this medication

Minipress can cause low blood pressure, especially when you first start taking the medication. This can cause you to become faint, dizzy, or lightheaded, particularly on standing up. You should avoid driving or any hazardous tasks where injury could occur for 24 hours after taking the first dose or after your dose has been increased.

Dizziness, fainting, or lightheadedness may also occur in hot weather, when exercising, or when standing for long periods of time. Ask your doctor what precautions you should take.

Possible food and drug interactions when taking this medication

Minipress can intensify the effects of alcohol. Be careful of the amount you drink.

If Minipress is taken with certain other drugs, the effects of either could be increased, decreased, or altered. It is especially important that you check with your doctor before combining Minipress with the following:

Beta blockers such as Inderal
Diuretics such as Dyazide
Estrogen-containing drugs
Other high blood pressure medications

Special information
if you are pregnant or breastfeeding

The effects of Minipress during pregnancy have not been adequately studied. If you are pregnant or plan to become pregnant, notify your doctor immediately. Minipress appears in breast milk and can affect a nursing infant. If this medication is essential to your health, your doctor may advise you to discontinue breastfeeding until your treatment is finished.

Recommended dosage

ADULTS

Dosages of this drug should be adjusted by your doctor according to each individual patient's blood pressure response.

The usual starting dose is 1 milligram, 2 or 3 times per day.

To determine an individual's regular dose, this medication may be slowly increased up to 20 milligrams per day, divided into smaller doses. The commonly prescribed daily dose is 6 milligrams to 15 milligrams per day, divided into smaller doses. Although doses higher than 20 milligrams per day have not been found to be effective, there are some patients who may benefit from a daily dose of 40 milligrams, divided into smaller doses.

If Minipress is used with a diuretic or other high blood pressure drug, the dose can be reduced to 1 to 2 milligrams, 3 times a day.

CHILDREN

The safety and effectiveness of this drug has not been established in children.

Overdosage

Any medication taken in excess can have serious consequences. If you suspect symptoms of a Minipress overdose, seek medical treatment immediately.

The symptoms of Minipress overdose may include:
Extreme drowsiness
Low blood pressure

Brand name:

MINOCIN

Generic name: Minocycline hydrochloride

Why is this drug prescribed?

Minocin is a form of the antibiotic tetracycline. It is given to help treat many different kinds of infection, including:

Acne
Amebic dysentery
Anthrax (a rare skin infection)
Cholera
Gonorrhea (when penicillin cannot be given)
Plague
Respiratory infections
Rocky Mountain spotted fever
Syphilis
Urinary tract infections caused by certain microbes

Most important fact about this drug

Some microbes, including many types of strep bacteria, cannot be killed by Minocin. For this reason, you should not be given Minocin to treat strep throat or any other strep infection unless a sensitivity test (e.g., a throat culture) shows that Minocin can kill the particular bacteria that have infected you.

How should you take this medication?

Take Minocin exactly as prescribed by your doctor. You may take the capsules with or without food. Your doctor will prescribe Minocin for a specific number of days according to the condition you are being treated for; keep taking the medication until you have used it all up.

Minocin may cause dizziness, lightheadedness, and feeling of whirling motion. You should use caution while driving or performing tasks that require mental alertness.

The liquid form of Minocin may be kept in the refrigerator. Do not freeze. Shake well before using.

To reduce the risk of throat irritation, take the tablet and capsule forms of minocycline with plenty of fluids.

Avoid prolonged exposure to sunlight.

You should avoid use of antacids such as Maalox and Mylanta, and iron preparations such as Feosol. If you must take these medicines, take them 2 to 3 hours before or after taking Minocin.

What side effects may occur?

Side effects cannot be anticipated. If any develop or change in intensity, inform your doctor as soon as possible. Only your doctor can determine if it is safe for you to continue taking Minocin.

■ *Side effects may include:*
Aching, inflamed joints, anal or genital sores with fungus infection, anaphylaxis (life-threatening allergic reaction), anemia, appetite loss, blurry vision, diarrhea, difficulty swallowing, discoloration of children's teeth, fluid retention, headache, hepatitis, hives, inflammation of the intestines, inflammation of the tongue, nausea, rash, sensitivity to light, skin coloration, skin inflammation and peeling, throat irritation, vomiting

Why should this drug not be prescribed?

Do not take Minocin if you have ever had an allergic reaction to it or to any other tetracycline antibiotic.

Although Minocin may be given to kill meningococcal (spinal) bacteria in people who are carriers, it should not be given to treat actual meningococcal meningitis (inflammation in the spinal canal).

Minocin is not a first-choice drug for treating any staphylococcal ("staph") infection.

Special warnings about this medication

If you have a kidney problem, a normal dose of Minocin may amount to an overdose for you. It is likely that you will need a lower-than-average dosage; if you need to take Minocin for an extended period of time, your doctor may order frequent blood tests to make sure you are not getting too much of the drug.

Because Minocin may make you dizzy or lightheaded, do not drive, climb, or perform hazardous tasks until you know how the medication affects you.

Minocin should not be given to children 8 years old or younger, since it may cause discoloration of the teeth. Occasionally, Minocin has also caused tooth discoloration in adults.

Like other tetracycline antibiotics, Minocin may cause a sensitivity to light, and you may sunburn very easily. Be careful in sun and under sunlamps. If your skin turns red and hot, stop taking Minocin immediately.

While taking Minocin you may be especially susceptible to fungus infections (e.g., vaginal yeast infection). If you do get a fungus infection, you should stop taking Minocin and seek treatment for the new infection.

If you get a headache and blurry vision while taking Minocin, or if an infant receiving Minocin develops bulging of the "soft spots" (fontanels) on the head, this could mean that the drug is causing a buildup of fluid within the skull. It is important to stop taking Minocin and see a doctor immediately.

Possible food and drug interactions when taking this medication

If Minocin is taken with certain other drugs, the effects of either could be increased, decreased, or altered. It is especially important to check with your doctor before combining Minocin with the following:

Oral contraceptives such as Ortho Novum
Blood thinners such as Coumadin and
   Panwarfin
Penicillin
Iron-containing preparations
Antacids containing aluminum, calcium, or
   magnesium
Penthrane, a general anesthetic

Special information if you are pregnant or breastfeeding

If you are pregnant or plan to become pregnant, inform your doctor immediately. If you take Minocin during the second half of pregnancy, it may cause permanent yellow, gray, or brown discoloration of your baby's teeth.

There is reason to believe that taking Minocin during pregnancy could also harm the baby in other ways. Therefore, Minocin should be taken during pregnancy only if an antibiotic is clearly needed and only if a non-tetracycline antibiotic cannot be used instead. Because Minocin does make its way into breast milk and could harm the baby, it should not be taken by a woman who is breastfeeding. If this drug is essential to your health, your doctor may advise you to discontinue breastfeeding until treatment is finished.

Recommended dosage

The usual dosage and number of times Minocin is taken per day differ from that of the other tetracyclines.

You may experience more side effects if you take more than the recommended dosage.

ADULTS

The usual dosage of Minocin is 200 milligrams to start with, followed by 100 milligrams every 12 hours. If your doctor wants you to take more frequent doses, he or she may prescribe two or four 50-milligram capsules initially, and then one 50-milligram capsule 4 times daily.

CHILDREN ABOVE 8 YEARS OF AGE

The usual dosage of Minocin is 4 milligrams per 2.2 pounds of bodyweight to start, followed by 2 milligrams per 2.2 pounds every 12 hours.

Overdosage

Although no specific information is available, any medication taken in excess can have serious consequences. If you suspect symptoms of an overdose of Minocin, seek medical attention immediately.

Generic name:

MINOCYCLINE HYDROCHLORIDE

See Minocin, page 385.

Generic name:

MINOXIDIL

See Rogaine, page 552.

Generic name:

MISOPROSTOL

See Cytotec, page 152.

Brand name:

MODICON

See Oral Contraceptives, page 437.

Brand name:

MODURETIC

Generic ingredients: Amiloride, Hydrochlorothiazide

Why is this drug prescribed?

Moduretic is a diuretic combination used in the treatment of high blood pressure and congestive heart failure, conditions which require the elimination of excess fluid (water) from the body. When used for high blood pressure, Moduretic can be used alone or with other high blood pressure medications. Diuretics help your body produce and eliminate more urine, which helps lower blood pressure. Amiloride, one of the ingredients, helps minimize the potassium loss that can be caused by the other component, hydrochlorothiazide.

Most important fact about this drug

This medication should be used only if your doctor has determined that the precise amount of each ingredient in Moduretic meets your specific needs.

Avoid potassium-containing salt substitutes, potassium supplements, or a potassium rich diet.

How should you take this medication?

Take this medication with food.

Take Moduretic exactly as prescribed by your doctor. Stopping Moduretic suddenly could cause your condition to worsen.

What side effects may occur?

Side effects cannot be anticipated. If any develop or change in intensity, inform your doctor as soon as possible. Only your doctor can determine if it is safe for you to continue taking Moduretic.

■ *More common side effects may include:*
Diarrhea, dizziness, elevated potassium levels, fatigue, headache, irregular heartbeat, itching, leg pain, loss of appetite, nausea, rash, shortness of breath, stomach and intestinal pain, weakness

■ *Less common or rare side effects may include:*
Anemia, appetite changes, back pain, bad taste, changes in liver function, changes in potassium levels leading to symptoms such as dry mouth, excessive thirst, weak or irregular heartbeat, muscle pain or cramps, chest pain, constipation, cough, decreased sex drive, dehydration, depression, dizziness on standing up, dry mouth, excessive perspiration, excessive urination at night, fainting, fever, fluid in lungs, flushing, frequent urination, fullness in abdomen, gas, gout, hair loss, heartburn, hiccups, hives, impotence, incontinence, indigestion, inflammation of blood vessels, inflammations of lungs, inflammation of the pancreas, inflammation of the salivary glands, insomnia, itching, joint pain, low sodium in blood, mental confusion, muscle cramps, nasal congestion, neck and shoulder ache, nervousness, numbness, painful or difficult urination, rapid heartbeat, ringing in ears, sensitivity to light, sleepiness, stomach and intestinal bleeding, stupor, sugar in blood or urine, thirst, tingling or pins and needles, tremors, vague feeling of bodily

discomfort, vertigo, vision changes, vomiting, yellow eyes and skin

Why should this drug not be prescribed?

If you are unable to urinate or have serious kidney disease, or if you have high potassium levels in your blood, you should not take this medication.

If you are sensitive to or have ever had an allergic reaction to amiloride, hydrochlorothiazide or similar drugs, or if you are sensitive to other sulfonamide-derived drugs, you should not take this medication. Make sure your doctor is aware of any drug reactions you may have experienced.

Potassium supplements, potassium-containing salt substitutes or other diuretics that minimize loss of potassium should not be used while taking Moduretic, unless specifically indicated by your doctor.

Special warnings about this medication

If you are taking Moduretic, a complete assessment of your kidney function should be done; kidney function should continue to be monitored.

If you are taking an ACE-inhibitor type of blood pressure medication such as Vasotec, this drug should be used with extreme caution.

If you have liver disease, diabetes, gout, or collagen vascular disease (lupus erythematosus), Moduretic should be used with caution.

If you have bronchial asthma or a history of allergies, you may be at risk for an allergic reaction to this medication.

Dehydration, excessive sweating, severe diarrhea or vomiting could deplete your fluids and cause your blood pressure to become too low. Be careful when exercising and in hot weather.

Notify your doctor or dentist that you are taking Moduretic if you have a medical emergency or before you have surgery.

Possible food and drug interactions when taking this medication

Moduretic may increase the effects of alcohol. Avoid alcohol while taking this medication.

If Moduretic is taken with certain other drugs, the effects of either could be increased, decreased, or altered. It is especially important to check with your doctor before combining Moduretic with the following:

ACE inhibitors such as Vasotec
Barbiturates such as phenobarbital
Corticosteroids such as prednisone
Insulin
Lithium
Narcotics such as Percocet
Nonsteroidal anti-inflammatory drugs
   such as Naprosyn
Norepinephrine (Levophed)
Oral drugs for treating diabetes such as
   Micronase, DiaBeta
Other high blood pressure medications
Skeletal muscle relaxants such as tubocurarine

Special information
if you are pregnant or breastfeeding

The effects of Moduretic during pregnancy have not been adequately studied. If you are pregnant or plan to become pregnant, inform your doctor immediately. Moduretic appears in breast milk and could affect a nursing infant. If this medication is essential to your health, your doctor may advise you to discontinue breastfeeding until your treatment is finished.

Recommended dosage

ADULTS

The usual starting dose is 1 tablet per day, which may be increased to 2 tablets per day taken at the same time or separately. Dosage can be adjusted to the individual patient's needs.

CHILDREN
The safety and effectiveness of Moduretic have not been established in children.

ELDERLY
Dosage should be determined by the particular needs of the elderly patient.

Each tablet of Moduretic contains 5 milligrams of amiloride hydrochloride and 50 milligrams of hydrochlorothiazide.

Overdosage
Any medication taken in excess can cause symptoms of overdose. If you suspect an overdose, seek medical attention immediately.

No specific information is available, but dehydration might be expected, along with loss of potassium, chloride, and sodium.

Generic name:

MOMETASONE FUROATE

See Elocon, page 231.

Brand name:

MONISTAT 3

Generic name: Miconazole nitrate

Why is this drug prescribed?
Monistat 3 vaginal suppositories are prescribed to treat candidiasis, a yeast-like fungal infection of the vulva and vagina.

Most important fact about this drug
Monistat 3 is effective only for an infection of the vulva or vagina caused by a Candida (yeast-like) species of fungus. Therefore, your doctor should perform a culture or smear before prescribing Monistat 3.

How should you use this medication?
Use this medication exactly as prescribed by your doctor.

What side effects may occur?
Side effects cannot be anticipated. If any develop or change in intensity, inform your doctor. Only your doctor can determine whether it is safe for you to continue taking Monistat 3.

■ *Side effects may include:*
   Cramping
   Headaches
   Hives
   Skin rash
   Vulval or vaginal burning
   Vulval or vaginal irritation
   Vulval or vaginal itching

Why should this drug not be prescribed?
If you have ever had an allergic reaction or are sensitive to miconazole nitrate, you should not take this medication. Make sure your doctor is aware of any drug reactions you have experienced.

Special warnings about this medication
If symptoms persist, or if an irritation or allergic reaction develops while you are using Monistat 3, notify your doctor.

The hydrogenated vegetable oil base of Monistat 3 may interact with certain latex products such as vaginal contraceptive diaphragms. The concurrent use of these two products is not recommended. Your doctor may prescribe Monistat 7 Vaginal Cream if you are using a diaphragm.

Possible food and drug interactions when taking this medication
No interactions have been reported.

Special Information
if you are pregnant or breastfeeding

Unless you are directed to do so by your doctor, do not use Monistat 3 during the first trimester (three months) of pregnancy because it is absorbed in small amounts from the vagina. It is not known whether miconazole appears in breast milk. If Monistat 3 is essential to your health, your doctor may advise you to discontinue breastfeeding until your treatment with this medication is finished.

Recommended dosage

The recommended dose is 1 suppository inserted into the vagina once daily at bedtime for 3 consecutive days.

Overdosage

Overdose of miconazole nitrate has not been reported. However any medication used in excess can have serious consequences. If you suspect an overdose, seek medical attention immediately.

Brand name:

MONOPRIL

Generic name: Fosinopril sodium

Why is this drug prescribed?

Monopril is a high blood pressure medication known as an ACE inhibitor. It is effective when used alone or in combination with other medications for the treatment of high blood pressure. Monopril works by inhibiting the salt and water retention associated with high blood pressure. Monopril also enhances blood flow throughout your blood vessels.

Most important fact about this drug

Since blood pressure lowers gradually, it may take several weeks for the full effect of Monopril to occur.

How should you take this medication?

Monopril is best taken one hour before meals; but it can be taken with food if it upsets your stomach.

Take this medication exactly as prescribed by your doctor.

Suddenly stopping Monopril could cause your blood pressure to increase. If you forget to take a dose, take it as soon as you remember. If it is almost time for your next dose, skip the one you missed and go back to your regular schedule. Never take two doses at the same time.

What side effects may occur?

Side effects cannot be anticipated. If any develop or change in intensity, inform your doctor as soon as possible. Only your doctor can determine if it is safe for you to continue taking Monopril.

■ *More common side effects may include:*
   Cough
   Diarrhea
   Dizziness
   Fatigue
   Headache
   Nausea
   Vomiting

■ *Less common or rare side effects may include:*
   Abdominal pain, changes in appetite and weight, changes in sexual performance, confusion, constipation, decreased sex drive, drowsiness, dry mouth, excessive sweating, eye irritation, gas, heartburn, itching, kidney failure, liver failure, muscle cramps, rash, ringing in ears, skin sensitivity to sunlight, sleep disturbances, tremors, vertigo, vision disturbances, weakness, yellow eyes and skin

If you develop swelling of your face, lips, tongue or throat, or arms and legs, or have difficulty swallowing, you should contact your doctor immediately. You may need emergency treatment.

Why should this drug not be prescribed?

If you are sensitive to or have ever had an allergic reaction to Monopril or similar drugs, you should not take this medication. Make sure that your doctor is aware of any drug reactions that you have experienced.

Special warnings about this medication

If you develop chest pain, rapid or irregular heartbeat, shortness of breath, a sore throat or fever and chills, you should contact your doctor immediately for medical attention.

If you are taking Monopril, your kidney function should get a complete assessment and should continue to be monitored.

If you have liver disease, Monopril should be used with caution.

If you are taking high doses of diuretic and Monopril, you may develop excessively low blood pressure.

Do not use potassium-containing salt substitutes without consulting your doctor.

If you have congestive heart failure, this drug should be started under close medical supervision. Your doctor should continue to monitor your progress for the first 2 weeks of treatment and whenever your dosage is increased.

Excessive sweating, dehydration, severe diarrhea, or vomiting could lead to excessive loss of water and cause your blood pressure to drop dangerously. Take precautions to avoid excessive water loss while exercising.

Possible food and drug interactions when taking this medication

If Monopril is taken with certain other drugs, the effects of either could be increased,

decreased, or altered. It is especially important to check with your doctor before combining Monopril with the following:

Antacids
Lithium
Potassium preparations
Potassium-sparing diuretics such as Moduretic and Aldactane
Thiazide diuretics

Special information if you are pregnant or breastfeeding

Monopril can cause birth defects, prematurity and death to the fetus and newborn. If you are pregnant or plan to become pregnant, inform your doctor immediately to discuss the potential hazard to your unborn child. Monopril appears in breast milk and could affect a nursing infant. If this medication is essential to your health, your doctor may advise you to discontinue breastfeeding until your treatment with this medication is finished.

Recommended dosage

ADULTS

Hypertension

The usual initial dose is 10 milligrams, taken once a day, both alone or when added to a diuretic. Dosage, after blood pressure is adjusted, should be 20 to 40 milligrams a day in a single dose.

Diuretic use should, if possible, be stopped before using Monopril. If not, your physician may give an initial dose of 10 milligrams under his supervision before any further medication is prescribed.

Patients with kidney disorders must be carefully monitored and dosages will be adjusted to the individual patient needs depending on their level of kidney function.

CHILDREN

The safety and effectiveness of Monopril have not been established in children.

ELDERLY

Dosage should be determined by the particular needs of the elderly patient.

Overdosage

Any medication taken in excess can cause symptoms of overdose. If you suspect an overdose, seek medical attention immediately.

A sudden drop in blood pressure is likely to be the primary effect of a Monopril overdose.

Generic name:

MORICIZINE HYDROCHLORIDE

See Ethmozine, page 243.

Generic name:

MORPHINE SULFATE

See MS Contin, page 352.

Brand name:

MOTRIN TABLETS

Generic name: Ibuprofen
Other Brand Names: Advil, Rufen

Why is this drug prescribed?

Ibuprofen, a nonsteroidal anti-inflammatory drug, is used to relieve the inflammation, swelling, stiffness, and joint pain associated with rheumatoid arthritis and osteoarthritis (the most common form of arthritis). It is also used in the treatment of menstrual and other types of pain.

Most important fact about this drug

You should have frequent check-ups with your doctor if you take ibuprofen regularly. Ulcers or internal bleeding can occur without warning.

How should you take this medication?

Your doctor may ask you to take ibuprofen with food or an antacid to avoid stomach upset.

Take this medication exactly as prescribed by your doctor.

If you are using ibuprofen for arthritis, you should take it regularly.

If you forget to take a dose, take it as soon as you remember. If it is almost time for your next dose, skip the one you missed and go back to your regular schedule. Never take two doses at the same time.

What side effects may occur?

Side effects cannot be anticipated. If any develop or change in intensity, inform your doctor as soon as possible. Only your doctor can determine if it is safe for you to continue taking ibuprofen.

■ *More common side effects may include:*
Abdominal cramps or pain, abdominal discomfort, bloating and gas, constipation, diarrhea, dizziness, fluid retention and swelling,, headache, heartburn, indigestion, itching, loss of appetite, nausea, nervousness, rash, ringing in ears, stomach pain, vomiting

■ *Less common or rare side effects may include:*
Abdominal bleeding, anemia, black stool, blood in urine, blurred vision, changes in heartbeat, chills, confusion, congestive heart failure, depression, dry eyes and mouth, fever, hair loss, hearing loss, hepatitis, high blood pressure, hives, inability to sleep, inflammation of nose,

inflammation of the pancreas, inflammation of the stomach, kidney failure, shortness of breath, skin eruptions, Stevens-Johnson syndrome (peeling skin), stomach or upper intestinal ulcer, ulcer of gums, vision loss, yellow eyes and skin

Why should this drug not be prescribed?

If you are sensitive to or have ever had an allergic reaction to ibuprofen, aspirin, or similar drugs, of if you have had asthma attacks caused by aspirin or other drugs of this type, or if you have angioedema, a condition whose symptoms are skin eruptions, you should not take this medication.

Make sure that your doctor is aware of any drug reactions that you have experienced.

Special warnings about this medication

Peptic ulcers and bleeding can occur without warning.

This drug should be used with caution if you have kidney or liver disease, and it can cause liver inflammation in some people.

Do not take aspirin or any other anti-inflammatory medications while taking ibuprofen unless your doctor tells you to do so.

Ibuprofen may cause vision problems. If you experience any changes in your vision, inform your doctor.

Ibuprofen may prolong bleeding time. If you are taking blood-thinning medication, this drug should be taken with caution.

This drug can cause water retention. It should be used with caution if you have high blood pressure or poor heart function.

Avoid the use of alcohol while taking this medication.

Ibuprofen may mask the usual signs of infection. Use with care in the presence of an existing infection.

Possible food and drug interactions when taking this medication

If ibuprofen is taken with certain other drugs, the effects of either could be increased, decreased, or altered. It is especially important to check with your doctor before combining ibuprofen with the following:

Anticoagulants
Aspirin
Diuretics such as Lasix and HydroDIURIL
Lithium
Methotrexate

Special information
if you are pregnant or breastfeeding

The effects of ibuprofen during pregnancy have not been adequately studied. If you are pregnant or plan to become pregnant, inform your doctor immediately. Ibuprofen may appear in breast milk and could affect a nursing infant. If this medication is essential to your health, your doctor may advise you to discontinue breastfeeding until your treatment with this medication is finished.

Recommended dosage

ADULTS

Rheumatoid Arthritis and Osteoarthritis
The usual dosage is 1,200 to 3,200 milligrams per day divided into 3 or 4 doses. Dosages will be tailored to the individual patient according to severity of symptoms, and the lowest possible dose should be used. Symptoms should be reduced within 2 weeks. Daily dosage should not be greater than 3,200 milligrams.

Mild to Moderate Pain
The usual dose is 400 milligrams every 4 to 6 hours as necessary.

Menstrual Pain
The usual dose is 400 milligrams every 4 hours as necessary. Begin treatment when symptoms first appear.

CHILDREN

The safety and effectiveness of ibuprofen in children have not been established.

ELDERLY

Dosage should be determined by the particular needs of the elderly patient.

Overdosage

Any medication taken in excess can cause symptoms of overdose. If you suspect an overdose, seek medical attention immediately.

Generic name:

MUPIROCIN

See Bactroban, page 56.

Brand name:

MYCELEX

See Lotrimin, page 344.

Brand name:

MYCO-TRIACET II

See Mycolog-II, page 395.

Brand name:

MYCOLOG-II

Generic ingredients: Nystatin, Triamcinolone acetonide
Other brand names: Myco-Triacet II, Mytrex

Why is this drug prescribed?

Mycolog-II Cream and Ointment are prescribed for the treatment of candidiasis (a yeast-like fungal infection) of the skin. The antifungal (nystatin)/steroid (triamcinolone acetonide) combination provides greater benefit than nystatin alone during the first few days of treatment.

Most important fact about this drug

Absorption of this drug through the skin can affect the whole body (systemic absorption) instead of just the surface of the skin being treated. Although unusual and most common if Mycolog-II is spread over large areas of the skin, symptoms of steroid excess such as weight gain, reddening and rounding of the face and neck, growth of excess body and facial hair, high blood pressure, emotional disturbances, hyperglycemia increases in blood sugar, and urinary excretion of glucose (increase in frequency of urination) may occur in some patients.

Use of this medication over large surface areas, or for prolonged periods or with airtight dressings or bandages may cause these problems, which are related to excessive systemic absorption. It is recommended that your doctor monitor your condition and periodically check for such problems.

How should you use this medication?

Use this medication exactly as prescribed by your doctor. It is for external use only. Avoid contact with the eyes.

What side effects may occur?

Side effects cannot be anticipated. If any develop or change in intensity, inform your doctor as soon as possible. Only your doctor can determine if it is safe for you to continue taking Mycolog-II.

■ *Side effects may include:*
Burning, dryness, eruptions resembling acne, excessive discoloring of the skin, excessive growth of hair, inflammation around the mouth, inflammation of hair follicles, irritation, itching, prickly heat, secondary infection, severe inflammation of the skin, softening of the skin, stretch marks, stretching or thinning of the skin

Why should this drug not be prescribed?
If you are sensitive to or have ever had an allergic reaction to nystatin, triamcinolone acetonide, or other drugs of these types (antifungals, steroids), you should not take this medication. Make sure that your doctor is aware of any drug reactions that you have experienced.

Special warnings about this medication
Do not use this drug for any disorder other than the one for which it was prescribed.

The use of tight-fitting diapers or plastic pants is not recommended for a child being treated in the diaper area with Mycolog-II. These garments may act in the same way as air tight dressings or bandages.

If an irritation or allergic reaction develops while using Mycolog-II, notify your doctor.

The treated skin area should not be bandaged, covered, or wrapped.

Apply Mycolog-II sparingly to the groin area and wear loose-fitting clothing.

Possible food and drug interactions when taking this medication
None.

Special information if you are pregnant or breastfeeding
If you are pregnant or plan to become pregnant, inform your doctor before using Mycolog-II.

It is not known whether this medication appears in breast milk. If this drug is essential to your health, your doctor may advise you to discontinue breastfeeding until your treatment with this medication is finished.

Recommended dosage

ADULTS

Mycolog-II Cream
Mycolog-II Cream is usually applied to the affected areas 2 times a day, in the morning and evening, by gently and thoroughly massaging the preparation into the skin. The cream should be discontinued if symptoms persist after 25 days of treatment.

Mycolog-II Ointment
A thin film of Mycolog-II Ointment is usually applied to the affected areas 2 times a day, in the morning and the evening. The ointment should be discontinued if symptoms persist after 25 days of treatment.

CHILDREN

Topical use of Mycolog-II for children should be limited to the least amount that is effective. Long-term treatment may interfere with the growth and development of children.

Overdosage
An acute overdosage is unlikely with the use of Mycolog-II; however, long-term or prolonged use can produce systemic (throughout the body) reactions.

Brand name:

MYSOLINE

Generic name: Primidone

Why is this drug prescribed?
Mysoline is used to treat epileptic and other seizures. Mysoline can be used alone or

with other anticonvulsant drugs. It is chemically similar to barbiturates.

Most important fact about this drug

Mysoline should not be stopped suddenly; this could cause you to have seizures. If the medication is no longer needed, the dosage should be reduced gradually.

How should you take this medication?

Mysoline should be taken exactly as prescribed by your doctor.

If using Mysoline Suspension, shake well before using.

If you miss a dose, take it as soon as you remember. If it is almost time for your next dose, skip the one you missed and go back to your regular schedule. Never take two doses at the same time.

Do not change from one manufacturer's product to another without consulting your doctor.

What side effects may occur?

Side effects cannot be anticipated. If any develop or change in intensity, inform your doctor as soon as possible. Only your doctor can determine if it is safe for you to continue taking Mysoline.

■ *More common side effects may include:*
Lack of muscle coordination
Vertigo or severe dizziness

■ *Less common side effects may include:*
Decreased sexual ability, double vision, drowsiness, emotional disturbances, exhaustion, hyperirritability, impotence, loss of appetite, nausea, rash that resembles measles, uncontrolled movement of the eyeballs, vomiting

Why should this drug not be prescribed?

Mysoline should not be taken if you have porphyria (an inherited metabolic disorder) or if you are allergic to phenobarbital.

Special warnings about this medication

Mysoline should not be stopped suddenly, which could cause you to have seizures. The dosage should be reduced gradually.

It can take several weeks before the full effectiveness of Mysoline occurs.

Since Mysoline is generally given for long periods of time, your doctor should check your blood count every 6 months.

Possible food and drug interactions when taking this medication

If Mysoline is taken with certain other drugs, the effects of either could be increased, decreased, or altered. It is especially important to check with your doctor before combining Mysoline with the following:

Estrogen-containing oral contraceptives such as Ortho-Novum, and Triphasil
Antidepressants called MAO inhibitors such as Parnate and Nardil
Blood-thinning drugs such as Coumadin and Panwarfin
Doxycycline (Doryx, Vibramycin)
Corticosteroids such as Decadron and prednisone
Griseofulvin (Fulvicin-U/F, Grifulvin V)

Avoid alcoholic beverages while you are taking Mysoline.

Special information if you are pregnant or breastfeeding

Although the effects of Mysoline in pregnancy and nursing infants is not known, recent studies show an increase in birth defects in infants born to epileptic women taking anticonvulsant medication (particularly Dilantin and phenobarbital). Although most pregnant women taking anticonvulsant medication give birth to normal, healthy babies, this possibility may also exist with Mysoline. If you are pregnant or plan to become pregnant, inform your doctor immediately. Mysoline appears in breast milk and can affect a nursing infant, causing excessive sleep and drowsiness. If this medication is essential to your health, your doctor may advise you to stop breastfeeding.

Recommended dosage

ADULTS

Patients 8 years of age and older who have received no previous treatment may be started on Mysoline according to the following regimen using either 50-milligram or scored 250-milligram Mysoline tablets.

Days 1 to 3: 100 to 125 milligrams at bedtime
Days 4 to 6: 100 to 125 milligrams 2 times a day
Days 7 to 9: 100 to 125 milligrams 3 times a day
Day 10 to maintenance: 250 milligrams 3 times a day

For most adults and children 8 years of age and over, the usual maintenance dosage is three to four 250-milligram Mysoline tablets daily in divided doses (250 milligrams 3 or 4 times a day). If required, an increase to five or six 250-milligram tablets daily may be taken, but daily doses should not exceed 500 milligrams 4 times a day.

In Patients Already Receiving Other Anticonvulsants
Mysoline should be started at 100 to 125 milligrams at bedtime and gradually increased to a maintenance level as the other drug is gradually decreased. This plan should be continued until a satisfactory dosage level is achieved for the combination, or the other medication is completely withdrawn. When Mysoline is to be used as a single drug the transition from two drugs should not be completed in less than 2 weeks.

CHILDREN UNDER AGE 8

Days 1 to 3: 50 milligrams at bedtime
Days 4 to 6: 50 milligrams 2 times a day
Days 7 to 9: 100 milligrams 2 times a day
Day 10 to maintenance: 125 milligrams 3 times a day to 250 milligrams 3 times a day

For children under 8 years of age, the usual maintenance dosage is 125 to 250 milligrams 3 times daily or 10 to 25 milligrams per 2.2 pounds of body weight per day in divided doses.

Overdosage

Any medication taken in excess can have serious consequences. If you suspect a Mysoline overdose, seek medical attention immediately.

Brand name:

MYTREX

See Mycolog II, page 395.

Generic name:

NADOLOL

See Corgard, page 135.

Generic name:

NADOLOL/ BENDROFLUMETHIAZIDE

See Corzide, page 138.

Brand name:

NALFON

Generic name: Fenoprofen calcium

Why is this drug prescribed?

Nalfon, a nonsteroidal anti-inflammatory drug, is used to relieve the inflammation, swelling, stiffness, and joint pain associated with rheumatoid arthritis and osteoarthritis (the most common form of arthritis). It is also used to relieve mild to moderate pain.

Most important fact about this drug

You should have frequent check-ups with your doctor if you take Nalfon regularly. Ulcers or internal bleeding can occur without warning.

How should you take this medication?

Your doctor may ask you to take Nalfon with food or an antacid or with a full glass of milk. Never take it on an empty stomach.

Take this medication exactly as prescribed by your doctor.

If you are using Nalfon for arthritis, it should be taken regularly.

If you forget to take a dose, take it as soon as you remember. If it is almost time for your next dose, skip the one you missed and go back to your regular schedule. Never take two doses at the same time.

What side effects may occur?

Side effects cannot be anticipated. If any develop or change in intensity, inform your doctor as soon as possible. Only your doctor can determine if it is safe for you to continue taking Nalfon.

■ *More common side effects may include:*
Abdominal pain, blurred vision, confusion, constipation, diarrhea, dizziness, fluid retention, headache, hearing loss, indigestion, itching, nausea, nervousness, rapid heartbeat, rash, ringing in ears, shortness of breath, sleepiness, sore throat, sweating, tiredness, tremors, upper respiratory infection, vomiting, weakness

■ *Less common or rare side effects may include:*
Abdominal bleeding, anemia, blood in urine, bloody stools, depression, disorientation, dry mouth, fluid in lungs, gas, hair loss, hemorrhage, hepatitis, inability to sleep, inflammation of the pancreas, inflammation of the skin, loss of appetite, painful urination, peptic ulcer, rapid heartbeat, red or purple spots on the skin, Stevens-Johnson syndrome (peeling skin), stomach inflammation, yellow eyes and skin

Why should this drug not be prescribed?

If you are sensitive to or have ever had an allergic reaction to Nalfon, aspirin, or similar drugs (anti-inflammatories), or if you have had asthma attacks caused by aspirin or other drugs of this type, you should not take this medication. If you have a history of decreased kidney function, you should not take this medication. Make sure that your doctor is aware of any drug reactions that you have experienced.

Special warnings about this medication

Peptic ulcers and bleeding can occur without warning.

This drug should be used with caution if you have kidney or liver disease. It can cause liver inflammation in some people.

Do not take aspirin or any other anti-inflammatory medications while taking Nalfon, unless your doctor tells you to do so.

Nalfon may cause vision problems. If you experience any changes in your vision, inform your doctor.

Nalfon may prolong bleeding time. If you are taking blood-thinning medication, this drug should be taken with caution.

This drug can increase water retention. Use with caution if you have heart disease or high blood pressure.

Nalfon may cause you to become drowsy or less alert; therefore, driving or operating dangerous machinery or participating in any hazardous activity that requires full mental alertness is not recommended.

Possible food and drug interactions while taking this medication
If Nalfon is taken with certain other drugs, the effects of either could be increased, decreased, or altered. It is especially important to check with your doctor before combining Nalfon with the following:

Anticoagulants
Aspirin
Phenytoin (Dilantin)
Loop diuretics such as Lasix
Phenobarbital
Steroids
Sulfonamides
Sulfonylureas (oral antidiabetic drugs such as Diabinese and Micronase)

Special information
if you are pregnant or breastfeeding
The effects of Nalfon during pregnancy have not been adequately studied. If you are pregnant or plan to become pregnant, inform your doctor immediately. Nalfon appears in breast milk and could affect a nursing infant. If this medication is essential to your health, your doctor may advise you to discontinue breastfeeding until your treatment with this medication is finished.

Recommended dosage
ADULTS

Mild to Moderate Pain
200 milligrams every 4 to 6 hours

Rheumatoid Arthritis and Osteoarthritis
Dosages should be tailored to the individual patient's needs; however, patients with rheumatoid arthritis generally seem to need larger doses than do those with osteoarthritis. The smallest dosage that provides control of pain should be used. The usual dosage is 300 to 600 milligrams, 3 to 4 times per day. Total daily dosage should not exceed 3,200 milligrams.

CHILDREN

The safety and effectiveness of Nalfon have not been established in children.

Overdosage
Any medication taken in excess can cause symptoms of overdose. If you suspect an overdose, seek medical attention immediately.

The most common symptoms of Nalfon overdose, which may appear within several hours, may include:

Abdominal pain, acute kidney failure, confusion, difficulty breathing, dizziness, drowsiness, extremely high temperature, headache, indigestion, lack of coordination, low blood pressure, nausea, rapid heartbeat, ringing in ears, tremors, vomiting

Generic name:

NAPHAZOLINE WITH PHENIRAMINE

See Naphcon-A, page 400.

Brand name:

NAPHCON-A

Generic ingredients: Naphazoline hydrochloride, Pheniramine maleate
Other brand name: Opcon-A

Why is this drug prescribed?
Naphcon-A, an eyedrop containing both a decongestant and an antihistamine, is used

to relieve eye redness caused by irritation, allergy, or inflammatory eye conditions.

Most important fact about this drug

To avoid contamination, never let the tip of the plastic dropper bottle touch your eye, your eyelid, the skin around your eye, or any other surface.

Do not use the solution if it becomes cloudy or changes color. Remove contact lenses before using this medication.

How should you use this medication?

Use this medication exactly as prescribed by your doctor.

To instill:

Hold your eye open with the fingers of one hand. With the other hand, position the dropper bottle slightly above your eye and gently squeeze out a drop or two, letting the solution fall onto your eyeball.

What side effects may occur?

Side effects cannot be anticipated. If any side effects develop or change in intensity, tell your doctor immediately. Only your doctor can determine whether it is safe to continue using this medicine.

Although you apply these drops to the surface of your eye, some of the ingredients may be absorbed from the eyeball into the bloodstream.

■ *Side effects may include:*
  Blood pressure increase
  Dilated pupils
  Drowsiness
  High blood-sugar level
  Increased pressure inside the eyeball
  Irregular heartbeat

Why should this drug not be prescribed?

Do not take Naphcon-A if you have ever had an allergic reaction to it or are sensitive to any of its ingredients.

Do not use this medication if you have glaucoma.

Special warnings about this medication

You should use this medication with caution in the following circumstances:

- If you are an older person and have severe heart disease (including any heartbeat irregularity),
- If you have high blood pressure that is not well controlled,
- If you have diabetes (especially if you are prone to diabetic ketoacidosis).

Do not give Naphcon-A to infants or children. This medication could cause stupor or coma and a serious drop in body temperature in a child.

Possible food and drug interactions when taking this medication

Do not use Naphcon-A simultaneously with an antidepressant of the monoamine oxidase inhibitor type, such as Marplan, Nardil, or Parnate. This drug combination could cause your blood pressure to rise suddenly and dangerously.

Special information if you are pregnant or breastfeeding

If you are pregnant or plan to become pregnant, inform your doctor immediately. This medication should be used during pregnancy only if the potential benefit to the mother outweighs the potential risk to the unborn child.

It is not known whether this medication can make its way into breast milk. To be safe, consult your doctor before using this medication while breastfeeding.

Recommended dosage

ADULTS

Place 1 or 2 drops in each eye every 3 to 4 hours or less to relieve symptoms.

Overdosage

Overdose from accidental oral use or excessive use can have serious consequences, especially in young children. If you suspect you may have used too much of this medication, seek medical attention immediately.

Common symptoms of Naphcon-A overdose may include:
Breathing irregularities
Coma
Slow heart rate
Severe drowsiness
Sweating

Brand name:

NAPROSYN

Generic name: Naproxen

Why is this drug prescribed?

Naprosyn, a nonsteroidal anti-inflammatory drug, is used to relieve the inflammation, swelling, stiffness, and joint pain associated with rheumatoid arthritis, osteoarthritis (the most common form of arthritis), juvenile arthritis, ankylosing spondylitis (spinal arthritis), tendinitis, bursitis, acute gout, menstrual cramps, and other types of mild to moderate pain.

Most important fact about this drug

You should have frequent check-ups with your doctor if you take Naprosyn regularly. Ulcers or internal bleeding can occur without warning.

How should you take this medication?

Naprosyn may be taken with food or an antacid, and with a full glass of water to avoid stomach upset. Never take it on an empty stomach.

Take this medication exactly as prescribed by your doctor.

If you are using Naprosyn for arthritis, it should be taken regularly.

What side effects may occur?

Side effects cannot be anticipated. If any develop or change in intensity, inform your doctor as soon as possible. Only your doctor can determine if it is safe for you to continue taking Naprosyn.

■ *More common side effects may include:*
Abdominal pain, bruising, constipation, diarrhea, difficult or labored breathing, dizziness, drowsiness, headache, hearing changes, heartburn, indigestion, inflammation of the mouth, itching, light-headedness, nausea, rapid heartbeat, red or purple spots on the skin, ringing in ears, skin eruptions, sweating, swelling due to fluid retention, thirst, vertigo, visual changes

■ *Less common or rare side effects may include:*
Abdominal bleeding, black stools, changes in hearing, changes in liver function, chills and fever, colitis, congestive heart failure, depression, dream abnormalities, hair loss, inability to concentrate, inability to sleep, inflammation of the lungs, kidney failure, menstrual disorders, muscle pain and weakness, peptic ulcer, shock, skin inflammation due to sensitivity to light, skin rashes, vomiting, vomiting of blood, yellow skin and eyes

Why should this drug not be prescribed?

If you are sensitive to or have ever had an allergic reaction to Naprosyn, Anaprox or Anaprox DS, aspirin, or similar drugs; or if you have had asthma attacks caused by aspirin or other drugs of this type, you should not take this medication. Make sure that your doctor is aware of any drug reaction that you have experienced.

Special warnings about this medication

Peptic ulcers and bleeding can occur without warning.

This drug should be used with caution if you have kidney or liver disease; and it can cause liver inflammation in some people.

Do not take aspirin or any other anti-inflammatory medications while taking Naprosyn, unless your doctor tells you to do so.

Naprosyn may prolong bleeding time. If you are taking blood-thinning medication, this drug should be used with caution.

This medication may cause vision problems. If you experience any changes in your vision, inform your doctor.

This drug can increase water retention. Use with caution if you have heart disease or high blood pressure. Naprosyn contains a significant amount of sodium. If you are on a low-sodium diet, discuss this with your doctor.

Naprosyn may cause you to become drowsy or less alert; therefore, driving or operating dangerous machinery or participating in any hazardous activity that requires full mental alertness is not recommended.

Possible food and drug interactions when taking this medication

If Naprosyn is taken with certain other drugs, the effects of either could be increased, decreased, or altered. It is especially important to check with your doctor before combining Naprosyn with the following:

Anticoagulants
Aspirin
Beta blockers such as Tenormin
Lithium
Loop diuretics such as Lasix
Methotrexate
Naproxen sodium
Phenytoin (Dilantin)
Probenecid (Benemid)
Sulfonamides
Sulfonylureas (oral antidiabetic drugs such as Diabinese and Micronase)

Special information if you are pregnant or breastfeeding

The effects of Naprosyn during pregnancy have not been adequately studied. If you are pregnant or plan to become pregnant, inform your doctor immediately. Naprosyn appears in breast milk and could affect a nursing infant. If this medication is essential to your health, your doctor may advise you to discontinue breastfeeding until your treatment with this medication is finished.

Recommended dosage

Use a teaspoon or the measuring cup marked in one-half teaspoon and 2.5 milliliter increments provided with Naprosyn to measure the correct dose.

ADULTS

(Available in both tablet and liquid form)

Rheumatoid Arthritis, Osteoarthritis, and Ankylosing Spondylitis
250 milligrams (10 milliliters or 2 teaspoons), 375 milligrams (15 milliliters or 3 teaspoons), or 500 milligrams (20 milliliters or 4 teaspoons) 2 times a day (morning and evening). Your dose may be adjusted by your doctor over your period of treatment. Improvement of symptoms should be seen in 2 to 4 weeks.

Acute Gout
Starting dose is 750 milligrams (30 milliliters or 6 teaspoons), followed by 250 milligrams

(10 milliliters or 2 teaspoons) every 8 hours until the symptoms are relieved.

Mild to Moderate Pain, Primary Dysmenorrhea, Acute Tendinitis and Bursitis
Starting dose is 500 milligrams (20 milliliters or 4 teaspoons), followed by 250 milligrams (10 milliliters or 2 teaspoons) every 6 to 8 hours as needed. The maximum daily dosage is 1,250 mg (50 milliliters or 10 teaspoons).

CHILDREN

Juvenile Arthritis
10 milligrams per 2.2 pounds of body weight, 2 times a day. Follow your doctor's directions carefully when giving a child this medicine.

The safety and effectiveness of Naprosyn have not been established in children under 2 years of age.

Overdosage

Any medication taken in excess can cause symptoms of overdose. If you suspect an overdose seek medical attention immediately.

The symptoms of Naprosyn overdose may include:
Drowsiness
Heartburn
Indigestion
Nausea
Vomiting

Generic name:

NAPROXEN

See Naprosyn, page 402.

Generic name:

NAPROXEN SODIUM

See Anaprox, page 27.

Brand name:

NARDIL

Generic name: Phenelzine sulfate

Why is this drug prescribed?

Nardil is a monoamine oxidase (MAO) inhibitor used to treat depression and anxiety and/or phobias mixed with depression. MAO is an enzyme responsible for breaking down certain neurotransmitters (chemical messengers) in the brain. By inhibiting MAO, Nardil helps restore more normal mood states. Unfortunately, MAO inhibitors such as Nardil also block MAO activity throughout the body, an action that can have many diverse and serious, even fatal, side effects—especially when MAO inhibitors are combined with other foods or drugs containing a substance called tyramine. As a result, Nardil is usually prescribed only after other antidepressant treatments have failed.

Most important fact about this drug

Avoid the following foods, beverages, and medications while taking Nardil and for 2 weeks following its discontinuation:

Food and beverages to avoid
Beer (including alcohol-free or reduced-alcohol beer)
Caffeine (in excessive amounts)
Cheese (except for cottage cheese and cream cheese)
Chocolate (in excessive amounts)
Dry sausage (including Genoa salami, hard salami, pepperoni, and Lebanon bologna)
Fava bean pods
Liver
Meat extract
Pickled herring
Pickled, fermented, aged, or smoked meat, fish, or dairy products
Sauerkraut

Spoiled or improperly stored meat, fish, or dairy products

Wine (including alcohol-free or reduced-alcohol wine)

Yeast extract (including large amounts of brewer's yeast)

Yogurt

Medications to avoid

"Pep" pills (amphetamines)

Antiappetite medications (Tenuate)

Antidepressants and medications derived from dibenzazepines (such as Prozac, Elavil, Triavil, Tegretol, Flexeril)

Asthma inhalants (Proventil, Ventolin)

Central nervous system stimulants

Cold and cough preparations (including those with dextromethorphan such as Robitussin DM)

Hay fever medications (Contact, Dristan, Sudafed)

L-tryptophan-containing products

Nasal decongestants (in tablet, drop, or spray form)

Sinus medications

Weight-loss medications

Taking Nardil with any of the above foods, beverages, or medications can cause serious, potentially fatal, high blood pressure. Therefore, when taking Nardil you should immediately report the occurrence of a headache, palpitations, or any other unusual symptom. In addition, make certain that you inform any other physician or dentist you see that you are currently taking Nardil or have taken Nardil within the last 2 weeks.

How should you take this medication?

Nardil may be taken with or without food.

Use of Nardil may complicate other medical treatment. Always carry a card that says you take Nardil, or wear a Medic Alert bracelet.

What side effects may occur?

Side effects cannot be anticipated. If any develop or change in intensity, inform your doctor as soon as possible. Only your doctor can determine if it is safe for you to continue taking Nardil.

- *Common side effects may include:*
  Constipation, dizziness, drowsiness, dry mouth, excessive sleeping, fatigue, disorders of the stomach and intestines, headache, insomnia, low blood pressure (especially when rising quickly from lying down or sitting up), muscle spasms, sexual difficulties, swelling due to fluid retention, tremors, twitching, weakness, weight gain

- *Less common or rare side effects may include:*
  Anxiety, blurred vision, coma, convulsions, euphoria, fever, glaucoma, jitteriness, lack of coordination, liver damage, mania, muscular rigidity, onset of schizophrenia, rapid breathing, rapid eye movements, rapid heart rate, skin rash, speech disorders, sweating, swelling in the throat, tingling sensation, urinary difficulties, yellowed skin and whites of eyes

Why should this drug not be prescribed?

You should not take this drug if you have pheochromocytoma (a small tumor of the adrenal gland), congestive heart failure, or a history of liver disease, or if you have had an allergic reaction to it.

You should not take Nardil if you are taking medications that may increase blood pressure (such as amphetamines, cocaine, allergy and cold medications, or Ritalin), other MAO inhibitors, L-dopa, methyldopa (Aldomet), phenylalanine, L-tryptophan, L-tyrosine, fluoxetine (Prozac), buspirone (BuSpar), bupropion (Wellbutrin), guanethidine (Ismelin), meperidine (Demerol), dextromethorphan, or central nervous system depressants such as alcohol and narcotics; or if you must consume the foods, beverages, or medications listed above in the "Most important fact about this drug" section.

Special warnings about this medication

You must follow the food and drug limitations established by your physician; failure to do so may lead to potentially fatal side effects. While taking Nardil, you should promptly report the occurrence of a headache or any other unusual symptoms.

Diabetic patients should use Nardil with caution, since it is not clear how MAO inhibitors affect blood sugar levels.

Patients taking Nardil should not undergo elective surgery requiring general anesthesia.

Rarely, withdrawal symptoms may occur following abrupt discontinuation of Nardil. These symptoms include nightmares, strange behavior, and convulsions.

Possible food and drug interactions when taking this medication

If Nardil is taken with certain other drugs, the effects of either could be increased, decreased, or altered. It is important that you closely follow your doctor's dietary and medication limitations when taking Nardil. Consult the "Most important fact about this drug" or "Why should this drug not be prescribed?" sections for lists of the foods, beverages, and medications that should be avoided while taking Nardil.

In addition, blood pressure medications (including diuretics and beta blockers) should be used with caution when taking Nardil, since excessively low blood pressure may result. Symptoms of low blood pressure include dizziness when rising

from a lying or sitting position, fainting, and tingling in the hands or feet.

Special information if you are pregnant or breastfeeding

The effects of Nardil during pregnancy have not been adequately studied. Nardil should be used during pregnancy only if the benefits of therapy clearly outweigh the potential risks to the fetus. If you are pregnant or plan to become pregnant, inform your doctor immediately. Nursing mothers should use Nardil only after consulting their physician, since it is not known whether Nardil appears in human milk.

Recommended dosage

ADULTS

The usual starting dose is 15 milligrams (1 tablet) 3 times a day. Dosage may be increased, if necessary, up to 90 milligrams per day.

After maximum benefit has been achieved, dosage may be reduced gradually. Maintenance doses as low as 15 milligrams daily or every 2 days may be possible.

CHILDREN

Nardil is not recommended, since safety and efficacy for children under the age of 16 have not been determined.

Overdosage

Any medication taken in excess can have serious consequences. An overdose of Nardil can be fatal. If you suspect an overdose, seek medical help immediately.

Symptoms of overdose may include:
Agitation, backward arching of the head, neck, and back, cool, clammy skin, coma, convulsions, difficult breathing, dizziness, drowsiness, faintness, hallucinations, high blood pressure, high fever, hyperactivity,

irritability, jaw muscle spasms, low blood pressure, pain in the heart area, rapid and irregular pulse, severe headache, sweating

Brand name:

NASALCROM

See Cromolyn sodium, page 144.

Brand name:

NAVANE

Generic names: Thiothixene

Why is this drug prescribed?
Navane is used to treat psychotic disorders (a severe sense of distorted reality). Researchers theorize that antipsychotic medications such as Navane work by lowering levels of dopamine, a neurotransmitter (or chemical messenger) in the brain. Excessive levels of dopamine are believed to be responsible for psychotic behavior.

Most important fact about this drug
Navane may cause tardive dyskinesia—a condition marked by involuntary muscle spasms and twitches in the face and body. This condition can be permanent and appears to be most common among the elderly, especially women. Ask your doctor for information about this possible risk.

How should you take this medication?
Navane may be taken in liquid or capsule form. In liquid form, a dropper is supplied.

Navane should not be taken with alcohol.

What side effects may occur?
Side effects cannot be anticipated. If any develop or change in intensity, inform your doctor as soon as possible. Only your doctor can determine if it is safe for you to continue taking this medication.

■ Side effects may include:
Abnormal muscle rigidity, abnormal secretion of milk, abnormalities in movements and posture, agitation, anemia, blurred vision, breast development in males, chewing movements, constipation, diarrhea, dizziness, drowsiness, dry mouth, excessive thirst, eyeball rotation or state of fixed gaze, fainting, fatigue, fever, fluid accumulation and swelling, headache, high or low blood sugar, hives, impotence, insomnia, intestinal blockage, irregular menstrual periods, itching, light-headedness, loss or increase of appetite, low blood pressure, narrow or dilated pupils of the eye, nasal congestion, nausea, painful muscle spasm, protruding tongue, puckering of mouth, puffing of cheeks, rapid heartbeat, rash, restlessness, salivation, sedation, seizures, sensitivity to light, skin inflammation and peeling, sweating, swelling of breasts, tremors, twitching in the body, neck, shoulders, and face, visual problems, vomiting, weakness, weight increase, worsening of psychotic symptoms

Why should this drug not be prescribed?
Do not give Navane to comatose individuals. Do not take Navane if you are known to be hypersensitive to it. Also, you should not be using Navane if you have a central nervous system depression due to any cause (such as taking sleeping medications), have had circulatory system collapse, or have an abnormal bone marrow or blood condition.

Special warnings about this medication
Navane may hide symptoms of brain tumor and intestinal obstruction. You should use Navane cautiously if you have or have ever had: a brain tumor, breast cancer, convulsive disorders, glaucoma, intestinal blockage, or heart disease; or if you are exposed to extreme heat or are recovering from alcohol addiction.

This drug may impair your ability to drive a car or operate potentially dangerous machinery. Do not participate in any activities that require full alertness if you are unsure of your ability.

Possible food and drug interactions when taking this medication

If Navane is taken with certain other drugs, the effects of either could be increased, decreased, or altered. It is especially important to check with your doctor before combining Navane with the following:

Antihistamines such as Benadryl
Atropine (Donnatal)

Extreme drowsiness and other potentially serious effects can result if Navane is combined with alcohol or other central nervous system depressants such as pain-killers, narcotics, or sleeping medications.

Special information
if you are pregnant or breastfeeding

If you are pregnant or plan to become pregnant, inform your doctor immediately; pregnant women should use Navane only if clearly needed. The drug can appear in breast milk and may affect a nursing infant.

Recommended dosage

Dosages of Navane should be tailored to the individual. Usually treatment begins with a small dose, which is increased if needed.

ADULTS

For Milder Conditions
The usual starting dosage is a daily total of 6 milligrams, divided into doses of 2 milligrams and taken 3 times a day. If necessary, this may be increased to a total daily dose of 15 milligrams.

For More Severe Conditions
The usual starting dosage is a daily total of 10 milligrams, taken in 2 doses of 5 milligrams each. If necessary, this dose may be increased to a total of 60 milligrams a day.

Taking more than 60 milligrams a day rarely increases the benefits of Navane.

Some people may find it beneficial to take Navane once a day. Check with your doctor.

CHILDREN

Navane is not recommended for children younger than 12 years old.

ELDERLY

In general, elderly people take dosages of Navane in the lower ranges. Because elderly people may develop low blood pressure while taking Navane, they should be closely monitored. Elderly people (especially elderly women) may be more susceptible to tardive dyskinesia—a possibly permanent condition that causes involuntary muscle spasms and twitches in the face and body. Elderly people should consult their doctor for information about these potential risks.

Overdosage

Any medication taken in excess can have serious consequences. If you suspect an overdose, seek medical help immediately.

Symptoms of Navane overdose may include:
Central nervous system depression, including
Coma
Difficulty swallowing
Head tilted to the side
Low blood pressure
Rigid muscles
Salivation
Tremors
Walking disturbances
Weakness

Brand name:

NEMBUTAL SODIUM CAPSULES

Generic name: Pentobarbital sodium

Why is this drug prescribed?

Nembutal is used as a sedative and may be prescribed to treat insomnia on a short-term basis.

After 2 weeks, Nembutal appears to lose its effectiveness as a sleep aid.

Most important fact about this drug

If taken for a long enough time, Nembutal can cause physical addiction. Taken in high enough amounts, it can be fatal. Nembutal should be used in the smallest possible amount, and it should always be stored in child-resistant containers.

How should you take this medication?

Nembutal should be taken at bedtime.

You should not take Nembutal with alcohol.

Take only the prescribed dose.

What side effects may occur?

Side effects cannot be anticipated. If any develop or change in intensity, inform your doctor as soon as possible. Only your doctor can determine if it is safe for you to continue taking Nembutal.

■ *More common side effects may include:*
Extreme sleepiness

■ *Less common or rare side effects may include:*
Agitation, anemia, anxiety, central nervous system depression, confusion, constipation, difficulty breathing, disturbed thinking, dizziness, fainting, fever, hallucinations, headache, inflammation and peeling, insomnia, lack of coordination, low blood pressure, nausea, nervousness, nightmares, overactivity, skin rash, slow heartbeat, temporary failure to breathe, vomiting

Why should this drug not be prescribed?

You should not take Nembutal if you have porphyria (a rare blood disorder).

Do not take Nembutal if you are known to be sensitive to barbiturates.

Special warnings about this medication

Do not abruptly stop taking Nembutal. This may result in withdrawal symptoms and even death. To reduce any possible withdrawal symptoms, follow your doctor's instructions closely when stopping Nembutal.

Minor withdrawal symptoms may include increased dreams or nightmares.

Other minor withdrawal symptoms usually occur in the following order: anxiety, muscle twitching, tremors of hands and fingers, progressive weakness, dizziness, visual problems, nausea, vomiting, insomnia, and light-headedness (especially on standing up).

Major withdrawal symptoms may include convulsions and delirium.

Use Nembutal cautiously if you have had liver disease or have a history of depression, suicidal tendencies, and drug or alcohol abuse.

Inform your doctor if you have chronic or episodic pain. Nembutal may hide pain-causing symptoms that require treatment.

Elderly people may become confused, depressed, or excited while taking Nembutal.

Nembutal may lessen the effectiveness of oral contraceptives. Women who take Nembutal may need to consider another type of birth control.

The 100-milligram strength of Nembutal contains a coloring agent that may cause allergic reactions in some people.

This drug may impair your ability to drive a car or operate potentially dangerous machinery. Do not participate in any activities that require full alertness if you are unsure of your ability.

Possible food and drug interactions when taking this medication

If Nembutal is taken with certain other drugs, the effects of either could be increased, decreased, or altered. It is especially important to check with your doctor before combining Nembutal with the following:

Anticoagulants such as Dicumarol and Coumadin
Antihistamines such as Benadryl
Corticosteroids such as Decadron, Prednisone
Doxycycline (Vibramycin)
Griseofulvin (Gris-PEG)
MAO inhibitors (antidepressant drugs such as Nardil)
Oral contraceptives
Phenytoin (Dilantin)
Steroidal hormones such as Progestrone and Premarin
Tranquilizers such as Xanax, Valium
Valproic acid (Depakene, Depakote)

Extreme drowsiness and other potentially serious effects can result if Nembutal is combined with alcohol or other central nervous system depressants (Percocet, Demerol).

Special information
if you are pregnant or breastfeeding

Nembutal causes fetal damage and withdrawal symptoms in newborns. It appears in breast milk, and should be used with caution by nursing mothers.

Recommended dosage

ADULTS

For Insomnia
The usual dose is 100 milligrams, taken at bedtime.

CHILDREN

Dosages for children should be based on the child's age and weight.

ELDERLY

Because elderly people may be more sensitive to Nembutal, it should be taken at lower dosages. People with impaired kidney function or liver disease should also take lower doses.

Overdosage

Any medication taken in excess can have serious consequences. An overdose of Nembutal can be fatal. If you suspect an overdose, seek medical help immediately.

Symptoms of Nembutal overdose may include:
Coma, constriction (or sometimes dilation) of pupils, difficulty breathing, fluid in the lungs, heart failure, kidney failure, lack of reflexes, low blood pressure, low body temperature, pneumonia, rapid or irregular heartbeat, reduced flow of urine

Brand name:

NEODECADRON OPHTHALMIC OINTMENT AND SOLUTION

Generic ingredients: Dexamethasone sodium phosphate, Neomycin sulfate

Why is this drug prescribed?

Neodecadron is a steroid and antibiotic combination that is used to treat inflammatory eye conditions in which there is also a bacterial infection or the possibility of a bacterial infection. Dexamethasone decreases inflammation. Neomycin, the antibiotic, kills some of the more common bacteria.

Most important fact about this drug
The prolonged use of Neodecadron may increase the possibility of developing additional eye infections, cause vision problems, or even result in glaucoma and cataracts. If you take this medication for 10 days or longer, your doctor will routinely check your eye pressure.

How should you use this medication?
A thin coating of Neodecadron Ophthalmic Ointment should be applied to the eye.

What side effects may occur?
Side effects cannot be anticipated. If any develop or change in intensity, notify your doctor as soon as possible. Only your doctor can determine whether it is safe to continue using Neodecadron.

■ *Side effects may include:*
 Allergic skin reactions
 Cataracts
 Delay in healing of wounds
 Development of additional eye infections
 Increased eye pressure with possible
  glaucoma and optic nerve damage

Why should this drug not be prescribed?
Neodecadron should be avoided if you have an inflammation of the cornea (lens); chickenpox; other bacterial, fungal, or viral eye infections; or if you have recently had a foreign body removed from your cornea. Do not use the ointment if you have ever had an allergic reaction or are sensitive to any of its ingredients.

Special warnings about this medication
Using Neodecadron for a long time may result in glaucoma, vision changes, and cataracts and increase the chances of developing an additional eye infection. The steroid component of Neodecadron (dexamethasone) may hide the symptoms of infection or cause an existing infection to worsen. If you use Neodecadron for 10 days or longer, your doctor should check your eye pressure regularly.

If you develop a skin rash or any other allergic reaction, stop using the ointment and contact your doctor.

Neodecadron may cause temporary blurring of vision or stinging.

This prescription should not be renewed unless your doctor has re-examined your eyes.

Using steroids for a long time may cause infections of the cornea.

Possible food and drug interactions when taking this medication
No interactions have been reported.

Special information
if you are pregnant or breastfeeding
No information is available about the safety of Neodecadron during pregnancy and when breastfeeding.

If you are pregnant or plan to become pregnant, inform your doctor immediately.

Recommended dosage
The length of treatment varies with the type of condition being treated. Treatment can take a few days or several weeks.

NEODECADRON OPHTHALMIC OINTMENT

Apply a thin coating of Neodecadron Ophthalmic Ointment 3 or 4 times a day. When the condition gets better, daily applications should be reduced to 2 and later to 1 if a maintenance dose is required to control the symptoms.

NEODECADRON OPTHALMIC SOLUTION

The recommended initial dose is to place 1 or 2 drops into the conjunctival sac every hour during the day and every 2 hours during the night.

Overdosage

Any medication taken in excess can have serious consequences. If you suspect a Neodecadron overdose, seek medical treatment immediately.

Generic name:

NEOMYCIN WITH DEXAMETHASONE

See NeoDecadron, page 410.

Brand name:

NEPTAZANE

Generic name: Methazolamide

Why is this drug prescribed?

Neptazane, a carbonic acid inhibitor, is used to treat chronic open-angle glaucoma. This type of glaucoma is caused by a gradual blockage of the outflow of fluid in the front compartment of the eye over a period of years, causing a slow rise in pressure. It rarely occurs before the age of 40. Neptazane is also used in acute angle-closure glaucoma when eye pressure must be lowered before surgery.

Most important fact about this drug

Neptazane should not be used by women during their childbearing years, or by pregnant women, especially during the first 3 months of pregnancy, unless a doctor has determined that the benefits outweigh the potential risks.

How should you take this medication?

Take Neptazane exactly as prescribed by your doctor.

It can be used with other eye medications.

What side effects may occur?

Side effects cannot be anticipated. If any occur or change in intensity, inform your doctor as soon as possible. Only your doctor can determine if it is safe for you to continue taking Neptazane. Most reactions to Neptazane have been mild and disappear when the medication is stopped or the dosage is adjusted.

■ *More common side effects may include:* Confusion, depression, diarrhea, dizziness, excessive urination, exhaustion or drowsiness, fever, general feeling of not being well, headache, hearing disfunction, loss of appetite, nausea, rash, ringing in the ears, severe allergic reaction, tingling in fingers, toes, hands or feet and occasionally the lips, mouth, and anus, vomiting

■ *Rare side effects may include:* Hives, increased sensitivity to sunlight, kidney stones

Why should this drug not be prescribed?

Neptazane should not be used if you have severe or absolute glaucoma, chronic noncongestive angle-closure glaucoma, kidney or liver disease, adrenal gland disorders, or low sodium or potassium.

Special warnings about this medication

This medication should not be used by women in their childbearing years or by pregnant women, especially during the first 3 months of pregnancy, unless a doctor has determined that the potential benefits outweigh the potential risks to the unborn child.

Neptazane initially causes your body to lose potassium and sodium. If you have liver or kidney disease, low potassium or sodium, or are on steroid therapy, this medication should be used cautiously.

Neptazane should not be used over a long period of time by people with angle-closure glaucoma, since it may cause organic closure of the angle.

Neptazane can aggravate acidosis, a disturbance in the acid-base balance in the blood where the blood is too acidic. If you have emphysema or a lung blockage, this drug should be used with care.

This medication is obtained from sulfonamide (sulfa drugs) and can cause allergic reactions, including fever, rash, redness of the skin, hives, difficulty breathing, serious skin and blood disorders, and even death. Make sure your doctor is aware of any drug reactions that you have experienced. Your doctor should do a complete blood count before starting treatment with Neptazane and should monitor your blood while you are taking this drug. Call your doctor immediately if you experience any allergic symptoms.

Possible food and drug interactions when taking this medication

If Neptazane is taken with certain other drugs, the effects of either could be increased, decreased, or altered.

Loss of body weight, rapid breathing, lethargy, coma, and death have been reported in cases where Neptazane and high-dose aspirin are taken at the same time.

Use of Neptazane with steroids may lead to a lowering of the blood's potassium level.

Special information if you are pregnant or breastfeeding

Neptazane should not be used by pregnant women, especially in the first 3 months of pregnancy. If you are pregnant or plan to become pregnant, inform your doctor immediately. Neptazane may appear in breast milk and could affect a nursing infant.

If this medication is essential to your health, your doctor may advise you to stop breastfeeding until your treatment with Neptazane is finished.

Recommended dosage

ADULTS

Dosage varies from 50 milligrams to 100 milligrams taken 2 to 3 times a day.

Overdosage

Any drug taken in excess can have serious consequences. If you suspect an overdose seek medical attention immediately.

Generic name:

NICARDIPINE HYDROCHLORIDE

See Cardene, page 91.

Brand name:

NICORETTE

Generic name: Nicotine polacrilex

Why is this drug prescribed?

Nicorette is used as a temporary aid by cigarette smokers who want to stop.

Nicorette is most effective when used in a medically supervised behavior modification program offering education, counseling, and psychological support.

Most important fact about this drug

Nicorette contains nicotine—an addicting and toxic substance. Nicorette is a powerful, potentially addicting medication that must be used according to your doctor's instructions.

How should you take this medication?

The following are general, medically approved guidelines for taking Nicorette, but you should carefully follow your doctor's instructions to avoid adverse effects and/or addiction to Nicorette.

1) You must give up smoking completely and immediately when you start using Nicorette.

2) When you want to smoke, put 1 piece of Nicorette in your mouth.

3) Chew Nicorette very slowly; chewing Nicorette too fast may release the nicotine in the product too quickly, causing the same effects as inhaling for the first time or smoking too fast (e.g. light-headedness, nausea, vomiting, throat and mouth soreness, hiccups, and upset stomach).

4) Stop chewing when you have a peppery taste or feel a slight tingling in your mouth. This usually happens after about 15 chews.

5) "Park" the gum by placing it between your cheek and gums.

6) Start SLOWLY chewing again when the peppery taste or tingling feeling is almost gone (about 1 minute). Stop chewing when the peppery taste or tingling returns.

7) "Park" the gum again in a different part of the mouth.

8) Repeat this procedure until most of the nicotine is gone from the gum (about 30 minutes).

9) Do not use more than 30 pieces of Nicorette a day.

10) As your urge to smoke fades, gradually use fewer pieces of Nicorette. This may be possible in 2 to 3 months.

11) Stop using Nicorette when you are satisfied with 1 or 2 pieces a day, unless your doctor tells you otherwise. If you have trouble reducing your use of Nicorette, contact your doctor. Do not use Nicorette for more than 6 months.

12) Carry Nicorette with you at all times in case you feel the urge to smoke again.

What side effects may occur?
Side effects cannot be anticipated. If any develop or change in intensity, inform your doctor as soon as possible. Only your doctor can determine if it is safe for you to continue taking this medication.

■ *More common side effects may include:*
Belching, dizziness, excessive saliva in mouth, headaches, hiccups, indigestion, inflammation of the gums, tongue, throat, injury to teeth or cheeks, insomnia (inability to sleep), irritability, jaw ache, light-headedness, loss of appetite, mouth sores and/or soreness, nausea, stomach and intestinal discomfort, throat soreness, vomiting

■ *Less common or rare side effects may include:*
Breathing difficulty, confusion, congestive heart failure, constipation, convulsions, cough, depression, diarrhea, dry mouth, erythemia (skin redness), exaggerated feeling of well-being, fainting, fluid retention, flushing, heart attack, high blood pressure, hives, hoarseness, irregular or rapid heartbeat, itching, nicotine poisoning, numbness, palpitations, rash, ringing in the ears, sneezing, stroke, tingling sensation, weakness, wheezing

Why should this drug not be prescribed?
You should not be using Nicorette if you are a non-smoker, have had a heart attack, have heart disease or abnormal heartbeat, or have disease of the joint of the jaw.

If you are pregnant or planning to become pregnant, you should not use Nicorette. If you become pregnant while using Nicorette, contact your doctor immediately as Nicorette should be discontinued.

Mothers who nurse their babies should not use Nicorette.

Special warnings about this medication

Using Nicorette on a long-term basis is not recommended because nicotine, if consumed for a long enough time, can be harmful and addicting.

You must chew Nicorette slowly and follow your doctor's instructions carefully to avoid adverse side effects and/or becoming addicted to Nicorette.

Before using Nicorette, tell your doctor if you have ever had asthma, Buerger's disease (disease of the arteries), endocrine (hormone) diseases, dental problems, diabetes, difficulty swallowing, heartburn, heart disease, high blood pressure, lung disease, pheochromocytoma (tumor of an adrenal gland), peptic ulcer, throat inflammation, or thyroid disease.

Nicorette may damage dentures.

Possible food and drug interactions when taking this medication

If Nicorette is taken with certain other drugs, the effects of either could be increased, decreased, or altered. It is especially important to check with your doctor before combining Nicorette with the following:

Adrenergic agonists (the asthma drugs
    Proventil, Ventolin)
Adrenergic blockers such as Tenormin
Furosemide (Lasix)
Glutethimide (the sedative drug Doriden)
Imipramine (Tofranil)
Pentazocine (Talwin)
Phenacetin, the pain and fever reducer
Propoxyphene (Darvon)

Propranolol (Inderal)
Theophylline (Theo-Dur)

Special information
if you are pregnant or breastfeeding

If you are pregnant or nursing your baby, you should not use Nicorette. If you become pregnant while using Nicorette, contact your doctor immediately, as Nicorette should be discontinued.

Recommended dosage

ADULTS

Chew 1 piece of Nicorette whenever you have the urge to smoke. Most adults require 10 to 12 pieces of Nicorette a day during the first month of treatment. Follow your doctor's advice to be sure you are using Nicorette correctly. Do not use more than 30 pieces a day. After three months, follow your doctor's plan for gradual withdrawal of Nicorette.

CHILDREN

Safety and effectiveness for children and adolescents who smoke have not been established. If a child swallows a piece of Nicorette accidentally, contact your doctor or local poison control center at once.

ELDERLY

Elderly patients should use Nicorette cautiously.

Overdosage

Any medication taken in excess can have serious consequences. Overdose may occur if you chew many pieces of Nicorette at one time and can result in serious adverse effects. Accidentally swallowing a piece of Nicorette will probably not cause side effects, but if you have any reason to suspect an overdose, seek medical help immediately.

Symptoms of Nicorette overdose are similar to symptoms of acute nicotine poisoning and may include:

Abdominal pain, circulatory collapse (followed by terminal convulsions and death), cold sweat, diarrhea, difficulty breathing, disturbed hearing and vision, dizziness, fainting, headache, low blood pressure, mental confusion, nausea, rapid, weak, and irregular pulse, respiratory failure followed by death, salivation, vomiting, weakness

Category:

NICOTINE PATCHES

Brand names: Habitrol, Nicoderm, Nicotrol, Prostep

Why is this drug prescribed?

Nicotine patches, which are available under several brand names, are designed to help you quit smoking by reducing your craving for tobacco. Each adhesive patch contains a specific amount of nicotine embedded in a pad or gel.

Nicotine, the habit-forming ingredient in tobacco, is a stimulant and a mood lifter. When you give up smoking, lack of nicotine makes you crave cigarettes and may also cause anger, anxiety, concentration problems, irritability, frustration, or restlessness.

When you wear a nicotine patch, a specific amount of nicotine steadily travels out of the patch, through your skin, and into your bloodstream, keeping a constant low level of nicotine in your body. Although the resulting level of nicotine is less than you would get from smoking, it may be enough to keep you from craving cigarettes or experiencing other withdrawal symptoms.

Habitrol patches are round and come in three strengths: 21, 14, or 7 milligrams of nicotine per patch. You wear a Habitrol patch 24 hours a day.

Nicoderm patches are rectangular and come in three strengths: 21, 14, or 7 milligrams of nicotine per patch. You wear a Nicoderm patch 24 hours a day.

Nicotrol patches are rectangular and come in three strengths: 15, 10, or 5 milligrams of nicotine per patch. You put on a Nicotrol patch in the morning, wear it all day, and remove it at bedtime. You do not use it when you sleep.

Prostep patches are round and come in two strengths: 22 or 11 milligrams of nicotine per patch. You wear a Prostep patch 24 hours a day.

Most important fact about this drug

Because a used nicotine patch still contains enough nicotine to poison a child or a pet, you must dispose of used patches with special care. Wrap each patch in the opened pouch or aluminum foil in which it came and throw it in a trash receptacle that is out of the reach of youngsters and animals.

How should you use this medication?

Nicotine patch therapy should be part of an overall stop-smoking program that also includes behavior modification, counseling, and support. The goal of the therapy should be complete cessation of smoking, not just "cutting down."

Do not smoke any form of tobacco while wearing a patch; doing so could give you an overdose of nicotine. Be aware that for several hours after you remove a patch, nicotine from the patch is still in your skin and passing into your bloodstream.

Use nicotine patches exactly as prescribed by your doctor. The general procedure is as follows:

■ Take a fresh patch out of its packaging and remove the protective liner from the adhesive.

- Stick the patch onto your outer upper arm or any other clean, nonhairy part of your body.
- Press the patch firmly onto your skin for about 10 seconds, making sure that the edges are sticking well.
- Wash your hands. Any nicotine sticking to your hands could get into your eyes or nose, causing irritation.
- After 16 or 24 hours (depending on the brand), remove that patch and apply a fresh patch to a different spot on your body. To reduce the chances of irritation, do not return to a previously used spot for at least a week.
- Fold the used patch in half, place it back in its own wrapper, and throw it in a trash container that cannot be reached by children or pets.

Water will not harm the nicotine patch. You may keep wearing your patch while bathing, showering, swimming, or using a hot tub.

If your patch does fall off, dispose of it carefully and apply a new patch.

As a memory aid, pick a specific time of day and always apply a fresh patch at that time. You may change the schedule if you need to. Just remember not to wear any single patch for more than the recommended time (16 or 24 hours), since after that time the patch will begin to lose strength and may begin to irritate your skin.

Do not remove a patch from its wrapping until you are ready to use it. Store your supply of patches at temperatures no higher than 86 degrees Fahrenheit; remember that in warm weather the inside of a car can get much hotter than this.

Do not change brands without consulting your doctor.

If you are unable to stop smoking by your fourth week of wearing nicotine patches, it is likely that patch treatment will not work for you. At this point, your doctor may stop prescribing the patches for you.

What side effects may occur?

Side effects cannot be anticipated. If any develop or change in intensity, inform your doctor as soon as possible. Only your doctor can determine if it is safe for you to continue using nicotine patches.

- *Most common side effects may include:*
Itching and burning at the application site
Rash
Redness of the skin

- *Less common side effects may include:*
Allergic reactions, back pain, chest pain, constipation, cough, diarrhea, dizziness, dreaming abnormalities, drowsiness, dry mouth, headache, indigestion, nausea, nervousness, numbness, pain, pins and needles sensation, sleeplessness, sore throat, stomach pain, sweating, taste perversion, tingling, vomiting, weakness

Why should this drug not be prescribed?

Do not take this medication if you are sensitive to or have ever had an allergic reaction to nicotine. Be cautious if you have ever had a bad reaction to a different brand of nicotine patch or to adhesive tape or other adhesive material.

Special warnings about this medication

The use of nicotine patches may aggravate certain medical conditions. Before you use any brand of nicotine patch, make sure your doctor knows if you have, or have ever had, any of the following conditions:

Allergies to drugs, adhesive tape, or bandages
Chest pain from a heart condition (angina)
Diabetes requiring insulin injections
Heart attack

High blood pressure (severe)
Irregular heartbeat (heart arrhythmia)
Kidney disease
Liver disease
Overactive thyroid
Skin disease
Stomach ulcer

Possible food and drug interactions when taking this medication

If nicotine patches are used with certain other drugs, the effects of either could be increased, decreased, or altered. It is especially important to check with your doctor before combining nicotine patches with the following:

Acetaminophen-containing drugs such as Tylenol
Adrenergic agonists such as Isuprel, Dristan, and Neo-Synephrine
Adrenergic antagonists such as Minipress, Trandate, and Normodyne
Caffeine-containing drugs such as No Doz
Imipramine (Tofranil)
Insulin
Oxazepam (Serex)
Pentazocine (Talwin)
Propranolol (Inderal)
Theophylline (Theo-Dur and others)

Special information
If you are pregnant or breastfeeding

If you are pregnant or plan to become pregnant, inform your doctor immediately. Ideally, a pregnant woman should not take nicotine in any form. Do your best to quit smoking with the aid of counseling and support and without drug therapy. If you are unable to quit, you and your doctor should discuss which is more likely to harm your unborn baby: continued smoking or use of nicotine patches to help you quit smoking. Because nicotine passes very readily into breast milk, ideally it should not be taken in any form during breastfeeding.

If you are breastfeeding and are unable to quit smoking, discuss with your doctor the pros and cons of using nicotine patches.

Remember that if you smoke while wearing a patch, you are giving your body a "double dose" of nicotine; if you are pregnant or breastfeeding, your baby will get the "double dose" too.

Recommended dosage

Nicotine patches come in two or three strengths, depending on the brand; larger patches contain higher doses of nicotine. The usual starting dose is 1 high-strength patch per day. If you weigh less than 100 pounds, however, or if you smoke less than half a pack of cigarettes a day or have heart disease, your doctor may start you on a lower-dose patch.

Your doctor will work closely with you to determine the best product and the most effective cessation program.

Overdosage

Any medication used in excess, including nicotine patches, can have serious consequences. If you suspect symptoms of an overdose of nicotine, either from a patch or from smoking while wearing a patch, seek medical attention immediately.

Symptoms of nicotine overdose may include: Abdominal pain, blurred vision, breathing abnormalities, cold sweat, confusion, diarrhea, dizziness, drooling, fainting, hearing difficulties, heart palpitations, low blood pressure, nausea, pallor, salivation, severe headaches, sweating, tremor, upset stomach, vision problems, vomiting, weakness

Generic name:

NICOTINE POLACRILEX

See Nicorette, page 413.

Generic name:

NIFEDIPINE

See Procardia, page 505.

Generic name:

NIMODIPINE

See Nimotop, page 419.

Brand name:

NIMOTOP

Generic name: Nimodipine

Why is this drug prescribed?

Nimotop belongs to a class of drugs known as calcium channel blockers.

It is used to treat neurological deficiencies or problems caused by ruptured blood vessels in the head (subarachnoid hemorrhage or ruptured aneurysm).

Most important fact about this drug

To be effective, treatment with Nimotop must begin within 96 hours of the rupture and continue for 21 days.

Nimotop, like other calcium channel blockers, may lower blood pressure to some extent. Therefore, your doctor should monitor your blood pressure during therapy.

How should you take this medication?

Take Nimotop exactly as prescribed by your doctor.

What side effects may occur?

Side effects cannot be anticipated. If any develop or change in intensity, inform

your doctor as soon as possible. Only your doctor can determine if it is safe for you to continue taking Nimotop.

Nimotop tends to cause low blood pressure.

■ *Other potential side effects include:*
Acne, depression, diarrhea, dizziness, fluid retention, flushing, headache, high blood pressure, indigestion, labored breathing, lightheadedness, muscle pains or cramps, nausea, rash, sweating, vomiting, wheezing, worsening of existing heart failure or heartbeat abnormality, yellow eyes and skin

Why should this drug not be prescribed?

There are no known reasons for avoiding the use of Nimotop.

Special warnings about this medication

If you have cirrhosis of the liver, your body will process Nimotop at a slower-than-average rate. Your dosage of Nimotop will need to be cut in half; your blood pressure and heart rate should be monitored closely.

Possible food and drug interactions when taking this medication

If you are already taking another calcium channel blocker (e.g., Calan or Isoptin) or a medication to lower your blood pressure, Nimotop could conceivably make your blood pressure drop too much and you might need a dosage adjustment.

If you are already taking the peptic ulcer medication Tagamet (cimetidine), you may need a lower-than-average dosage of Nimotop.

Special information
if you are pregnant or breastfeeding

If you are pregnant or plan to become pregnant, inform your doctor immediately.

Nimotop should be used during pregnancy only if the potential benefit to the mother outweighs the potential risk to the unborn child.

It is not known whether Nimotop appears in breast milk. Therefore, new mothers are advised not to breastfeed while taking this drug.

Recommended dosage

ADULTS

The usual recommended dose of Nimotop is 60 milligrams every 4 hours for 21 consecutive days.

CHILDREN

It is not known whether Nimotop is safe and effective for children.

Overdosage

Although no specific information is available, an overdose of Nimotop would be expected to cause a severe drop in blood pressure, possibly requiring life-support measures.

Any medication taken in excess can have serious consequences. If you suspect an overdose of Nimotop, seek medical attention immediately.

Generic name:

NITROFURANTOIN

See Macrodantin, page 354.

Generic name:

NITROGLYCERIN

Brand names: Nitro-Bid, Nitro-Dur, Nitrolingual Spray, Nitrostat Tablets, Transderm-Nitro

Why is this drug prescribed?

Nitroglycerin is prescribed to prevent and treat angina pectoris (suffocating chest pain). This condition occurs when the arteries and veins become constricted and are not able to carry sufficient oxygen to the heart. Apparently, nitroglycerin improves oxygen flow by relaxing the muscles of arteries and veins, thus allowing them to dilate.

Nitroglycerin is used in different forms. As a patch or ointment, nitroglycerin may be applied to the skin. The patch is for prevention of chest pain. The ointment is used for both prevention and treatment.

Swallowed in capsule or tablet form, nitroglycerin helps to *prevent* chest pain from occurring.

In the form of sublingual (held under the tongue) or buccal (held in the cheek) tablets, or in oral spray (sprayed on or under the tongue), nitroglycerin helps relieve chest pain that has *already occurred*. The spray can also *prevent* anginal pain. The type of nitroglycerin you use will depend on your condition.

Most important fact about this drug

Nitroglycerin may cause severe low blood pressure (possibly marked by dizziness or light-headedness), especially if you are in an upright position. You may also find your heart rate slowing and your chest pain increasing. People taking diuretic medication, or who have low systolic blood pressure (less than 90 mm Hg) should use nitroglycerin with caution.

How should you take this medication?

Since nitroglycerin is available in many forms, it is crucial for you to follow your doctor's directions for taking the type of nitroglycerin prescribed for you. Never interchange brands.

Ideally, you should take nitroglycerin while sitting down—especially if you feel dizzy or light-headed—so as to avoid a fall.

What side effects may occur?

Side effects cannot be anticipated. If any develop or change in intensity, inform your doctor as soon as possible. Only your doctor can determine if it is safe for you to continue taking nitroglycerin.

If your vision becomes blurred or your mouth becomes dry, nitroglycerin should be discontinued. Contact your doctor immediately.

■ *More common side effects may include:*
Dizziness
Flushed skin (neck and face)
Headache
Light-headedness
Worsened angina pain

■ *Less common, or rare side effects may include:*
Diarrhea, fainting, heart pounding, low blood pressure, nausea, numbness, pallor, restlessness, sweating, vertigo, vomiting, weakness

Why should this drug not be prescribed?

You should not be using nitroglycerin if you are allergic to it or to the adhesive in the patch, if you have a head injury, or if you have any condition caused by increased fluid pressure in your head. Nitroglycerin should not be taken if you have severe anemia or if you recently had a heart attack. The capsule form should not be used if you have closed-angle glaucoma postural hypotension.

Special warnings about this medication

If your vision becomes blurry or your mouth becomes dry while taking nitroglycerin, it should be discontinued. Contact your doctor immediately if these symptoms develop.

You may develop acute headaches if you take nitroglycerin excessively. Also, some people may develop a tolerance to nitroglycerin, and

it may become less beneficial over time, especially if used in excess.

Take no more than the smallest possible amount needed to relieve pain.

Daily headaches may be an indicator of the drug's activity. Do not change your dose to avoid the headache, because you may reduce the drug's effectiveness at the same time.

Before taking nitroglycerin, tell your doctor if you have had a recent heart attack, head injury, or stroke; or if you have anemia, glaucoma, or heart, kidney, liver, or thyroid disease.

If you use a patch, dispose of it carefully. There is enough drug left in a used patch to be harmful to children and pets.

Since nitroglycerin can cause dizziness, you should observe caution while driving, operating machinery, or performing other tasks that demand concentration.

Possible food and drug interactions when taking this medication

If nitroglycerin is taken with certain other drugs, the effects of either could be increased, decreased, or altered. It is important to check with your doctor before combining nitroglycerin with the following:

Taken with many high blood pressure drugs, nitroglycerin may cause extreme low blood pressure (dizziness, fainting, numbness).

Alcohol may interact with nitroglycerin and cause a swift decrease in blood pressure, possibly causing dizziness and fainting.

Special information if you are pregnant or breastfeeding

It has not been determined whether nitroglycerin might harm a fetus or a pregnant woman. As a result, nitroglycerin should be used only when the benefits of therapy clearly outweigh the potential risks to the fetus and woman. It is not known if nitroglycerin appears in breast milk; therefore, nursing mothers should use nitroglycerin with caution.

Recommended dosage

The following section is intended to provide guidelines for taking nitroglycerin. Follow your doctor's instructions carefully for using nitroglycerin in the form prescribed for you.

ADULTS

Sublingual or Buccal Tablets
At the first sign of chest pain, 1 tablet should be dissolved under the tongue or inside the cheek. You may repeat the dose every 5 minutes until the pain is relieved. If your pain continues after you have taken 3 tablets in a 15-minute period, notify your doctor or seek medical attention immediately.

You may take sublingual or buccal nitroglycerin from 5 to 10 minutes before starting activities that may cause chest pain.

Patch Form
A patch is applied to the skin for 12 to 14 hours. After this time, the patch is removed; it is not applied again for 10 to 12 hours (a "patch-off" period).

Spray Form
At the first sign of chest pain, spray 1 or 2 premeasured doses onto or under the tongue. You should not use more than 3 doses within a 15-minute period. If your chest pain continues, you should contact your doctor or seek medical attention immediately.

The spray can be used 5–10 minutes before activity that might precipitate an attack.

Ointment Form
Your initial dose may be a daily total of 1 inch of ointment. Apply one-half inch on rising in the morning, and the remaining one-

half inch 8 hours later. If needed, follow your doctor's instructions for increasing your dosage. Apply in a thin, uniform layer, regardless of the amount of your dosage. There should be a daily period where no ointment is applied. Usually, the "ointment-off" period will last from 10 to 12 hours.

Absorption varies with site of application—more is absorbed through the chest.

Sustained-Release Capsules or Tablets
The smallest effective amount should be taken 2 or 3 times a day at 8- to 12-hour intervals.

CHILDREN

The safety and effectiveness of nitroglycerin have not been established for children.

ELDERLY

In general, dosages less than the above adult dosages are recommended, since the elderly may be more susceptible to low blood pressure and headaches.

Overdosage

Any medication taken in excess can have serious consequences. Severe overdosage of nitroglycerin may result in death. If you suspect an overdose, seek medical attention immediately.

Symptoms of overdose may include:
Bluish skin, clammy skin, colic, coma, confusion, diarrhea (may be bloody), difficult and/or slow breathing, dizziness, fainting, fever, flushed skin, headache (persistent, throbbing), increased pressure within the skull, irregular pulse, loss of appetite, nausea, palpitations (an abnormally rapid throbbing or fluttering of the heart), paralysis, rapid decrease in blood pressure, seizures, slow pulse/heartbeat, sweating, vertigo, visual disturbances, vomiting

Generic name:

NIZATIDINE

See Axid, page 50.

Brand name:

NIZORAL

Generic name: Ketoconazole

Why is this drug prescribed?

Nizoral, a broad-spectrum antifungal drug available in tablet form, may be given to treat several systemic fungal infections, including oral thrush and candidiasis.

It may also be given to treat severe, hard-to-treat fungal skin infections that have not cleared up after treatment with the drug griseofulvin, including Fulvicin, Grisactin, and others.

Most important fact about this drug

In some people, Nizoral may cause serious or even fatal damage to the liver. Before starting to take Nizoral, and at frequent intervals while you are taking it, you should have blood tests to evaluate your liver function. Tell your doctor immediately if you experience any signs or symptoms suggestive of liver damage: these include unusual fatigue, loss of appetite, nausea or vomiting, dark urine, or pale stools.

Serious and sometime fatal reactions involving the heart have been reported in patients taking Nizoral and Seldane. You should not take these two drugs together.

How should you take this medication?

Before you start to take Nizoral, you should have tests as well as a physical examination to determine that you do in fact have a fungal infection.

Take Nizoral exactly as prescribed by your doctor.

You should take Nizoral until tests show that your fungal infection has subsided. Be sure to keep taking the medication until you have used it all; if you stop too soon, the infection might return.

You may want to take Nizoral Tablets with meals to avoid stomach upset.

Do not take with antacids. If necessary, you should wait 2 to 3 hours before taking antacids.

What side effects may occur?

Side effects from Nizoral cannot be anticipated. If any develop or change in intensity, inform your doctor as soon as possible. Only your doctor can determine if it is safe for you to continue taking Nizoral.

■ *More common side effects may include:*
Abdominal pain
Itching
Nausea
Vomiting

■ *Less common side effects may include:*
Breast swelling (in men), bulging fontanel (soft areas on a baby's scalp), decreased sperm count, depression, diarrhea, dizziness, drowsiness, fever and chills, headache, impotence, light-sensitivity, rash

Why should this drug not be prescribed?

Do not take Nizoral if you are sensitive to it or have ever had an allergic reaction to it.

Nizoral is ineffective in treating meningitis caused by a fungus and should not be prescribed for this purpose.

Special warnings about this medication

A few people have had anaphylaxis (a life-threatening allergic reaction) after taking their first dose of Nizoral. Observe caution when driving or performing other tasks requiring alertness, due to potential side effects of headache, dizziness, and drowsiness.

Possible food and drug interactions when taking this medication

If Nizoral is taken with alcoholic beverages or certain other drugs, the effects of either could be increased, decreased, or altered. It is especially important to check with your doctor before combining Nizoral with the following:

Alcoholic beverages
Antacids such as Di-Gel, Maalox, Mylanta, and others
Anticoagulants such as Coumadin, Dicumarol, and others
Antidiabetic drugs such as Diabinese, Tolinase, and others
Anti-ulcer medications such as Axid, Pepcid, Tagamet, and Zantac
Benzodiazepines such as Dalmane, Valium, Xanax, and others
Corticosteroids such as Celestone, Florinef, Medrol, and others
Cyclosporine A (Sandimmune)
Isoniazid (Nydrazid)
Phenytoin (Dilantin)
Rifampin (Rifadin, Rifamate, and Rimactane)
Terfenadine (Seldane)
Theophyllines such as Bronkodyl, Elixicon, Theo-Dur, and others

Special information if you are pregnant or breastfeeding

If you are pregnant or plan to become pregnant, inform your doctor immediately. Nizoral should be taken during pregnancy only if the benefit outweighs the possible harm to your unborn child.

Since Nizoral can probably make its way into breast milk, it should not be taken during breastfeeding. If you are a new mother, you may need to stop breastfeeding while you are taking Nizoral.

Recommended dosage

ADULTS

The recommended starting dose of Nizoral is a single daily dose of 200 milligrams (1 tablet).

In very serious infections, or if the patient's response is insufficient within the expected time, the dose of Nizoral may be increased to 400 milligrams (2 tablets) once daily.

CHILDREN

In small numbers of children over 2 years of age, a single daily dose of 3.3 to 6.6 milligrams per 2.2 pounds of body weight has been used.

Nizoral has not been studied in children under 2 years of age.

Overdosage

Although no specific information is available, any medication taken in excess can have serious consequences. If you suspect an overdose of Nizoral, seek medical attention immediately.

Brand name:

NOLAMINE

Generic ingredients: Phenindamine tartrate, Chlorpheniramine maleate, Phenylpropanolamine hydrochloride

Why is this drug prescribed?

Nolamine is a nasal decongestant that relieves stuffiness caused by the common cold, inflamed sinuses, or hay fever and other allergies. Nolamine's ingredients include antihistamines (chlorpheniramine maleate and phenindamine tartrate), that reduce itching and swelling and dry up secretions from the nose, eyes, and throat, and a decongestant (phenylpropanolamine hydrochloride), that improves breathing.

Most important fact about this drug

Nolamine can cause drowsiness. Driving or operating dangerous machinery or participating in any hazardous activity that requires full mental alertness is not recommended until know how you react to Nolamine.

How should you take this medication?

Nolamine should be taken exactly as prescribed by your doctor.

What side effects may occur?

Side effects cannot be anticipated. If any develop or change in intensity, inform your doctor as soon as possible. Only your doctor can determine if it is safe for you to continue taking Nolamine.

■ *Side effects may include:*
Difficulty sleeping
Dizziness
Drowsiness
Nervousness
Tremors

Why should this drug not be prescribed?

Nolamine should not be taken if you are sensitive to or have ever had an allergic reaction to any of its ingredients, or if you are taking MAO inhibitor medications such as the antidepressant drugs Nardil and Parnate.

Special warnings about this medication

Nolamine should be used cautiously if you have high blood pressure, cardiovascular disease, diabetes, overactive thyroid, glaucoma, or an enlarged prostate.

Before getting behind the wheel, remember that Nolamine can make you drowsy.

Possible food and drug interactions when taking this medication

If Nolamine is taken with certain other drugs, the effects of either could be increased, decreased, or altered. It is especially important to check with your doctor before combining Nolamine with the following:

MAO inhibitor medication such as the antidepressants Parnate, Nardil, and Marplan

Recommended dosage

ADULTS

The usual dose is 1 tablet every 8 hours. The dosage in mild cases is 1 tablet every 10 to 12 hours.

Overdosage

Although there are no reports of overdose, any medication taken in excess can have serious consequences. If you suspect an overdose, seek medical attention immediately.

Brand name:

NOLEX LA

See Entex LA, page 237.

Brand name:

NOLVADEX

Generic name: Tamoxifen citrate

Why is this drug prescribed?

Nolvadex, an anticancer drug, may be given after mastectomy to help delay a recurrence of breast cancer. It also has proved effective when breast cancer has spread to other parts of the body. Nolvadex is most effective in thwarting the kind of breast cancer that thrives on estrogen.

Most important fact about this drug

In a few women Nolvadex has caused overgrowth of, or polyps within, the endometrium (lining of the uterus). If you experience unexplained bleeding from the vagina while taking Nolvadex, report this to your doctor immediately.

How should you take this medication?

Take Nolvadex exactly as prescribed by your doctor.

Medical researchers are still investigating how long Nolvadex should be taken following breast-cancer surgery. In one ongoing study, women who have undergone mastectomy will be taking the drug twice a day for five years.

Birth control measures are recommended during treatment with Nolvadex. However, methods other than "the Pill" must be employed.

What side effects may occur?

Side effects from Nolvadex are usually mild and rarely require the drug to be stopped. Some women experience adverse effects on their vision, such as cataracts or problems with the cornea or retina. Some get overgrowth of, or polyps within, the lining of the uterus. In others, Nolvadex may produce hypercalcemia, an abnormally high level of calcium in the blood.

- *More common side effects may include:*
  Hot flashes
  Nausea
  Vomiting

- *Less common side effects may include:*
  Bone pain, menstrual irregularities, skin rash, tumor pain, vaginal bleeding, vaginal discharge

- *Rare side effects may include:*
  Depression, distaste for food, dizziness, headache, swelling of arms or legs, vaginal itching, visual problems

Why should this drug not be prescribed?

Do not take Nolvadex if you are sensitive to it or have ever had an allergic reaction to it.

Special warnings about this medication

In a few women Nolvadex may raise the level of cholesterol and other fats in the blood. Your doctor may periodically do blood tests to check your cholesterol and triglyceride levels.

If you are also taking a blood thinner such as Coumadin, Nolvadex may cause the drug to thin your blood too much. To guard against this, your doctor will probably do frequent tests to check the time it takes your blood to clot.

If tests while you are taking Nolvadex show that your blood contains too few white blood cells or platelets, your doctor should monitor you with special care. Low white blood cell or platelet counts have sometimes been found in women taking Nolvadex; whether the drug caused the blood-cell abnormalities is uncertain.

Possible food and drug interactions when taking this medication

If Nolvadex is taken with certain other drugs, the effects of either could be increased, decreased, or altered. It is especially important to check with your doctor before combining Nolvadex with blood thinners such as Coumadin.

Special information if you are pregnant or breastfeeding

It is important to avoid pregnancy while taking Nolvadex, because the drug could harm the unborn child. Since Nolvadex is an anti-estrogen drug, you will need to use a non-hormonal form of contraception, such as a condom and/or diaphragm, and not birth control pills. If you accidentally become pregnant while taking Nolvadex, discuss this with your doctor right away.

Because Nolvadex might cause serious harm to a nursing infant, you should not breastfeed your baby while taking this drug. If you are a new mother, you may need to choose between taking Nolvadex and breastfeeding your baby.

Recommended dosage

ADULT

One or two 10-milligram tablets in the morning and evening.

Overdosage

Although no specific information is available, any medication taken in excess can have serious consequences. If you suspect an overdose of Nolvadex, seek medical attention immediately.

Brand name:

NORCET

See Vicodin, page 678.

Brand name:

NORDETTE

See Oral Contraceptives, page 437.

Brand name:

NORETHIN

See Oral Contraceptives, page 437.

Generic name:

NORFLOXACIN

See Noroxin, page 431.

Brand name:

NORGESIC FORTE

Generic ingredients: Orphenadrine citrate, Aspirin, Caffeine
Other brand name: Norgesic

Why is this drug prescribed?

Norgesic Forte is prescribed, along with rest, physical therapy, and other measures, for the relief of mild-to-moderate pain of severe skeletal muscle disorders.

Most important fact about this drug

Because the safety of continuous, long-term therapy with Norgesic Forte has not been established, your doctor should monitor your blood, urine, and liver function if you use this drug for a prolonged period of time.

How should you take this medication?

Take Norgesic Forte exactly as prescribed by your doctor.

What side effects may occur?

Side effects cannot be anticipated. If any develop or change in intensity, inform your doctor as soon as possible. Only your doctor can determine if it is safe for you to continue taking Norgesic Forte.

■ *Side effects, usually associated with the aspirin or caffeine content of Norgesic Forte, may include:*
Blurred vision, confusion (in the elderly), constipation, difficulty in urinating, dilation of the pupils, dizziness, drowsiness, dry mouth, fainting, hallucinations, headache, hives, light-headedness, nausea, palpitations, rapid heart rate, skin diseases, stomach and intestinal bleeding, vomiting, weakness

Why should this drug not be prescribed?

If you are sensitive to or have ever had an allergic reaction to orphenadrine, aspirin, caffeine, or drugs of this type, you should not take this medication. Make sure that your doctor is aware of any drug reactions that you have experienced.

You should not be taking Norgesic Forte if you have glaucoma, a stomach or intestinal blockage, an enlarged prostate gland, bladder neck obstruction, achalasia (failure of stomach or intestinal muscles to relax), or myasthenia gravis (muscle weakness and fatigue).

Because there is a possible association between aspirin and Reye's syndrome, Norgesic Forte should not be given to any person who has chickenpox or flu.

Special warnings about this medication

Norgesic Forte may impair your ability to drive a car or operate dangerous machinery. Participation in potentially hazardous activities is not recommended until you know how you react to this medication.

Because Norgesic Forte contains aspirin, you should be careful taking it if you have a peptic ulcer or problems with blood clotting.

Possible food and drug interactions when taking this medication

If Norgesic Forte is taken with certain other drugs, the effects of either could be increased, decreased, or altered. It is especially important to check with your doctor before combining Norgesic Forte with Propoxyphene (Darvon).

Confusion, anxiety, and tremors have been reported occasionally when the orphenadrine component of Norgesic Forte is used in combination with Darvon.

Special information if you are pregnant or breastfeeding

The effects of Norgesic Forte during pregnancy have not been adequately studied. If you are pregnant or plan to become pregnant, inform your doctor immediately. This drug may appear in breast milk and could affect a nursing infant. If this medication is essential to your health, your doctor may advise you to discontinue breastfeeding until your treatment is finished.

Recommended dosage

ADULTS

The usual recommended dosage of Norgesic Forte is one-half to 1 tablet, taken 3 or 4 times per day.

CHILDREN

The safety and effectiveness of orphenadrine have not been established in children under 12 years of age.

ELDERLY

The usual recommended dosage of Norgesic is 1 to 2 tablets 3 or 4 times per day. Norgesic is exactly half the strength of Norgesic Forte.

Some elderly patients have experienced confusion when taking this drug. Therefore, the doctor will prescribe a dose individualized to the elderly patient's needs.

Overdosage

Any medication taken in excess can have serious consequences. If you suspect an overdose, seek emergency medical treatment immediately.

Brand name:

NORINYL

See Oral Contraceptives, page 437.

Brand name:

NORMODYNE

Generic name: Labetalol hydrochloride
Other brand name: Trandate

Why is this drug prescribed?

Normodyne is used in the treatment of high blood pressure. It is effective when used alone or in combination with other high blood pressure medications, especially thiazide and loop diuretics (types of water pills).

Most important fact about this drug

Normodyne must be taken regularly for it to be effective. Even if you are feeling well, you must continue to take this medication. It is needed to maintain control of your blood pressure.

How should you take this medication?

Normodyne can be taken with or without food. The amount of Normodyne absorbed into your bloodstream is actually increased with food.

This medication should be taken exactly as prescribed by your doctor, even if your symptoms have disappeared.

Try not to miss any doses. If Normodyne is not taken regularly, your condition may worsen.

What side effects may occur?

Side effects cannot be anticipated. If any develop or change in intensity, inform your doctor as soon as possible. Only your doctor can determine if it is safe for you to continue taking Normodyne.

■ *More common side effects may include:*
Changes in taste, dizziness, dizziness when standing, ejaculation failure, fatigue, fluid retention, headache, impotence, indigestion, nausea, rash, shortness of breath, stuffy nose, tingling or pins and needles, vertigo, vision changes, weakness

■ *Less common or rare side effects may include:*
Aching, sore throat,* closure of the larynx, colitis (inflammation of the colon),* depression, diarrhea, difficulty breathing,* difficulty urinating, disorientation,* drowsiness, dry eyes, emotional instability,* fainting, fever, heart block (condition disorder), hives, increased sweating, low blood pressure, lupus erythematosus (collagen vascular disease), muscle cramps, muscle disease, rash, short-term memory loss,* slow heartbeat, tingling scalp, weakness, wheezing or asthma-like symptoms, vomiting, yellow eyes and skin

*These side effects have been reported with other medications of this type and may occur with Normodyne.

Why should this drug not be prescribed?

Normodyne should not be used if you have bronchial asthma, active congestive heart failure, heart block (conduction disorder), inadequate blood supply to the circulatory system (cardiogenic shock), or a severely slow heartbeat.

Special warnings about this medication

Normodyne has caused severe liver damage in some patients. Although this is a rare occurrence, if you develop any symptoms of abnormal liver function—itching, dark urine, continuing loss of appetite, yellow eyes and skin, or unexplained "flu-like" symptoms—contact your doctor immediately.

If you have a history of congestive heart failure or kidney disease, Normodyne should be used with caution.

Normodyne should not be stopped suddenly. This can cause chest pain and heart attack. Dosage should be gradually reduced.

If you suffer from asthma, chronic bronchitis, emphysema, or other bronchial diseases, Normodyne should be used cautiously.

If you suffer from adrenal tumors, treatment with Normodyne may cause your blood pressure to rise. Your doctor should monitor you carefully while you are on this medication.

This medication may mask the symptoms of low blood sugar or alter blood sugar levels. If you are diabetic, discuss this with your doctor.

Notify your doctor or dentist that you are taking Normodyne if you have a medical emergency, and before you have surgery or dental treatment.

Possible food and drug interactions when taking this medication

If Normodyne is taken with certain other drugs, the effects of either could be increased, decreased, or altered. It is especially important to check with your doctor before taking Normodyne with the following:

Adrenergic bronchodilators such as Proventil and Ventolin
Cimetidine (Tagamet)
Halothane, an anesthetic (Fluothane)
Nitroglycerin products such as Transderm-Nitro
Medications for depression called tricyclic antidepressants (for example, Elavil)

Special information if you are pregnant or breastfeeding

The effects of Normodyne during pregnancy have not been adequately studied. If you are pregnant or plan to become pregnant, inform your doctor immediately. Normodyne appears in breast milk and could affect a nursing infant. If this medication is essential to your health, your doctor may advise you to discontinue breastfeeding until your treatment is finished.

Recommended dosage

ADULTS

Dosages of this medication should be adjusted to the individual patient's needs. Your doctor may observe its effect in his office over a 1- to 3-hour period after you begin taking the drug, and then check your pressure again at regular office visits (12 hours after a dose) to make sure that the medicine is effective.

The usual starting dose is 100 milligrams, 2 times per day, alone or with a diuretic drug. After 2 to 3 days of checking your blood pressure, your doctor may begin increasing your dose by 100 milligrams, 2 times per day, at intervals of 2 to 3 days.

The regular dose ranges from 200 to 400 milligrams, 2 times per day. Some patients may require total daily dosage of as much as 1,200 to 2,400 milligrams, either alone or with a thiazide diuretic. In these cases, your doctor will observe the drug's effect and adjust your dose accordingly.

Your doctor may also adjust your dosage if this drug is used with a diuretic since this may increase the blood pressure-lowering effect more than is needed.

CHILDREN

The safety and effectiveness of this drug in children have not been established.

ELDERLY

This drug should be used with caution in elderly patients.

Overdosage

Any medication taken in excess can have serious consequences. If you suspect an overdose, seek medical treatment immediately.

The symptoms of Normodyne overdose may include:
Dizziness when standing up
Severely low blood pressure
Severely slow heartbeat

Brand name:

NOROXIN

Generic name: Norfloxacin

Why is this drug prescribed?

Noroxin is an antibacterial used to treat infections of the urinary tract, including cystitis (inflammation of the inner lining of the bladder caused by a bacterial infection), and certain sexually transmitted diseases, such as gonorrhea.

Most important fact about this drug

Noroxin is not given for the treatment of syphilis. When used in high doses for a short period of time to treat gonorrhea, it may actually mask or delay the symptoms of syphilis. Your doctor may perform certain tests for syphilis at the time of diagnosing gonorrhea, and after treatment with Noroxin.

How should you take this medication?

Noroxin should be taken, with a glass of water, either 1 hour *before* or 2 hours *after* eating a meal. Do not take more than the dosage prescribed by your doctor.

It is important to drink plenty of fluids while taking Noroxin.

You must continue the use of Noroxin until all the prescribed medicine has been taken. Failure to do so may result in incomplete elimination of the infection, causing a relapse.

What side effects may occur?

Side effects cannot be anticipated. If any develop or change in intensity, inform your doctor as soon as possible. Only your doctor can determine whether it is safe for you to continue taking this medication.

■ *More common side effects may include:*
Dizziness
Fatigue
Headache
Nausea

■ *Other side effects may include:*
Abdominal cramping, arthritis, back pain, bitter taste, confusion, constipation, convulsions, dead skin, depression, diarrhea, dizziness, dry mouth, double vision, extreme sleepiness, fever, flushed, reddish skin, gas, hallucinations, headache, heartburn, hives, indigestion, insomnia, itching, joint pain, kidney failure (symptoms may include reduced amount of urine, drowsiness, nausea, vomiting, coma, and death), lack of coordination, light-headedness, loss of appetite, muscle pain, nausea, peeling skin, psychotic reactions, rash (such as pimples, blisters, and nodules) on skin and mucous membranes, reduced blood platelets causing bleeding disorders (such as bleeding into the skin), restlessness, severe blisters and bleeding in genitals and in mucous membranes of eyes, lips, mouth, and nasal passages, severe skin reaction to sun, shock, shortness of breath, stomach pain, sweating, temporary hearing loss, tingling (pins and needles sensation), vomiting, weakness, yellow eyes and skin

Why should this drug not be prescribed?

You should not be using Noroxin if you are sensitive to it or to other drugs of the same type, such as Cipro.

Special warnings about this medication

Noroxin should NOT be used by:

Adolescents (under the age of 18)
Children
Nursing mothers
Pregnant women

People with disorders such as epilepsy, severe cerebral arteriosclerosis, and other conditions that might lead to seizures should use Noroxin cautiously.

There have been reports of convulsions in some people taking Noroxin.

Some people taking drugs chemically similar to Noroxin have experienced severe, sometimes fatal reactions, possibly occurring after only one dose.

These reactions may include:
Confusion, convulsions, difficulty breathing, hallucinations, heart collapse, hives, increased pressure in the head, itching, light-headedness, loss of consciousness, psychosis, rash, restlessness, shock, swelling in the face or throat, tingling, tremors

If you experience any of these reactions you should immediately stop taking Noroxin and seek medical help, if necessary.

Some patients may find needle-shaped crystals in their urine after taking Noroxin. Drink plenty of fluids while taking Noroxin to help you produce sufficient urine and thus avoid dehydration.

Noroxin may cause dizziness or light-headedness and might impair your ability to drive a car or operate potentially dangerous machinery. Do not participate in any activities that require full alertness if you are unsure about your ability.

You should avoid excessive exposure to direct sunlight while taking Noroxin. Stop taking Noroxin immediately if you have a severe reaction to sunlight, such as a skin rash.

Possible food and drug interactions when taking this medication

If Noroxin is taken with certain other drugs, the effects of either could be increased, decreased, or altered. It is especially important to check with your doctor before combining Noroxin with the following:

Antacids, such as Maalox and Tums
Caffeine (including coffee, tea, and some soft drinks)
Calcium supplements
Cyclosporine (Sandimmune)
Nitrofurantoin (Macrodantin, Macrobid)
Oral anticoagulants, such as warfarin (Coumadin)
Probenecid (Benemid)
Sucralfate (Carafate)
Theophylline (Theo-Dur)
Vitamins or products containing iron or zinc

Special information if you are pregnant or breastfeeding

Pregnant women and women who breastfeed an infant should not use Noroxin.

Recommended dosage

Take Noroxin with a full glass of water 1 hour before, or 2 hours after, eating a meal. Drink plenty of liquids while taking Noroxin.

Uncomplicated Urinary Tract Infections
The suggested dose is 800 milligrams per day. 400 milligrams should be taken twice a day for 3 to 10 days, depending upon the kind of bacteria causing the infection. People with impaired kidney function may take 400 milligrams once a day for 3 to 10 days.

Complicated Urinary Tract Infections
The suggested dose is 800 milligrams per day. 400 milligrams should be taken twice a day for 10 to 21 days.

Sexually Transmitted Diseases (Gonorrhea)
The recommended usual dose is one single dose of 800 milligrams for 1 day.

The maximum total daily dosage of Noroxin should not be more than 800 milligrams.

Overdosage

The symptoms of overdose with Noroxin are not known. However, any medication taken in excess can have serious consequences. If you suspect Noroxin overdose, seek medical help immediately.

Brand name:

NORPACE

Generic name: Disopyramide phosphate

Why is this drug prescribed?

Norpace is used to treat severe irregular heartbeat (arrhythmias). Arrhythmias are generally divided into two main types: heartbeats that are faster than normal (tachycardia) and heartbeats that are slower than normal (bradycardia). Arrhythmias are often caused by drugs or disease but can occur in otherwise healthy people with no history of heart disease or other illness. Norpace is similar to procainamide and quinidine, two other antiarrhythmic medications.

Most important fact about this drug

Your doctor should carefully monitor your heartbeat to make sure the medication is producing the desired effect. Norpace and Norpace CR are not recommended for mildly irregular heart rhythms and should be used only when other medications have been ineffective.

How should you take this medication?

Take this medication exactly as prescribed by your doctor.

Do not stop taking this medication without your doctor's approval.

What side effects may occur?

Side effects cannot be anticipated. If any develop or change in intensity, inform your doctor as soon as possible. Only your doctor can determine if it is safe for you to continue taking Norpace or Norpace CR.

■ *More common side effects may include:*
Abdominal pain, bloating, and gas, aches and pains, blurred vision, chest pain, congestive heart failure, constipation, diarrhea, dizziness, dry eyes, nose, and throat, dry mouth, fainting, fatigue, fluid retention, headache, impotence, increased urinary frequency and urgency, itching, loss of appetite, low blood pressure, muscle weakness, nausea, nervousness, rash, shortness of breath, urinary difficulty, vague feeling of bodily discomfort, vomiting, weight gain

■ *Less common or rare side effects may include:*
Breast development in males, depression, difficulty breathing, difficulty sleeping, low blood sugar (hypoglycemia), numbness or tingling, painful urination, severe psychosis, yellow eyes and skin

Why should this drug not be prescribed?

This drug should not be used if you have an inadequate blood supply to the heart (cardiogenic shock), heart block (without a pacemaker) or other cardiac conduction disorders, or if you are sensitive to or have ever had an allergic reaction to Norpace or Norpace CR.

Special warnings about this medication

If you have structural heart disease, inflammation of the heart muscle, or other heart disorders, this medication should be used with extreme caution.

Norpace or Norpace CR may cause or worsen congestive heart failure and can cause severe low blood pressure. If you have a history of heart failure, your doctor should carefully monitor your heart function while you are taking this medication.

Low blood sugar (hypoglycemia) can occur, especially if you have congestive heart failure; poor nutrition; or kidney, liver, or other diseases; or if you are taking beta blockers (Tenormin) or alcohol.

Norpace or Norpace CR should be used with other antiarrhythmic drugs, such as quinidine, procainamide, encainide, flecainide, propafenone, and/or propranolol, only when the irregular rhythm is considered life-threatening and other antiarrhythmic medication has not worked.

If you have glaucoma, myasthenia gravis, or difficulty urinating (particularly men with prostate conditions), use this drug cautiously.

Dosage levels should be reduced if you have liver or kidney disease.

Your doctor should check your potassium levels before starting you on Norpace or Norpace CR. High potassium levels may make this drug ineffective or increase its toxic effects.

Possible food and drug interactions when taking this medication

If Norpace or Norpace CR is taken with certain other drugs, the effects of either could be increased, decreased, or altered. It is especially important to check with your doctor before combining Norpace or Norpace CR with the following:

Phenytoin (Dilantin)
Other antiarrythmics such as quinidine (Quinidex), procainamide (Procan SR), lidocaine (Xylocaine), propranolol (Inderal)

Special information
if you are pregnant or breastfeeding

The effects of Norpace and Norpace CR during pregnancy have not been adequately studied. If you are pregnant or plan to become pregnant, inform your doctor immediately. Norpace and Norpace CR

appear in breast milk and may affect a nursing infant. If this medication is essential to your health, your doctor may advise you to discontinue breastfeeding until your treatment with this medication is finished.

Recommended dosage

Treatment with Norpace and Norpace CR should be started in the hospital.

ADULTS

Your doctor will adjust your dosage according to your own response to, and tolerance of, Norpace or Norpace CR.

The usual dosage of Norpace and Norpace CR is 400 milligrams to 800 milligrams per day, divided into smaller doses.

The recommended dosage for most adults is 600 milligrams per day, divided into smaller doses (either 150 milligrams every 6 hours for immediate-release Norpace or 300 milligrams every 12 hours for Norpace CR).

For patients whose body weight is less than 110 pounds, the recommended dosage is 400 milligrams per day, divided into smaller doses (either 100 milligrams every 6 hours for immediate-release Norpace or 200 milligrams every 12 hours for Norpace CR).

For patients with severe heart disease, initial doses should be limited to 100 milligrams of immediate-release Norpace every 6 to 8 hours. Dosage adjustments should be made gradually, and your doctor will monitor you closely for any signs of low blood pressure or heart failure.

For patients with moderately reduced kidney or liver function, the recommended dosage is 400 milligrams per day, divided into smaller doses (either 100 milligrams every 6 hours for immediate-release Norpace or 200 milligrams every 12 hours for Norpace CR).

For patients with severe kidney impairment, the recommended dosage of immediate-release Norpace is 100 milligrams at various times, depending on the degree of kidney dysfunction. The dose will be determined by your doctor.

Norpace CR is not recommended for patients with severe kidney disease.

CHILDREN

Dosage in children to age 18 is based on body weight. The total daily dosage should be divided into equal doses administered orally every 6 hours or at intervals according to the individual patient's needs. Your doctor will determine the correct dosage.

ELDERLY

Dosages for elderly patients should be individualized and monitored carefully.

Overdosage

Any medication taken in excess can have serious consequences. If you suspect symptoms of a Norpace or Norpace CR overdose, seek medical treatment immediately.

The symptoms of Norpace or Norpace CR overdose may include:
Cessation of breathing
Irregular heartbeat
Loss of consciousness

Deaths have occurred following overdosage.

Brand name:

NORPRAMIN

Generic name: Desipramine hydrochloride

Why is this drug prescribed?
Norpramin is used in the treatment of depression. It is one of a family of drugs called tricyclic antidepressants. Drugs in this class are thought to work by affecting the levels of the brain's natural chemical messengers (called neurotransmitters), and adjusting the brain's response to them.

Most important fact about this drug
If taken in large enough amounts, Norpramin can be fatal. It should be prescribed in the smallest possible amount, and it should always be stored in child-resistant containers.

How should you take this medication?
Norpramin should be taken exactly as prescribed.

It increases the affect of alcohol, so you should avoid alcoholic beverages.

Do not be discouraged if the medication has no immediate effect; improvement may not be seen for 2 to 3 weeks. You should not discontinue Norpramin unless instructed by your doctor.

What side effects may occur?
Side effects cannot be anticipated. If any develop or change in intensity, inform your doctor as soon as possible. Only your doctor can determine if it is safe for you to continue taking Norpramin.

■ *Side effects may include:*
Abdominal cramps, agitation, anxiety, black tongue, black, red, or blue spots on skin, blurred vision, breast development in males, confusion, constipation, delusions, diarrhea, dilated pupils, disorientation, dizziness, drowsiness, dry mouth, excessive or spontaneous flow of milk, fatigue, fever, sore throat, flushing, frequent urination or difficulty or delay in urinating, hallucinations, headache, heart attack, hepatitis, high or low blood pressure, high or low blood sugar, hives, impotency, increased or decreased libido, inflammation of the mouth, insomnia, intestinal blockage, lack of coordination, light-headedness (especially

when rising from lying down), loss of appetite, loss of hair, nausea, stomach pain, vomiting, nightmares, odd taste in mouth, painful ejaculation, palpitations, restlessness, ringing in the ears, seizures, sensitivity to light, skin itching and rash, stroke, sweating, swelling due to fluid retention (especially in face or tongue), swelling of breasts, swelling of testicles, swollen glands, tingling and numbness in hands and feet, tremors, urinating at night, visual problems, weakness, weight gain or loss, yellowed skin and whites of eyes

Why should this drug not be prescribed?

Norpramin should not be used if you are known to be hypersensitive to it, or if you have had a recent heart attack.

People who take antidepressant drugs known as MAO inhibitors (including Nardil, Parnate, and Marplan) should not take Norpramin.

Special warnings about this medication

Before using Norpramin, tell your doctor if you have heart or thyroid disease, a seizure disorder, or a history of urinary retention.

Nausea, headache, and malaise can result if you suddenly stop taking Norpramin. Consult your doctor and follow instructions closely when discontinuing Norpramin.

This drug may impair your ability to drive a car or operate potentially dangerous machinery. Do not participate in any activities that require full alertness if you are unsure about your ability.

Tell your doctor if you develop a fever and sore throat while you are taking Norpramin. He may want to do some blood tests.

Possible food and drug interactions when taking this medication

People who take antidepressant drugs known as MAO inhibitors (including Nardil, Parnate and Marplan) should not take Norpramin.

If Norpramin is taken with certain other drugs, the effects of either could be increased, decreased, or altered. It is especially important to check with your doctor before combining Norpramin with the following:

Cimetidine (Tagamet)
Drugs that improve breathing such as Proventil
Drugs that relax certain muscles such as Bentyl
Fluoxetine (Prozac)
Guanethidine (Ismelin)
Sedatives/hypnotics (Halcion, Valium)
Thyroid medications (Synthroid)

Extreme drowsiness and other potentially serious effects can result if Norpramin is combined with alcohol or other depressants such as narcotics, painkillers, sleeping medications, and tranquilizers (Valium).

Special information if you are pregnant or breastfeeding

Pregnant women or mothers who are nursing an infant should use Norpramin only when the potential benefits clearly outweigh the potential risks. If you are pregnant or planning to become pregnant, inform your doctor immediately.

Recommended dosage

Doses should be tailored to the individual and should start at a low level. No more than the minimum effective amount should be used.

ADULTS

The usual dose ranges from 100 to 200 milligrams per day. If needed, dosages may gradually be increased to 300 milligrams a day.

CHILDREN

Norpramin is not recommended for children.

ELDERLY AND ADOLESCENTS

The usual dose ranges from 25 to 100 milligrams per day. If needed, dosages may gradually be increased to 150 milligrams a day.

Overdosage

Any medication taken in excess can have serious consequences. An overdosage of Norpramin can be fatal. If you suspect an overdose, seek medical help immediately.

Symptoms of overdose may include:
Agitation, bluish or yellowish skin, coma, extremely low blood pressure, fever, irregular heart rate, kidney failure, palpitations, rigid muscles, seizures, shock, stupor, vomiting

Generic name:

NORTRIPTYLINE HYDROCHLORIDE

See Pamelor, page 450.

Brand name:

NOVOLIN

See Insulin, page 297.

Generic name:

NYSTATIN WITH TRIAMCINOLONE

See Mycolog II, page 395.

Generic name:

OFLOXACIN

See Floxin, page 263.

Generic name:

OLSALAZINE SODIUM

See Dipentum, page 202.

Generic name:

OMEPRAZOLE

See Prilosec, page 501.

Brand name:

OPCON-A

See Naphcon-A, page 400.

Brand name:

OPTICROM

See Cromolyn Sodium, page 144.

Category:

ORAL CONTRACEPTIVES

Brand names:

Demulen	Norethin
Levlen	Norinyl
Loestrin	Ortho-Novum
Lo/Ovral	Ovcon
Modicon	Ovral
Nordette	Triphasil

Why is this drug prescribed?

Oral contraceptives (also known as "The Pill") are highly effective means of preventing pregnancy. Oral contraceptives consist of synthetic forms of two hormones produced naturally in the body: either progestin alone or estrogen and progestin. Estrogen and progestin regulate a woman's menstrual cycle, and the fluctuating levels of these hormones play an essential role in pregnancy.

To reduce side effects, oral contraceptives are available in a wide range of estrogen and progestin concentrations. Progestin-only products (such as Micronor) are usually prescribed for women who should avoid estrogens; however, they may not be as effective as estrogen/progestin contraceptives.

Most important fact about this drug

Cigarette smoking increases the risk of serious heart-related side effects (stroke, heart attack, blood clots, etc.) in women who use oral contraceptives. This risk increases with heavy smoking (15 or more cigarettes per day) and with age. There is an especially significant increase in heart disease risk in women over 35 years old who smoke and use oral contraceptives.

How should you take this medication?

Oral contraceptives should be taken every day, preferably no more than 24 hours apart, and according to your physician's instructions. Ideally, you should take your pill at the same time every day to reduce the chance of forgetting a dose.

If you neglect to take only one estrogen/ progestin pill, take it as soon as you remember and continue taking the rest of the medication cycle. The risk of pregnancy is small if you miss only one combination pill per cycle. If you miss more than one tablet, do not take the missed tablets; instead you should resume the normal medication cycle while *employing another form of contraceptive for the duration of that medication cycle.*

Missing a single progestin-only tablet increases the chance of pregnancy. Therefore, you should consult with your doctor immediately if you miss a single dose.

What side effects may occur?

Side effects cannot be anticipated. If any develop or change in intensity, inform your doctor as soon as possible. Only your doctor can determine if it is safe for you to continue taking an oral contraceptive.

■ *Side effects may include:*
Abdominal cramps, acne, appetite changes, bleeding in spots during a menstrual period, bloating, blood clots, breast tenderness or enlargement, cataracts, chest pain, contact lens discomfort, decreased flow of milk when given immediately after birth, depression, difficulty breathing, dizziness, fluid retention, gallbladder disease, growth of face, back, chest, or stomach hair, hair loss, headache, heart attack, high blood pressure, inflammation of the large intestine, kidney trouble, liver tumors, lumps in the breast, menstrual pattern changes, migraine, muscle, joint, or leg pain, nausea, nervousness, premenstrual syndrome (PMS), secretion of milk, sex drive changes, skin rash or discoloration, stomach cramps, stroke, unexplained bleeding in the vagina, vaginal discharge, vaginal infections (and/or burning and itching), visual disturbances, vomiting, weight gain or loss, yellow skin or whites of eyes

Why should this drug not be prescribed?

You should not take oral contraceptives if you have had an allergic reaction to them or if you are pregnant (or think you might be).

If you have ever had breast cancer or cancer in the reproductive organs or liver tumors, you should not take oral contraceptives.

If you have or have ever had a stroke, heart disease, angina (severe chest pain), or blood clots, you should not take oral contraceptives. Women who have had pregnancy-related jaundice or jaundice stemming from previous use of oral contraceptives should not take them.

If you have undiagnosed and/or unexplained abnormal genital bleeding, do not take oral contraceptives.

Special warnings about this medication

Oral contraceptives should be used with caution if you are over 40 years old; smoke tobacco; have liver, heart, gallbladder, kidney, or thyroid disease; or have high blood pressure, high cholesterol, diabetes, epilepsy, asthma, or porphyria (a blood disorder).

In addition, you should use oral contraceptives with caution if you have a family history of breast cancer or other cancers, or you have a personal history of depression, migraine or other headaches, irregular menstrual periods, or visual disturbances.

Since the blood's clotting ability may be affected by oral contraceptives, your doctor may take you off them prior to surgery. If bleeding lasts more than 8 days while you are on a progestin-only oral contraceptive, be sure to let your doctor know.

Possible food and drug interactions when taking this medication

If oral contraceptives are taken with certain other drugs, the effects of either could be increased, decreased, or altered. It is especially important to check with your doctor before combining oral contraceptives with the following:

Amitriptyline (Elavil, Endep)
Ampicillin (Polycillin, Principen)
Barbiturates (phenobarbital, etc.)
Carbamazepine (Tegretol)
Certain antibiotics
Chloramphenicol (Chloromycetin)

Clomipramine (Anafranil)
Diazepam (Valium)
Doxepin (Sinequan)
Glipizide (Glucotrol)
Griseofulvin (Fulvicin, Grisactin)
Imipramine (Trofranil, Janimine)
Lorazepam (Ativan)
Metoprolol (Lopressor)
Oxazepam (Serax)
Penicillin (Veetids, Pen-Vee K)
Phenylbutazone (Butazolidin)
Phenytoin (Dilantin)
Prednisolone (Delta-Cortef, Prelone)
Prednisone (Deltasone)
Primidone (Mysoline)
Propranolol (Inderal)
Rifampin (Rifadin, Rimactane)
Sulfonamides (Gantanol, Septra)
Tetracycline (Achromycin V)
Theophylline (Theo-Dur)
Warfarin (Coumadin, Panwarfin)

In addition, oral contraceptives may affect tests for blood sugar levels and thyroid function and may cause an increase in blood cholesterol levels.

Special Information
if your are pregnant or breastfeeding

If you are pregnant (or think you might be), you should not use oral contraceptives, since they are not safe during pregnancy.

In general, nursing mothers should not use oral contraceptives, since these drugs can appear in breast milk and may cause jaundice and enlarged breasts in nursing infants. Your doctor may advise you to use a different form of contraception while you are nursing your baby.

Recommended dosage

If you have any questions about how you should take oral contraceptives, consult your doctor or the patient instructions that come in the drug package. The following is a partial list of instructions for taking oral contraceptives; it should not be used as a substitute for consultation with your doctor.

Oral contraceptives are supplied in 21-day and 28-day packages.

For a 21-day schedule:
Oral contraceptives are taken for a 3-week period, followed by 1 week of no oral contraceptives.

1) Starting on the first Sunday after the beginning of your menstrual period, take one tablet daily (preferably at the same time each day) for the next 20 or 21 days (depending upon the brand of oral contraceptive used). Note: If your period begins on Sunday, take the first tablet that day.

2) Wait 1 week before taking any tablets. Your menstrual period should occur during this time.

3) Following this 1-week waiting time, begin taking tablets again for the next 20 or 21 days.

For a 28-day schedule:
Starting on the first Sunday after the beginning of your menstrual period, take one tablet daily (preferably at the same time each day) for the next 28 days. Continue taking the oral contraceptives according to your physician's instructions. Note: If your period begins on Sunday, take the first tablet that day.

For both 21- and 28-day regimens:
If the first Sunday falls more than 5 days after the beginning of your period, it is important to use an alternate means of contraception while taking oral contraceptives until your physician indicates it is no longer necessary.

Progestin-only tablets should be taken every day of the year.

Overdosage
While any medication taken in excess can cause overdose, the risk associated with oral contraceptives is minimal. Even young children who have taken large amounts of oral contraceptives have not experienced serious adverse effects. However, if you suspect an overdose, seek medical help immediately.

Symptoms of overdose may include:
Nausea
Withdrawal bleeding in females

Brand name:

ORAP

Generic name: Pimozide

Why is this drug prescribed?
Orap is an oral medication available in tablet form. Orap is prescribed for people with severe Tourette's disorder (Tourette's syndrome) who have not been helped sufficiently by Haldol (haloperidol), the first-choice medication. Orap helps suppress the physical and verbal tics—twitches, jerks, and bizarre outbursts—that are associated with Tourette's disorder.

Most important fact about this drug
Because Orap may cause several serious side effects, it should not be given to suppress tics that are merely annoying. Treatment with Orap should be considered only if the tics make normal functioning impossible and if Haldol or other tic-suppressant medications have not worked.

How should you take this medication?
Take Orap exactly as prescribed by your doctor.

Do not exceed the prescribed dose of Orap. Sudden and unexpected fatalities have occurred in patients taking high doses of Orap for disorders other than Tourette's syndrome.

What side effects may occur?
Side effects cannot be anticipated. If any develop or change in intensity, notify your doctor immediately. Only your doctor can determine whether it is safe to continue taking Orap.

■ *Side effects may include:*
Altered mental status, appetite increase, behavioral changes, belching, blood pressure changes, blurred vision, changes in heart rhythm, chewing movements, constant trembling of hands, constipation, diarrhea, dizziness, drooling, drowsiness, dry mouth, excessive thirst, fine worm-like movement of the tongue, handwriting change, headache, impotence, inability to sit still, increased body heat, involuntary movements of tongue, face, mouth, or jaw, irregular pulse, light-headedness, loss of libido, loss of movement, nausea, parkinson-like symptoms, pounding in chest, protrusion of tongue, puckering of mouth, puffing of cheeks, rash, rigid stoop, sedation, speech disorder, stiff, shuffling, overbalancing walk, stiffness, stomach upset, sweating, swelling around eyes, tremors, unblinking fixed expression, uncontrollable jerking or twitching, visual disturbances, vomiting, weakness

Why should this drug not be prescribed?
You should not take Orap if you have ever had an allergic reaction to it or are sensitive to its ingredients. If you have ever had a bad reaction to any other antipsychotic medication, be sure your doctor knows about it.

Your doctor may not prescribe Orap if you have a history of abnormal heart rhythm, or if you have simple tics.

Your doctor may not give you Orap if you are taking a medication that may cause tics. Such medications include Ritalin, Dexedrine, and Cylert.

Special warnings about this medication
Treatment with Orap has serious risks. If your doctor decides to prescribe Orap, he or she will discuss them with you.

Orap may cause drowsiness. Be careful while driving or performing tasks that require mental alertness.

Orap and related drugs used over a long-term have been associated with two potentially serious syndromes, tardive dyskinesia and neuroleptic malignant syndrome (NMS). Be sure to report any side effects to your doctor immediately.

Possible food and drug interactions when taking this medication
If Orap is taken with certain other drugs, the effects of either could be increased, decreased, or altered. It is especially important to check with your doctor before combining Orap with the following:

Alcohol
Anticonvulsants such as Dilantin
Antiarrhythmic heart drugs such as Calan, Pronestyl, and others
Other central nervous system depressants such as Percocet, Valium, Dalmane, and Xanax
Phenothiazines such as Thorazine, Mellaril, Stelazine, and others
Tricyclic antidepressants such as Elavil, Tofranil, and others

Special information if you are pregnant or breastfeeding
If you are pregnant or plan to become pregnant, inform your doctor immediately.

Because of the possibility of harm to the fetus, Orap should not be taken during pregnancy unless the potential benefit to the mother outweighs the potential risk to the child.

If Orap is essential to your health, your doctor may advise you to stop breast-feeding your baby.

Recommended dosage

ADULTS

Your doctor will carefully tailor your individual dose of Orap. The recommended initial dose is 1 to 2 milligrams a day in divided doses.

Your doctor may later adjust the dose to a point where the suppression of tics is balanced against the side effects.

CHILDREN

Reliable dosage information concerning the effects of Orap on tics in Tourette's disorder patients under the age of 12 is not available.

Overdosage

Any medication taken in excess can have serious consequences. If you suspect an overdose of Orap, seek medical attention immediately.

Symptoms of Orap overdose may include:
Coma with slowed breathing
Heartbeat irregularities
Low blood pressure
Severe involuntary movements

Brand name:

ORASONE

See Deltasone, page 172.

Brand name:

ORINASE

Generic name: Tolbutamide

Why is this drug prescribed?

Orinase is an oral antidiabetic medication used to treat Type II (non-insulin-dependent) diabetes. Diabetes occurs when the body does not make enough insulin, or when the insulin that is produced no longer works properly.

Insulin works by helping sugar get inside the cell, where it is then used for energy.

There are two forms of diabetes: Type I (insulin-dependent) and Type II (non-insulin-dependent). Type I diabetes usually requires taking insulin injections for life, while Type II diabetes can usually be treated by dietary changes, exercise, and/or oral antidiabetic medications such as Orinase. Orinase controls diabetes by stimulating the pancreas to secrete more insulin and by helping insulin work better.

Occasionally, Type II diabetics must take insulin injections, sometimes temporarily during stressful periods or times of illness. When diet, exercise, and an oral antidiabetic medication fail to reduce symptoms and/or blood sugar levels, a patient with Type II diabetes may require long-term insulin injections.

Most important fact about this drug

Orinase-type drugs may possibly lead to more heart problems than diet treatment alone or treatment with diet and insulin. If you have heart problems, discuss them with your doctor.

Always consider Orinase an addition to, not a substitute for, diet therapy. The safest and most desirable way to control Type II diabetes is to keep your weight and blood sugar down through diet and exercise. Orinase or another antidiabetic drug should be considered only if a diet and exercise program fail to correct your high blood sugar.

How should you take this medication?

In general, Orinase should be taken 30 minutes before a meal to achieve the best control over blood sugar levels. However, the exact dosing schedule as well as the dosage amount must be determined by your physician. Ask your doctor when it is best for you to take this medication.

To help prevent low blood sugar levels (hypoglycemia) you should:
Understand the symptoms of hypoglycemia.
Know how exercise affects your blood sugar levels.
Maintain an adequate diet.
Keep a product containing quick-acting sugar with you at all times.

Limit alcohol intake. If alcohol is ingested, it may cause breathlessness and facial flushing.

What side effects may occur?

Side effects cannot be anticipated. If any develop or change in intensity, inform your doctor as soon as possible. Only your doctor can determine if it is safe for you to continue taking Orinase.

Side effects from Orinase are rare and seldom require discontinuation of the medication.

■ *More common side effects may include:*
Bloating
Heartburn
Nausea

■ *Less common or rare side effects may include:*
Anemia and other blood disorders, blistering, changes in taste, headache,

hepatic porphyria (a condition frequently characterized by sensitivity to light, stomach pain, and nerve damage, caused by excessive levels of porphyrin in the liver), hives, itching, redness of the skin, skin eruptions, skin rash

Orinase, like all oral antidiabetics, may cause hypoglycemia (low blood sugar). The risk of hypoglycemia can be increased by missed meals, alcohol, other medications, fever, trauma, infection, surgery, or excessive exercise. To avoid hypoglycemia, you should closely follow the dietary and exercise plan suggested by your physician.

Symptoms of mild hypoglycemia may include:
Cold sweat, fast heartbeat, drowsiness, headache, nausea, nervousness.

Symptoms of more severe hypoglycemia may include:
Coma, pale skin, seizures, shallow breathing.

Contact your doctor immediately if these symptoms of severe low blood sugar occur.

Ask your doctor what you should do if you experience mild hypoglycemia. Severe hypoglycemia should be considered a medical emergency, and prompt medical attention is essential.

Why should this drug not be prescribed?

You should not take Orinase if you have had an allergic reaction to it.

Orinase should not be taken if you are suffering from diabetic ketoacidosis (a life-threatening medical emergency caused by insufficient insulin and marked by excessive thirst, nausea, fatigue, pain below the breastbone, and fruity breath).

In addition, Orinase should not be used as the sole therapy in treating Type I (insulin-dependent) diabetics.

Special warnings about this medication
If you are taking Orinase, you should check your blood or urine periodically for abnormal sugar (glucose) levels.

It is important that you closely follow the diet and exercise plan recommended by your doctor.

Even patients with well-controlled diabetes may find that stress, illness, surgery or fever results in a loss of control over their diabetes. In these cases, the patient's physician may recommend that Orinase be discontinued temporarily and injected insulin administered.

In addition, the effectiveness of any oral antidiabetic, including Orinase, may decrease with time. This may occur either because of a diminished responsiveness to the medication or a worsening of the diabetes.

Like other antidiabetic drugs, Orinase may produce severe low blood sugar if the dosage is wrong. While taking Orinase, you are particularly susceptible to episodes of low blood sugar if:

You suffer from a kidney or liver problem;
You have a lack of adrenal or pituitary hormone;
You are elderly, run-down, malnourished, hungry, exercising heavily, drinking alcohol, or using more than one glucose-lowering drug.

Possible food and drug interactions when taking this medication
If Orinase is taken with certain other drugs, the effects of either could be increased, decreased or altered. It is especially important to check with your doctor before combining Orinase with the following:

Adrenal corticosteroids such as prednisone and cortisone
Anabolic steroids such as testosterone and danazol
Barbiturates such as Amobartibal, Seconal, and phenobarbital
Beta blockers such as Inderal and Tenormin
Calcium channel blockers such as Cardizem and Procardia
Chloramphenicol (Chloromycetin)
Coumarins such as Coumadin
Epinephrine
Estrogens
Furosemide (Lasix)
Isoniazid such as Laniazid, Rifamate, and Tubizid
MAO inhibitors such as Nardil and Parnate
Nicotinic acid (Niacin, Nicobid, Nicolar)
Nonsteroidal anti-inflammatory agents such as Advil, aspirin, Butazolidin, Motrin, Naprosyn, and Nuprin
Miconazole
Oral contraceptives
Phenytoin (Dilantin)
Phenothiazines such as Stelazine and Mellaril
Probenecid (Benemid, ColBENEMID)
Sulfonamides such as Sulfacetamide
Sympathomimetics such as Proventil and epinephrine
Thiazide and other diuretics such as Diuril, HydroDIURIL, and Lasix
Thyroid medication such as Synthroid and Proloid

Alcohol must be used carefully, since excessive alcohol can cause low blood sugar.

**Special information
if you are pregnant or breastfeeding**
The effects of Orinase during pregnancy have not been adequately established in humans. Since Orinase has caused birth defects in rats, it is not recommended for use by pregnant women. Therefore, if you are pregnant or planning to become pregnant, you should

only take Orinase on the advice of your physician. Since studies suggest the importance of maintaining normal blood sugar (glucose) levels during pregnancy, your physician may prescribe injected insulin during pregnancy.

While it is not known if Orinase enters breast milk, other similar medications do. Therefore, patients should discuss with their doctors whether to discontinue the medication or to stop breastfeeding. If the medication is discontinued, and if diet alone does not control glucose levels, then insulin injections should be considered.

Recommended dosage

Dosage levels must be based on each patient's needs.

ADULTS

Usually an initial daily dose of 1 to 2 grams is recommended. Maintenance therapy usually ranges from 0.25 to 3 grams daily. Daily doses greater than 3 grams are not recommended.

CHILDREN

Safety and effectiveness have not been established in children.

ELDERLY

Elderly, malnourished, or debilitated patients, or patients with impaired kidney and liver function, usually receive lower initial and maintenance doses to minimize the risk of low blood sugar (hypoglycemia).

Overdosage

Any medication taken in excess can have serious consequences. An overdose of Orinase can cause low blood sugar (see "Special warnings about this medication"). Eating sugar, or a sugar-based product will often correct mild hypoglycemia. If you

suspect an overdose, seek medical attention immediately.

Brand name:

ORTHO-NOVUM

See Oral Contraceptives, page 437.

Brand name:

ORUDIS

Generic name: Ketoprofen

Why is this drug prescribed?

Orudis, a nonsteroidal anti-inflammatory drug, is used to relieve the inflammation, swelling, stiffness and joint pain associated with rheumatoid arthritis and osteoarthritis (the most common form of arthritis). It is also used to relieve menstrual pain and other mild to moderate pain.

Most important fact about this drug

You should have frequent check-ups with your doctor if you take Orudis regularly. Ulcers or internal bleeding can occur without warning.

How should you take this medication?

To minimize side effects, Orudis may be taken with food, an antacid, or milk, if your physician recommends.

Take this medication exactly as prescribed by your doctor.

If you are using Orudis for arthritis, it should be taken regularly.

What side effects may occur?

Side effects cannot be anticipated. If any develop or change in intensity, inform your doctor as soon as possible. Only your doctor can determine if it is safe for you to continue taking Orudis.

■ *More common side effects may include:*
Changes in kidney function, constipation, depression, diarrhea, dizziness, fatigue, gas, headache, inability to sleep, indigestion, inflammation of the mouth, loss of appetite, nausea, nervousness, rash, ringing in the ears, sleepiness, stomach pain, visual disturbance, vomiting

■ *Less common or rare side effects may include:*
Allergic reaction, anemia, asthma, belching, bloody or black stools, change in taste, chills, confusion, congestive heart failure, decrease in white blood cells, dry mouth, eye pain, facial swelling due to fluid retention, forgetfulness, hair loss, high blood pressure, hives, impaired hearing, impotence, increase in appetite, increased salivation, inflammation of eyelids, itching, kidney failure, loosening of fingernails, migraine, muscle pain, nosebleed, peptic or intestinal ulcer, prickling, rapid heartbeat, rectal bleeding, sensitivity to light, shock, shortness of breath, skin discoloration, skin inflammation and eruptions, stomach inflammation, sweating, swelling of the throat, thirst, vertigo, vomiting blood, weight gain or loss

Why should this drug not be prescribed?

If you are sensitive to or have ever had an allergic reaction to Orudis, aspirin, or similar drugs, or if you have had asthma attacks caused by aspirin or other drugs of this type, you should not take this medication. Make sure that your doctor is aware of any drug reactions that you have experienced.

Special warnings about this medication

Stomach ulcers and bleeding can occur without warning.

This drug should be used with caution if you have kidney or liver disease, and it can cause kidney inflammation in some people.

Do not take aspirin or any other anti-inflammatory medications while taking Orudis, unless your doctor tells you to do so.

If you are taking Orudis for an extended period of time, your doctor should check your blood for anemia.

Orudis prolongs bleeding time. If you are taking blood-thinning medication, this drug should be used with caution.

This drug can increase water retention. Use with caution if you have heart disease or high blood pressure.

Possible food and drug interactions when taking this medication

If Orudis is taken with certain other drugs, the effects of either could be increased, decreased, or altered. It is especially important to check with your doctor before combining Orudis with the following:

Anticoagulants (blood thinners such as Coumadin)
Aspirin
Lithium
Methotrexate
Probenecid (given with several antibiotics)
The diuretic hydrochlorothiazide

Special information if you are pregnant or breastfeeding

The effects of Orudis during pregnancy have not been adequately studied. If you are pregnant or plan to become pregnant, inform your doctor immediately. Orudis may appear in breast milk and could affect a nursing infant. If this medication is essential to your health, your doctor may advise you to discontinue breastfeeding until your treatment with this medication is finished.

Recommended dosage

ADULTS

Rheumatoid Arthritis and Osteoarthritis
The starting dose is 75 milligrams, 3 times a day or 50 milligrams 4 times a day. The usual daily dose is 150 to 300 milligrams, divided into 3 or 4 doses. (Note: Some side effects, such as headache or upset stomach, are dose-related with this medication. Smaller people may need smaller doses.)

Mild to Moderate Pain and Menstrual Pain
The usual dose is 25 to 50 milligrams every 6 to 8 hours as needed. Dosages may need to be adjusted for smaller patients or those with kidney or liver disease.

The lowest dose that proves beneficial should be used.

CHILDREN

The safety and effectiveness of Orudis have not been established in children.

ELDERLY

Lower dosages may be needed; dosage should be determined by the particular needs of the elderly patient.

Overdosage

Reports of overdose are rare. The most common symptom is vomiting; drowsiness has also been reported. If you suspect an overdose, seek medical attention immediately.

Brand name:

OVCON

See Oral Contraceptives, page 437.

Brand name:

OVRAL

See Oral Contraceptives, page 437.

Generic name:

OXAZEPAM

See Serax, page 575.

Generic name:

OXICONAZOLE NITRATE

See Oxistat, page 447.

Brand name:

OXISTAT CREAM

Generic name: Oxiconazole nitrate

Why is this drug prescribed?
Oxistat is used to treat fungal skin diseases commonly called ringworm (tinea). Oxistat Cream is prescribed for athlete's foot (tinea pedis), jock itch (tinea cruris), and ringworm of the entire body (tinea corporis).

Most important fact about this drug
Oxistat Cream should not be used in, on, or near the eyes.

How should you use this medication?
Use Oxistat Cream exactly as prescribed by your doctor.

Oxistat is for external use only.

Wash and dry the area to be treated before applying Oxistat and then apply the cream so that it covers the entire affected area.

Be careful when applying to raw, blistered, or oozing skin.

What side effects may occur?

Side effects cannot be anticipated. If any develop or change in intensity, notify your doctor as soon as possible. Only your doctor can determine whether it is safe for you to continue using Oxistat.

■ *Side effects may include:*
Allergic skin inflammation, burning, grooves in the skin, irritation, itching, rash, skin redness, skin softening, small, firm, raised skin eruptions (similar to those of chickenpox), small tissue lump protruding from the skin, stinging

Why should this drug not be prescribed?

Do not use Oxistat Cream if you have ever had an allergic reaction or are sensitive to oxiconazole or any other ingredients in the cream.

Special warnings about this medication

If you develop an irritation or sensitivity to the medication, notify your doctor.

Possible food and drug interactions when taking this medication

No interactions have been reported.

Special information
if you are pregnant or breastfeeding

Oxistat has not been proved safe during pregnancy. If you are pregnant or plan to become pregnant, inform your doctor immediately.

Oxistat appears in breast milk and could affect a nursing infant. If Oxistat is essential to your health, your doctor may advise you to stop breastfeeding until your treatment is finished.

Recommended dosage

ADULTS AND CHILDREN

Apply Oxistat Cream to cover the affected area once a day, in the evening. Athlete's foot (tinea pedis) is treated for 1 month. Jock itch (tinea cruris) and ringworm of the body (tinea corporis) are treated for 2 weeks.

Overdosage

Overdose of Oxistat has not been reported. However, if you suspect an overdose, seek medical attention immediately.

Generic name:

OXTRIPHYLLINE

See Choledyl, page 107.

Generic name:

OXYCODONE WITH ACETAMINOPHEN

See Percocet, page 465.

Brand name:

PBZ-SR

Generic name: Tripelennamine hydrochloride

Why is this drug prescribed?

PBZ-SR is an antihistamine that relieves nasal stuffiness and inflammation and red, inflamed eyes caused by hay fever and other allergies. It is also used to treat: itching, swelling, and redness from hives and other rashes that are caused by mild allergic reactions; allergic reactions to blood transfusions; and, with other medications, anaphylactic shock (severe allergic reaction). Antihistamines work by decreasing the effects of histamine, a chemical the body releases in response to certain irritants. Histamine narrows air passages in the lungs and contributes to inflammation. Antihistamines reduce itching and swelling and dry up secretions from the nose, eyes, and throat.

Most important fact about this drug

PBZ-SR often produces drowsiness and reduces mental alertness.

How should you take this medication?

PBZ-SR should be taken exactly as prescribed by your doctor.

The tablets should be swallowed whole, not crushed or chewed.

What side effects may occur?

Side effects cannot be anticipated. If any develop or change in intensity, inform your doctor as soon as possible. Only your doctor can determine if it is safe for you to continue taking PBZ-SR.

■ *More common side effects may include:*
Disturbed coordination
Dizziness
Drowsiness
Dry mouth, nose, and throat
Extreme calm (sedation)
Increased chest congestion
Sleepiness
Stomach upset

■ *Less common or rare side effects may include:*
Allergic reactions (including rash, hives, anaphylactic shock—severe allergic reaction), an exaggerated sense of well-being, blood disorders, blurred vision, chills, confusion, constipation, convulsions, diarrhea, difficulty sleeping, difficulty urinating, double vision, excitation, fatigue, frequent urination, headache, hysteria, irritability, loss of appetite, low blood pressure, nausea, nervousness, pounding heartbeat, rapid heartbeat, restlessness, ringing in the ears, stuffy nose, tightness in chest, urinary retention, vertigo, vomiting, wheezing

Why should this drug not be prescribed?

PBZ-SR should not be used in newborn or premature infants or in mothers who are breastfeeding their infants.

Do not take this medication if you are taking MAO inhibitor drugs such as the antidepressants Nardil, Parnate, and Marplan; or if you have narrow-angle glaucoma, peptic ulcer, symptoms of an enlarged prostate, bladder or stomach obstruction, or asthma or other breathing disorders. Also, you should not take this drug if you are sensitive to or have ever had an allergic reaction to tripelennamine or other medications with a similar chemical composition.

Special warnings about this medication

Antihistamines can cause drowsiness or excitation in children.

Antihistamines can also cause drowsiness in adults. Driving or operating dangerous machinery or participating in any hazardous activity that requires full mental alertness is not recommended until you know how you react to PBZ-SR.

Antihistamines can cause dizziness, extreme calm (sedation), and low blood pressure in the elderly (over age 60).

PBZ-SR should be used cautiously if you have glaucoma, an overactive thyroid, cardiovascular disease, high blood pressure, or a history of bronchial asthma.

Possible food and drug interactions when taking this medication

PBZ-SR may increase the effects of alcohol. Do not drink alcohol while taking this medication.

If PBZ-SR is taken with certain other drugs, the effects of either could be increased, decreased, or altered. It is especially important to check with your doctor before combining PBZ-SR with the following:

MAO inhibitors (including antidepressants such as Marplan and Nardil)
Medications for anxiety such as Librium and Buspar
Sedatives/hypnotics such as Nembutal and Seconal

Special information
If you are pregnant or breastfeeding

The effects of PBZ-SR during pregnancy have not been adequately studied. If you are pregnant or plan to become pregnant, inform your doctor immediately. PBZ-SR should be used during pregnancy only if clearly needed. Antihistamines are not advised for nursing mothers. If this medication is essential to your health, your doctor may advise you to discontinue breastfeeding until your treatment is finished.

Recommended dosage

ADULTS

Dosage should be individualized according to the needs and response of the patient.

One 100-milligram PBZ-SR tablet in the morning and 1 in the evening is usually adequate. In more difficult cases, one 100-milligram PBZ-SR tablet every 8 hours may be required.

CHILDREN

PBZ-SR tablets are not intended for use by children.

Overdosage

Any medication taken in excess can have serious consequences. An antihistamine overdose can be fatal especially in infants and children. If you suspect an overdose, seek medical treatment immediately.

Symptoms of a PBZ-SR overdose may include:
Cardiovascular collapse
Coma
Decreased alertness
Drowsiness

Symptoms more common in children may include:
Convulsions
Dry mouth
Excitement
Fever
Fixed, dilated pupils
Flushing
Hallucinations
Involuntary wringing of the hands
Lack of coordination
Stimulation

Brand name:

PCE

See *Erythromycin, Oral, page 239.*

Brand name:

PAMELOR

Generic name: Nortriptyline hydrochloride
Other brand name: Aventyl

Why is this drug prescribed?

Pamelor is prescribed for the relief of symptoms of depression; it is most effective in endogenous depression (depression due to physical causes inside the body). Pamelor is in the class of drugs known as tricyclic antidepressants.

Most important fact about this drug

Extremely high fever, severe convulsions, and death have occurred when drugs such as Pamelor have been taken in combination with another type of antidepressant known as MAO inhibitors, including brands such as

Nardil, Parnate, and Marplan. Discontinuance of a MAO inhibitor for at least 2 weeks is recommended before starting treatment with Pamelor. Inform your doctor of any prescription or nonprescription drugs you are taking before starting treatment with Pamelor.

How should you take this medication?
Pamelor should be taken exactly as prescribed by your doctor.

What side effects may occur?
Side effects cannot be anticipated. If any develop or change in intensity, inform your doctor as soon as possible. Only your doctor can determine if it is safe for you to continue taking Pamelor.

■ *Side effects may include:*
Abdominal cramps, agitation, anxiety, black tongue, blurred vision, breast development in males, breast enlargement, confusion, constipation, diarrhea, dilation of pupils, disorientation, dizziness, drowsiness, dry mouth, excessive or spontaneous flow of milk, excessive urination at night, fatigue, fluid retention, flushing, hair loss, hallucinations, headache, heart attack, high or low blood pressure, high or low blood sugar, hives, impotence, inability to sleep, increased or decreased sex drive, inflammation of the mouth, intestinal blockage, itching, loss of appetite, loss of coordination, nausea, nightmares, numbness, panic, perspiration, problems with urination, rapid, pounding or irregular heartbeat, rash, reddish or purplish spots on skin, restlessness, ringing in the ears, sensitivity to light, stomach upset, strange taste, stroke, swelling of the testicles, tingling, tremors, urinary frequency, vomiting, weight gain or loss, yellow eyes and skin

■ *Side effects due to rapid decrease or abrupt withdrawal from Pamelor include:*
Headache

Nausea
Vague feeling of bodily discomfort

These side effects do not indicate addiction to this drug.

Why should this drug not be prescribed?
If you are sensitive to or have ever had an allergic reaction to Pamelor or similar drugs, you should not take this medication. Make sure that your doctor is aware of any drug reactions that you have experienced.

Do not take Pamelor if you are taking an MAO inhibitor, or have taken one within the past 14 days. (See "Most important fact about this drug.")

Unless you are directed to do so by your doctor, do not take this medication if you are recovering from a heart attack or are taking other antidepressant drugs.

Special warnings about this medication
Pamelor may cause you to become drowsy or less alert; therefore, driving or operating dangerous machinery or participating in any hazardous activity that requires full mental alertness is not recommended.

Notify your doctor or dentist that you are taking this drug if any emergency occurs and before surgery.

Pamelor should be used with caution if you have a history of seizures, urinary retention, or glaucoma or other chronic eye conditions; or if you have cardiovascular (heart and circulatory) disease or are receiving thyroid medication. You should discuss all of your medical problems with your doctor before taking this medication.

If you are being treated for a severe mental disorder (schizophrenia or manic depression), consult with your doctor before taking Pamelor.

Possible food and drug interactions when taking this medication

Combining Pamelor and MAO inhibitors can be fatal.

Pamelor may intensify the effects of alcohol. Do not drink alcohol while taking this medication.

If Pamelor is taken with certain other drugs, the effects of either could be increased, decreased, or altered. It is especially important to check with your doctor before combining Pamelor with the following:

Cimetidine (Tagamet)
Drugs that control certain muscle contractions such as Bentyl
Drugs to improve breathing such as Ventolin
High blood pressure drugs
Other antidepressants such as Prozac
Quinidine (Quinaglute)
Thyroid medication

Special information
if you are pregnant or breastfeeding

The effects of Pamelor during pregnancy have not been adequately studied. If you are pregnant or planning to become pregnant, inform your doctor immediately. Also consult your doctor before breastfeeding.

Recommended dosage

This medication is available in tablet and liquid form. Only tablet dosages are listed. Consult your doctor if you cannot take the tablet form of this medication.

ADULTS

Your doctor should supervise your response to this medication carefully. Dosages will be increased or decreased gradually to suit each individual patient's needs.

The usual starting dosage is 25 milligrams, 3 or 4 times per day. This dose can be increased gradually by your doctor if necessary.

Your doctor may prescribe that the total daily dose be taken once a day as an alternative.

Doses above 150 milligrams per day are not recommended.

Your doctor may want to perform a blood test to help in deciding the best dose you should receive.

CHILDREN

The safety and effectiveness of Pamelor have not been established for use in children and its use is not recommended. However, adolescent patients may be given 30 to 50 milligrams per day, either in a single dose or divided into 2 doses, as determined by your doctor.

ELDERLY

The usual dose is 30 to 50 milligrams taken in a single dose or divided into 2 doses, as determined by your doctor.

Overdosage

Deaths have occurred from overdosage with drugs of this class.

Overdose symptoms include:
Agitation, coma, confusion, congestive heart failure, convulsions, decreased breathing, excessive reflexes, extremely high fever, rapid heartbeat, restlessness, rigid muscles, shock, stupor, vomiting

If you suspect a Pamelor overdose, seek medical attention immediately.

Brand name:

PANADOL

See Tylenol, page 661.

Brand name:

PANCREASE

Generic name: Pancrelipase

Why is this drug prescribed?

Pancrease is used to treat pancreatic enzyme deficiency. It is often prescribed for people with cystic fibrosis, chronic inflammation of the pancreas, blockages of the pancreas or common bile duct caused by cancer, or for individuals who have had their pancreas removed or have had gastrointestinal bypass surgery. Pancrease is taken to help with digestion of proteins, starches, and fats.

Most important fact about this drug

Pancrease should not be chewed or crushed.

How should you take this medication?

Take this medication exactly as prescribed by your doctor.

If swallowing the Pancrease capsule is difficult, open the capsule and shake the contents (microspheres) onto a small amount of soft food, such as applesauce or gelatin, that does not require chewing and swallow immediately.

Pancrease should be taken with meals or snacks.

What side effects may occur?

Side effects cannot be anticipated. If any develop or change in intensity, inform your doctor as soon as possible. Only your doctor can determine if it is safe for you to continue taking Pancrease.

- *More common side effects may include:*
  Abdominal upset

- *Less common or rare side effects may include:*
  Allergic-type reactions

Why should this drug not be prescribed?

Pancrease should not be used if you are sensitive to or have ever had an allergic reaction to pork protein.

Special warnings about this medication

If you develop a sensitivity or allergic reaction to Pancrease, stop taking the medication and inform your doctor immediately.

Possible food and drug interactions when taking this medication

No interactions have been reported.

Special information if you are pregnant or breastfeeding

The effects of Pancrease during pregnancy have not been adequately studied. If you are pregnant or plan to become pregnant, inform your doctor immediately. Pancrease may appear in breast milk and could affect a nursing infant. If this medication is essential to your health, your doctor may advise you to stop breastfeeding until your treatment with Pancrease is finished.

Recommended dosage

ADULTS

One or 2 capsules during each meal and 1 capsule with snacks. Occasionally a third capsule may be required with meals, depending on the individual.

Overdosage

Although no specific information is available, any medication taken in excess can have serious consequences. If you suspect an overdose seek medical treatment immediately.

Generic name:

PANCRELIPASE

See Pancrease, page 453.

Brand name:

PARAFON FORTE DSC

Generic name: Chlorzoxazone

Why is this drug prescribed?

Parafon Forte DSC is prescribed, along with rest and physical therapy, for the relief of discomfort associated with severe, painful skeletal muscle disorders.

Most important fact about this drug

This drug should be used with caution if you have a known allergy or a history of allergies to drugs. If a sensitivity reaction such as hives, redness, or itching of skin occurs while you are taking Parafon Forte DSC, or if you notice any signs of liver problems, such as yellowing of the skin or the whites of the eyes, notify your doctor immediately.

How should you take this medication?

Take Parafon Forte DSC exactly as prescribed by your doctor. Do not increase the dose or take more often than prescribed. Parafon Forte DSC may discolor urine orange or purple red.

What side effects may occur?

Parafon Forte DSC is generally well tolerated and rarely produces undesirable side effects. However, if any develop or change in intensity, inform your doctor as soon as possible. Only your doctor can determine if it is safe for you to continue taking Parafon Forte DSC.

■ Uncommon and rare side effects may include:

Bruises, dizziness, drowsiness, feeling of illness, fluid retention, light-headedness, overstimulation, red or purple spots on the skin, skin rashes, stomach or intestinal disturbances or bleeding, urine discoloration

Why should this drug not be prescribed?

If you have had any reaction to this drug, notify your doctor. Make sure that your doctor is aware of any drug reactions that you have experienced.

Possible food and drug interactions when taking this medication

Parafon Forte DSC may intensify the effects of alcohol. Do not drink alcohol while taking this medication.

If Parafon Forte DSC is taken with certain other drugs, the effects of either could be increased, decreased, or altered. It is especially important to check with your doctor before combining Parafon Forte DSC with central nervous system depressants such as Percocet, Valium, and Xanax.

Special information if you are pregnant or breastfeeding

The effects of Parafon Forte DSC during pregnancy have not been adequately studied. If you are pregnant or plan to become pregnant, inform your doctor immediately. This drug may appear in breast milk and could affect a nursing infant. If this medication is essential to your health, your doctor may advise you to discontinue breastfeeding until your treatment is finished.

Recommended dosage

ADULTS

The usual recommended dosage of Parafon Forte DSC is 1 caplet taken 3 or 4 times per day. If you do not respond to this dosage, your doctor may increase it to 1½ caplets (750 milligrams) taken 3 or 4 times per day.

Overdosage

Any medication taken in excess can have serious consequences. If you suspect an overdose, seek medical treatment immediately.

Symptoms of Parafon Forte DSC overdose may include:
Diarrhea
Dizziness

Drowsiness
Headache
Light-headedness
Nausea
Vomiting

*Symptoms that may develop after a period
of time include:*
Feeling of illness
Loss of muscle tone
Sluggishness
Troubled or rapid breathing

Brand name:

PARLODEL

Generic name: Bromocriptine mesylate

Why is this drug prescribed?

Parlodel mimics the action of dopamine, a
chemical lacking in the brain of someone with
Parkinson's disease. It also inhibits the
secretion of the hormone prolactin from the
pituitary gland, thereby preventing production
of breast milk. It is used to treat a variety
of medical conditions, including:

Growth hormone overproduction
Infertility in some women
Menstrual problems such as the abnormal
    stoppage or absence of flow
Parkinson's disease
Pituitary gland tumors
To control excessive or spontaneous flow of
    milk
To interrupt milk production in women who
    do not want to breastfeed or should not
    breastfeed for medical reasons

This drug has sometimes been used to reduce
"cravings" in patients attempting to recover
from cocaine abuse. With these "cravings"
under control, patients are more likely to
avoid relapse.

Most important fact about this drug

Since Parlodel can restore fertility and
pregnancy can result, women who do not
want to become pregnant should use a
mechanical or "barrier" method of
contraception during treatment with this
medication. Do not use the "Pill" or oral
contraceptives, as they may prevent Parlodel
from working properly.

If you become pregnant while taking Parlodel,
notify your doctor immediately.

How should you take this medication?

Parlodel should be taken with food. Take the
first dose while lying down. Dizziness or
fainting may occur due to diminished blood
pressure, especially following the first dose.

What side effects may occur?

The number and severity of side effects
depend on many factors including the
condition being treated, dosage, and duration
of treatment. Side effects cannot be
anticipated. If any develop or change in
intensity, inform your doctor as soon as
possible. Only your doctor can determine if
it is safe for you to continue taking Parlodel.

■ *More common side effects may include:*
    Abdominal cramps, constipation, depression,
    diarrhea, dizziness, drop in blood pressure
    on rising, drowsiness, dry mouth, fainting,
    fatigue, hallucinations (particularly in
    Parkinson's patients), headache, indigestion,
    light-headedness, loss of appetite, loss of
    coordination, nasal congestion, nausea,
    shortness of breath, uncontrolled body
    movement, vertigo, vomiting

■ *Less common side effects may include:*
    Abdominal bleeding, anxiety, closing of
    eyelids, confusion, difficulty swallowing,
    fluid retention in feet and ankles, frequent
    urination, mottling of skin, nervousness,
    seizures, stroke, urinary incontinence

Some of the above side effects are also symptoms of Parkinson's disease.

- *Rare side effects may include:*
  Abnormal heart rhythm, black, tarry stools, bloody vomit, blurred vision or temporary blindness, cold feet, continuing loss of appetite, continuous runny nose, fast or slow heartbeat, hair loss, increase in blood pressure, increased sweating, lower back pain, numbness, paranoia, prickling or tingling, severe chest pain, severe nausea or vomiting, severe or continuous headache, severe stomach pain, sluggishness, sudden weakness, weakness

Why should this drug not be prescribed?
You should not be using Parlodel if you have uncontrolled high blood pressure, toxemia of pregnancy, or sensitivity to Parlodel or any other drugs considered to be ergot alkaloids.

Special warnings about this medication
Your doctor should do a complete evaluation of your pituitary system before you are treated with Parlodel.

If pregnancy occurs while you are being treated with Parlodel, you should be carefully monitored by your doctor.

If you have kidney or liver disease, consult with your doctor before taking Parlodel.

If you are being treated with Parlodel for endocrine problems related to a tumor and stop taking this medication, rapid regrowth of the tumor may occur.

If you are being treated for Parkinson's disease, the use of Parlodel alone or Parlodel with levodopa may cause hallucinations. If this happens, notify your doctor immediately.

If you have an abnormal heartbeat rhythm caused by a previous heart attack, consult with your doctor before taking Parlodel.

If you experience a persistent watery nasal discharge while taking Parlodel, notify your doctor.

This drug may impair your ability to drive a car or operate potentially dangerous machinery. Do not participate in any activities that require full alertness if you are unsure about your ability to do so.

Your first dose of Parlodel may cause dizziness. If so, check with your doctor.

Use with caution when taking other medications that lower blood pressure.

You may not feel the full effect of this medication for a few weeks. Do not stop taking Parlodel without first checking with your doctor.

Possible food and drug interactions when taking this medication
Parlodel may intensify the effects of alcohol. Do not drink while taking this medication.

Certain drugs used for psychotic conditions, including Thorazine or other phenothiazines and Haldol, inhibit the action of Parlodel. It is important that you consult with your doctor before taking these drugs while on Parlodel therapy.

Other drugs that may interact with Parlodel include:

Blood pressure lowering drugs
Oral contraceptives
Other ergot derivatives

Special information if you are pregnant or breastfeeding
The use of Parlodel during pregnancy should be discussed thoroughly with your doctor. If Parlodel is essential to your treatment, you should be carefully monitored throughout your pregnancy.

Because Parlodel can be used to prevent milk flow, it should not be used by mothers who wish to breastfeed their infants.

Recommended dosage

ADULTS

Parlodel is available as 2.5 and 5 milligram tablets. Dosage information given is for 2.5 milligram tablets.

Excessive or Unwanted Milk Production
If you are being treated for excessive milk production, the usual starting dose is ½ to 1 tablet daily. An additional tablet may be added every 3 to 7 days, until the correct treatment dose is obtained. The usual treatment dose is 5 to 7.5 milligrams per day and ranges from 2.5 to 15 milligrams per day.

The usual dose for the prevention of milk flow is 1 tablet 2 times a day. Therapy should be discontinued after 14 days but if necessary may be given up to 21 days.

Growth Hormone Overproduction
Treatment for the overproduction of growth hormones is usually ½ to 1 tablet with food at bedtime for 3 days. An additional ½ to 1 tablet can be added every 3 to 7 days until the correct dose is obtained. The usual treatment dose varies from 20 to 30 milligrams per day. The dose should not exceed 100 milligrams per day. A monthly re-evaluation should be performed by your doctor.

Parkinson's Disease
Parodel given in combination with levodopa may provide additional treatment benefits to patients with Parkinson's disease who are currently taking high doses of levodopa, those who are beginning to develop a tolerance to levodopa, or those who are experiencing "end of dose failure" on levodopa therapy.

The usual starting dose of Parlodel is ½ tablet twice a day with meals. Your dose should be monitored by your doctor at 2-week intervals. If necessary, the dose may be increased every 14 to 28 days by 1 tablet per day.

CHILDREN

The safety and effectiveness of Parlodel have not been established in children under 15 years of age.

Overdosage

Any medication taken in excess can have serious consequences. If you suspect an overdose, contact your doctor immediately or seek other medical attention.

Brand name:

PEDIAPRED

Generic ingredients: Prednisolone sodium phosphate

Why is this drug prescribed?

Pediapred, a corticosteroid drug, is used to reduce inflammation and improve symptoms in a variety of disorders, including rheumatic arthritis, acute gouty arthritis, and severe cases of asthma. It may be given to people to treat primary or secondary adrenal cortex insufficiency (lack of or insufficient adrenal cortical hormone in the body). It is also given to help treat following disorders:

Severe allergic conditions (e.g., drug-induced allergic state)
Blood disorders (e.g., leukemia and various anemias)
Certain cancers (along with other drugs)
Skin diseases (e.g., severe psoriasis)
Collagen (connective tissue) diseases (e.g., systemic lupus erythematosus)

Digestive tract diseases (e.g., ulcerative colitis)

High serum levels of calcium associated with cancer

Fluid retention due to nephrotic syndrome (a condition in which damage to the kidney causes a loss of protein in the urine)

Eye diseases of various kinds

Lung diseases (e.g., tuberculosis)

Studies have shown that high doses of Pediapred are effective in controlling severe symptoms of multiple sclerosis. The studies do not show that they affect the ultimate outcome or natural history of the disease.

Most important fact about this drug

Pediapred decreases your resistance to infection; thus it is possible for you to get a new infection while taking this medication. Pediapred may also mask some of the signs and symptoms of new infection, which makes it difficult for a doctor to diagnose the actual problem.

How should you take this medication?

Take this medication exactly as prescribed by your doctor.

Pediapred may cause stomach upset and should be taken with food.

What side effects may occur?

Side effects cannot be anticipated. If any develop or change in intensity, inform your doctor as soon as possible. Only your doctor can determine if it is safe for you to continue taking Pediapred.

■ *Side effects may include:*

Abnormal loss of bony tissue causing fragile bones, abnormal redness of the face, backbone break that collapses the spinal column, bruising, cataracts, convulsions, dizziness, fluid retention (edema), fracture of long bones, glaucoma (increased eye pressure), headache, high blood pressure, increased sweating, loss of muscle mass, menstrual irregularities, mental capacity changes, muscle disease, muscle weakness, peptic (stomach) ulcer with possible bleeding, protrusion of eyeball, salt retention, slow growth in children, slow wound healing, sugar diabetes, swelling of the abdomen, thinning of the skin

Why should this drug not be prescribed?

This drug should not be used for fungal infections of the body.

Special warnings about this medication

Patients should not be vaccinated against smallpox while being treated with Pediapred. Other immunization procedures should not be undertaken in patients who are taking corticosteroids, especially if they are taken in high doses, because of the possible hazards of nervous system complications and a lack of natural antibody response.

If you are taking Pediapred, (a corticosteroid), and are subjected to unusual stress, notify your doctor. He or she may increase your dosage of this rapidly acting corticosteroid before, during, and after the stressful situation.

Prolonged use of corticosteroids may produce posterior subcapsular cataracts (disorder under the envelope-like structure at the back of the eye that causes the lens to become less transparent) or glaucoma (disease of the eye, producing visual defects) and may intensify additional eye infections due to fungi or viruses.

Average and high doses of this medication may cause an increase in blood pressure, salt and water retention, and an increased loss of potassium. Decreasing your salt intake and increasing your potassium intake may be necessary.

Pediapred should only be used with an appropriate antituberculosis regimen in patients with suddenly occurring or spreading tuberculosis.

The effects of Pediapred may intensify if you have an underactive thyroid or long-term liver disease.

This drug should be used with caution in patients with ocular herpes simplex (virus causing painful blisters of the eye) because of the possibility of corneal perforation (puncture of the outer, transparent part of the eye).

The lowest possible dose of this medication should be used to control the condition under treatment, and when reduction in the dose is possible, the reduction should be gradual.

The use of Pediapred may cause mood swings, feelings of elation, insomnia, personality changes, severe depression, or severe mental disorders. Also, existing emotional instability may be made worse by corticosteroids.

If you are being treated for a blood clotting factor deficiency, aspirin should be used with caution when taking Pediapred. Do not use this drug for any disorder other than that for which it was prescribed.

This medication should be used with caution if you have ulcerative colitis (inflammation and breaks in the skin of the colon and rectum) where there is a possibility of a puncture, abscess, or other infection; diverticulitis (inflammation of a sac formed at weak points of the colon); fresh intestinal anastomoses (a surgical connection between two separate parts of the colon); active or inactive peptic (stomach) ulcer; unsatisfactory kidney function; high blood pressure; osteoporosis (brittle bones that may fracture); and myasthenia gravis (long-term disease characterized by abnormal fatigue and weakness of certain muscles).

The growth and development of infants and children taking Pediapred for a prolonged period of time should be monitored by their doctor.

Do not discontinue the use of Pediapred abruptly or without medical supervision.

If you should develop a fever or other signs of infection while taking Pediapred, notify your doctor immediately.

Possible food and drug interactions when taking this medication

If Pediapred is taken with certain other drugs, the effects of either could be increased, decreased, or altered. It is especially important to check with your doctor before combining Pediapred with barbiturates such as Phenobarbital and Seconal.

Special information if you are pregnant or breastfeeding

The effects of Pediapred during pregnancy have not been adequately studied. If you are pregnant or plan to become pregnant, inform your doctor immediately. This medication may appear in breast milk and could affect a nursing infant. If this drug is essential to your health, your doctor may advise you to discontinue breastfeeding until your treatment is finished.

Recommended dosage

The starting dosage of Pediapred may vary from 5 milliliters to 60 milliliters, depending on the specific disease being treated.

In less severe conditions lower doses will generally be adequate, while in certain patients higher starting doses may be required.

The starting dosage should be maintained or adjusted until the desired response is achieved. If the condition does not improve after a reasonable period of time, Pediapred should be stopped and the patient switched to another medication.

Dosage requirements are variable and must be individualized on the basis of the disease being treated and the response of the patient.

Once a favorable response occurs, the maintenance dosage should be determined by gradually decreasing the starting dosage by small amounts until the lowest dosage which will keep an adequate response is reached.

Drug dosage should be constantly monitored.

If Pediapred is stopped after long-term therapy, it should be withdrawn slowly rather than abruptly.

In the treatment of acute flare-ups of multiple sclerosis (MS), doses of 200 milligrams per day of Pediapred for one week followed by 80 milligrams every other day or 4 to 8 milligrams of dexamethasone every other day for one month have been effective.

Overdosage

Although no specific information is available, any medication taken in excess can have serious consequences. If you suspect an overdose of Pediapred seek medical treatment immediately.

Brand name:

PEDIAZOLE

Generic ingredients: Erythromycin ethylsuccinate, Sulfisoxazole acetyl

Why is this drug prescribed?

Pediazole is prescribed for the treatment of severe middle ear infections in children.

Most important fact about this drug

Sulfisoxazole is one of a group of drugs called sulfonamides, which prevent the growth of certain bacteria in the body. However, sulfonamides have been known to cause fatalities due to severe reactions such as Stevens-Johnson syndrome (a rare skin condition characterized by severe blisters and bleeding in the mucous membrane of the lips, mouth, nose, and eyes), sudden and severe liver damage, a severe blood disorder (agranulocytosis), and a lack of red and white blood cells because of a bone marrow disorder.

It is therefore very important that you notify your doctor at the first sign of a side effect such as skin rash, sore throat, fever, joint pain, cough, shortness of breath, abnormal skin paleness, reddish or purplish skin spots, or yellowing of the skin or whites of the eyes.

Your doctor should perform complete blood counts regularly while sulfonamides are being used.

How should you take this medication?

Pediazole can be taken with or without food.

It is important to drink plenty of fluids while taking this medication in order to prevent sediment in the urine and the formation of stones.

What side effects may occur?

Side effects cannot be anticipated. If any develop or change in intensity, inform your doctor as soon as possible. Only your doctor can determine if it is safe to continue taking Pediazole.

■ *More common side effects may include:*
Abdominal cramping and discomfort

■ *Less common or rare side effects may include:*
Chills, convulsions, depression, diarrhea,

difficulty in urinating or inability to urinate, fever, hallucinations, headache, hepatitis, hives, inability to fall or stay asleep (insomnia), increased urine, inflammation of heart muscle, inflammation of the mouth, itching, joint pain, lack of muscle coordination, lack or loss of appetite, nausea, redness and swelling of the tongue, reversible hearing loss, ringing in the ears, scaling of dead skin due to inflammation, sensitivity to light, severe allergic reactions, severe skin welts or swelling, skin eruptions, skin rash, Stevens-Johnson syndrome, swelling around the eye, vertigo, vomiting

Why should this drug not be prescribed?

If your child is sensitive to or has ever had an allergic reaction to erythromycin, sulfonamides, or drugs of this type, he or she should not take this medication. Make sure that your doctor is aware of any drug reactions that your child has experienced.

This medication should not be prescribed for infants under 2 months of age.

Special warnings about this medication

If your child has impaired kidney or liver function or a history of severe allergies or bronchial asthma, caution should be exercised when giving Pediazole. Consult with your doctor.

Your doctor may recommend frequent urine tests while your child is taking Pediazole.

Possible food and drug interactions when taking this medication

If Pediazole is taken with certain other drugs, the effects of either could be increased, decreased, or altered. It is especially important to check with your doctor before combining Pediazole with high doses of theophylline (Theo-Dur), a bronchodilator used to treat asthma, bronchitis, or emphysema.

Special information if you are pregnant or breastfeeding

This drug is not prescribed for adults, and should never be taken at term of pregnancy or when breastfeeding.

Recommended dosage

CHILDREN

The recommended dose for children 2 months of age or older is determined by weight. The following table is a guideline for this dosage, which is given every 6 hours (four times daily) for 10 days:

Less than 18 pounds	Determined by doctor
18 pounds	½ teaspoonful
35 pounds	1 teaspoonful
53 pounds	1½ teaspoonfuls
Over 100 pounds	2 teaspoonfuls

Overdosage

Any medication taken in excess can have serious consequences.

If you suspect an overdose, seek medical treatment immediately.

Generic name:

PEMOLINE

See Cylert, page 150.

Brand name:

PEN-VEE K

See Penicillin V, page 462.

Generic name:

PENICILLIN V

Brand names: Beepen VK, Betapen-VK, Pen-Vee K, V-cillin K, Veetids

Why is this drug prescribed?

Penicillin V is used to treat infections including:
Dental infection
Infections in the heart
Middle ear infections
Rheumatic fever
Scarlet fever
Skin infections
Upper and lower respiratory tract infections

Penicillin V works only against certain types of bacteria—it is ineffective against fungi, viruses, and parasites.

Most important fact about this drug

Penicillin V should not be taken by people who are allergic to penicillin or cephalosporin antibiotics (Ceclor), since serious reactions—even death—can result.

How should you take this medication?

The dose of oral solution of penicillin V must be measured with a calibrated measuring spoon.

Penicillin V may be taken on a full or empty stomach.

The oral solution must be kept under refrigeration for 14 days. Do not freeze. Shake well before using. Penicillin V must be taken for the full time of treatment.

What side effects may occur?

Side effects cannot be anticipated. If any develop or change in intensity, inform your doctor as soon as possible. Only your doctor can determine if it is safe for you to continue taking this medication.

■ *Side effects may include:*
Anemia
Black, hairy tongue
Diarrhea
Fever
Hives
Nausea
Skin eruptions
Stomach upset or pain
Swelling in throat
Vomiting

Why should this drug not be prescribed?

You should not be using penicillin V if you have had an allergic reaction to penicillin or cephalosporin antibiotics.

Special warnings about this medication

If any allergic reactions occur, stop taking penicillin V and contact your doctor immediately.

If new infections (called superinfections) occur, consult your doctor.

If you have ever had allergic reactions such as rashes, hives or hay fever, consult with your doctor before taking penicillin V.

Before taking penicillin, tell your doctor if you have ever had asthma, colitis (inflammatory bowel disease), diabetes, or kidney or liver disease.

For infections such as strep throat, it is important to take penicillin V for the entire amount of time your doctor has prescribed. Even if you feel better, you need to continue taking this medication. If you stop taking this medication before your treatment time is complete, your infection may recur.

Possible food and drug interactions when taking this medication

If penicillin V is taken with certain other drugs, the effects of either could be increased, decreased, or altered. It is especially important to check with your doctor before combining penicillin V with the following:

Tetracyclines (Sumycin)
Oral contraceptives (Ortho-Novum)

Special Information
if you are pregnant or breastfeeding

The effects of penicillin V in pregnancy have not been adequately studied. If you are pregnant or planning to become pregnant, inform your doctor immediately.

Penicillin V should be used during pregnancy only if your doctor determines the potential benefit justifies the potential risk to the fetus.

Since penicillin V appears in breast milk, you should consult with your doctor if you plan to breastfeed your baby. If this medication is essential to your health, your doctor may advise you to discontinue breastfeeding until your treatment is finished.

Recommended dosage

ADULTS AND CHILDREN 12 YEARS OLD AND OVER

Continue taking penicillin V for the full time of treatment, even if you begin to feel better after a few days. Failure to take a full course of therapy may prevent complete elimination of the infection. It is best to take the doses at evenly spaced times, around the clock.

For mild to moderately severe streptococcal infections of the upper respiratory tract and skin, and scarlet fever
The usual dosage is 125 to 250 milligrams every 6 to 8 hours for 10 days.

For mild to moderately severe pneumococcal infections of the respiratory tract, including middle ear infections
The usual dosage is 250 milligrams every 6 hours until the patient has been without a fever for at least 2 days.

For mild staph infections of skin
The usual dosage is 250 milligrams every 6 to 8 hours.

For mild to moderately severe gum infections known as Vincent's gingivits
The usual dosage is 250 milligrams every 6 to 8 hours.

To prevent recurring rheumatic fever and/or chorea (infective disorder of the nervous system)
The usual dosage is 125 milligrams 2 times a day on a continuing basis.

Prevention of bacterial endocarditis in patients with heart disease who are undergoing dental or surgical procedures
For oral therapy, the usual dose is 2 grams of penicillin V ½ to 1 hour before the procedure, then 500 milligrams every 6 hours for 8 doses.

For combined oral-injectable therapy, the usual dose of injectable form is determined by your doctor. The oral dose after the procedure is 500 milligrams every 6 hours for 8 doses.

Overdosage

Any medication taken in excess can cause symptoms of overdose. If you suspect an overdose, seek medical attention immediately.

Symptoms of overdose may include:
Diarrhea
Nausea
Vomiting

Generic name:

PENTAZOCINE HYDROCHLORIDE WITH ASPIRIN

See Talwin, page 602.

Generic name:

PENTOBARBITAL SODIUM

See Nembutal, page 409.

Generic name:

PENTOXIFYLLINE

See Trental, page 646.

Brand name:

PEPCID

Generic name: Famotidine

Why is this drug prescribed?

Pepcid is an anti-ulcer drug prescribed for the short-term treatment of active duodenal ulcer (4 to 8 weeks) and active, benign gastric ulcer (6 to 8 weeks), and as maintenance therapy, at reduced dosage, after a duodenal ulcer has healed. It is also prescribed for short-term treatment of GERD, a condition in which the contents of the stomach flow back into the esophagus, and for resulting inflammation of the esophagus. It is also used for certain diseases that cause the stomach to produce excessive quantities of acid, such as Zollinger-Ellison syndrome. Pepcid belongs to a class of drugs known as Histamine H2 blockers.

Most important fact about this drug

Although Pepcid can be used for up to 8 weeks to heal ulcers, most are healed within 4 weeks.

How should you take this medication?

Take this medication exactly as prescribed by your doctor.

You can take an antacid for pain while you are taking Pepcid.

This medication is available for home use in tablets and in an oral suspension form. The unused portion of the oral suspension should be discarded after 30 days. An intravenous form may be used in the hospital.

What side effects may occur?

Side effects cannot be anticipated. If any develop or change in intensity, inform your doctor as soon as possible. Only your doctor can determine if it is safe for you to continue taking Pepcid.

- *More common side effects may include:*
  Constipation
  Diarrhea
  Dizziness
  Headache

- *Less common or rare side effects may include:*
  Abdominal discomfort, acne, altered taste, anxiety, changes in blood count, changes in liver function, confusion, decrease in white blood cells, decreased sex drive, difficulty sleeping, dry mouth, dry skin, facial swelling due to fluid retention, fatigue, fever, flushing, grand mal seizures, hair loss, hallucinations, hives, hypersensitivity reaction, impotence, irregular heartbeat, itching, loss of appetite, muscle, bone or joint pain, nausea, pounding heartbeat, prickling, tingling, rash, reversible behavior changes, ringing in ears, sleepiness, vomiting, weakness, wheezing, yellow eyes and skin

Why should this drug not be prescribed?

If you are sensitive to or have ever had an allergic reaction to Pepcid or similar drugs, you should not take this medication. Make sure that your doctor is aware of any drug reactions that you have experienced.

Special warnings about this medication
A stomach malignancy could be present, even if your symptoms have been relieved by Pepcid.

If you have severe kidney disease, this medication should be used with caution.

Possible food and drug interactions when taking this medication
No drug interactions have been identified.

Special information
if you are pregnant or breastfeeding
The effects of Pepcid during pregnancy have not been adequately studied. If you are pregnant or plan to become pregnant, inform your doctor immediately. Pepcid may appear in breast milk and could affect a nursing infant. If this medication is essential to your health, your doctor may advise you to discontinue breastfeeding until your treatment with this medication is finished.

Recommended dosage
ADULTS

For Duodenal Ulcer
The usual starting dose is 40 milligrams or 5 milliliters (1 teaspoonful) 1 time a day at bedtime. Results should be seen within 4 weeks, and this medication should not be used at high dosage longer than 6 to 8 weeks. You may be prescribed 20 milligrams or 2.5 milliliters (one-half teaspoonful) 2 times per day. The normal maintenance dose after healing is 20 milligrams or 2.5 milliliters (one-half teaspoonful) at bedtime.

Benign Gastric Ulcer
The usual dose is 40 milligrams or 5 milliliters (1 teaspoonful) 1 time a day at bedtime.

Gastroesophageal Reflux Disease (GERD)
The recommended dose is 20 milligrams or 2.5 milliliters (one-half teaspoonful) 2 times a day for up to 6 weeks. For inflammation of the esophagus due to GERD, the recommended oral dosage is 20 or 40 milligrams 2 times a day for up to 12 weeks.

Other Hypersecretory Conditions (such as Zollinger-Ellison Syndrome)
Dosages are adjusted to individual patient needs. Your doctor will advise you of the proper dosage.

The recommended starting dose is 20 milligrams every six hours. In some patients, a higher starting dose may be required.

Dosages in patients with reduced kidney function will be adjusted by their doctor.

CHILDREN

The safety and effectiveness of Pepcid have not been established in children.

ELDERLY

Dosage should be determined by the particular needs of the elderly patient.

Overdosage
Any medication taken in excess can have serious consequences. If you suspect an overdose, seek medical attention immediately.

Brand name:

PERCOCET

Generic ingredients: Acetaminophen, Oxycodone hydrochloride
Other brand names: Roxicet, Tylox

Why is this drug prescribed?
Percocet, a narcotic analgesic, is used to treat moderate to moderately severe pain. It contains two drugs—acetaminophen and oxycodone. Acetaminophen is used to reduce

both pain and fever. Oxycodone, a narcotic analgesic, is used to treat moderate to severe pain.

People who are allergic to aspirin can take Percocet.

Most important fact about this drug

Percocet contains a narcotic (oxycodone) and, even if taken in prescribed amounts, can cause physical and psychological dependence when taken for a long time.

How should you take this medication?

Percocet may be taken with meals or with milk but never with alcohol.

What side effects may occur?

Side effects cannot be anticipated. If any develop or change in intensity, inform your doctor as soon as possible. Only your doctor can determine if it is safe for you to continue taking Percocet.

■ *More common side effects may include:*
Dizziness
Lightheadedness
Nausea
Sedation
Vomiting

■ *Less common or rare side effects may include:*
Constipation, depressed feeling, exaggerated feeling of well-being, itchy skin, skin rash

Why should this drug not be prescribed?

You should not use Percocet if you are sensitive to either acetaminophen or oxycodone.

Special warnings about this medication

Psychological and physical dependence may result if Percocet is taken for a long enough time. You should take Percocet cautiously and according to your doctor's instructions, as you would take any medication containing a narcotic. Make sure your doctor is aware of any history of drug or alcohol addiction you may have.

If you have experienced a head injury, consult with your doctor before taking Percocet. The effects of Percocet may be stronger for people with head injuries, and using it may delay recovery.

If you have stomach problems, such as an ulcer, check with your doctor before taking Percocet. Percocet may hide the symptoms of stomach problems, making them difficult to diagnose and treat.

If you have ever had liver, kidney, thyroid, or Addison's disease (adrenal insufficiency), difficulty urinating, or a prostate condition, consult with your doctor before taking Percocet.

Elderly people should take Percocet cautiously.

This drug may impair your ability to drive a car or operate potentially dangerous machinery. Do not participate in any activities that require full alertness if you are unsure about your ability.

Possible food and drug interactions when taking this medication

Alcohol may increase the sedative effects of Percocet. You should not take Percocet with alcohol.

If Percocet is taken with certain other drugs, the effects of either could be increased, decreased, or altered. It is especially important to check with your doctor before combining Percocet with the following:

Anticholinergic drugs (Cogentin)
Drugs for severe mental disorders such as Thorazine
General anesthetics
MAO inhibitors (Nardil)

Other narcotic painkillers such as Darvon
Other tranquilizers such as Xanax and Valium
Sedative/hypnotics and other central nervous
   system depressants (phenobarbital, Seconal)
Tricyclic antidepressants (Elavil, Pamelor)

Taking Percocet with anticholinergic drugs
(e.g., Donnatal, Bentyl) may cause obstruction
of the small intestine.

Special information
if you are pregnant or breastfeeding

It is not known whether Percocet could injure
a fetus or affect a woman's reproductive
capacity. Using any medication that contains
a narcotic during pregnancy may cause
physical addiction for your newborn baby.
If you are pregnant or plan to become
pregnant, inform your doctor immediately.
As with other narcotic painkillers, taking
Percocet shortly before delivery (especially at
higher dosages) may cause some degree of
impaired breathing in the mother and
newborn. Because it is not known if Percocet
appears in breast milk and thus may harm
a nursing infant, nursing mothers should use
Percocet only under a doctor's directions.

Recommended dosage

ADULTS

The usual dose is 1 tablet ever 6 hours as
needed.

CHILDREN

The safety and effectiveness of Percocet have
not been established in children.

ELDERLY

This drug should be used with caution in
elderly patients.

Overdosage

Severe overdose of Percocet can cause death.
If you suspect an overdose, seek medical help
immediately.

Symptoms of Percocet overdose may include:
Bluish skin, eyes or skin with yellow tone,
cold and clammy skin, decreased or irregular
breathing (stoppage in severe overdose),
extreme sleepiness progressing to stupor or
coma, heart attack, low blood pressure,
muscle weakness/softness, nausea, slow heart
beat, sweating, vague bodily discomfort,
vomiting

Generic name:

PERGOLIDE MESYLATE

See Permax, page 470.

Brand name:

PERIACTIN

Generic name: Cyproheptadine hydrochloride

Why is this drug prescribed?

Periactin is an antihistamine available in the
form of tablets or syrup that is given to
help relieve cold- and allergy-related symptoms
such as stuffy nose, red eyes, hives, and
swelling. Periactin may also be given after
epinephrine to help treat anaphylaxis, a
life-threatening allergic reaction. Periactin is
under study for use as an appetite
stimulant.

Most important fact about this drug

Like other antihistamines, Periactin may make
you feel sleepy and sluggish. However,
some people, particularly children, may have
the opposite reaction and become excited.

How should you take this medication?

Take Periactin exactly as prescribed by your
doctor.

Avoid drinking alcohol.

Be careful when driving or performing tasks
that require alertness.

What side effects may occur?

Side effects cannot be anticipated. If any side effects develop or change in intensity, tell your doctor immediately. Only your doctor can determine whether it is safe for you to continue taking Periactin.

■ *Side effects may include:*
Anaphylaxis (life-threatening allergic reaction), anemia, appetite (increased), blood-cell abnormalities, burning, chest tightness, chills, confusion, constipation, convulsions, diarrhea, dizziness, dry mouth, nose, or throat, earlier-than-expected menstrual period, euphoria, excitation, faintness, fatigue, headache, heart problems, hallucinations, hives, hysteria, insomnia, irritability, lack of coordination, light sensitivity, low blood pressure, nausea, vomiting, nervousness, rash and swelling, restlessness, ringing in the ears, sleepiness, stomach pain, stuffy nose, sweating, tingling in arms or legs, urinary frequency, retention, or difficulty, vertigo, vision problems (double vision, blurred vision), weight gain, wheezing, yellow eyes and skin

Older people, in particular, are likely to become confused, faint, nervous, dizzy, or drowsy, or to develop low blood pressure in response to Periactin.

Why should this drug not be prescribed?

Do not take Periactin if you are sensitive to it, or if you have ever had an allergic reaction to or are sensitive to cyproheptadine or a similar antihistamine.

Do not take Periactin if you have bronchial asthma, hyperthyroidism, heart disease, high blood pressure, angle-closure glaucoma, a stenosing peptic ulcer, an enlarged prostate, obstruction of the neck of the bladder, obstruction of the outlet of the stomach, or Parkinson's disease.

Special warnings about this medication

Like other antihistamines, Periactin may make you drowsy or impair your coordination. Be very careful about driving, climbing, or operating machinery, or doing hazardous tasks until you know how you react to this medication.

Possible food and drug interactions when taking this medication

If Periactin is taken with certain other drugs, the effects of either could be increased, decreased, or altered. It is especially important to check with your doctor before combining Periactin with the following:

Alcohol
Anti-anxiety drugs such as Valium
MAO inhibitor antidepressants such as
    Marplan, Nardil, and Parnate
Sedatives such as Xanax and Halcion
Tranquilizers such as Librium

Special information if you are pregnant or breastfeeding

Because of possible harm to the unborn baby, Periactin should not be used during pregnancy unless it is clearly needed. Periactin should not be taken by a woman who is breastfeeding. If you have just given birth, you will need to choose between breast-feeding and taking Periactin.

Recommended dosage

Your doctor will tailor a dosage according to your individual needs and response to treatment.

Each Periactin tablet contains 4 milligrams of cyproheptadine hydrochloride.

Each 5 milliliters of Periactin syrup contains 2 milligrams of cyproheptadine hydro-chloride. Although intended primarily for administration to children, the syrup is also useful for adults who cannot swallow tablets.

ADULTS

The usual recommended initial dose is 4 milligrams (1 tablet or 2 teaspoonfuls) 3 times daily. For most patients the recommended daily dosage is 12 to 16 milligrams. Some patients may require up to 32 milligrams a day for adequate relief of symptoms.

CHIILDREN

Age 2 to 6 Years
The usual recommended dose is 2 milligrams (one-half tablet or 1 teaspoon) 2 or 3 times a day, adjusted as necessary according to the size and response of the patient. The dose is not to exceed 12 milligrams a day.

Age 7 to 14 Years
The usual dose is 4 milligrams (1 tablet or 2 teaspoons) 2 or 3 times a day, adjusted as necessary according to the size and response of the patient. The dose is not to exceed 16 milligrams a day.

Overdosage

Any drug taken in excess may have serious consequences. If you suspect an overdose of Periactin, seek medical attention immediately. Call your local poison center or your doctor for assistance.

Symptoms of Periactin overdose may include:
Dilated pupils
Dry mouth
Extreme excitement and agitation
Fever
Flushing
Stomach or bowel distress
Stupor or coma

Overdosage in children may produce hallucinations and convulsions.

Brand name:

PERIDEX

Generic name: Chlorhexidine gluconate

Why is this drug prescribed?

Peridex is an oral rinse used to treat gingivitis, a condition in which the gums become red and swollen. Peridex is also used to control gum bleeding caused by gingivitis.

Most important fact about this drug

If you are sensitive to or have ever had an allergic reaction to Peridex or similar drugs, you should not use Peridex. Make sure that your doctor is aware of any drug reactions that you have experienced.

How should you take this medication?

Treatment with Peridex should start following a thorough dental cleaning and examination.

After brushing, thoroughly rinsing, and flossing your teeth, rinse with Peridex by swishing one-half fluid ounce (marked in cap) around in your mouth for 30 seconds, then spit it out. Do not dilute Peridex and do not eat or drink for several hours after using this medication.

What side effects may occur?

Side effects cannot be anticipated. If any develop or change in intensity, inform your doctor as soon as possible. Only your doctor can determine if it is safe for you to continue.

■ *More common side effects may include:*
Change in taste
Increase in plaque
Staining of teeth, mouth, tooth fillings, and dentures or other appliances in the mouth

■ *Less common or rare side effects may include:*
Irritation of the mouth

Why should this drug not be prescribed?

Unless you are directed to do so by your doctor, do not use Peridex if you have shown a sensitivity to or are allergic to Peridex.

Special warnings about this medication

If you have both gingivitis and periodontitis (disease of the tissue that supports and attaches the teeth), Peridex should be used for the treatment of gingivitis only. Periodontitis may require additional treatment by your doctor or dentist.

The use of Peridex may leave a bitter aftertaste. Rinsing your mouth with or drinking water after using Peridex may increase the bitterness.

The use of Peridex can cause staining of your teeth, fillings, and the back of your tongue. It can also cause an excess of tartar build-up on your teeth. It is recommended that you have your teeth cleaned at least every 6 months.

Foods may taste different to you for up to 4 hours after rinsing with Peridex. In most cases, this effect becomes less noticeable after continued use. Taste should return to normal when treatment with Peridex is finished.

Possible food and drug interactions when taking this medication

No interactions with other drugs have been reported.

Special information
if you are pregnant or breastfeeding

The effects of Peridex during pregnancy have not been adequately studied. If you are pregnant or plan to become pregnant, inform your doctor immediately. It is not known whether this medication appears in breast milk. If it is essential for you to use Peridex, your doctor may advise you to stop breastfeeding until your treatment is finished.

Recommended dosage

ADULTS

The usual dose of undiluted Peridex is one-half fluid ounce. Peridex should be spit out after rinsing and never swallowed.

CHILDREN

The effectiveness and safety of Peridex have not been established in children under 18 years of age.

Overdosage

If you suspect that a child of 22 pounds or less has swallowed 4 or more ounces of Peridex, seek medical attention immediately.

Also seek immediate medical attention if any child shows signs of stomach distress, including nausea or signs of alcohol intoxication such as slurred speech, staggering, or sleepiness, and you suspect he or she has swallowed Peridex.

Brand name:

PERMAX

Generic name: Pergolide mesylate

Why is this drug prescribed?

Permax, a drug derived from the fungus called ergot, is given to help relieve symptoms of Parkinson's disease.

In Parkinson's disease, the brain cells receive too little of a natural chemical messenger called dopamine. This results in tremor, rigid muscles, difficulty with walking and talking, and other distressing symptoms.

People with Parkinson's disease are given medication to increase the amount of dopamine reaching their brain; the medication may be levodopa, such as Dopar or Larodopa, or, more commonly, a levodopa-carbidopa combination, such as Sinemet.

Side effects from Sinemet include nausea, loss of appetite, and involuntary movements. The role of Permax is to increase the effectiveness of Sinemet so that patients need less of it and may thus avoid some of the side effects.

Most important fact about this drug

In some people, Permax causes confusion and hallucinations, which may be severe. Sometimes the confusion and hallucinations appear only when the person suddenly stops taking Permax. Thus, if you have been taking Permax but need to stop, you should taper off gradually rather than quitting all at once. When one starts taking Permax, one may become drowsy, dizzy, or less alert; use caution when driving. Your body will adjust, and these effects will usually go away.

How should you take this medication?

Take Permax exactly as prescribed by your doctor—most likely on a 3-times-a-day schedule.

The usual procedure is to start with a small dose of Permax and work up to an effective dose over the next 12 days, with a dosage increase approximately every 3 days. During this same time, your Sinemet dosage will gradually be decreased.

What side effects may occur?

Side effects cannot be anticipated. If any develop or change in intensity, inform your doctor as soon as possible. Only your doctor can determine if it is safe for you to continue taking Permax.

■ *More common side effects may include:*
Anxiety, common-cold symptoms, confusion, constipation, diarrhea, dizziness or light-headedness, hallucinations, insomnia, nausea, sleepiness, tremor, uncontrolled movements of face, tongue, arms, hands, head, or upper body, upset stomach

■ *Less common side effects include:*
Abdominal pain, abnormal dreams, abnormal gait, abnormal heartbeat rhythm, abnormal sense of taste, abnormal vision, aching joints, aching muscles, ankle swelling, appetite loss, back pain, bloody urine, bursitis, chest pain, chills, depression, double vision, dry mouth, eye problems, face, arm, or leg twitching, facial swelling, fainting, flu syndrome, fluid retention, flushing, frequent urination, headache, heart attack, heart palpitations, hiccups, high blood pressure, infection, lack of coordination, lethargy, low blood pressure upon standing up, neck pain, nerve pain, nosebleed, pain, personality disorder, psychosis, rash, restlessness, shortness of breath, speech problems, sweating, temporary paralysis, tense muscles, tingling or numbness, twitching, urinary tract infection, vomiting, weight gain

Why should this drug not be prescribed?

Do not take this medication if you are sensitive to it or have ever had an allergic reaction to it or to any other medication derived from ergot, such as Hydergine.

Special warnings about this medication

If you are apt to have abnormal heartbeat rhythms, be sure to inform your doctor. Permax may make your condition worse.

When you first begin taking Permax, you may discover that you feel weak or faint, particularly when you stand up suddenly. This effect is likely to wear off once your body becomes accustomed to the drug.

Possible food and drug interactions when taking this medication

If Permax is taken with certain other drugs, the effects of either could be increased, decreased, or altered. It is especially important to check with your doctor before combining Permax with the following:

Antipsychotics such as Haldol, Navane, Stelazine, and Thorazine
Reglan (metoclopramide)

Special information if you are pregnant or breastfeeding

The effects of Permax during pregnancy have not been adequately studied. If you are pregnant or plan to become pregnant, notify your doctor immediately. Permax should be taken during pregnancy only if it is clearly needed. Since it may interfere with the production of breast milk or appear in breast milk, your doctor may advise you to stop breastfeeding until your treatment is finished.

Recommended dosage

The usual starting daily dosage is 0.05 milligram for the first 2 days, to be gradually increased by 0.1 or 0.15 milligram per day every third day over the next 12 days of therapy.

Your doctor may increase the dosage by 0.25 milligram per day every third day until the desired effect is achieved.

Permax is usually divided into smaller, equal doses and given 3 times per day.

The effectiveness of Permax at doses above 5 milligrams per day has not been totally studied.

Overdosage

Any medication taken in excess can have serious consequences. If you suspect symptoms of a Permax overdose, seek medical attention immediately.

Symptoms of Permax overdose may include:
Agitation, convulsions, dizziness or light-headedness (especially when standing up from a lying or sitting position), hallucinations, heart palpitations, irregular heartbeat, low blood pressure, nausea, severe involuntary movements, tingling in the arms and legs, vomiting

Generic name:

PERPHENAZINE WITH AMITRIPTYLINE

See Triavil, page 648.

Brand name:

PERSANTINE

Generic name: Dipyridamole

Why is this drug prescribed?

Persantine helps reduce the formation of blood clots in patients who have had heart valve surgery. It is used in combination with coumarin anticoagulants (blood thinners) such as Coumadin to prevent complications after heart valve surgery.

Most important fact about this drug

Unless you are directed to do so by your doctor, do not take aspirin or any medication that contains aspirin while taking Persantine.

Do not change from one brand of dipyridamole to another without consulting your doctor or pharmacist. Products manufactured by different companies may not be equally effective.

How should you take this medication?

Persantine must be taken exactly as your doctor prescribes, at regularly scheduled times.

If you forget to take a dose, take it as soon as you remember. If it is within 4 hours of your next scheduled dose, skip it and go back to your regular schedule. Never take two doses at the same time.

What side effects may occur?

Side effects cannot be anticipated. If any develop or change in intensity, inform your doctor as soon as possible. Only your doctor can determine if it is safe for you to continue taking Persantine.

■ *More common side effects may include:*
Abdominal distress
Dizziness

■ *Less common or rare side effects may include:*
Diarrhea, feeling flushed, headache, itching, nausea and vomiting, skin rash

Why should this drug not be prescribed?

Unless you are directed to do so by your doctor, do not take this medication if you have low blood pressure.

Special warnings about this medication

Persantine is indicated only for use after heart valve replacement. Consult with your doctor if this drug has been prescribed for other reasons.

If your doctor has prescribed aspirin to be taken with Persantine, take only the amount prescribed.

Notify your doctor or dentist that you are taking Persantine if you have a medical emergency or before you have surgery or dental treatment.

Possible food and drug interactions when taking this medication

If Persantine is taken with certain other drugs, the effects of either could be increased, decreased, or altered. It is especially important to check with your doctor before combining Persantine with the following:

Aspirin
Blood thinners (Coumadin)

Special information
if you are pregnant or breastfeeding

The effects of Persantine during pregnancy have not been adequately studied. If you are pregnant or plan to become pregnant, inform your doctor immediately. This drug appears in breast milk and may affect a nursing infant. If this medication is essential to your health, your doctor may advise you to discontinue breastfeeding until your treatment with this medication is finished.

Recommended dosage

ADULTS

The usual recommended dose is 75 milligrams to 100 milligrams, 4 times a day.

CHILDREN

The safety and effectiveness of this medication have not been established in children under 12 years of age.

Overdosage

Low blood pressure is the most common symptom of overdose and usually lasts for a short period of time. If this occurs, contact your doctor or emergency room immediately.

Brand name:

PHENAPHEN WITH CODEINE

See Tylenol with Codeine, page 662.

Generic name:

PHENAZOPYRIDINE HYDROCHLORIDE

See Pyridium, page 527.

Generic name:

PHENELZINE SULFATE

See Nardil, page 404.

Brand name:

PHENERGAN

Generic name: Promethazine hydrochloride

Why is this drug prescribed?

Phenergan is an antihistamine that relieves nasal stuffiness and inflammation and red, inflamed eyes caused by hay fever and other allergies; itching, swelling, and redness from hives and other rashes; allergic reactions to blood transfusions; and, with other medications, anaphylactic shock (severe allergic reaction).

Phenergan is also used as a sedative and sleep aid for both children and adults, and is prescribed to prevent and control nausea and vomiting before and after surgery and to prevent and treat motion sickness.

Antihistamines work by decreasing the effects of histamine, a chemical the body releases in response to certain irritants. Histamine narrows air passages in the lungs and contributes to inflammation. Antihistamines reduce itching and swelling and dry up secretions from the nose, eyes, and throat.

Most important fact about this drug

Phenergan may cause considerable drowsiness. Driving or operating dangerous machinery or participating in any hazardous activity that requires full mental alertness is not recommended until you know how you react to Phenergan. Children should be carefully supervised while bike-riding, roller-skating, or playing until the drug's effect on them is established.

How should you take this medication?

Phenergan should be taken exactly as prescribed by your doctor.

Suppositories should be stored in the refrigerator, in a closed container.

What side effects may occur?

Side effects cannot be anticipated. If any develop or change in intensity, inform your doctor as soon as possible. Only your doctor can determine if it is safe for you to continue taking Phenergan.

■ *More common side effects may include:*
Blurred vision
Dizziness
Dry mouth
Increased/decreased blood pressure
Nausea
Rash
Sedation (extreme calm)
Sleepiness
Vomiting

■ *Rare side effects may include:*
Abnormal eye movements, blood disorders, confusion, disorientation, protruding tongue, sensitivity to light, stiff neck

Why should this drug not be prescribed?

Phenergan should not be used if you have asthma or other breathing difficulties or if you are sensitive to or have ever had an allergic reaction to promethazine or to other phenothiazine medications, such as Thorazine, Mellaril, Stelazine, or Prolixin.

Special warnings about this medication

If you are taking other medications that cause sedation, your doctor may reduce the dosage of these medications or eliminate them while you are using Phenergan.

If you have a seizure disorder, Phenergan may cause your seizures to occur more often.

Avoid this medication if you have sleep apnea (periods when breathing stops).

Antihistamines should be used cautiously if you have cardiovascular disease, liver problems, narrow-angle glaucoma, narrowing peptic ulcer or other abdominal obstructions, or urinary bladder obstruction due to an enlarged prostate.

Phenergan may affect the results of pregnancy tests and glucose tolerance tests.

There have been reports of jaundice (yellow eyes and skin) with this medication.

Tell your doctor if you have any uncontrolled movements or seem to be unusually sensitive to sunlight.

Remember that Phenergan can cause drowsiness.

Possible food and drug interactions when taking this medication

Phenergan may increase the effects of alcohol. Do not drink alcohol, or at least substantially reduce the amount you drink, while taking this medication.

If Phenergan is taken with certain other drugs, the effects of either could be increased, decreased, or altered. It is especially important to check with your doctor before combining Phenergan with the following:

Narcotic analgesics such as Demerol and Dilaudid
Sedative/hypnotics such as Halcion, Dalmane, and Seconal
Tranquilizers such as Xanax and Valium
Tricyclic antidepressants such as Elavil

Special information if you are pregnant or breastfeeding

The effects of Phenergan during pregnancy have not been adequately studied. If you are pregnant or plan to become pregnant, inform your doctor immediately. Phenergan may appear in breast milk and may affect a nursing infant. If this medication is essential to your health, your doctor may advise you to discontinue breastfeeding until your treatment is finished.

Recommended dosage

Phenergan is available in tablet, syrup, and suppository form. Phenergan tablets and suppositories are not recommended for children under 2 years of age.

ALLERGY

Adults
The average oral dose is 25 milligrams taken before bed; however, 12.5 milligrams may be taken before meals and before bed, if necessary.

Children
The usual dose is a single 25-milligram dose at bedtime, or 6.25 to 12.5 milligrams 3 times daily.

After treatment begins in children or adults, dosage should be adjusted to the smallest amount needed to relieve symptoms. Doses of 25 milligrams will control minor allergic reactions.

MOTION SICKNESS

Adults
The average adult dose is 25 milligrams taken twice daily. The first dose should be taken one-half to 1 hour before you plan to travel, and it should be repeated 8 to 12 hours later, if necessary. On travel days after that, the recommended dose is 25 milligrams when you get up and again before the evening meal.

Children
Phenergan tablets, syrup, or rectal suppositories, 12.5 to 25 milligrams twice daily, may be given for motion sickness.

NAUSEA AND VOMITING

The average effective dose of Phenergan for nausea and vomiting in children or adults is 25 milligrams. When oral medication cannot be tolerated, the dose should be given by rectal suppository. Doses of 12.5 to 25 milligrams may be repeated as necessary at 4- to 6-hour intervals.

For nausea and vomiting in children, the dose is usually calculated at 0.5 milligram per pound of body weight. It should also be adjusted to the age of the patient and the severity of the condition being treated.

SEDATION

This product relieves anxiety, leading to a quiet sleep from which the patient can be easily aroused.

Adults
The usual dose is 25 to 50 milligrams for nighttime sedation.

Children
A dose of 12.5 to 25 milligrams of Phenergan by tablets or rectal suppository at bedtime will provide sedation in children.

Overdosage
Any medication taken in excess can have serious consequences. If you suspect an overdose, seek medical treatment immediately.

Symptoms of Phenergan overdose may include:
Cardiovascular depression
Difficulty breathing
Dry mouth
Fixed, dilated pupils
Flushing
Loss of consciousness
Mild central nervous system depression
Stomach and intestinal problems
Very low blood pressure

Children may become overstimulated or become overexcited and have nightmares; rarely, they may have convulsions. The elderly may also become overstimulated.

Brand name:

PHENERGAN WITH CODEINE

Generic ingredients: Promethazine hydrocholoride, Codeine phosphate

Why is this drug prescribed?
Phenergan with Codeine is used to relieve coughs and the symptoms of allergies and the common cold. Promethazine, an antihistamine, helps reduce itching and swelling and dries up secretions from the nose, eyes, and throat. It also has sedative effects and helps control nausea and vomiting. Codeine, a narcotic analgesic, helps relieve pain and stops coughing.

Most important fact about this drug
Phenergan with Codeine may cause considerable drowsiness. Driving or operating dangerous machinery or participating in any hazardous activity that requires full mental alertness is not recommended until you know how you react to this medication. Children should be carefully supervised while bike-riding, roller-skating, or playing until the drug's effect on them is established.

How should you take this medication?
Take this medication exactly as prescribed by your doctor.

What side effects may occur?
Side effects cannot be anticipated. If any develop or change in intensity, inform your doctor as soon as possible. Only your doctor can determine if it is safe for you to continue taking Phenergan with Codeine.

■ *Side effects may include:*
Allergic reactions, blurred vision, constipation, convulsions, decreased amount of urine, difficulty breathing, disorientation, dizziness, dizziness on standing, dry mouth, exaggerated sense of well-being, fainting, faintness, feeling of anxiety, restlessness, flushing, headache, hives, increased/decreased blood pressure, itching, light-headedness, nausea, passing hallucinations, pounding heartbeat, rapid heartbeat, rash, sedation (extreme calm), sleepiness, slow heartbeat, sweating, swelling due to fluid retention (including the throat), urinary retention, vision changes, vomiting, weakness, yellowed skin or whites of eyes

■ *Side effects seen rarely include:*
Abnormal eye movements, blood disorders, confusion, disorientation, skin sensitivity to light, protruding tongue, stiff neck

Why should this drug not be prescribed?
Phenergan with Codeine should not be used if you have asthma or other breathing difficulties or if you are sensitive to or have ever had an allergic reaction to codeine, promethazine, or other phenothiazine medications, such as Thorazine, Mellaril, Stelazine, or Prolixin. Do not use the product if you have a high fever associated with productive cough.

Special warnings about this medication
Psychological and physical dependence have occurred with codeine use. Although the likelihood of abuse with oral codeine is quite low, be cautious if you have a history of drug abuse or dependence.

Never take more cough syrup than has been prescribed. If your cough does not seem better within 5 days, check back with your doctor.

Codeine can cause or worsen constipation.

Phenergan with Codeine should be used with extreme caution in young children.

People suffering from head injuries, narrow-angle glaucoma, peptic ulcer or other abdominal obstructions, urinary bladder obstruction due to an enlarged prostate and narrowing of the bladder neck, cardiovascular disease, liver or kidney disease, fever, seizures, an underactive thyroid, intestinal inflammation, or Addison's disease (a disorder of the adrenal glands) should be carefully monitored while using this medication. Caution should also be exercised with people who have had recent gastrointestinal or urinary surgery, and with the very young, elderly, or debilitated.

This medication may make you dizzy when you stand up. Getting up slowly can help prevent this problem.

If you are taking other medications that cause sedation (extreme calm), your doctor may reduce the dosage of these medications or eliminate them altogether while you are using Phenergan with Codeine.

If you have a seizure disorder, this medication may cause your seizures to occur more often.

Avoid using Phenergan with Codeine if you have sleep apnea (periods when breathing stops).

Phenergan with Codeine may affect the results of pregnancy tests and glucose tolerance tests.

Tell your doctor if you have any involuntary muscle movements or seem to be unusually sensitive to sunlight.

Possible food and drug interactions when taking this medication
Phenergan with Codeine may increase the effects of alcohol. Do not drink alcohol, or at least substantially reduce the amount you drink, while taking this medication.

If Phenergan with Codeine is taken with certain other drugs, the effects of either could be increased, decreased, or altered. It is especially important to check with your doctor before combining Phenergan with Codeine with the following:

MAO inhibitors (antidepressant drugs such as Marplan and Nardil)
Other medications for depression (Elavil, Prozac)
Other narcotic analgesics (Demerol, Dilaudid)
Sedative/hypnotics (Seconal, Halcion, Dalmane)
Tranquilizers (Xanax, Valium)

Special information
If you are pregnant or breastfeeding
The effects of Phenergan with Codeine during pregnancy have not been adequately studied. If you are pregnant or plan to become pregnant, inform your doctor immediately. Phenergan with Codeine may appear in breast milk and may affect a nursing infant. If this medication is essential to your health, your doctor may advise you to discontinue breastfeeding until your treatment is finished.

Recommended dosage
ADULTS

The usual dosage is 1 teaspoon (5 milliliters) every 4 to 6 hours, not to exceed 6 teaspoons, or 30 milliliters, in 24 hours.

CHILDREN 6 YEARS TO UNDER 12 YEARS

The usual dose is one-half to 1 teaspoon (2.5 to 5 milliliters) every 4 to 6 hours, not to exceed 6 teaspoons, or 30 milliliters, in 24 hours.

CHILDREN UNDER 6 YEARS (40 POUNDS)

The usual dose is one-quarter to one-half teaspoon (1.25 to 2.5 milliliters) every 4 to 6 hours, not to exceed 9 milliliters in 24 hours.

CHILDREN UNDER 6 YEARS (35 POUNDS)

The usual dose is one-quarter to one-half teaspoon (1.25 to 2.5 milliliters) every 4 to 6 hours, not to exceed 8 milliliters in 24 hours.

CHILDREN UNDER 6 YEARS (30 POUNDS)

The usual dose is one-quarter to one-half teaspoon (1.25 to 2.5 milliliters) every 4 to 6 hours, not to exceed 7 milliliters in 24 hours.

CHILDREN UNDER 6 YEARS (25 POUNDS)

The usual dose is one-quarter to one-half teaspoon (1.25 to 2.5 milliliters) every 4 to 6 hours, not to exceed 6 milliliters in 24 hours.

Phenergan with Codeine is not recommended for children under 2 years of age.

Overdosage
Any medication taken in excess can have serious consequences. Deaths have occurred with codeine overdose. If you suspect an overdose, seek medical treatment immediately.

Symptoms of an overdose of Phenergan with Codeine may include:
Bluish skin, cold, clammy skin, coma, difficulty breathing, dry mouth, extreme sleepiness, low blood pressure, muscle weakness, softness, slow heartbeat, small pupils, stupor

Generic name:

PHENOBARBITAL

Why is this drug prescribed?
Phenobarbital is given to produce sedation (calmness) and as an anticonvulsant to treat certain seizures, such as generalized or grand mal seizures and partial seizures. It is also given in combination with an

antispasmodic drug to treat irritable bowel syndrome (irregular bowel habits combined with stomach pain).

Most important fact about this drug
Phenobarbital can be habit-forming. Tolerance (needing more and more of the drug to achieve the same effect) and physical and psychological dependence may occur with continued use. Never increase the amount of phenobarbital you take without checking with your doctor.

How should you take this medication?
Take this medication exactly as prescribed by your doctor.

If you are given phenobarbital for seizures, do not stop this medication abruptly.

What side effects may occur?
Side effects cannot be anticipated. If any develop or change in intensity, notify your doctor as soon as possible. Only your doctor can determine whether it is safe to continue taking phenobarbital.

■ *Side effects may include:*
Abnormal thinking, aggravation of existing emotional disturbances and phobias, agitation, angioedema (chest pain, swelling of face around lips, tongue, and throat and around arms and legs, sore throat, fever, chills, difficulty breathing), allergic reactions (localized swelling, especially of the eyelids, cheeks, or lips, skin redness [like sunburn]), anxiety, chronic inflammation of the skin with redness and flakiness, circulatory collapse, confusion, constipation, decreased breathing, depression of central nervous system function (brain and spinal cord), difficulty sleeping, diffuse muscle, nerve, or arthritic pain, especially in people with insomnia, dizziness, excitement, fainting, fever, hallucinations, headache, increased physical activity and muscle movement, irritability and

hyperactivity in children, lack of muscle coordination, low blood pressure, nausea, nervousness, nightmares, psychiatric disturbances, rash, residual "hangover" or drowsiness, restlessness, excitement, and delirium when given for pain, shallow breathing, sleepiness, slow heartbeat, softening of bones, temporary cessation of breathing, tiredness, vomiting

Why should this drug not be prescribed?
Phenobarbital should not be used if you suffer from porphyria (an inherited metabolic disorder), liver disease, or a lung disease that causes blockages or breathing difficulties, or if you have ever had an allergic reaction or are sensitive to phenobarbital or similar medications.

Special warnings about this medication
Phenobarbital may be habit-forming. Tolerance and physical and psychological dependence may occur with continued use. Make sure you take the medication exactly as prescribed by your doctor.

Phenobarbital should be used with extreme caution, or not at all, by people who are depressed, have suicidal tendencies, or have a history of drug abuse.

Phenobarbital may cause excitement, depression, or confusion in an elderly or weakened person, and excitement in children.

Phenobarbital should be used carefully if you have liver disease or impaired adrenal functioning.

Barbiturates, such as phenobarbital, may cause you to become tired or less alert. Be careful driving, operating machinery, or doing any activity that requires full mental alertness until you know how you react to this medication.

Possible food and drug interactions when taking this medication

Phenobarbital may increase the effects of alcohol. Do not drink alcohol while taking phenobarbital.

If phenobarbital is taken with certain other drugs, the effects of either could be increased, decreased, or altered. It is especially important to check with your doctor before combining phenobarbital with the following:

Antidepressant drugs known as MAO
  inhibitors, such as Marplan and Nardil
Antihistamines such as Benadryl
Blood-thinning medications such as Coumadin
  and Panwarfin
Corticosteroids such as Medrol and Deltasone
Doxycycline (Doryx, Vibramycin)
Griseofulvin (Fulvicin-U/F, Grifulvin V)
Other sedatives/hypnotics such as Nembutal and
  Seconal
Phenytoin (Dilantin)
Sodium valproate
Steroidal hormones such as oral contraceptives
Tranquilizers such as Xanax and Valium
Valproic acid (Depakene)

Special information
if you are pregnant or breastfeeding

Barbiturates such as phenobarbital may cause damage to the fetus during pregnancy. Withdrawal symptoms may occur in an infant whose mother took barbiturates during the last 3 months of pregnancy. If you are pregnant or plan to become pregnant, inform your doctor immediately.

Phenobarbital appears in breast milk and could affect a nursing infant. If phenobarbital is essential to your health, your doctor may advise you to stop breastfeeding until your treatment is finished.

Recommended dosage

Your doctor will individualize your dose by taking into consideration your age, weight, and condition.

ADULTS

Sedation

The usual recommended initial dose of phenobarbital is a single dose of 30 to 120 milligrams. Your doctor may repeat this dose at intervals, depending on how you respond to this medication.

The maximum phenobarbital dose should not exceed 400 milligrams during a 24-hour period.

Daytime Sedation

The usual recommended dose is 30 to 120 milligrams a day in 2 to 3 divided doses.

To Induce Sleep

The usual recommended dose is 100 to 200 milligrams.

Anticonvulsant Use

For use as an anticonvulsant, phenobarbital dosage must be individualized on the basis of specific laboratory tests. Your doctor will determine the correct doses.

The usual recommended dose is 60 to 200 milligrams daily.

Convulsions Due to Fever

Usual doses may be 60 to 200 milligrams per day.

CHILDREN

Anticonvulsant Use

For use as an anticonvulsant, the phenobarbital dosage must be individualized on the basis of specific laboratory tests. Your doctor will determine the correct doses.

The usual recommended dose is 3 to 6 milligrams per 2.2 pounds of body weight per day.

Convulsions Due to Fever
Usual doses may be 3 to 6 milligrams per 2.2 pounds per day.

ELDERLY

If you are elderly or debilitated, your dose may be lower than the regular adult dose. Patients with liver disease and impaired kidneys may require a lower dose of phenobarbital.

Overdosage
Any medication taken in excess can have serious consequences. Deaths have occurred with barbiturate overdose. If you suspect an overdose, seek medical treatment immediately.

Symptoms of phenobarbital overdose may include:
Congestive heart failure, depressed breathing, depression of central nervous system function (brain and spinal cord), extremely low body temperature, fluid in lungs, involuntary eyeball movements, irregular heartbeat, kidney failure, lack of muscle coordination, low blood pressure, poor reflexes, skin reddening or bloody blisters at pressure points.

Generic name:

PHENOBARBITAL WITH BELLADONNA ALKALOIDS

See Donnatal, page 212.

Generic name:

PHENTERMINE HYDROCHLORIDE

See Fastin, page 249.

Generic name:

PHENTERMINE RESIN

See Ionamin, page 301.

Generic name:

PHENYLBUTAZONE

See Butazolidin, page 76.

Generic name:

PHENYLPROPANOLAMINE WITH GUAIFENESIN

See Entex LA, page 237.

Generic name:

PHENYTOIN SODIUM

See Dilantin, page 195.

Brand name:

PHOSPHOLINE IODIDE

Generic name: Echothiophate iodide

Why is this drug prescribed?
Phospholine Iodide is used to treat chronic open-angle glaucoma by helping reduce fluid pressure in the eye.

In chronic open-angle glaucoma, a partial loss of vision or blindness results from a gradual increase in pressure of fluid in the eye. Because the vision loss occurs slowly, people often do not experience any symptoms and do not realize that their vision has worsened. By the time the loss is noticed, it may be irreversible.

It is also used to treat secondary glaucoma (such as glaucoma following surgery to remove cataracts), for subacute or chronic angle-closure glaucoma after iridectomy (surgical removal of a portion of the iris), when surgery is refused or contraindicated, and to treat children with accommodative esotropia ("cross-eye").

Most important fact about this drug

Before using Phospholine Iodide, you should have an eye exam that includes an examination with a gonioscope (an instrument that examines the area of the eye in front of the lens).

While using Phospholine Iodide, you should have regular eye examinations to determine whether your eye lens is clear.

How should you use this medication?

Phospholine Iodide may cause vision problems. Be careful when driving at night or performing tasks in dim or poor light.

Keep eyedrops in refrigerator for 6 months or at room temperature if used within a month.

Avoid exposure to certain pesticides or insecticides. If you work with these chemicals, wear respiratory masks and wash and change your clothing frequently.

To use Phospholine Iodide:
1. To minimize drainage of Phospholine Iodide into your nose, your doctor may instruct you to apply pressure with the middle finger to the inside corner of the eye for one to two minutes after placing drops in your eyes.
2. Wipe off any excess Phospholine Iodide around the eye with a tissue.
3. Wash off any Phospholine Iodide that may get onto your hands.

What side effects may occur?

Side effects cannot be anticipated. If any side effects develop or change in intensity, tell your doctor immediately. Only your doctor can determine whether it is safe to continue taking this medication.

■ *Side effects may include:*
Ache above the eyes, blurred vision, burning, clouded eye lens, decreased pupil size, decreased visual sharpness, excess tears, eye pain, increased eye pressure, inflamed iris, lid muscle twitching, nearsightedness, red eyes, stinging

Why should this drug not be prescribed?

You should not use Phospholine Iodide if you have inflamed eyes.

Most people with angle-closure glaucoma (a condition in which there is a sudden increase in pressure of fluid in the eye) should not use Phospholine Iodide.

If you have ever had an allergic reaction to or are sensitive to Phospholine Iodide or its preservative (chlorobutanol), you should not use this medication.

Special warnings about this medication

Drugs such as Phospholine Iodide should be used cautiously (if at all) if you have a history of:

Bronchial asthma
Detached retina
Epilepsy
Extreme low blood pressure
Parkinson's disease
Peptic ulcer
Recent heart attack
Slow heartbeat
Stomach or intestinal problems
Surgery to treat a peptic ulcer

Possible food and drug interactions when taking this medication

If Phospholine Iodide is taken with certain other drugs, the effects of either could be increased, decreased, or altered. It is especially important to check with your doctor before combining Phospholine Iodide with the following:

Succinylcholine (Anectine), a muscle-relaxing drug used during surgery

Drugs such as Enlon, Mestinon, or Tensilon, used to treat myasthenia gravis, a condition of muscle weakness that usually affects muscles in the eyes, face, limbs, and throat

Special information if you are pregnant or breastfeeding

If you are pregnant or plan to become pregnant, inform your doctor immediately. No information is available about the safety of Phospholine Iodide during pregnancy.

Phospholine Iodide should not be used by women who are breastfeeding.

Recommended dosage

ADULTS

For Chronic Simple Glaucoma, Advanced Chronic Simple Glaucoma, and Glaucoma Secondary to Cataract Surgery

A dose of 0.03 percent should be used 2 times a day, in the morning and at bedtime. Doses may be increased if necessary.

CHILDREN

For Accommodative Estropia

One drop of 0.125 percent may be placed in both eyes at bedtime for 2 or 3 weeks, to diagnose the condition.

If treatment is successful, dosages may be gradually reduced to the lowest amount that produces a favorable response.

The maximum dose usually recommended is 0.125 percent once daily.

Surgery should be considered if the eyedrops are slowly withdrawn after a year or two of treatment and the eye problem returns.

Overdosage

Any medication used in excess can have serious consequences. If you suspect an overdose, seek medical help immediately.

Brand name:

PILOCAR

Generic name: Pilocarpine hydrochloride
Other brand name: Isopto Carpine

Why is this drug prescribed?

Pilocar causes constriction of the pupils (miosis). It is used to treat open-angle glaucoma and to lower eye pressure before surgery for acute angle-closure glaucoma. It can be used alone or in combination with other medications. Glaucoma, one of the leading causes of blindness in the United States, is an eye disease that causes increased pressure in the eye, damaging the optic nerve and causing loss of vision.

Most important fact about this drug

Pilocar may make it difficult for your eyes to adjust to the dark; be careful driving at night or performing any hazardous activities in dim light.

How should you use this medication?

Pilocar should not be taken by mouth.

To avoid contaminating the dropper and solution, do not touch the eyelids or surrounding areas with the tip of the dropper.

Keep the bottle tightly closed when it is not being used.

Do not use if the solution is discolored.

What side effects may occur?

Side effects cannot be anticipated. If any develop or change in intensity, inform your doctor as soon as possible. Only your doctor can determine if it is safe for you to continue using Pilocar.

■ *More common side effects may include:*
Cloudy vision
Detached retina
Difficulty seeing at a distance
    (nearsightedness)
Eye muscle spasms (eyelids)
Headache over your eye
Tearing eyes

■ *Rare side effects may include:*
Breathing difficulty, diarrhea, excessive salivation, fluid in lungs, high blood pressure, nausea, rapid heartbeat, sweating, vomiting

Why should this drug not be prescribed?

Pilocar should not be used if you are sensitive to or have ever had an allergic reaction to any of the components of this solution.

Special warnings about this medication

Pilocar may make it difficult for you to see in the dark. Be careful driving at night, or doing any hazardous activity in dim light.

Possible food and drug interactions when using this medication

No interactions have been reported.

Special information if you are pregnant or breastfeeding

The effects of Pilocar during pregnancy have not been adequately studied. If you are pregnant or plan to become pregnant, inform your doctor immediately. Pilocar may appear in breast milk and could affect a nursing infant. If this medication is essential to your health, your doctor may advise you to stop breastfeeding until your treatment with Pilocar is finished.

Recommended dosage

ADULTS

The initial recommended dose is 1 or 2 drops, which can be repeated up to 6 times daily, depending on the severity of the glaucoma and your response. During an acute attack, put drops into the unaffected eye to prevent an attack of narrow-angle glaucoma.

Overdosage

If you suspect an overdose seek medical attention immediately.

Any medication taken in excess can have serious consequences.

Symptoms of Pilocar overdose may include:
Difficulty breathing
Excessive salivation
Flushing
Loss of bowel or bladder control
Pinpoint pupils
Slowed heart rate
Tearing

Generic name:

PILOCARPINE HYDROCHLORIDE

See Pilocar, page 483.

Generic name:

PIMOZIDE

See Orap, page 440.

Generic name:

PINDOLOL

See Visken, page 680.

Generic name:

PIROXICAM

See Feldene, page 250.

Brand name:

PLAQUENIL

Generic name: Hydroxychloroquine sulfate

Why is this drug prescribed?

Plaquenil is prescribed for the treatment and prevention of certain forms of malaria.

Also, if milder drugs (that may have less serious side effects) have not been effective, Plaquenil may be prescribed for the treatment of some forms of arthritis. These include: discoid lupus erythematosus (DLE—an immune system abnormality causing scaly red lesions on the face and occasionally other areas); systemic lupus erythematosus (SLE—an inflammatory skin disease similar to DLE but affecting the whole body, whose symptoms include arthritis, weakness, fatigue, and skin lesions); and severe or long-lasting rheumatoid arthritis (inflammation and destruction of joints).

Most important fact about this drug

Children are especially sensitive to Plaquenil. Relatively small doses of this medication have caused fatalities. Keep this drug in a child-proof container and out of the reach of children.

How should you take this medication?

Dose and duration of therapy depends on the patient's age and the condition being treated. Take Plaquenil specifically as prescribed for the full course of therapy.

If your doctor prescribes Plaquenil for rheumatoid arthritis, it will take several weeks for beneficial effects to appear.

Consult your doctor if you experience any change in vision, or ringing in the ears, or hearing problems.

If your doctor has prescribed this medication for rheumatoid arthritis, each dose should be taken with a meal or a glass of milk.

What side effects may occur?

Side effects cannot be anticipated. If any develop or change in intensity, inform your doctor as soon as possible. Only your doctor can determine if it is safe for you to continue taking Plaquenil.

■ *Side effects of treatment for an acute malarial attack may include:*
Abdominal cramps
Diarrhea
Dizziness
Lack or loss of appetite
Mild headache
Nausea
Vomiting

■ *Side effects of treatment for lupus erythematosus and rheumatoid arthritis may include:*
Abdominal cramps, abnormal eye pigmentation, anemia, bleaching of hair, blood disorders, blurred vision, convulsions, decreased vision, diarrhea, difficulty focusing (eye), emotional changes, excessive coloring of the skin, eye muscle paralysis, eye swelling due to fluid retention, "foggy vision," halos around lights, headache, hearing loss, hives, involuntary eyeball movement, irritability, itching, lack of muscle coordination, light flashes and streaks, light intolerance, loss of hair, loss or lack of appetite, muscle weakness, nausea, nervousness, nightmares, psoriasis (dry, scaly, red skin patches), reading difficulties, ringing in the ears, skin eruptions, skin peeling, skin rash, vertigo, vomiting, weariness, weight loss

Why should this drug not be prescribed?

If you are sensitive to or have ever had an allergic reaction to Plaquenil or drugs of this type (e.g. Aralen, Chloroquin), you should not take this medication. Make sure that your doctor is aware of any drug reactions that you have experienced.

Plaquenil should not be prescribed if you have had retinal or visual field changes (small areas of partial or complete loss of vision) while taking this medication or drugs of this type. Notify your doctor of any past or present visual changes that you have experienced.

This drug should not be prescribed for long-term therapy in children.

Special warnings about this medication

Unless you are directed to do so by your doctor, do not take this medication if you have psoriasis (a recurrent skin disorder characterized by patches of red, dry, scaly skin) or porphyria (an inherited metabolic disorder affecting the liver or bone marrow). The use of Plaquenil may cause a severe attack of psoriasis and may increase the severity of porphyria.

Disorders of the retina causing impairment or loss of vision may be related to the length of time and the dose of Plaquenil given for lupus and rheumatoid arthritis. Problems have occurred within several months to several years of daily therapy. Specified symptoms of retinal change may or may not occur. When prolonged therapy is prescribed, eye examinations should be performed by your doctor at the beginning of treatment and every 3 months after that. Retinal changes and visual disturbances may progress, even after treatment with this drug has been discontinued.

All patients on long-term therapy with this drug should have a physical examination periodically, including testing of knee and ankle reflexes, to detect any evidence of muscular weakness.

If you are being treated for rheumatoid arthritis and have shown no improvement (such as reduced joint swelling or increased mobility) within 6 months, your doctor may decide to discontinue this drug.

This drug has not been proved safe for treatment of juvenile arthritis.

Plaquenil should be used with caution in alcoholics and patients with liver disease.

Your doctor should conduct periodic blood cell counts if you are on prolonged therapy with this medication. If any severe blood disorder appears that is not attributed to the disease you are being treated for, your doctor may discontinue use of this drug.

Consult with your doctor if you are taking a drug that has a tendency to produce dermatitis (inflammation of the skin), because you may have some skin reactions while taking Plaquenil.

Possible food and drug interactions when taking this medication

If Plaquenil is taken with certain other drugs, the effects of either could be increased, decreased, or altered. It is especially important to check with your doctor before combining Plaquenil with the following:

Any medication that may cause liver damage
Aurothioglucose (Solganal)
Cimetidine (Tagamet)
Digoxin (Lanoxin)

Special information if you are pregnant or breastfeeding

Use of this drug during pregnancy should be avoided except in the suppression or treatment of malaria when, in the judgment of your doctor, the benefit outweighs the possible hazard. This drug may appear in breast milk and could affect a nursing infant. If this medication is essential to your health, your doctor may advise you to discontinue breastfeeding until your treatment is finished.

Recommended dosage

ADULTS

Restraint or Prevention of Malaria
The recommended dose is 400 milligrams taken on exactly the same day of each week. If circumstances permit, preventive therapy should begin 2 weeks prior to exposure. If this is not possible, a starting dose of 800 milligrams may be divided into 2 doses, taken 6 hours apart. Suppressive therapy should be continued for 8 weeks after leaving the area where malaria occurs.

Acute Attack of Malaria
The recommended starting dose is 800 milligrams, to be followed by 400 milligrams in 6 to 8 hours and 400 milligrams on each of 2 consecutive days.

Alternatively, your doctor may prescribe a single dose of 800 milligrams.

Lupus Erythematosus
The recommended initial dose for adults is 400 milligrams once or twice daily. This dose will be continued for several weeks or months depending on your response. For longer-term maintenance therapy, the dose may be reduced to a total of 200 to 400 milligrams per day.

Rheumatoid Arthritis
The recommended initial dose for adults is 400 to 600 milligrams per day taken with a meal or a glass of milk. If a good response is obtained, usually within 4 to 12 weeks, the dose will be reduced to a maintenance level of 200 to 400 milligrams daily.

CHILDREN

For treatment of malaria, dosage is calculated on the basis of weight.

Overdosage

Any medication taken in excess can have serious consequences. If you suspect an overdose, seek emergency medical treatment immediately.

Symptoms of an overdose of Plaquenil may occur within 30 minutes. They include:
Convulsions
Drowsiness
Headache
Heart and blood vessel failure
Inability to breathe
Visual disturbances

Brand name:

PLENDIL

Generic name: Felodipine

Why is this drug proscribed?

Plendil, a type of medication called a calcium channel blocker, is prescribed for the treatment of high blood pressure. It is effective alone or in combination with other high blood pressure medications. Calcium channel blockers ease the workload of the heart by slowing down the muscle contractions of the heart and the passage of nerve impulses through the heart. This improves blood flow through the heart and throughout the body, reduces blood pressure, and helps prevent angina pain (chest pain, often accompanied by a feeling of choking, usually caused by lack of oxygen in the heart due to clogged arteries).

Most important fact about this drug

You must take Plendil regularly for it to be effective. Even if you are feeling well, you must continue to take it. If you stop taking the drug, your high blood pressure will return.

How should you take this medication?

Plendil can be taken with or without food.

Tablets should be swallowed whole, not crushed or chewed.

Plendil should be taken exactly as prescribed by your doctor, even if your symptoms have disappeared.

Try not to miss any doses. If Plendil is not taken regularly, your blood pressure may increase.

What side effects may occur?
Side effects cannot be anticipated. If any develop or change in intensity, inform your doctor as soon as possible. Only your doctor can determine if it is safe for you to continue taking Plendil.

■ *More common side effects may include:*
Abdominal pain, back pain, chest pain, constipation, cough, diarrhea, dizziness, flushing, headache, indigestion, muscle cramps, nausea, pounding heartbeat, rash, runny nose, sore throat, swelling of the legs and feet, tingling sensation, upper respiratory infection, weakness

■ *Less common or rare side effects may include:*
Anemia, angina pectoris (chest pain), ankle pain, anxiety disorders, arm pain, arthritis, blurred vision, bronchitis, bruising, decreased sex drive, depression, difficulty sleeping, dry mouth, excessive nighttime urination, excessive perspiration, facial swelling, fainting, fatigue, flu, foot pain, frequent urination, gas, generalized muscle pain, heart attack, hip pain, hives, impotence, inflammation of the gums, inflammation of the nose, irregular heartbeat, irritability, itching, joint pain, knee pain, leg pain, low blood pressure, neck pain, nervousness, nosebleeds, painful or difficult urination, rapid heartbeat, respiratory infections, ringing in the ears, shortness of breath, shoulder pain, sinus inflammation, sleepiness,

sneezing, stomach and intestinal pain, tremor, unusual redness of the skin, urgent urination, vomiting, warm sensation

Why should this drug not be prescribed?
If you are sensitive to or have ever had an allergic reaction to Plendil or other calcium channel blockers, you should not take this medication. Make sure your doctor is aware of any drug reactions you have experienced.

Special warnings about this medication
Plendil can cause your blood pressure to become too low. If you feel light-headed or faint, or if you feel your heart racing or you experience chest pain, contact your doctor immediately.

If you have congestive heart failure, Plendil should be used with caution, especially if you are also taking a drug in the "beta-blocker" family, such as Inderal or Tenormin.

Your legs and feet may swell when you start taking Plendil, usually within the first 2 to 3 weeks of treatment.

If you have liver disease or are over age 65, your doctor should monitor your blood pressure carefully while adjusting your dosage of Plendil.

Your gums may become swollen and sore while you are taking Plendil. Good dental hygiene will help control this problem.

Possible food and drug interactions when taking this medication
If Plendil is taken with certain other drugs, the effects of either could be increased, decreased, or altered. It is especially important to check with your doctor before combining Plendil with the following:

Beta blockers such as Lopressor, Inderal, and Tenormin
Cimetidine (Tagamet)
Digoxin (Lanoxin)

Special information
if you are pregnant or breastfeeding

Although the effects of Plendil during pregnancy have not been adequately studied in humans, birth defects have occurred in animal studies. If you are pregnant or plan to become pregnant, inform your doctor immediately. Plendil may appear in breast milk and can affect a nursing infant. If this medication is essential to your health, your doctor may advise you to discontinue breastfeeding until your treatment is finished.

Recommended dosage

ADULTS

Dosages should be adjusted to each individual patient's response to the drug.

The usual starting dose is 5 milligrams once a day; the dose should be adjusted at intervals of not less than 2 weeks.

The usual dosage range is 5 to 10 milligrams once daily.

The maximum recommended daily dose is 20 milligrams once a day.

Patients with reduced liver function should be monitored closely, and doses over 10 milligrams per day are not recommended.

CHILDREN

The safety and effectiveness of Plendil in children have not been established.

ELDERLY

Patients over 65 years of age should have their blood pressure monitored closely during dosage adjustment. In general, doses above 10 milligrams should not be considered in the elderly.

Overdosage

Any medication taken in excess can have serious consequences. If you suspect an overdose, seek medical treatment immediately.

Symptoms of Plendil overdose may include:
Severely low blood pressure
Slow heartbeat

Brand name:

POLARAMINE

Generic name: Dexchlorpheniramine maleate

Why is this drug prescribed?

Polaramine is an antihistamine that relieves allergy symptoms, including: nasal stuffiness and inflammation and red, inflamed eyes caused by hay fever and other allergies; itching, swelling, and redness from hives and other rashes; allergic reactions to blood transfusions; and, with other medications, anaphylactic shock (severe allergic reaction). Antihistamines work by decreasing the effects of histamine, a chemical the body releases in response to certain irritants. Histamine narrows air passages in the lungs and contributes to inflammation. Antihistamines reduce itching and swelling and dry up secretions from the nose, eyes, and throat.

Most important fact about this drug

Polaramine may cause mild to moderate drowsiness. Driving or operating dangerous machinery or participating in any hazardous activity that requires full mental alertness is not recommended until you know how you react to this medication.

How should you take this medication?

Polaramine should be taken exactly as prescribed by your doctor. Never take two doses at the same time.

What side effects may occur?

Side effects cannot be anticipated. If any develop or change in intensity, inform your doctor as soon as possible. Only your doctor can determine if it is safe for you to continue taking Polaramine.

■ *The most common side effect is:*
Mild to moderate drowsiness

■ *Less common or rare side effects may include:*
Acute inflammation of the inner ear, anaphylactic shock (severe allergic reaction), anemia, blood disorders, blurred vision, chest congestion, chills, confusion, constipation, convulsions, diarrhea, difficulty sleeping, difficulty urinating, disturbed coordination, dizziness, dry mouth, nose, and throat, early menustration, excessive perspiration, excitement (especially in children), extreme fatigue, exaggerated sense of well-being, frequent urination, headache, hives, hysteria, irritability, loss of appetite, low blood pressure, nausea, nervousness, pounding heartbeat, premature heart contractions, rapid heartbeat, restlessness, ringing in ears, sedation (extreme calm), sensitivity to light, stomach upset, stuffy nose, tightness in chest, tingling or pins and needles, tremor, urinary retention, vertigo, vomiting, wheezing

Why should this drug not be prescribed?
Polaramine should not be used in newborn or premature infants.

Do not take this medication if you are taking antidepressant drugs known as MAO inhibitors (Parnate, Nardil), if you have asthma or other breathing difficulties, or if you are sensitive to or have ever had an allergic reaction to dexchlorpheniramine or other medications with a similar chemical composition.

Special warnings about this medication
Polaramine should be used with care if you have narrow-angle glaucoma, narrowing peptic ulcer or other stomach problems, symptoms of an enlarged prostate, difficulty urinating, a history of bronchial asthma, increased eye pressure, an overactive thyroid, cardiovascular disease, or high blood pressure.

Antihistamines may cause dizziness, sedation (extreme calm), and low blood pressure in the elderly (age 60 and over).

Remember that Polaramine may make you feel drowsy.

Possible food and drug interactions when taking this medication
Polaramine can cause extremely low blood pressure when taken with MAO inhibitor drugs such as the antidepressants Nardil and Parnate, and should never be taken with them.

Alcohol may increase the effects of Polaramine. Avoid alcohol while taking this medication.

If Polaramine is taken with certain other drugs, the effects of either could be increased, decreased, or altered. It is especially important to check with your doctor before combining Polaramine with the following:

Antidepressants
Blood-thinning medications (Coumadin)
Sedatives/hypnotics (Nembutal, Seconal, Halcion)
Tranquilizers (Xanax, Valium)

Special information if you are pregnant or breastfeeding
The effects of Polaramine during pregnancy have not been adequately studied. The drug definitely should not be used in third trimester. If you are pregnant or plan to become pregnant, inform your doctor immediately. Polaramine may appear in breast milk and could affect a nursing infant. If this medication is essential to your health, your doctor may advise you to discontinue breastfeeding until your treatment is finished.

Recommended dosage
All dosages should be individualized according to the needs and response of the patient.

POLARAMINE REPETABS TABLETS

Adults and Children 12 Years or Older
The usual dose is one 4- or 6-milligram POLARAMINE REPETABS tablet at bedtime or every 8 to 10 hours during the day.

Children 6 to 12 Years
The usual dose is one 14-milligram REPETABS tablet daily, usually at bedtime.

POLARAMINE TABLETS

Adults and Children 12 Years of Age and Over
The usual dose is 1 tablet every 4 to 6 hours.

Childern 6 Through 11 Years
The usual dose is one-half tablet every 4 to 6 hours.

Children 2 Through 5 Years
The usual dose is one-quarter tablet every 4 to 6 hours.

POLARAMINE SYRUP

Adults and Children 12 Years of Age and Over
The usual dose is 1 teaspoonful (2 milligrams) every 4 to 6 hours.

Children 6 Through 11 Years
The usual dose is one-half teaspoonful (1 milligram) every 4 to 6 hours.

Children 2 Through 5 Years
The usual dose is one-quarter teaspoonful (one-half milligram) every 4 to 6 hours.

Overdosage

Any medication taken in excess can have serious consequences. Antihistamine overdose may cause hallucinations, convulsions, and death, especially in infants and children. If you suspect an overdose, seek medical treatment immediately.

Symptoms of Polaramine overdose may include:
Blurred vision, cardiovascular collapse, convulsions, death, decreased alertness, difficulty sleeping, dizziness, hallucinations, lack of muscle coordination, low blood pressure, ringing in ears, sedation (extreme calm), temporary failure to breathe, tremors

Overdose symptoms more common in children include:
Dry mouth
Extremely high body temperature
Fixed, dilated pupils
Flushing
Stimulation
Stomach and intestinal problems

Brand name:

POLY-VI-FLOR

Generic ingredients: Vitamins A, B_6, B_{12}, C, D, E, Folic acid, Thiamine, Riboflavin, Niacin, Fluoride

Why is this drug prescribed?

Poly-Vi-Flor is a multivitamin and fluoride supplement with 10 essential vitamins plus the mineral fluoride. It is prescribed for children aged 2 and older to provide fluoride where the drinking water contains less than the amount recommended by the American Dental Association to build strong teeth and prevent cavities. Poly-Vi-Flor supplies significant amounts of other vitamins to avoid deficiencies. The American Academy of Pediatrics recommends that children up to age 16 take a fluoride supplement if they live in areas where the drinking water contains less than the recommended amount of fluoride.

Most important fact about this drug

Do not give your child more than the recommended dose. Too much fluoride can cause discoloration and pitting of teeth.

How should you take this medication?

Do not give your child more than your doctor prescribes.

Poly-Vi-Flor should be chewed or crushed before swallowing.

What side effects may occur?

An allergic rash has occurred rarely.

Why should this drug not be prescribed?

Children should not take Poly-Vi-Flor if they are getting significant amounts of fluoride from other medications or sources.

Special warnings about this medication

Do not give your child more than the recommended dosage. Your child's teeth should be checked periodically for discoloration or pitting. Notify your doctor if white, brown, or black spots appear on your child's teeth.

The fluoride level of your drinking water should be determined before Poly-Vi-Flor is prescribed.

Let your doctor know if you change drinking water or filtering systems.

Fluoride does not replace proper dental habits, such as brushing, flossing, and having dental checkups.

Recommended dosage

The usual dose is 1 tablet every day as prescribed by the doctor.

Overdosage

Although overdose is unlikely, any medication taken in excess can have serious consequences. If you suspect an overdose, seek medical treatment immediately.

Generic name:

POLYETHYLENE GLYCOL WITH ELECTROLYTES

See Colyte, page 130.

Brand name:

POLYMOX

See Amoxil, page 23.

Brand name:

PONSTEL

Generic name: Mefenamic acid

Why is this drug prescribed?

Ponstel, a nonsteroidal anti-inflammatory drug, is used for the relief of moderate pain (when treatment will not last for more than 7 days) and for the treatment of menstrual pain.

Most important fact about this drug

You should have frequent check-ups with your doctor if you take Ponstel regularly. Ulcers or internal bleeding can occur without warning.

How should you take this medication?

Take with food if possible. If stomach upset occurs, be sure to take with food or an antacid or with a full glass of milk.

Take Ponstel exactly as prescribed by your doctor.

What side effects may occur?

Side effects cannot be anticipated. If any develop or change in intensity, inform your doctor as soon as possible. Only your doctor can determine if it is safe for you to continue taking Ponstel.

■ *More common side effects may include:*
Abdominal pain
Diarrhea
Nausea
Upset stomach
Vomiting

■ *Less common or rare side effects may include:*
Anemia, blurred vision, changes in liver function, constipation, decrease in white blood cells, dizziness, drowsiness, ear pain, eye irritation, facial swelling due to fluid retention, gas, headache, heartburn, hives, inability to sleep, increased need for insulin in a diabetic, kidney failure, labored breathing, loss of appetite, nervousness, rapid heartbeat, rash, red or purple spots on the skin, sweating, ulcers and internal bleeding

Why should this drug not be prescribed?
If you are sensitive to or have ever had an allergic reaction to Ponstel, aspirin, or similar drugs; or if you have had asthma attacks caused by aspirin or other drugs of this type, you should not take this medication. Make sure that your doctor is aware of any drug reactions that you have experienced.

Do not take Ponstel if you have ulcerations (sores) or frequently recurring inflammation of your stomach and intestines.

Avoid this drug if you have serious kidney disease.

Special warnings about this medication
If you develop rash, diarrhea or other stomach problems, you should stop taking this medication and contact your doctor.

Stomach ulcers and bleeding can occur without warning.

Ponstel should be used with caution if you have kidney disease or liver disease; it can cause liver inflammation in some people.

Ponstel may cause visual disturbances. If you experience any changes in your vision, inform your doctor.

This drug may prolong bleeding time. If you are taking blood-thinning medication, this drug should be taken with caution.

Ponstel may cause you to become drowsy or less alert; therefore, driving or operating dangerous machinery or participating in any hazardous activity that requires full mental alertness is not recommended.

Possible food and drug interactions when taking this medication
If Ponstel is taken with certain other drugs, the effects of either could be increased, decreased, or altered. It is especially important to check with your doctor before combining Ponstel with the following:

Anticoagulants (blood thinners)
Aspirin
Methotrexate

Special information if you are pregnant or breastfeeding
The effects of Ponstel during pregnancy have not been adequately studied. If you are pregnant or plan to become pregnant, inform your doctor immediately. Ponstel may appear in breast milk and could affect a nursing infant. If this medication is essential to your health, your doctor may advise you to discontinue breastfeeding until your treatment with this medication is finished.

Recommended dosage
Take Ponstel with food, if possible.

ADULTS AND CHILDREN OVER 14

Acute Pain
The usual starting dose is 500 milligrams, followed by a regular dose of 250 milligrams every 6 hours for one week.

Menstrual Pain
The usual starting dose, once symptoms appear, is 500 milligrams, followed by 250 milligrams every 6 hours for 2 to 3 days.

CHILDREN

The safety and effectiveness of Ponstel have not been established in children under 14.

ELDERLY

Dosage should be determined by the particular needs of the elderly patient.

Overdosage

Any medication taken in excess can cause symptoms of overdose. If you suspect an overdose, seek medical attention immediately.

There is no specific overdose information available for this medication.

Generic name:

POTASSIUM CHLORIDE

See Micro-K, page 376.

Brand name:

PRAVACHOL

Generic name: Pravastatin sodium

Why is this drug prescribed?

Pravachol is a cholesterol-lowering drug. Your doctor may prescribe it along with a cholesterol-lowering diet if your blood cholesterol level is dangerously high, and if you have not been able to lower it by diet alone.

The drug works by helping to clear harmful low-density lipoprotein (LDL) cholesterol out of the blood and by limiting the body's ability to form new LDL cholesterol.

Most important fact about this drug

Pravachol should be an addition to, not a substitute for, a cholesterol-lowering diet. Like most other medications, Pravachol may produce side effects. The diet, on the other hand, will produce no side effects; in addition, it may help improve your overall health.

How should you take this medication?

Before starting Pravachol, you should try to lower your cholesterol by diet alone. Ask your doctor for an official cholesterol-lowering diet, then follow the diet faithfully for 3 to 6 months.

After this time, if your cholesterol level is still too high despite your best efforts at diet, your doctor may prescribe Pravachol. Take the drug exactly as prescribed.

Continue your cholesterol-lowering diet, and consider Pravachol merely an addition to the diet. Do not think of Pravachol as a substitute for a cholesterol-lowering diet.

You will get an even greater cholesterol-lowering effect if you take Pravachol in tandem with a different kind of lipid-lowering drug such as Questran or Colestid. However, you must not take Pravachol at the same time of day as the other cholesterol-lowering drug. Take Pravachol at least 1 hour before or 4 hours after taking the other drug.

Studies have shown that Pravachol works best when it is taken in the evening. You may take Pravachol with or without food.

What side effects may occur?

Side effects from Pravachol cannot be anticipated. If any develop or change in intensity, inform your doctor as soon as possible. Only your doctor can determine if it is safe for you to continue taking Pravachol.

■ *Side effects may include:*
Abdominal pain, allergic reaction, altered sense of taste, appetite loss, breast swelling (in men), chest pain, cold, constipation, cough, diarrhea, dizziness, eye movement difficulties, fatigue, flu, gas, headache, heartburn, inflammation of nasal passages, jaundice (yellowing of skin and whites of eyes), lowered sex drive, memory loss, mild stomach or bowel discomfort, muscle aches or pain, nausea, nerve pain or twitching, numbness or tingling, penile erection problems, rash, sluggish facial muscles, tremor, urinary difficulties, vomiting

Why should this drug not be prescribed?
Do not take Pravachol if you are sensitive or have ever had an allergic reaction to it.

Do not take Pravachol if you have a disease of the liver.

Special warnings about this medication
Pravachol should **not** be used to try to lower high cholesterol that stems from a medical condition such as alcoholism, poorly controlled diabetes, an underactive thyroid gland, or a kidney or liver problem.

Because Pravachol may cause damage to the liver, your doctor will test your blood regularly. Your doctor should monitor you especially closely if you have ever had liver disease or if you are or have ever been a heavy drinker.

Since Pravachol may cause damage to muscle tissue, promptly report to your doctor any unexplained muscle pain, tenderness, or weakness, especially if you also have a fever or you just generally do not feel well.

The doctor may want to do a blood test to check for signs of muscle damage.

Possible food and drug interactions when taking this medication
If Pravachol is taken with certain other drugs, the effects of either could be increased, decreased, or altered. It is especially important to check with your doctor before combining Pravachol with the following:

Cholestyramine (Questran)
Cimetidine (Tagamet)
Colestipol (Colestid)
Erythromycin drugs such as E.E.S., Erythrocin, and others
Gemfibrozil (Lopid)
Immunosuppressive drugs such as Sandimmune
Ketoconazole (Nizoral)
Niacin
Warfarin (Coumadin, Panwarfin)

Special information if you are pregnant or breastfeeding
You must not become pregnant while taking Pravachol. Because this drug lowers cholesterol, and because cholesterol is necessary for the proper development of an unborn baby, there is some suspicion that Pravachol might cause birth defects. Your doctor will prescribe Pravachol only if you understand this risk, and only if you are highly unlikely to become pregnant while taking the drug. If you do become pregnant while taking Pravachol, inform your doctor immediately.

Because Pravachol does find its way into breast milk, and because its cholesterol-lowering effects might prove harmful to a nursing baby, you should not take Pravachol while you are breastfeeding.

Recommended dosage
Patients taking this medication should be on a standard cholesterol-lowering diet for

at least 3 to 6 months before therapy begins. This diet should continue as the drug is taken. Pravachol can be taken with or without meals.

Blood tests for cholesterol levels should be done every 4 weeks to determine the effectiveness of the dose.

ADULTS

The usual starting dose is 10 to 20 milligrams once a day at bedtime.

The recommended maintenance dose is 10 to 40 milligrams, 1 time a day at bedtime.

ELDERLY

The usual starting dose is 10 milligrams a day at bedtime; the maintenance dose is 20 milligrams per day or less.

Overdosage
Although no specific information is available, any medication taken in excess can have serious consequences. If you suspect symptoms of an overdose of Pravachol, seek medical attention immediately.

Generic name:

PRAVASTATIN SODIUM

See Pravachol, page 494.

Generic name:

PRAZEPAM

See Centrax, page 105.

Generic name:

PRAZOSIN HYDROCHLORIDE

See Minipress, page 383.

Brand name:

PRED FORTE

Generic name: Prednisolone acetate

Why is this drug prescribed?
Pred Forte contains an anti-inflammatory steroid that is 3 to 5 times as potent as hydrocortisone. The drops may be applied to ease certain inflammations of the eye, the conjunctiva (the mucous membrane that lines the inner eyelid and eyeball), or the front portion of the eyeball.

Most important fact about this drug
Pred Forte works to reduce inflammation, but has no power to kill microbes. In fact, the drops could conceivably conceal or aggravate a pus-forming infection—which is why you should use this medication only if a doctor has prescribed it for your particular condition. If your eye inflammation is caused by an infection, you will need other medication to kill the infectious microorganisms.

How should you use this medication?
Use Pred Forte exactly as prescribed by your doctor.

Vigorously shake the plastic dropper bottle before each use. To avoid contaminating the whole bottle with your germs, do not let the tip of the dropper actually touch your eye; always keep it poised slightly above the place where you want the drops to fall.

What side effects may occur?
Side effects cannot be anticipated. If any develop or change in intensity, inform your doctor as soon as possible. Only your doctor can determine if it is safe for you to continue taking Pred Forte.

■ *Side effects may include:*
Cataract formation
Increased pressure inside the eyeball
Perforation of the eyeball
Secondary infection with fungi or viruses

Since any one of these developments could affect your vision temporarily or permanently, it is important to keep in close contact with your doctor while using Pred Forte eyedrops, and to use the drops only as directed.

Occasionally, long-term use of Pred Forte eyedrops may cause whole-body side effects due to an overload of cortisone-like hormone. Such side effects may include a "moonfaced" appearance, obese trunk, humped upper back, wasted limbs, and purple stretch marks on the skin. These effects are likely to disappear once the medication is withdrawn. If systemic side effects have occurred, you will need to stop using the eyedrops gradually rather than all at once.

Why should this drug not be prescribed?
Do not use Pred Forte if you have an undiagnosed, pus-forming eye infection.

Pred Forte is probably inappropriate for you if your eye condition is caused solely by a virus, a fungus, or the tuberculosis microbe.

Do not use if you are allergic to prednisolone.

Special warnings about this medication
You must stay in close touch with your doctor while using this medication, for the following reasons:

If you use Pred Forte eyedrops extensively and/or for an extended period of time, you may be at increased risk for cataracts.

If you use Pred Forte eyedrops for a condition that causes thinning of the cornea, you are at increased risk for perforation of the eyeball.

If you have a persistent ulceration of the cornea of your eye while using Pred Forte eyedrops, the problem may be a secondary fungus infection which Pred Forte cannot cure. An eye doctor should evaluate this possibility.

While you are using Pred Forte eyedrops, an eye doctor should check your intraocular pressure (pressure inside the eyeball) frequently. If increased pressure is allowed to continue, it may cause loss of vision.

Pred Forte contains sodium bisulfite, a sulfite that may cause allergic-type reactions, including life-threatening or less severe asthmatic episodes. Sulfite sensitivity is seen more frequently in asthmatic than non-asthmatic people.

Possible food and drug interactions when using this medication
Prednisolone acetate, the active ingredient in Pred Forte eyedrops, is also available in tablet and injectable forms for the treatment of other disorders. According to reports in the medical literature, if these other forms of prednisolone acetate are taken with certain other drugs, the effects of either could be increased, decreased, or altered. Therefore, check with your doctor before combining Pred Forte with other medications.

Special information if you are pregnant or breastfeeding
If you are pregnant or plan to become pregnant, inform your doctor immediately. Pred Forte eyedrops should be used during pregnancy only if the benefit outweighs the potential risk to the unborn baby.

It is not known whether the cortisone-like hormone from Pred Forte eyedrops can make its way into breast milk. If it can, the small quantity involved would be unlikely to harm a breastfeeding baby. Nevertheless, caution is advised in using Pred Forte eyedrops while breastfeeding.

Recommended dosage

ADULTS

Shake well before using. Instill 1 to 2 drops into the eyelid 2 to 4 times daily. During the first 24 to 48 hours, your doctor may want you to use more frequent doses. Give the drug time to work properly.

Overdosage

A one-time accidental overdose of Pred Forte eyedrops ordinarily will not cause acute problems. Over time, however, overdosage may have serious consequences. If you suspect symptoms of a chronic overdose with Pred Forte eyedrops, seek medical attention immediately.

If you accidentally swallow Pred Forte eyedrops, drink fluids to dilute the medication. Call your local poison center or your doctor for assistance.

Generic name:

PREDNISOLONE ACETATE

See Pred Forte, page 496.

Generic name:

PREDNISOLONE SODIUM PHOSPHATE

See Pediapred, page 457.

Generic name:

PREDNISONE

See Deltasone, page 172.

Brand name:

PREMARIN

Generic name: Conjugated estrogens

Why is this drug prescribed?

Premarin, a mixture of estrogens (female hormones) from natural sources, comes in tablets of five different strengths. It is given to reduce menopausal symptoms, such as feelings of warmth in the face, neck, and chest or sudden intense episodes of heat and sweating ("hot flashes"). It is also prescribed to prevent brittle bones, treat certain types of abnormal uterine bleeding due to hormonal imbalance, treat atrophic vaginitis (itching, burning, or dryness in or around the vagina), treat atrophic urethritis (which may cause difficulty or burning on urination), and treat certain cancers.

Most important fact about this drug

Although menopause, the female "change of life," may produce physical discomforts and emotional upsets, Premarin cannot relieve nervousness or depression associated with menopause and should not be prescribed for that purpose.

How should you take this medication?

Take Premarin exactly as prescribed by your doctor.

Your doctor has prescribed this drug for you and you alone. Do not share your Premarin with anyone else.

If you are taking calcium supplements as a part of the treatment to help prevent brittle bones, check with your doctor about how much to take.

You should see your doctor regularly to reduce the risk of estrogen use. If you have a family history of breast cancer or have ever had an abnormal mammogram, you need to have more frequent breast examinations.

You should read the patient package insert provided with the prescription of Premarin.

What side effects may occur?
Side effects cannot be anticipated. If any develop or change in intensity, inform your doctor immediately. Only your doctor can determine whether it is safe to continue taking Premarin.

■ *Side effects may include:*
Abdominal cramps, abnormal vaginal bleeding, bloating, breast swelling and tenderness, depression, dizziness, enlargement of benign tumors in the uterus, fluid retention, gallbladder disease, hair loss from the scalp, increased body hair, intolerance to contact lenses, migraine headache, nausea, vomiting, sex-drive changes, skin darkening, especially on the face, skin rash or redness, swelling of wrists and ankles, vaginal yeast infection, weight gain or loss, yellow eyes and skin

Why should this drug not be prescribed?
Do not take Premarin if you have ever had a bad reaction to it.

Do not take Premarin if you have undiagnosed abnormal vaginal bleeding.

Except in certain special circumstances, you should not be given Premarin if you have breast cancer or any other "estrogen-dependent" cancer.

Do not take Premarin if you have had any heart or circulation problem including a tendency for abnormal blood clotting.

Special warnings about this medication
The risk of cancer of the uterus increases when estrogen is used for a long time or taken in large doses.

There may be an increased risk of breast cancer in women who take estrogen for a long time.

Women who take Premarin after menopause are more likely to develop gallbladder disease.

Premarin also increases the risk of blood clots. These blood clots can cause stroke, heart attack, or other serious disorders.

While taking Premarin, get in touch with your doctor right away if you notice any of the following:

Abdominal pain, tenderness, or swelling
Abnormal bleeding from the vagina
Breast lumps
Coughing up blood
Pain in your chest or calves
Severe headache, dizziness, or faintness
Sudden shortness of breath
Vision changes
Yellowing of the skin

Possible food and drug interactions when taking this medication
If Premarin is taken with certain other drugs, the effects of either could be increased, decreased, or altered. It is especially important to check with your doctor before combining Premarin with the following:

Barbiturates such as phenobarbital
Blood thinners such as Coumadin
Drugs used for epilepsy, such as Dilantin
Rifampin (Rifadin)

Tricyclic antidepressants such as Elavil and
 Tofranil

Special information
if you are pregnant or breastfeeding

If you are pregnant or plan to become
pregnant, notify your doctor immediately.
Premarin should not be taken during
pregnancy because of the possibility of
harm to the unborn child. Premarin can not
prevent a miscarriage.

Recommended dosage

Your doctor will start therapy with Premarin
at a low dose. He or she will want to
check you periodically at 3- to 6-month
intervals to determine the need for
continued therapy.

PREMARIN TABLETS

*Vasomotor Symptoms (Hot Flashes
Associated with Menopause)*
The usual recommended dosage is 0.3 to 1.25
milligrams daily. If the patient has not
menstruated within the last two months or
more, therapy is started arbitrarily. If the
patient is menstruating, cyclic (3 weeks on
and 1 week off) therapy is started on day
5 of bleeding.

*Atrophic Vaginitis and Atrophic Urethritis
(Tissue Degeneration in the Vagina or
Urethra)*
The usual recommended dosage is 0.3
to 1.25 milligrams or more daily, depending
upon the response of the individual patient.
The drug is taken cyclically (3 weeks on
and 1 week off).

*Hypoestrogenism (Low Estrogen Levels) Due
to Reduced Ovary Function*
The usual dosage is 2.5 to 7.5 milligrams
daily, in divided doses for 20 days, followed
by a 10-day rest period. If bleeding does not
occur by the end of this period, the same
dosage schedule is repeated. The number of

courses of estrogen therapy necessary to
produce bleeding may vary depending on the
responsiveness of the endometrium (lining
of the uterus).

If bleeding occurs before the end of the
10-day period, a 20-day estrogen-progestin
cyclic regimen should be begun with Premarin:
2.5 to 7.5 milligrams daily in divided
doses for 20 days. During the last 5 days of
estrogen therapy, an oral progestin should
be given.

If bleeding occurs before this course is
concluded, therapy is discontinued and
may be resumed on the 5th day of bleeding.

Ovary Removal or Ovarian Failure
The usual dosage is 1.25 milligrams daily,
cyclically (3 weeks on and 1 week off).
Dosage is adjusted upward or downward,
according to severity of symptoms and
your response to treatment. For maintenance,
the dosage should be adjusted to the
lowest level that will provide effective control.

Osteoporosis (Loss of Bone Mass)
The usual dosage is 0.625 milligram daily.
Administration should be cyclic (3 weeks
on and 1 week off).

*Advanced Androgen-Dependent Cancer of the
Prostate, for Relief of Symptoms Only*
The usual dosage is 1.25 to 2.5 milligrams
3 times daily. The effectiveness of therapy
can be judged by laboratory tests as well as
by improvement of symptoms.

*Breast Cancer (for Relief of Symptoms Only)
in Appropriately Selected Women and Men
with Metastatic Disease*
The suggested dosage is 10 milligrams 3 times
daily for a period of at least 3 months.
Patients with an intact uterus are monitored
closely for signs of endometrial cancer,
and appropriate diagnostic tests are run
to rule out malignancy in the event of

persistent or recurring abnormal vaginal bleeding.

PREMARIN VAGINAL CREAM

Given cyclically for short-term use only.

Atrophic Vaginitis or Kraurosis Vulva (Degeneration of Genital Tissue or Severe Itching)

The lowest dose that will control symptoms should be used, with treatment discontinued as soon as possible. Administration should be cyclic (3 weeks on and 1 week off). Attempts to discontinue or taper medication should be made at 3- to 6-month intervals.

The recommended dosage is 2 to 4 grams (one-half to 1 applicator of cream) daily, inserted into the vagina, depending on the severity of the condition. Patients with an intact uterus should be monitored closely for signs of endometrial cancer, with appropriate diagnostic measures taken to rule out malignancy in the event of persistent or recurring abnormal vaginal bleeding.

Instructions for use of applicator:

1. Remove cap from tube.
2. Screw nozzle end of applicator onto tube.
3. Gently squeeze tube from the bottom to force sufficient cream into the barrel to provide the prescribed dose.
4. Unscrew applicator from tube.
5. Lie on back with knees drawn up. Gently insert applicator deeply into the vagina and press plunger downward to its original position.

To cleanse:

Pull plunger out from barrel. Wash with mild soap and warm water. *Do not boil or use hot water.*

Overdosage

Any medication taken in excess can have serious consequences. If you suspect an overdose of Premarin, seek medical attention immediately.

Brand name:

PRILOSEC

Generic name: Omeprazole

Why is this drug prescribed?

Prilosec is an antiulcer medication prescribed for the short-term treatment (4 to 8 weeks) of active duodenal ulcer, gastroesophageal reflux disease (backflow of acid stomach contents), and severe erosive esophagitis. It is also used for the long-term treatment of hypersecretory conditions such as Zollinger-Ellison syndrome, multiple endocrine adenomas (benign tumors), and systemic mastocytosis.

Most important fact about this drug:

Prilosec should not be used for long-term therapy after an ulcer has healed.

How should you take this medication?

Prilosec works best when taken before meals. It can be taken with an antacid.

Take this medication exactly as prescribed by your doctor.

The capsule should be swallowed whole. It should not be opened, chewed or crushed.

What side effects may occur?

Side effects cannot be anticipated. If any develop or change in intensity, inform your doctor as soon as possible. Only your doctor can determine if it is safe for you to continue taking Prilosec.

■ *More common side effects may include:*
Abdominal pain, back pain, constipation, cough, diarrhea, dizziness, gas, headache, nausea, rash, upper respiratory infection, vomiting, weakness

■ *Less common or rare side effects
may include:*
Abdominal swelling, aggression, anemia,
anxiety, breast development in males,
blood in urine, changes in liver function,
chest pain, confusion, depression,
difficulty sleeping, discolored feces, dry
mouth, dry skin, fatigue, fever, hair
loss, hallucinations, hepatitis, hives,
irritable colon, itching, joint and leg
pain, low blood sugar, loss of appetite,
muscle cramps and pain, nervousness,
nosebleeds, pain, pain in testicles, pounding
heartbeat, rapid heartbeat, rash,
ringing in ears, sleepiness, slow heartbeat,
taste distortion, tingling or pins and
needles, throat pain, urinary frequency,
urinary tract infection, vertigo, weight
gain, yellow eyes and skin

Why should this drug not be prescribed?
If you are sensitive to or have ever had an
allergic reaction to Prilosec or similar
drugs, you should not take this medication.
Make sure that your doctor is aware of
any drug reactions that you have experienced.

Special warnings about this medication
The safety of long-term use of this drug has
not been established.

A stomach malignancy could be present, even
if your symptoms have been relieved by
Prilosec.

Possible food and drug interactions
when taking this medication
If Prilosec is taken with certain other drugs,
the effects of either could be increased,
decreased, or altered. It is especially important
to check with your doctor before
combining Prilosec with the following:

Ampicillins such as Spectrobid
Cyclosporine (Sandimmune)
Diazepam (Valium)
Disulfiram (Antabuse)

Iron
Ketoconazole (Nizoral)
Phenytoin (Dilantin)
Warfarin (Coumadin)

Special information
if you are pregnant or breastfeeding
The effects of Prilosec during pregnancy have
not been adequately studied. If you are
pregnant or plan to become pregnant, inform
your doctor immediately. Prilosec may
appear in breast milk and could affect a
nursing infant. If this medication is
essential to your health, your doctor may
advise you to discontinue breastfeeding
until your treatment with this medication is
finished.

Recommended dosage

ADULTS

*Short-term Treatment of Active
Duodenal Ulcer*
The usual dose is 20 milligrams once a day.
Most people heal within 4 weeks.

*Severe Erosive Esophagitis or Poorly
Responsive Gastroesophageal Reflux
Disease (GERD)*
The usual dose is 20 milligrams daily for 4
to 8 weeks.

Pathological Hypersecretory Conditions
The usual starting dose is 60 milligrams once
a day. Dosage of more than 80 milligrams
per day should be divided into smaller doses.
Dosing should be individualized according
to the patient's needs.

CHILDREN

The safety and effectiveness of Prilosec in
children have not been established.

ELDERLY

Dosage should be determined by the particular
needs of the elderly patient.

Overdosage

Any medication taken in excess can cause symptoms of overdose. If you suspect an overdose, seek medical attention immediately.

No specific symptoms of Prilosec overdose are known.

Generic name:

PRIMIDONE

See Mysoline, page 396.

Brand name:

PRINIVIL

See Zestril, page 696.

Generic name:

PROBENECID WITH COLCHICINE

See ColBENEMID, page 124.

Generic name:

PROBUCOL

See Lorelco, page 340.

Brand name:

PROCAN SR

Generic name: Procainamide hydrochloride

Why is this drug prescribed?

Procan SR is used to treat severe irregular heartbeats (arrhythmias) and, in some instances, certain types of less severe irregular heartbeats. Arrhythmias are generally divided into two main types: heartbeats that are faster than normal (tachycardia), and heartbeats that are slower than normal (bradycardia). Irregular heartbeats are often caused by drugs or disease but can occur in otherwise healthy people with no history of heart disease or other illness.

Most important fact about this drug

Serious side effects have occurred with Procan SR treatment. It should be used only if its benefits clearly outweigh its risks. Your doctor should carefully monitor your heartbeat to make sure the medication is producing the desired effect.

How should you take this medication?

Take this medication exactly as prescribed by your doctor.

Procan SR should be swallowed whole. Do not break or chew the tablet. The tablet matrix of Procan SR may be seen in the stool, since it does not disintegrate following release of procainamide.

Try not to miss any doses. Skipping doses, changing the intervals between doses, or "making up" missed doses by doubling up later may cause your condition to worsen and could be dangerous.

Never take two doses at the same time.

What side effects may occur?

Side effects cannot be anticipated. If any develop or change in intensity, inform your doctor as soon as possible. Only your doctor can determine if it is safe for you to continue taking Procan SR.

■ *More common side effects may include:*
Abdominal pain
Bitter taste
Diarrhea
Enlarged liver
Loss of appetite
Nausea

Symptoms similar to those of lupus erythematosus (collagen vascular disease): joint pain, abdominal or chest pain, fever, chills, muscle pain, skin lesions
Vomiting

■ *Less common side effects may include:*
Depression, dizziness, fluid retention, flushing, giddiness, hallucinations, hives, itching, rash, weakness

■ *Rare side effects may include:*
Anemia, changes in blood counts, low blood pressure

Why should this drug not be prescribed?

Procan SR should not be taken if you have complete heart block (conduction disorder) or have had an allergic reaction to procaine or similar local anesthetics.

If you have been diagnosed with lupus erythematosus (collagen vascular disease) or torsades de pointes (an unusual arrhythmia), do not take Procan SR.

Special warnings about this medication

Extended treatment with Procan SR can cause a positive ANA test (used to diagnose lupus erythematosus). If a positive ANA test develops, your doctor may decide to stop treatment with Procan SR.

Serious blood disorders can develop, especially during the first 3 months of therapy. Your doctor should take a complete blood count weekly for the first 12 weeks and should continue to monitor your blood count carefully.

If you develop a fever, chills, sore throat or mouth, bruising or bleeding, infections, chest or abdominal pain, loss of appetite, weakness, muscle or joint pain, skin rash, nausea, pounding heartbeat, vomiting, diarrhea, hallucinations, dizziness,

depression, wheezing, yellow eyes and skin, or dark urine, contact your doctor immediately. It could indicate a serious illness.

Procan SR should be used cautiously if you have ever had congestive heart failure or other types of heart disease.

Procan SR should be used with other antiarrhythmic drugs, such as quinidine or disopyramide, only if they have been tried and have not worked when used alone.

If you have ever had kidney disease, liver disease, or myasthenia gravis (a disease that causes muscle weakness, especially in the face and neck), you should be carefully monitored while taking Procan SR.

Make sure your doctor is aware of any drug reactions you have experienced, especially to procaine, other local anesthetics, or aspirin.

Possible food and drug interactions when taking this medication

If Procan SR is taken with certain other drugs, the effects of either could be increased, decreased, or altered. It is especially important to check with your doctor before combining Procan SR with the following:

Other antiarrhythmics such as quinidine (Quinidex), propranolol (Inderal), and mexiletine (Mexitil)
Lidocaine
Drugs that ease muscle spasms (anticholinergies such as Cogentin and Artane)
Neuromuscular blocking agents such as Tensilon

Special information if you are pregnant or breastfeeding

The effects of Procan SR during pregnancy have not been adequately studied. If you are pregnant or plan to become pregnant, inform your doctor immediately. Procan SR appears in breast milk and may affect a nursing infant. If this medication is essential to your health, your doctor may advise you to discontinue breastfeeding until your treatment is finished.

Recommended dosage

ADULTS

Dosages and intervals between doses should be adjusted for each individual patient, based on your doctor's assessment of the degree of underlying heart disease, your age, and the way your kidneys are functioning.

Younger patients with normal kidney function should start with a total daily oral dose of up to 50 milligrams per 2.2 pounds of body weight, divided into smaller doses given every 6 hours.

For older patients, especially those over 50 years of age, or for patients with reduced kidney, liver, or heart function, lower doses or longer intervals between doses may produce adequate results and decrease the probability of dose-related side effects.

CHILDREN

The safety and effectiveness of this drug have not been established in children.

ELDERLY

Dosages should be adjusted according to body weight and level of kidney, liver, and heart function.

Overdosage

Any medication taken in excess can have serious consequences. If you suspect an overdose, seek medical treatment immediately.

Symptoms of Procan SR overdose may include:
Changes in heart function and heartbeat

Brand name:

PROCARDIA

Generic name: Nifedipine
Other brand name: Adalat

Why is this drug prescribed?

Procardia, a type of medication called a calcium channel blocker, is prescribed for the treatment of angina (chest pain, often accompanied by a feeling of choking, usually caused by lack of oxygen to the heart due to clogged arteries). Calcium channel blockers ease the workload of the heart by slowing down passage of nerve impulses through the heart and hence the contractions of the heart muscle, and by dilating the arteries. This improves blood flow through the heart and throughout the body, reduces blood pressure, and helps prevent angina pain.

Most important fact about this drug

Procardia can reduce or eliminate angina pain caused by exertion or exercise. If you are feeling better, be careful not to do too much until you discuss with your doctor how much exertion is appropriate.

How should you take this medication?

Procardia can be taken with or without food. It should be swallowed whole.

Take Procardia exactly as prescribed by your doctor, even if your symptoms have disappeared.

If you miss a dose, take it as soon as you remember. If it is almost time for your next dose, skip the one you missed and go back to your regular schedule. Never take two doses at the same time.

What side effects may occur?

Side effects cannot be anticipated. If any develop or change in intensity, inform your doctor as soon as possible. Only your doctor can determine if it is safe for you to continue taking Procardia.

■ *More common side effects may include:*
Cough, dizziness, flushing, giddiness, headache, heartburn, heat sensation, light-headedness, low blood pressure, mood changes, muscle cramps, nasal congestion, nausea, nervousness, pounding heartbeat, shortness of breath, sore throat, swelling of arms, legs, hands, and feet due to water retention, tremors, weakness, wheezing

■ *Less common side effects may include:*
Blurred vision, chest congestion, chills, constipation, cramps, diarrhea, difficulties in balance, excessive sweating, fever, gas, hives, inflammation, itching, jitteriness, muscle cramps, sexual difficulties, shakiness, skin inflammation, sleep disturbances, stiff joints

■ *Rare side effects may include:*
Anemia, arthritis, blood disorders, brief, temporary blindness, burning pain, heat, redness in the feet, depression, fainting, gum disorders, hepatitis, paranoia, reddish or purplish spots below the skin

Why should this drug not be prescribed?
If you are sensitive to or have ever had an allergic reaction to Procardia or other calcium channel blockers, you should not take this medication. Make sure your doctor is aware of any drug reactions you have experienced.

Special warnings about this medication
Procardia can cause your blood pressure to become too low, which can make you feel light-headed or faint. This is more likely to happen when you start taking the medication and when the amount you take is increased. Your doctor should check your blood pressure when you start taking Procardia and continue to monitor it while your dosage is being adjusted.

If you experience increased angina pain when you start taking Procardia or when your dosage is increased, contact your doctor immediately.

Angina pain and withdrawal symptoms can occur if you suddenly stop taking beta blockers to begin Procardia therapy. If your doctor has decided to take you off beta blockers, they should be gradually withdrawn before beginning Procardia therapy.

If you have tight aortic stenosis (a narrowing of the aortic valve that obstructs blood flow from the heart to the body) and are taking a beta blocker, you should be carefully monitored while taking Procardia.

Mild to moderate swelling of the legs and feet can occur with use of Procardia. Your doctor can prescribe a diuretic (water pill) to avoid this problem.

Procardia may prolong the time it takes for your blood to clot. If you notice unusual bruising, contact your doctor.

Notify your doctor or dentist that you are taking Procardia if you have a medical emergency, and before you have surgery or dental treatment.

Possible food and drug interactions when taking this medication
If Procardia is taken with certain other drugs, the effects of either could be increased, decreased, or altered. It is especially important to check with your doctor before combining Procardia with the following:

Beta-blocking heart and blood pressure
    medications such as Inderal and
    Lopressor

Digitalis (Lanoxin)
Blood thinners such as Coumadin
Cimetidine (Tagamet)
Fentanyl (Innovar) anesthesia

Special information
if you are pregnant or breastfeeding

The effects of Procardia during pregnancy have not been adequately studied. If you are pregnant or plan to become pregnant, inform your doctor immediately. It is not known if Procardia appears in breast milk and can affect a nursing infant. If this medication is essential to your health, your doctor may advise you to discontinue breastfeeding until your treatment is finished.

Recommended dosage

ADULTS

Dosages of this drug must be carefully adjusted to each patient's needs. Too much of this medication can result in light-headedness and fainting. Your doctor will gradually change your dose over a 7- to 14-day period to achieve the desired effect. In some cases, your doctor may increase your doses before the 7- to 14-day period is over.

The usual starting dose of Procardia or Adalat is one 10-milligram capsule, 3 times per day. The usual range is 10 to 20 milligrams 3 times a day. In some patients, a higher dose of 20 to 30 milligrams, 3 or 4 times per day may be needed. Most daily doses will not exceed 120 milligrams per day and doses above 180 milligrams a day are not recommended.

The usual starting dose of Procardia XL, an extended-release form of the drug, is one 30-milligram or 60-milligram tablet per day. Doses above 120 milligrams per day are not recommended.

CHILDREN

There is no recommended use in children.

ELDERLY

This drug should be used with caution in elderly patients.

Overdosage

Any medication taken in excess can cause symptoms of overdose. If you suspect an overdose, seek medical treatment immediately.

Symptoms of Procardia overdose may include:
Severe low blood pressure
Peripheral vasodilation

Brand name:

PROCARDIA XL

Generic name: Nifedipine

Why is this drug prescribed?

Procardia XL is a type of medication called a calcium channel blocker that is used to treat angina (chest pain, often accompanied by a feeling of choking, usually caused by lack of oxygen to the heart due to clogged arteries or spasm of arteries) and high blood pressure. Calcium channel blockers ease the workload of the heart by interfering with the normal role of calcium in muscle contraction and transmission of nerve impulses. Calcium channel blockers dilate arteries. This improves blood flow through the heart and throughout the body, reduces blood pressure, and helps prevent angina. Procardia XL is taken once a day and provides a steady rate of medication over a 24-hour period.

Most important fact about this drug

Some patients with certain heart conditions may experience an increase in frequency and duration of angina attacks when starting Procardia XL or during a dosage increase.

How should you take this medication?

Procardia XL should be taken exactly as prescribed by your doctor, even if your symptoms have disappeared.

Procardia XL Tablets are specially designed to slowly release the medication into your bloodstream. As a result, something that looks like a tablet may occasionally appear in your stool. This is normal and simply means that the medication has been released, and the shell that contains the medication has been eliminated from your body.

Procardia XL tablets should be swallowed whole. Do not break, crush, or chew.

Procardia XL can be taken with or without food.

This medication should be taken once a day.

What side effects may occur?

Side effects cannot be anticipated. If any develop or change in intensity, inform your doctor as soon as possible. Only your doctor can determine whether it is safe for you to continue taking Procardia XL.

■ *Most common side effects may include:*
Constipation
Dizziness
Fatigue
Fluid retention (ankle or leg swelling)
Headache
Nausea

■ *More common side effects may include:*
Abdominal pain, diarrhea, difficulty sleeping, drowsiness, dry cough, dry mouth, flushing, gas, impotence, itching, joint pain, leg cramps, nervousness, non-specific chest pain, pain, pounding heartbeat, production of large amounts of pale urine, rash, shortness of breath, tingling or pins and needles, upset stomach, weakness

■ *Less common or rare side effects may include:*
Abnormal or terrifying dreams, anxiety, back pain, belching, breast pain, breathing disorders, coughing, dark stools containing blood, decreased sex drive, depression, diffuse muscle pain, distorted taste, dizziness, dulled sense of touch, excessive urination at night, facial swelling, fainting, feelings of hot and cold, fever, gout, gum irritation, hair loss, heartburn, hives, hot flashes, increased sweating, increased angina, inflammation of the sinuses, irregular heartbeat, itching, low blood pressure, migraine, muscle incoordination, muscle tension, nosebleeds, painful or difficult urination, rapid heartbeat, reddish or purplish spots under the skin, ringing in the ears, swelling around the eyes, tearing eyes, tremor, upper respiratory tract infection, vague feeling of weakness, vision changes, vomiting, weight gain

Why should this drug not be prescribed?

Procardia XL should not be used if you have ever had an allergic reaction or are sensitive to nifedipine.

Special warnings about this medication

Procardia XL may cause your blood pressure to become too low, which may make you feel light-headed or faint. This is more likely to happen when you start taking the medication and when the amount you take is increased. It is also more likely to occur if you are also taking beta blockers (such as Tenormin). Your doctor should check your blood pressure when you start taking Procardia XL and continue monitoring it while your dosage is being adjusted.

If you experience increased angina pain when you start taking Procardia XL, or when your dosage is increased, contact your doctor immediately.

Angina pain and withdrawal symptoms can occur if you suddenly stop taking beta blockers to begin Procardia XL therapy. If your doctor has decided to take you off beta blockers, they should be gradually withdrawn before beginning Procardia XL.

If you have tight aortic stenosis (a narrowing of the aortic valve that obstructs blood flow from the heart to the body) and are taking a beta blocker, you should be carefully monitored while taking Procardia XL.

Mild to moderate swelling of the legs and feet can occur with use of Procardia XL. Your doctor can prescribe a diuretic (water pill) to avoid this problem.

Procardia XL should be used cautiously if you have any stomach or intestinal narrowing.

The tablet coating may occasionally appear in your stool. This is normal and should not be a concern.

Possible food and drug interactions when taking this medication

If Procardia XL is taken with certain other drugs, the effects of either could be increased, decreased, or altered. It is especially important to check with your doctor before combining Procardia XL with the following:

Blood thinners such as Coumadin and
  Panwarfin
Cimetidine (Tagamet)
Digitalis (Lanoxin)
Fentanyl (Innovar)
Other heart and blood pressure medications
  such as Inderal and Lopressor

Special information
if you are pregnant or breastfeeding

The effects of Procardia XL during pregnancy have not been adequately studied. If you are pregnant or plan to become pregnant, inform your doctor immediately. It is not known whether Procardia XL appears in breast milk and can affect a nursing infant. If this medication is essential to your health, your doctor may advise you to discontinue breastfeeding until your treatment with Procardia XL is finished.

Recommended dosage

ADULTS

The starting dose is usually the 30- or 60-milligram tablet given once daily. The dose may be increased over 1 to 2 weeks if the response to the starting dose is not adequate.

Procardia XL is available in 30-, 60-, and 90-milligram tablets.

Doses above 120 milligrams per day are not recommended.

Although no serious side effects have been reported when Procardia XL is stopped, it is recommended that doses be lowered gradually under close supervision of a physician.

Overdosage

Any medication taken in excess can have serious consequences. If you suspect an overdose, seek medical treatment immediately.

Symptoms of Procardia XL overdose may include:
Dizziness
Extremely low blood pressure
Flushing
Nervousness
Pounding heartbeat

Generic name:

PROCHLORPERAZINE

See Compazine, page 132.

Brand name:

PROLIXIN

Generic name: Fluphenazine hydrochloride

Why is this drug prescribed?

Prolixin is used to reduce the symptoms of psychotic disorders such as schizophrenia.

Most important fact about this drug

Prolixin may cause tardive dyskinesia—a condition marked by involuntary muscle spasms and twitches in the face and body. This condition may be permanent and appears to be most common among the elderly, especially women. Ask your doctor for information about this possible risk.

How should you take this medication?

If you are taking Prolixin in a liquid form, (Elixir) examine it first. The flavoring oils may have separated from the solutions, causing globs or a wispy appearance. If this happens, gently shake the bottle. The oil should blend in, and the solution should look clear. If the solution is not clear, do not take it.

Avoid use of alcohol when taking Prolixin.

If you are taking Prolixin Concentrate, you can mix it with water, homogenized milk, or fruit juice. Do *not* mix with caffeine-containing beverages or apple juice.

What side effects may occur?

Side effects cannot be anticipated. If any develop or change in intensity, inform your doctor as soon as possible. Only your doctor can determine if it is safe for you to continue taking this medication.

■ *Side effects may include:*
A large mass of hard feces, abnormal muscle rigidity, abnormal secretion of milk, abnormalities of movements and posture, asthma, blood disorders, blurred vision, breast development in males, changed mental state, chewing movements, complete or almost complete loss of movement, constipation, dizziness, drowsiness, dry mouth, excessive or spontaneous flow of milk, excessive urine, excitement, eye problems, eyeball rotation or state of fixed gaze, fluid accumulation and swelling, fluid accumulation in the brain, glaucoma, headache, heart attack, high blood pressure, high fever, hives, impotence, inability to sit still, increased sex drive in women, intestinal blockage, irregular blood pressure, pulse, and heartbeat, irregular menstrual periods, loss of appetite, masklike face and rigidity, muscle spasms, nasal congestion, nausea, oily scalp, painful muscle spasm, protruding tongue, puckering of mouth, puffing of cheeks, rapid heartbeat, red blood spots, restlessness, salivation, sensitivity to light, skin inflammation and peeling, skin itching, pigmentation, rash, skin lesions, crusts, sluggishness, sore throat, mouth and gums, strange dreams, sweating, swelling of the throat, twitching in the body, neck, shoulders, and face, visual problems, weight change, yellowing of skin and whites of eyes

Why should this drug not be prescribed?

Do not give Prolixin to someone in a comatose state. Do not take the drug if you are also taking central nervous system depressants (alcohol, barbiturates, or narcotics), of if you have had brain or liver damage, or have an abnormal bone marrow or blood condition.

Special warnings about this medication

You should use Prolixin cautiously if you have ever had: breast cancer; convulsive disorders; heart or kidney disease; seizures; or certain tumors, or if you are exposed to extreme heat or pesticides.

Stomach inflammation, dizziness, nausea, vomiting, and tremors can result if you suddenly stop taking Prolixin. Follow your doctor's instructions closely when discontinuing Prolixin.

Your doctor should periodically check your liver, kidneys, and blood while you are taking Prolixin.

This drug may impair your ability to drive a car or operate potentially dangerous machinery. Do not participate in any activities that require full alertness if you are unsure of your ability.

Prolixin 2.5-, 5-, and 10-milligram tablets contain a coloring agent that can cause an allergic reaction in some people.

Possible food and drug interactions when taking this medication
If Prolixin is taken with certain other drugs, the effects of either could be increased, decreased, or altered. It is especially important to check with your doctor before combining Prolixin with the following:

Analgesics such as Percocet
Antihistamine such as Benadryl
Atropine
Barbiturates such as phenobarbital

Drugs such as Prolixin should not be used with epinephrine (EpiPen).

Extreme drowsiness and other potentially serious effects can result if Prolixin is combined with alcohol or other depressants such as narcotics and sleeping medications.

Special information
if you are pregnant or breastfeeding
Pregnant women should use Prolixin only if clearly needed. If you are pregnant or plan to become pregnant, inform your doctor immediately. Prolixin may appear in breast milk and might affect a nursing infant.

Recommended dosage
The smallest effective dose of Prolixin should be used. This dose should be tailored to the individual.

ADULTS

The usual beginning total daily dose is 2.5 to 10 milligrams. This amount should be divided into 3 or 4 equal doses and given 6 or 8 hours apart.

If necessary, total dosage may be increased to 40 milligrams daily.

Dosage may be decreased when symptoms are controlled. A daily maintenance dose may range from 1 to 5 milligrams, usually given in a single dose.

CHILDREN

It has not been determined whether Prolixin is safe for children to use.

ELDERLY

Elderly patients may start with a daily dose of 1 to 2.5 milligrams. In general, elderly people take dosages of Prolixin in the lower ranges. Elderly people (especially elderly women) may be more susceptible to tardive dyskinesia—a possibly permanent condition characterized by involuntary muscle spasms and twitches in the face and body. Elderly people should consult their doctor for information about these potential risks.

Overdosage
Any medication taken in excess can have serious consequences. If you suspect an overdose of Prolixin, seek medical help immediately.

Brand name:

PROLOID

Generic name: Thyroglobulin

Why is this drug prescribed?
Proloid, a medication made from hog thyroid glands, contains the two thyroid hormones T_3 and T_4. Your doctor may prescribe Proloid

for you if your own thyroid gland is not making enough hormone.

Most important fact about this drug

Although Proloid will speed up your metabolism, it is not effective as a weight-loss drug, and you should not take it for that purpose. Too much Proloid may cause life-threatening side effects, especially if you take it along with an amphetamine-like appetite suppressant medication.

How should you take this medication?

If your thyroid gland does not make enough hormone or has been removed, it is likely that you will need to take thyroid medication indefinitely.

Take Proloid exactly as prescribed by your doctor. There is no "typical" dosage; the amount you need will depend on how much thyroid hormone your body produces on its own. (Take no more or less than the prescribed amount. Take your dose at the same time every day for consistent effect.)

Your doctor will probably start you on low-dose Proloid, increasing the amount every 2 or 3 weeks until you reach your ideal maintenance dosage. Periodically the doctor will order a blood test to make sure the dosage is still correct for you.

What side effects may occur?

When Proloid is given at the correct dosage, adverse effects are rare.

However, excessive dosage or a too-rapid increase in dosage may lead to overstimulation of the thyroid gland. Symptoms of overstimulation may include:

Diarrhea, changes in appetite, fever, headache, increased heart rate, irritability, nausea, nervousness, sleeplessness, sweating, weight loss

Children who take Proloid may initially lose some hair, but this effect is usually temporary.

Why should this drug not be prescribed?

You should not take Proloid:
- If you have ever had an allergic reaction to it
- If your thyroid gland is making too much thyroid hormone
- If your adrenal glands are not making enough corticosteroid hormones

Special warnings about this medication

If you are elderly, and/or suffer from angina (chest pain due to a heart condition), you should take Proloid at low dosage and under very close medical supervision.

Since elderly people are more sensitive to Proloid than younger patients, they should receive lower dosages.

If you have diabetes mellitus or diabetes insipidus, or if your body makes too little adrenal corticosteroid hormone, Proloid will tend to make your symptoms worse. If you take medication for any of these disorders, the dosage will probably have to be adjusted once you begin taking Proloid.

Your thyroid status should be tested and your treatment evaluated periodically while you are taking Proloid.

Possible food and drug interactions when taking this medication

If Proloid is taken with certain other drugs, the effects of either could be increased, decreased, or altered. It is especially important to check with your doctor before combining Proloid with the following:

Antidiabetic drugs (Diabinese, Glucotrol, others)
Blood thinners (Coumadin, Dicumarol, others)
Cholestyramine (Questran)

Colestipol (Colestid)
Contraceptive pills containing estrogen (Ortho
  Novum, Ovral, others)
Estrogen (Estinyl, Premarin, others)
Insulin

If you are having a blood test to determine
whether your dosage of Proloid is correct,
make sure your doctor knows about other
medications you may be taking. Any of the
following drugs may interfere with the results
of the thyroid-level test:

Androgens
Corticosteroids such as prednisone
Contraceptive pills with estrogen
Estrogens
Iodine-containing drugs
Salicylate-containing drugs

Special information
if you are pregnant or breastfeeding
If you need to take Proloid because of a
thyroid hormone deficiency, you should
continue to take the medication during
pregnancy. Once your baby is born, you may
breastfeed while taking the drug. However,
as with any medication taken during
breastfeeding, caution is recommended.

Recommended dosage
Your doctor will tailor dosage to meet your
individual requirements, taking into consideration the status of your thyroid gland
and other medical conditions you may have.

Overdosage
An excess of thyroid hormone may produce
serious or even life-threatening effects. If
you experience any of these symptoms,
seek medical attention immediately.

*Symptoms of overdosage with Proloid may
include any or all of the following:*

Chest pain
Excessive sweating
Heart palpitations
Heat intolerance
Increased pulse
Nervousness
Racing heart

Generic name:

PROMETHAZINE HYDROCHLORIDE

See Phenergan, page 474.

Generic name:

PROMETHAZINE WITH CODEINE

See Phenergan with Codeine, page 476.

Generic name:

PROPAFENONE HYDROCHLORIDE

See Rythmol, page 561.

Brand name:

PROPINE

Generic name: Dipivefrin hydrochloride

Why is this drug prescribed?
Propine is used to treat chronic open-angle
glaucoma. It belongs to a class of medication
called "prodrugs," drugs that generally are
not active by themselves, but are
converted in the body to an active form.

Most important fact about this drug
Your eye pressure should be checked regularly
by your doctor.

How should you use this medication?

Use this medication exactly as prescribed by your doctor. If you use too much, or use it too often, Propine may cause side effects.

Wash your hands before and after you use the eyedrops. Once the drops are in your eye, keep your eye closed for 1 to 2 minutes so the medicine can be properly absorbed.

A number appears on the cap of the dropper bottle to tell you what dose you are taking. After each dose, replace the cap and rotate it to the next number. Turn until you hear a click.

If you forget to use the medicine, apply the missed dose as soon as possible. If it's almost time for your next dose, skip the missed dose and go back to your normal dosage schedule. Never apply more than one dose at a time.

What side effects may occur?

Side effects cannot be anticipated. If any develop or change in intensity, inform your doctor as soon as possible. Only your doctor can determine if it is safe for you to continue taking Propine.

■ *More common side effects may include:*
Burning and stinging
Red eye

■ *Less common or rare side effects may include:*
Allergic reactions, change in heart rhythm, conjunctivitis, extreme dilation of pupils, increased heart rate or blood pressure, increased sensitivity to light

Why should this drug not be prescribed?

If you are sensitive to or have ever had an allergic reaction to Propine or similar drugs, you should not use this medication. Make sure that your doctor is aware of any drug reactions that you have experienced.

Unless you are directed to do so by your doctor, do not use this medication if you have narrow-angle glaucoma.

Special warnings about this medication

Propine may cause vision problems, including blurry vision, for a short time after the eyedrops are applied. If this occurs, make sure you do not drive, use machinery, or participate in any hazardous activity that requires clear vision.

Possible food and drug interactions when taking this medication

No significant interactions have been reported.

Special information if you are pregnant or breastfeeding

The effects of Propine during pregnancy have not been adequately studied. If you are pregnant or plan to become pregnant, inform your doctor immediately. Propine may appear in breast milk and could affect a nursing infant. If this medication is essential to your health, your doctor may advise you to discontinue breastfeeding your baby until your treatment is finished.

Recommended dosage

ADULTS

The usual dose is 1 drop in the eye(s) every 12 hours. It usually takes about 30 minutes for Propine to start working. You should feel the maximum effects of the drug within 1 hour.

CHILDREN

The safety and effectiveness of Propine have not been established in children under 12 years of age.

Overdosage

Any medication taken in excess can have serious consequences. If you suspect an overdose, seek medical attention immediately.

Generic name:

PROPOXYPHENE HYDROCHLORIDE

See Darvon, page 163.

Generic name:

PROPOXYPHENE NAPSYLATE WITH ACETAMINOPHEN

See Darvocet-N, page 161.

Generic name:

PROPRANOLOL HYDROCHLORIDE

See Inderal, page 290.

Generic name:

PROPRANOLOL WITH HYDROCHLOROTHIAZIDE

See Inderide, page 293.

Brand name:

PROSCAR

Generic name: Finasteride

Why is this drug prescribed?

Proscar, which is available in tablet form, is prescribed to help shrink an enlarged prostate.

The prostate, a chestnut-shaped gland present in males, produces secretions that form part of the semen. This gland completely encloses the upper part of the urethra, the tube through which urine flows out of the bladder. Many men over age 50 suffer from a benign (noncancerous) enlargement of the prostate. The enlarged gland squeezes the urethra, obstructing the normal flow of urine. Resulting problems may include difficulty in starting urination, weak flow of urine, the need to urinate frequently, and leakage of urine. Sometimes surgical removal of the prostate is necessary.

By shrinking the enlarged prostate, Proscar may alleviate the various associated urinary problems, making surgery unnecessary.

Most important fact about this drug

Benign enlargement of the prostate is not the only condition that can cause male urinary inefficiency and discomfort. Other possibilities include infection, obstruction, cancer of the prostate, and bladder disorders. Before prescribing Proscar, your doctor will want to do various tests to determine the cause of your urinary problems.

How should you take this medication?

Take Proscar exactly as prescribed by your doctor. The recommended dosage is 1 tablet per day. You may take Proscar either with a meal or between meals.

Different men have different responses to Proscar:

- You may experience early relief from your urinary problems.
- You may need to take the drug for 6 months or even a year before noticing any improvement.
- Or you may find that, even after a year of treatment, Proscar simply has not helped you.

Even if Proscar does relieve your urinary symptoms, periodic checkups are necessary to test for possible development of cancer of the prostate. Proscar is not an effective treatment for prostate cancer.

PDR FAMILY GUIDE TO PRESCRIPTION DRUGS

What side effects may occur?
Side effects cannot be anticipated. If any develop or change in intensity, inform your doctor as soon as possible. Only your doctor can determine if it is safe for you to continue taking Proscar.

■ *Side effects may include:*
  Decreased amount of semen per ejaculation
  Decreased sex drive
  Impotence

Why should this drug not be prescribed?
Proscar should never be taken by a woman or a child.

Do not take Proscar if you are sensitive to it or have ever had an allergic reaction to it.

Special warnings about this medication
If accidentally absorbed by a pregnant woman who is carrying a male fetus, Proscar may cause abnormal development of the unborn baby's genital organs. Thus, a woman who is pregnant or who may become pregnant should never even touch a crushed Proscar tablet. If she is going to have intercourse with a man who is taking Proscar, she should insist that he wear a condom to protect her from his semen, which may contain small amounts of the medication.

Possible food and drug interactions when taking this medication
No significant drug interactions have been reported.

Special information
If you are pregnant or breastfeeding
As noted above, if a pregnant woman who is carrying a male fetus absorbs Proscar accidentally, the drug may cause defective development of the baby's genital organs. Any woman of childbearing age should be careful never to touch a crushed Proscar tablet. If her sexual partner is taking Proscar,

he should always wear a condom when they have intercourse to avoid any possible transfer of the drug to her body via his semen.

Recommended dosage
ADULTS

The recommended dosage is one 5-milligram tablet per day.

Overdosage
Although no specific information is available, any medication taken in excess can have serious consequences. If you suspect symptoms of an overdose of Proscar, seek medical attention immediately.

Brand name:

PROSOM

Generic name: Estazolam

Why is this drug prescribed?
ProSom, a sleeping pill, is given for the short-term treatment of insomnia. Insomnia may involve difficulty falling asleep, frequent awakenings during the night, or too-early morning awakening.

Most important fact about this drug
As a chemical cousin of Valium and similar tranquilizers, ProSom is potentially addictive; thus, you should plan on taking this drug only as a temporary sleeping aid. Even after relatively short-term use of ProSom, you may experience some withdrawal symptoms when you stop taking the medication.

How should you take this medication?
Take ProSom exactly as prescribed by your doctor. A typical schedule is 1 tablet every night at bedtime. For small, physically run-down, or older people, ½ a tablet may be a safer starting dose.

Avoid drinking alcoholic beverages while taking ProSom.

If you have ever had seizures, do not abruptly stop taking ProSom, even if you are taking antiseizure medication. Instead, taper off from ProSom under your doctor's supervision.

Even if you have never had seizures, it is better to taper off from ProSom than to stop taking the medication abruptly. Experience suggests that tapering off can help prevent drug withdrawal symptoms.

Typically, the only withdrawal symptoms caused by ProSom are mild and temporary insomnia or irritability. Occasionally, however, withdrawal can involve considerable discomfort or even danger, with symptoms such as abdominal and muscle cramps, convulsions, sweating, tremors, and vomiting.

What side effects may occur?
Side effects cannot be anticipated. If any develop or change in intensity, inform your doctor as soon as possible. Only your doctor can determine whether it is safe for you to continue taking ProSom.

■ *More common side effects may include:*
Daytime sleepiness
Dizziness
Lack of coordination
Sluggishness

■ *Less common side effects may include:*
Abdominal pain, acne, allergic reactions, appetite changes, back pain, body pain, chest pain, chills, confusion, cough, drowsiness, depression, dreaming abnormality, dry mouth, dry skin, ear pain, excitement, eye pain, fever, gas, hangover, headache, hostility, indigestion, itching, joint pain, lack of coordination, memory loss, muscle pain, muscle stiffness, nausea, nervousness, pounding

heartbeat, rash, runny nose, penile discharge, shortness of breath, sore throat, symptoms resembling a cold, thinking abnormality, tingling, urinary problems, unexpected behavior changes, vaginal itching, vague feeling of being sick, vomiting, weakness, weight changes

Why should this drug not be prescribed?
Do not take ProSom if you are sensitive or allergic to it, or if you have ever had an adverse reaction to another Valium-type medication.

Do not take ProSom if you are pregnant or planning to become pregnant. Drugs in this class may cause damage to the unborn child.

Special warnings about this medication
Since ProSom may cloud your thinking, impair your judgment, or interfere with your normal physical coordination, do not drive, climb, or perform hazardous tasks until you know your reaction to this medication. It is important to remember that the tablet you took in the evening may continue to affect you well into the following day.

If you are older or physically run-down, or if you have liver or kidney damage or breathing problems, you will be particularly vulnerable to side effects from ProSom, and you should use this medication with special caution.

Possible food and drug interactions when taking this medication
Do not drink alcohol while you are taking ProSom; this combination could make you comatose or dangerously slow your breathing.

For the same reason, do not combine ProSom with any other medication that might calm or slow the functioning of your central nervous system. Among such drugs are:

Anticonvulsants such as Dilantin, Tegretol, Depakene, or others

Antihistamines such as Benadryl or Chlortrimeton

Antipsychotics such as Haldol, Mellaril, or others

Barbiturates such as phenobarital

MAO inhibitor antidepressants such as Marplan, Nardil, or Parnate

Narcotics such as Percodan or Tylox

Sedatives such as Valium

If you smoke, you will tend to process and eliminate ProSom fairly quickly compared with a nonsmoker.

Special information
if you are pregnant or breastfeeding

If you are pregnant, you must not take ProSom; it could cause birth defects in your child.

When a pregnant woman takes ProSom or a similar medication shortly before giving birth, her baby is likely to have poor muscle tone (flaccidity) and/or experience drug withdrawal symptoms.

Because ProSom is thought to pass into breast milk, you should not take this medication while breastfeeding.

Recommended dosage

ADULTS

The recommended initial dose is 1 milligram at bedtime; however, some patients may need a 2-milligram dose.

CHILDREN

There is no information on the safety or effectiveness of ProSom in patients under age 18.

ELDERLY

The recommended usual dosage for the elderly is 1 milligram. However, some patients may require 0.5 milligram.

Overdosage

Any medication takes in excess can have serious consequences. If you suspect symptoms of an overdose of ProSom, seek medical attention immediately.

Symptoms of a ProSom overdose may include:
Confusion
Depressed breathing
Drowsiness and eventually coma
Lack of coordination
Slurred speech

Brand name:

PROSTEP

See Nicotine Patches, page 416.

Brand name:

PROVENTIL

Generic name: Albuterol sulfate
Other brand name: Ventolin

Why is this drug prescribed?

Albuterol is prescribed for the prevention and relief of bronchial spasms. This especially applies to the treatment of asthma. This medication is also used for the prevention of bronchial spasm due to exercise.

Most important fact about this drug

Albuterol's effects may last up to 6 to 8 hours or longer; therefore, it should not be used more frequently than your doctor recommends. Increasing the number of doses can be dangerous and may actually make symptoms of asthma worse.

If the dose your doctor recommends does not provide relief of your symptoms, or if your symptoms become worse, consult with your doctor immediately.

How should you take this medication?

If you are using a metered-dose inhaler, follow the instructions carefully. If you skip a dose of albuterol, take it as soon as you remember. Do not double the dose.

What side effects may occur?

Side effects cannot be anticipated. If any develop or change in intensity, inform your doctor as soon as possible. Only your doctor can determine if it is safe for you to continue taking albuterol.

■ *More common side effects may include:*
Aggression, agitation, cough, diarrhea, dizziness, excitement, general bodily discomfort, headache, heartburn, increased appetite, increased blood pressure, indigestion, irritability, labored breathing, light-headedness, muscle cramps, nausea, nervousness, nightmares, nosebleed, overactivity, palpitations, rapid heartbeat, rash, ringing in the ears, shakiness, sleeplessness, stomachache, stuffy nose, throat irritation, tooth discoloration, tremors, vomiting, wheezing, worsening bronchospasm

■ *Less common side effects may include:*
Chest pain (sometimes crushing) or discomfort, difficulty urinating, dry mouth and throat, flushing, high blood pressure, muscle spasm, restlessness, sweating, unusual taste, vertigo, weakness

■ *Rare side effects following the use of inhaled albuterol include:*
Hoarseness, increased breathing or wheezing, skin rash or hives, unusual and unexpected swelling of mouth and throat

Why should this drug not be prescribed?

If you are sensitive to or have ever had an allergic reaction to albuterol or other bronchodilators, you should not take this medication. Make sure that your doctor is aware of any drug reactions that you have experienced.

Special warnings about this medication

When taking albuterol inhalation aerosol, you should not use other inhaled medications before checking with your doctor.

Consult with your doctor before using this medication if you have a cardiovascular or convulsive disorder, high blood pressure, abnormal heartbeat, overactive thyroid gland, or diabetes.

Do not exceed your doctor's recommended dose of albuterol.

Possible food and drug interactions when taking this medication

Albuterol inhalation aerosol should not be used with other aerosol bronchodilators.

If albuterol is taken with certain other drugs, the effects of either could be increased, decreased, or altered. It is especially important to check with your doctor before combining albuterol with the following:

Antidepressants such as Elavil and Nardil
Epinephrine
Heart medications (e.g., beta blockers)
Other sympathomimetics

Special information if you are pregnant or breastfeeding

The effects of albuterol during pregnancy have not been adequately studied. If you are pregnant or plan to become pregnant, inform your doctor immediately. It is not known whether albuterol appears in breast milk. If this drug is essential to your health, your doctor may advise you to stop nursing your baby until your treatment is finished.

Recommended dosage

ADULTS

Inhalation Aerosol
Patient instructions are available with both products.

If you are being treated for a sudden or severe bronchial spasm or the prevention of asthma symptoms, the usual dosage of albuterol inhalation aerosol for adults and children aged 4 and over (Ventolin) or 12 and over (Proventil) is 2 inhalations repeated every 4 to 6 hours. More frequent use is not recommended. In some patients, 1 inhalation every 4 hours may be sufficient.

The recommended dose of Proventil Inhalation Aerosol for prevention of recurring symptoms is 2 inhalations, 4 times a day.

For exercise-induced bronchial spasm, the usual dosage for adults and children 12 years and older is 2 inhalations, 15 minutes prior to exercise.

Tablets
The usual starting dose for adults and children 12 years of age and older is 2 or 4 milligrams 3 to 4 times a day.

Syrup
The usual starting dose for adults and children over 14 years of age is 1 or 2 teaspoonfuls 3 or 4 times a day.

Ventolin Rotacaps for Inhalation
The usual dosage for adults and children 4 years and older is the contents of one 200-microgram capsule inhaled every 4 to 6 hours using a Rotahaler inhalation device. Some patients may require two 200-microgram capsules every 4 to 6 hours.

Inhalation Solution
The usual dosage for adults and children 12 years of age and older is 2.5 milligrams administered 3 to 4 times daily by nebulization. To administer 2.5 milligrams, dilute 0.5 milliliter of the 0.5 percent solution for inhalation with 2.5 milliliters of sterile normal saline solution.

Ventolin Nebules Inhalation Solution
The usual dosage for adults and children 12 years and older is 2.5 milligrams of Ventolin taken 3 to 4 times a day by nebulization.

Proventil Repetabs Tablets
The usual starting dosage for adults and children 12 years and over is 1 or 2 tablets (4 or 8 milligrams) every 12 hours.

CHILDREN

Inhalation Aerosol
Safety and effectiveness in children below the age of 12 (Proventil) and below the age of 4 (Ventolin) have not been established. For dosage in children above these ages, see adult section.

Tablets
The usual starting dose for children 6 to 12 years of age is 2 milligrams 3 or 4 times a day. The dose can be increased with caution but should not exceed 24 milligrams per day.

Syrup
The usual starting dose for children 6 to 14 years of age is 1 teaspoonful 3 to 4 times a day. For children 2 to 6 years of age, the starting dose is 0.1 milligram per 2.2 pounds of body weight, to a maximum of 4 milligrams, 3 times a day.

ELDERLY

Oral Dosage
For elderly patients, the usual starting dose of tablets or syrup is 2 milligrams 3 or 4 times a day.

Overdosage

Symptoms of albuterol overdose may include:
High blood pressure
Low potassium level
Radiating chest pain

Exaggerated side effects may also be a sign of an overdose. If you suspect an overdose, seek medical attention immediately.

Brand name:

PROVERA

Generic name: Medroxyprogesterone Acetate

Why is this drug prescribed?

Provera is derived from the female hormone progestrone. You may be given Provera if a female-hormone imbalance is keeping you from having menstrual periods or is causing your uterus to bleed abnormally.

Most important fact about this drug

You should never take Provera during the first four months of pregnancy. During this formative period, even a few days' treatment with Provera might put your unborn baby at increased risk for birth defects. If you take Provera and later discover that you were pregnant when you took it, discuss this with your doctor right away.

How should you take this medication?

Before starting to take Provera you should have a complete physical exam, including examination of your breasts and pelvic organs. You should also have a cervical smear (Pap test).

Provera may cause some degree of fluid retention. If you have a medical condition that could be made worse by fluid retention— such as epilepsy, migraine, asthma, or a heart or kidney problem—make sure your doctor knows about it.

Do not change from one brand to another without consulting your doctor or pharmacist.

If you are diabetic, you should monitor blood and urine sugar closely, since Provera decreases glucose tolerance.

Your doctor will probably have you take Provera for 10 days and then stop; you should have your period within 3 to 7 days after the last dose.

If you are being treated for lack of regular menstrual periods, your doctor may have you start taking Provera at any time. If you are being treated for abnormal uterine bleeding due to a female-hormone imbalance, your doctor will probably have you start taking Provera on day 16 or 21 of your menstrual cycle (i.e., 16 days or 21 after the start of your last period). You should have your period within 3 to 7 days after the last dose.

What side effects may occur?

Side effects from Provera cannot be anticipated. If any develop or change in intensity, inform your doctor as soon as possible. Only your doctor can determine if it is safe for you to continue taking Provera.

■ *Side effects may include:*
Acne, anaphylaxis (life-threatening allergic reaction), blood clot in a vein, lungs, or brain, breakthrough bleeding (between menstrual periods), breast tenderness or sudden flow of milk, cervical erosion or secretion changes, depression, drowsiness, fever, fluid retention, headache, hives, insomnia, itching, jaundice, menstrual flow changes; spotting, nausea, rash, skin discoloration, weight gain or weight loss

Why should this drug not be prescribed?

Do not take Provera if you are sensitive to it or have ever had an allergic reaction to it.

If you suspect you may have become pregnant unintentionally, do not take Provera as a test for pregnancy. Doctors once prescribed Provera for this purpose, but no longer do so for two reasons:

1. Quicker, safer pregnancy tests are now available.
2. If you are in fact pregnant, Provera might injure the baby.

Do not take Provera during your first 4 months of pregnancy. In the past, Provera was sometimes given to try to prevent miscarriage. However, doctors now believe that this treatment is not only ineffective but also potentially harmful to the baby.

Do not take Provera if you have:

Cancer of the breast or genital organs
Liver disease or a liver condition
"Missed abortion" (dead embryo or fetus still
   in the uterus)
Undiagnosed bleeding from the vagina

Do not take Provera if you have, or ever had, a blood clot in a vein.

Special warnings about this medication

Provera may mask the onset of menopause. In other words, while taking Provera you may continue to experience regular menstrual bleeding even if your menopause has started.

Provera may make you depressed, especially if you have suffered from depression in the past. If you become seriously depressed, you should probably stop taking Provera.

If you are diabetic, Provera could make your diabetes worse; your doctor should monitor you closely while you are taking this drug.

There is some concern that Provera, like birth control pills, might increase your risk for a blood clot in a vein. If you experience any symptoms that might suggest the onset of such a condition—pain with swelling, warmth and redness in a leg vein, coughing or shortness of breath, vision problems, migraine, weakness or numbness in an arm or leg—see your doctor right away.

Possible food and drug interactions when taking this medication

If Provera is taken with certain other drugs, the effects of either may be increased, decreased, or altered. It is especially important to check with your doctor before combining Provera with aminoglutethimide (Cytadren).

Special information if you are pregnant or breastfeeding

If you are pregnant or plan to become pregnant, inform your doctor immediately. You should not take Provera during pregnancy.

Provera does find its way into breast milk. Thus, if you are a new mother, you may need to choose between taking Provera and breastfeeding your baby.

Recommended dosage

ADULTS

To Restore Menstrual Periods
Provera Tablets are taken in dosages of 5 to 10 milligrams daily for 5 to 10 days. Make sure you discuss what effect this will have on your menstrual cycle with your doctor.

*Abnormal Uterine Bleeding Due to
Hormonal Imbalance*
Beginning on the calculated 16th or 21st day

of the menstrual cycle, 5 to 10 milligrams are taken daily for from 5 to 10 days. Make sure you discuss what effect this will have on your menstrual cycle with your doctor.

Overdosage
Although no specific information is available, any medication taken in excess can have serious consequences. If you suspect an overdose of Provera, seek medical attention immediately.

Brand name:

PROZAC

Generic name: Fluoxetine hydrochloride

Why is this drug prescribed?
Prozac is prescribed for the treatment of major depression, that is, a continuing depression that interferes with daily functioning. The symptoms usually include changes in appetite, sleep habits and mind/body coordination, decreased sex drive, increased fatigue, feelings of guilt or worthlessness, difficulty concentrating, slowed thinking, and suicidal thoughts.

Most important fact about this drug
Serious, sometimes fatal reactions have occurred when Prozac is used in combination with other antidepressant drugs known as MAO inhibitors, including Nardil, Parnate, and Marplan; and when Prozac is discontinued and a MAO inhibitor is started. Never take Prozac with one of these drugs or within 14 days of discontinuing therapy with one of them. If you are taking any prescription or nonprescription drugs, notify your doctor before taking Prozac.

Allow at least 5 weeks between stopping Prozac and starting a MAO inhibitor.

How should you take this medication?
Prozac should be taken exactly as prescribed by your doctor.

Because this medication may need to be taken for several weeks before you feel better, your doctor should check your progress periodically.

What side effects may occur?
Side effects cannot be anticipated. If any develop or change in intensity, inform your doctor as soon as possible. Only your doctor can determine if it is safe for you to continue taking Prozac.

■ *More common side effects may include:* Abnormal dreams, agitation, anxiety, bronchitis, chills, diarrhea, dizziness, drowsiness and fatigue, hay fever, inability to fall or stay asleep, increased appetite, lack or loss of appetite, light-headedness, nausea, nervousness, sweating, tremors, weakness, weight loss, yawning

■ *Less common side effects may include:* Abnormal ejaculation, abnormal gait, abnormal stoppage of menstrual flow, acne, amnesia, apathy, arthritis, asthma, belching, bone pain, breast cysts, breast pain, brief loss of consciousness, bursitis, chills and fever, conjunctivitis, convulsions, dark, tarry stool, difficulty in swallowing, dilation of pupils, dimness of vision, dry skin, ear pain, eye pain, exaggerated feeling of well-being, excessive bleeding, facial swelling due to fluid retention, fluid retention, hair loss, hallucinations, hangover effect, hiccups, high or low blood pressure, hives, hostility, impotence, increased sex drive, inflammation of the esophagus, inflammation of the gums, inflammation of the stomach lining, inflammation of the tongue, inflammation of the vagina, intolerance of light, involuntary movement, irrational ideas, irregular heartbeat, jaw or neck pain, lack of muscle coordination, low blood pressure upon standing, low blood sugar, migraine headache, mouth inflammation, neck pain and rigidity, nosebleed, ovarian disorders, paranoid reaction, pelvic pain, pneumonia, rapid breathing, rapid heartbeat, ringing in the ears, severe chest pain, skin inflammation, skin rash, thirst, twitching, uncoordinated movements, urinary disorders, vague feeling of bodily discomfort, vertigo, weight gain

■ *Rare side effects may include:*
Abortion, antisocial behavior, blood in urine, bloody diarrhea, bone disease, breast enlargement, cataracts, colitis, coma, deafness, decreased reflexes, dehydration, double vision, drooping of eyelids, duodenal ulcer, enlarged abdomen, enlargement of liver, enlargement or increased activity of thyroid gland, excess growth of coarse hair on face, chest etc., excess uterine or vaginal hemorrhage, extreme muscle tension, eye bleeding, female milk production, fluid accumulation and swelling in the head, fluid buildup in larynx and lungs, gallstones, glaucoma, gout, heart attack, hepatitis, high blood sugar, hysteria, inability to control bowel movements, increased salivation, inflammation of eyes and eyelids, inflammation of fallopian tubes, inflammation of testes, inflammation of the gallbladder, inflammation of the small intestine, inflammation of tissue below skin, kidney disorders, lung inflammation, menstrual disorders, mouth sores, muscle inflammation or bleeding, muscle spasms, painful sexual intercourse for women, psoriasis, rashes, reddish or purplish spots on the skin, reduction of body temperature, rheumatoid arthritis, seborrhea, shingles, skin discoloration, skin

inflammation and disorders, slowing of heart rate, slurred speech, spitting blood, stomach ulcer, stupor, suicidal thoughts, taste loss, temporary cessation of breathing, tingling sensation around the mouth, tongue discoloration and swelling, urinary tract disorders, vomiting blood, yellow eyes and skin

Why should this drug not be prescribed?
If you are sensitive to or have ever had an allergic reaction to Prozac or similar drugs, you should not take this medication. Make sure that your doctor is aware of any drug reactions that you have experienced.

Do not take this drug while using a MAO inhibitor. (See "Most important fact about this drug.")

Special warnings about this medication
Unless you are directed to do so by your doctor, do not take this medication if you are recovering from a heart attack or if you have kidney or liver disease or diabetes.

Prozac may cause you to become drowsy or less alert and may affect your judgment. Therefore, driving or operating dangerous machinery or participating in any hazardous activity that requires full mental alertness is not recommended.

While taking this medication, you may feel dizzy or light-headed or actually faint when getting up from a lying or sitting position. If getting up slowly doesn't help or if this problem continues, notify your doctor.

If you develop a skin rash or hives while taking Prozac, discontinue use of the medication and notify your doctor immediately.

Prozac should be used with caution if you have a history of seizures. You should discuss all of your medical problems with your doctor before taking this medication.

Possible food and drug interactions when taking this medication

Combining Prozac with MAO inhibitors has caused fatalities.

Do not drink alcohol while taking this medication.

If Prozac is taken with certain other drugs, the effects of either could be increased, decreased, or altered. It is especially important to check with your doctor before combining Prozac with the following:

Diazepam (Valium)
Digitalis (Lanoxin)
Drugs that act on the central nervous system (brain and spinal cord) such as Xanax and Valium
Lithium
Other antidepressants (Elavil)
Tryptophan
Warfarin (Coumadin)

Special information if you are pregnant or breastfeeding

The effects of Prozac during pregnancy have not been adequately studied. If you are pregnant or planning to become pregnant, inform your doctor immediately. This medication may appear in breast milk. If this medication is essential to your health, your doctor may advise you to discontinue breastfeeding your baby until your treatment with Prozac is finished.

Recommended dosage

ADULTS

The usual starting dose is 20 milligrams per day, taken in the morning. Your doctor may increase your dose after several weeks if no improvement is observed. Patients with kidney or liver disease and those taking

other drugs may have their dosages adjusted by their doctor.

Dosages above 20 milligrams daily should be divided into 2 doses per day. Dosage should not exceed 80 milligrams per day.

CHILDREN

The safety and effectiveness of Prozac have not been established in children.

ELDERLY

Your dose should be determined by your doctor.

Overdosage

Any medication taken in excess or in combination with other drugs can cause symptoms of overdose. If you suspect an overdose, seek medical attention immediately.

Symptoms of Prozac overdose include:
Agitation
Nausea
Restlessness
Vomiting

Brand name:

PSORCON

Generic name: Diflorasone diacetate

Why is this drug prescribed?

Psorcon is prescribed for the relief of the inflammatory and itching symptoms of skin disorders that respond to the topical application (applied directly to the skin) of corticosteroids (hormones produced by the body that have potent anti-inflammation effects).

Most important fact about this drug

Absorption of Psorcon through the skin can affect the whole body instead of just the surface of the skin being treated. Although unusual (most common if Psorcon is spread over large areas of the skin), symptoms of corticosteroid hormone excess such as weight gain, reddening and rounding of the face and neck, growth of excess body and facial hair, high blood pressure, emotional disturbances, high blood sugar (loss of energy), and urinary excretion of glucose (increase in frequency of urination) may occur.

The use of this medication over large surface areas, or for prolonged periods, or with airtight dressings or bandages may cause these problems related to excessive systemic absorption. It is recommended that your doctor monitor your condition and periodically check for such problems.

How should you use this medication?
Use this medication exactly as prescribed by your doctor. It is for external use only. Avoid contact with the eyes.

What side effects may occur?
Side effects cannot be anticipated. If any develop or change in intensity, inform your doctor as soon as possible. Only your doctor can determine if it is safe for you to continue taking Psorcon.

■ *Side effects may include:*
Burning, dryness, eruptions resembling acne, excessive discoloring of the skin, excessive growth of hair, inflammation of hair follicles, inflammation around the mouth, irritation, itching, prickly heat, secondary infection, severe inflammation of the skin, softening of the skin, stretch marks, stretching or thinning of the skin

Why should this drug not be prescribed?
If you are sensitive to or have ever had an allergic reaction to diflorasone diacetate or other drugs of this type (antifungals, steroids), you should not take this

medication. Make sure that your doctor is aware of any drug reactions that you have experienced.

Special warnings about this medication
Do not use this drug for any other disorder.

The treated skin area should not be bandaged, covered, or wrapped unless otherwise directed by your doctor.

The use of tight-fitting diapers or plastic pants is not recommended for a child being treated in the diaper area with Psorcon. These garments may act as airtight dressings or bandages.

If an irritation or allergic reaction develops while using Psorcon, notify your doctor.

Possible food and drug interactions when taking this medication
No interactions with food or other drugs have been reported.

Special information if you are pregnant or breastfeeding
If you are pregnant or plan to become pregnant, inform your doctor before using Psorcon. It is not known whether this medication appears in breast milk. If this drug is essential to your health, your doctor may advise you to discontinue breastfeeding until treatment with this medication is finished.

Recommended dosage
ADULTS

A thin film of Psorcon ointment should be applied to the affected area from 1 to 3 times a day, depending on the severity or resistant nature of the condition.

Your doctor may recommend airtight bandages for the management of psoriasis (chronic skin disorder) or stubborn skin conditions. If an infection develops, the

use of airtight dressings should be
discontinued.

CHILDREN

Topical use of Psorcon for children should
be limited to the least amount that is
effective. Long-term treatment may interfere
with the growth and development of
children.

Overdosage

An acute overdosage is unlikely with the use
of Psorcon; however, long-term or
prolonged use can produce systemic effects.
If you suspect an overdose, seek medical
attention immediately.

Brand name:

PYRIDIUM

*Generic name: Phenazopyridine
hydrochloride*

Why is this drug prescribed?

Pyridium is a urinary tract analgesic that helps
relieve the pain, burning, urgency,
frequency, and irritation caused by infection,
trauma, catheters, or various surgical
procedures in the lower urinary tract.
Pyridium is indicated for short-term use
and can only relieve symptoms; it is not a
treatment for the underlying cause of the
symptoms.

Most important fact about this drug

Pyridium produces an orange to red color
in urine and tears, and may stain fabric
and contact lenses.

How should you take this medication?

Pyridium should be taken exactly as
prescribed by your doctor.

Take Pyridium after meals.

If you miss a dose, take it as soon as you
remember. If it is almost time for your
next dose, skip the one you missed and go
back to your regular schedule. Never take
two doses at the same time.

What side effects may occur?

Side effects cannot be anticipated. If any occur
or change in intensity, inform your doctor
as soon as possible. Only your doctor can
determine if it is safe for you to continue
taking Pyridium.

■ *Side effects may include:*
   Abdominal upset
   Headache
   Itching
   Rash
   Severe allergic reaction (rash, difficulty
      breathing, fever, rapid heartbeat,
      convulsions)

Why should this drug not be prescribed?

Pyridium should be avoided if you have
kidney disease, or if you are sensitive to
or have ever had an allergic reaction to
phenazopyridine hydrochloride.

Special warnings about this medication

If your skin or the white of your eyes
develops a yellowish tone, it may indicate
that your kidneys are not eliminating the
medication as they should (especially in
the elderly). Notify your doctor immediately.

Possible food and drug interactions
when taking this medication

No interactions have been reported.

Special information
if you are pregnant or breastfeeding

The effects of Pyridium during pregnancy have
not been adequately studied. If you are
pregnant or plan to become pregnant, inform
your doctor immediately. To date, there
is no available information on the secretion
of Pyridium into human breast milk. If

this medication is essential to your health, your doctor may advise you to stop breastfeeding until your treatment with Pyridium is finished.

Recommended dosage

ADULTS

The usual dose is two 100-milligram tablets, 3 times a day after meals or one 200-milligram tablet, 3 times a day after meals.

Treatment with Pyridium should not last for more than 2 days when used concurrently with an antibacterial medication for the treatment of a urinary tract infection.

Overdosage

Any medication taken in excess can have serious consequences. If you suspect symptoms of a Pyridium overdose, seek medical treatment immediately.

Symptoms of Pyridium overdose may include: Changes in kidney, liver, and blood functioning

Generic name:

QUAZEPAM

See Doral, page 214.

Brand name:

QUESTRAN

Generic name: Cholestyramine

Why is this drug prescribed?

Questran is used to lower cholesterol levels in the blood of patients with primary hypercholesterolemia (too much LDL cholesterol). Hypercholesterolemia is a genetic condition characterized by a lack of the

low-density lipoprotein (LDL) receptors that remove cholesterol from the bloodstream.

This drug is also prescribed for patients with hypertriglyceridemia, a condition in which an excess of fat is stored in the body.

However, Questran is usually prescribed only when a low-fat, low-sugar, and low-cholesterol diet does not lower cholesterol levels enough.

This drug may also be prescribed for itching associated with gallbladder obstruction.

It is available in two forms: Questran and Questran Light. The same instructions apply to both.

Most important fact about this drug

Questran should be considered for use only when reasonable attempts to lower cholesterol levels through a regular routine of diet and exercise have failed. However, taking this medication does not reduce the importance of adhering to a diet and exercise program prescribed for you by your doctor.

Excess body weight may be an important risk factor leading to an unusually high concentration of lipoproteins (cholesterol) in the blood. A low-calorie diet for weight reduction should begin prior to therapy with this drug.

How should you take this medication?

Drink plenty of fluids and mix each packet or level scoopful of this medication in at least 2 to 6 ounces of water or other beverage before taking.

Questran should not be taken in its dry form.

What side effects may occur?

Side effects cannot be anticipated. If any develop or change in intensity, inform your doctor as soon as possible. Only your doctor can determine if it is safe for you to continue taking Questran.

■ *More common side effects include:*
Constipation

■ *Less common or rare side effects may include:*
Abdominal discomfort, anemia, anxiety, arthritis, asthma, backache, black stools, bleeding around the teeth, blood in the urine, brittle bones, burnt odor to urine, diarrhea, difficulty swallowing, dizziness, drowsiness, fainting, fatigue, fluid retention, gas, headache, heartburn, hiccups, hives, increased sex drive, increased tendency to bleed due to vitamin K deficiency, indigestion, inflammation of the eye, inflammation of the pancreas, irritation around the anal area, irritation of the skin and tongue, joint pain, lack or loss of appetite, muscle pain, nausea, night blindness due to vitamin A deficiency, painful or difficult urination, rash, rectal bleeding and/or pain, ringing in the ears, shortness of breath, sour taste, swollen glands, tingling sensation, ulcer attack, vertigo, vitamin D deficiency, vomiting, weight gain or loss, wheezing

Why should this drug not be prescribed?
If you are sensitive to or have ever had an allergic reaction to Questran or similar drugs, you should not take this medication. Make sure that your doctor is aware of any drug reactions that you have experienced.

Unless you are directed to do so by your doctor, do not take this medication if you are being treated for gallbladder obstruction.

Special warnings about this medication
If you have phenylketonuria, a genetic disorder, check with your doctor before taking Questran because this product contains phenylalanine.

If you are being treated for any disease that contributes to increased blood cholesterol, such as hypothyroidism (reduced thyroid function), diabetes, nephrotic syndrome (kidney and blood vessel disorder), dysproteinemia, or obstructive liver disease, consult with your doctor before taking this medication.

Questran should begin to reduce cholesterol levels during the first month of therapy. If adequate reduction of cholesterol is not obtained, this medication should be discontinued. Therefore, it is important that your doctor check your progress regularly.

The use of this medication may produce or worsen constipation and aggravate hemorrhoids. If this happens, inform your doctor. Only your doctor can determine if your dose needs to be reduced or discontinued.

The prolonged use of Questran may change acidity in the bloodstream, especially in younger and smaller patients in whom the doses are relatively higher. Again, it is important that you or your child be checked by your doctor on a regular basis.

Possible food and drug interactions when taking this medication
If Questran is taken with certain other drugs, the effects of either could be increased, decreased, or altered. It is especially important to check with your doctor before taking Questran with the following:

Digitalis (Lanoxin)
The diuretic drug chlorothiazide (Diuril)
Penicillin G
Phenobarbital
Phenylbutazone (Butazolidin)
Propranolol (Inderal)
Sulfonylureas (oral diabetes drugs such as DiaBeta and Diabinese)
Tetracycline (Achromycin V)

Thyroid medication (Synthroid)
Warfarin (Coumadin)

Your doctor may recommend that you take other medication at least 1 hour before or 4 to 6 hours after you take Questran.

If you are taking a potentially harmful drug such as digitalis (Lanoxin) and your dose was adjusted to a maintenance level while taking Questran, stopping Questran could be hazardous, since you might experience exaggerated effects of the digitalis. Consult with your doctor before discontinuing Questran.

This drug may interfere with normal digestion and absorption of fats, including fat-soluble vitamins such as A, D, and K. If supplements of vitamins A, D, and K are essential to your health, your doctor may prescribe an alternative form of these vitamins.

There are no special considerations regarding alcohol use with this medication.

Special information
if you are pregnant or breastfeeding
The effects of Questran during pregnancy have not been adequately studied. If you are pregnant or plan to become pregnant, inform your doctor immediately. Because this medication can interfere with vitamin absorption, it may have an effect on nursing infants. If this drug is essential to your health, your doctor may advise you to discontinue breastfeeding until your treatment is finished.

Recommended dosage

ADULTS

The recommended starting dose is 1 single-dose packet or 1 level scoopful, 1 to 2 times daily. The usual maintenance dosage is a total of 2 to 4 packets or scoopfuls

daily divided into 2 doses. The maximum daily dose is 6 packets or scoopfuls. Although the recommended dosing schedule is 2 times daily, your doctor may ask you to take Questran in 1 to 6 doses per day.

CHILDREN

Experience with the use of Questran in infants and children is limited. If this medication is essential to your child's health, follow your doctor's recommended dosing schedule.

ELDERLY

This drug should be used with caution in elderly patients.

Overdosage
There have been no reported cases of overdose with Questran. However, should you suspect an overdose, seek medical attention immediately.

The main potential harm of an overdose would be obstruction of the stomach and intestines.

Brand name:

QUINIDEX EXTENTABS

Generic name: Quinidine sulfate

Why is this drug prescribed?
Quinidex Extentabs is used to treat specific types of irregular heartbeat rhythms (arrhythmias). They are generally divided into two main types: heartbeats that are faster than normal (tachycardia) and heartbeats that are slower than normal (bradycardia). Arrhythmias are often caused by drugs or disease but can occur in otherwise healthy people with no history of heart disease or other illness.

Most important fact about this drug
This medication must be swallowed whole to insure its controlled-release effect.

How should you take this medication?

Quinidex Extentabs should be taken exactly as prescribed by your doctor.

They should be taken whole, not crushed or chewed, with a full glass of water, milk, or other liquid.

You should take this medication while you are sitting up or standing. This will make it easier to swallow the tablets.

What side effects may occur?

Side effects cannot be anticipated. If any develop or change in intensity, inform your doctor as soon as possible. Only your doctor can determine if it is safe for you to continue taking Quinidex Extentabs.

■ *More common side effects include:*
Abdominal pain
Cinchonism (a sensitivity reaction.
    Symptoms include: ringing in the
    ears, loss of hearing, dizziness,
    light-headedness, headache,
    nausea, and/or disturbed vision)
Diarrhea
Hepatitis
Inflammation of the esophagus (gullet)
Loss of appetite
Nausea
Vomiting

■ *Less common or rare side effects may*
include:
Allergic reaction (symptoms include:
swelling of face, lips, tongue, throat,
arms, and legs, sore throat, fever and chills,
difficulty swallowing, chest pain),
anemia, apprehension, asthma attack,
blood clots, blurred vision, changes
in skin pigmentation, collagen vascular
disease (lupus erythematosus),
confusion, delirium, depression, dilated
pupils, disturbed color perception,
double vision, eczema, excitement,
fainting, fever, fluid retention,
flushing, headache, hearing changes,
hives, inability to breathe, intense
itching, intolerance of light, joint pain,
lack of coordination, low blood
pressure, mental decline, muscle pain,
night blindness, psoriasis, rash,
reddish or purplish spots below the skin,
severe asthma attack, skin eruptions,
skin sensitivity to light, vertigo, vision
changes

Why should this drug not be prescribed?

Quinidex Extentabs should not be taken if you have heart block (conduction disorder), myasthenia gravis (abnormal muscle weakness), or if you are sensitive to or have ever had an allergic reaction to quinidine or cinchona derivatives. (Quinidine comes from the bark of the cinchona tree.)

Special warnings about this medication

Concentrations of digoxin in your blood may increase or even double when digoxin is taken with Quinidex Extentabs. Your doctor may need to reduce the amount of digoxin you take.

If you have poorly controlled cardiovascular disease, Quinidex Extentabs should be used cautiously. It can cause low blood pressure, slow heartbeat, or heart block.

This medication should be carefully monitored if you have partial heart block. It can produce complete heart block (heart disorder that causes an irregular heartbeat).

Quinidex Extentabs should be used cautiously if you have kidney, heart, or liver disease. Your doctor should check your blood count and liver and kidney function periodically during long-term therapy.

There have been cases of liver damage due to quinidine sensitivity. If you develop an unexplained fever, especially when you begin taking quinidine, your doctor should monitor your liver function for the first 4 to 8 weeks of therapy. Symptoms usually disappear when quinidine is stopped.

There have been cases of severe allergic reaction to quinidine, especially during the first few weeks of therapy. Discuss any allergic reactions you have experienced with your doctor.

Possible food and drug interactions when taking this medication

If Quinidex Extentabs is taken with certain other drugs, the effects of either could be increased, decreased, or altered. It is especially important to check with your doctor before combining Quinidex Extentabs with the following:

Amiodarone (Cordarone)
Anticholinergics such as Bentyl
Blood thinners such as Coumadin
Carbonic anhydrase inhibitors such as Diamox
Cholinergics such as Physostigmine
Cimetidine (Tagamet)
Decamethonium
Digoxin (Lanoxin)
Nifedipine (Procardia)
Phenobarbital
Phenothiazine products such as the major tranquilizer Thorazine
Phenytoin (Dilantin)
Ranitidine (Zantac)
Reserpine (Serpasil)
Rifampin (Rifadin)
Sodium bicarbonate
Succinylcholine (Anectine)
Thiazide diuretics such as Dyazide and HydroDIURIL
Tubocurarine
Verapamil (Calan)

Special information if you are pregnant or breastfeeding

The effects of Quinidex Extentabs during pregnancy have not been adequately studied.

If you are pregnant or plan to become pregnant, inform your doctor immediately. Quinidex Extentabs appears in breast milk and can affect a nursing infant. If this medication is essential to your health, your doctor may advise you to discontinue breastfeeding until your treatment is finished.

Recommended dosage

ADULTS

The usual dosage is 1 or 2 Quinidex Extentabs tablets every 8 to 12 hours.

CHILDREN

The safety and effectiveness of this drug in children have not been established.

ELDERLY

This drug should be used with caution in elderly patients. Your doctor will adjust your medication.

Overdosage

Any medication taken in excess can have serious consequences. If you suspect an overdose, seek medical treatment immediately.

The symptoms of Quinidex Extentabs overdose may include:
Abnormal heart rhythms
Changes in heart function
Coma
Decreased breathing
Decreased production of urine
Fluid in the lungs
Low blood pressure
Seizures

Generic name:

QUINIDINE SULFATE

See Quinidex, page 530.

Generic name:

QUININE SULFATE

See Quinamm, page 533.

Brand name:

QUINAMM

Generic name: Quinine sulfate

Why is this drug prescribed?

Quinamm is frequently prescribed to help prevent painful leg cramps at night.

Most important fact about this drug

The active ingredient of Quinamm is cinchona alkaloid. It can cause harm to the fetus when given to a pregnant woman. Repeated doses or overdosage of quinine may cause ringing in the ears, headache, nausea, and disturbed vision.

How should you take this medication?

Take Quinamm exactly as prescribed by your doctor.

Once you have had several consecutive nights free of leg cramps, you may no longer need Quinamm. At this point, your doctor may ask you to stop taking the medication for a trial period.

What side effects may occur?

Side effects cannot be anticipated. If any develop or change in intensity, inform your doctor as soon as possible. Only your doctor can determine if it is safe for you to continue taking Quinamm.

■ *Side effects may include:*
Angina, apprehension, asthma, blurred vision, confusion, deafness, double vision, facial swelling, fainting, fever, flushing, headache, hepatitis, hives, intolerance to light, itching, nausea, purplish "bruises," rash, restlessness, ringing in the ears, stomach pain, sweating, vertigo, vision disturbances, vomiting.

Why should this drug not be prescribed?

Do not take this medication if you have ever had an allergic reaction to it or to quinine.

Special warnings about this medication

Typical symptoms of quinine allergy are breathing difficulty, fever, extreme flushing, intense skin itching, skin rashes, ringing in the ears, upset stomach, and vision disturbances. More rarely, quinine allergy causes asthma or damage to the red blood cells. If you develop any such symptoms, you should immediately stop taking Quinamm and seek medical attention.

Possible food and drug interactions when taking this medication

If Quinamm is taken with certain other drugs, the effects of either could be increased, decreased, or altered. It is especially important to check with your doctor before combining Quinamm with the following:

Acetazolamide (Diamox)
Aluminum-containing antacids such as
    ALternaGEL, Basaljel, and others
Baking soda (used as an antacid)
Digitoxin (Crystodigin)
Digoxin (Lanoxin, Lanoxicaps)
Warfarin (Coumadin, Panwarfin, other blood
    thinners)

Special information
if you are pregnant or breastfeeding

Quinine may cause birth defects or stillbirth. Be very sure you are not pregnant before you start taking Quinamm and avoid getting pregnant while you are taking it. Quinine may appear in breast milk and could affect a nursing infant. If this medication is essential to your health, your doctor may advise you to discontinue breastfeeding until your treatment is finished.

Recommended dosage

ADULTS

The usual dose is 1 tablet taken at bedtime. If needed, however, 2 tablets may be taken nightly—1 following the evening meal and 1 at bedtime.

Overdosage

Any medication taken in excess can have serious consequences. If you suspect an overdose, seek medical attention immediately.

Symptoms of mild Quinamm overdose may include:
Dizziness
Intestinal cramps
Rash
Ringing in the ears

Symptoms of large Quinamm overdose may include:
Apprehension
Confusion
Convulsions
Fever
Headache
Vomiting

In several instances, a large overdose of quinine has caused temporary blindness, with some residual permanent vision loss.

Generic name:

RAMIPRIL

See Altace, page 18.

Generic name:

RANITIDINE HYDROCHLORIDE

See Zantac, page 692.

Brand name:

REGLAN

Generic name: Metoclopramide hydrochloride

Why is this drug prescribed?

Reglan increases the contractions of the stomach and small intestine, helping the passage of food. It is given to treat the symptoms of diabetic gastroparesis (such as vomiting, nausea, heartburn, feeling of indigestion, persistent fullness after meals, and appetite loss). It is also given to treat nausea and vomiting caused by cancer chemotherapy and surgery. Reglan is also used, for short periods, to treat symptoms of heartburn in patients with gastroesophageal reflux disorder (backflow of stomach contents into the esophagus).

Reglan may also be used to facilitate certain medical procedures, such as threading a tube into the small bowel or taking a barium X-ray of the stomach or intestine.

Reglan is available in tablet, syrup, or injectable form.

Most important fact about this drug

Reglan may cause severe depression and thoughts of suicide. If you have suffered from depression in the past, you should take Reglan only if the expected benefit outweighs the potential risk.

How should you take this medication?

Take Reglan exactly as prescribed. Take the medication 30 minutes before a meal. Do not freeze Reglan syrup.

If you suffer from heartburn that occurs only intermittently or only at certain times of day, your doctor may want you to schedule your Reglan therapy around those times.

You will probably take Reglan for only 4 to 12 weeks. Continuous treatment beyond 12 weeks is not recommended.

If you have diabetic "lazy stomach" (gastric stasis) that tends to recur, your doctor may want you to take Reglan at the first sign of a recurrence.

What side effects may occur?
Side effects cannot be anticipated. If any develop or change in intensity, inform your doctor as soon as possible. Only your doctor can determine if it is safe for you to continue taking Reglan.

■ *More common side effects may include:*
Drowsiness
Fatigue
Lassitude
Restlessness

■ *Less common side effects may include:*
Asthma, blistering, blood pressure changes (higher or lower), breast enlargement (in men), confusion, continual discharge of milk from the breasts, depression, diarrhea, dizziness, fluid retention, headache, hives, impotence, insomnia, menstrual irregularities, nausea, pounding or slow heartbeat, rash, slow movement, swollen tongue or larynx, tremor, urinary frequency, urinary incontinence, vision problems

Rarely, Reglan may cause hallucinations.

Reglan may cause symptoms similar to Parkinson's disease, such as slow movements, rigidity, tremor, or a mask-like facial appearance.

Reglan may produce tardive dyskinesia, a syndrome of involuntary facial movements.

Reglan may produce involuntary movements of the arms and legs, grimacing, tongue-thrusting, locking of the jaw, and sometimes loud or labored breathing.

Reglan may cause intense restlessness with associated symptoms such as anxiety, foot-tapping, pacing, inability to sit still, jitteriness, and insomnia. These symptoms may disappear as your body gets used to Reglan, or if your dosage is reduced.

Why should this drug not be prescribed?
Do not take Reglan if you are sensitive to it or have ever had an allergic reaction to it.

You should not take Reglan if you have a condition such as obstruction, perforation, or hemorrhage of the stomach or small bowel that might be aggravated by increased stomach and small-bowel movement.

If you have pheochromocytoma (a nonmalignant tumor that causes hypertension), do not take Reglan; it could trigger a dangerous jump in blood pressure.

Do not take Reglan if you have epilepsy; it could increase the frequency and severity of seizures.

If you are taking a drug that is likely to cause extrapyramidal side effects (tremors, jerks, grimaces, or writhing movements), do not take Reglan; it could make such symptoms more severe.

If you have Parkinson's disease, you should be given Reglan cautiously or not at all, since the drug may make your Parkinson's symptoms worse.

Special warnings about this medication
Because Reglan may make you drowsy and impair your coordination, you should not drive, climb, or perform hazardous tasks until you know how the medication affects you.

Reglan should be used with caution if you have high blood pressure.

Possible food and drug interactions when taking this medication

If Reglan is taken with certain other drugs, the effects of either could be increased, decreased, or altered. It is especially important to check with your doctor before combining Reglan with the following:

Acetaminophen (Panadol, Tylenol, and others)
Alcoholic beverages
Anticholinergic drugs such as Bentyl and
    Pro-Banthine
Cimetidine (Tagamet)
Digoxin (Lanoxin)
Hypnotic drugs
Insulin
MAO inhibitor antidepressants such as
    Marplan, Nardil, and Parnate
Levodopa (Dopar, Sinemet)
Narcotic painkillers such as Percocet,
    Demerol, and others
Sleeping pills such as Dalmane, Halcion,
    Restoril, and others
Tetracycline (Achromycin, Panmycin, Tetracyn
    and others)
Tranquilizers such as Paxipam, Valium, Xanax,
    and others

If you take insulin for diabetes, your insulin dosage or dosing schedule may have to be adjusted while you are taking Reglan.

Special information if you are pregnant or breastfeeding

If you are pregnant or plan to become pregnant, inform your doctor immediately. Reglan should be used during pregnancy only if it is clearly needed. Reglan does find its way into human milk. Thus, caution is advised when Reglan is taken during breastfeeding.

Recommended dosage

ADULTS

Relief of Symptomatic Gastroesophageal Reflux
The usual recommended dose is 10 milligrams to 15 milligrams of Reglan by mouth, up to 4 times a day, 30 minutes before each meal and at bedtime, depending upon symptoms being treated and effectiveness of this dose. Usual time of treatment is 12 weeks.

If symptoms occur only intermittently or at specific times of the day, your doctor may give you a single dose of up to 20 milligrams as a preventive measure.

Relief of Symptoms Associated with Diabetic Gastric Stasis
The usual recommended dose is 10 milligrams 30 minutes before each meal and at bedtime for 2 to 8 weeks.

ELDERLY

Relief of Symptomatic Gastroesophageal Reflux
The usual recommended dose is 5 milligrams per dose by mouth.

Overdosage

Although no specific information is available, any medication taken in excess can have serious consequences. If you suspect an overdose of Reglan, seek medical attention immediately.

Generic name:

RESERPINE, HYDRALAZINE AND HYDROCHLOROTHIAZIDE

See Ser-Ap-Es, page 573.

Brand name:

RESTORIL

Generic name: Temazepam

Why is this drug prescribed?
Restoril is used for the relief of insomnia (difficulty in falling asleep, waking up frequently at night or waking up early in the morning). It belongs to a class of drugs known as benzodiazepines.

Most important fact about this drug
Tolerance and dependence can occur with the long-term use of Restoril. This drug should be withdrawn gradually. You may experience withdrawal symptoms if you stop using it abruptly; your insomnia may worsen. Discontinue or change your dose only on advice of your doctor.

How should you take this medication?
There are no special instructions.

Take this medication exactly as prescribed by your doctor.

What side effects may occur?
Side effects cannot be anticipated. If any develop or change in intensity, inform your doctor as soon as possible. Only your doctor can determine if it is safe for you to continue taking Restoril.

■ *More common side effects may include:*
Confusion
Dizziness
Drowsiness
Exaggerated feeling of well-being
Relaxed feeling
Sluggishness or unresponsiveness

■ *Less common or rare side effects may include:*
Diarrhea, excitement, falling, hallucinations, hyperactivity, involuntary eye movement, lack of concentration, lack of coordination, loss of appetite, loss of equilibrium, rapid, strong heartbeat, tremors, weakness

■ *Side effects due to rapid decrease in or abrupt withdrawal from Restoril:*
Abdominal and muscle cramps, convulsions, feeling of discomfort, inability to fall asleep or stay asleep, sweating, tremors, vomiting

Why should this drug not be prescribed?
If you are pregnant or plan to become pregnant, you should not take this medication because of the potential risk to the fetus.

Special warnings about this medication
Restoril may cause you to become drowsy or less alert; therefore, driving or operating dangerous machinery or participating in any hazardous activity that requires full mental alertness is not recommended.

If you are severely depressed or have suffered from severe depression, consult with your doctor before taking this medication.

If you have impaired kidney or liver function or chronic respiratory or lung disease, use of this drug should be discussed with your doctor.

Possible food and drug interactions when taking this medication
Restoril may intensify the effects of alcohol. Do not drink alcohol while taking this medication.

If Restoril is taken with certain other drugs, the effects of either could be increased, decreased, or altered. It is especially important to check with your doctor before combining Restoril with the following:

Antihistamines such as Benadryl

Drugs for anxiety or sleep disorders, such as Valium or Xanax.

Special information
if you are pregnant or breastfeeding

Do not take Restoril if you are pregnant or planning to become pregnant. There is an increased risk of birth defects. This drug may appear in breast milk and could affect a nursing infant. If this medication is essential to your health, your doctor may advise you to discontinue breastfeeding until your treatment with this medication is finished.

Recommended dosage

ADULTS

The usual recommended dose is 30 milligrams at bedtime; however, 15 milligrams may be all that is necessary. Your dose should be individualized to your needs by your doctor.

CHILDREN

The safety and effectiveness of Restoril have not been established in children under 18 years of age.

ELDERLY

Dosage should be limited to the smallest effective amount to avoid oversedation, dizziness, confusion or lack of muscle coordination. The usual recommended initial dose is 15 milligrams.

Overdosage

Any medication taken in excess can cause symptoms of overdose. If you suspect an overdose, seek medical attention immediately.

The symptoms of Restoril overdose may include:
Coma
Confusion
Diminished reflexes

Loss of coordination
Low blood pressure
Labored or difficult breathing
Seizures
Sleepiness
Slurred speech

Brand name:

RETIN-A

Generic name: Tretinoin

Why is this drug prescribed?

Retin-A is prescribed for the treatment of acne vulgaris (an inflammatory disease of the skin, usually affecting persons in puberty or early adult years).

Most important fact about this drug

While using Retin-A, exposure to sunlight, including sunlamps, should be kept to a minimum. If you have a sunburn, do not use this medication until you have fully recovered. Use of sunscreen products and protective clothing over treated areas is recommended when exposure to the sun cannot be avoided. Weather extremes, such as wind and cold, should also be avoided while using Retin-A.

How should you use this medication?

Retin-A gel, cream, or liquid should be applied once a day, at bedtime, to the skin where acne appears, using enough to lightly cover the affected area. The liquid may be applied using a fingertip, gauze pad, or cotton swab. If gauze or cotton is used, avoid oversaturation, which might cause the liquid to run into areas where treatment is not intended.

You may use cosmetics while being treated with Retin-A; however, you should thoroughly cleanse the areas to be treated before applying the medication.

What side effects may occur?

If you have sensitive skin, the use of this medication may cause your skin to become excessively red, puffy, blistered, or crusted. If this happens, notify your doctor, who may recommend that you discontinue Retin-A until your skin returns to normal, or adjust the medication to a level that you can tolerate.

An unusual darkening of the skin or lack of color of the skin may occur temporarily with repeated application of Retin-A.

Why should this drug not be prescribed?

If you are sensitive to or have ever had an allergic reaction to any of the ingredients in Retin-A, you should not use this medication. Make sure that your doctor is aware of any drug reactions that you have experienced.

The safety and effectiveness of long-term use of this product in the treatment of disorders other than acne have not been established.

Special warnings about this medication

Retin-A should be kept away from the eyes, mouth, angles of the nose, and mucous membranes.

If use of this medication causes an abnormal redness or peeling of the skin where it has been applied, notify your doctor. He may suggest that you use Retin-A less frequently, discontinue use temporarily, or discontinue use altogether.

If you have eczema (skin inflammation consisting of itching and small blisters that ooze and crust over), use this medication with extreme caution, as it may cause severe irritation.

If a sensitivity reaction or chemical irritation occurs, notify your doctor. He may suggest that you discontinue using this medication.

Retin-A may cause a brief feeling of warmth or slight stinging when applied.

During the early weeks of therapy, a worsening of acne lesions may occur due to the action of the medication on deep, previously unseen lesions. This is not a reason to discontinue therapy, but do notify your doctor if it occurs.

Possible food and drug interactions when taking this medication

If Retin-A is taken with certain other drugs, the effects of either could be increased, decreased, or altered. It is especially important to check with your doctor before combining Retin-A with the following:

Preparations containing sulfur (ointments and other preparations used to treat skin disorders and infections)
Resorcinol (a drug, used in ointments to treat acne, that causes skin to peel)
Salicylic acid (a drug that causes skin to peel and kills bacteria and fungi)

"Resting" a patient's skin is recommended after treatment with one of the above preparations and before treatment with Retin-A.

Caution should be exercised when using Retin-A in combination with other topical medications, medicated or abrasive soaps and cleansers, soaps and cosmetics that have a strong drying effect, and products with high concentrations of alcohol, astringents, spices, or lime.

Special information if you are pregnant or breastfeeding

There are no adequate and well-controlled studies in pregnant women. If you are pregnant or plan to become pregnant, inform your doctor immediately. It is not known if this drug appears in breast milk. If Retin-A is essential to your treatment, your doctor may advise you to discontinue breastfeeding until your treatment is finished.

Recommended dosage

ADULTS

Any change in formulation, drug concentration, or dose frequency should be closely monitored by your doctor for response and skin tolerance.

Results should be noticed after 2 to 3 weeks of treatment with this medication. More than 6 weeks of treatment may be needed before definite beneficial effects are seen.

Once acne has responded satisfactorily, it may be possible to maintain the improvement with less frequent applications or other dosage forms.

Overdosage

If medication is applied excessively, no faster or better results will be obtained, and marked redness, peeling, or discomfort may occur.

Brand name:

RETROVIR

Generic name: Zidovudine

Why is this drug prescribed?

Retrovir is prescribed for adult patients with human immunodeficiency virus (HIV). HIV causes the immune system to break down so that it can no longer respond effectively to infection. This virus leads to the fatal disease known as acquired immune deficiency syndrome (AIDS) or AIDS-related complex (ARC). Retrovir slows down the progress of HIV.

This drug is also prescribed for HIV-infected children over 3 months of age who have symptoms of HIV or who have no symptoms but, through testing, have shown evidence of impaired immunity.

Signs and symptoms consistent with HIV disease are significant weight loss, fever, diarrhea, secondary infections, and problems with the nervous system.

Most important fact about this drug

The long-term effects of treatment with zidovudine are unknown. However, treatment with this drug may lead to blood diseases, including granulocytopenia (a severe blood disorder characterized by a sharp decrease of certain types of white blood cells called granulocytes) and severe anemia requiring blood transfusions. This is especially true in patients with more advanced disease and those who start treatment later in the course of their infection.

Also, because Retrovir is not a cure for HIV infections or AIDS, patients may continue to develop complications, including opportunistic infections (infections not usually seen in humans that develop when the immune system falters). Therefore, frequent blood counts by your doctor are strongly advised. Notify your doctor immediately of any changes in your general health.

How should you take this medication?

Take this medication exactly as prescribed by your doctor. Do not share this medication with anyone and do not exceed your recommended dosage. Take it at even intervals every four hours around the clock.

What side effects may occur?

Side effects cannot be anticipated. If any develop or change in intensity, inform your doctor as soon as possible. Only your doctor can determine if it is safe for you to continue taking Retrovir.

The frequency and severity of side effects associated with the use of Retrovir are greater in patients whose infection is more advanced when treatment is started. Sometimes it is difficult to distinguish side effects from underlying signs of HIV disease or infections caused by HIV.

■ *More common side effects may include:*
Inability to fall or stay asleep
Nausea
Severe headache
Muscle pain

■ *Less common side effects may include:*
Changes in taste, diarrhea, difficulty breathing, dizziness, excessive perspiration, fatigue, fever, general feeling of illness, indigestion, lack or loss of appetite, pins and needles sensation, rash, shortness of breath, sleepiness, stomach or intestinal pain, vomiting, weakness

■ *Rare side effects may include:*
Acne, anxiety, back pain, belching, bleeding from the rectum, bleeding gums, body odor, changeable emotions, chest pain, chills, confusion, constipation, cough, decreased mental sharpness, depression, dimness of vision, excess sensitivity to pain, fainting, flu-like symptoms, frequent urination, gas, generalized swelling of lymph nodes ("glands"), hearing loss, hives, hoarseness, inability or difficulty swallowing, increase in urine volume, inflammation of the sinuses or nose, itching, joint pain, light intolerance, mouth sores, muscle spasm, nervousness, nosebleed, painful or difficult urination, sore throat, swelling of the lip, swelling of the tongue, tremor, twitching, vertigo

Why should this drug not be prescribed?
If you have ever had a life-threatening allergic reaction to Retrovir, you should not be prescribed this drug.

Special warnings about this medication
This drug has been studied for only a limited period of time. Long-term safety and effectiveness are not known, especially for patients who are in a less advanced stage of AIDS or ARC, and for those using the drug over a prolonged period of time.

If you develop a blood disease, you may require a blood transfusion, and your doctor may reduce your dose or take you off the drug altogether. Make sure that your doctor monitors your blood count on a regular basis.

The use of Retrovir has *not* been shown to reduce the risk of transmission of HIV to others through sexual contact or blood contamination.

Retrovir should be used with extreme caution in patients who have a bone marrow disease.

Sensitization reactions (development of antibodies that weaken or destroy a particular substance) have occurred in patients taking Retrovir. If you develop a rash, notify your doctor.

Because there are not much data available concerning the use of this drug in patients with impaired kidney or liver function, check with your doctor before using Retrovir if you have either problem.

Possible food and drug interactions when taking this medication
If Retrovir is taken with certain other drugs, the effects of either could be increased, decreased, or altered. It is especially important to check with your doctor before combining Retrovir with the following:

Acetaminophen (Tylenol)
Amphotericin B (Fungizone, a drug used to treat fungal infections)
Doxorubicin (Adriamycin, a cancer drug)
Aspirin
Dapsone (a drug used to treat leprosy)
Flucytosine (Ancobon)
Indomethacin (Indocin)
Interferon (Intron A, Roferon)
Pentamidine (NebuPent, Pentam)

Phenytoin (Dilantin, an anticonvulsant)
Probenecid (Benemid, an antigout drug)
Vinblastine (Velban, a cancer drug)
Vincristine (Oncovin, a cancer drug)

The use of drugs such as acetaminophen may increase the risk of Retrovir becoming poisonous to your system.

The combined use of phenytoin and Retrovir should be monitored by your doctor because of the possibility of seizures.

Special Information
if you are pregnant or breastfeeding

The effects of Retrovir during pregnancy have not been adequately studied. If you are pregnant or plan to become pregnant, inform your doctor immediately. This drug may appear in breast milk and could affect a nursing infant. If this medication is essential to your health, your doctor may advise you to discontinue breastfeeding until your treatment is finished.

Recommended dosage

ADULTS

All dosages of Retrovir must be very closely monitored by your physician. The following dosages are general in nature; your physician will tailor the dose to your specific condition.

Capsules and Syrup
For adults who have symptoms of HIV infection, including AIDS, the recommended starting dose is 200 milligrams (two 100-milligram capsules or 4 teaspoonfuls of syrup) taken every 4 hours. After 1 month, your doctor may reduce your dose to 100 milligrams taken every 4 hours.

For adults with asymptomatic HIV infection (HIV infection with no symptoms), the recommended dose is 100 milligrams taken every 4 hours while awake.

CHILDREN

The recommended starting dose for children 3 months to 12 years of age is determined by body size. While the dose should not exceed 200 milligrams every 6 hours, it must still be individually determined. Safety and efficacy have not been determined for infants under 3 months of age.

Overdosage

Any medication taken in excess can have serious consequences. If you suspect an overdose, seek emergency medical treatment immediately.

Symptoms of Retrovir overdose may include:

Nausea
Vomiting

Brand name:

RHEUMATREX

See Methotrexate, page 368.

Brand name:

RIDAURA

Generic name: Auranofin

Why is this drug prescribed?

Ridaura, a gold preparation, is given to help treat rheumatoid arthritis. Ridaura is taken by mouth, unlike other gold compounds, which are given by injection. It is only recommended for people who have not been helped sufficiently by other anti-inflammatory drugs (Anaprox, Dolobid, Indocin, Motrin, and others). Ridaura should be part of a comprehensive arthritis treatment program that also includes non-drug forms of therapy.

You are most likely to benefit from Ridaura if you have active, early-stage joint inflammation.

Most important fact about this drug

Unlike the anti-inflammatory medications, Ridaura does not take effect immediately. In fact, you may have to wait for 3 to 6 months to get any benefit from Ridaura. Ridaura prevents or suppresses joint swelling, but does not cure rheumatoid arthritis.

How should you take this medication?

Take Ridaura exactly as prescribed by your doctor.

You should read the patient information sheet provided with the prescription of Ridaura.

You should observe good oral hygiene during therapy with Ridaura.

Gold dermatitis (inflammation of skin) with rash may develop with this drug and could lead to actinic rash (rash aggravated by sunlight). Minimize exposure to artificial ultraviolet light or sunlight.

What side effects may occur?

Side effects cannot be anticipated. If any side effects develop or change in intensity, tell your doctor immediately. Only your doctor can determine whether it is safe for you to continue taking Ridaura. Ridaura causes loose stools or diarrhea in about half of all people who take it; there may also be indigestion, stomach pain and gas, loss of appetite, vomiting, or nausea.

■ *Other commonly reported side effects include:*
Blood-cell abnormalities which may result in bleeding, bloody or black stools, easy bruising, fever, gold dermatitis (inflammation of skin), hair loss, hives, itching, metallic taste, "pinkeye," rash, sores in the mouth

Why should this drug not be prescribed?

Do not take Ridaura if you have ever had any of the following reactions to a medication containing gold:

Anaphylaxis (life-threatening allergic reaction)
Blood or bone marrow abnormality
Fibrosis (scar tissue formation) of the lungs
Serious bowel inflammation
Skin disorder in which skin peeled off in sheets

Special warnings about this medication

You are at risk for various adverse effects from Ridaura, and should be monitored especially closely while taking the medication if you have any of the following:

History of a blood-cell abnormality
Inflammatory bowel disease
Kidney disease
Liver disease
Skin rash

Your doctor may order periodic blood and urine tests to check for unwanted effects. Like other medications containing gold, Ridaura may cause serious blood abnormalities. If you start to bruise easily, or develop small red or purplish skin discolorations, you should immediately stop taking Ridaura and have blood tests, including a platelet count.

Ridaura may cause protein or microscopic amounts of blood to spill into your urine. If a urine test shows that this is happening, you should stop taking Ridaura immediately.

Gold compounds may cause your skin to become more sensitive to sunlight, so you may need to limit your exposure to the sun and wear a sunscreen.

Possible food and drug interactions when taking this medication

If Ridaura is taken with certain other drugs, the effects of either could be increased, decreased, or altered. It is especially important to check with your doctor before combining Ridaura with phenytoin (Dilantin).

Special information if you are pregnant or breastfeeding

If you are pregnant or plan to become pregnant, inform your doctor immediately. Because Ridaura may cause birth defects, it should not be taken during pregnancy.

Likewise, Ridaura should not be taken during breastfeeding, because the gold that it contains finds its way into breast milk. If you are a new mother, you may have to choose between taking Ridaura and breastfeeding your baby.

Recommended dosage

ADULTS

The usual recommended dosage of Ridaura is 6 milligrams daily in a single dose or 2 small doses.

Overdosage

Any medication taken in excess can have serious consequences. If you suspect an overdose of Ridaura, seek medical attention immediately.

Brand name:

RIFADIN

Generic name: Rifampin
Other brand name: Rimactane

Why is this drug prescribed?

Rifadin is an antituberculosis drug used to treat all forms of tuberculosis. Rifadin is always used in combination with at least one other antituberculosis drug, usually either isoniazid, pyrazinamide, or ethambutol. Rifadin is also used to eliminate a bacteria that causes meningitis in people who are carriers of the disease but have no symptoms of the illness. Rifadin is not effective as a treatment for active meningitis.

Most important fact about this drug

Rifadin may cause your urine, feces, saliva, sputum, sweat, and tears to turn a red-orange color. This is to be expected and is not harmful. It may also permanently discolor soft contact lenses.

How should you take this medication?

Take Rifadin exactly as prescribed by your doctor. Do not stop taking Rifadin without consulting your doctor.

Rifadin should be taken on an empty stomach, either one hour before or two hours after a meal.

If you are taking Rifadin for tuberculosis, treatment usually lasts for 6 months to 2 years.

If you are unable to swallow the capsule, you may mix content of the capsule with soft foods, such as applesauce or jelly.

Avoid alcoholic beverages.

What side effects may occur?

Side effects cannot be anticipated. If any develop or change in intensity, tell your doctor immediately. Only your doctor can determine whether it is safe for you to continue taking Rifadin.

■ *More common side effects may include:* Behavioral changes, cramps, decrease in blood pressure, diarrhea, dizziness, drowsiness, fatigue, fever, "flu-like" symptoms (fever, chills, headache, dizziness, bone pain), flushing and itching (with or without rash), gas, headache, heartburn, inability to concentrate, loss of appetite, menstrual changes, mental confusion, muscular weakness or incoordination, nausea, pain and numbness in arms and legs, shortness of breath, stomach upset, swelling of the face, arms and legs, vision changes, vomiting, wheezing, yellow eyes and skin

■ *Less common or rare side effects may include:*
Blisters, bloodshot eyes, hives, itching, rash, sore mouth/tongue

Why should this drug not be prescribed?
Do not take this medication if you have ever had an allergic reaction or are sensitive to any rifamycin drugs.

Special warnings about this medication
Rifadin can cause problems with liver function. If you have liver disease, Rifadin should be used with extreme caution and be carefully monitored by your doctor.

If you are taking Rifadin because your doctor has determined you are a carrier of the meningitis bacteria, the drug must be used only for short-term treatment.

When Rifadin is given at high doses (more than 600 milligrams) once or twice a week, there is a high incidence of side effects, including "flu-like" symptoms, upset stomach, blood disorders, and liver and kidney reactions.

Rifadin may decrease the effectiveness of birth control pills. Talk to your doctor about alternative methods.

Possible food and drug interactions when taking this medication
If Rifadin is taken with certain other drugs, the effects of either could be increased,

decreased, or altered. It is especially important to check with your doctor before combining Rifadin with the following:

Analgesics such as Darvon and Tylenol
Anticonvulsants such as Tegretol, Klonopin, and Dilantin
Antidiabetics such as Diabeta, Glucotrol, and Diabinese
Barbiturates such as phenobarbital and Nembutal
Benzodiazepines such as Valium and Xanax
Beta blockers such as Inderal and Tenormin
Birth control pills such as Ortho-Novum and Norinyl
Blood thinners such as Coumadin
Cardiac glycosides such as Lanoxin
Chloramphenicol (Chloromycetin)
Clofibrate (Atromid-S)
Corticosteroids such as Deltasone, Decadron, and Medrol
Cyclosporine (Sandimmune)
Dapsone
Disopyramide (Norpace)
Estrogens such as Premarin
Ketoconazole (Nizoral)
Methadone
Mexiletine (Mexitil)
Narcotics such as Morphine and Demerol
Probenecid (Benemid)
Progestins such as Megace
Quinidine (Quinidex, Duraquin)
Theophylline (Theolair, Slo-Phyllin, Theo-Dur)
Tocainide (Tonocard)
Verapamil (Calan, Isoptin)
Vitamin D

**Special information
if you are pregnant or breastfeeding**
If you are pregnant or plan to become pregnant, inform your doctor immediately. No information is available about the safety of Rifadin during pregnancy.

Rifadin may appear in breast milk and could affect a nursing infant. If Rifadin is essential to your health, your doctor may recommend you stop breastfeeding until your treatment with Rifadin is finished.

Recommended dosage

Rifadin can be administered by mouth or by intravenous infusion.

A liquid suspension may be prepared for lower doses or for pediatric and adult patients who have trouble swallowing capsules. Ask your doctor or pharmacist about this dosage form.

TUBERCULOSIS

Adults

The usual recommended dosage is 600 milligrams in a single daily dose either orally or intravenously.

In the treatment of tuberculosis, Rifadin should always be administered with at least one other antituberculosis drug.

In general, treatment for tuberculosis should be continued for 6 to 9 months.

MENINGITIS CARRIERS

Adults

It is recommended that 600 milligrams of Rifadin be given twice daily for 2 days. Alternatively, 600 mg may be given once daily for 4 days.

CHILDREN

10 to 20 milligrams for each 2.2 pounds of body weight, not to exceed 600 milligrams per day, orally or intravenously.

For Children 1 Month of Age or Older
10 milligrams for each 2.2 pounds of body weight every 12 hours for 2 days, or once daily for 4 days (not to exceed 600 milligrams per day).

For Children Under 1 Month of Age
5 milligrams for each 2.2 pounds of body weight every 12 hours for 2 days.

Overdosage

Any medication taken in excess can have serious consequences. If you suspect an overdose, seek medical attention immediately.

Symptoms of Rifadin overdose may include:
Brownish-red or orange discoloration of skin, urine, sweat, saliva, tears, and feces (the intensity of color is proportional to the amount ingested)
Increasing tiredness
Liver enlargement and tenderness
Nausea
Unconsciousness
Vomiting
Yellow eyes and skin

Generic name:

RIFAMPIN

See Rifadin, page 544.

Brand name:

RIMACTANE

See Rifadin, page 544.

Brand name:

RITALIN

Generic name: Methylphenidate hydrochloride

Why is this drug prescribed?

Ritalin is a mild central nervous system stimulant and is used in the treatment of attention deficit disorders. (This is a general term for several behavior problems previously known as minimal brain dysfunction in children. Other names being used are hyperkinetic child syndrome, minimal brain damage, minimal cerebral dysfunction, and minor cerebral dysfunction.) Ritalin is also used to treat narcolepsy (an uncontrollable desire to sleep).

This drug should be used as an integral part of a total treatment program that includes psychological, educational, and social measures. Symptoms of attention deficit disorder include a chronic history of moderate to severe distractibility, short attention span, hyperactivity, emotional changeability, and impulsiveness.

Most important fact about this drug
Ritalin should be given with caution to emotionally unstable patients, such as those with a history of drug dependence or alcoholism, because such patients may increase dosage on their own. Long-term abuse can lead to tolerance and mental dependence with varying degrees of abnormal behavior. Careful supervision by your doctor is required during drug withdrawal, because severe depression and the effects of chronic overactivity may become evident.

How should you take this medication?
Dosage should be individualized according to the needs and response of the patient and should be taken exactly as prescribed by the doctor. Ritalin is available in standard and sustained-release tablets (Ritalin-SR).

It is recommended that Ritalin tablets be taken 30 to 45 minutes before meals. Ritalin-SR tablets should be swallowed whole, never crushed or chewed.

What side effects may occur?
Side effects cannot be anticipated. If any develop or change in intensity, inform your doctor as soon as possible. Only your doctor can determine if it is safe for you to continue taking Ritalin.

■ *More common side effects may include:*
Inability to fall or stay asleep
Nervousness

These side effects can usually be controlled by reducing the dosage and omitting the drug from the afternoon or evening dosing schedule.

In children, loss of appetite, abdominal pain, weight loss during long-term therapy, inability to fall or stay asleep, and abnormally fast heartbeat are more common side effects.

■ *Less common or rare side effects may include:*
Abdominal pain, abnormal heartbeat, abnormal muscular movements, blood pressure changes, chest pain, dizziness, drowsiness, fever, headache, hives, jerking, joint pain, lack or loss of appetite, nausea, palpitations (pounding heartbeat), pulse changes, rapid heartbeat, reddish or purplish skin spots, skin inflammation with peeling, skin rash, Tourette's syndrome (severe and multiple twitching), uncontrollable twitching, weight loss during long-term treatment, writhing movements

Why should this drug not be prescribed?
This drug should not be prescribed if you are experiencing anxiety, tension, and agitation, since the drug may aggravate these symptoms.

If you are sensitive to or have ever had an allergic reaction to methylphenidate or drugs of this type, you should not take this medication. Make sure that your doctor is aware of any drug reactions that you have experienced.

Unless you are directed to do so by your doctor, do not take this medication if you have glaucoma, tics (repeated, involuntary twitches), or a family history of Tourette's syndrome (severe and multiple tics).

Ritalin is not intended for use in children whose symptoms may be caused by stress or a psychiatric disorder.

Ritalin should not be used for the prevention or treatment of normal fatigue, nor should it be used for the treatment of depression traced to a specific event or caused by biochemical, psychological, or genetic factors.

Special warnings about this medication

Treatment with Ritalin should be considered only after a complete history and evaluation is performed by your doctor. Duration and severity of symptoms, as well as a patient's age, should be considered prior to treatment with this medication.

Ritalin should not be used in children under 6 years of age; safety and effectiveness in this age-group have not been established.

Information regarding the safety and effectiveness of long-term Ritalin treatment in children of all ages is not available. However, because suppression of growth has been reported with the long-term use of stimulants, it is recommended that patients be carefully monitored by their doctor during treatment.

Blood pressure should be monitored in all patients taking Ritalin, especially those with high blood pressure.

Visual disturbances such as blurred vision have occurred while being treated with Ritalin.

The use of Ritalin in patients with seizure disorders is not recommended. Be sure your doctor is aware of any problem in this area.

Possible food and drug interactions when taking this medication

If Ritalin is taken with certain other drugs, the effects of either could be increased, decreased, or altered. It is especially important to check with your doctor before combining Ritalin with the following:

Guanethidine, a drug used to reduce high blood pressure (Ismelin)

MAO inhibitors (antidepressant drugs such as Nardil, Parnate, and Marplan)

Coumarin anticoagulants (blood thinners such as Coumadin)

Anticonvulsants (phenobarbital, Dilantin, Tegretol)

Phenylbutazone (the anti-inflammatory drug Butazolidin)

Tricyclic antidepressant drugs such as Tofranil, and Norpramin

Special information
if you are pregnant or breastfeeding

The effects of Ritalin during pregnancy have not been adequately studied. If you are pregnant or plan to become pregnant, inform your doctor immediately. It is not known if Ritalin appears in breast milk. If this medication is essential to your health, your doctor may advise you to discontinue nursing your baby until your treatment with this medication is finished.

Recommended dosage

Dosage should be individualized according to the needs and responses of each patient.

ADULTS

Tablets

The average dosage is 20 to 30 milligrams, divided into 2 or 3 doses per day, preferably 30 to 45 minutes before meals. Some patients may require 40 to 60 milligrams daily, and others may require only 10 to 15 milligrams daily. Your dose should be determined by your doctor. If you are unable to sleep, check with your doctor, who may recommend that you take the last dose before 6:00 p.m.

SR Tablets

Ritalin-SR tablets have a duration of action of 8 hours. Therefore, Ritalin-SR tablets may be used in place of Ritalin tablets when the 8-hour dosage of Ritalin-SR corresponds to the divided 8-hour dose of Ritalin. Ritalin-SR tablets must be swallowed whole and never crushed or chewed.

CHILDREN

Ritalin should not be used in children under 6 years of age.

Ritalin should be started in small doses with gradual weekly increases; daily dosage above 60 milligrams is not recommended.

If improvement is not observed over a period of 1 month, check with your doctor. He may wish to discontinue the drug.

Tablets
The recommended starting dose is 5 milligrams taken 2 times a day, before breakfast and lunch, with gradual increases of 5 to 10 milligrams weekly.

SR Tablets
Ritalin-SR tablets have a duration of action of 8 hours. SR tablets may be used in place of tablets when the 8-hour dosage of Ritalin-SR corresponds to the divided 8-hour dosage of Ritalin.

This drug should be periodically discontinued by your doctor in order to re-assess the child's condition. Drug treatment should not, and need not, be indefinite and usually may be discontinued after puberty.

Overdosage
Symptoms of Ritalin overdose may include: Agitation, confusion, convulsions (may be followed by coma), delirium, dryness of mucous membranes, enlarging of the pupil of the eye, exaggerated feeling of elation, extremely elevated body temperature, flushing, hallucinations, headache, high blood pressure, irregular heartbeat, muscle twitching,

palpitations, rapid heartbeat, sweating, tremors, vomiting

If you suspect an overdose, seek medical attention immediately.

Brand name:

ROBAXIN

Generic name: Methocarbamol

Why is this drug prescribed?
Robaxin is prescribed, along with rest, physical therapy and other measures, for the relief of discomfort associated with severe, painful skeletal muscle conditions due to injury, sprain, or strain.

Most important fact about this drug
Robaxin is not a substitute for the rest or physical therapy needed for proper healing.

Robaxin makes an injury temporarily feel better; but do not push your recovery. Lifting or exercising too soon may further damage the muscle.

Robaxin may lessen the normal activity of the central nervous system (brain and spinal cord) and hence the level of other body functions. Therefore, caution should be exercised when taking Robaxin in combination with alcohol or other central nervous system depressants such as barbiturates, sedatives, and tranquilizers.

How should you take this medication?
Take Robaxin exactly as prescribed by your doctor. Do not take a larger dose or use more often than prescribed.

Robaxin causes drowsiness and blurred vision. Exercise extra caution while driving or performing tasks that require mental alertness.

Avoid alcoholic beverages.

Robaxin may darken urine to brown, green, or black.

What side effects may occur?
Side effects cannot be anticipated. If any develop or change in intensity, inform your doctor as soon as possible. Only your doctor can determine if it is safe for you to continue taking Robaxin.

■ *Side effects may include:*
  Blurred vision, dizziness, drowsiness, fever, headache, hives, itching, light-headedness, nasal congestion, nausea, pinkeye, rash

Why should this drug not be prescribed?
If you are sensitive to or have ever had an allergic reaction to methocarbamol or other drugs of this type (Parafon Forte, Norgesic Forte), you should not take this medication. Make sure that your doctor is aware of any drug reactions that you have experienced.

Possible food and drug interactions when taking this medication
If Robaxin is taken with certain other drugs, the effects of either could be increased, decreased, or altered. It is especially important to check with your doctor before combining Robaxin with the following:

Central nervous system depressants such as Xanax, Halcion, Valium, Benadryl, Percocet, Tylenol with Codeine, alcohol, and others

Special information if you are pregnant or breastfeeding
The effects of Robaxin during pregnancy have not been adequately studied. If you are pregnant or plan to become pregnant, inform your doctor immediately. It is not known if this drug appears in breast milk. If this medication is essential to your health, your doctor may advise you to discontinue breastfeeding your baby until your treatment is finished.

Recommended dosage
ADULTS

Robaxin-500
The usual starting dosage is 3 tablets taken 4 times a day. The usual maintenance dosage is 2 tablets taken 4 times a day.

Robaxin-750
The usual starting dosage is 2 tablets taken 4 times a day. The usual maintenance dosage is 1 tablet taken every 4 hours or 2 tablets taken 3 times a day.

CHILDREN

The safety and effectiveness of Robaxin have not been established in children under 12 years of age.

Overdosage
Any drug taken in excess can have dangerous consequences. If you suspect an overdose, seek emergency medical treatment immediately.

Brand name:

ROCALTROL

Generic name: Calcitriol

Why is this drug prescribed?
Rocaltrol is a synthetic form of vitamin D used to treat people on dialysis who have hypocalcemia (abnormally low blood calcium levels) and resulting bone damage.
Rocaltrol is also prescribed to treat low blood calcium levels in people who have hypoparathyroidism (decreased functioning of the parathyroid glands). When functioning correctly, these glands help control the level of calcium in the blood.

Most important fact about this drug
Rocaltrol is the most potent form of vitamin D available. Additional amounts of vitamin D in any form are dangerous and may cause serious side effects (such as

irregular heartbeats) that may require emergency medical care.

How should you take this medication?
People with normally functioning kidneys who take Rocaltrol should be sure they are getting enough fluids and do not become dehydrated while taking this drug.

What side effects may occur?
Side effects cannot be anticipated. If any develop or change in intensity, inform your doctor as soon as possible. Only your doctor can determine if it is safe for you to continue taking Rocaltrol.

■ *More common side effects occurring early may include:*
Bone pain
Constipation
Dry mouth
Extreme drowsiness
Headache
Metallic taste
Muscle pain
Nausea
Vomiting
Weakness

■ *More common side effects occurring later may include:*
Abnormal thirst, decreased libido, dislike of bright lights, ectopic calcification (abnormal bone formation), elevated blood cholesterol levels, excessive urination, extremely high body temperature, eye discharge, high blood pressure, irregular heartbeat, itchy eyes, itchy skin, kidney problems, liver problems, loss of appetite, nighttime urination, red eye, runny nose, severe stomach pain, weight loss, yellowish skin

■ *Rare side effects may include:*
Psychosis, red patches (irregular or circular shape) on arms and hands

Excessive amounts of Vitamin D may cause hypercalcemia (abnormally high calcium levels in the blood).

Why should this drug not be prescribed?
You should not use Rocaltrol if you have hypercalcemia (high blood levels of calcium), or if you have vitamin D poisoning.

Special warnings about this medication
You should not take additional doses of vitamin D while taking Rocaltrol. People who are on dialysis should not take antacids containing magnesium (such as Maalox) while taking Rocaltrol.

Your calcium levels should be monitored while taking Rocaltrol.

You should use Rocaltrol cautiously if you take digitalis (Lanoxin)

Your doctor will prescribe the lowest possible dose of Rocaltrol at the beginning of treatment. He or she will also monitor your blood calcium levels if the dosage is increased.

While taking Rocaltrol, you should have an adequate daily intake of calcium, either from foods (such as milk and dairy products) or from a calcium supplement. Your daily calcium intake should be estimated before you take this drug to see if you will require more calcium.

People with normally functioning kidneys who take Rocaltrol should be sure they are getting enough fluids, and that they do not become dehydrated while taking this drug.

Possible food and drug interactions when taking this medication
If Rocaltrol is taken with certain other drugs, the effects of either could be increased, decreased, or altered. It is especially important to check with your doctor before combining Rocaltrol with the following:

Antacids containing magnesium, such as
  Maalox
Calcium supplements
Cholestyramine (Questran)
Digitalis (Lanoxin)
Vitamin D pills

Special information
if you are pregnant or breastfeeding
The effects of Rocaltrol during pregnancy have
not been adequately studied. If you are
pregnant or plan to become pregnant, inform
your doctor immediately. Pregnant women
should use Rocaltrol only if the possible
benefit outweighs possible risk to the
unborn baby.

Women should not use Rocaltrol while
nursing a baby.

Recommended dosage
Blood calcium levels should be monitored in
anyone who takes Rocaltrol.

ADULTS

For People on Dialysis
The suggested beginning dose is 0.25
microgram daily. If needed, this dosage
may be increased.

People with normal or slightly low blood
calcium levels may find it helpful to take
0.25 microgram every other day.

*To Treat Low Blood Calcium Levels in People
Who Have Hypoparathyroidism
(Decreased Functioning of the Parathyroid
Glands)*
The suggested beginning dose is 0.25
microgram daily, given in the morning.
If needed, this dosage may be increased.

For most adults, dosages ranging from 0.5
to 2 micrograms daily are effective.

CHILDREN

*To Treat Low Blood Calcium Levels in
Children Who Have Hypoparathyroidism*
For most children 6 years and older, dosages
ranging from 0.5 to 2 micrograms per
day are effective.

Children from 1 to 5 years old usually are
given from 0.25 to 0.75 microgram each
day.

Overdosage
Any medication taken in excess can have
serious consequences. Severe overdosage
of Rocaltrol may cause serious effects, such
as extremely high blood levels of calcium.
If you suspect a Rocaltrol overdose, seek
medical help immediately.

Symptoms of Rocaltrol overdose may include:
Coma
Confusion
Extreme drowsiness
High calcium levels in blood
High calcium levels in urine
High phosphate levels in blood

Brand name:

ROGAINE

Generic name: Minoxidil

Why is this drug prescribed?
Rogaine is a topical (applied directly to the
scalp) hair growth stimulant that treats
baldness in men and thinning hair in women.

Most important fact about this drug
Rogaine must be used twice a day for at least
4 months before new hair growth can
be expected. If you stop using Rogaine you
will probably shed the new hair within
a few months. Larger or more frequent doses
do not speed up or increase hair growth,
but do increase the possibility of side effects.

How should you use this medication?

Use this medication exactly as prescribed by your doctor. Do not use more than is recommended.

Hair and scalp should be dry before applying the medication.

If you use your fingertips to apply Rogaine, be sure to wash your hands thoroughly when you are finished.

What side effects may occur?

Side effects cannot be anticipated. If any develop or change in intensity, inform your doctor as soon as possible. Only your doctor can determine if it is safe for you to continue using Rogaine.

■ *Side effects may include:*
Aches and pains, arthritis symptoms, anxiety, back pain, blood disorders, bone fractures, bronchitis, changes in blood pressure, changes in pulse rate, chest pain, depression, diarrhea, dizziness, dry skin/scalp flaking, ear infections, eczema, exhaustion, facial swelling, faintness, fluid retention, genital infections and irritation, growth of excess body hair, headache, hives, increased hair loss, itching, lightheadedness, menstrual and breast changes, nausea, pink eye (conjunctivitis), pounding heartbeat, redness of skin, runny nose, sexual dysfunction, sinus inflammation, skin irritation and other allergic reactions, vision changes, vomiting, weight gain

Why should this drug not be prescribed?

Rogaine should not be used if you are sensitive or have ever had an allergic reaction to any of its ingredients.

Special warnings about this medication

Rogaine is for external use only.

You should have a healthy, normal scalp before starting treatment with Rogaine.

Scalp irritations or cardiovascular disease will increase the absorption of Rogaine and increase the chance of side effects developing.

Even though Rogaine is applied to your skin, it is absorbed into your bloodstream. If you use more medication than is recommended, systemic side effects can occur. In tablet form, minoxidil, a high blood pressure medication, can cause salt and water retention, generalized and local fluid retention, rapid heartbeat, angina (crushing pain, usually in the chest, accompanied by a choking feeling), and inflammation of the sac that surrounds the heart. Although the likelihood is very small, these symptoms could possibly occur with the use of Rogaine, and people with heart disease would be at particular risk. Rogaine could also have adverse effects when used by people taking medications to lower their blood pressure.

You should have a checkup after you have been using Rogaine for 1 month and every 6 months thereafter.

Rogaine contains alcohol. Be careful not to get it in your eyes.

Rogaine should not be used with other topical medications, such as steroids, that increase skin absorption, or with petroleum jelly.

Possible food and drug interactions while using this medication

No interactions with Rogaine have been reported.

Special information if you are pregnant or breastfeeding

The effects of Rogaine during pregnancy have not been adequately studied. However, minoxidil may cause birth defects, and the use of Rogaine during pregnancy is not recommended. If you are pregnant or plan to become pregnant, inform your doctor immediately. Minoxidil appears in breast milk and could affect a nursing infant. Rogaine is not recommended for use by nursing mothers.

Recommended dosage

ADULTS

Apply 1 milliliter of Rogaine to the total affected areas of the scalp 2 times a day. The total daily dosage should not be more than 2 milliliters. Make sure the hair and scalp are dry before applying the medication. It could take up to 4 months of twice-daily use to see results. If hair regrowth occurs, continue to apply Rogaine 2 times a day for additional or continued hair regrowth.

CHILDREN

Safety and effectiveness in children under 18 have not been established.

Overdosage

Any medication taken in excess can have serious consequences. If you suspect an overdose, seek medical attention immediately.

Brand name:

RONDEC

Generic ingredients: Carbinoxamine maleate, Pseudoephedrine hydrochloride

Why is this drug prescribed?

Rondec is an antihistamine/decongestant that relieves runny nose and the symptoms of hay fever and other allergies. Carbinoxamine, the antihistamine in this combination, fights the effects of histamine, a chemical released by the body in response to certain irritants. Histamine narrows air passages in the lungs and contributes to inflammation. Antihistamines reduce itching and swelling and dry up secretions from the nose, eyes, and throat. Pseudoephedrine, the decongestant,

reduces nasal congestion and makes breathing easier.

Most important fact about this drug

Rondec may cause mild to moderate drowsiness. Driving or operating dangerous machinery or participating in any hazardous activity that requires full mental alertness is not recommended until you know how you react to this medication.

How should you take this medication?

Rondec is available in four forms. Rondec Drops, Syrup, and Tablets can be taken up to 4 times a day. Rondec-TR Tablets can be taken twice a day.

What side effects may occur?

Side effects cannot be anticipated. If any develop or change in intensity, inform your doctor as soon as possible. Only your doctor can determine if it is safe for you to continue taking Rondec.

■ *Side effects may include:*
Convulsions, diarrhea, difficulty breathing, difficulty sleeping (Insomnia), dizziness, double vision, dry mouth, excitability in children (rare), hallucinations, headache, heartburn, increased blood pressure, increased heart rate, increased production of urine, irregular heartbeat, loss of appetite, nausea, nervousness, painful or difficult urination, pallor, sedation (extreme calm), stimulation, tremors, vomiting, weakness

Why should this drug not be prescribed?

Rondec should be avoided if you are taking antidepressants known as MAO inhibitors (Nardil, for example), if you are undergoing an asthma attack, or if you have narrow-angle glaucoma, difficulty urinating, peptic ulcer, severe high blood pressure, or coronary artery disease.

Do not take this medication if you are sensitive to or have ever had an allergic reaction to any of its ingredients.

Special warnings about this medication

Rondec should be used with care if you have high blood pressure, heart disease, asthma, an overactive thyroid, increased eye pressure, diabetes, or an enlarged prostate.

This medication should be used cautiously if you are age 60 or over.

If you are sensitive to antihistamines, Rondec can cause moderate to severe drowsiness. Be careful driving, operating machinery, or using appliances.

Possible food and drug interactions when taking this medication

Rondec may increase the effects of alcohol. Do not drink alcohol while taking this medication.

If Rondec is taken with certain other drugs, the effects of either may be increased, decreased, or altered. It is important that you consult with your doctor before combining Rondec with the following:

Beta blockers such as Tenormin and Inderal
Drugs for depression such as Elavil and Nardil
High blood pressure drugs such as Aldomet, Serpasil, and Inversine
Sedatives/hypnotics such as Halcion and Restoril
Tranquilizers such as Xanax and Valium

Special information if you are pregnant or breastfeeding

The effects of Rondec during pregnancy have not been adequately studied. If you are pregnant or plan to become pregnant, notify your doctor immediately. Rondec may appear in breast milk and could affect a nursing infant. If this medication is essential to your health, your doctor may advise you to discontinue breastfeeding until your treatment is finished.

Recommended dosage

RONDEC ORAL DROPS

Children
The usual dosage is:
1 to 3 months old, one-quarter dropperful (one-quarter milliliter), 4 times a day.

3 to 6 months old, one-half dropperful (one-half milliliter), 4 times a day.

6 to 9 months old, three-quarters dropperful (three-quarters milliliter), 4 times a day.

9 to 18 months old, 1 dropperful (1 milliliter), 4 times a day.

RONDEC SYRUP AND TABLETS

Children
The usual dosage for children 18 months to 6 years old is ½ teaspoonful (2.5 milliliters), 4 times a day.

Adults and Children 6 Years and Over
The usual dosage is 1 teaspoonful (5 milliliters) or 1 tablet, 4 times a day.

RONDEC-TR TABLETS

Adults and Children 12 Years and Over
The usual dose is 1 tablet, 2 times a day.

(In mild cases or in particularly sensitive patients, less frequent or reduced doses may be adequate.)

Overdosage

Any medication taken in excess can have serious consequences. If you suspect an overdose, seek medical attention immediately.

Although no information is available for Rondec, the following symptoms have been reported with antihistamine and ephedrine overdose:
Abdominal cramps, coma, convulsions, diarrhea, difficulty sleeping (insomnia), difficulty urinating, dizziness, drowsiness, dry

mouth, excitement, fever, flushing, headache, high blood pressure with subsequent low blood pressure, irregular heartbeat, irritability, loss of appetite, metallic taste, nausea, pounding heartbeat, restlessness, talkativeness, tremor, vomiting

Symptoms more common in children are:
Coma
Convulsions
Death
Excitement
Fever
Fixed and dilated pupils
Flushed face
Hallucination
Lack of muscle coordination
Tremors

Brand name:

ROWASA

Generic name: Mesalamine

Why is this drug prescribed?
Rowasa Suspension Enema is used to treat mild to moderate distal ulcerative colitis (inflammation of the large intestine and rectum), inflammation of the lower colon, and inflammation of the rectum.

Rowasa Suppositories are used to treat inflammation of the rectum.

Most important fact about this drug
Mesalamine, an ingredient in Rowasa Suppositories and Rowasa Suspension Enema, has sometimes caused side effects such as:

Bloody diarrhea
Cramping
Fever
Rash
Severe headache
Sudden, severe stomach pain

It is recommended that anyone who experiences any of these effects should stop taking drugs such as Rowasa Suspension Enema and Rowasa Suppositories that contain mesalamine.

How should you use this medication?
To Use Rowasa Suspension Enema
1. Rowasa Suspension Enema should be stored at controlled room temperatures from 59 to 86 degrees Fahrenheit.
2. Rowasa Suspension Enema comes in boxes of 7 bottles each. After the foil on the box has been unwrapped, all Rowasa Suspension Enemas should be used promptly, following your doctor's instructions. The Suspension Enema is normally off-white to tan in color, but may darken over time once its foil cover is unwrapped. You may still use the enema if it is slightly discolored, but do not use Rowasa Suspension Enema if it is dark brown. If you have any questions about using Rowasa Suspension Enema, contact your doctor.
3. Rowasa Suspension Enema should be used at bedtime.
4. Shake the bottle thoroughly.
5. Uncover the applicator tip.
6. You may find it easier to use Rowasa Suspension Enema if you lie down on your left side, extending your left leg and bending your right leg forward for a comfortable balance. An alternative position is to squat with your knees to your chest.
7. Pointing the applicator tip up, gently insert the tip into the rectum.
8. Squeeze the bottle steadily to discharge the contents.
9. The enema should be retained all night (8 hours) for best results.

To Use Rowasa Suppositories

1. Rowasa Suppositories should be stored at controlled room temperatures from 66 to 79 degrees Fahrenheit.
2. Rowasa Suppositories should be used twice a day.
3. You should handle the suppositories as little as possible, because they are designed to melt at body temperature.
4. Remove one suppository from the strip of suppositories.
5. While holding the suppository upright, carefully remove the foil wrapper.
6. Using gentle pressure, insert the suppository (with the pointed end first) completely into the rectum.
7. The suppository should be retained for 1 to 3 hours or longer for best results.

What side effects may occur?

Side effects cannot be anticipated. If any side effects develop or change in intensity, tell your doctor immediately. Only your doctor can determine whether it is safe to continue using this medication.

■ *More common side effects of Rowasa Suspension Enema may include:*
Flu-like symptoms
Gas
Headache
Nausea
Stomach pain/cramps

■ *Less common side effects of Rowasa Suspension Enema may include:*
Back pain, bloating, diarrhea, dizziness, fever, hemorrhoids, itching, leg/joint pain, pain on insertion of enema tip, rash, rectal pain, sore throat, tiredness, weakness

■ *Rare side effects of Rowasa Suspension Enema may include:*
Constipation, hair loss, insomnia, swelling of the arms or legs, urinary burning

■ *More common side effects of Rowasa Suppositories may include:*
Diarrhea
Dizziness
Gas
Headache
Stomach pain

■ *Less common side effects of Rowasa Suppositories may include:*
Acne, cold symptoms, fever, inflammation of the colon, nausea, rash, rectal pain, swelling, weakness

Why should this drug not be prescribed?

Rowasa Suspension Rowasa Suppositories and Rowasa Suspension Enemas should not be used by anyone who is allergic or sensitive to mesalamine or to other ingredients in the suppositories or enemas.

Special warnings about this medication

Anyone using Rowasa Suspension Enema (especially people with a history of kidney disease and people using other anti-inflammatory drugs, such as Dipentum) should have urine and blood tests to check kidney function.

You should use Rowasa Suspension Enema and Rowasa Suppositories cautiously if you are allergic to sulfasalazine (Azulfidine). If you develop a rash or fever, you should stop using Rowasa and notify your doctor.

Some people using Rowasa Suspension Enema have developed flare-ups of their colitis.

Rare cases of pericarditis, in which the membrane surrounding the heart becomes inflamed, have been reported with products containing mesalamine, including Rowasa Suppositories and Suspension Enema. Symptoms may include chest, neck, and shoulder pain, and shortness of breath.

Rowasa Suspension Enema contains a sulfite that may cause allergic reactions in some people. These reactions may include shock and severe, possibly fatal asthma attacks. Most people aren't sensitive to sulfites. However, some people with asthma might be sensitive and should take any medication containing sulfites cautiously.

Rowasa Suspension Enema may stain clothes, fabrics, granite, marble, painted surfaces, vinyl, and other surfaces.

Possible food and drug interactions when taking this medication

If Rowasa Suspension Enema or Rowasa Suppositories is taken with certain other drugs, the effects of either could be increased, decreased, or altered. It is especially important to check with your doctor before combining Rowasa Suspension Enema or Rowasa Suppositories with the following:

Sulfasalazine (Azulfidine)
Other anti-inflammatory drugs such as Dipentum.

Special information
if you are pregnant or breastfeeding

Pregnant women should use Rowasa Suppositories or Rowasa Suspension Enema only if clearly required. It is not known whether mesalamine appears in breast milk, and if it might affect a nursing infant.

Recommended dosage

ADULTS

Rowasa Suspension Enema
The usual dose is 1 rectal enema (60 milliliters) per day, preferably used at bedtime and retained for about 8 hours. Treatment time usually lasts from 3 to 6 weeks, although improvement may be seen within 3 to 21 days.

Rowasa Suppositories
The usual dose is one rectal suppository (500 milligrams) 2 times a day. To get the most benefit from a Rowasa Suppository, it should

be retained for 1 to 3 hours or longer. Treatment time usually lasts from 3 to 6 weeks, although improvement may be seen within 3 to 21 days.

CHILDREN

Safety and effectiveness in children have not been established.

Overdosage

There have been no proven reports of serious effects resulting from overdoses of mesalamine, the main ingredient of Rowasa Suspension Enema and Rowasa Suppositories. However, any medication taken in excess can have serious consequences. If you suspect an overdose, seek medical attention immediately.

Brand name:

ROXICET

See Percocet, page 465.

Brand name:

RU-TUSS TABLETS

Generic ingredients: Phenylephrine hydrochloride, Phenylpropanolamine hydrochloride, Chlorpheniramine maleate, Hyoscyamine sulfate, Atropine sulfate, Scopolamine hydrobromide

Why is this drug prescribed?

Ru-Tuss is an antihistamine/decongestant that relieves the runny, stuffy nose, nasal drip, itching, watery eyes, and scratchy, itchy throat caused by allergies, colds, and other irritations of the sinus, nose, and upper respiratory tract. Chlorpheniramine, the antihistamine, reduces itching and swelling and dries up secretions from the nose, eyes, and throat. Phenylephrine and phenylpropanolamine combine to reduce congestion and make breathing easier. Hyoscyamine, atropine, and scopolamine, commonly called belladonna alkaloids, enhance the drying effects of Ru-Tuss.

Most important fact about this drug

Ru-Tuss tablets may cause drowsiness. Driving or operating dangerous machinery or participating in any hazardous activity that requires full mental alertness is not recommended until you know how you react to this medication.

How should you take this medication?

Take this medication exactly as prescribed by your doctor. The tablets act continuously for 10 to 12 hours. Tablets should be swallowed whole, not crushed or chewed.

What side effects may occur?

Side effects cannot be anticipated. If any develop or change in intensity, inform your doctor as soon as possible. Only your doctor can determine if it is safe for you to continue taking Ru-Tuss.

■ *Side effects may include:*
Allergic reactions (rash, hives), blood disorders, blurred vision, constipation, diarrhea, difficulty sleeping (insomnia), dilated pupils, dizziness, drowsiness, dry mouth, dry nose and other mucous membranes, exhaustion, faintness, frequent urination, giddiness, headache, hyper-irritability, increased chest congestion, loss of appetite, low blood pressure/high blood pressure, nausea, nervousness, painful or difficult urination, pounding heartbeat, rapid heartbeat, ringing in the ears, stomach upset, tightness in the chest, uncoordination, vision changes, vomiting

Why should this drug not be prescribed?

Ru-Tuss should be avoided if you are pregnant, if you are sensitive to or have ever had an allergic reaction to antihistamines or any of the ingredients in this medication, if you have glaucoma or bronchial asthma, or if you are taking antidepressant drugs known as MAO inhibitors (Nardil, for example). Ru-

Tuss should not be given to children under 12 years of age.

Special warnings about this medication

This medication can make you feel drowsy. Be careful driving, operating machinery, or using appliances.

Ru-Tuss should be used with care if you have a bladder obstruction, high blood pressure, cardiovascular disease, or an overactive thyroid.

Possible food and drug interactions when taking this medication

Ru-Tuss may increase the effects of alcohol. Do not drink alcohol while taking this medication.

If Ru-Tuss is taken with certain other drugs, the effects of either could be increased, decreased, or altered. It is especially important to check with your doctor before combining Ru-Tuss with the following:

Hypnotics such as Halcion and Dalmane
Tranquilizers such as Xanax and Valium

Special information if you are pregnant or breastfeeding

Ru-Tuss is not recommended for use by pregnant women. If you are pregnant or plan to become pregnant, notify your doctor immediately.

Recommended dosage

ADULTS AND CHILDREN 12 YEARS OR OLDER

The usual dosage is 1 tablet in the morning and 1 tablet in the evening. This drug is not recommended for children under 12.

Overdosage

Any medication taken in excess can have serious consequences. Convulsions and death may occur from antihistamine overdose in children and infants. If you suspect an overdose, seek medical treatment immediately.

Symptoms of Ru-Tuss overdose may include:
Coma
Delirium
Fever
Rapid breathing
Respiratory failure
Stupor

Brand name:

RUFEN

See Motrin, page 393.

Brand name:

RYNATAN

Generic ingredients: Phenylephrine tannate, Chlorpheniramine tannate, Pyrilamine tannate

Why is this drug prescribed?
Rynatan is an antihistamine/decongestant that relieves runny nose and nasal congestion caused by the common cold, inflamed sinuses, hay fever, and other upper respiratory conditions. Chlorpheniramine and pyrilamine, the antihistamines in the combination, reduce itching and swelling and dry up secretions from the eyes, nose, and throat. Phenylephrine, the decongestant, reduces congestion and makes breathing easier.

Most important fact about this drug
This medication can make you drowsy. Driving or operating dangerous machinery or participating in any hazardous activity that requires full mental alertness is not recommended until you know how you react to Rynatan.

How should you take this medication?
Take this medication exactly as indicated.

What side effects may occur?
Side effects cannot be anticipated. If any develop or change in intensity, inform your doctor as soon as possible. Only your doctor can determine if it is safe for you to continue taking Rynatan.

■ *Side effects may include:*
Drowsiness
Dry nose, mouth, and throat
Extreme calm (sedation)
Stomach and intestinal problems

Why should this drug not be prescribed?
Rynatan should not be given to newborn babies, nursing mothers, or people who are sensitive to or have ever had an allergic reaction to any of its ingredients or to similar medications.

Special warnings about this medication
If you are taking antidepressant drugs known as MAO inhibitors (Nardil, for example), avoid Rynatan or use with caution.

Rynatan should be used with care if you have high blood pressure, cardiovascular disease, an overactive thyroid, diabetes, narrow-angle glaucoma, or an enlarged prostate.

Possible food and drug interactions when taking this medication
Rynatan may increase the effects of alcohol. Do not drink alcohol while taking this medication.

If Rynatan is taken with certain other drugs, the effects of either could be increased, decreased, or altered. It is especially important to check with your doctor before combining Rynatan with the following:

MAO inhibitor drugs such as Nardil and Marplan
Sedative/hypnotics such as Halcion and Dalmane
Tranquilizers such as Xanax and Valium

Special information if you are pregnant or breastfeeding
The effects of Rynatan during pregnancy have not been adequately studied. If you are

pregnant or plan to become pregnant, notify your doctor immediately. Rynatan should not be taken if you are breastfeeding.

Recommended dosage

RYNATAN TABLETS

Adults
The usual dosage is 1 or 2 tablets every 12 hours.

RYNATAN PEDIATRIC SUSPENSION

Children Over 6:
The usual dosage is 1 to 2 teaspoonfuls (5 to 10 milliliters) every 12 hours.

Children 2 to 6:
The usual dosage is ½ to 1 teaspoonful (2.5 to 5 milliliters) every 12 hours.

Children under 2:
Doctor will determine.

Overdosage

Any medication taken in excess can have serious consequences. Antihistamine overdose in young children may lead to convulsions and death. If you suspect an overdose, seek medical treatment immediately.

Symptoms of Rynatan overdose may vary from central nervous system depression to stimulation (restlessness to convulsions).

Brand name:

RYTHMOL

Generic name: Propafenone

Why is this drug prescribed?

Rythmol is used to help correct certain life-threatening heartbeat irregularities (ventricular arrhythmias).

Most important fact about this drug

Because Rythmol sometimes causes heartbeat irregularities, you should only take it if your doctor believes your medical condition is severe enough that the benefits of Rythmol outweigh the risks of treatment.

How should you take this medication?

Take Rythmol exactly as prescribed by your doctor. The usual starting dosage is 1 tablet 3 times a day. Depending on how you respond to Rythmol, your doctor may gradually increase the dosage. If you are older or have extensive heart damage, any dosage increase should be very gradual.

If you have the heartbeat irregularity known as "sustained ventricular tachycardia," your Rythmol treatment should be started in the hospital so that you can be monitored closely.

Rythmol may be taken with food or on an empty stomach.

What side effects may occur?

Side effects cannot be anticipated. If any develop or change in intensity, inform your doctor as soon as possible. Only your doctor can determine if it is safe for you to continue taking Rhythmol.

The most common side effects affect the digestive system. The most serious are heartbeat abnormalities caused by Rythmol. About 20 percent of all people treated with Rythmol must stop taking this drug because of the side effects.

■ *More common side effects may include:*
Constipation
Dizziness
Heartbeat abnormalities
Nausea, vomiting
Unusual taste in the mouth

■ *Other side effects may include:*
Abdominal pain, cramps, or gas, angina (chest pain), anxiety, blood disorders, blurred vision, breathing difficulties,

bruising, cardiac arrest, coma, confusion, congestive heart failure, depression, diarrhea, dreaming abnormalities, drowsiness, dry mouth, eye irritation, fainting or near fainting, fatigue, fever, flushing, hair loss, headache, heart palpitations, heartbeat abnormalities (rapid, irregular, slow), hot flashes, impotence, increased blood sugar, indigestion, inflamed esophagus or stomach, insomnia, itching, kidney disease, kidney failure, loss of appetite, loss of balance, low blood pressure, memory loss, morbid sensations, muscle cramps, muscle weakness, numbness, pain, psychosis, rash, ringing in the ears, seizures, speech abnormalities, sweating, swollen wrists and ankles, tremor, unusual smell sensations, vertigo, vision abnormalities, weakness

Why should this drug not be prescribed?

Do not take Rythmol if you have ever had an allergic reaction or are sensitive to it. Your doctor will not prescribe Rythmol if you are suffering from any of the following conditions:

Abnormally slow heartbeat
Atrioventricular block or "sick sinus" syndrome not corrected by a pacemaker
Cardiogenic shock
Chronic bronchitis or emphysema
Congestive heart failure that is not well controlled
Mineral (electrolyte) imbalance
Severe low blood pressure

Special warnings about this medication

Since Rythmol may cause new or worsened heartbeat irregularities, you must have a physical exam and an electrocardiogram before you start taking this medication, and again during the course of treatment.

If you have congestive heart failure, this condition must be brought under full medical control before you start taking Rythmol.

If you have a pacemaker, the pacemaker's settings must be monitored—and possibly reprogrammed—while you are taking Rythmol.

There is some risk that Rythmol may interfere with your body's normal ability to manufacture blood cells. Too few white blood cells may cause signs and symptoms that mimic infection. If you experience fever, chills, or sore throat while taking Rythmol—especially during the first three months of treatment—notify your doctor right away.

Rythmol may cause a lupus-like illness. If you have been taking Rythmol and testing shows that your blood contains ANA (antinuclear antibodies), your doctor may want you to go off the medication.

Possible food and drug interactions when taking this medication

If Rythmol is taken with certain other drugs, the effects of either could be increased, decreased, or altered. It is especially important to check with your doctor before combining Rythmol with the following:

Beta blockers such as Inderal, and Lopressor, Cimetidine (Tagamet)
Digitalis (Lanoxin)
Local anesthetics (such as during dental work)
Quinidine (Quinora, Cardioquin,)
Warfarin (blood thinners such as Coumadin and Panwarfin)

Special information if you are pregnant or breastfeeding

If you are pregnant or plan to become pregnant, inform your doctor immediately. Because of a possible risk of birth defects, Rythmol is not recommended during pregnancy unless the benefit to the mother outweighs the potential risk to the unborn baby.

It is not known whether Rythmol appears in breast milk. You are advised not to take Rythmol if you are nursing a baby. If treatment with Rhthmol is essential to your health, you may need to choose between taking the drug and breastfeeding.

Recommended dosage

ADULTS

In some cases, treatment with Rythmol begins in the hospital.

Your doctor will tailor your dosage according to your individual condition and the presence of other disorders.

The usual initial dose of Rythmol is 150 milligrams every 8 hours. Your doctor may increase the dosage depending on how you respond to the initial dosage. The recommended maximum daily dosage of Rythmol is 900 milligrams.

ELDERLY

Dosages should be increased more slowly at the beginning of treatment, especially in patients with heart attack or other heart damage.

Overdosage

Any medication taken in excess can have serious consequences. If you suspect an overdose of Rythmol, seek medical attention immediately.

Symptoms of Rythmol overdose, which are usually most severe within the first three hours of taking the medication, may include:
Convulsions (rarely)
Drowsiness
Heartbeat irregularities
Low blood pressure

Generic name:

SALSALATE

See Disalcid, page 204.

Brand name:

SANDIMMUNE

Generic name: Cyclosporine

Why is this drug prescribed?

Sandimmune, an immunosuppresant drug, is given after organ transplant surgery to help prevent rejection of organs (kidney, heart, or liver) by dampening the body's immune system. It is also used to treat chronic (long-term) rejection in patients previously treated with other immunosuppresant drugs, such as Imuran. Sandimmune is being studied for the treatment of arthritis and certain other diseases.

Sandimmune is often given simultaneously with prednisone or a similar corticosteroid. It is available in capsules, liquid, or as an injection.

Most important fact about this drug

If you take Sandimmune orally over a period of time, your doctor will monitor your blood levels of cyclosporine to make sure your body is receiving the correct amount of Sandimmune. The reason for this repeated testing is that the absorption of this drug in the body is erratic. Constant monitoring is necessary to prevent toxicity due to overdosing or to prevent possible organ rejection due to underdosing. It is important to note that Sandimmune may need to be taken by mouth for an indefinite period following surgery.

How should you take this medication?

Take Sandimmune exactly as prescribed by your doctor.

Take the Sandimmune capsule or oral liquid at the same time every day. You may take the medication either with a meal or between meals, but be consistent.

To make Sandimmune oral liquid more palatable, you may mix it with room-temperature milk, chocolate milk, or orange juice. Be sure to use the same type of beverage every day. Use a container made of glass, not plastic. Never let the mixture stand; drink it as soon as you prepare it. To make sure you get your full dose, rinse the glass with a little more liquid and drink that too.

You should maintain good dental hygiene and see your dentist frequently for teeth cleaning to prevent tenderness, bleeding, and gum enlargement.

If you are taking the liquid form of Sandimmune, do not store the medication in the refrigerator. Once opened, the contents must be used within 2 months.

What side effects may occur?
Side effects cannot be anticipated. If any appear or change in intensity, inform your doctor immediately. Only your doctor can determine if it is safe for you to continue taking Sandimmune. The principal adverse effects of Sandimmune are high blood pressure, hirsutism (excessive hairiness), kidney damage, overgrowth of the gums, and tremor.

■ *Other common side effects may include:*
Abdominal discomfort, acne, breast swelling (in men), convulsions, cramps, diarrhea, flushing, headache, infection, liver damage, nausea or vomiting, numbness or tingling, sinus inflammation

■ *Less common side effects may include:*
Allergic reactions, anemia, appetite loss, confusion, conjunctivitis, fever, fingernail brittleness, fluid retention, hearing loss, hiccups, high blood sugar, muscle pain, peptic ulcer, ringing in the ears, upset stomach

■ *Rare side effects may include:*
Chest pain, constipation, depression, hair breaking, joint pain, lethargy, mouth sores, heart attack, night sweats, itching, swallowing difficulty, visual disturbance, weakness, weight loss

Why should this drug not be prescribed?
You should not receive Sandimmune by injection if you have ever had an allergic reaction to injected cyclosporine and/or you are especially sensitive to castor oil.

Special warnings about this medication
When your immune system is suppressed by Sandimmune, you are at increased risk of infection and of certain malignancies, including skin cancer and lymph-system cancer.

High-dose Sandimmune is toxic to the kidneys and may cause serious kidney damage. Because this toxicity has symptoms similar to kidney transplant rejection, you must be monitored closely. If your body is trying hard to reject a transplanted organ, your doctor will probably allow the rejection to occur rather than give you very high dose of Sandimmune.

If you take large doses of a prednisone-like drug called methylprednisolone (Depo-Medrol, Medrol, Solu-Medrol) along with Sandimmune, you may be at increased risk of convulsions.

Possible food and drug interactions when taking this medication
Avoid getting vaccinations and immunizations while you are taking Sandimmune. The drug may make vaccinations less effective, or increase your risk of getting an illness from a live vaccine.

If Sandimmune is taken with certain other drugs, the effects of either could be increased, decreased, or altered. It is especially important to check with your doctor before combining Sandimmune with the following:

Amphotericin B (Fungizone I.V.)
Azapropazon
Bromocriptine (Parlodel)
Calcium antagonists such as Calan and Cardene
Carbamazepine (Tegretol)
Cimetidine (Tagamet)
Danazol (Danocrine)
Diclofenac (Voltaren)
Digoxin (Lanoxin, Lanoxicaps)
Erythromycin (E.E.S., Erythrocin, and others)
Fluconazole (Diflucan)
Gentamicin (Garamycin)
Ketoconazole (Nizoral)
Lovastatin (Mevacor)
Melphalan (Alkeran)
Methylprednisolone (Depo-Medrol, Medrol, Solu-Medrol)
Metoclopramide (Reglan)
Phenobarbital (Luminal)
Phenytoin (Dilantin)
Potassium-sparing diuretics (Dyrenium, Midamor, and others)
Prednisolone (Delta-Cortef, Metricortelone)
Ranitidine (Zantac)
Rifampin (Rifadin, Rifamate, Rimactane)
Tobramycin (Nebcin)
Trimethoprim/sulfamethoxazole (Bactrim, Septra)
Vancomycin (Vancocin)

Special information
if you are pregnant or breastfeeding

If you are pregnant or plan to become pregnant, inform your doctor immediately. Sandimmune should be used during pregnancy only if the benefit justifies the potential risk to the unborn child. Since Sandimmune appears in breast milk, it should not be used during breastfeeding. If you are a new mother, you may need to choose between

taking Sandimmune and breastfeeding your baby.

Recommended dosage

Your doctor will tailor your dosage in accordance with your body's response. Special instructions are given elsewhere in this drug profile for mixing the medication with liquids to make it easier to take.

Overdosage

Although no specific information is available, an overdose of Sandimmune would be expected to cause liver and kidney problems. Any medication taken in excess can have serious consequences. If you suspect an overdose of Sandimmune, seek medical attention immediately.

Brand name:

SANSERT

Generic name: Methysergide maleate

Why is this drug prescribed?

Sansert tablets are prescribed to prevent or partly prevent severe "vascular" headaches (the kind caused by constriction and dilation of arteries within the head). Your doctor may consider treating you with Sansert if you have one or more severe headaches per week, or if your headaches are extremely severe and uncontrollable.

Sansert is preventive medication. Sansert is not a painkiller and cannot diminish a headache that has already developed.

Most important fact about this drug

Long-term treatment with Sansert may cause abnormal tissue growth in the lungs, around the ureters, or around the blood vessels. This may result in chest pain, kidney failure, or leg cramps. Therefore, Sansert is used as a preventive measure in patients whose headaches are frequent and/or severe and uncontrollable, and who are under close medical supervision.

How should you take this medication?

You may take Sansert with food to avoid stomach upset.

Sansert may cause weight gain. You should watch your caloric intake.

Take Sansert exactly as prescribed by your doctor. To reduce the risk of serious side effects, you should take Sansert no longer than six consecutive months, gradually reducing the dosage during the last two or three weeks to prevent "rebound" headaches. After completing the six-month course of treatment, you should take a three- or four-week break and then begin taking Sansert for another six-month stretch if your doctor so advises.

If you miss a dose of Sansert, skip the missed dose and go back to your regular dosing schedule. Do not take double doses.

What side effects may occur?

Side effects from Sansert cannot be anticipated. If any develop or change in intensity, inform your doctor as soon as possible. Only your doctor can determine if it is safe for you to continue taking Sansert.

Diarrhea, nausea or vomiting, abdominal pain, and heartburn are typical early reactions to Sansert; you can avoid these symptoms if you start with a lower dosage of Sansert and increase the amount gradually, and if you always take the medication with meals.

■ *Other potential side effects include:*
  Aching joints or muscles, blood cell abnormalities, constipation, dizziness, drowsiness, euphoria (mild), fluid retention, flushing, hair loss (may be temporary), hallucinations or "unworldly" feelings, lack of muscular coordination,

light-headedness, rash, redness around nose and cheeks, sleeplessness, stomach disorders, unsteady movement, weakness, weight gain

If fluid retention develops, it may disappear following a dosage reduction, a low-salt diet, or treatment with diuretics.

If you use Sansert for a long time, there is a risk that fibrotic tissue will develop within the abdomen, lungs, heart valves, or in other parts of the body. Because of this danger, you should immediately contact your doctor if you experience any of the following:

Abdominal pain
Backache
Breathing difficulty
Chest pain or tightness
Cold, numb, painful hands or feet
Fatigue
General malaise
Intermittent limping because of pain in the
  thigh or buttocks
Leg swelling or pain
Low-grade fever
Painful or difficult urination
Weight loss

Why should this drug not be prescribed?

Do not take Sansert if you have any of the following conditions:

Arteriosclerosis (severe)
Collagen disease
Coronary artery disease
Debilitation from chronic illness
Fibrotic conditions
Heart valve disease
High blood pressure (severe)
Infection (serious)
Kidney abnormality
Leg phlebitis or cellulitis
Liver abnormality
Lung disease
Pregnancy

Special warnings about this medication

As noted under "What side effects may occur?," long-term use of Sansert may cause unwanted fibrotic changes in various body tissues. Be especially alert for the following symptoms:

Cold, numb, painful hands and feet
Cramps in the legs while walking
Pain in the chest, flank, or loin

If you develop any of these symptoms, stop taking Sansert and see your doctor right away.

If fibrotic changes do occur, there is a good chance the condition will disappear when you stop taking Sansert. Thus, corrective surgery may not be necessary.

Sansert tablets contain a food coloring called tartrazine (Yellow No. 5). In some people, tartrazine may cause an allergic reaction that includes bronchial asthma. You are at increased risk for this reaction if you are allergic to aspirin.

Possible food and drug interactions when taking this medication

No information is available regarding interactions with Sansert.

Special information
if you are pregnant or breastfeeding

Sansert should not be used during pregnancy. If you are pregnant or plan to become pregnant, inform your doctor immediately. It is not known whether Sansert appears in breast milk. If this drug is essential to your health, your doctor may advise you to stop breastfeeding until your tratment is finished.

Recommended dosage

ADULTS

The usual recommended dose is 4 to 8 milligrams daily, given with meals.

CHILDREN

Sansert is not recommended for use in children.

Overdosage

Although no specific information is available, any medication taken in excess can have serious consequences. If you suspect an overdose of Sansert, seek medical attention immediately.

Generic name:

SECOBARBITAL SODIUM

See Seconal, page 567.

Brand name:

SECONAL

Generic name: Secobarbital sodium

Why is this drug prescribed?

Seconal is a barbiturate used to treat insomnia on a short-term basis.

After 2 weeks, Seconal appears to lose its effectiveness as a sleep aid. Because of the risk of addiction and overdose associated with barbiturates, other drugs are now often prescribed in their place.

Most important fact about this drug

If taken for a long enough time, Seconal can cause physical addiction, and if taken in a large enough amount, it can cause death.

How should you take this medication?

Seconal should be taken at bedtime.

You should not take Seconal with alcohol.

Take only the prescribed dose.

What side effects may occur?

Side effects cannot be anticipated. If any develop or change in intensity, inform your doctor as soon as possible. Only your doctor can determine if it is safe for you to continue taking Seconal.

■ *More common side effects may include:*
Extreme sleepiness

■ *Less common or rare side effects may include:*
Agitation, anemia, anxiety, confusion, constipation, difficulty breathing, disturbed thinking, dizziness, fever, fluid retention, hallucinations, headache, insomnia, irregular pulse, lack of coordination, low blood pressure, nausea, nervousness, nightmares, overactivity, slow heartbeat, skin rash, inflammation, and/or peeling, temporary interruptions of breathing, vomiting

Why should this drug not be prescribed?

You should not take Seconal if you have porphyria (a rare blood disorder), liver damage, or lung disease that causes difficult breathing.

Do not take Seconal if you are known to be hypersensitive to drugs of this type.

Special warnings about this medication

You should not stop taking Seconal suddenly, since this may result in withdrawal symptoms and even death. To reduce the possibility of withdrawal symptoms, follow your doctor's instructions closely when discontinuing Seconal.

Minor withdrawal symptoms may include an increase in dreams or nightmares.

Other minor withdrawal symptoms include (in order of occurrence): Anxiety, muscle twitching, tremors of hands and fingers, progressive weakness, dizziness, visual problems, nausea, vomiting, insomnia, and light-headedness (especially when rising from a horizontal position).

Major withdrawal symptoms include convulsions and delirium.

Use Seconal cautiously if you have had liver disease or have a history of depression, suicidal tendencies, and drug or alcohol abuse.

Inform your doctor if you have chronic or acute pain. Seconal may hide pain-causing disorders that require treatment.

Children may become excited while taking Seconal.

Elderly people may become confused, depressed, or excited while taking Seconal.

Seconal may lessen the effectiveness of oral contraceptives. Women who take Seconal may need to consider another type of birth control.

This drug may impair your ability to drive a car or operate potentially dangerous machinery. Do not participate in any activities that require full alertness if you are unsure about your ability.

Possible food and drug interactions when taking this medication

If Seconal is taken with certain other drugs, the effects of either could be increased, decreased, or altered. It is especially important to check with your doctor before combining Seconal with the following:

Anticoagulants (blood thinners such as Dicumarol and Coumadin)
Antihistamines such as Benadryl
Corticosteroids such as prednisone
Doxycycline (Vibramycin)
Griseofulvin (Gris-PEG)
MAO inhibitors (antidepressants such as Nardil)
Oral contraceptives
Phenytoin (Dilantin)
Sedatives/hypnotics such as Halcion
Sodium valproate (Depakoate)

Steroidal hormones such as Premarin
Tranquilizers such as Xanax and Valium
Valproic acid (Depakene)

Extreme drowsiness and other potentially
serious effects can result if Seconal is
combined with alcohol and other central
nervous system depressants.

Special information
if you are pregnant or breastfeeding

Studies have shown Seconal to have a
potentially harmful effect on the unborn child.
If you are pregnant or plan to become
pregnant, inform your doctor immediately.
Use this drug during pregnancy only if clearly
needed and if potential benefits outweigh
possible risks. Small amounts of Seconal
appear in breast milk; consult your doctor
before you begin breastfeeding.

Recommended dosage

ADULTS

For Insomnia
The usual dosage is 100 milligrams, taken
at bedtime.

CHILDREN

Dosages for children should be based on the
child's condition, age, and weight.

ELDERLY

Because elderly people may be more sensitive
to Seconal, they should take lower dosages;
this is also true for people with impaired
kidney function or liver disease.

Overdosage

Any medication taken in excess can have
serious consequences. An overdose of Seconal
can be fatal. If you suspect an overdose, seek
medical help immediately.

*Symptoms of Seconal overdose may be seen
within 15 minutes and may include:*
Blood blisters

Difficulty breathing
Extreme drowsiness
Extreme low body temperature
Fluid in the lungs
Low blood pressure

Brand name:

SECTRAL

Generic name: Acebutolol hydrochloride

Why is this drug prescribed?

Sectral, a type of medication known as a beta
blocker, is used in the treatment of high
blood pressure and abnormal heart rhythms.
When used to treat high blood pressure,
it is effective used alone or in combination
with other high blood pressure
medications, particularly with a thiazide-type
diuretic. Beta blockers decrease the force
and rate of heart contractions.

Most important fact about this drug

If you have high blood pressure, you must
take Sectral regularly for it to be effective.
Even if you are feeling well, you need the
medication to keep your blood pressure
under control.

How should you take this medication?

Sectral can be taken with or without food.

Take this medication exactly as prescribed by
your doctor, even if your symptoms have
disappeared.

Try not to miss any doses. If this medication
is not taken regularly, your condition may
worsen.

If you forget to take a dose, take it as soon
as you remember. If it's within 4 hours
of your next scheduled dose, skip the one
you missed and go back to your regular
schedule. Never take two doses at the same
time.

What side effects may occur?

Side effects cannot be anticipated. If any develop or change in intensity, inform your doctor as soon as possible. Only your doctor can determine if it is safe for you to continue taking Sectral.

■ *More common side effects may include:*
Abnormal vision, chest pain, constipation, cough, decreased sexual ability, depression, diarrhea, dizziness, fatigue, frequent urination, gas, headache, indigestion, joint pain, nasal inflammation, nausea, shortness of breath or difficulty breathing, strange dreams, swelling due to fluid retention, trouble sleeping, weakness

■ *Less common or rare side effects may include:*
Abdominal pain, anxiety, back pain, burning eyes, cold hands and feet, conjunctivitis, dark urine, excessive urination at night, eye pain, fever, heart failure, impotence, itching, loss of appetite, low blood pressure, muscle pain, nervousness, painful or difficult urination, rash, slow heartbeat, throat inflammation, vomiting, wheezing

Why should this drug not be prescribed?

If you have heart failure; inadequate blood supply to the circulatory system (cardiogenic shock); heart block (conduction disorder); or a severely slow heartbeat, you should not take this medication.

Special warnings about this medication

If you have had severe congestive heart failure in the past, Sectral should be used with caution.

Sectral should not be stopped suddenly. This can cause increased chest pain and heart attack. Dosage should be gradually reduced.

If you suffer from asthma, seasonal allergies or other bronchial conditions, coronary artery disease or kidney or liver disease, this medication should be used with caution.

Ask your doctor if you should check your pulse while taking Sectral. This medication can cause your heartbeat to become too slow.

This medication may mask the symptoms of low blood sugar or alter blood sugar levels. If you are diabetic, discuss this with your doctor.

Notify your doctor or dentist that you are taking Sectral if you have a medical emergency, or before you have any surgery.

Tell your doctor if you are taking over-the-counter cold medications and nasal drops. They may interact with Sectral.

If you experience difficulty breathing, or develop hives or large areas of swelling, seek medical attention immediately. You may be having a serious allergic reaction to the medicine.

Possible food and drug interactions when taking this medication

If Sectral is taken with certain other drugs, the effects of either could be increased, decreased, or altered. It is especially important to check with your doctor before combining Sectral with the following:

Catecholamine-depleting drugs such as reserpine
Alpha-adrenergic stimulants commonly found in over-the-counter cold remedies and nasal drops such as Afrin, Neo-Synephrine, Sudafed
Nonsteroidal anti-inflammatory drugs such as Motrin and Voltaren

Special information if you are pregnant or breastfeeding

The effects of Sectral during pregnancy have not been adequately studied. If you are pregnant or plan to become pregnant, inform your doctor immediately. Sectral appears in breast milk and could affect a nursing infant. If this medication is essential to your health, your doctor may advise you to discontinue breastfeeding until your treatment with Sectral is finished.

Recommended dosage

ADULTS

Hypertension
The usual initial dose for mild to moderate high blood pressure is 400 milligrams per day. It may be given in a single daily dose, or as 200 milligrams taken 2 times a day. The usual daily dosage ranges from 200 to 800 milligrams.

Patients with severe high blood pressure may receive a dosage of up to 1,200 milligrams per day divided into 2 doses. It may be given alone or in combination with another high blood pressure medication.

Irregular heartbeat
The usual starting dosage is 400 milligrams per day divided into 2 doses. The dose may be gradually increased to 600 to 1,200 milligrams per day. If this medication is stopped, it should be gradually withdrawn over a period of 2 weeks.

CHILDREN

The safety and effectiveness of Sectral have not been established in children.

ELDERLY

Dosage should be determined by the particular needs of the elderly patient but should not exceed 800 milligrams per day.

Overdosage

Any medication taken in excess can cause symptoms of overdose. If you suspect an overdose, seek medical attention immediately.

There is no specific information available; however, overdose symptoms seen with other beta blockers include:
Bronchospasm
Extremely slow heartbeat
Heart block
Heart conduction problems
Low blood pressure
Low blood sugar
Seizures
Severe congestive heart failure

Brand name:

SELDANE

Generic name: Terfenadine

Why is this drug prescribed?
Seldane is an antihistamine that relieves the sneezing, runny nose, stuffiness, itching, and tearing eyes caused by hay fever. Seldane is chemically different from other antihistamines and causes significantly less drowsiness. Antihistamines work by decreasing the effects of histamine, a chemical the body releases in response to certain irritants. Histamine narrows air passages in the lungs and contributes to inflammation. Antihistamines reduce itching and swelling and dry up secretions from the nose, eyes, and throat.

Most important fact about this drug
Seldane should be taken only as needed. Do not take more than your doctor has indicated.

Rare, serious, heart-related side effects have been reported when Seldane is used with erythromycin (PCE, E-Mycin) or ketoconazole (Nizoral), a medicine for fungal infections. If you are taking Seldane you should not take these drugs.

How should you take this medication?
Take Seldane exactly as prescribed by your doctor.

What side effects may occur?

Side effects cannot be anticipated. If any develop or change in intensity, inform your doctor as soon as possible. Only your doctor can determine if it is safe for you to continue taking Seldane.

■ *More common side effects may include:*
Change in bowel habits, cough, dizziness, drowsiness, dry mouth, nose, throat, fatigue, headache, hives, itching, nausea, nervousness, rash, sore throat, stomach and intestinal problems, vomiting

■ *Less common or rare side effects may include:*
Confusion, depression, difficulty sleeping, excessive or spontaneous flow of milk, fainting, frequent urination, hair thinning or loss, irregular heartbeat, insomnia, low blood pressure, menstrual disorders and pain, nightmares, nosebleed, palpitations, rapid heartbeat, seizures, sensitivity to light, severe allergic reaction (anaphylactic shock), sweating, tingling or pins and needles, tremor, vision changes, wheezing

Why should this drug not be prescribed?

Do not take Seldane if you are sensitive to or have ever had an allergic reaction to it.

Special warnings about this medication

Seldane should be used cautiously if you have liver disease or heart disease. An irregular heartbeat can develop.

Cases of irregular heartbeat have occurred when erythromycin, ketoconazole (Nizoral), or troleandomycin (Tao Capsules) have been taken in combination with Seldane.

Possible food and drug interactions when taking this medication

If Seldane is taken with certain other drugs, the effects of either could be increased, decreased, or altered. It is especially important to check with your doctor before combining Seldane with the following:

Amiodarone (Cordarone)
Disopyramide (Norpace)
Erythromycin (PCE, E-Mycin)
Ketoconazole (Nizoral)
Procainamide (Pronestyl)
Quinidine (Quinaglute, Quinidex)
Troleandomycin (Tao Capsules)

Special information
if you are pregnant or breastfeeding

The effects of Seldane during pregnancy have not been adequately studied. If you are pregnant or plan to become pregnant, inform your doctor immediately. Seldane is not recommended if you are breastfeeding. Animal studies have shown decreased weight gain in babies exposed to this drug. If this medication is essential to your health, your doctor may recommend that you stop breastfeeding until your treatment with Seldane is finished.

Recommended dosage

ADULTS AND CHILDREN 12 AND OLDER

The usual dose is 1 tablet (60 milligrams) 2 times a day.

CHILDREN

Safety and effectiveness in children below the age of 12 have not been established.

Overdosage

Any medication taken in excess can have serious consequences. If you suspect an overdose, seek medical attention immediately.

Symptoms of Seldane overdose may include:
Changes in heartbeat
Confusion
Fainting
Headache
Irregular heartbeat
Nausea
Seizures

Generic name:

SELEGILINE HYDROCHLORIDE

See Eldepryl, page 229.

Brand name:

SEPTRA

See Bactrim, page 53.

Brand name:

SER·AP·ES

Ingredients: Serpasil (reserpine), Apresoline (hydralazine hydrochloride), Esidrix (hydrochlorothiazide)

Why is this drug prescribed?

Ser-Ap-Es is a combination drug used in the treatment of high blood pressure. It combines two high blood pressure medications—Serpasil and Apresoline— with a thiazide diuretic Esidrix. Serpasil and Apresoline improve blood flow throughout your body. Esidrix helps your body produce and eliminate more urine, which also helps lower blood pressure.

Most important fact about this drug

This medication should be used only if your doctor has determined that the precise amount of each ingredient in Ser-Ap-Es meets your specific needs.

Diuretics can cause your body to lose too much potassium. Ask your doctor for the warning signs of too much potassium loss, and whether you should eat specific foods that are rich in potassium or take a potassium supplement to avoid this problem.

How should you take this medication?

Take Ser-Ap-Es exactly as prescribed by your doctor, even if your symptoms have disappeared.

Try not to miss any doses. If this medication is not taken regularly, your condition may worsen.

What side effects may occur?

Side effects cannot be anticipated. If any develop or change in intensity, inform your doctor as soon as possible. Only your doctor can determine if it is safe for you to continue taking Ser-Ap-Es.

■ *Side effects may include:*
Anemia, anxiety, blood disorders, blurred vision, breast development in males, breast engorgement, change in potassium levels (dry mouth, excessive thirst, weak or irregular heartbeat, muscle pain or cramps), chills, conjunctivitis, constipation, cramping (stomach and intestinal), crushing chest pain (angina), deafness, decreased sex drive, depression, diarrhea, difficult or labored breathing, difficult or painful urination, disorientation, dizziness, dizziness when standing up, drowsiness, dry mouth, enlarged spleen, eye disorders, fainting, fever, fluid in the lungs, fluid retention, flushing, glaucoma, headache, hepatitis, high blood sugar, hives, impotence, inflammation of the lungs, inflammation of the pancreas, inflammation of the salivary glands, irregular heartbeat, irritation of the stomach, itching, joint pain, loss of appetite, low blood pressure, muscle aches, muscle cramps, muscle spasm, nasal congestion, nausea, nervousness, nightmares, nosebleeds, numbness, paralysis of intestines, parkinsonian syndrome (tremors, muscle weakness, shuffling walk, stooped posture, drooling), pounding heartbeat, rapid heartbeat, rash, respiratory distress, restlessness, skin peeling, skin sensitivity to light, slow heartbeat, sugar in the urine, teary eyes, tingling or pins and needles, tremors, vertigo, vision changes, vomiting,

weakness, weight gain, yellow eyes and skin

Why should this drug not be prescribed?
If you are being treated for depression you should avoid this medication.

Ser-Ap-Es should not be prescribed if you have an active peptic ulcer, ulcerative colitis (chronic inflammation of the large intestine and rectum), coronary artery disease, or mitral valve prolapse, rheumatic heart disease, or if you are unable to urinate, or are receiving electroshock therapy. Make sure your doctor is aware of all your medical problems.

If you are sensitive to or have ever had an allergic reaction to Ser-Ap-Es, any of its ingredients, or sulfa drugs, do not take this medication. Inform your doctor of any drug reactions you have experienced.

Special warnings about this medication
If you have a history of depression, Ser-Ap-Es should be used with extreme caution. Depression caused by the medication can last for several months after you have stopped taking Ser-Ap-Es, and it can be severe. If you develop any signs of depression—despondency, waking early in the morning, loss of appetite, impotence, loss of self-esteem—contact your doctor immediately.

If you have a history of peptic ulcer, ulcerative colitis, or gallstones you should use this medication cautiously.

Some people have developed symptoms similar to those of lupus erythematosus, a disease characterized by rash, fever, and sometimes the symptoms of arthritis. These symptoms usually disappear when the Ser-Ap-Es is discontinued.

If you have lupus erythematosus, Ser-Ap-Es may activate or worsen its symptoms.

If you have coronary artery, kidney, or liver disease, you should be carefully monitored while taking Ser-Ap-Es.

This medication may mask the symptoms of low blood sugar or alter blood sugar levels. If you are diabetic, discuss this with your doctor.

Allergic reactions are more likely to occur if you have a history of allergies or bronchial asthma.

Abnormal amounts of uric acid in the blood may develop while taking this medication, leading to an attack of gout.

Notify your doctor or dentist that you are taking Ser-Ap-Es if you have a medical emergency, or before you have surgery or dental treatment.

Possible food and drug interactions when taking this medication
If Ser-Ap-Es is taken with certain other drugs, the effects of either could be increased, decreased, or altered. It is especially important to check with your doctor before combining Ser-Ap-Es with the following:

ACTH (adrenal hormone)
Amphetamines such as Dexedrine
Central nervous system stimulants such as Cylert and Desoxyn
Digitalis (Lanoxin)
Drugs for depression such as Elavil
Drugs that stimulate the nervous system (epinephrine, ephedrine, isoproterenol, metaraminol, tyramine, phenylephrine)
Insulin
Lithium (Eskalith)
MAO inhibitors (antidepressant drugs, such as Nardil)
Methyldopa (Aldomet)
Nonsteroidal anti-inflammatory drugs (arthritis drugs and pain killers, such as Motrin)
Norepinephrine (Levophed)

Other high blood pressure drugs such as
    Vasotec
Quinidine (Quinidex)
Steroids such as prednisone
Tubocurarine

Special information
if you are pregnant or breastfeeding

The effects of Ser-Ap-Es during pregnancy
have not been adequately studied. If you
are pregnant or plan to become pregnant,
notify your doctor immediately. Ser-Ap-Es
appears in breast milk and could seriously
affect a nursing infant. If this medication
is essential to your health, your doctor may
advise you to discontinue breastfeeding
until your treatment is finished.

Recommended dosage

ADULTS

Dosages of this drug should be adjusted to
each individual patient's needs.

CHILDREN

The safety and effectiveness of this drug
in children have not been established.

ELDERLY

This drug should be used with caution in
elderly patients.

Overdosage

Any medication taken in excess can cause
symptoms of overdose. If you suspect an
overdose, seek medical attention immediately.

*Symptoms of Ser-Ap-Es overdose may
include:*
Coma, confusion, constricted pupils, cramps
of the calf muscles, ecreased amounts of
urine, diarrhea, dizziness, drowsiness,
fatigue, flushing, headache, heart attack,
inability to urinate, increased amounts
of urine, increased salivation, irregular
heartbeat, low blood pressure, low body
temperature, nausea, rapid heartbeat,

severe loss of fluid, shock, slow heartbeat,
slowed breathing, thirst, tingling or pins
and needles, vomiting, weakness

Brand name:

SERAX

Generic name: Oxazepam

Why is this drug prescribed?

Serax is used in the treatment of anxiety
disorders. Anxiety associated with
depression is also responsive to Serax.

This drug can also be used in the
management of anxiety, tension, agitation
and irritability in older patients and to relieve
symptoms of acute alcohol withdrawal.

Serax is in a class of drugs known as
benzodiazepines.

Most important fact about this drug

Tolerance and dependence can occur with
the long-term use of Serax. You may
experience withdrawal symptoms if you stop
using the drug abruptly. If the drug is
stopped, the dosage should be decreased
gradually over 4 to 8 weeks. Discontinue
or change your dose only on advice of your
doctor.

How should you take this medication?

There are no special instructions. Always take
medications exactly as prescribed by your
doctor.

What side effects may occur?

Side effects cannot be anticipated. If any
develop or change in intensity, inform
your doctor as soon as possible. Only your
doctor can determine if it is safe for you
to continue taking Serax. Your doctor should
periodically reassess the need for this
drug.

■ *More common side effects may include:*
Drowsiness

■ *Less common or rare side effects may include:*
Blood disorders, change in sex drive, dizziness, headache, loss or lack of muscle control, nausea, skin rashes, sluggishness or unresponsiveness, slurred speech, swelling due to fluid retention, tremors

If you experience contradictory side effects such as stimulation, rage, muscle spasticity, menstrual irregularities, hallucinations, acute blood disorders, double or blurred vision, loss of urinary control, fever, or excessive optimism or euphoria, contact your doctor immediately. It may be necessary to discontinue the use of this drug.

■ *Side effects due to rapid decrease or abrupt withdrawal from Serax:*
Abdominal and muscle cramps, convulsions, depressed mood, inability to fall or stay asleep, sweating, tremors, vomiting

Why should this drug not be prescribed?

If you are sensitive to or have ever had an allergic reaction to Serax or similar drugs, you should not take this medication. Make sure that your doctor is aware of any drug reactions that you have experienced.

Anxiety or tension related to everyday stress usually does not require treatment with Serax. Discuss your symptoms thoroughly with your doctor.

Serax should not be prescribed if you are being treated for mental disorders more serious than anxiety.

Special warnings about this medication

Serax may cause you to become drowsy or less alert; therefore, driving or operating dangerous machinery or participating in any hazardous activity that requires full mental alertness is not recommended.

This medication may cause your blood pressure to drop. If you have heart disease, consult with your doctor before taking this medication.

The 15 milligram tablet of this drug contains FD&C Yellow No. 5, which may cause an allergic reaction. If you are sensitive to aspirin or susceptible to allergies, consult with your doctor before taking this dose form.

If you have liver or kidney disease, this drug should be used with caution.

Possible food and drug interactions when taking this medication

Serax may intensify the effects of alcohol. Do not drink alcohol while taking this medication.

If Serax is taken with certain other drugs, the effects of either could be increased, decreased, or altered. It is especially important to check with your doctor before combining Serax with the following:

Antihistamines such as Benadryl
Central nervous system depressants such as
  narcotics

Special information if you are pregnant or breastfeeding

Do not take Serax if you are pregnant or planning to become pregnant. There is an increased risk of birth defects. Serax may appear in breast milk and could affect a nursing infant. If this drug is essential to your health, your doctor may advise you to stop breastfeeding until your treatment with this medication is finished.

Recommended dosage

Your dose should be individualized to your needs by your doctor.

ADULTS

The usual recommended dose is 10 to 15 milligrams 3 or 4 times per day.

Severe Anxiety
The usual recommended dose is 15 to 30 milligrams, 3 or 4 times per day.

Acute Alcohol Withdrawal
The usual recommended dose is 15 to 30 milligrams 3 or 4 times per day.

CHILDREN

This medication is not intended for use in children under 6 years of age. Dosage for children 6 to 12 years of age has not been established. Consult with your doctor.

ELDERLY

The usual starting dose is 10 milligrams, 3 times per day. Your doctor may increase the dose to 15 milligrams 3 or 4 times per day, according to individual need.

Overdosage

Any medication taken in excess can cause symptoms of overdose. If you suspect an overdose, seek medical attention immediately.

No specific information on Serax overdose is available.

Brand name:

SEROPHENE

See Clomiphene Citrate, page 117.

Generic name:

SERTRALINE HYDROCHLORIDE

See Zoloft, page 702.

Brand name:

SILVADENE CREAM 1%

Generic name: Silver sulfadiazine

Why is this drug prescribed?

Silvadene Cream 1% is a topical medicine that is applied directly to the skin. The cream is used along with other medications to prevent and treat wound infections in people with second- and third-degree burns. It is effective against a variety of bacteria as well as yeast.

Most important fact about this drug

Silvadene is a sulfa derivative. If you have ever had an allergic reaction to sulfa drugs, such as Bactrim or Septra, you may have a similar reaction to this medication. Make sure your doctor is aware of any drug reactions you have experienced.

If burn wounds cover extensive areas of the body, Silvadene may be absorbed to a significant extent. This could lead to systemic side effects related to sulfa drugs.

How should you use this medication?

Silvadene is for external use only.

Bathe the burned area daily.

Continue using Silvadene Cream until healing occurs or until the site is ready for skin grafting.

Clean your skin and apply Silvadene with a sterile, gloved hand. Apply a thin layer (about one-sixteenth inch) to the affected area.

Keep the burn areas covered with Silvadene at all times. Reapply the medicine if it is rubbed or washed off.

What side effects may occur?

Side effects cannot be anticipated. If any side effects develop or change in intensity, tell your doctor immediately. Only your doctor can determine whether it is safe for you to continue using Silvadene.

- *More common side effects may include:*
  Burning sensation
  Itching
  Rash

- *Less common or rare side effects may include:*
  Dead skin (skin necrosis), red, raised rash on the body, skin discoloration

Why should this drug not be prescribed?

Silvadene should not be used at the end of pregnancy, on premature infants, or on newborn infants during the first 2 months of life. Sulfa drugs may cause a substance called bilirubin to build up in the bloodstream of newborns. This buildup can lead to complications.

Special warnings about this medication

If kidney or liver function becomes impaired, and the amount of Silvadene being eliminated from the body decreases, it may be necessary to stop using the medication.

Silvadene should be used with extreme caution if you have a history of sensitivity to Silvadene or other sulfa drugs.

Possible food and drug interactions when using this medication

If Silvadene is used with certain other drugs, the effects of either could be increased, decreased, or altered. It is especially important to check with your doctor before combining Silvadene with topical enzyme preparations containing collagenase, papain, or sutilains.

Special information
if you are pregnant or breastfeeding

If you are pregnant or plan to become pregnant, inform your doctor immediately.

No information is available about the safety of Silvadene during pregnancy.

Although it is not known whether Silvadene appears in breast milk, sulfa drugs are excreted in breast milk and can cause harm to a nursing infant. If this medication is essential to your health, your doctor may advise you to stop breastfeeding until your treatment is finished.

Recommended dosage

Silvadene Cream 1% is applied to the affected area once or twice daily to a thickness of one-sixteenth of an inch. Treatment with Silvadene should be continued until satisfactory healing has occurred or until the burn site is ready for grafting.

Overdosage

Any medication taken in excess can have serious consequences. If you suspect an overdose, seek medical treatment immediately.

Generic name:

SILVER SULFADIAZINE

See Silvadene, page 577.

Generic name:

SIMVASTATIN

See Zocor, page 699.

Brand name:

SINEMET CR

Generic ingredients: Carbidopa, Levodopa

Why is this drug prescribed?

Sinemet CR is a controlled-release tablet that may be given to help relieve the muscle stiffness, tremor, and weakness caused by

Parkinson's disease. It may also be given to relieve Parkinson-like symptoms caused by encephalitis (brain fever), carbon monoxide poisoning, or manganese poisoning.

Sinemet CR contains two drugs, carbidopa and levodopa. The drug that actually produces the anti-Parkinson effect is levodopa. Carbidopa prevents vitamin B_6 from destroying levodopa, thus allowing levodopa to work more efficiently and enabling you to get more out of a given amount.

Most important fact about this drug

There is also a regular, non-controlled-release form of this medication, which is called Sinemet. Over a period of hours, Sinemet CR, the controlled-release form, gives a smoother release of the drug than regular Sinemet. If you have been taking regular Sinemet, be aware that you may need a somewhat higher dosage of Sinemet CR to get the same degree of relief. Your first morning dose of Sinemet CR may take as much as an hour longer to start working than your first morning dose of regular Sinemet.

How should you take this medication?

Take Sinemet CR exactly as prescribed by your doctor. Swallow the tablets without chewing or crushing them.

Sinemet CR releases its ingredients slowly over a period of 4 to 6 hours. It is important to follow a careful schedule, taking your doses at the same time every day.

You should not change the prescribed dosage or add another product for Parkinson's disease without first consulting your doctor.

What side effects may occur?

Side effects from Sinemet CR cannot be anticipated. If any develop or change in intensity, inform your doctor immediately.

Only your doctor can determine if it is safe for you to continue taking Sinemet CR.

■ *Side effects may include:*

Abdominal or stomach pain, agitation, anxiety, back pain, bitter taste, bizarre breathing patterns, blurred vision, burning sensation of tongue, chest pain, clumsiness in walking, common cold, constipation, cough, dark sweat, delusions, depression, diarrhea, disorientation, dizziness, dizziness upon rising from a sitting or lying position, dream abnormalities, drooling, drowsiness, dry mouth, euphoria, eyelid twitching, faintness, falling, fatigue, fever, flatulence, fluid retention, flushing, hair loss, hallucinations, headache, heart attack, heart palpitations, heartburn, hiccups, high or low blood pressure, hoarseness, increased hand tremor, insomnia or other sleep problems, irregular heartbeat, leg pain, locked jaw, loss of appetite, malignant melanoma, memory problems, mental changes, muscle cramps, muscle twitching, nausea, nervousness, numbness, "on-off" phenomena, paralysis of certain muscles and unwanted movement of others, paranoia, persistent erection, rash, shortness of breath, shoulder pain, slowed physical movements, sore throat, speech impairment, stomach ulcer, swallowing difficulties, sweating, teeth-grinding, tingling or pins and needles, uncontrollable twitching or jerking, upper respiratory infection, upset stomach, urinary frequency, urinary incontinence, urinary retention, urinary tract infections, weakness, weight loss or gain, writhing or flailing movements, vomiting

Why should this drug not be prescribed?

Do not take Sinemet CR if you are sensitive to or have ever had an allergic reaction to its ingredients.

Special warnings about this medication

Sinemet CR should be prescribed cautiously if you have any of the following:

Bronchial asthma
Cardiovascular or lung disease (severe)
Endocrine (glandular) disorder
History of heart attack or heartbeat
   irregularity
History of active peptic ulcer
Kidney disorder
Liver disorder

Periodic evaluation of liver, blood, kidney, and heart function are recommended during extended therapy with Sinemet CR.

If you have been taking levodopa alone, you should stop taking levodopa for at least 8 hours before starting to take Sinemet CR.

The carbidopa contained in Sinemet CR cannot eliminate side effects caused by levodopa. Since carbidopa helps levodopa reach your brain, Sinemet CR may, in fact, produce some levodopa side effects— particularly twitching, jerking, or writhing— sooner and at a lower dosage than levodopa alone or even regular Sinemet. If such involuntary movements develop while you are taking Sinemet CR, you may need a dosage reduction.

Like levodopa, Sinemet CR may cause depression and suicidal feelings. This medication should be prescribed with caution if you have a psychotic disorder or a history of psychosis.

Sinemet CR should not be used in patients with suspicious, undiagnosed skin lesions or a history of melanoma.

Possible food and drug interactions when taking this medication

If Sinemet CR is taken with certain other drugs, the effects of either could be in- creased, decreased, or altered. It is especially important to check with your doctor before combining Sinemet CR with the following:

Antacids such as Di-Gel, Maalox, Mylanta,
   and others
Anticholinergics such as Artane, Cogentin,
   Disipal, and others
Antihypertensives
Antipsychotics such as Haldol and Moban
Benzodiazepines such as Dalmane, Valium,
   Xanax and others
Clonidine (Catapres)
Hydantoins such as Dilantin
Methionines such as Odor-Scrip and Pedameth
Methyldopa (Aldomet)
Metoclopramide (Reglan)
MAO inhibitor antidepressants such as
   Marplan, Nardil, and Parnate
Papaverine (Pavabid)
Phenothiazines such as Mellaril and Serentil
Pyridoxine (Vitamin B_6)
Tricyclic antidepressants such as Elavil,
   Tofranil, and others

If you have been taking an MAO inhibitor antidepressant such as Marplan, Nardil, or Parnate, you must discontinue it at least 2 weeks before starting to take Sinemet CR.

Take Sinemet CR after meals, rather than before or between meals.

Special information if you are pregnant or breastfeeding

If you are pregnant or plan to become pregnant, inform your doctor immediately. Sinemet CR should be used during pregnancy only if the benefit outweighs the potential risk to the unborn child.

It is not known whether Sinemet CR can make its way into breast milk. Caution is advised when this drug is used by a mother who is breastfeeding.

Recommended dosage

Your doctor will tailor your individual dosage carefully, depending on your response to previous therapy and symptoms.

ADULTS

In patients with mild to moderate disease, the initial recommended dose is 1 tablet of Sinemet CR taken 2 times a day.

Starting dose should be spaced out every 6 hours and then adjusted to each patient's individual response.

The usual dose is 2 to 8 tablets per day, taken in divided doses every 4 to 8 hours during the waking day.

Higher doses (12 or more tablets per day) and shorter intervals (less than 4 hours) have been used, but are not usually recommended.

When doses of Sinemet CR are given at intervals of less than 4 hours, and/or if the divided doses are not equal, it is recommended that the smaller doses be given at the end of the day.

An interval of at least 3 days between dosage adjustments is recommended.

Dosage adjustment of Sinemet CR may be necessary when other drugs are added. A dose of Sinemet (carbidopa-levodopa) 25-100 or 10-100 (one half or a whole tablet) can be added to the dosage regimen of Sinemet CR in selected patients with advanced disease who need additional levopoda for a brief time during daytime hours.

Patients should be observed carefully if abrupt reduction or discontinuation of Sinemet CR is required.

CHILDREN

Use of Sinemet CR in children under 18 is not recommended.

Overdosage

Too much Sinemet CR may cause muscle twitches, inability to open the eyes, or other symptoms of levodopa overdosage. Like other medications, Sinemet CR taken in excess can have serious consequences. If you suspect symptoms of a Sinemet CR overdose, seek medical attention immediately.

Brand name:

SINEQUAN

*Generic name: Doxepin hydrochloride,
Other brand name: Adapin*

Why is this drug prescribed?

Sinequan is used in the treatment of depression and anxiety. It helps relieve tension, improve sleep, elevate mood, increase energy and generally ease the feelings of fear, guilt, apprehension and worry most people experience. It is effective in treating people whose depression and/or anxiety is psychological, associated with alcoholism, or a result of another disease (cancer, for example) or psychotic depressive disorders (severe mental illness). It is in the family of drugs called tricyclic antidepressants.

Most important fact about this drug

Serious, sometimes fatal, reactions have occurred when Sinequan is used in combination with another type of antidepressant called MAO inhibitors. Any drug of this type should be discontinued at least 2 weeks prior to starting treatment with Sinequan, and you should be carefully monitored by your doctor.

If you are taking any prescription or non-prescription drugs, consult with your doctor before taking Sinequan.

How should you take this medication?

Take this medication exactly as prescribed by your doctor. It may take several weeks for you to feel better.

What side effects may occur?

Side effects cannot be anticipated. If any develop or change in intensity, inform your doctor as soon as possible. Only your doctor can determine if it is safe for you to continue taking Sinequan.

■ *More common side effects may include:* Drowsiness

■ *Less common or rare side effects may include:*
Blurred vision, breast development in males, buzzing or ringing in the ears, changes in sex drive, chills, confusion, constipation, diarrhea, difficulty urinating, disorientation, dizziness, dry mouth, enlarged breasts, eye pain, fatigue, fluid retention, flushing, fragmented or incomplete movements, hair loss, hallucinations, headache, high fever, high or low blood sugar, inappropriate breast milk secretion, indigestion, inflammation of the mouth, itching and skin rash, lack of muscle control, loss of appetite, loss of coordination, nausea, nervousness, numbness, poor bladder control, rapid heartbeat, red or brownish spots on the skin, seizures, sensitivity to light, severe muscle stiffness, sore throat, sweating, swelling of the testicles, taste disturbances, tingling sensation, tremors, vomiting, weakness, weight gain, worsening of asthma, yellow eyes and skin

Why should this drug not be prescribed?

If you are sensitive to or have ever had an allergic reaction to Sinequan or similar drugs, you should not take this medication. Make sure that your doctor is aware of any drug reactions that you have experienced.

Unless you are directed to do so by your doctor, do not take this medication if you have glaucoma or difficulty urinating.

Special warnings about this medication

Sinequan may cause you to become drowsy or less alert; therefore, driving or operating dangerous machinery or participating in any hazardous activity that requires full mental alertness is not recommended.

Notify your doctor or dentist that you are taking Sinequan if you have a medical emergency, and before you have surgery or dental treatment.

It can take up to a week for the effects of Sinequan to wear off.

Possible food and drug interactions when taking this medication

Alcohol increases the danger in a Sinequan overdose. Do not drink alcohol while taking this medication.

If Sinequan is taken with certain other drugs, the effects of either could be increased, decreased, or altered. It is especially important to check with your doctor before combining Sinequan with the following:

Cimetidine (Tagamet)
MAO inhibitors (antidepressants such as Nardil)
Tolazamide (Tolinase)

Special information if you are pregnant or breastfeeding

The effects of Sinequan during pregnancy have not been adequately studied. If you are pregnant or planning to become pregnant, inform your doctor immediately. Sinequan may appear in breast milk and could affect a nursing infant. If this medication is essential to your health, your doctor may advise you to discontinue breastfeeding your baby until your treatment is finished.

Recommended dosage
ADULTS

The starting dose for mild to moderate illness is usually 75 milligrams per day. This dose can be increased or decreased by your doctor according to individual need. The usual ideal dose ranges from 75 milligrams per day to 150 milligrams per day, although it can be as low as 25 to 50 milligrams per day. The total daily dose can be given once a day or divided into smaller doses. If you are taking this drug once a day, the recommended dose is 150 milligrams at bedtime.

The 150-milligram capsule strength is intended for maintenance therapy only and is not recommended as a starting dose.

For more severe illness, gradually increased doses of up to 300 milligrams may be required as determined by your doctor.

CHILDREN

Safety and effectiveness have not been established for use in children under 12 years of age.

ELDERLY

A once-a-day dosage should be carefully adjusted by your doctor, depending upon the severity of your illness.

Sinequan capsules come in strengths of 10, 25, 50, 75, 100, and 150 milligrams. Sinequan Oral Concentrate is supplied in 120-milliliter bottles.

Overdosage
Symptoms of Sinequan overdose may include:
Blurred vision, coma, convulsions, decreased intestinal movement, dilated pupils, drowsiness, excessive dryness of mouth, high or low body temperature, irregular or rapid heartbeat, low or high blood pressure, overactive reflexes, severe breathing problems, stupor, urinary problems

If you experience any of these symptoms, seek medical attention immediately.

Brand name:

SLOW-K

See Micro-K, page 376.

Generic name:

SODIUM FLUORIDE

See Luride, page 351.

Brand name:

SODIUM SULAMYD

Generic name: *Sulfacetamide sodium*
Other brand name: *Bleph-10*

Why is this drug prescribed?
Sodium Sulamyd is available as eyedrops or ointment, for the treatment of conjunctivitis ("pinkeye"), corneal ulcer, and other eye infections. Sodium Sulamyd may be used along with an oral sulfa drug to treat a serious eye infection called trachoma.

Most important fact about this drug
Sodium Sulamyd is a medication similar to oral sulfa drugs such as Bactrim, Gantranol, Gantrisin, Suladyne, and Microsul. If you are allergic to any of these medications, you may also be allergic to Sodium Sulamyd. In addition, if you have taken one of these medications in the past, you may have developed a "hidden" allergy to sulfa drugs that might show up when you take Sodium Sulamyd. Be alert for a rash, itching, or other signs of allergy;

if any of these symptoms develop, stop taking Sodium Sulamyd immediately and consult your doctor.

How should you use this medication?

Sodium Sulamyd is available as an ophthalmic solution or an ophthalmic ointment.

Use Sodium Sulamyd exactly as prescribed by your doctor. If you are using the eyedrops, place 1 or 2 drops in the eye every 2 or 3 hours, or less often, as directed. If you are using the ointment, apply it to the eye 4 times per day, and again at bedtime. Your doctor may tell you to use both the eyedrops and the ointment. Sodium Sulamyd should be applied into the lower conjunctival sac (under the lower eyelid).

To avoid contaminating the eyedrops or the ointment, do not touch your eye with the dropper bottle or the tip of the tube. Keep the dropper bottle or tube poised slightly above your eye as you instill the drops or squeeze out the ointment.

What side effects may occur?

Side effects cannot be anticipated. Sodium Sulamyd may irritate your eye, causing stinging and burning. The irritation usually lasts only a short time. If it is very painful or lasts for a long time, you may have to stop using the medication.

In rare cases, people using Sodium Sulamyd have developed a blistering skin rash or a fatal lupus-like syndrome. Be alert for skin reactions. If a rash appears, stop using Sodium Sulamyd and call your doctor.

Why should this drug not be prescribed?

Do not use Sodium Sulamyd if you have ever had an allergic reaction to or are sensitive to this medication or any other sulfa drug.

Special warnings about this medication

Stay in close touch with your doctor while using Sodium Sulamyd. In some cases, an eye ointment may actually delay healing of the cornea. If you have a pus-producing eye infection, the pus may inactivate Sodium Sulamyd. Since sulfa drugs do not kill fungi, it is possible to get a fungus infection in your eye while using Sodium Sulamyd.

Possible food and drug interactions when taking this medication

If you use Sodium Sulamyd with another eye medication, the effect of either medication may be increased, decreased, or altered. Check with your doctor before using Sodium Sulamyd simultaneously with any other eyedrops or eye ointment.

Special information if you are pregnant or breastfeeding

If you are pregnant or plan to become pregnant, inform your doctor immediately. There is no information about the safety of Sodium Sulamyd during pregnancy.

It is not known whether Sodium Sulamyd appears in breast milk. If Sodium Sulamyd is essential to your health, it may be necessary to stop breastfeeding during treatment.

Recommended dosage

SODIUM SULAMYD OPHTHALMIC SOLUTION 30%

Conjunctivitis or Corneal Ulcer
Place 1 drop in lower conjunctival sac (eyelid) every 2 hours or less frequently according to severity of infection.

Trachoma (Contagious Conjunctivitis)
Use 2 drops every 2 hours.

SODIUM SULAMYD OPHTHALMIC SOLUTION 10%

Place 1 or 2 drops in the lower conjunctival sac (eyelid) every 2 or 3 hours during the day, less often at night.

SODIUM SULAMYD OPHTHALMIC
OINTMENT 10%

Apply a small amount of the ointment 4 times
daily and at bedtime. The ointment may
be used at the same time as either of the
solution forms.

Overdosage

Although no specific information is available,
any medication used in excess can
have serious consequences. If you suspect you
may have used too much Sodium
Sulamyd, seek medical attention immediately.

Brand name:

SOMA

Generic name: Carisoprodol

Why is this drug prescribed?

Soma is prescribed, along with rest, physical
therapy, and other measures, for the relief
of pain and discomfort associated with severe
disorders of skeletal muscle (muscle that is
attached to the skeleton and responsible for
the movement of bones).

Most important fact about this drug

Occasionally, the first dose of Soma may cause
unusual symptoms that appear within minutes
or hours of taking the medication.

Symptoms reported include: Agitation,
confusion, disorientation, dizziness, double
vision, enlargement of pupils, extreme
weakness, exaggerated feeling of well-being,
lack of coordination, speech problems,
temporary loss of vision, temporary paralysis
of arms and legs

Symptoms usually subside within a few hours.
If you experience any of these symptoms,
consult with your doctor immediately.

How should you take this medication?

Take Soma exactly as prescribed by your
doctor.

What side effects may occur?

Side effects cannot be anticipated. If any
develop or change in intensity, inform your
doctor as soon as possible. Only your doctor
can determine if it is safe for you to continue
taking Soma.

■ *Side effects may include:*
Agitation, dizziness, drowsiness, facial
flushing, fainting, headache, hiccups,
inability to fall or stay asleep, irritability,
loss of coordination, nausea, rapid heart
rate, tremors, vertigo, vomiting

Allergic reactions usually seen between the
first and fourth doses of Soma in patients
who have never taken this drug include:
itching, red welts on skin, and skin rash.

■ *Severe allergic reactions may include:*
Asthmatic attacks, dizziness, fever, low
blood pressure, stinging of the eyes,
swelling due to fluid retention, weakness

Why should this drug not be prescribed?

If you are sensitive to or have ever had an
allergic reaction to Soma or drugs of this type,
such as meprobamate (Miltown), mebutamate,
or tybamate (Tybatran), you should not take
this medication. Make sure that your doctor
is aware of any drug reactions that you
have experienced.

Unless you are directed to do so by your
doctor, do not take this medication if you
have porphyria (an inherited blood metabolism
disorder).

Special warnings about this medication

Soma may impair the mental or physical
abilities you need to drive a car or operate
dangerous machinery. Participation in
hazardous activities is not recommended.

If you have a history of drug dependence,
consult with your doctor before taking this
medication.

Caution should be exercised when taking this drug if you have impaired kidney or liver function. Consult with your doctor.

Withdrawal symptoms, including abdominal cramps, chilliness, headache, insomnia, and nausea, have occurred in people who suddenly stop taking Soma.

Possible food and drug interactions when taking this medication

Soma may intensify the effects of alcohol. Use caution while taking this medication.

If Soma is taken with certain other drugs, the effects of either could be increased, decreased, or altered. It is especially important to check with your doctor before combining Soma with the following:

Central nervous system depressants such as Nembutal or Restoril
Psychotropic drugs (drugs that affect mood, such as tranquilizers and antidepressants)

Special information
if you are pregnant or breastfeeding

The effects of Soma during pregnancy have not been adequately studied. If you are pregnant or plan to become pregnant, inform your doctor immediately. This drug appears in breast milk and could affect a nursing infant. If this medication is essential to your health, your doctor may advise you to discontinue breastfeeding until your treatment is finished.

Recommended dosage

ADULTS

The usual recommended dosage of Soma is one 350-milligram tablet, taken 3 times daily and at bedtime.

CHILDREN

The safety and effectiveness of this drug have not been established in children under 12 years of age.

Overdosage

An overdose of Soma can be fatal.

Symptoms of Soma overdose may include:
A state of unresponsiveness or
   unconsciousness
Breathing difficulty
Coma
Shock

If you suspect an overdose, seek medical attention immediately.

Brand name:

SORBITRATE

See Isordil, page 303.

Brand name:

SPECTAZOLE CREAM

Generic name: Econazole nitrate

Why is this drug prescribed?

Spectazole cream is prescribed for fungal skin diseases commonly called ringworm (tinea). It is used to treat athlete's foot (tinea pedis), "jock itch" (tinea cruris), a fungus infection of the entire body (tinea corporis), and tinea versicolor (yellow- or brown-colored skin eruptions). It is also prescribed for yeast infections caused by candida fungus (cutaneous candidiasis).

Most important fact about this drug

Spectazole is not for use in or near the eyes.

How should you use this medication?

Use Spectazole Cream exactly as prescribed by your doctor.

When applied, the cream should completely cover the affected area.

What side effects may occur?

Side effects cannot be anticipated. If any develop or change in intensity, inform your doctor as soon as possible. Only your doctor can determine whether it is safe for you to continue using Spectazole.

■ *More common side effects may include:*
Burning
Itching
Skin redness
Stinging

■ *Less common or rare side effects may include:*
Itching rash

Why should this drug not be prescribed?

Spectazole Cream should not be used if you are sensitive to it or have ever had an allergic reaction to any of its ingredients.

Special warnings about this medication

If you develop an irritation or an allergic reaction to Spectazole, stop using the cream and inform your doctor.

Possible food and drug interactions when taking this medication

No interactions have been reported.

Special information if you are pregnant or breastfeeding

Spectazole should be used during the first trimester (3 months) of pregnancy only if it is essential to your health; Spectazole should be used during the remainder of your pregnancy only if your doctor feels it is clearly needed. If you are pregnant or plan to become pregnant, inform your doctor immediately. Spectazole may appear in breast milk and could affect a nursing infant. If this medication is essential to your health, your doctor may advise you to stop breastfeeding until your treatment with Spectazole is finished.

Recommended dosage

ATHLETE'S FOOT, JOCK ITCH, TINEA CORPORIS, TINEA VERSICOLOR

Apply sufficient Spectazole Cream to completely cover the affected area once a day. Athlete's foot is treated for 1 month; jock itch and tinea corporis are treated for 2 weeks. Tinea versicolor usually clears up after 2 weeks.

CUTANEOUS CANDIDIASIS

Apply sufficient Spectazole Cream to completely cover the affected area 2 times a day, once in the morning and once in the evening. Cutaneous candidiasis is treated for 2 weeks.

Overdosage

Although no specific information is available on Spectazole Cream overdosage, any medication used in excess can have serious consequences. If you suspect an overdose, seek medical attention immediately.

Generic name:

SPIRONOLACTONE

See Aldactone, page 13.

Generic name:

SPIRONOLACTONE WITH HYDROCHLOROTHIAZIDE

See Aldactazide, page 11.

Brand name:

SPIROZIDE

See Aldactazide, page 11.

Brand name:

STELAZINE

Generic name: Trifluoperazine hydrochloride

Why is this drug prescribed?

Stelazine is used to treat psychotic disorders as well as anxiety that does not respond to ordinary tranquilizers.

Most important fact about this drug

Stelazine may cause tardive dyskinesia—a condition marked by involuntary muscle spasms and twitches in the face and body. This condition may be permanent and appears to be most common among the elderly, especially women. Ask your doctor for information about this possible risk.

How should you take this medication?

If taking Stelazine in a liquid concentrate form, you will need to dilute it with a liquid such as a carbonated beverage, coffee, fruit juice, milk, orange syrup, simple syrup, tea, tomato juice, or water. Puddings, soups, and other semisolid foods may also be used. Stelazine should be diluted immediately prior to use.

You should not take Stelazine with alcohol.

What side effects may occur?

Side effects cannot be anticipated. If any develop or change in intensity, inform your doctor as soon as possible. Only your doctor can determine if it is safe for you to continue taking Stelazine.

■ *Side effects may include:*
Abnormal secretion of milk, abnormal sugar in urine, abnormalities in movement and posture, agitation, allergic reactions, anemia, asthma, blood disorders, blurred vision, breast development in males, catatonic states, chewing movements, constipation, difficulty swallowing, dizziness, drowsiness, dry mouth, ejaculation problems, exaggerated reflexes, excessive or spontaneous flow of milk, excessive reflexes, eye problems causing a state of fixed gaze, eye spasms, fatigue, fever, flu-like symptoms, fluid accumulation and swelling (including the brain), fragmented movements, head bent back onto back, headache, heart attack, high or low blood sugar, hives, impotence, increase in appetite and weight, infections, insomnia, intestinal blockage, involuntary movements of arms and legs, irregular blood pressure, pulse, and heartbeat, irregular or no menstrual periods, light-headedness (especially when standing up), loss of appetite, low blood pressure, mask-like face, muscle stiffness and rigidity, narrow or dilated pupils, nasal congestion, nausea, pain and stiffness in neck, persistent, painful erections, pill-rolling movement, protruding tongue, psychotic symptoms, puckering of mouth, puffing of cheeks, rapid heartbeat, red blood spots, restlessness, rigid arms, feet, head, and muscles, seizures, sensitivity to light, shock, shuffling walk, skin inflammation and peeling, skin itching, pigmentation, rash, spasms in jaw, face, tongue, back, and mouth, sweating, swelling of the throat, tremors, twisted neck, weakness, yellowing of skin and whites of eyes

Why should this drug not be prescribed?

You should not be using Stelazine if you have liver damage, or if you are taking central nervous system depressants such as alcohol, barbiturates, or narcotics. Stelazine should not be used if you have an abnormal bone marrow or blood condition. Do not give Stelazine to someone in a comatose state.

Special warnings about this medication

You should use Stelazine cautiously if you have ever had: a brain tumor, breast cancer, intestinal blockage, glaucoma, heart, or liver disease, seizures, or if you are exposed to pesticides or extreme heat. Be aware that Stelazine may obscure diagnosis of intestinal obstruction, brain tumor, and Reye's syndrome.

Appetite loss, dizziness, nausea, vomiting, and tremors can result if you suddenly stop taking Stelazine. Follow your doctor's instructions when discontinuing Stelazine.

Tell your doctor immediately if you experience symptoms such as a fever or sore throat, mouth, or gums. These signs of infection may signal the need to stop Stelazine treatment.

This drug may impair your ability to drive a car or operate potentially dangerous machinery. Do not participate in any activities that require full alertness if you are unsure about your ability.

Stelazine concentrate contains a sulfite that may cause allergic reactions in some people.

Possible food and drug interactions when taking this medication

If Stelazine is taken with certain other drugs, the effects of either could be increased, decreased, or altered. It is especially important to check with your doctor before combining Stelazine with the following:

Anticonvulsants such as Dilantin
Anticoagulants/blood thinners such as
  Dicumarol
Atropine (Donnatal)
Guanethidine (Ismelin)
Propranolol (Inderal)
Thiazide diuretics such as Dyazide

Extreme drowsiness and other potentially serious effects can result if Stelazine is combined with alcohol or other mental depressants, narcotics and painkillers such as Percocet, antihistamines such as Benadryl, and barbiturates such as Phenobarbital.

Special information if you are pregnant or breastfeeding

Pregnant women should use Stelazine only if clearly needed. The effects of Stelazine during pregnancy have not been adequately studied. If you are pregnant or plan to become pregnant, inform your doctor immediately. Stelazine appears in breast milk and may affect a nursing infant.

Recommended dosage

Doses should be tailored to the individual. The minimum effective amount should be used.

ADULTS

Non-Psychotic Anxiety
Doses usually range from 2 to 4 milligrams daily. This amount should be divided into 2 equal doses and taken 2 times per day. Dosage should not exceed 6 milligrams a day or be given for more than 12 weeks.

Psychotic Disorders
The usual starting dose is 4 to 10 milligrams a day, divided into 2 equal doses; doses range from 15 to 40 milligrams daily.

CHILDREN

Doses are based on the child's weight and the severity or his or her symptoms.

Psychotic Children 6 to 12 Years Old Who Are Closely Monitored or Hospitalized
Doses range from 1 to 15 milligrams daily.

ELDERLY

Elderly people usually take Stelazine at lower doses. Because they may develop low blood pressure while taking Stelazine, they should be closely monitored. Elderly people (especially elderly women) may be more susceptible to tardive dyskinesia—a possibly permanent condition characterized by involuntary muscle spasms and twitches in the face and body. Elderly people should consult their doctor for information about these potential risks.

Overdosage

Any medication taken in excess can have serious consequences. If you suspect an overdose, seek medical help immediately.

Symptoms of Stelazine overdose may include: Agitation, coma, convulsions, difficulty breathing, difficulty swallowing, dry mouth, extreme sleepiness, fever, intestinal blockage, irregular heart rate, low blood pressure, restlessness

Brand name:

STUARTNATAL 1 + 1

Generic name: Maternal vitamin and mineral supplement

Why is this drug prescribed?

Stuartnatal 1 + 1 contains vitamins and minerals including iron, calcium, zinc, and folic acid. The tablets are given during pregnancy and after childbirth to assure an adequate supply. They may also be prescribed to improve a woman's nutritional status before she becomes pregnant.

Most important fact about this drug

Though Stuartnatal 1 + 1 contains folic acid for the blood, you should not take if for pernicious anemia which is caused by a lack of vitamin B_{12}. Folic acid will not correct nerve damage caused by pernicious anemia.

How should you take this medication?

Take Stuartnatal 1 + 1 exactly as prescribed by your doctor. The usual dosage is 1 tablet per day.

Why should this drug not be prescribed?

Do not take Stuartnatal 1 + 1 if you have pernicious anemia.

Special warnings about this medication

Stuartnatal 1 + 1 is available only by prescription. As with all medications, keep it out of the reach of children.

Special information if you are pregnant or breastfeeding

Pregnancy and breastfeeding impose special nutritional demands on the mother. A vitamin and mineral supplement can help ensure that there are enough nutrients for both you and your baby.

Recommended dosage

ADULTS

Before, during, and after pregnancy, 1 tablet daily, or as directed by your doctor.

Overdosage

Although no specific overdose information is available, any medication taken in excess—including a nutritional supplement—can have serious consequences. If you suspect an overdose of Stuartnatal 1 + 1, seek medical attention immediately.

Generic name:

SUCRALFATE

See Carafate, page 90.

Generic name:

SULFACETAMIDE SODIUM

See Sodium Sulamyd, page 583.

Generic name:

SULFASALAZINE

See Azulfidine, page 51.

Generic name:

SULFISOXAZOLE

See Gantrisin, page 267.

Generic name:

SULINDAC

See Clinoril, page 115.

Brand name:

SUMYCIN

See Achromycin V Capsules, page 3.

Brand name:

SUPRAX

Generic name: Cefixime

Why is this drug prescribed?
Suprax, a cephalosporin antibiotic, is prescribed for bacterial infections of the chest, ears, urinary tract, and throat.

Most important fact about this drug
If you are sensitive to or have ever had an allergic reaction to penicillin, cephalosporins, or similar drugs, notify your doctor before taking this medication. Severe allergic reactions have been reported in penicillin-sensitive patients.

How should you take this medication?
Suprax can be taken with or without food. If the medication causes stomach upset, take it with meals. Food, however, will slow down the rate at which medication is absorbed into your bloodstream.

If you are taking a liquid form of Suprax, use the specially marked measuring spoon to measure each dose accurately. Shake well before using. Suprax liquid may be kept for 14 days, either at room temperature or in the refrigerator. Discard any unused portion after 14 days.

It is important that you finish taking all of this medication even if you are feeling better, in order to obtain the medicine's maximum benefit.

If you are taking this medication once a day and you forget to take a dose, take it as soon as you remember. Wait at least 10 to 12 hours before taking your next dose. Then return to your regular schedule.

If you are taking this medication 2 times a day and you forget to take a dose, take it as soon as you remember and take your next dose 5 to 6 hours later. Then go back to your regular schedule.

If you are taking this medication 3 times a day and you forget to take a dose, take it as soon as you remember and take your next dose 2 to 4 hours later. Then return to your regular schedule.

What side effects may occur?
Side effects cannot be anticipated. If any develop or change in intensity, inform your doctor as soon as possible. Only your doctor can determine if it is safe for you to continue taking Suprax.

■*More common side effects may include:*
Abdominal pain
Gas
Indigestion
Loose stools
Mild diarrhea
Nausea
Vomiting

■*Less common side effects may include:*
Colitis, dizziness, fever, headaches, hives, itching, skin rashes, vaginitis

■ *Rare side effects may include:*
Bleeding, decrease in urine output, seizures, severe abdominal or stomach cramps, severe diarrhea (sometimes accompanied by blood), shock, skin redness

Why should this drug not be prescribed?
If you are sensitive to or have ever had an allergic reaction to Suprax or similar drugs, you should not take this medication. Make sure that your doctor is aware of any drug reactions that you have experienced.

Special warnings about this medication
Notify your doctor if you have had allergic reactions to penicillins or other cephalosporin antibiotics.

If you have a history of stomach or intestinal disease such as colitis, check with your doctor before taking Suprax.

If your symptoms of infection do not improve within a few days, or if they get worse, notify your doctor immediately.

If nausea, vomiting, or severe diarrhea occurs while taking Suprax, check with your doctor before taking diarrhea medication. Certain diarrhea medications (Lomotil, Paregoric) may make your diarrhea worse or cause it to last longer.

If you are a diabetic, it is important to note that Suprax may cause false urine-sugar test results. Notify your doctor that you are taking this medication before being tested for sugar in the urine. Do not change diet or dosage of diabetes medication without first consulting with your doctor.

Do not give this medication to other people or use it for other infections. Some bacteria will not respond to this medication.

If you have a kidney disorder, check with your doctor before taking Suprax. You may need a reduced dose of this medication because of your medical condition.

Repeated use of Suprax may result in an overgrowth of bacteria that do not respond to the medication and can cause a secondary infection. Therefore, do not save this medication for use at another time. Take this medication only when directed to do so by your doctor.

Possible food and drug interactions when taking this medication
No interactions with other drugs have been reported.

Special information if you are pregnant or breastfeeding
The effects of Suprax during pregnancy have not been adequately studied. If you are pregnant or plan to become pregnant, inform your doctor immediately. Suprax may appear in breast milk and could affect a nursing infant. If this medication is essential to your health, your doctor may advise you to discontinue breastfeeding your baby until your treatment with this medication is finished.

Recommended dosage

ADULTS

The usual adult dose is 400 milligrams daily. This may be taken as a single 400 milligram tablet once a day or as a 200 milligram tablet every 12 hours.

CHILDREN

The safety and effectiveness of Suprax in children less than 6 months old have not been established. The usual child's dose is 8 milligrams of liquid per 2.2 pounds of body weight per day. This may be given as a single dose or in 2 half doses every 12 hours. Children weighing more than 110 pounds or older than 12 years of age should be treated with an adult dose.

ELDERLY

Your doctor may wish to start you on a low dosage because this drug is eliminated from your body by the kidneys and kidney function tends to decrease with age.

Overdosage

Any medication taken in excess can cause symptoms of overdose. If you suspect an overdose, seek medical attention immediately.

Symptoms of Suprax overdose may include:
Blood in the urine
Diarrhea
Nausea
Upper abdominal pain
Vomiting

Brand name:

SURMONTIL

Generic name: Trimipramine maleate

Why is this drug prescribed?

Surmontil is used to treat depression. It is a member of the family of drugs known as tricyclic antidepressants.

Most important fact about this drug

If taken in high enough amounts, Surmontil can be fatal. It should be prescribed in the smallest amount, and it should always be stored in child-resistant containers.

It is important to take Surmontil exactly as prescribed by your doctor, even if the drug seems to have no effect. It may take 2 or 3 weeks for its benefits to appear.

How should you take this medication?

Surmontil may be taken in one dose at bedtime, or the total daily dosage may be divided into smaller amounts taken during the day.

If you are on maintenance therapy with Surmontil, a single bedtime dose is preferred.

You should not take Surmontil with alcohol.

What side effects may occur?

Side effects cannot be anticipated. If any develop or change in intensity, inform your doctor as soon as possible. Only your doctor can determine if it is safe for you to continue taking Surmontil.

■ *Side effects may include:*
Abdominal cramps, agitation, anxiety, black tongue, blocked intestine, blood disorders, blurred vision, breast development in the male, confusion (especially in elderly people), constipation, delusions, diarrhea, difficulty urinating, dilated pupils, disorientation, dizziness, drowsiness, dry mouth, excessive or spontaneous milk excretion, fatigue, fever, flushing, frequent urination, hair loss, hallucinations, headache, heart attack, high blood pressure, high blood sugar, hives, impotence, increased or decreased sex drive, increased psychotic symptoms, inflamed lymph gland under tongue, inflammation of the mouth, insomnia, irregular heart rate, lack of coordination, loss of appetite, low blood pressure, low blood sugar, nausea, nightmares, numbness, pounding heartbeat, peculiar taste in mouth, purple or reddish-brown spots on skin, rapid heartbeat, restlessness, ringing in the ears, seizures, skin itching, skin rash, sore throat, stomach upset, stroke, sensitivity to light, sweating, swelling of breasts, swelling of face and tongue, swelling of testicles, swollen glands, tingling, pins and needles, tremors, visual problems, vomiting, weakness, weight gain or loss, yellowing of the skin and whites of the eyes

Why should this drug not be prescribed?

Surmontil should not be used if you have had a recent heart attack.

Do not use Surmontil if you are taking antidepressant drugs known as MAO inhibitors, including those such as Parnate and Nardil.

You should not take Surmontil if you are known to be hypersensitive to it.

Special warnings about this medication

People who have had seizures, glaucoma, or heart, liver, or thyroid disease, or who are taking thyroid medication, or who have a history of urinary retention should take Surmontil cautiously.

Nausea, headache, and a general feeling of illness may result if you suddenly stop taking Surmontil. Follow your doctor's instructions closely when discontinuing the drug.

This drug may impair your ability to drive a car or operate potentially dangerous machinery. Do not participate in any activities that require full alertness if you are unsure about your ability.

Possible food and drug interactions when taking this medication

People who take the antidepressants known as MAO inhibitors (Parnate, Nardil, Marplan) should not take Surmontil.

If Surmontil is taken with certain other drugs, the effects of either could be increased, decreased, or altered. It is especially important to check with your doctor before combining Surmontil with the following:

Anticholinergic drugs such as Cogentin
Catecholamines such as EpiPen
Cimetidine (Tagamet)
Guanethidine (Ismelin)
Local anesthetics
Local decongestants such as Dristan Nasal
    Spray
Oral nasal decongestants such as Sudafed
Thyroid medications

Extreme drowsiness and other potentially serious effects may result if you combine Surmontil with alcohol.

Special information
if you are pregnant or breastfeeding

Pregnant women should use Surmontil only when the potential benefits clearly outweigh the potential risks.

Recommended dosage

Dosages should start at a low level and be gradually increased if needed.

ADULTS

The usual starting dose is 75 milligrams per day, divided into equal smaller doses. If needed, this amount may be gradually increased to 150 milligrams per day, divided into smaller doses. Doses over 200 milligrams a day are not recommended. Maintenance dosages may range from 50 to 150 milligrams daily. This total daily dosage may be taken at bedtime, or spread throughout the day.

CHILDREN

Surmontil is not recommended for children.

ELDERLY AND ADOLESCENTS

Dosages usually start at 50 milligrams per day. This amount may be gradually increased to 100 milligrams a day, if needed.

Overdosage

Any medication taken in excess can have serious consequences. An overdose of Surmontil can be fatal. If you suspect an overdose, seek medical help immediately.

Symptoms of Surmontil overdose may include: Agitation, coma, convulsions, difficulty breathing, dilated pupils, discolored bluish skin, drowsiness, fever, heart failure, involuntary movement, irregular heart rate, lack of coordination, low blood pressure, muscle rigidity, rapid heartbeat, restlessness, shock, stupor, sweating, vomiting

Brand name:

SYMADINE

See Symmetrel, page 595.

Brand name:

SYMMETREL

Generic name: Amantadine hydrochloride
Other brand names: Symadine

Why is this drug prescribed?

Symmetrel is an oral medication that comes in capsules or syrup. Symmetrel is used to treat or prevent flu caused by the *Influenza A* virus; to treat Parkinson's disease; and to relieve tremors, jerks, or writhing caused by treatment with other drugs.

We do not know how Symmetrel works. The drug is known to have an effect on the brain and nervous system. It also appears to keep *Influenza A* virus particles from releasing their contents into healthy cells.

If you work in a hospital or in close contact with someone who has or is likely to get flu caused by the *Influenza A* virus, you should have a flu shot each year. If a flu shot is impossible or contraindicated, preventive treatment with Symmetrel may be advisable. You may get a flu shot even after starting to take Symmetrel. Once your body has manufactured enough antibodies to the *Influenza A* virus, you will no longer need to take Symmetrel.

Most important fact about this drug

If you are going to take Symmetrel to treat flu caused by the *Influenza A* virus, you should start taking the drug as soon as possible after your flu symptoms develop—preferably within 24 to 48 hours—and continue taking it for 24 to 48 hours after your flu symptoms disappear.

How should you take this medication?

Take Symmetrel exactly as prescribed by your doctor. It may be as long as 48 hours before the drug takes effect.

If you take Symmetrel for Parkinson's disease, the drug may become less effective after several months of treatment. At this point, your doctor may increase your dosage slightly or tell you to stop taking the medication for several weeks and then start again. Either approach may help restore Symmetrel's effectiveness. If it does not, your doctor may need to prescribe an additional anti-Parkinson medication. If you stop taking Symmetrel abruptly, you may experience a sudden worsening of your symptoms.

What side effects may occur?

Side effects cannot be anticipated. If any develop or change in intensity, inform your doctor imemdiately. Only your doctor can determine whether it is safe for you to continue taking Symmetrel.

■ *More common side effects may include:*
Dizziness (light-headedness)
Insomnia
Nausea

■ *Less common or rare side effects may include:*
Agitation, anxiety, appetite loss, breathing difficulties, confusion, congestive heart failure (shortness of breath, swollen ankles), constipation, decreased sexual desire, depression, diarrhea, dizziness upon arising from a sitting position, dream abnormality, dry mouth or nose, fatigue, feeling of extreme happiness, hallucinations, headache, high blood pressure, irritability, loss of coordination, loss of memory, nervousness, psychosis, purplish mottling of the lower legs, rash, slurred speech, swollen ankles, urinary retention, vision problems, vomiting, weakness

Why should this drug not be prescribed?

Do not take Symmetrel if you have ever had an allergic reaction to it, or are sensitive to it.

Special warnings about this medication

If you have epilepsy, Symmetrel may increase your risk of having a seizure.

If you have swollen ankles or a history of congestive heart failure, your doctor should monitor you especially closely. Symmetrel has caused congestive heart failure in some people.

If you take Symmetrel for Parkinson's disease and begin feeling better, resume your normal activities gradually. Keep in mind any other medical problems that may pose a danger, such as osteoporosis (brittle bones) or inflamed veins where a blood clot might form.

If Symmetrel causes blurred vision, makes you drowsy, or impairs your coordination, you should avoid driving, climbing, and performing hazardous tasks as long as you are taking the medication.

If you are older than 65 or have kidney problems, your dosage of Symmetrel should be reduced.

Possible food and drug interactions when taking this medication

If Symmetral is taken with certain other drugs, the effects of either could be increased, decreased, or altered. It is especially important to check with your doctor before combining Symmetral with the following:

Anticholinergic drugs such as Cogentin, Akineton, Artane, and others
Central nervous system stimulants such as Dexedrine, Desoxyn, and others

Special information
if you are pregnant or breastfeeding

If you are pregnant or plan to become pregnant, notify your doctor immediately.

Symmetrel should not be used during pregnancy unless the benefit outweighs the potential risks to the unborn baby. Because Symmetrel appears in breast milk, caution is advised when taking this medication while breastfeeding.

Recommended dosage

FOR PARKINSONISM

Adults

The usual adult dose of Symmetrel is 100 milligrams twice a day when used alone. Symmetrel usually begins to work within 48 hours.

FOR DRUG-INDUCED TREMORS

Adults

The usual adult dose of Symmetrel is 100 milligrams twice a day. Occasionally patients who do not respond to Symmetrel at 200 milligrams daily may benefit if the dosage is increased up to 300 milligrams daily in divided doses.

FOR INFLUENZA A

For prophylaxis of Influenza A virus illness and treatment of uncomplicated Influenza A virus illness in patients with normal renal function.

Adults

The daily adult dosage of Symmetrel is 200 milligrams, given as single daily dose of two 100-milligram capsules (or 4 teaspoonfuls of syrup), or as 1 capsule of 100 milligrams (or 2 teaspoonfuls of syrup) twice a day. If central nervous system side effects develop on once-a-day dosage, a split dosage schedule may reduce such complaints.

Children 9 to 12 years of age

The total daily dose is 200 milligrams, given as one capsule of 100 milligrams (or 2 teaspoonfuls of syrup) twice a day.

Children 1 to 9 years of age
The total daily dose is calculated on the basis of 2 to 4 milligrams per pound of body weight, but should not exceed 150 milligrams per day.

Elderly
The daily dosage of Symmetrel is 100 milligrams for people 65 years of age or older.

Overdosage

Too much Symmetrel may cause hyperactivity, convulsions, stupor, kidney failure, and coma. Heartbeat abnormalities, very low blood pressure, and urinary retention may also occur. An overdose of Symmetrel may be fatal. If you suspect an overdose, seek medical attention immediately.

Brand name:

SYNALGOS-DC

Generic ingredients: Dihydrocodeine bitartrate, Aspirin, Caffeine

Why is this drug prescribed?

Synalgos-DC is a narcotic analgesic prescribed for the relief of moderate to moderately severe pain.

Most important fact about this drug

Mental and physical dependence can occur with the use of narcotics such as Synalgos-DC when taken over long periods of time.

How should you take this medication?

Take Synalgos-DC exactly as prescribed by your doctor. Do not increase the amount you take without your doctor's approval.

Avoid or reduce use of alcohol while taking Synalgos-DC.

What side effects may occur?

Side effects cannot be anticipated. If any develop or change in intensity, inform your doctor as soon as possible. Only your doctor can determine if it is safe for you to continue taking Synalgos-DC.

■ *Side effects may include:*
Constipation
Dizziness
Drowsiness
Itching
Light-headedness
Nausea
Sedation
Skin reactions
Vomiting

Why should this drug not be prescribed?

If you are sensitive to or have ever had an allergic reaction to Synalgos-DC, narcotic pain relievers, or aspirin, you should not take this medication. Make sure that your doctor is aware of any drug reactions that you have experienced.

Special warnings about this medication

Synalgos-DC may cause you to become drowsy or less alert; therefore, driving or operating dangerous machinery or participating in any hazardous activity that requires full mental alertness is not recommended.

If you have a history of drug dependence, consult with your doctor before taking Synalgos-DC.

If you are being treated for a stomach ulcer or blood-clotting disorder, consult with your doctor before taking this medication.

Possible food and drug interactions when taking this medication

Synalgos-DC is a central nervous system depressant and intensifies the effects of alcohol. Therefore, use of alcohol should be reduced or avoided.

If Synalgos-DC is taken with certain other drugs, the effects of either could be increased, decreased, or altered. It is especially important to check with your doctor before combining Synalgos-DC with the following:

Central nervous system depressants
   Narcotic pain relievers such as Percocet
   and Demerol
Sedative/hypnotics such as Halcion
Tranquilizers such as Valium and Xanax

The use of anticoagulants (blood thinners such as Coumadin) in combination with Synalgos-DC may cause internal bleeding. If you are taking an anticoagulant, consult with your doctor before taking this drug.

The use of Synalgos-DC in combination with uricosuric drugs (antigout medications such as Benenid) may alter the effects of this drug. Consult with your doctor.

Special information
if you are pregnant or breastfeeding
The effects of Synalgos-DC during pregnancy have not been adequately studied. If you are pregnant or plan to become pregnant, inform your doctor immediately. This drug may appear in breast milk and could affect a nursing infant. If this medication is essential to your health, your doctor may advise you to discontinue breastfeeding until your treatment is finished.

Recommended dosage

ADULTS

Your doctor will prescribe a dosage according to the severity of pain and your individual response to this medication. The usual dose of Synalgos-DC is 2 capsules taken every 4 hours as needed.

CHILDREN

The safety and effectiveness of this medication have not been established in children 12 years of age and under.

ELDERLY

Synalgos-DC should be given with caution to elderly patients. Therefore, your doctor will prescribe a dose individualized to your needs.

Overdosage
Although no specific information is available, any medication taken in excess can have serious consequences. If you suspect an overdose, seek medical atention immediately.

Brand name:

SYNTHROID

Generic name: Levothyroxine
Other brand names: Levothroid, Levoxine

Why is this drug prescribed?
Synthroid, a synthetic thyroid hormone available in tablet or injectable form, may be given in any of the following cases:

  If your own thyroid gland is not making
    enough hormone
  If you have a goiter or are at risk for
    developing goiter
  If you need a "suppression test" to
    determine whether your thyroid gland
    is making too much hormone
  If you have received neck irradiation for
    cancer, to prevent development of
    thyroid gland cancer.

Most important fact about this drug
Although Synthroid will speed up your metabolism, it is not effective as a weight-loss drug and should not be used as such. An overdose may cause life-threatening side effects, especially if you take Synthroid with an appetite-suppressant medication.

How should you take this medication?
Take Synthroid exactly as prescribed.

If children cannot swallow whole tablets, you may crush a Synthroid tablet and mix it into a spoonful of liquid. Give this mixture while it is very fresh; never store it for future use.

Take no more or less than the prescribed amount. Take your dose at the same time every day for consistent effect.

If you are taking Synthroid because your thyroid gland does not make enough hormone, you may need the medication indefinitely.

While taking Synthroid, you should have periodic blood tests to determine whether you are getting the right amount.

What side effects may occur?
Side effects from Synthroid, other than overdose symptoms, are rare. Children who are treated with Synthroid may initially lose some hair, but this effect is temporary. However, excessive dosage or a too rapid increase in dosage may lead to overstimulation of the thyroid gland. Symptoms of overstimulation may include:

Changes in appetite, diarrhea, fever, headache, increased heart rate, irritability, nausea, nervousness, sleeplessness, sweating, weight loss

Why should this drug not be prescribed?
You should not be treated with Synthroid if:

You have ever had an allergic reaction to it;
Your thyroid gland is making too much thyroid hormone; or
Your adrenal glands are not making enough corticosteroid hormone.

Special warnings about this medication
You should receive low doses of Synthroid, under very close supervision, if you are an older person, or if you suffer from angina (chest pain caused by a heart condition).

If you have diabetes mellitus or diabetes insipidus, or if your body makes insufficient adrenal corticosteroid hormone, Synthroid will tend to make your symptoms worse. If you take medication for any of these disorders, the dosage will probably have to be adjusted once you begin taking Synthroid.

Possible food and drug interactions when taking this medication
If Synthroid is taken with certain other drugs, the effects of either could be increased, decreased or altered. It is especially important to check with your doctor before combining Synthroid with the following:

Amiodarone medications such as Cordarone
Antidiabetic drugs such as Diabinese, Glucotrol, and others
Beta blockers such as Inderal, Tenormin, and others
Blood thinners such as Coumadin, Dicumarol, and others
Cholestyramine drugs such as Questran
Colestipol (Colestid)
Estrogen or contraceptive pills with estrogen such as Ortho-Novum, Ovral, and others
Digitalis drugs such as Lanoxin, Crystodigin, and others
Insulin
Ketamine (Ketalar)
Lovastatin (Mevacor)
Theophylline (Bronkodyl, Theo-Dur, and others)
Tricyclic antidepressants such as Elavil, Tofranil, and others

If you are having a blood test to determine whether your dosage of Synthroid is correct, make sure your doctor knows about other medications you may be taking. Any of the following drugs may interfere with the results of the thyroid-level test:

Androgens
Corticosteroids such as Decadron and
    prednisone
Estrogens such as Premarin
Iodine-containing drugs
Oral contraceptive pills containing estrogen
Salicylate-containing drugs such as aspirin

Special information
if you are pregnant or breastfeeding

If you need to take synthroid because of a
thyroid hormone deficiency, you should
continue to take the medication during
pregnancy. Once your baby is born, you
may breastfeed while continuing to take
Synthroid; in fact, you will probably need
the medication in order to produce enough
breast milk for your baby.

Recommended dosage

Your doctor will tailor the dosage to meet
your individual requirements, taking into
consideration the status of your thyroid gland
and other medical conditions you may
have.

Overdosage

If you suspect symptoms of a Synthroid
overdose, seek medical attention
immediately. Taken in excess, Synthroid may
have serious consequences.

Symptoms of Synthroid overdose may include:
Changes in appetite, changes in menstrual
periods, chest pain, diarrhea, excessive
sweating, hand tremors, heat intolerance,
increased pulse, irregular heartbeat,
nervousness, shortness of breath, trouble
sleeping, weight loss

Brand name:

T-STAT

See Erythromycin, Topical, page 242.

Brand name:

TAGAMET

Generic name: Cimetidine

Why is this drug prescribed?

Tagamet is prescribed for the treatment of
certain kinds of stomach ulcers and
related conditions. These include: active
duodenal ulcers; active benign gastric
ulcers; erosive gastroesophageal reflux disease
(backflow of acid stomach contents);
reduction of upper abdominal bleeding in
critically ill patients, and pathological
hypersecretory conditions such as Zollinger-
Ellison syndrome (a form of peptic ulcer
with too much acid) usually caused by
tumors. It is also used for maintenance
therapy following the healing of active ulcers.
Tagamet is known as a histamine blocker.

Most important fact about this drug

Short-term treatment with Tagamet can result
in complete healing of a duodenal ulcer.
Starting treatment of the duodenal ulcer at
the onset of pain will not prevent
recurrence of the ulcer after Tagamet has been
discontinued.

The rate of ulcer recurrence may be slightly
higher in patients healed with Tagamet
rather than other forms of therapy. However,
Tagamet is usually prescribed for more
severe disease.

How should you take this medication?

Tagamet should be taken with or immediately
following meals to obtain the full effect
of this medication.

What side effects may occur?

Side effects cannot be anticipated. If any
develop or change in intensity, inform
your doctor as soon as possible. Only your
doctor can determine if it is safe for you
to continue taking Tagamet.

■ *More common side effects may include:*
Agitation, anxiety, breast development
in males, depression, diarrhea,
disorientation, dizziness, hallucinations,
headache, impotence, mental confusion,
psychosis, sexual dysfunction, sleepiness

Less common adverse reactions may appear
in severely ill patients who have been
treated for 1 month or longer. However, these
reactions are reversible and have cleared
within 3 to 4 days of discontinuation of the
drug.

■ *Less common or rare side effects may
include:*
Allergic reactions, anemia, blood disorders,
fever, joint pain, kidney disorders,
liver disorders, mild rash, muscle
inflammation, muscle pain, pancreas
inflammation, rapid heartbeat, skin
reactions, slow heartbeat

Why should this drug not be prescribed?
If you are allergic to Tagamet, do not take
this medication. If you are being treated
for a liver or kidney disorder, consult with
your doctor before taking Tagamet. If you
are taking other prescription or non-
prescription drugs, this should be
discussed with your doctor to determine if
these drugs would interact with Tagamet.

Special warnings about this medication
Ulcers may be more difficult to heal if you
smoke cigarettes.

You may experience abnormal heart rhythm
and low blood pressure following the
rapid administration of Tagamet. Do not take
more of this drug than is prescribed.

If you are over 50 years old, have liver or
kidney disease or are severely ill, you may
experience temporary mental confusion while
taking Tagamet. Notify your doctor.

Possible food and drug interactions when taking this medication
Tagamet may reduce or increase the effects
of warfarin (blood thinner), phenytoin
(Dilantin), propranolol, nifedipine,
chlordiazepoxide, diazepam, some tricyclic
antidepressants (Elavil), lidocaine, theophylline,
and metronidazole. When Tagamet is
given with any of these drugs, there may be
a greater than usual risk of side effects.
You should discuss all your medication with
your doctor.

Antacids can reduce the effect of Tagamet
when taken at the same time. If an
antacid is needed, the doses should be
separated by 3 hours.

Special information if you are pregnant or breastfeeding
The effects of Tagamet during pregnancy have
not been adequately studied. If you are
pregnant or plan to become pregnant, notify
your doctor immediately. Tagamet appears
in breast milk and could affect a nursing
infant. If this medication is essential to
your health, your doctor may advise you to
discontinue breastfeeding until treatment
with this drug is finished.

Recommended dosage

ADULTS

Active Duodenal Ulcer
The usual dose is 400 milligrams to 1,600
milligrams once daily at bedtime.
However, other doses shown to be effective
are:

300 milligrams 4 times a day with meals and
at bedtime
400 milligrams 2 times a day, in the morning
and at bedtime

If you require maintenance therapy, the
recommended dose is 400 milligrams at
bedtime. However, 800 milligrams at bedtime
is the dose of choice for most patients.

Active Benign Gastric Ulcer
The usual dose is 800 milligrams once a day at bedtime or 300 milligrams taken 4 times a day with meals and at bedtime.

Erosive Gastroesophageal Reflux Disease
The usual dosage is a total of 1,600 milligrams daily divided into doses of 800 milligrams 2 times a day or 400 milligrams 4 times a day for 12 weeks. The beneficial use of Tagamet beyond 12 weeks has not been firmly established.

Pathological Hypersecretory Condition
The usual dosage is 300 milligrams 4 times a day with meals and at bedtime. Doses should be adjusted to meet individual needs but should not usually exceed 2,400 milligrams per day.

CHILDREN

Safety and effectiveness have not been established in children under 16 years old. However, your doctor may decide that the potential benefits of Tagamet use may outweigh the potential risks.

ELDERLY

Dosage in the elderly is generally the same as that for other adults. However, many elderly patients require reduced doses of a variety of drugs. Your doctor will decide if any dosage adjustment of Tagamet is needed due to your age or other existing medical condition.

Overdosage

Information concerning overdosage is limited. However, respiratory failure, an increased heartbeat, or exaggerated side effect symptoms are signs of Tagamet overdose. If you experience any of these symptoms, notify your doctor immediately.

Brand name:

TALWIN COMPOUND

Generic ingredients: Pentazocine hydrochloride, Aspirin

Why is this drug prescribed?
Talwin Compound combines the strong analgesic properties of Pentazocine and the analgesic, anti-inflammatory, and fever-reducing properties of aspirin. It is used for the relief of moderate pain.

Most important fact about this drug
Talwin Compound should be used with extreme caution in patients being treated by a doctor for a head injury. This medication may cause troubled breathing and pressure on the skull from increased brain and spinal fluid—which can be exaggerated by a head injury. This drug may also mask or hide the pain from head injury, making it difficult for your doctor to treat.

Talwin Compound can cause dependence. Do not share Talwin Compound with other people.

How should you take this medication?
Take Talwin Compound exactly as prescribed by your doctor. Do not increase the amount you take without your doctor's approval.

What side effects may occur?
Side effects cannot be anticipated. If any develop or change in intensity, inform your doctor as soon as possible. Only your doctor can determine if it is safe for you to continue taking Talwin.

■ *More common side effects may include:*
Confusion, disorientation, dizziness, feelings of elation, hallucinations, headache, light-headedness, nausea, sedation, sweating, vomiting

If any of these side effects occur, it may help if you lie down after taking the medication.

■ *Less common side effects may include:* Blurred vision, constipation, depression, difficulty in focusing, disturbed dreams, fainting, flushing, inability to fall or stay asleep, lowered blood pressure, rapid heart rate, rash, weakness

■ *Rare side effects may include:* Abdominal distress, chills, diarrhea, excitement, facial swelling, fluid retention, hives, inability to urinate, irritability, lack or loss of appetite, ringing in the ears, skin peeling, tingling sensation, tremors, troubled or slowed breathing

Why should this drug not be prescribed?
If you are sensitive to or have ever had an allergic reaction to pentazocine or salicylates (anti-inflammatory drugs such as aspirin), or other drugs of this type, you should not take this medication. Make sure that your doctor is aware of any drug reactions that you have experienced.

Because there is a possible association between aspirin and Reye's syndrome, Talwin should not be given to children and teenagers who have chickenpox or flu unless your doctor specifically prescribes it.

Special warnings about this medication
Drug dependence and withdrawal symptoms can occur with the use of pentazocine. If you have a history of drug dependence, Talwin should be used only under the close supervision of your doctor.

Talwin Compound may cause you to become drowsy, dizzy, or less alert; therefore, driving or operating dangerous machinery or participating in any hazardous activity that requires full mental alertness is not recommended.

Talwin Compound contains aspirin. If you have a stomach ulcer, consult with your doctor before taking this medication. Aspirin may irritate the stomach lining and may cause bleeding.

If you have a kidney or liver disorder, or if you are prone to seizures, consult with your doctor before taking Talwin.

Talwin Compound may cause breathing difficulties. If you have severe bronchial asthma or other respiratory problems, check with your doctor before taking this medication.

Talwin should be used with caution if you are recovering from a heart attack.

Possible food and drug interactions when taking this medication
Talwin Compound depresses activity of the central nervous system and intensifies the effects of alcohol. Do not drink alcohol while taking this medication.

If Talwin Compound is taken with certain other drugs, the effects of either could be increased, decreased, or altered. It is especially important to check with your doctor before combining Talwin Compound with the following:

Benzodiazepines such as Valium and Xanax
MAO inhibitors (antidepressants such as
    Nardil)
Other analgesics (pain relievers)
Sleep aids such as Dalmane and Halcion

The use of these drugs with Talwin Compound increases their sedative or calming effects and may lead to overdose symptoms.

The use of anticoagulants (blood thinners) in combination with Talwin Compound may cause bleeding. If you are taking an anticoagulant, consult with your doctor before taking this drug.

The use of narcotics, including methadone (prescribed for the daily treatment of drug dependence), with Talwin Compound may produce withdrawal symptoms.

Special information if you are pregnant or breastfeeding

The effects of Talwin Compound during pregnancy have not been adequately studied. Consult your physician before taking Talwin Compound when pregnant. It is not known whether Talwin Compound appears in breast milk. If this medication is essential to your health, your doctor may advise you to discontinue breastfeeding until your treatment is finished.

Recommended dosage

ADULTS

The usual dose of Talwin Compound is 2 caplets, 3 or 4 times per day.

CHILDREN

The safety and effectiveness of Talwin Compound have not been established in children under 12 years of age.

ELDERLY

Your doctor will prescribe a dose individualized to suit your needs.

Overdosage

Symptoms of an overdose of Talwin Compound, because of its aspirin content, may include:
Coma, confusion, convulsions, diarrhea, dizziness, gasping, headache, heavy perspiration, nausea, rapid breathing, rapid heart rate, ringing in the ears, thirst, vomiting

Death may occur.

If you suspect an overdose, seek emergency medical treatment immediately.

Brand name:

TAMBOCOR

Generic name: Flecainide acetate

Why is this drug prescribed?

Tambocor is prescribed to treat certain heart rhythm disturbances, including paroxysmal atrial fibrillation (a sudden attack or worsening of irregular heartbeat in which the upper chamber of the heart beats irregularly and very rapidly). Tambocor is also given to treat paroxysmal supraventricular tachycardia (a sudden attack or worsening of an abnormally fast but regular heart rate that occurs in intermittent episodes).

Most important fact about this drug

Tambocor may sometimes cause or worsen heartbeat irregularities. It may worsen certain heart conditions, such as heart failure (the inability of the heart to sustain its workload of pumping blood). Before prescribing Tambocor, your doctor will explain the risks and benefits of Tambocor and how he or she will monitor your condition.

How should you take this medication?

In almost every case, your doctor will initiate Tambocor therapy in the hospital.

Take Tambocor exactly as prescribed by your doctor. Serious heartbeat disturbances may result if you do not follow your doctor's instructions, if you miss any regular doses, or if you increase or decrease the dosage.

Your doctor may order regular blood tests to monitor your therapy.

What side effects may occur?

Tambocor has a wide variety of possible cardiac side effects, including new or worsened heartbeat abnormalities, congestive heart failure, and heart block. If any develop, inform your doctor immediately. Only your doctor can determine whether it is safe for you to continue taking Tambocor.

■ *Other side effects may include:*
Abdominal pain, anxiety, appetite loss, breathing difficulties, chest pain, confusion, constipation, depression, diarrhea, dizziness, drowsiness, dry mouth, edema (accumulation of fluid in the tissues), fainting, fatigue, fever, fluid retention, flushing, gas, headache, heart palpitations (pounding heartbeat), impotence, insomnia, malaise (feeling unwell or ill), muscle pain, nausea, numbness or tingling of the extremities, rash, ringing in the ears, skin peeling, speech problems, sweating, swollen lips, tongue, and mouth, taste changes, tremor, upset stomach, vertigo, vision problems, vomiting, weakness

Why should this drug not be prescribed?

Your doctor should not prescribe Tambocor if you have ever had an allergic reaction to it, or if you are sensitive to it, if you have heart block (without a pacemaker), or if you have certain types of irregular heartbeat.

Special warnings about this medication

If you have a pacemaker, you should be monitored very closely while taking Tambocor—your pacemaker may need to be adjusted.

If you have liver disease, you should take Tambocor only if your doctor believes the benefits outweigh the risks. In addition, you should have frequent blood tests to make sure your dosage is not too high.

If you have a history of congestive heart failure or a weak heart, you may be at increased risk for dangerous cardiac side effects from Tambocor.

If you have very alkaline urine, perhaps caused by a kidney condition or by a strict vegetarian diet, your body will tend to process and eliminate Tambocor rather slowly and you may need a lower-than-average dosage.

Possible food and drug interactions when taking this medication

If Tambocor is taken with certain other drugs, the effects of either could be increased, decreased, or altered. It is especially important to check with your doctor before combining Tambocor with the following:

Amiodarone (Cordarone)
Beta blockers (cardiovascular drugs such as Inderal, Tenormin, and Sectral)
Carbamazepine (Tegretol)
Cimetidine (Tagamet)
Diltiazem (Cardizem)
Disopyramide (Norpace)
Nifedipine (Procardia)
Phenobarbital
Phenytoin (Dilantin)
Verapamil (Calan, Isoptin)

Special information if you are pregnant or breastfeeding

If you are pregnant or plan to become pregnant, inform your doctor immediately. Tambocor should be used during pregnancy only if the benefit justifies the potential risk to the unborn child. Tambocor appears in breast milk. Because the drug can harm a nursing infant, a decision must be made between taking Tambocor and breastfeeding your baby.

Recommended dosage

ADULTS

Treatment with Tambocor almost always begins in the hospital.

The usual recommended initial dose is 50 to 100 milligrams every 12 hours, depending on the condition under treatment. Every four days, your doctor may increase your dose by 50 milligrams every 12 hours until desired results are obtained.

Overdosage

An overdose of Tambocor is likely to cause slowed heartbeat, other cardiac problems, low blood pressure, and, eventually, death from heart or respiratory failure. Taken even in moderate excess, Tambocor may have serious consequences. If you suspect an overdose of Tambocor, seek medical attention immediately.

Generic name:

TAMOXIFEN CITRATE

See Nolvadex, page 425.

Brand name:

TAVIST

Generic name: Clemastine fumarate

Why is this drug prescribed?

Tavist is an antihistamine. Both Tavist and Tavist-1 are prescribed to treat the sneezing, runny nose, itching, and watery eyes caused by hay fever. Tavist Tablets (2.68 milligrams) also relieve mild allergic skin reactions such as hives and swelling. Antihistamines reduce itching and swelling and dry up secretions from the eyes, nose, and throat.

Most important fact about this drug

Tavist may cause drowsiness. Driving or operating dangerous machinery or participating in any hazardous activity that requires full mental alertness is not recommended until you know how you react to this medication.

How should you take this medication?

Tavist should be taken exactly as prescribed by your doctor.

Avoid alcoholic beverages.

What side effects may occur?

Side effects cannot be anticipated. If any develop or change in intensity, inform your doctor as soon as possible. Only your doctor can determine if it is safe for you to continue taking Tavist.

■ *More common side effects may include:*
Disturbed coordination
Dizziness
Drowsiness
Extreme calm (sedation)
Sleepiness
Upset stomach

■ *Less common or rare side effects may include:*
Acute inflammation of the inner ear, anemia, blurred vision, chills, confusion, constipation, convulsions, diarrhea, difficulty sleeping, difficulty urinating, double vision, dry mouth, nose, and throat, early menstruation, exaggerated sense of well-being, excessive perspiration, excitement, fatigue, frequent urination, headache, hives, hysteria, increased chest congestion, irregular heartbeat, irritability, loss of appetite, low blood pressure, nausea, nerve inflammation, nervousness, palpitations, rapid heartbeat, rash, restlessness, ringing in the ears, sensitivity to light, severe allergic reaction (anaphylactic shock), sleepiness, stuffy nose, tightness of chest, tingling or pins and needles, tremor, urinary retention, vertigo, vomiting, wheezing

Why should this drug not be prescribed?

Tavist should be avoided if you are breast-feeding, if you are taking antidepressant drugs known as MAO inhibitors (Nardil, Parnate, Marplan), or if you have asthma or other breathing problems. If you are sensitive to or have ever had an allergic reaction to clemastine fumarate or other antihistamines with a similar chemical composition, do not take this medication.

Special warnings about this medication

Antihistamines should be used very cautiously if you have narrow-angle glaucoma, a narrowing peptic ulcer or other stomach problems, intestinal blockage, a bladder obstruction, or an enlarged prostate.

Antihistamines are more likely to cause dizziness, extreme calm (sedation), and low blood pressure in the elderly (over age 60).

Tavist should be used with care if you have a history of bronchial asthma, increased eye pressure, an overactive thyroid, cardiovascular disease, or high blood pressure.

Possible food and drug interactions when taking this medication

Tavist may increase the effects of alcohol. Do not drink alcohol while taking this medication.

If Tavist is taken with certain other drugs, the effects of either could be increased, decreased, or altered. It is especially important to check with your doctor before combining Tavist with the following:

Antidepressant drugs known as MAO
   inhibitors such as Nardil, Marplan,
   and others
Sedatives/hypnotics such as Nembutal,
   Seconal, and others
Tranquilizers such as Xanax, Valium,
   and others

Special information if you are pregnant or breastfeeding

The effects of Tavist during pregnancy have not been adequately studied. If you are pregnant or plan to become pregnant, inform your doctor immediately. Tavist should not be used if you are breastfeeding.

Recommended dosage

TAVIST-1 TABLETS

The recommended starting dose is 1 tablet twice daily. Dosage may be increased as required, but should not exceed 6 tablets daily.

TAVIST TABLETS

The maximum recommended dosage is 1 tablet 3 times daily. Many patients respond favorably to a single dose, which may be repeated as required up to a total of 3 tablets daily.

TAVIST SYRUP

All dosage should be individualized according to the needs and response of the patient.

Adults and Children 12 years and over

For Symptoms of Allergic Rhinitis
The starting dose of Tavist Syrup is 2 teaspoonfuls (1 milligram) 2 times a day. Dosage may be increased as required but should not exceed 12 teaspoonfuls daily (6 milligrams).

For Urticaria and Angioedema
The starting dose of Tavist Syrup is 4 teaspoonfuls (2 milligrams) 2 times a day, not to exceed 12 teaspoonfuls daily (6 milligrams).

Children 6 to 12

For Symptoms of Allergic Rhinitis
The starting dose of Tavist Syrup is 1 teaspoonful (0.5 milligram) 2 times per day. Since single doses of up to 2.25 milligrams are well tolerated by this age-group, dosage may be increased as required, but should not exceed 6 teaspoonfuls daily (3 milligrams).

For Urticaria and Angioedema
The starting dose of Tavist Syrup is
2 teaspoonfuls (1 milligram) 2 times a
day, not to exceed 6 teaspoonfuls daily
(3 milligrams).

Overdosage
Any medication taken in excess can have
serious consequences. If you suspect an
overdose, seek medical treatment immediately.

Symptoms of Tavist overdose may include:
Central nervous system depression
Dry mouth
Fixed, dilated pupils
Flushing
Stimulation, especially in children
Stomach and intestinal problems

Brand name:

TEGRETOL

Generic name: Carbamazepine
Other brand names: Epitol, Atretol

Why is this drug prescribed?
Tegretol is used in the treatment of seizure
disorders, including certain types of
epilepsy, as well as trigeminal neuralgia
(pain of the tongue and throat). It is
sometimes used in the treatment of certain
psychiatric disorders but has not received
FDA approval for this purpose.

Most important fact about this drug
There are potentially fatal side effects
associated with improper use of
Tegretol. If you experience symptoms
such as fever, sore throat, ulcers in the
mouth, easy bruising or reddish or purplish
spots on the skin, indicating hemorrhage,
you should notify your doctor immediately.
These symptoms could reflect a potential
blood disorder brought on by the drug.

How should you take this medication?
A detailed medical history and physical
examination should be made by your
doctor before this medication is prescribed.
Your doctor should monitor your blood
regularly while you are taking Tegretol.

This medication should only be taken with
food, never on an empty stomach.

What side effects may occur?
■ *There are some common side effects
associated with the use of
Tegretol, especially when dosing is first
started. They may include:*
Dizziness
Drowsiness
Nausea
Unsteadiness
Vomiting

■ *The most severe side effects involve the
blood, the skin, and the cardiovascular
system. They may include:*
Abdominal pain, abnormal heartbeat and
rhythm, abnormal involuntary
movements, aching joints and muscles,
acute skin inflammation, agitation,
aplastic anemia, blood clots, blurred vision,
bone marrow depression, chills,
confusion, congestive heart failure,
conjunctivitis, constipation,
depression, diarrhea, double vision, dry
mouth and throat, fainting, fatigue,
fever, fluid retention, frequent urination,
hair loss, hallucinations, headache,
hepatitis, high blood pressure (aggravation
of), hives, impotence, inflammation of
the lungs, inflammation of the mouth and
tongue, kidney failure, labored
breathing, leg cramps, liver disorders, loss
of appetite, loss of coordination, low
blood pressure, pneumonia, reddish or
purplish spots on the skin, reduced
urinary volume, ringing in the ears,
sensitivity to light, skin peeling, skin

rashes, skin pigmentation changes, speech difficulties, stomach problems, sweating, talkativeness, tingling sensation, yellow eyes and skin

If you experience any of these side effects or reactions, inform your doctor immediately. Only your doctor can determine if it is safe for you to continue taking this medication.

Why should this drug not be prescribed?

If you have a history of bone marrow depression, a sensitivity to Tegretol, a sensitivity to tricyclic drugs such as amitriptyline (Elavil), or MAO inhibitors such as selegiline (Eldepryl) or phenelzine (Nardil), use of this drug is not recommended.

Tegretol is not a simple pain reliever and should not be used for the relief of minor aches and pains.

Special warnings about this medication

If you have a history of heart, liver, or kidney damage, an adverse blood reaction to any drug, glaucoma, or serious reactions to other drugs, you should discuss this history thoroughly with your doctor before taking this medication.

Anticonvulsant drugs such as Tegretol should not be discontinued if you are taking the medication to prevent major seizures. There exists the strong possibility of continuous epileptic attacks without return to consciousness, leading to possible severe brain damage and death. Only your doctor should determine if and when you should stop taking this medication.

Since dizziness and drowsiness may occur while taking Tegretol, you should refrain from operating machinery or driving an automobile or participating in any high-risk activity that requires full mental alertness until you know how this drug affects you.

Possible food and drug interactions when taking this medication

The use of the anti-seizure medications phenobarbital (Donnatal), phenytoin (Dilantin), or primidone (Mysoline) may reduce the effectiveness of Tegretol. Take other anticonvulsants along with Tegretol only if your doctor advises it. The use of Tegretol with other anticonvulsants may change thyroid gland function.

The effectiveness of haloperidol (Haldol) and valproic acid (Depakene) may be reduced when these drugs are taken with Tegretol.

The use of erythromycin, cimetidine (Tagamet), propoxyphene (Darvon), isoniazid or calcium channel blockers such as Calan may cause Tegretol to become toxic.

Lithium used with Tegretol may cause harmful nervous system side effects.

If you are taking an oral contraceptive and Tegretol, you may experience blood spotting and the reliability of your contraceptive may be adversely affected.

The activity of theophylline, doxycycline, phenytoin, and the blood thinner warfarin (Coumadin) may be affected significantly by Tegretol.

Special information if you are pregnant or breastfeeding

There are no adequate safety studies regarding the use of Tegretol in pregnant women. However, there have been reports of congenital malformations, including spina bifida, in infants. Therefore, this medication should be used during pregnancy only if the potential benefits justifies the potential risk to the fetus. If you are pregnant or plan on becoming pregnant, you should discuss this with your doctor.

Tegretol appears in breast milk. If you are breastfeeding, your doctor may advise you to discontinue doing so if taking Tegretol is essential to your health.

Recommended dosage

ADULTS

Seizures
The usual dose for adults and children over 12 years of age is one 200-milligram tablet taken twice daily or 1 teaspoon 4 times a day. This can be increased by your doctor at weekly intervals by adding 200-milligram or 2-teaspoon doses to a total of 3 or 4 times per day. Dosage should generally not exceed 1,000 milligrams daily in children 12 to 15 years old and 1,200 milligrams daily for adults and children over 15. The usual daily dosage range is 800 to 1,200 milligrams.

Trigeminal Neuralgia
The usual dose is one 100-milligram tablet twice or ½ teaspoon 4 times on the first day. This dose may be increased by your doctor using increments of 100 milligrams every 12 hours or ½ teaspoon 4 times daily only as needed to achieve freedom from pain. Doses should not exceed 1,200 milligrams daily and are usually in the range of 400 to 800 milligrams a day.

CHILDREN

Seizures
The usual dose for children 6 to 12 years old is one 100-milligram tablet twice daily or ½ teaspoon 4 times a day. This can be increased at weekly intervals by adding 100 milligrams or 1 teaspoon 3 or 4 times a day. Total daily dosage should generally not exceed 1,000 milligrams and should be divided into 3 or 4 doses. The usual daily

dosage range is 400 to 800 milligrams. Safety and effectiveness in children under 6 years of age have not been established.

ELDERLY

This drug may cause confusion or agitation in elderly patients. Your doctor may want to monitor the amount of Tegretol in your blood to help make decisions about the best dosage you should take. For this test, you will have blood drawn from a vein in your arm.

Overdosage

Any medication taken in excess can cause symptoms of overdose. If you suspect an overdose, seek medical attention immediately. The first signs and symptoms of an overdose of Tegretol appear after 1 to 3 hours.

The most prominent signs of a Tegretol overdose include:
Coma, convulsions, dizziness, drowsiness, involuntary rapid eye movements, irregular or reduced breathing, lack or absence of urine, lack of coordination, low or high blood pressure, muscular twitching, nausea, pupil dilation, rapid heartbeat, restlessness, severe muscle spasm, shock, tremors, unconsciousness, vomiting

Cardiovascular symptoms of overdosage are generally milder than nervous system symptoms. Severe heart complications have occurred when very high doses (over 60 grams) have been taken.

Generic name:

TEMAZEPAM

See Restoril, page 537.

Brand name:

TEMOVATE

Generic name: Clobetasol propionate

Why is this drug prescribed?

Temovate is a topical steroid (applied directly to the skin) that relieves itching and inflammation of moderate to severe skin conditions. Temovate Scalp Application is used for short-term treatment of scalp conditions; Temovate Cream and Ointment are used for short-term treatment of skin conditions on the body.

Most important fact about this drug

Treatment should not last for more than 2 weeks.

How should you use this medication?

Temovate should be used exactly as directed by your doctor.

Temovate is for external use only. It should not touch your eyes.

A thin layer of cream or ointment should be gently rubbed into the affected area.

The affected area should not be covered or bandaged.

What side effects may occur?

Side effects cannot be anticipated. If any develop or change in intensity, inform your doctor as soon as possible. Only your doctor can determine if it is safe for you to continue using Temovate. This medication is generally well tolerated when used for 2 weeks. However, some localized (at the site of the affected area) side effects have been reported.

TEMOVATE CREAM

■ *More common side effects may include:*
Localized stinging or burning

■ *Less common side effects may include:*
Cracks and fissures (grooves) in skin, itching

TEMOVATE OINTMENT

■ *More common side effects may include:*
Burning sensation
Irritation
Itching

■ *Less common side effects may include:*
Cracking of skin, inflammation of the hair follicles, localized red spots that become pale or white with pressure, numbness of fingers, stinging, unusual redness of skin

TEMOVATE SCALP APPLICATION

■ *More common side effects may include:*
Burning and/or stinging sensation
Scalp pustules
Tingling

■ *Less common side effects may include:*
Eye irritation, hair loss, headache, itching, skin inflammation, tenderness, tightness of scalp

■ *Rare side effects for all forms of Temovate may include:*
Acne, additional infections, allergic contact skin reactions, dryness, excessive hair growth, prickly heat, skin softening

Why should this drug not be prescribed?

All forms of Temovate should be avoided if you are sensitive to or have ever had an allergic reaction to clobetasol propionate, other corticosteroids, or any of their ingredients. Temovate Scalp Application should not be used if you have a scalp infection.

Special warnings about this medication

Temovate is a strong corticosteroid that can be absorbed into the bloodstream. It has caused Cushing's syndrome (a disorder characterized by a moon-shaped face, emotional disturbances, high blood pressure, weight gain, and, in women, abnormal growth of facial and body hair) and changes in blood sugar.

This medication should not be used for any condition other than the one for which it was prescribed.

If you develop any localized side effects, report them to your doctor.

Temovate should not be used by children under 12 years of age.

Possible food and drug interactions when using this medication

No interactions have been reported.

Special information if you are pregnant or breastfeeding

Although Temovate is applied to the skin, there is no way of knowing how much medication is absorbed into the bloodstream. Strong corticosteroids have caused birth defects in animals. Temovate, a strong corticosteroid, should be used only if the potential benefits outweigh the potential risks to the unborn baby; limit use to small amounts, on a limited area, for a short period of time. If you are pregnant or plan to become pregnant, inform your doctor immediately.

It is not known whether topical steroids are absorbed in sufficient amounts to appear in breast milk. If your doctor considers Temovate to be essential to your health, he or she may advise you to stop breastfeeding until your treatment with the medication is finished.

Recommended dosage

ADULTS AND CHILDREN 12 YEARS AND OLDER

Temovate Cream or Ointment
Gently rub the medication into the affected area 2 times a day, once in the morning

and once at night. Treatment should not last for more than 2 consecutive weeks, and the affected area should not be covered with a bandage. No more than 50 grams per week (approximately one large tube) should be used.

Temovate Scalp Application
Apply to the affected scalp areas 2 times a day, once in the morning and once at night. Treatment should not last for more than 2 consecutive weeks, and the affected areas should not be covered with a bandage. No more than 50 grams per week (approximately one large bottle) should be used.

Overdosage

Temovate is a strong corticosteroid that can be absorbed into the bloodstream, especially when it is used over a large area, for an extended period of time, or when the affected areas are covered. It can cause increases in blood sugar and Cushing's syndrome, a condition characterized by a moon-shaped face, emotional disturbances, high blood pressure, weight gain, and, in women, growth of body and facial hair. If you suspect symptoms of an overdose of Temovate, seek medical attention immediately or call your local poison center.

Brand name:

TENEX

Generic name: Guanfacine hydrochloride

Why is this drug prescribed?

Tenex, an oral medication in tablet form, is given to help control high blood pressure. This medication reduces nerve impulses to the heart and arteries; this slows the heartbeat, relaxes the blood vessels, and thus reduces blood pressure. Tenex is designed to work with a thiazide diuretic, such as Diuril, Esidrix, Naturetin, and others.

Most important fact about this drug

If you have been taking Tenex for a while, do not stop taking it without consulting your doctor. Discontinuing abruptly may result in high blood pressure, nervousness, rapid pulse, anxiety, and heartbeat irregularities. Tenex helps to control your blood pressure; it does not cure high blood pressure.

How should you take this medication?

Take Tenex exactly as prescribed by your doctor—usually 1 dose per day. Tenex should be taken at bedtime, since it will probably cause drowsiness.

After 3 or 4 weeks, if your blood pressure is still too high, your doctor may raise the dosage of Tenex. In some cases, you may take 2 evenly spaced doses per day rather than a single dose at bedtime.

If you have been taking Tenex and must stop, it is better to taper off gradually. Stopping abruptly may cause nervousness, anxiety, and/or so-called rebound high blood pressure (higher than before you started taking Tenex). If you do have rebound high blood pressure, it will probably develop 2 to 4 days after your last dose of Tenex. Rebound high blood pressure, if it occurs, will usually diminish and then disappear over a period of 2 to 4 days.

What side effects may occur?

Side effects cannot be anticipated. If any develop or change in intensity, inform your doctor as soon as possible. Only your doctor can determine whether it is safe for you to continue taking Tenex. This medication will probably make you drowsy, especially when you first begin to take it.

■ *Side effects may include:*
Abdominal pain, amnesia, breathing difficulties, chest pain, confusion, conjunctivitis (red, puffy eyes), constipation, decreased sex drive, depression, diar-rhea, difficulty swallowing, dizziness, dry mouth, extreme sleepiness, fainting, fatigue, headaches, heart palpitations, impotence, indigestion, insomnia, itching, leg cramps, malaise (vague feeling of being sick), nausea, numbness or tingling of the skin, purplish spots on the skin, rash and peeling, ringing in the ears, "runny" nose, skin inflammation, slow heartbeat, stuffy nose, sweating, taste alterations, upset stomach, urinary incontinence, vision disturbance, weakness

Some of these side effects may lessen or disappear as your body gets used to Tenex.

Why should this drug not be prescribed?

Do not take Tenex if you are sensitive to it or have ever had an allergic reaction to it.

Tenex is not recommended for controlling the severe high blood pressure that accompanies toxemia of pregnancy (a disorder of pregnant women characterized by a rise in blood pressure, swelling, and leakage of protein into urine).

Special warnings about this medication

While taking Tenex, you should be monitored very closely by your doctor if you have any of the following medical conditions:

Atherosclerosis
Chronic kidney or liver failure
Heart disease
History of stroke
Recent heart attack

Since Tenex causes drowsiness and may also make you dizzy, do not drive, climb, or perform hazardous tasks until you find out exactly how the medication affects you.

While taking Tenex, use alcoholic beverages with care; you may feel intoxicated after drinking only a small amount of alcohol.

If you have kidney damage and also take the antiseizure drug phenytoin (Dilantin), your body may process and eliminate Tenex rather quickly; in that case, you may need fairly frequent doses of Tenex to lower your blood pressure adequately.

Possible food and drug interactions when taking this medication

If Tenex is taken with certain other drugs, the effects of either could be increased, decreased, or altered. It is especially important to check with your doctor before combining Tenex with the following:

Barbiturates such as Amytal, Tuinal, Seconal, and others
Benzodiazepines such as Tranxene, Valium, Xanax, and others
Phenothiazines such as Mellaril, Stelazine, Thorazine, and others
Phenytoin (Dilantin)

Special information if you are pregnant or breastfeeding

If you are pregnant or plan to become pregnant, notify your doctor immediately. Tenex should be taken during pregnancy only if clearly needed.

It is not known whether Tenex can make its way into breast milk. Caution is advised when using Tenex during breastfeeding.

Recommended dosage

ADULTS

You should already be taking a thiazide-type diuretic such as HydroDIURIL when you begin taking Tenex.

The usual recommended dose of Tenex is 1 milligram daily, taken at bedtime. If necessary, after 3 to 4 weeks your doctor may increase the daily dosage to 2 milligrams, and later to 3 milligrams.

Overdosage

Any medication taken in excess can have serious consequences. If you suspect an overdose of Tenex, seek medical attention immediately.

Symptoms of Tenex overdose may include:
Drowsiness
Lethargy
Slowed heartbeat
Very low blood pressure

Brand name:

TENORETIC

Generic ingredients: Atenolol, Chlorthalidone

Why is this drug prescribed?

Tenoretic is a combination product used in the treatment of high blood pressure. It combines a beta-blocker drug and a diuretic. In patients with more severe high blood pressure, Tenoretic can be used alone or in combination with other high blood pressure medications. Atenolol, the beta blocker, decreases the force and rate of heart contractions. Chlorthalidone, the thiazide diuretic, helps your body produce and eliminate more urine, which helps in lowering blood pressure.

Most important fact about this drug

Since blood pressure drops gradually, it may take several weeks for the full effect of Tenoretic to occur. Even if you are feeling well, you must continue to take this medication to control your blood pressure.

How should you take this medication?

Tenoretic can be taken with or without food.

Take this medication exactly as prescribed by your doctor, even if your symptoms have disappeared.

Try not to miss any doses. If this medication is not taken regularly, your condition may worsen.

If you forget to take a dose, take it as soon as you remember. If it's within 8 hours of your next scheduled dose, skip the one you missed and go back to your regular schedule. Never take two doses at the same time.

What side effects may occur?
Side effects cannot be anticipated. If any develop or change in intensity, inform your doctor as soon as possible. Only your doctor can determine if it is safe for you to continue taking Tenoretic.

■ *More common side effects may include:*
Decreased sexual ability, diarrhea, dizziness, dizziness when getting up, fatigue, light-headedness, low potassium leading to symptoms like dry mouth, excessive thirst, weak or irregular heartbeat, muscle pain or cramps, nausea, slow heartbeat, sluggishness or unresponsiveness, vertigo

■ *Less common or rare side effects may include:*
Changes in liver function, constipation, depression, drowsiness, dry eyes, fever and sore throat, high blood sugar, loss of appetite, reddish or purplish spots on skin, shortness of breath, skin sensitivity to light, tingling or prickling, tiredness, vomiting, yellow eyes and skin

Why should this drug not be prescribed?
If you have a slow heartbeat; heart block (conduction disorder); inadequate blood supply to the circulatory system (cardiogenic shock); heart failure; or inability to urinate; or if you are sensitive to or have ever had an allergic reaction to Tenoretic, its ingredients or similar drugs, or to other sulfonamide-derived drugs, you should not take this medication.

Special warnings about this medication
If you have a history of congestive heart failure, Tenoretic should be used with caution.

Tenoretic should not be stopped suddenly. It can cause increased chest pain and heart attack. Dosage should be gradually reduced.

If you suffer from asthma, seasonal allergies or other bronchial conditions, or liver or kidney disease, this medication should be used with caution.

Ask your doctor if you should check your pulse while taking Tenoretic. This medication can cause your heartbeat to become too slow.

This medication may mask the symptoms of low blood sugar or alter blood sugar levels. If you are diabetic, discuss this with your doctor.

Tenoretic can cause you to become drowsy or less alert; therefore, activity that requires full mental alertness is not recommended until you know how you respond to the drug.

Notify your doctor that you are taking Tenoretic if you have a medical emergency, and before you have surgery.

Possible food and drug interactions when taking this medication
If Tenoretic is taken with certain other drugs, the effects of either could be increased, decreased, or altered. It is especially important to check with your doctor before combining Tenoretic with the following:

Other blood pressure drugs
Catecholamine-depleting drugs such as
    reserpine
Norepinephrine (Levophed)
Tubocurarine

Lithium
Clonidine (Catapres)
Epinephrine (Epipen)

Special Information
if you are pregnant or breastfeeding

The effects of Tenoretic during pregnancy have not been adequately studied. If you are pregnant or plan to become pregnant, inform your doctor immediately. Tenoretic appears in breast milk and could affect a nursing infant. If this medication is essential to your health, your doctor may advise you to discontinue breastfeeding until your treatment with this medication is finished.

Recommended dosage

ADULTS

Dosage must be individualized.

The usual starting dosage is a single 50 milligram dose of Tenoretic 50 each day. Dosage may be gradually increased to a maximum of 1 tablet Tenoretic 100 per day. Other high blood pressure medications may be added to this drug in a gradual fashion.

Dosages will also be adjusted for patients with reduced kidney function.

CHILDREN

The safety and effectiveness of Tenoretic have not been established in children.

Overdosage

Any medication taken in excess can cause symptoms of overdose. If you suspect an overdose, seek medical attention immediately.

No specific information on Tenoretic is available, but common symptoms of overdose with the drug's atenolol component are:
Bronchospasm
Congestive heart failure

Low blood pressure
Low blood sugar
Slow heartbeat
Sluggishness
Wheezing

Brand name:

TENORMIN

Generic name: Atenolol

Why is this drug prescribed?

Tenormin, a type of medication known as a beta blocker, is used in the treatment of high blood pressure, angina pectoris (chest pain, usually caused by lack of oxygen to the heart due to clogged arteries), and heart attack. When used for high blood pressure it is effective alone or combined with other high blood pressure medications, particularly with a thiazide-type diuretic. Beta blockers decrease the force and rate of heart contractions.

Most important fact about this drug

If you have high blood pressure, you must take Tenormin regularly for it to be effective. Even if you are feeling well, you must continue to take the medication. It's needed to keep your blood pressure under control.

How should you take this medication?

Tenormin can be taken with or without food.

Take this medication exactly as prescribed by your doctor, even if your symptoms have disappeared.

Try not to miss any doses, especially if you are taking Tenormin once a day. If this medication is not taken regularly, your condition may worsen.

If you forget to take a dose, take it as soon as you remember. If it's within 8 hours of your next scheduled dose, skip the one you missed and go back to your regular schedule. Never take two doses at the same time.

What side effects may occur?

Side effects cannot be anticipated. If any develop or change in intensity, inform your doctor as soon as possible. Only your doctor can determine if it is safe for you to continue taking Tenormin.

■ *More common side effects may include:*
Diarrhea
Dizziness
Fatigue
Headache
Light-headedness
Low blood pressure on standing
Nausea
Slow heartbeat
Vertigo

■ *Less common or rare side effects may include:*
Depression, dry eyes, fever, hallucinations, impotence, rash, red or purple spots on the skin, shortness of breath, sore throat, tiredness, vision changes

Why should this drug not be prescribed?

If you have heart failure, inadequate blood supply to the circulatory system (cardiogenic shock), heart block (conduction disorder), or a severely slow heartbeat, you should not take this medication.

Special warnings about this medication

If you have a history of severe congestive heart failure, Tenormin should be used with caution.

Tenormin should not be stopped suddenly. It can cause increased chest pain and heart attack. Dosage should be gradually reduced.

If you suffer from asthma, seasonal allergies, or other bronchial conditions, coronary artery disease or kidney disease, this medication should be used with caution.

Ask your doctor if you should check your pulse while taking Tenormin. This medication can cause your heartbeat to become too slow.

This medication may mask the symptoms of low blood sugar or alter blood sugar levels. If you are diabetic, discuss this with your doctor.

Notify your doctor or dentist that you are taking Tenormin if you have a medical emergency, and before you have surgery or dental surgery.

Possible food and drug interactions when taking this medication

If Tenormin is taken with certain other drugs, the effects of either could be increased, decreased, or altered. It is especially important to check with your doctor before combining Tenormin with the following:

Catecholamine-depleting drugs such as reserpine
Clonidine (Catapres)
Epinephrine (Epipen)
Verapamil (Calan)

Special information if you are pregnant or breastfeeding

The effects of Tenormin during pregnancy have not been adequately studied. If you are pregnant or plan to become pregnant, inform your doctor immediately. Tenormin appears in breast milk and could affect a nursing infant. If this medication is essential to your health, your doctor may advise you to discontinue breastfeeding until your treatment is finished.

Recommended dosage

ADULTS

Hypertension
The usual starting dose is 50 milligrams a
day in 1 dose, alone or with a diuretic.
Full effects should be seen in 1 to 2 weeks.
Dosage may be increased to a maximum
of 100 milligrams per day. Your doctor can
and may use this medication with other
high blood pressure medications.

Angina Pectoris
The usual starting dose is 50 milligrams given
as 1 tablet a day. Full effects should be
seen in 1 week. Dosage may be increased to
a maximum of 100 milligrams per day.
In some cases, a single dose of 200 milligrams
per day may be given. Dosage will be
individualized by your doctor.

Heart Attack
This medication may be used in the acute
treatment of heart attack in both
injectable and tablet form. Your doctor will
determine the proper dosage.

CHILDREN

The safety and effectiveness of Tenormin have
not been established in children.

ELDERLY

Dosage should be determined by the particular
needs of the elderly patient, especially if
the patient has reduced kidney function.

Overdosage

Any medication taken in excess can cause
symptoms of overdose. If you suspect an
overdose, seek medical attention immediately.

*Symptoms of Tenormin overdose may
include:*
Bronchospasm
Changes in breathing
Congestive heart failure
Low blood pressure
Low blood sugar
Slow heartbeat
Sluggishness
Wheezing

Brand name:

TENUATE

Generic name: Diethylpropion hydrochloride

Why is this drug prescribed?
Tenuate, an appetite suppressant, is prescribed
for short-term use (a few weeks) as part
of an overall diet plan for weight reduction.
Tenuate should be used with a behavior
modification program.

Most important fact about this drug
Loss of effectiveness (tolerance) of Tenuate
and other related drugs develops within
a few weeks. When Tenuate becomes less
effective, you should discontinue the
medicine rather than increase the dosage.

How should you take this medication?
Take this medication exactly as prescribed by
your doctor.

Tenuate may be habit-forming and can be
addicting.

You should not share Tenuate with others.

Avoid alcoholic beverages while taking this
medicine.

If you are taking Tenuate Dospan (the
controlled release formulation), do not
crush or chew the tablets. Swallow the
medication whole.

What side effects may occur?
Side effects cannot be anticipated. If any
develop or change in intensity, inform
your doctor as soon as possible. Only your
doctor can determine if it is safe for you
to continue using Tenuate.

■ *Side effects may include:*
Abdominal discomfort, abnormal redness of the skin, anxiety, blood pressure elevation, blurred vision, bruising, changes in sex drive, chest pain, constipation, depression, diarrhea, difficulty with voluntary movements, dizziness, drowsiness, dryness of the mouth, excessive male breast development, feelings of discomfort, feelings of elation, hair loss, headache, hives, impotence, inability to fall or stay asleep, increased heart rate, increased sweating, increased volume of diluted urine, irregular heartbeat, jitteriness, menstrual upset, muscle pain, nausea, nervousness, overstimulation, painful urination, palpitations, pupil dilation, rash, restlessness, shortness of breath or labored breathing, sluggishness, tremors, unpleasant taste, vomiting

Why should this drug not be prescribed?

If you are sensitive to or have ever had an allergic reaction to diethylpropion hydrochloride or similar drugs (anorectics), you should not take this medication. Make sure that your doctor is aware of any drug reactions that you have experienced.

Unless directed to do so by your doctor, do not take this drug if you have hardening of the arteries, an overactive thyroid, glaucoma, or severe high blood pressure, or if you are in an agitated state, have a history of drug abuse or are taking or have taken MAO inhibitors (antidepressant drugs such as Nardil) within the last 14 days.

Special warnings about this medication

Tenuate or Tenuate Dospan may impair your ability to engage in potentially hazardous activities. Therefore, make sure you know how you react to this medication before you drive, operate dangerous machinery, or do anything else that requires alertness or concentration.

If you have heart disease or high blood pressure, caution should be exercised when taking this medication.

This drug may increase convulsions in some epileptics. Therefore, epileptics receiving Tenuate or Tenuate Dospan should be carefully monitored by their doctor.

Psychological dependence has occurred while taking this drug. Consult with your doctor if you rely on this drug to maintain a state of well-being.

The abrupt withdrawal of this medication following prolonged usage of high doses may result in extreme fatigue, mental depression, and sleep disturbances.

Possible food and drug interactions when taking this medication

Tenuate or Tenuate Dospan may interact with alcohol unfavorably. Do not drink alcohol while taking this medication.

If Tenuate or Tenuate Dospan is taken with certain other drugs, the effects of either could be increased, decreased, or altered. It is especially important that you consult with your doctor before combining Tenuate with the following:

Antidiabetic drugs such as Insulin, Micronase, and others
General anesthetics
Antihypertensive drugs such as Ismelin
Phenothiazines such as Thorazine, Phenergan

Special information
if you are pregnant or breastfeeding

The effects of Tenuate or Tenuate Dospan during pregnancy have not been adequately studied. If you are pregnant or plan to become pregnant, inform your doctor immediately. This drug appears in breast milk. If the medication is essential to your health, your doctor may advise you to discontinue breastfeeding until your treatment is finished.

Recommended dosage

ADULTS

Tenuate Immediate-Release
The recommended dosage is one 25-milligram tablet taken 3 times a day, 1 hour before meals and in the midevening, if desired, to overcome night hunger.

Tenuate Dospan Controlled-Release
The recommended dosage is one 75-milligram tablet taken once daily, swallowed whole, in midmorning.

CHILDREN

Safety and effectiveness have not been established in children below 12 years of age.

Overdosage

If you suspect a Tenuate overdose, seek emergency medical treatment immediately.

Symptoms of Tenuate overdose may include:
Assaultiveness, confusion, depression, diarrhea, elevated blood pressure, excessive vomiting, fatigue, hallucinations, irregular heartbeat, lowered blood pressure, nausea, overreactive reflexes, panic state, rapid breathing, restlessness, tremors

Brand name:

TERAZOL 3

Generic name: Terconazole

Why is this drug prescribed?

Terazol 3 Vaginal Cream and Suppositories are prescribed to treat candidiasis (a yeast-like fungal infection) of the vulva and vagina. This diagnosis, however, should be confirmed by your doctor before starting treatment with Terazol 3.

Most important fact about this drug

If your infection does not clear up, notify your doctor. Appropriate testing should be repeated to confirm the diagnosis.

How should you use this medication?

Use this medication exactly as prescribed by your doctor.

A patient instruction sheet is available with the product.

The use of Terazol 3 is not affected by menstruation. If you are menstruating, do not use tampons, because the tampon may soak up some of the medication.

What side effects may occur?

Side effects cannot be anticipated. If any develop or change in intensity, inform your doctor as soon as possible. Only your doctor can determine if it is safe to continue using Terazol 3.

■ *More common side effects may include:*
Headache
Menstrual pain

■ *Less common side effects may include:*
Abdominal pain, burning, fever, flu-like illness (fever, chills, headache 1 to 3 hours after administration), itching

Why should this drug not be prescribed?

If you have ever had an allergic reaction to or are sensitive to terconazole, you should not use this medication. Make sure your doctor is aware of any drug reactions you have experienced.

Special warnings about this medication

If irritation, an allergic reaction, fever, chills, or flu-like symptoms develop while using this medication, notify your doctor.

Possible food and drug interactions when taking this medication

No interactions have been reported.

Special information
if you are pregnant or breastfeeding

Since Terazol 3 Cream is absorbed from the vagina, it should not be used during the first trimester (first three months) of pregnancy unless your doctor considers it essential to your health. It is not known whether this drug appears in breast milk. Your doctor may advise you to discontinue breastfeeding your baby while using this medication.

Recommended dosage

ADULTS

Terazol 3 Vaginal Cream

The recommended dose is 1 full applicator (5 grams) of cream inserted into the vagina once daily at bedtime for 3 consecutive days. Before prescribing another course of treatment, it is recommended that your doctor reconfirm the diagnosis.

Terazol 3 Vaginal Suppositories

The recommended dose is 1 suppository inserted into the vagina once daily at bedtime for 3 consecutive days.

CHILDREN

Safety and effectiveness have not been established in children.

Overdosage

There has been no reported overdose of this medication. Any medication used in excess, however, can have serious consequences. If you suspect an overdose with Terazol 3, seek medical attention immediately.

Generic name:

TERAZOSIN HYDROCHLORIDE

See Hytrin, page 286.

Generic name:

TERBUTALINE SULFATE

See Brethine, page 69.

Generic name:

TERCONAZOLE

See Terazol, page 620.

Generic name:

TERFENADINE

See Seldane, page 571.

Brand name:

TESSALON

Generic name: Benzonatate

Why is this drug prescribed?

Tessalon is a nonnarcotic cough medication that acts within 15 to 20 minutes. Its effect lasts from 3 to 8 hours.

Most important fact about this drug

Tessalon should be swallowed whole, not chewed.

How should you take this medication?

Tessalon perles (soft capsule form) should be swallowed whole. If chewed, they can produce a temporary numbness of the mouth and throat that could cause choking.

What side effects may occur?

Side effects cannot be anticipated. If any occur or change in intensity, inform your doctor as soon as possible. Only your doctor can determine if it is safe to continue taking Tessalon.

■ *Side effects may include:*
Allergic reactions, burning sensation in the eyes, constipation, extreme calm (sedation), headache, itching and skin rashes, mild dizziness, nausea, numbness in chest, stuffy nose, upset stomach, vague "chilly" feeling

Why should this drug not be prescribed?
Tessalon should not be used if you are sensitive to or have ever had an allergic reaction to benzonatate or similar drugs (such as local anesthetics).

Special warnings about this medication
If Tessalon perles are chewed, they can cause numbness in the mouth and throat that may cause choking. They must be swallowed whole.

Possible food and drug interactions when taking this medication
None.

Special information if you are pregnant or breastfeeding
The effects of Tessalon during pregnancy have not been studied adequately. Tessalon should be used during pregnancy only if clearly needed. If you are pregnant or plan to become pregnant, notify your doctor immediately. It is unknown if Tessalon appears in breast milk and could affect a nursing infant. If this medication is essential to your health, your doctor may advise you to stop breastfeeding until your treatment with Tessalon ends.

Recommended dosage

CHILDREN OVER AGE 10 AND ADULTS

The usual dose is a 100-milligram perle 3 times per day, as needed. Maximum dose is 600 milligrams a day.

Overdosage
If capsules are chewed or allowed to dissolve in the mouth, anesthesia (numbness) of the mouth and throat will develop rapidly. Difficulty breathing due to blockage of the airway may occur.

Keep out of reach of children. If you suspect symptoms of a Tessalon overdose, seek medical attention immediately.

Generic name:

TETRACYCLINE HYDROCHLORIDE

See Achromycin V Capsules, page 3.

Brand name:

THALITONE

See Hygroton, page 284.

Brand name:

THEO-DUR

Generic name: Theophylline

Why is this drug prescribed?
Theo-Dur, an oral bronchodilator medication, is given to prevent or relieve symptoms of asthma, chronic bronchitis, and emphysema. The active ingredient of Theo-Dur, theophylline, is a chemical cousin of caffeine. It relieves bronchospasm by relaxing the smooth muscle of the airways and blood vessels in the lungs.

This drug is available in two forms. If you take Theo-Dur extended-release capsules, you should swallow the capsule whole. If you take Theo-Dur Sprinkle sustained-release capsules, you may either swallow the capsule whole or open the capsule and sprinkle the granules on a spoonful of soft food before swallowing.

Most important fact about this drug

Theo-Dur is a controlled-release medication. For an acute episode of severe bronchospasm, you should take an immediate-release medication instead of more Theo-Dur. If you develop *status asthmaticus* (severe breathing difficulty that does not clear up with your usual medications), do not take extra Theo-Dur; instead, seek medical treatment immediately. Since even a little extra Theo-Dur may constitute an overdose, you should be treated in a setting where close monitoring is possible.

Individual doses are determined by a patient's response (a decrease in symptoms of asthma). Your doctor will perform tests to determine blood levels regularly in order to avoid overdosing or underdosing.

You should not change from Theo-Dur to another brand without first consulting your doctor or pharmacist. Products manufactured by different companies may not be equally effective.

How should you take this medication?

Take Theo-Dur exactly as prescribed by your doctor.

With the extended-release capsules that are to be swallowed whole, you will most likely need 2 doses per day (1 dose every 12 hours). You may take these capsules with or without food.

With the sprinkle capsules, which must be taken either *one hour before or two hours after a meal*, it may be more convenient to take 3 somewhat smaller doses per day (1 dose every 8 hours). Sprinkle the granules onto a spoonful of food that is soft but not hot. Without chewing, immediately swallow the spoonful of food and follow it with a glass of cool water or juice. Never subdivide the contents of a capsule (i.e., do not try to take half a capsule of granules).

You should avoid large amounts of caffeine-containing beverages, such as tea or coffee.

What side effects may occur?

Side effects from Theo-Dur cannot be anticipated. Nausea and restlessness may occur when you first start to take Theo-Dur, but will probably disappear as your body becomes used to the drug. If side effects persist, see your doctor; the dosage may be too high.

■ *Other side effects may include:* Convulsions, diarrhea, disturbances of heart rhythm, fluid retention, flushing, frequent urination, hair loss, headache, heart pounding, irritability, low blood pressure, muscle twitching, nausea, nosebleed, rapid breathing, rash, restlessness, sleeplessness, stomach pain, vomiting

Theo-Dur may cause or worsen heartbeat abnormalities. While you are taking this medication, any significant change in your heartbeat rate or rhythm should be investigated promptly and thoroughly.

Why should this drug not be prescribed?

Do not take Theo-Dur if you are sensitive to it or have ever had an allergic reaction, to it.

Do not take Theo-Dur if you have an active peptic ulcer. If you have epilepsy, you should take the correct dosage of antiseizure medication before you start treatment with Theo-Dur.

Special warnings about this medication

If you are a tobacco or marijuana smoker, your body will tend to process and get rid of Theo-Dur rather quickly; thus, you may need to take more frequent doses than a nonsmoker. Even if you quit smoking, this quick-clearance effect may linger for 6 months to 2 years.

You should take Theo-Dur cautiously and under close medical supervision if you are over 55, especially if you are a male with chronic lung disease.

You should also take Theo-Dur cautiously and under close supervision if you have had a sustained high fever, or if you have heart disease or liver failure, high blood pressure, low blood oxygen, alcoholism, or a history of stomach ulcers.

It is very important not to take too much Theo-Dur. This medication may produce serious signs of overdose without warning.

Possible food and drug interactions when taking this medication

If Theo-Dur is taken with certain other drugs, the effects of either could be increased, decreased, or altered. It is especially important to check with your doctor before combining Theo-Dur with the following:

Allopurinol (Lopurin, Zyloprim)
Cimetidine (Tagamet)
Ciprofloxacin (Cipro)
Ephedrine
Erythromycin (E.E.S., ERYC, Erythrocin, and others)
Lithium carbonate (Eskalith, Lithobid, and others)
Oral contraceptive pills
Phenytoin (Dilantin)
Propranolol (Inderal)
Rifampin (Rifadin, Rifamate, Rimactane)
Troleandomycin (Tao)

Special information if you are pregnant or breastfeeding

If you are pregnant or plan to become pregnant, inform your doctor immediately. Theo-Dur should not be taken during pregnancy unless it is clearly needed, and unless the benefits to the mother outweigh the potential risk to the unborn child.

Theo-Dur does find its way into breast milk; it may make a nursing baby irritable or harm the baby in other ways. If you are a new mother, you will probably need to choose between breastfeeding and taking Theo-Dur.

Recommended dosage

Theo-Dur (200, 300, and 450 milligrams) Extended-Release Tablets may be taken with or without meals.

CHILDREN UNDER 55 POUNDS

It is recommended that for children under 55 pounds proper dosage be established with a liquid preparation to permit gradual increase in dosages.

CHILDREN OVER 55 POUNDS AND ADULTS

The average initial dose is 1 Theo-Dur 200 milligram tablet every 12 hours.

If the desired response is not achieved with the above average initial dose recommendations, there are no side effects and other laboratory tests are negative, dosages can be adjusted by approximately 25% increments at 3-day intervals. Following each adjustment, if the clinical response is satisfactory, that dosage level should be maintained.

Once-daily Dosing
The slow action and effect of this form of Theo-Dur may allow once-daily dosing in adult nonsmokers with appropriate laboratory tests. Once-daily dosing should be considered only after the patient has been gradually adjusted to the medication. It is not recommended that Theo-Dur, when used as a once-a-day product, be taken at night. Theo-Dur, when used as a once-a-day product, must be taken whole and not broken.

Overdosage

Most of the symptoms listed in the "side effects" section are actually caused by slight overdosage.

Be aware that a flu shot, or influenza itself, may make your usual dose of Theo-Dur act like an overdose. Consult your doctor if you anticipate getting a flu shot, or if you think you have the flu; you may need a temporary dosage reduction.

A mild overdose of Theo-Dur may cause nausea and restlessness. A larger overdose may not give any warning before causing serious heartbeat irregularities, convulsions, or even death. If at any time you suspect symptoms of an overdose of Theo-Dur, seek medical attention immediately.

Generic name:

THEOPHYLLINE

See Theo-Dur, page 622.

Brand name:

THEROXIDE

See Desquam-E, page 181.

Generic name:

THIORIDAZINE HYDROCHLORIDE

See Mellaril, page 365.

Generic name:

THIOTHIXENE

See Navane, page 407.

Brand name:

THORAZINE

Generic name: Chlorpromazine

Why is this drug prescribed?

Thorazine is used for the reduction of symptoms of psychotic disorders such as schizophrenia; for the short-term treatment of severe behavioral disorders in children, including explosive hyperactivity and combativeness; and for the symptoms of manic-depressive illness (severely exaggerated moods).

Thorazine is also used to control nausea and vomiting, and to relieve restlessness and apprehension before surgery. It is used as an aid in the treatment of tetanus, and is prescribed for severe hiccups and acute intermittent porphyria (attacks of pain sometimes accompanied by psychiatric disturbances).

Most important fact about this drug

Thorazine may cause tardive dyskinesia—a condition marked by involuntary muscle spasms and twitches in the face and body. This condition may be permanent, and appears to be most common among the elderly, especially women. Ask your doctor for information about this possible risk.

How should you take this medication?

If taking Thorazine in a liquid concentrate form, you will need to dilute it with a liquid such as a carbonated beverage, coffee, fruit juice, milk, orange syrup, simple syrup, tea, tomato juice, or water. Puddings, soups, and other semisolid foods may also be used. Thorazine will taste best if it is diluted immediately prior to use. Since the liquid concentrate form of Thorazine is light-sensitive, it should be stored in a dark place, but it does not need to be refrigerated.

You should not take Thorazine with alcohol.

Do not take antacids such as Gelusil at the same time as Thorazine. Leave at least 1 to 2 hours between doses of the two drugs.

What side effects may occur?
Side effects cannot be anticipated. If any develop or change in intensity, inform your doctor as soon as possible. Only your doctor can determine if it is safe for you to continue taking Thorazine.

■ *More common side effects may include:*
Abnormal secretion of milk, abnormal sugar in urine, agitation, anemia, asthma, blood disorders, breast enlargement in males, chewing movements, constipation, difficulty breathing, difficulty swallowing, drooling drowsiness, ejaculation problems, eye problems causing fixed gaze, fever, flu-like symptoms, fluid accumulation and swelling, headache, heart attack, high or low blood sugar, hives, impotence, infections, intestinal blockage, involuntary movements of arms and legs, tongue, face, mouth, or jaw, irregular blood pressure, pulse, and heartbeat, irregular or no menstrual periods, jitteriness, mask-like face, muscle stiffness and rigidity, narrow or dilated pupils, nasal congestion, nausea, pain and stiffness in the neck, persistent, painful erections, pill-rolling motion, protruding tongue, puckering of the mouth, puffing of the cheeks, rigid arms, feet, head, and muscles (including the back), seizures, sensitivity to light, severe allergic reactions, shuffling walk, sore throat, spasms in jaw, face, tongue, neck, mouth, and feet, sweating, swelling of breasts in women, tremors, twitching in the body, neck, shoulders and face, visual problems

■ *Less common and rare side effects may include:*
Abnormalities in movement and posture, dizziness, dry mouth, fainting, increase of appetite and weight, insomnia, light-headedness (on standing up), rapid heartbeat, skin inflammation and peeling, twisted neck, yellowed skin and whites of eyes

Why should this drug not be prescribed?
You should not be using Thorazine if you are taking mental depressants such as alcohol, barbiturates, or narcotics.

Do not give Thorazine to a comatose individual.

Special warnings about this medication
You should use Thorazine cautiously if you have ever had: asthma; a brain tumor; breast cancer; intestinal blockage; emphysema; glaucoma; heart, kidney, or liver disease; seizures; or an abnormal bone marrow or blood condition; or if you are exposed to pesticides or extreme heat. Be aware that Thorazine can mask symptoms of brain tumor, intestinal blockage, and Reye's syndrome.

Stomach inflammation, dizziness, nausea, vomiting, and tremors may result if you suddenly stop taking Thorazine. Follow your doctor's instructions closely when discontinuing Thorazine.

Thorazine can suppress the cough reflex. Tell your doctor immediately if you experience symptoms such as a fever or sore throat, mouth, or gums. They may signal the need to discontinue Thorazine therapy.

This drug may impair your ability to drive a car or operate potentially dangerous machinery. Do not participate in any activities that require full alertness if you are unsure about your ability.

This drug can increase your sensitivity to light. Avoid being out in the sun too long.

Thorazine may cause a false-positive test result for pregnancy and for phenylketonuria (a birth defect involving damage to the central nervous system).

If you are on Thorazine for prolonged therapy, you should see your doctor for regular evaluations, since side effects can get worse over time.

Possible food and drug interactions when taking this medication

If Thorazine is taken with certain other drugs, the effects of either could be increased, decreased, or altered. It is especially important to check with your doctor before combining Thorazine with the following:

Anesthetics
Antacids such as Gelusil
Anticoagulants such as Dicumarol
Anticonvulsants such as Dilantin
Atropine (Donnatal)
Barbiturates such as phenobarbital
Cimetidine (Tagamet)
Diuretics such as Dyazide
Guanethidine (Ismelin)
Narcotics such as Percocet
Propranolol (Inderal)

Extreme drowsiness and other potentially serious effects can result if Thorazine is combined with alcohol and other mental depressants such as narcotics and painkillers.

Because Thorazine prevents vomiting, it can hide the signs and symptoms of overdose of other drugs.

Special information if you are pregnant or breastfeeding

Pregnant women should use Thorazine only if clearly needed. Thorazine is excreted in breast milk and may affect a nursing infant.

Recommended dosage

Doses should be tailored to the individual. Enough Thorazine should be used to control symptoms, but dosage should be decreased to the smallest effective amount as treatment continues.

ADULTS

Psychotic Disorders
Dosages should be gradually increased until symptoms are controlled. You may not see full improvement for weeks or even months.

Initial dosages may range from 30 to 75 milligrams daily. The amount should be divided into equal doses and taken 3 or 4 times a day. If needed, dosages may be increased by 20 to 50 milligrams at semiweekly intervals.

Nausea and Vomiting
The usual tablet dosage is 10 to 25 milligrams, taken every 4 or 6 hours, as needed.

One 100-milligram suppository can be used every 6 to 8 hours.

Severe Hiccups
Dosages may range from 75 to 200 milligrams daily, divided into 3 or 4 equal doses.

Acute Intermittent Porphyria
Dosages may range from 75 to 200 milligrams daily, divided into 3 or 4 equal doses.

CHILDREN

Thorazine is generally not prescribed for children younger than 6 months.

Severe Behavior Problems and Vomiting
Dosages are based on the child's weight.

Oral: The daily dose is one-quarter milligram for each pound of the child's weight, taken every 4 to 6 hours, as needed.

Rectal: the usual dose is one-half milligram per pound of body weight, taken every 6 to 8 hours, as necessary.

ELDERLY

In general, elderly people take lower dosages of Thorazine, and any increase in dosage should be gradual. Because they may develop low blood pressure while taking Thorazine, they should be closely monitored. Elderly people (especially elderly women) may be more susceptible to tardive dyskinesia—a possibly permanent condition characterized by involuntary muscle spasms and twitches in the face and body. Elderly people should consult their doctor for information about these potential risks.

Overdosage

Any medication taken in excess can have serious consequences. An overdose of Thorazine can be fatal. If you suspect an overdose, seek medical help immediately.

Symptoms of Thorazine overdose may include: Agitation, coma, convulsions, difficulty breathing, difficulty swallowing, dry mouth, extreme sleepiness, fever, intestinal blockage, irregular heart rate, restlessness

Generic name:

THYROGLOBULIN

See *Proloid,* page 511.

Generic name:

THYROID HORMONES

See *Armour thyroid,* page 34.

Brand name:

TIGAN

Generic name: Trimethobenzamide hydrochloride

Why is this drug prescribed?
Tigan is prescribed for the control of nausea and vomiting.

Most important fact about this drug
Antiemetics (drugs that prevent or lessen nausea and vomiting) are not recommended for the treatment of simple vomiting in children. Use of Tigan in children should be limited to prolonged vomiting caused by a known disease.

Caution should always be exercised when using this drug in children, since there may be a link between the use of antiemetic drugs to treat symptoms of viral illnesses and the development of Reye's syndrome, which is a potentially fatal childhood disease of the brain.

How should you take this medication?
Take this medication exactly as prescribed by your doctor.

If you must use this medicine regularly, and you miss a dose, use it as soon as possible. However, if it is almost time for your next dose, skip the missed dose, and go back to your regular dosing schedule. Do not double doses.

What side effects may occur?
Side effects cannot be anticipated. If any develop or change in intensity, inform your doctor as soon as possible. Only your doctor can determine if it is safe for you to continue taking Tigan.

■ *Side effects may include:*
   Allergic-type skin reactions, blurred vision, coma, convulsions, diarrhea,

disorientation, dizziness, drowsiness, headache, jaundice (liver disorder causing yellowish skin), mood of depression, muscle cramps, severe muscle spasm, tremors

Why should this drug not be prescribed?

If you are sensitive to or have ever had an allergic reaction to trimethobenzamide (antinausea medication), benzocaine (local anesthetic), or similar drugs, do not take this medication. Make sure that your doctor is aware of any drug reactions you have experienced.

Unless you are directed to do so by your doctor, do not administer suppositories to premature or newborn infants.

Special warnings about this medication

Tigan may cause you to become drowsy or less alert; therefore, driving or operating dangerous machinery or participating in any hazardous activity that requires full mental alertness is not recommended until you know how you respond to this drug.

Reye's syndrome has been associated with the use of Tigan; it may appear abruptly following an illness that is accompanied by a high fever. Reye's syndrome is characterized by severe, persistent vomiting, sluggishness, irrational behavior, and a progressive brain disorder leading to coma, convulsions, and death.

Caution should be exercised, especially with children and the elderly, when taking Tigan if you have a severe illness accompanied by high fever, inflammation of the brain encephalitis), inflammation of the stomach and intestines (gastroenteritis), or an electrolyte imbalance due to dehydration.

Severe vomiting should not be treated with Tigan alone. Your doctor should emphasize restoration of body fluids, the relief of fever, and the relief of the disease causing the vomiting. However, the over-consumption of fluids may result in cerebral edema (excessive accumulation of fluid in the brain).

The anti-nausea/vomiting effects of Tigan may make it difficult to diagnose such conditions as appendicitis and may mask signs of drug poisoning due to overdosage of other drugs.

Tigan suppositories contain benzocaine, and patients known to be sensitive to this or similar local anesthetics should not use these products.

Possible food and drug interactions when taking this medication

The use of alcohol in combination with this drug may produce an unfavorable reaction.

Caution should be exercised when taking Tigan in combination with central nervous system drugs such as phenothiazines (tranquilizers and antiemetics), barbiturates such as Phenobarbital, and drugs derived from belladonna, such as Donnatal.

Special information if you are pregnant or breastfeeding

The effects of Tigan during pregnancy or breastfeeding have not been adequately studied. If you are pregnant or plan to become pregnant, inform your doctor immediately. If you are breastfeeding your baby, consult with your doctor before taking this medication.

Recommended dosage

Dosage is adjusted by your doctor according to your illness, severity of symptoms, and response.

ADULTS

Capsules
The usual dosage is one 250-milligram capsule taken 3 or 4 times per day, as determined by your doctor.

Suppositories
The recommended dosage is 1 suppository (200 milligrams) inserted into the rectum 3 or 4 times per day, as determined by your doctor.

CHILDREN

Capsules
The usual dosage for children weighing 30 to 90 pounds is one or two 100-milligram capsules taken 3 or 4 times per day, as determined by the doctor.

Suppositories
The usual dosage for children weighing under 30 pounds is 100 milligrams inserted into rectum 3 or 4 times a day, as determined by your doctor.

The usual dosage for children weighing 30 to 90 pounds is one half to one 200-milligram suppository (100 milligrams to 200 milligrams) rectally 3 or 4 times a day, as determined by the doctor.

Pediatric Suppositories
The usual dosage for children weighing under 30 pounds is 1 suppository (100 milligrams) rectally 3 or 4 times a day, as determined by the doctor.

The usual dosage for children weighing 30 to 90 pounds is 1 to 2 suppositories (100 milligrams to 200 milligrams) rectally 3 or 4 times a day, as determined by the doctor.

Overdosage

Although no specific information is available, any medication taken in excess can have serious consequences. If you suspect a Tigan overdose, seek medical attention immediately.

Generic name:

TIMOLOL MALEATE (OPHTHALMIC)

See Timoptic, page 630.

Brand name:

TIMOPTIC

Generic name: Timolol maleate

Why is this drug prescribed?
Timoptic is a topical medication (applied directly in the eye) that effectively reduces internal pressure in the eye. Timoptic is used in the treatment of glaucoma to lower elevated eye pressure that could damage vision and, with other glaucoma medications, to further reduce pressure in the eye.

Most important fact about this drug
Although Timoptic is applied directly to the eye, the drug can still be absorbed into the bloodstream. Timoptic is a beta-blocker drug and should be used cautiously—or not at all—with similar medications taken by mouth or applied topically.

How should you use this medication?
Timoptic should be used exactly as prescribed by your doctor.

If you are using Timoptic in Ocudose, use the medication as soon as you open the individual unit and throw out any leftover solution.

What side effects may occur?
Side effects cannot be anticipated. If any side effects develop or change in intensity, tell your doctor immediately. Only your doctor can determine whether it is safe to continue using this medication. If Timoptic

is absorbed into the bloodstream, it can cause additional side effects.

■ *Side effects may include:*
Breathing failure, burning, prickling, or tingling, chest pain, cough, depression, diarrhea, dizziness, double vision, eye irritation (pinkeye, inflammation of the eyelids, inflammation of the cornea, drooping eyelids), fainting, fatigue and weakness of muscles (especially those in the face and neck), hair loss, headache, heart failure, hives, irregular heartbeat, low blood pressure, nausea, pounding heartbeat, rash, shortness of breath, slow heartbeat, stroke, stuffy nose, vision changes, weakness, wheezing

Why should this drug not be prescribed?
Do not use Timoptic if you have bronchial asthma, a history of bronchial asthma, or other serious breathing disorders such as emphysema, slow heartbeat, heart block (conduction disorder), active heart failure, or inadequate blood supply to the circulatory system (cardiogenic shock), or if you have ever had an allergic reaction or are sensitive to Timoptic or any of its ingredients.

Special warnings about this medication
Use Timoptic cautiously if you have a history of heart failure or poor cerebral circulation.

Timoptic may mask the symptoms of low blood sugar. If you are diabetic, discuss this possibility with your doctor.

Tell your doctor or dentist that you are using Timoptic if you have a medical emergency or before you have surgery or dental treatment.

Timoptic should not be used with other topical beta blockers and should be used with caution if you are taking oral beta blockers.

Timoptic may mask symptoms of an overactive thyroid. If your doctor suspects you have hyperthyroidism, he or she will manage your case carefully to avoid such symptoms as rapid heartbeat, which can occur when the drug is withdrawn too abruptly.

Timoptic's anti-glaucoma effects may decrease if you use the medication for a long time.

Possible food and drug interactions when using this medication
If Timoptic is used with certain other drugs, the effects of either could be increased, decreased, or altered. It is especially important to check with your doctor before combining Timoptic with the following:

Epinephrine (Epipen)
Catecholamine-depleting drugs, such as blood pressure drugs that contain reserpine (Serpasil)
Calcium antagonists such as Cardizem and Isoptin
Digitalis (Lanoxin)

Special information
if you are pregnant or breastfeeding
If you are pregnant or plan to become pregnant, inform your doctor immediately. No information is available about the safety of using Timoptic during pregnancy.

Timolol appears in breast milk and may harm a nursing infant. If using Timoptic is essential to your health, your doctor may advise you to stop breastfeeding until your treatment is finished.

Recommended dosage
ADULTS

Your doctor will tailor an individual Timoptic dosage depending on your medical condition and how you responded to any previous glaucoma treatment.

The usual recommended initial dose is to place 1 drop of 0.25 percent Timoptic in the affected eye(s) twice a day. If you do not respond satisfactorily to this dosage, your doctor may tell you to place 1 drop of 0.5 percent Timoptic in the affected eye(s) twice a day.

Overdosage

Although there is no information available on Timoptic overdose, you should seek medical treatment immediately if you think you might have used too much Timoptic. Call your local poison control center or your doctor for assistance.

The following overdose symptoms have been reported with other beta blockers:

Extremely slow heartbeat
Heart block (conduction problems)
Low blood pressure
Seizures and, in some cases, wheezing
Severe heart failure

Generic name:

TOBRAMYCIN

See Tobrex, page 632.

Brand name:

TOBREX

Generic name: Tobramycin

Why is this drug prescribed?

This medication is a topical antibiotic used to treat external bacterial infections of the eye.

Most important fact about this drug

The dropper tip or tube should not touch the eye. Keep them from touching any surface as this may contaminate the contents.

How should you use this medication?

Use Tobrex exactly as prescribed by your doctor. It is important that you finish using all of your prescription to obtain the maximum benefit.

To apply the ointment form of this medication:
1. Tilt your head back.
2. Place a finger on your cheek just under your eye and gently pull down until a "V" pocket is formed between your eyeball and your lower lid.
3. Place a small amount of Tobrex in the "V" pocket. Do not let the tip of the tube touch the eye.
4. Look downward before closing your eye.

If you forget a dose of this medication, use it as soon as you remember.

What side effects may occur?

Side effects cannot be anticipated. If any develop or change in intensity, inform your doctor as soon as possible. Only your doctor can determine if it is safe for you to continue to take Tobrex.

■ *Side effects may include:*
  Abnormal redness of eye tissue
  Lid itching
  Swelling

Why should this drug not be prescribed?

If you are sensitive to or have ever had an allergic reaction to Tobrex or similar drugs, you should not use this medication. Make sure that your doctor is aware of any drug reactions that you have experienced.

Special warnings about this medication

Your response to this medication should be monitored by your doctor.

If you experience a sensitivity reaction to this medication, discontinue use and inform your doctor.

Continued or prolonged use of Tobrex may result in a growth of bacteria that do not respond to this medication and can cause a secondary infection.

Ophthalmic ointments may retard corneal wound healing.

Possible food and drug interactions when taking this medication

If you are taking any other prescription or non-prescription topical antibiotics for your eyes, check with your doctor before using Tobrex. Using this medication with certain other antibiotics in your system may produce side effects or interactions.

Special information if you are pregnant or breastfeeding

The effects of Tobrex during pregnancy have not been adequately studied. If you are pregnant or plan to become pregnant, inform your doctor immediately. Tobrex may appear in breast milk. Your doctor may advise you to discontinue breastfeeding until your treatment with this medication is finished.

Recommended dosage

ADULTS

Solution

If the infection is mild to moderate, place 1 or 2 drops into the affected eye(s) every 4 hours. In severe infections, place 2 drops into the eye(s) every hour until there is improvement. Treatment should be reduced before stopping altogether.

Ointment

If the infection is mild to moderate, apply a ½-inch ribbon into the affected eye(s) 2 or 3 times per day. In severe infections, apply a ½-inch ribbon into the affected eye(s) every 3 or 4 hours until there is improvement. Treatment should be reduced before stopping altogether.

CHILDREN

Tobrex is safe and effective for use in children. Consult with your doctor for a child's dosing information.

Overdosage

Symptoms of an overdose may be similar to side effects. They include:
Corneal redness and inflammation
Excessive eye tearing
Fluid retention
Lid itching

If you suspect an overdose, seek medical attention immediately.

Generic name:

TOCAINIDE HYDROCHLORIDE

See Tonocard, page 640.

Brand name:

TOFRANIL

Generic name: Imipramine hydrochloride
Other brand names: Janimine

Why is this drug prescribed?

Tofranil is used to treat depression. It is a member of the family of drugs called tricyclic antidepressants.

Also, Tofranil may be used along with other behavioral therapies to treat bedwetting in children on a short-term basis. Its effectiveness may decrease with longer use.

Most important fact about this drug

If taken in high enough amounts, Tofranil can be fatal, especially in children. It should be prescribed in the smallest possible amount, and it should always be stored in child-resistant containers.

How should you take this medication?

Tofranil may be taken with or without food.

You should not take Tofranil with alcohol.

What side effects may occur?

Side effects cannot be anticipated. If any develop or change in intensity, inform your doctor as soon as possible. Only your doctor can determine if it is safe for you to continue taking Tofranil.

■ *Side effects may include:*
Abdominal cramps, agitation, anxiety, black tongue, bleeding sores, blood disorders, blurred vision, breast development in males, confusion, constipation or diarrhea, cough, fever, sore throat, delusions, dilated pupils, disorientation, dizziness, drowsiness, dry mouth, episodes of elation or irritability, excessive or spontaneous flow of milk, fatigue, fever, flushing, frequent urination or difficulty or delay in urinating, hair loss, hallucinations, headache, heart attack, heart failure, high blood pressure, high or low blood sugar, high pressure of fluid in the eyes, hives, impotence, increased or decreased sex drive, inflammation of the mouth, insomnia, intestinal blockage, lack of coordination, light-headedness (especially when rising from lying down), loss of appetite, nausea, stomach pain, vomiting, nightmares, odd taste in mouth, pounding heart, purple or reddish-brown spots on skin, rapid heartbeat, restlessness, ringing in the ears, seizures, sensitivity to light, skin itching and rash, stroke, sweating, swelling due to fluid retention (especially in face or tongue), swelling of breasts, swelling of testicles, swollen glands, tendency to fall, tingling, pins and needles, and numbness in hands and feet, tremors, visual problems, weakness, weight gain or loss, yellowed skin and whites of eyes

■ *The most common side effects in children being treated for bedwetting are:*
Nervousness, sleep disorders, stomach and intestinal problems, tiredness

■ *Other side effects in children are:*
Anxiety, collapse, constipation, convulsions, emotional instability, fainting

Why should this drug not be prescribed?

Tofranil should not be used if you have had a recent heart attack.

People who take antidepressant drugs known as MAO inhibitors, such as Nardil and Parnate, should not take Tofranil. You should not take Tofranil if you have a known hypersensitivity to it.

Special warnings about this medication

You should use Tofranil cautiously if you have or have ever had: narrow-angle glaucoma or increased pressure in the eye; urinary retention; heart, liver, kidney, or thyroid disease; or seizures, or if you are taking thyroid medication. General feelings of illness, headache, and nausea can result if you suddenly stop taking Tofranil. Follow your doctor's instructions closely when discontinuing Tofranil.

Tell your doctor if you develop a sore throat or fever while taking Tofranil.

This drug may impair your ability to drive a car or operate potentially dangerous machinery. Do not participate in any activities that require full alertness if you are unsure about your ability.

This drug can make you sensitive to light. Try to stay out of the sun as much as possible while you are taking it.

Possible food and drug interactions when taking this medication

If Tofranil is taken with certain other drugs, the effects of either could be increased, decreased, or altered. It is especially important to check with your doctor before combining Tofranil with the following:

Albuterol (Proventil, Ventolin)
Anticholinergics such as Cogentin
Antihypertensives such as Wytensin
Carbamazepine (Tegretol)
Central nervous system depressants such as
   Xanax and Valium
Cimetidine (Tagamet)
Clonidine (Catapres)
Decongestants such as Sudafed
Desipramine (Norpramin)
Epinephrine (Epipen)
Fluoxetine (Prozac)
Guanethidine (Ismelin)
Methylphenidate (Ritalin)
Thyroid medications

Extreme drowsiness and other potentially serious effects can result if Tofranil is combined with alcohol or other mental depressants, such as narcotic painkillers (Percocet), sleeping medications (Halcion), or tranquilizers (Valium).

Special information
if you are pregnant or breastfeeding

Pregnant women should use Tofranil only when the potential benefits clearly outweigh the potential risks. If you are pregnant or plan to become pregnant, inform your doctor immediately. Tofranil may appear in breast milk and could affect a nursing infant. If this medication is essential to your health, your doctor may advise you to stop breast-feeding until your treatment is finished.

Recommended dosage

Doses should be tailored to the individual. The minimum effective amount needed should be used.

ADULTS

Usual doses range from 50 to 150 milligrams per day. The total daily dosage should not exceed 200 milligrams.

CHILDREN

It has been reported that children are more sensitive than adults to overdoses of Tofranil.

Tofranil should not be used in children to treat any condition but bedwetting, and use should be limited to short-term therapy.

Total daily dosages for children should not exceed 2.5 milligrams for each 2.2 pounds of the child's weight.

Safety and effectiveness in children under the age of 6 have not been established.

To Treat Bedwetting for Children 6 through 11 Years Old
Doses usually begin at 25 milligrams per day. This amount should be taken an hour before bedtime. If needed, this dose may be increased after 1 week to 50 milligrams, taken in one dose at bedtime or divided into 2 doses, 1 taken at midafternoon and 1 at bedtime.

Children over 12 years old
The dose may be raised to 75 milligrams in a single bedtime dose or divided into 2 doses, taken at midafternoon and bedtime.

ADOLESCENTS AND ELDERLY

People in these two age groups should take lower doses. Dosage starts out at 40 milligrams per day and can go up to no more than 100 milligrams a day.

Overdosage

Any medication taken in excess can have serious consequences. An overdose of Tofranil can cause death. If you suspect an overdose, seek medical help immediately.

Symptoms of Tofranil overdose may include: Agitation, bluish skin, coma, convulsions, difficulty breathing, dilated pupils, drowsiness, heart failure, high fever, involuntary writhing or jerky movements, irregular or rapid heartbeat, lack of coordination, overactive reflexes, restlessness, rigid muscles, shock, stupor, sweating, vomiting

Generic name:

TOLAZAMIDE

See Tolinase, page 638.

Generic name:

TOLBUTAMIDE

See Orinase, page 442.

Brand name:

TOLECTIN

Generic name: Tolmetin sodium

Why is this drug prescribed?
Tolectin is a nonsteroidal anti-inflammatory drug used to relieve the inflammation, swelling, stiffness and joint pain associated with rheumatoid arthritis and osteoarthritis (the most common form of arthritis). It is used for both acute episodes and long-term treatment. It is also used to treat juvenile arthritis and other kinds of pain.

Most important fact about this drug
You should have frequent checkups with your doctor if you take Tolectin regularly. Ulcers or internal bleeding can occur without warning.

How should you take this medication?
Tolectin may be taken with food or an antacid, and with a full glass of water, if necessary, to avoid stomach upset.

Take this medication exactly as prescribed by your doctor.

If you are using Tolectin for arthritis, it should be taken regularly.

If you forget to take a dose, take it as soon as you remember. If it is almost time for your next dose, skip the one you missed and go back to your regular schedule. Never take two doses at the same time.

What side effects may occur?
Side effects cannot be anticipated. If any develop or change in intensity, inform your doctor as soon as possible. Only your doctor can determine if it is safe for you to continue taking Tolectin.

■ *More common side effects may include:*
Abdominal pain, change in weight, chest pain, constipation, depression, diarrhea, dizziness, drowsiness, gas, headache, heartburn, high blood pressure, indigestion, nausea, peptic ulcer, ringing in ears, skin irritation, stomach inflammation, stomach upset, swelling due to fluid retention, urinary tract infections, visual disturbances, vomiting, weakness

■ *Less common or rare side effects may include:*
Anemia, blood and protein in urine, congestive heart failure, fever, hepatitis, hives, inflammation of the mouth or tongue, kidney failure, painful urination, purple or reddish spots on skin, stomach or intestinal bleeding, yellow eyes or skin

Why should this drug not be prescribed?
If you are sensitive to or have ever had an allergic reaction to Tolectin, aspirin, or similar drugs, or if you have had asthma attacks caused by aspirin or other drugs of this type, you should not take this medication. Make sure that your doctor is aware of any drug reactions that you have experienced.

Special warnings about this medication

Peptic ulcers and bleeding can occur without warning.

This drug should be used with caution if you have kidney or liver disease. It can cause liver reactions in some people.

Do not take aspirin or any other anti-inflammatory medications while taking Tolectin unless your doctor tells you to do so.

Tolectin can cause visual disturbances. If you experience a change in your vision, inform your doctor.

Tolectin prolongs bleeding time. If you are taking blood-thinning medication, this drug should be taken with caution.

Tolectin may intensify the effects of alcohol. Do not drink alcohol while taking this medication.

This drug can increase water retention. Use with caution if you have heart disease or high blood pressure.

Tolectin causes some people to become drowsy or less alert. If it has this effect on you, driving or operating dangerous machinery or participating in any hazardous activity that requires full mental alertness is not recommended.

Possible food and drug interactions when taking this medication

If Tolectin is taken with certain other drugs, the effects of either could be increased, decreased, or altered. It is especially important to check with your doctor before combining Tolectin with the following:

Anticoagulants (blood thinners such as
   Coumadin)
Aspirin

Methotrexate
Probenecid (Benemid)

**Special information
if you are pregnant or breastfeeding**

The effects of Tolectin during pregnancy have not been adequately studied. If you are pregnant or plan to become pregnant, inform your doctor immediately. Tolectin appears in breast milk and could affect a nursing infant. If this medication is essential to your health, your doctor may advise you to discontinue breastfeeding until your treatment is finished.

Recommended dosage

ADULTS

Rheumatoid Arthritis or Osteoarthritis
The starting dosage is usually 1,200 milligrams a day divided into 3 doses of 400 milligrams. Take 1 dose when you wake up and 1 at bedtime, and 1 sometime in between. Dosages are often adjusted after 1 to 2 weeks. Most patients will take a total daily dosage of 600 to 1,800 milligrams in divided doses, usually 3 times a day.

You should see the benefits of Tolectin in a few days to a week. The lowest dose that proves beneficial should be used.

CHILDREN

The starting dose for children 2 years and older is usually a total of 20 milligrams per 2.2 pounds of body weight, divided into 3 or 4 smaller doses. Your doctor will advise you on use in children. The usual dose ranges from 15 to 30 milligrams per 2.2 pounds per day.

The safety and effectiveness of Tolectin have not been established in children under 2 years of age.

ELDERLY

Dosage should be determined by the particular needs of the elderly patient.

Overdosage

Any medication taken in excess can cause symptoms of overdose. If you suspect an overdose, seek medical attention immediately.

No specific symptoms of Tolectin overdose have been documented.

Brand name:

TOLINASE

Generic name: Tolazamide

Why is this drug prescribed?

Tolinase is an oral antidiabetic drug available in tablet form. It lowers the blood sugar level by stimulating the pancreas to release insulin. Tolinase may be given as a supplement to diet therapy to help control Type II (non-insulin-dependent) diabetes.

Most important fact about this drug

Drugs such as Tolinase may possibly lead to more heart problems than diet treatment alone, or treatment with diet and insulin. If you have heart problems, you may want to discuss this with your doctor.

Always consider Tolinase an addition to, not a substitute for, diet therapy. The safest and most desirable way to control Type II diabetes is to keep your weight down through diet and exercise. Tolinase or another antidiabetic drug should be considered only if a diet and exercise program fails to correct your high blood sugar.

How should you take this medication?

Remember that if you are diligent about diet and exercise, you may need Tolinase for only a short period of time.

Take Tolinase exactly as prescribed by your doctor.

While taking Tolinase, your blood and urine glucose levels should be monitored regularly.

Your doctor may also want you to have a periodic glycosylated hemoglobin blood test, which will show how well you have kept your blood sugar down during the weeks preceding the test.

What side effects may occur?

Side effects cannot be anticipated. If any appear or change in intensity, inform your doctor as soon as possible. Only your doctor can determine if it is safe for you to continue taking Tolinase. The most frequently encountered side effects from Tolinase—nausea, a full, bloated feeling, and heartburn—may disappear if the dosage is reduced.

Hives, itching, and rash may appear initially and then disappear as you continue to take the drug. If a skin reaction persists, you should stop taking Tolinase.

■ *Less common side effects may include:*
Blistering on sun-exposed skin, photosensitivity

■ *Rare side effects may include:*
Dizziness, fatigue, headache, malaise, vertigo, weakness

Why should this drug not be prescribed?

Do not take Tolinase if you are sensitive to it or have ever had an allergic reaction to it; if you are suffering from diabetic ketoacidosis; or if you have Type I (insulin-dependent) diabetes and are not taking insulin.

Special warnings about this medication

Like other oral antidiabetic drugs, Tolinase may produce severe low blood sugar (hypoglycemia) if the dosing is wrong. While taking Tolinase, you are particularly susceptible to episodes of low blood sugar if:

You suffer from a kidney or liver problem;
You have a lack of adrenal or pituitary hormones; or

You are elderly, run-down, or malnourished.

You are at increased risk for a low-blood-sugar episode if you are hungry, exercising heavily, drinking alcohol, or using more than one glucose-lowering drug.

Mild stress such as fever, trauma, infection, or surgery may also cause lowering of blood sugar.

Note that an episode of low blood sugar may be difficult to recognize if you are elderly or if you are taking a beta-blocker drug (Inderal, Lopressor, Tenormin, and others).

If switching to Tolinase from chlorpropamide (Diabinese), you should take special care to avoid an episode of low blood sugar.

Possible food and drug interactions when taking this medication

If Tolinase is taken with certain other drugs, the effects of either could be increased, decreased, or altered. It is especially important to check with your doctor before combining Tolinase with the following:

Alcohol
Aspirin or related drugs
Beta blockers such as Inderal, Lopressor, Tenormin, and others
Calcium channel blockers such as Calan, Isoptin, and others
Chloramphenicol (Chloromycetin)
Corticosteroids such as Cortef, Decadron, Medrol, and others
Coumarin (Coumadin, Dicumarol)
Diuretics such as Esidrix, Diuril, Naturetin, and others
Estrogens (Premarin)
Isoniazid (Nydrazid)
MAO inhibitors (antidepressants such as Marplan, Nardil, and Parnate)
Miconazole (Monistat)
Nicotinic acid (Nicobid)
Nonsteroidal anti-inflammatory drugs such as Motrin, Naprosyn, and others
Oral contraceptives such as Enovid, Ovral, and others
Phenothiazines (antipsychotic drugs such as Haldol, Mellaril, Prolixin, and others)
Phenytoin (Dilantin)
Probenecid (Benemid)
Rifampin (Rifadin)
Sulfonamides such as Bactrim, Gantrisin, and others
Sympathomimetics such as Isuprel, Neo-Synephrine, and others
Thyroid drugs such as Proloid, Euthroid, Synthroid, and others

Special information if you are pregnant or breastfeeding

If you are pregnant or plan to become pregnant, inform your doctor immediately. Tolinase is not recommended for use during pregnancy, and should not be prescribed if you might become pregnant while taking it.

Control of diabetes during pregnancy is very important, but in most cases should be accomplished with insulin injections rather than oral antidiabetic drugs.

Tolinase should not be used during breastfeeding because of possible harmful effects on the baby. If you are a new mother, you may need to choose between taking Tolinase and breastfeeding your baby.

Recommended dosage

Dosage levels are determined by each patient's needs.

ADULTS

The usual starting dose of Tolinase Tablets for the mild to moderately severe Type II diabetic patient is 100 to 150 milligrams daily taken with breakfast or the first main meal.

ELDERLY

If the patient is malnourished, underweight, elderly, or not eating properly, initial dose is usually 100 milligrams once a day. Failure to follow an appropriate dosage regimen may precipitate hypoglycemia. Patients who do not stick to their prescribed dietary regimen are more likely to have an unsatisfactory response to this medication.

Overdosage

An overdose of Tolinase can cause an episode of low blood sugar. Mild low blood sugar without loss of consciousness should be treated with oral glucose, an adjusted meal pattern, and possibly a reduction in the Tolinase dosage. Severe low blood sugar, which may cause coma or seizures, is a medical emergency and must be treated in a hospital.

Any medication taken in excess can have serious consequences. If you suspect an overdose of Tolinase, seek medical attention immediately.

Generic name:

TOLMETIN SODIUM

See Tolectin, page 636.

Brand name:

TONOCARD

Generic name: Tocainide hydrochloride

Why is this drug prescribed?

Tonocard is used to treat severe irregular heartbeat (arrhythmias). Arrhythmias are generally divided into two main types: heartbeats that are faster than normal (tachycardia), or heartbeats that are slower than normal (bradycardia). Irregular heartbeats are often caused by drugs or disease but can occur in otherwise-healthy people with no history of heart disease or other illness. Tonocard works differently from other antiarrhythmic drugs, such as quinidine (Quinidex), procainamide (Procan SR), and disopyramide (Norpace). It is similar to lidocaine (Xylocaine) and is effective in treating ventricular arrhythmias (irregular heartbeats that occur in a particular part of the heart).

Most important fact about this drug

Serious blood disorders and lung disorders have occurred with Tonocard treatment. It should be used only if its benefits clearly outweigh its risks.

How should you take this medication?

Take this medication exactly as prescribed by your doctor.

Try not to miss any doses. If this medication is not taken regularly, your condition may worsen.

What side effects may occur?

Side effects cannot be anticipated. If any develop or change in intensity, inform your doctor as soon as possible. Only your doctor can determine if it is safe for you to continue taking Tonocard.

■ *More common side effects may include:*
Confusion/disorientation, dizziness/vertigo, diarrhea/loose stools, excessive sweating, hallucinations, increased irregular heartbeat, lack of coordination, loss of appetite, nausea, nervousness, rash/skin eruptions, tingling or pins and needles, tremor, vision disturbances, vomiting

■ *Less common side effects may include:*
Arthritis, anxiety, chest pain, conduction disorders, congestive heart failure, drowsiness, exhaustion, fatigue, headache, hearing loss, hot/cold feelings, involuntary eyeball movement, joint pain, low blood pressure, muscle pain, pounding heartbeat, rapid heartbeat, ringing in ears, sleepiness, slow heartbeat,

sluggishness, tiredness, unsteadiness, walking disturbances

■ *Rare side effects may include:*
Abdominal pain/discomfort, agitation, allergic reactions, anemia, angina, blood clots in lungs, blood disorders, changes in blood counts, changes in heart function, chills, cinchonism (a sensitivity reaction with symptoms including ringing in the ears, loss of hearing, dizziness, light-headedness, headache, nausea, and/or disturbed vision), cold hands and feet, coma, constipation, decreased mental ability, decreased urination, depression, difficulty breathing, difficulty speaking, difficulty sleeping, difficulty swallowing, disturbed behavior, disturbed dreams, dizziness on standing, double vision, dry mouth, earache, enlarged heart, fainting, fever, fluid in lungs, fluid retention, flushing, general bodily discomfort, hair loss, heart attack, hepatitis, hiccups, high blood pressure, hives, inflammation of the pancreas, increased stuttering, increased urination, lung disorders, memory loss, muscle cramps, muscle twitching/spasm, myasthenia gravis, neck pain or pain extending from the neck, pallor, pneumonia, seizures, skin peeling, slurred speech, smell disturbance, stomach upset, taste disturbance, thirst, weakness, yawning, yellow eyes and skin

Why should this drug not be prescribed?

If you have heart block (conduction disorder) and do not have a pacemaker, or if you are sensitive to or have ever had an allergic reaction to Tonocard or certain local anesthetics such as Xylocaine, do not take this medication.

Special warnings about this medication

Serious blood disorders can occur while taking Tonocard, especially within the first 3 months of treatment. Any unexplained bruising or bleeding or signs of infection such as fever, chills, sore throat, or sores or soreness in your mouth, should be reported to your doctor immediately. A complete blood count should be done each week for the first 12 weeks of therapy, and your blood count should be monitored frequently.

Serious lung disorders are also a possibility while taking Tonocard. If you develop a fever, cough, wheezing, or rash, or you have difficulty breathing, contact your doctor immediately. A chest x-ray should be done to determine the cause of the symptoms.

If you have congestive heart failure, Tonocard should be used cautiously. It could worsen your condition.

You should be carefully monitored if you have severe liver or kidney disease.

Possible food and drug interactions when taking this medication

If Tonocard is taken with certain other drugs, the effects of either could be increased, decreased, or altered. It is especially important to check with your doctor before combining Tonocard with any of the following:

The anesthetic Lidocaine (Xylocaine)
Metoprolol (Lopressor)
Other anti-arrhythmics such as Quinidex, Inderal, Mexitil

Special information if you are pregnant or breastfeeding

The effects of Tonocard during pregnancy have not been adequately studied. However, animal studies have shown an increase in stillbirths and spontaneous abortions. If you are pregnant or plan to become pregnant, inform your doctor immediately. Tonocard may appear in breast milk and could affect a nursing infant. If this medication is essential to your health, your doctor may advise you to discontinue breastfeeding until your treatment is finished.

Recommended dosage

ADULTS

Dosages of Tonocard must be adjusted to its effects on each individual. Your doctor should monitor you carefully to determine if the dosage you are taking is working properly. He may divide your doses further or make other changes, such as shortening the time between doses, if side effects occur.

The usual starting dose is 400 milligrams every 8 hours.

The usual dose range is between 1,200 and 1,800 milligrams total per day divided into 3 doses. This medication can be taken in 2 doses a day with careful monitoring by your doctor.

Doses beyond 2,400 milligrams per day are rarely used.

Some patients, particularly those with reduced kidney or liver function, may be treated successfully with less than 1,200 milligrams per day.

CHILDREN

The safety and effectiveness of this drug in children have not been established.

ELDERLY

This drug should be used with caution in elderly patients.

Overdosage

Any medication taken in excess can cause symptoms of overdose. If you suspect an overdose, seek medical attention immediately.

There are no specific reports of Tonocard overdose. However, the first and most important signs of overdose would be

expected to appear in the central nervous system. Disorders of the stomach and intestines might follow. Convulsions and heart and lung slowing or stopping might occur.

Brand name:

TOPICORT

Generic name: Desoximetasone

Why is this drug prescribed?

Topicort is a topical (applied directly to the skin) synthetic cortisone-like steroid that relieves the inflammation and itching caused by a variety of skin conditions.

Most important fact about this drug

Although it is applied to the skin, when you use Topicort cream, gel, or ointment, you inevitably absorb some of the steroid through the skin and into the bloodstream. After applying Topicort, leave the skin exposed to the air or, at most, covered only by clothing. If you use an airtight bandage, Topicort will get into your blood; this could lead to un-desirable effects.

How should you use this medication?

Topicort should be used exactly as prescribed by your doctor.

This medication is for external use only. It should not touch your eyes.

Apply a thin coating of Topicort to the affected area. Rub in gently.

The treated area should not be covered unless your doctor has told you to do so.

If Topicort is being used for an infant or toddler with a genital rash, make sure the diapers or plastic pants are not too tight, so that air can circulate.

What side effects may occur?

Side effects cannot be anticipated. If any develop or change in intensity, inform your doctor as soon as possible. Only your doctor can determine if it is safe for you to continue using Topicort. The side effects listed below occur infrequently, but may occur more often if the treated area is covered with a bandage.

■ *Side effects may include:*
Acne-like pimples, burning of the skin, "broken" capillaries (fine reddish lines under the skin), dryness, excessive growth of hair, inflammation of the hair follicles, irritation, itching, loss of skin pigmentation, prickly heat, skin inflammation around the mouth, rash, redness, stretch marks on the skin, thinning of the skin

Using too much Topicort, or using Topicort for too long, may produce additional adverse effects: see the "Overdosage" section.

Do not use Topicort if you are sensitive to it or have ever had an allergic reaction to any of its ingredients.

Special warnings about this medication

Topicort is for external use only. Avoid getting it into your eyes. Do not use Topicort to treat any condition other than the one for which it was prescribed.

Possible food and drug interactions when using this medication

No interactions have been reported.

Special information if you are pregnant or breastfeeding

Topicort should not be used during pregnancy unless the benefit outweighs the potential risks to the unborn child. If you are pregnant or plan to become pregnant, inform your doctor immediately.

It is not known whether topical steroids are absorbed in sufficient amounts to appear in breast milk. If your doctor considers Topicort essential to your health, he may advise you to stop breastfeeding until your treatment with the medication is finished.

Recommended dosage

ADULTS

Apply a thin film of Topicort to the affected area 2 times a day.

CHILDREN

Topicort Ointment is not recommended for use in children under 10 years old.

Overdosage

Large doses of topical steroids applied over a large area, and long-term use of topical steroids, especially when the treated area is covered, can cause increases in blood sugar and Cushing's syndrome, a condition characterized by a moon-shaped face, emotional disturbances, high blood pressure, weight gain and, in women, baldness or growth of body and facial hair.

Cushing's Syndrome may also trigger the development of sugar diabetes (diabetes mellitis). If left uncorrected, Cushing's Syndrome may become serious. If you suspect your use of Topicort has led to Cushing's Syndrome, seek medical attention immediately.

Brand name:

TRANDATE

See Normodyne, page 429.

Brand name:

TRANSDERM NITRO

See Nitroglycerin, page 420.

Brand name:

TRANXENE

Generic name: Clorazepate dipotassium
Other brand names: Tranxene-SD,
Tranxene-SD Half Strength

Why is this drug prescribed?

Tranxene belongs to a class of drugs known as benzodiazepines. It is used in the treatment of anxiety disorders and for short-term relief of the symptoms of anxiety.

It is also used to relieve the symptoms of acute alcohol withdrawal and as an adjunct in treatment of certain convulsive disorders such as epilepsy.

Most important fact about this drug

Tranxene can be habit-forming if taken regularly over a long period. You may experience withdrawal symptoms if you stop using this drug abruptly. Only your doctor should advise you to discontinue or change your dose.

Do not exceed the prescribed dose. Discuss overuse with your doctor.

How should you take this medication?

Tranxene should be taken exactly as prescribed by your doctor. Never take two doses at the same time.

What side effects may occur?

Side effects cannot be anticipated. If any develop or change in intensity, inform your doctor as soon as possible. Only your doctor can determine if it is safe for you to continue taking Tranxene.

■ *More common side effects may include:*
Drowsiness

■ *Less common or rare side effects may include:*
Blurred vision, depression, difficulty in sleeping or falling asleep, dizziness, dry mouth, double vision, fatigue, genital and urinary tract disorders, headache, irritability, lack of muscle coordination, mental confusion, nervousness, tremors, skin rashes, slurred speech, stomach and intestinal disorders

■ *Side effects due to rapid decrease or abrupt withdrawal from Tranxene include:*
Diarrhea, difficulty in sleeping or falling asleep, hallucinations, impaired memory, irritability, muscle aches, nervousness, tremors

Why should this drug not be prescribed?

If you are sensitive to or have ever had an allergic reaction to Tranxene or similar drugs, you should not take this medication. Make sure that your doctor is aware of any drug reactions that you have experienced.

Unless you are directed to do so by your doctor, do not take this medication if you have acute narrow-angle glaucoma.

Anxiety or tension related to everyday stress usually does not require treatment with a medication of this type. Discuss your symptoms thoroughly with your doctor.

Tranxene is not recommended for use in more serious conditions such as depression or psychosis.

Special warnings about this medication

Tranxene may cause you to become drowsy or less alert; therefore, driving or operating dangerous machinery or participating in any hazardous activity that requires full mental alertness is not recommended.

If you are being treated for anxiety associated with depression, your doctor may recommend the lowest dose of this medication. Do not increase your dose without consulting with your doctor.

Possible food and drug interactions when taking this medication

Tranxene is a central nervous system depressant and may intensify the effects of alcohol. Do not drink alcohol while taking this medication.

If Tranxene is taken with certain other drugs, the effects of either could be increased, decreased, or altered. It is especially important to check with your doctor before combining Tranxene, with the following:

Antidepressant drugs known as MAO
   inhibitors
Barbiturates
Narcotics
Other antidepressants
Phenothiazine-type tranquilizers

If you are taking any of the above or other prescription or non-prescription drugs, consult with your doctor before taking Tranxene.

Special information if you are pregnant or breastfeeding

The effects of Tranxene during pregnancy have not been adequately studied. However, because there is an increased risk of birth defects associated with this class of drugs, their use during pregnancy should be avoided. Tranxene may appear in breast milk and could affect a nursing infant. If this medication is essential to your health, your doctor may advise you to discontinue breastfeeding until your treatment with this medication is finished.

Recommended dosage

ADULTS

Anxiety
The usual recommended daily dosage is 30 milligrams divided into several smaller doses. A normal daily dose can be as little as 15 milligrams. Dosage may be increased gradually by your doctor to as much as 60 milligrams, according to your individual needs.

Tranxene is also available in a single bedtime dose. The initial dose is 15 milligrams, but dosage can be adjusted by your doctor to your individual needs.

Tranxene-SD, a 22.5 milligram tablet, can be taken once daily every 24 hours. This dose should not be used when starting treatment with this drug.

Tranxene-SD Half Strength, an 11.25 milligram tablet, can be taken once daily every 24 hours. This dose should not be used when starting treatment with this drug.

Acute Alcohol Withdrawal:
Tranxene is often used in a multi-day program for relief of the symptoms of acute alcohol withdrawal.

Dosages are usually increased in the first 2 days from 30 to 90 milligrams and then reduced over the next 2 days to lower levels. This medication should be used for this purpose only under strict medical supervision.

WHEN USED WITH ANTIEPILEPTIC DRUGS

Tranxene can be used in conjunction with antiepileptic drugs. The recommended dosages should be followed carefully to avoid drowsiness.

ADULTS AND CHILDREN OVER 12 YEARS OLD

The starting dose is 7.5 milligrams 3 times a day. Dosages can be increased by 7.5 milligrams per week to a maximum of 90 milligrams a day.

CHILDREN 9 TO 12 YEARS OLD

The starting dose should be no more than 7.5 milligrams 2 times a day. Dosages can be increased by 7.5 milligrams a week to a maximum of 60 milligrams a day.

Safety and effectiveness in children under 9 years of age have not been established.

ELDERLY

The usual starting dose in treating elderly patients for anxiety is 7.5 to 15 milligrams per day.

Overdosage

Any medication taken in excess can have serious consequences. If you suspect an overose, seek medical treatment immediately.

Symptoms of Tranxene overdose may include:
Coma
Low blood pressure
Sedation

Generic name:

TRAZODONE HYDROCHLORIDE

See Desyrel, page 182.

Brand name:

TRENTAL

Generic name: Pentoxifylline

Why is this drug prescribed?

Trental is a medication that reduces the viscosity or "stickiness" of your blood, allowing your blood to flow more freely. It helps relieve the painful leg cramps caused by "intermittent claudication," a condition resulting from poor blood supply to the leg muscles caused by hardening of the arteries.

Most important fact about this drug

Trental can ease the pain in your legs and make walking easier but should not replace other treatments such as physical therapy or surgery.

How should you take this medication?

Trental should be taken exactly as prescribed by your doctor.

Never take two doses at the same time.

What side effects may occur?

Side effects cannot be anticipated. If any develop or change in intensity, inform your doctor as soon as possible. Only your doctor can determine if it is safe for you to continue taking Trental.

■ *More common side effects may include:*
Belching
Bloating
Dizziness
Gas
Headache
Indigestion
Nausea

■ *Less common side effects may include:*
Abdominal discomfort, agitation/nervousness, allergic reaction (symptoms include: swelling of face, lips, tongue, throat, arms, or legs, sore throat, fever and chills, difficulty swallowing, chest pain), anxiety, bad taste in the mouth, blind spot in vision, blurred vision, brittle fingernails, chest pain (sometimes crushing), confusion, conjunctivitis (pink eye), constipation, diarrhea, difficult or labored breathing, difficulty sleeping, drowsiness, dry mouth/thirst, earache, excessive salivation, flu-like symptoms, fluid retention, flushing, general body discomfort, hives, inflammation of the gallbladder, irregular heartbeat, itching, laryngitis, loss of appetite, low blood pressure, nosebleeds, palpitations, rash, sore throat/swollen neck glands, stuffy nose, tremor, vomiting, weight change

■ *Rare side effects may include:*
Anemia, rapid heartbeat, yellow eyes and skin

Why should this drug not be prescribed?
If you are sensitive to or have ever had an allergic reaction to Trental, caffeine, theophylline (medication for asthma or other breathing disorders), or theobromine, do not take this medication. They are all chemically similar. Make sure that your doctor is aware of any drug reactions that you have experienced.

Special warnings about this medication
Most people tolerate Trental well, but there have been occasional cases of crushing chest pain, low blood pressure, and irregular heartbeat in patients with heart disease and brain disorders.

Possible food and drug interactions when taking this medication
If Trental is taken with certain other drugs, the effects of either could be increased, decreased, or altered. It is especially important to check with your doctor before combining Trental with the following:

Blood-thinning drugs such as Coumadin
Platelet aggregation inhibitors such as Persantin

Special information if you are pregnant or breastfeeding
The effects of Trental during pregnancy have not been adequately studied. If you are pregnant or plan to become pregnant, inform your doctor immediately. Trental appears in breast milk and could affect a nursing infant. If this medication is essential to your health, your doctor may advise you to discontinue breastfeeding until your treatment with this medication is finished.

Recommended dosage

ADULTS

The usual dosage of Trental in controlled-release tablets is one 400-milligram tablet 3 times a day with meals.

While the effect of Trental may be seen within 2 to 4 weeks, it is recommended that treatment be continued for at least 8 weeks.

Any stomach or central nervous system (affecting the brain and spinal cord) side effects are related to the dose. If any of these side effects occur, the dosage should be lowered to 1 tablet, 2 times a day, for a total of 800 milligrams a day. If side effects persist at this lower dosage, your doctor may consider stopping this drug.

CHILDREN

The safety and effectiveness of this drug in children under age 18 have not been established.

ELDERLY

This drug should be used with caution in elderly patients.

Overdosage
Any medication taken in excess can have serious consequences. If you suspect symptoms of a Trental overdose, seek medical attention immediately. Symptoms have appeared within 4 to 5 hours and have lasted for 12 hours.

Symptoms of Trental overdose may include:
Agitation
Convulsions
Fever
Flushing
Loss of consciousness
Low blood pressure,
Sleepiness

Generic name:

TRETINOIN

See Retin-A, page 538.

Generic name:

TRIAMTERENE WITH HYDROCHLOROTHIAZIDE

See Dyazide, page 219,
and Maxzide, page 357.

Brand name:

TRIAVIL

Generic ingredients: Amitriptyline,
Perphenazine

Why is this drug prescribed?
Triavil is used to treat anxiety and depression
in schizophrenics (people with a distorted
sense of reality) and non-schizophrenic people.
Triavil is a combination of a tricyclic
antidepressant (amitriptyline) and
perphenazine.

Most important fact about this drug
Triavil may cause tardive dyskinesia—a
condition marked by involuntary muscle
spasms and twitches in the face and body.
This condition may be permanent and appears
to be most common among the elderly,
especially women. Ask your doctor for
information about this possible risk.

How should you take this medication?
Triavil may be taken with or without food.
You should not take Triavil with alcohol.

What side effects may occur?
Side effects cannot be anticipated. If any
develop or change in intensity, inform your
doctor as soon as possible. Only your doctor
can determine if it is safe for you to continue
taking Triavil.

■ Side effects may include:
Abnormal secretion of milk, abnormalities
of movements and posture, anxiety, asthma,
black tongue, blood disorders, blurred
vision, body rigidly arched backward, breast
development in males, coma, confusion,
constipation, convulsions, delusions,
diarrhea, difficulty breathing, difficulty
concentrating, difficulty swallowing, dilated
pupils, disorientation, dizziness, drowsiness,
dry mouth, eating abnormal amounts of
food, ejaculation failure, episodes of elation
or irritability, excessive or spontaneous flow
of milk, excitement, exhaustion, eye
problems, eye spasms, eyes in a fixed
position, fatigue, fever, fluid accumulation
and swelling (including throat and brain,
face and tongue), frequent urination,
hallucinations, headache, heart attacks, high
blood pressure, high or low blood sugar,
hives, impotence, increased or decreased sex
drive, inflammation of the mouth, insomnia,
intestinal blockage, intolerance to light,
involuntary jerky movements of tongue,
face, mouth, lips, jaw, body, or arms and
legs, irregular blood pressure, pulse, and
heartbeat, irregular menstrual periods, lack
of coordination, liver problems, lockjaw,
loss or increase of appetite, low blood
pressure, muscle stiffness, nasal congestion,
nausea, nightmares, odd taste in the mouth,
overactive reflexes, pain and stiffness around
neck, palpitations, protruding tongue,
purple-reddish-brown spots on skin, rapid
heartbeat, restlessness, rigid arms, feet, head,
and muscles, ringing in the ears, salivation,
sedation, seizures, sensitivity to light, severe
allergic reactions, skin itching, pigmentation,
rash, inflammation, scaling, spasms in the

hands and feet, speech problems, stomach upset, stroke, sweating, swelling of breasts, swelling of testicles, swollen glands, tingling, pins and needles, and numbness in hands and feet, tremors, twisted neck, twitching in the body, neck, shoulders, and face, uncontrollable and involuntary urination, urinary problems, visual problems, vomiting, weakness, weight gain or loss, yellowed skin and whites of eyes

Why should this drug not be prescribed?

You should not be using Triavil if you are taking central nervous system depressants such as alcohol, barbiturates, analgesics, antihistamines, or narcotics. Triavil should not be used if you have had a recent heart attack, or if you have an abnormal bone marrow or blood condition. Avoid Triavil if you are known to be hypersensitive to it.

People who take antidepressant drugs known as MAO inhibitors (including such as Nardil and Parnate) should not take Triavil.

Special warnings about this medication

Before using Triavil, tell your doctor if you have ever had: glaucoma; urinary retention; breast cancer; convulsive disorders; heart, liver, or thyroid disease; or if you are exposed to extreme heat or pesticides. Be aware that Triavil may mask signs of brain tumor and intestinal blockage.

Nausea, headache, and a general ill feeling can result if you suddenly stop taking Triavil. Follow your doctor's instructions closely when discontinuing Triavil.

This drug may impair your ability to drive a car or operate potentially dangerous machinery. Do not participate in any activities that require full alertness if you are unsure about your ability.

Possible food and drug interactions when taking this medication

People who take antidepressant drugs known as MAO inhibitors should not take Triavil.

If Triavil is taken with certain other drugs, the effects of either could be increased, decreased, or altered. It is especially important to check with your doctor before combining Triavil with the following:

Anticonvulsants such as Dilantin
Anticholinergics such as Bentyl
Anticoagulants such as Dicumarol
Antihistamines such as Benadryl
Atropine (Donnatal)
Barbiturates such as phenobarbital
Cimetidine (Tagament)
Disulfiram (Antabuse)
Epinephrine (Epipen)
Ethchlorvynol (Placidyl)
Fluoxetine (Prozac)
Furazolidone (Furoxone)
Guanethidine (Ismelin)
Narcotic analgesics such as Percocet
Thyroid medications

Extreme drowsiness and other potentially serious effects can result if Triavil is combined with alcohol or other central nervous system depressants such as narcotics, painkillers, and sleep medications.

Special information
if you are pregnant or breastfeeding

Triavil may cause false-positive results on pregnancy tests. Triavil should not be used by pregnant women or mothers who are breastfeeding.

Recommended dosage

Your doctor will individualize your dose.

You should not take more than 4 tablets of Triavil 4-50 or 8 tablets of any other strength in one day. It may be a few days to a few weeks before you notice any change.

ADULTS

For Non-Psychotic Anxiety and Depression
The usual dose is 3 or 4 tablets of Triavil 2-25 or 4-25 daily, divided into 3 or 4 doses, or 2 tablets of Triavil 4-50 daily, divided into 2 doses.

For Anxiety in People with Schizophrenia
The usual dose is 6 tablets of Triavil 4-25 daily (2 tablets 3 times a day). Your doctor may tell you to take another tablet of Triavil 4-25 at bedtime, if needed.

If you need to keep taking Triavil, your doctor will probably gradually reduce your dosage to 1 tablet of Triavil 2-25 or 4-25 2 to 4 times a day or 1 tablet of Triavil 4-50 twice a day.

CHILDREN

Children should not use Triavil.

ELDERLY AND ADOLESCENTS

For Anxiety
The usual dose is 3 or 4 tablets of Triavil 4-10 daily, divided into 3 or 4 doses. People in these age groups usually take Triavil at lower doses.

Overdosage

Any medication taken in excess can have serious consequences. An overdose of Triavil can be fatal. If you suspect an overdose, seek medical help immediately.

Symptoms of Triavil overdose may include:
Abnormalities of posture and movements, agitation, coma, confusion, convulsions, dilated pupils, drowsiness, extreme low body temperature, eye movement problems, high fever, heart failure, overactive reflexes, rapid or irregular heartbeat, rigid muscles, stupor, very low blood pressure, vomiting

Generic name:

TRIAZOLAM

See Halcion, page 275.

Brand name:

TRIDESILON

Generic name: Desonide
Other brand name: DesOwen

Why is this drug prescribed?
Tridesilon is a topical (applied directly to the skin) corticosteroid that relieves the itching and inflammation of a variety of skin problems.

Most important fact about this drug
Do not use this medication for any other condition than the one for which it was prescribed.

How should you use this medication?
Tridesilon should be used exactly as directly by your doctor.

It is for external use only. It should not touch your eyes.

The treated area should not be covered or wrapped with bandages or other coverings unless your doctor has told you to do so.

If Tridesilon is being used on an infant or toddler with a genital rash, be careful that diapers are not too tight and that plastic pants are not worn, so that air can circulate.

What side effects may occur?
Side effects cannot be anticipated. If any develop or change in intensity, notify your doctor as soon as possible. Only your doctor can determine if it is safe for you to continue using Tridesilon. The side effects listed below are rare, but may occur more

often if the affected area is covered with a bandage or treated for a long time.

■ *Side effects may include:*
Acne, additional infections, allergic reactions of the skin, burning, dryness, excessive hair growth, inflammation of the hair follicles, irritation, itching, loss of skin color, prickly heat, rash, skin inflammation around the mouth, skin loss, skin softening, stretch marks

■ *Side effects that may occur in children include:*
Delayed weight gain, headaches, slowed growth

Why should this drug not be prescribed?

You should not take this medication if you are sensitive or allergic to any of its ingredients.

Because drugs of this type may interfere with their growth and development, children should use the lowest strength of topical corticosteroid that provides effective therapy.

Special warnings about this medication

If an irritation develops, inform your doctor.

Large doses of corticosteroids (steroids) when applied over a large area, and long-term use of topical steroids, especially when the treated areas are covered, can cause increases in blood sugar or sugar in the urine, Cushing's syndrome (a condition characterized by a moon-shaped face), emotional disturbances, high blood pressure, weight gain, and, in women, growth of body hair, and effects on the adrenal gland, pituitary, and hypothalamus.

Possible food and drug interactions when using this medication

No interactions have been reported.

Special information
if you are pregnant or breastfeeding

Although Tridesilon is applied to the skin, there is no way of knowing how much medication is absorbed into the bloodstream. The more powerful corticosteroids have caused birth defects in animals. In general, topical steroids should not be used extensively on pregnant patients, in large amounts, or for prolonged periods of time. They should only be used if the potential benefits outweigh the potential risks to the unborn baby. If you are pregnant or plan to become pregnant, inform your doctor immediately.

It is not known whether topical steroids are absorbed in sufficient amounts to appear in breast milk. If your doctor considers Tridesilon essential to your health, he may advise you to stop breastfeeding until your treatment with the medication is finished.

Recommended dosage

ADULTS AND CHILDREN

Tridesilon should be applied to the affected area as a thin film, from 2 to 4 times a day, depending on the severity of the condition.

A bandage or other covering may be prescribed by your doctor to apply over the affected area for psoriasis or conditions that are not responding as well as expected.

Overdosage

Any medication taken in excess can have serious consequences. Overuse or misuse of Tridesilone Cream can result in too much medicine entering the body, which can cause increases in blood sugar and Cushing's syndrome, a condition characterized by a moon-shaped face, emotional disturbances, high blood pressure, weight gain, and, in women, growth of body and facial hair.

Brand name:

TRIDIONE

Generic name: Trimethadione

Why is this drug prescribed?

Tridione is a medication given to people who experience absence seizures (petit mal seizures) that have proved difficult to treat. The drug may be given in tablet form or as a liquid.

Although absence seizures occur most often in children, adults may have them too. The typical absence seizure lasts for 10 seconds or less and may be very subtle, involving merely a blinking or rolling of the eyes, a blank stare, and slight movements of the mouth. If not treated, a person may have as many as 100 absence seizures per day. It is possible for an absence seizure to develop into a grand mal seizure (collapse and convulsions).

Most important fact about this drug

Because Tridione may produce a variety of very serious side effects, it should only be given to people who have not been helped by more traditional antiseizure medications.

How should you take this medication?

Take Tridione exactly as prescribed by your doctor.

Do not change the dose or stop taking Tridione without first consulting with your doctor.

To avoid stomach upset, you may want to take this drug with food.

Tridione may cause drowsiness. You should exercise extra caution while driving or performing tasks requiring mental alertness.

You should carry identification listing your medical condition (seizures) and the medications you are taking.

What side effects may occur?

Side effects cannot be anticipated. If any develop or change in intensity, inform your doctor immediately. Only your doctor can determine if it is safe for you to continue taking Tridione.

Since Tridione may cause serious side effects, including some that are potentially fatal, you should be alert for certain symptoms that may signal trouble. You may need to stop taking Tridione temporarily or even permanently.

See your doctor immediately if you experience any of the following symptoms.

■ *Side effects may include:*
Abdominal pain, bleeding gums, blurred vision caused by bright light, burst blood vessel in eye, changes in blood pressure, difficulty sleeping, dizziness, double vision, drowsiness, easy bruising, fatigue, fever, hair loss, headache, hepatitis, hiccups, impaired vision (e.g., blind spots), increased irritability, itching, jaundice, loss of appetite, lupus erythematosus (a disease of the immune system), muscle weakness, nausea, nephrosis (kidney disease), nosebleed, personality changes, reddish or purplish spots on skin, seizures, sensitivity to light, sensitivity to the sun, skin rash (even a minor rash), sore throat, swollen glands, tingling or pins and needles, upset stomach, vaginal bleeding, vague feeling of being sick, vertigo, vomiting, weight loss

Why should this drug not be prescribed?

Do not take Tridione if you are sensitive to it or have ever had an allergic reaction to it.

Special warnings about this medication

You should not take Tridione if you have impaired liver or kidney function or a blood-cell abnormality. Before you start to take this medication, your doctor will order liver and kidney function tests and a complete blood-cell count (all of these are blood tests). The tests should be repeated once a month while you are taking Tridione.

Tridione has a strong sedative action, at least at the beginning of therapy. If the dosage is too high, the medication may cause drowsiness or affect your balance. Do not drive, swim, climb, or operate dangerous machinery until you know how Tridione affects you.

Over time, as your body adjusts to Tridione, the sedative effect should end. If it persists, tell your doctor; you may need a reduced dosage.

Abrupt discontinuation of Tridione can trigger absence seizures. Thus, if you must stop taking this medication, it is mandatory to taper off over a period of days. Your doctor may give you another antiseizure medication as you are gradually withdrawing from Tridione.

Possible food and drug interactions when taking this medication

If Tridione is taken with certain other drugs, the effects of either could be increased, decreased, or altered. It is especially important to check with your doctor before combining Tridione with any other drugs that are known to cause dizziness, drowsiness, nausea, staggering, or visual disturbances.

Special information if you are pregnant or breastfeeding

If taken by a pregnant woman, Tridione may cause birth defects. Thus, it is important to use an effective contraceptive while taking Tridione. If you are taking the drug and become pregnant, see your doctor immediately.

No information is available about the use of Tridione by a nursing mother.

Recommended dosage

ADULTS

Usual dose is 0.9 to 2.4 grams daily in 3 or 4 equally divided doses (i.e., 300 to 600 milligrams 3 or 4 times daily). Your doctor will begin with 0.9 gram daily and increase this dose by 300 milligrams at weekly intervals until desired results are seen or until serious (toxic) symptoms appear.

Maintenance dosage should be the minimum amount of Tridione required to maintain control.

CHILDREN

Usual dose is 0.3 to 0.9 gram daily in 3 or 4 equally divided doses.

Overdosage

Any medication taken in excess can have serious consequences. If you suspect symptoms of a Tridione overdose, seek medical attention immediately.

■ *Symptoms of Tridione overdose may include:*
Dizziness
Drowsiness
Nausea
Staggering gait
Vision problems

Generic name:

TRIFLUOPERAZINE HYDROCHLORIDE

See Stelazine, page 588.

Generic name:

TRIHEXYPHENIDYL HYDROCHLORIDE

See Artane, page 36.

Brand name:

TRILISATE

*Generic name: Choline magnesium
trisalicylate*

Why is this drug prescribed?

Trilisate, a nonsteroidal, anti-inflammatory medication, is prescribed for the relief of the signs and symptoms of rheumatoid arthritis (chronic joint inflammation disease), osteoarthritis (degenerative joint disease), and other forms of arthritis. This drug is also used in the long-term management of these diseases, especially for severe rheumatoid arthritis that comes on suddenly.

Trilisate may be prescribed for the treatment of acute painful shoulder, for mild to moderate pain in general, and for fever.

In children, this medication is prescribed for severe conditions—such as juvenile rheumatoid arthritis—requiring an anti-inflammatory (reduces inflammation) or an analgesic (pain reliever).

Most important fact about this drug

Because there is a possible association between the development of the rare but serious Reye's syndrome and the use of medicines containing salicylates or aspirin, Trilisate should not be used by children or teenagers who have chickenpox, influenza, or flu symptoms unless otherwise advised by their doctor.

How should you take this medication?

Trilisate is available in tablet or liquid form. Take Trilisate exactly as prescribed by your doctor.

What side effects may occur?

Side effects cannot be anticipated. If any develop or change in intensity, inform your doctor as soon as possible. Only your doctor can determine if it is safe for you to continue taking Trilisate.

■ *More common side effects may include:*
Constipation
Diarrhea
Heartburn
Indigestion
Nausea
Ringing in the ears
Stomach pain and upset
Vomiting

■ *Less common side effects may include:*
Dizziness, drowsiness, headache, hearing impairment, light-headedness, sluggishness

■ *Rare side effects may include:*
Asthma, blood in the stool, confusion, distorted sense of taste, hallucinations, hearing loss, hepatitis, hives, inflammation of the esophagus, itching, loss of appetite, nosebleed, rash, skin eruptions or discoloration, stomach or intestinal ulcers, swelling due to fluid accumulation, weight gain

Why should this drug not be prescribed?

If you are sensitive to or have ever had an allergic reaction to Trilisate or drugs of this type, you should not take this medication. Make sure that your doctor is aware of any drug reactions that you have experienced.

Special warnings about this medication

Trilisate should be used with caution if you have severe or recurring kidney or liver disorder, gastritis (inflammation of the stomach lining), or a stomach ulcer. Consult with your doctor regarding any medical problems you may have.

If you are an asthmatic allergic to aspirin, check with your doctor before taking Trilisate.

It may be 2 to 3 weeks before you feel the effect of this medication.

Possible food and drug interactions when taking this medication

If Trilisate is taken with certain other drugs, the effects of either could be increased, decreased, or altered. It is especially important to check with your doctor before combining Trilisate with the following:

Antacids such as Gaviscon and Maalox
Anticoagulants (blood-thinners such as
    Coumadin)
Antigout medications
Carbonic anhydrase inhibitors such as
    acetazolamide (Diamox) used to treat heart
    failure, glaucoma, and certain convulsive
    disorders
Corticosteroids
Insulin
Methotrexate, an anticancer drug
Other salicylates used to reduce fever,
    inflammation, and pain (aspirin)
Phenytoin (the anticonvulsant Dilantin)
Sulfonylureas (drugs used to treat diabetes,
    such as Tolinase and Orinase)
Valproic acid (the anticonvulsant Depakene)

Special information
if you are pregnant or breastfeeding

The effects of Trilisate during pregnancy have not been adequately studied. If you are pregnant or plan to become pregnant, inform your doctor immediately. This drug does appear in breast milk and could affect a nursing infant. If this medication is essential to your health, your doctor may advise you to discontinue breastfeeding until your treatment is finished.

Recommended dosage

ADULTS

In rheumatoid arthritis, osteoarthritis, more severe arthritis, and acute painful shoulder, the recommended starting dose is 1,500 milligrams taken 2 times a day or 3,000 milligrams taken once a day. Your dosage should be adjusted by your doctor according to your response to this medication.

If you have a kidney disorder, your doctor will monitor you and adjust your dose accordingly.

For mild to moderate pain or to reduce a high fever, the usual dosage is 2,000 to 3,000 milligrams per day divided into 2 equal doses as recommended by your doctor.

CHILDREN

For reduction of inflammation or pain, the recommended dose for children is determined by weight. The usual dose for children who weigh 81 pounds or less is 50 milligrams per 2.2 pounds of body weight, given 2 times a day. For heavier children, the usual dose is 2,250 milligrams per day.

Trilisate liquid is available for the treatment of younger patients and for adults who are unable to swallow a tablet.

ELDERLY

The usual recommended dosage is 2,250 milligrams divided into 3 doses of 750 milligrams each.

Overdosage

Any medication taken in excess can have serious consequences. If you suspect an overdose, seek medical treatment immediately. Death has occurred from an overdose of Trilisate.

Symptoms of Trilisate overdose may include: Confusion, diarrhea, dizziness, drowsiness, headache, hearing impairment, rapid breathing, ringing in the ears, sweating, vomiting

Generic name:

TRIMETHADIONE

See Tridione, page 652.

Generic name:

TRIMETHOBENZAMIDE HYDROCHLORIDE

See Tigan, page 628.

Generic name:

TRIMETHOPRIM WITH SULFAMETHOXAZOLE

See Bactrim, page 53.

Generic name:

TRIMIPRAMINE MALEATE

See Surmontil, page 593.

Brand name:

TRIMOX

See Amoxil, page 23.

Brand name:

TRINALIN REPETABS

Generic ingredients: Azatadine maleate, Pseudoephedrine sulfate

Why is this drug prescribed?

Trinalin Repetabs is a long-acting antihistamine/decongestant that relieves nasal stuffiness and middle ear congestion caused by allergies, including hay fever and the common cold. It can be used alone or with antibiotics and analgesics such as aspirin or acetaminophen. Azatadine, the antihistamine in the combination, reduces itching and swelling and dries up secretions from the nose, eyes, and throat. Pseudoephedrine, the decongestant, reduces nasal congestion and makes breathing easier.

Most important fact about this drug

Trinalin Repetabs may cause drowsiness. Driving or operating dangerous machinery or participating in any hazardous activity that requires full mental alertness is not recommended until you know how you react to this medication.

How should you take this medication?

Take this medication as indicated; do not take more than your doctor has prescribed.

Never take two doses at the same time.

What side effects may occur?

Side effects cannot be anticipated. If any develop or change in intensity, inform your doctor as soon as possible. Only your doctor can determine if it is safe for you to continue taking Trinalin.

■ *Side effects may include:*
Abdominal cramps, acute inflammation of the inner ear, anemia, anxiety, blood disorders, blurred vision, chest pain, chills, confusion, constipation, convulsions, diarrhea, difficulty breathing, dilated pupils, disturbed coordination, dizziness, dry mouth, nose, and throat, early menstruation, exaggerated feeling of well-being, excessive perspiration, excitement, extreme calm (sedation), fatigue, fear, frequent urination, hallucinations, headache, high blood pressure, hives, hysteria, increased chest congestion, increased sensitivity to light, insomnia, irregular heartbeat, irritability, loss of appetite, low blood pressure, nausea, nervousness, painful or difficult urination, pale skin, pounding heartbeat, rapid heartbeat, rash, restlessness, ringing in the ears, severe allergic reaction, sleepiness, stuffy nose, tension, tightness in chest, tingling or pins and needles, tremor, upset stomach, urinary retention, vertigo, vomiting, weakness, wheezing

Why should this drug not be prescribed?

Trinalin should be avoided if you have narrow-angle glaucoma or difficulty urinating, if you are taking antidepressant drugs known as MAO inhibitors or have stopped taking them within the past 10 days, if you have severe high blood pressure, severe heart disease, or an overactive thyroid, or if you are sensitive to or have ever had an allergic reaction to any of its ingredients.

This drug should not be used to treat asthma and other lower respiratory tract diseases.

Special warnings about this medication

Trinalin should be used with care if you have peptic ulcer due to narrowing of the duct or other upper intestinal obstruction or other stomach problems, bladder obstruction due to an enlarged prostate or other bladder problems, a history of bronchial asthma, heart disease, high blood pressure, increased eye pressure, or diabetes.

If you are taking digitalis (Lanoxin) or blood-thinning medications (Coumadin), use Trinalin cautiously.

Pseudoephedrine can cause tolerance and dependence at high doses. Remember that this medication can make you feel drowsy. Be careful driving, operating machinery, or using appliances.

Antihistamines may cause dizziness, extreme calm (sedation), and low blood pressure in the elderly (age 60 and over). Decongestants are more likely to cause side effects—such as confusion, convulsions, hallucinations, and death—in the elderly.

Trinalin should not be given to children under 12 years old.

Possible food and drug interactions when taking this medication

Trinalin may increase the effects of alcohol. Do not drink alcohol while taking this medication.

If Trinalin is taken with certain other drugs, the effects of either could be increased, decreased, or altered. It is especially important to check with your doctor before combining Trinalin with the following:

Antacids such as Maalox
Anticoagulants such as Coumadin
Barbiturates such as phenobarbital
Beta blockers such as Tenormin and Inderal
Digitalis (Lanoxin)
Drugs for depression such as Prozac and Elavil
High blood pressure drugs such as Aldomet and Inversine
Kaolin (Kaopectate)
MAO inhibitor drugs (antidepressants such as Marplan and Nardil)
Sedatives/hypnotics such as Nembutal and Seconal
Tranquilizers such as Xanax and Valium

Special information if you are pregnant or breastfeeding

Although the effects of Trinalin during pregnancy have not been adequately studied, antihistamines have caused severe reactions in premature and newborn babies when used in the last 3 months of pregnancy. If you are pregnant or plan to become pregnant, notify your doctor immediately. Trinalin may appear in breast milk and could affect a nursing infant. If this medication is essential to your health, your doctor may advise you to discontinue breastfeeding until your treatment with Trinalin is finished.

Recommended dosage

ADULTS AND CHILDREN OVER 12:

The usual dosage is 1 tablet twice a day.

Overdosage

Any medication taken in excess can have serious consequences. Deaths have occurred from overdose. If you suspect an overdose, seek medical attention immediately.

Symptoms of Trinalin overdose may include:
Anxiety, bluish color caused by lack of
oxygen, blurred vision, coma, convulsions,
decreased mental alertness, difficulty sleeping,
difficulty urinating, dizziness, excitement,
extreme calm (sedation), exaggerated sense
of well-being, giddiness, hallucinations,
headache, high blood pressure/low blood
pressure, lack of muscle coordination, muscle
tenseness, muscle weakness, nausea,
perspiration, pounding heartbeat, rapid
heartbeat, restlessness, ringing in the ears,
temporary interruption of breathing, thirst,
tremors, vomiting

*Overdose symptoms more common in
children may include:*
Dry mouth, fixed, dilated pupils, flushing,
stimulation, stomach and intestinal problems,
very high body temperature

Generic name:

TRIPELENNAMINE HYDROCHLORIDE

See PBZ, page 448.

Brand name:

TRIPHASIL

See Oral Contraceptives, page 437.

Brand name:

TUSSI-ORGANIDIN DM

*Generic ingredients: Organidin (iodinated
glycerol), Dextromethorphan hydrobromide*

Why is this drug prescribed?
Tussi-Organidin DM is a non-narcotic cough
medicine that relieves dry, irritating coughs
associated with bronchitis, bronchial asthma,
the common cold, and other respiratory-
tract infections including laryngitis, sore
throat, croup, whooping cough and
emphysema.

Most important fact about this drug
Do not use Tuss-Organidin DM if you are
pregnant or breastfeeding. This medication
contains iodides, which can damage thyroid
development in the fetus. If you become
pregnant while using Tussi-Organidin DM,
stop taking it and contact your doctor
immediately.

How should you take this medication?
Tussi-Organidin DM should be taken as
prescribed by your doctor.

It should be stored at room temperature in
a tightly closed bottle.

What side effects may occur?
Side effects cannot be anticipated. If any develop
or change in intensity, inform your doctor
immediately. Only your doctor can determine
whether it is safe to continue using Tussi-
Organidin DM. Side effects have been rare.

■ *Rare side effects may include:*
   Allergic reactions to iodides
   Drowsiness
   Rash
   Stomach and intestinal irritation or
      disturbances

Why should this drug not be prescribed?
Tussi-Organidin DM should not be used if
you have ever had an alergic reaction or
are sensitive to inorganic iodides or any of
the other ingredients in this medication.
Avoid this medication if you are pregnant
or breastfeeding. Do not give this medication
to newborn infants.

Special warnings about this medication
Stop using this medication if a rash or allergic
reaction develops.

Tussi-Organidin DM should be used cautiously (or not at all) if you have thyroid disease.

This medication should be used with care by children with cystic fibrosis, because these children are more likely to develop an enlarged thyroid.

Medications that contain iodides, such as Tussi-Organidin DM, may cause flare-ups of adolescent acne.

Skin inflammations have occurred with long-term use of iodides.

Possible food and drug interactions when taking this medication

If Tussi-Organidin DM is taken with certain other drugs, the effects of either could be increased, decreased, or altered. It is especially important to check with your doctor before combining Tussi-Organidin DM the following:

Lithium (Lithobid, Cibalith-S Syrup)
Antithyroid drugs such as propylthiouracil, methimazole

Special information if you are pregnant or breastfeeding

Tussi-Organidin DM should not be used during pregnancy. It can damage the thyroid in the developing fetus. If you are pregnant or plan to become pregnant, stop taking it and inform your doctor immediately. Tussi-Organidin DM may appear in breast milk and can harm a nursing infant. It should not be used if you are breastfeeding.

Recommended dosage

ADULTS

The usual dose is 1 to 2 teaspoonfuls every 4 hours.

CHILDREN

The usual dose is ½ to 1 teaspoonful every 4 hours.

Overdosage

Reports of overdose with Tussi-Organidin DM are rare, and include no serious problems. Nevertheless, any medication used in excess can have serious consequences. If you suspect an overdose, seek medical advice immediately.

Brand name:

TUSSIONEX

Generic ingredients: Hydrocodone polistirex, Chlorpheniramine polistirex

Why is this drug prescribed?

Tussionex Extended-Release Suspension is a cough-suppressant/antihistamine combination used to relieve coughs and the upper respiratory symptoms of colds and allergies. Hydrocodone, a mild narcotic similar to codeine, is believed to work directly on the cough center. Chlorpheniramine, an antihistamine, reduces itching and swelling and dries up secretions from the eyes, nose, and throat.

Most important fact about this drug

This medication can cause considerable drowsiness and make you less alert. Driving or operating machinery or participating in any activity that requires full mental alertness is not recommended until you know how you react to Tussionex.

How should you take this medication?

Tussionex should be taken exactly as prescribed by your doctor.

It should not be diluted with other liquids or mixed with other drugs. Shake well before using.

What side effects may occur?

Side effects cannot be anticipated. If any develop or change in intensity, inform your doctor as soon as possible. Only your doctor can determine if it is safe for you to continue taking Tussionex.

■ *Side effects may include:*
Anxiety, constipation, decreased mental and physical performance, difficulty breathing, dizziness, drowsiness, dry throat, emotional dependence, exaggerated feeling of depression, extreme calm (sedation), exaggerated sense of well-being, fear, itching, mental clouding, mood changes, nausea, rash, restlessness, sluggishness, tightness in chest, urinary retention, urinary spasms, vomiting

Why should this drug not be prescribed?
Do not take Tussionex if you are sensitive to or have ever had an allergic reaction to hydrocodone or chlorpheniramine. Make sure your doctor is aware of any drug reactions you have experienced.

Special warnings about this medication
Tussionex contains a mild narcotic that can cause dependence and tolerance when the drug is used for several weeks. However, it is unlikely that dependence will develop when Tussionex is used for the short-term treatment of a cough.

As with all narcotics, Tussionex may produce irregular breathing. If you have lung disease or a breathing disorder, this medication should be used cautiously.

Tussionex should be used with care if you have narrow-angle glaucoma, asthma, an enlarged prostate, urinary difficulties, an intestinal disorder, liver or kidney disease, an underactive thyroid, or Addison's disease (a disorder of the adrenal glands), or if you have recently suffered a head injury.

Extra caution should be used when giving Tussionex to young children and the elderly.

Remember that Tussionex can cause drowsiness.

Possible food and drug interactions when taking this medication
Tussionex may increase the effects of alcohol. Do not drink alcohol while taking this medication.

If Tussionex is taken with certain other drugs, the effects of either could be increased, decreased, or altered. It is especially important to check with your doctor before combining Tussionex with the following:

Antipsychotics such as Thorazine and Compazine
MAO inhibitor drugs (antidepressant drugs such as Nardil and Parnate)
Medications for anxiety such as Xanax and Valium
Medications for depression such as Elavil and Prozac
Other antihistamines such as Benadryl
Other narcotics such as Percocet and Demerol

Special information if you are pregnant or breastfeeding
The safety of Tussionex during pregnancy has not been adequately studied. However, babies born to mothers who have been taking narcotics regularly before delivery will be born addicted. If you are pregnant or plan to become pregnant, inform your doctor immediately. Tussionex may appear in breast milk and could affect a nursing infant. If this medication is essential to your health, your doctor may recommend that you stop breastfeeding until your treatment with Tussionex is finished.

Recommended dosage

ADULTS

The usual dose is 1 teaspoonful (5 milliliters) every 12 hours. Do not take more than 2 teaspoonfuls in 24 hours.

CHILDREN AGED 6 TO 12

The usual dose is ½ teaspoonful every 12 hours. Do not take more than 1 teaspoonful in 24 hours.

Tussionex is not recommended for children under 6 years old.

Overdosage

Any medication taken in excess can have serious consequences. Death can occur with narcotic overdose. If you suspect an overdose, seek medical treatment immediately.

Symptoms of Tussinoex overdose may include:
Blue skin color due to lack of oxygen
Cardiac arrest
Cold and clammy skin
Decreased or difficult breathing
Extreme sleepiness leading to stupor or coma
Low blood pressure
Slow heartbeat
Temporary cessation of breathing

Brand name:

TYLENOL

Generic name: Acetaminophen
Other brand names: Panadol, Aspirin Free Anacin

Why is this drug prescribed?

Tylenol is a fever- and pain-reducing medication that is widely used to relieve simple headaches and muscle aches; the minor aches and pains of bursitis, arthritis, rheumatism, neuralgia (nerve inflammation), sprains, overexertion, and menstrual cramps; and the discomfort of fever due to colds and the flu.

Most important fact about this drug

Do not use Tylenol to relieve pain for more than 10 days, or to reduce fever for more than 3 days unless your doctor has specifically told you to do so.

How should you take this medication?

Follow the dosing instructions on the label. Do not take more Tylenol than is recommended.

Tylenol is sold in tamper-resistant bottles with a printed red neck wrap. If the wrapping is broken or missing, do not use the medication.

What side effects may occur?

Tylenol is relatively free of side effects. Rarely, an allergic reaction may occur. If you develop any allergic symptoms such as rash, hives, swelling, or difficulty breathing, stop taking Tylenol immediately.

Special warnings about this medication

Tylenol should not be used for more than 10 days for pain, or 3 days for fever. If your fever remains, or your pain persists, contact your doctor. These symptoms could indicate a more serious illness.

Possible food and drug interactions when taking this medication

No interactions with Tylenol have been noted.

Special information
if you are pregnant or breastfeeding

As with all medications, ask your doctor or healthcare professional whether it is safe for you to use Tylenol while you are pregnant or breastfeeding.

Recommended dosage

For Tylenol Regular Strength tablets and caplets, use the following dosage recommendations.

ADULTS AND CHILDREN 12 YEARS AND OLDER

1 to 2 tablets, 3 or 4 times daily.

CHILDREN 6 TO 12 YEARS OLD
One-half to 1 tablet 3 or 4 times a day.

CHILDREN UNDER 6 YEARS OLD
Consult your physician or healthcare professional

Overdosage
Any medication taken in excess can have serious consequences. If you suspect an overdose, seek medical attention immediately. Massive doses of Tylenol may cause liver poisoning.

Symptoms of Tylenol overdose may include:
Excessive perspiration
Exhaustion
Nausea
Vomiting

Brand name:

TYLENOL WITH CODEINE

Generic ingredients: Acetaminophen, Codeine phosphate
Other brand name: Phenaphen with Codeine

Why is this drug prescribed?
Tylenol with Codeine, a narcotic analgesic, is used to treat moderate to moderately severe pain. It contains two drugs—acetaminophen and codeine. Acetaminophen, an antipyretic (fever reducing) analgesic, is used to reduce pain and fever. Codeine, a narcotic analgesic, is used to treat pain that is moderate to severe.

People who are allergic to aspirin can take Tylenol with Codeine.

Most important fact about this drug
Tylenol with Codeine contains a narcotic (codeine) and, even if taken in prescribed amounts, can cause physical and psychological addiction if taken for a long enough time.

Addiction may be more of a risk for a person who has been addicted to alcohol or drugs. Be sure to follow your doctor's instructions carefully when taking Tylenol with Codeine (or any other drugs that contain a narcotic).

How should you take this medication?
Tylenol with Codeine may be taken with meals or with milk (but not with alcohol).

What side effects may occur?
Side effects cannot be anticipated. If any develop or change in intensity, inform your doctor as soon as possible. Only your doctor can determine if it is safe for you to continue taking Tylenol with Codeine.

■ *More common side effects may include:*
Dizziness
Light-headedness
Nausea
Sedation
Shortness of breath
Vomiting

■ *Less common side effects may include:*
Abdominal pain, allergic reactions, constipation, depressed feeling, exaggerated feeling of well-being, itchy skin

■ *Rare side effects may include:*
Decreased breathing (when Tylenol with Codeine is taken at higher doses)

Why should this drug not be prescribed?
You should not use Tylenol with Codeine if you are sensitive to either acetaminophen (Tylenol) or codeine.

Special warnings about this medication
You should take Tylenol with Codeine cautiously and only according to your doctor's instructions, as you would take any medication containing a narcotic. Make sure your doctor is aware of any history of drug or alcohol addiction you have.

Tylenol with Codeine tablets contain a sulfite that may cause allergic reactions in some people. These reactions may include shock and severe, possibly fatal, asthma attacks. People with asthma are more likely to be sensitive to sulfites.

If you have experienced a head injury, consult with your doctor before taking Tylenol with Codeine.

If you have stomach problems, such as an ulcer, check with your doctor before taking Tylenol with Codeine. Tylenol with Codeine may obscure the symptoms of stomach problems, making them difficult to diagnose and treat.

If you have ever had liver, kidney, thyroid, or Addison's disease, difficulty urinating, or a prostate condition, consult with your doctor before taking Tylenol with Codeine.

This drug may cause drowsiness and impair your ability to drive a car or operate potentially dangerous machinery. Do not participate in any activities that require full attention when using this drug until you are sure of its effect on you.

Possible food and drug interactions when taking this medication

Alcohol may increase the sedative effects of Tylenol with Codeine. Therefore, do not drink alcohol while you are taking this medication.

If Tylenol with Codeine is taken with certain other drugs, the effects of either could be increased, decreased, or altered. It is especially important to check with your doctor before combining Tylenol with Codeine with the following:

Antipsychotic drugs such as Clozaril and
   Thorazine

Anticholinergic drugs such as Cogentin
General anesthetics
MAO inhibitors such as Nardil and Eldepryl
Other narcotic painkillers such as Darvon
Tranquilizers such as Xanax and Valium
Tricyclic antidepressants such as Elavil
   and Tofranil

Special information if you are pregnant or breastfeeding

It is not known if Tylenol with Codeine could injure a fetus, or if it could affect a woman's reproductive capacity. Using any medication that contains a narcotic during pregnancy may cause babies to be born with a physical addiction to the narcotic. If you are pregnant or plan to become pregnant, you should not take Tylenol with Codeine unless the potential benefits clearly outweigh the possible dangers. As with other narcotic painkillers, taking Tylenol with Codeine shortly before delivery (especially at higher dosages) may cause some degree of respiratory depression in the mother and newborn.

Some studies (but not all) have reported that codeine appears in breast milk and might affect a nursing infant. Therefore, nursing mothers should use Tylenol with Codeine only if the potential gains are greater than the potential hazards.

Recommended dosage

ADULTS

Dosage will depend on how severe your pain is and how you respond to the drug.

To Relieve Pain
A single dose may contain from 15 milligrams to 60 milligrams of codeine phosphate and from 300 to 1,000 milligrams of acetaminophen. The maximum dose in a 24-hour period should be 360 milligrams of codeine phosphate and 4,000 milligrams of acetaminophen. Your doctor will

determine the amounts of codeine phosphate and acetaminophen taken in each dose. Doses may be repeated up to every 4 hours.

Single doses above 60 milligrams of codeine do not give enough pain relief to balance the increased number of side effects.

Adults may also take Tylenol with Codeine elixir (liquid). Tylenol with Codeine elixir contains 120 milligrams of acetaminophen and 12 milligrams of codeine phosphate per teaspoonful.

The usual adult dose is 1 tablespoonful every 4 hours as needed.

CHILDREN

The safety of Tylenol with Codeine elixir has not been established in children under 3 years old.

Children 3 to 6 years old may take 1 teaspoonful 3 or 4 times daily.

Children 7 to 12 years old may take 2 teaspoonsful 3 or 4 times daily.

ELDERLY

Elderly patients should use Tylenol with Codeine cautiously.

Overdosage

Any medication taken in excess can cause symptoms of overdose. Severe overdosage of Tylenol with Codeine can cause death. If you suspect an overdose, seek medical attention immediately.

Symptoms of Tylenol with Codeine overdose may include:
Bluish skin, cold and clammy skin, coma due to low blood sugar, decreased, irregular, or stopped breathing, extreme sleepiness progressing to stupor or coma, general bodily discomfort, heart attack, kidney failure,

liver failure, low blood pressure, muscle weakness, nausea, slow heartbeat, sweating, vomiting

Brand name:

TYLOX

See Percocet, page 465.

Brand name:

ULTRACEF

See Duricef, page 218.

Brand name:

URISED

Generic ingredients: Methenamine, Methylene blue, Phenyl salicylate, Benzoic acid, Atropine sulfate, Hyoscyamine

Why is this drug prescribed?
Urised relieves lower urinary tract discomfort caused by inflammation or diagnostic procedures. It is used to treat urinary tract infections including cystitis (inflammation of the bladder and ureters), urethritis (inflammation of the urethra), and trigonitis (inflammation of the mucous membrane of the bladder). Methenamine, the major component of this drug, acts as a mild antiseptic by changing into formaldehyde in the urinary tract when it comes in contact with acidic urine.

Most important fact about this drug
Urised may give a blue to blue-green color to urine and discolor stools as well.

How should you take this medication?
If dry mouth occurs, use of sugarless hard candy or gum, saliva substitute, or crushed ice may provide temporary relief.

Take this medication exactly as prescribed by your doctor. Do not take more than the recommended dose.

Drugs and foods that produce alkaline urine (such as sodium bicarbonate, antacids, and orange juice) should be limited.

Your doctor may ask you to check your urine with phenaphthazine paper to see if it is acidic. Urine acidifiers, such as vitamin C, may be recommended if the urine is not acidic enough.

Drinking plenty of fluids will help the medication work better and relieve discomfort.

What side effects may occur?

Side effects cannot be anticipated. If any develop or change in intensity, inform your doctor as soon as possible. Only your doctor can determine if it is safe for you to continue taking Urised.

Side effects with long-term use may include:
Acute urinary retention (in men with an enlarged prostate)
Blurry vision
Difficulty urinating
Dizziness
Dry mouth
Flushing
Rapid pulse
Skin rash

Why should this drug not be prescribed?

Urised should be avoided if you have glaucoma, a bladder or abdominal blockage, cardiospasm (a disorder that prevents the passage of food into the stomach), or if you are sensitive to or have ever had an allergic reaction to any of Urised's ingredients.

Special warnings about this medication

Urised should be used cautiously if you have heart disease or have ever had a reaction to medications that are chemically similar to atropine.

Possible food and drug interactions when taking this medication

If Urised is taken with certain other drugs, the effects of either could be increased, decreased, or altered. It is especially important to check with your doctor before combining Urised with the following:

Sulfa drugs such as Gantrisin, Gantanol, Bactrim, and Septra

Special information if you are pregnant or breastfeeding

The effects of Urised during pregnancy have not been adequately studied. If you are pregnant or plan to become pregnant, inform your doctor immediately. Urised may appear in breast milk and could affect a nursing infant. If this medication is essential to your health, your doctor may advise you to stop breastfeeding until your treatment with Urised ends.

Recommended dosage

ADULTS

The usual dose is 2 tablets, 4 times a day.

CHILDREN 6 YEARS AND OLDER

The dosage must be determined by your doctor.

CHILDREN UNDER 6 YEARS

Use is not recommended in children under 6 years old.

Overdosage

Any medication taken in excess can have serious consequences. Deaths can occur from an overdose of atropine and hyoscyamine, two of the ingredients in Urised. If you suspect symptoms of Urised overdose, seek medical treatment immediately.

Symptoms of Urised overdose may include:
Abdominal pain, bladder and abdominal irritation, bloody diarrhea, bloody urine, burning pain in throat and mouth, circulatory collapse, coma, dilated pupils (large pupils), dizziness, dry nose, mouth, and throat, elevated blood pressure, extremely high body temperature, headache, hot, dry, flushed skin, painful and frequent urination, pallor (paleness), pounding heartbeat (pounding sensation against the chest), rapid heartbeat (increased pulse rate), respiratory failure, ringing in ears, sweating, vomiting, weakness, white sores in mouth

Brand name:

URISPAS

Generic name: Flavoxate hydrochloride

Why is this drug prescribed?

Urispas prevents spasms in the urinary tract and relieves the painful or difficult urination, urinary urgency, excessive nighttime urination, pubic area pain, frequency of urination, and inability to hold urine caused by urinary tract infections including cystitis (inflammation of the bladder and ureters), prostatitis (inflammation of the prostate gland), and urethritis (inflammation of the urethra). Urispas is used in combination with antibiotics to treat the infection.

Most important fact about this drug

Urispas can cause blurred vision and drowsiness. Be careful driving, operating machinery, or performing any activity that requires complete mental alertness until you know how you will react to this medication.

How should you take this medication?

Take this medication exactly as prescribed by your doctor.

What side effects may occur?

Side effects cannot be anticipated. If any develop or change in intensity, notify your doctor as soon as possible. Only your doctor can determine whether it is safe for you to continue taking Urispas.

■ *Side effects may include:*
Allergic skin reactions, including hives, blurred vision and vision changes, drowsiness, dry mouth, headache, high body temperature, mental confusion (especially in the elderly), nausea, nervousness, painful or difficult urination, pounding heartbeat, rapid heartbeat, vertigo, vomiting

Why should this drug not be prescribed?

Urispas should not be taken if you have stomach or intestinal blockage, muscle relaxation problems (especially the sphincter muscle), abdominal bleeding, or urinary tract blockage.

Special warnings about this medication

Urispas should be used cautiously if you might have glaucoma.

Possible food and drug interactions when taking this medication

No interactions involving Urispas have been noted.

Special information
if you are pregnant or breastfeeding

The effects of Urispas during pregnancy have not been adequately studied. If you are pregnant or plan to become pregnant, inform your doctor immediately. Urispas may appear in breast milk and could affect a nursing infant. If this medication is essential to your health, your doctor may advise you to stop breastfeeding until your treatment is finished.

Recommended dosage

ADULTS AND CHILDREN OVER AGE 12

The usual dose of Urispas is one or two 100-milligram tablets 3 or 4 times a day.

When your symptoms have improved, your doctor may reduce the dosage.

CHILDREN

Urispas is not recommended for children under 12 years of age.

Overdosage

Any medication taken in excess can have serious consequences. If you suspect an overdose of Urispas, seek medical attention immediately.

Symptoms of Urispas overdose may include:
Convulsions
Decreased ability to sweat
   (warm, red skin, dry mouth, and
   increased body temperature)
Hallucinations
Increased heart rate and blood pressure
Mental confusion

Generic name:

URSODIOL

See Actigall, page 7.

Brand name:

V-CILLIN K

See Penicillin V, page 462.

Brand name:

VALIUM

Generic name: Diazepam

Why is this drug prescribed?

Valium is used in the treatment of anxiety disorders and for short-term relief of the symptoms of anxiety. It belongs to a class of drugs known as benzodiazepines.

It is also used to relieve the symptoms of acute alcohol withdrawal, to relax muscles, to relieve the uncontrolled muscle movements caused by cerebral palsy and paralysis of the lower limbs, to control involuntary movement of the hands (athetosis), to relax the tight, aching muscles of stiff-man syndrome, and, along with other medications, to treat convulsive disorders such as epilepsy.

Most important fact about this drug

Tolerance and dependence can occur with the use of Valium. You may experience withdrawal symptoms if you stop using this drug abruptly. Discontinue or change your dose only on your doctor's advise.

How should you take this medication?

Take this medication exactly as prescribed by your doctor.

If you're taking Valium for epilepsy, make sure you take it every day at the same time.

If you forget to take a dose, take it as soon as you remember. If it is almost time for your next dose, skip the one you missed and go back to your regular schedule. Never take two doses at the same time.

What side effects may occur?

Side effects cannot be anticipated. If any develop or change in intensity, inform your doctor as soon as possible. Only your doctor can determine if it is safe for you to continue taking Valium.

■ *More common side effects may include:*
   Drowsiness
   Light-headedness
   Loss of muscle coordination
   Mild fatigue

■ *Less common or rare side effects may include:*
   Anxiety, blurred vision, changes in salivation, changes in sex drive,

confusion, constipation, contradictory over-excitation, depression, dizziness, double vision, hallucinations, headache, incontinence, low blood pressure, nausea, seizures (mild changes in brain wave patterns), skin rash, sleep disturbances, slow heartbeat, slurred speech, tremors, urinary retention, yellowing of eyes and skin

■ *Side effects due to rapid decrease or abrupt withdrawal from Valium:*
Abdominal and muscle cramps, convulsions, sweating, tremors, vomiting

Why should this drug not be prescribed?
If you are sensitive to or have ever had an allergic reaction to Valium or similar drugs, you should not take this medication.

Unless you are directed to do so by your doctor, do not take this medication if you have acute narrow-angle glaucoma.

Anxiety or tension related to everyday stress usually does not require treatment with Valium. Discuss your symptoms thoroughly with your doctor.

Valium should not be prescribed if you are being treated for mental disorders more serious than anxiety.

Special warnings about this medication
Valium may cause you to become drowsy or less alert; therefore, driving or operating dangerous machinery or participating in any hazardous activity that requires full mental alertness is not recommended.

Possible food and drug interactions when taking this medication
Valium is a central nervous system depressant and may intensify the effects of alcohol. Do not drink alcohol while taking this medication.

If Valium is taken with certain other drugs, the effects of either could be increased, decreased, or altered. It is especially important to check with your doctor before combining Valium with any of the following:

Anticonvulsants such as Dilantin
Barbiturates such as phenobarbital
Cimetidine (Tagamet)
Disulfiram
Fluoxetine (Prozac)
Isoniazid
Levodopa
MAO inhibitors (antidepressant drugs such as Nardil)
Narcotics such as Percocet
Oral contraceptives
Propoxyphene (Darvon)
Ranitidine (Zantac)
Rifampin

Special information if you are pregnant or breastfeeding
Do not take Valium if you are pregnant or planning to become pregnant. There is an increased risk of birth defects. This drug may appear in breast milk and could affect a nursing infant. If this medication is essential to your health, your doctor may advise you to discontinue breastfeeding until your treatment is finished.

Recommended Dosage

ADULTS

Treatment of Anxiety Disorders and Short-Term Relief of the Symptoms of Anxiety
The usual dose, depending upon severity of symptoms, is 2 milligrams to 10 milligrams 2 to 4 times daily.

Acute Alcohol Withdrawal
The usual dose is 10 milligrams 3 or 4 times during the first 24 hours, then 5 milligrams 3 or 4 times daily as needed.

Relief of Muscle Spasm
The usual dose is 2 milligrams to 10 milligrams 3 or 4 times daily.

Convulsive Disorders
The usual dose is 2 milligrams to 10 milligrams 2 to 4 times daily.

CHILDREN

Valium should not be prescribed for children under 6 months of age.

The usual starting dose for children over 6 months is 1 to 2.5 milligrams 3 or 4 times a day. The dosage may be increased gradually.

ELDERLY

The usual dosage is 2 milligrams to 2.5 milligrams 1 or 2 times a day, increased as needed. The dosage should be limited to the smallest effective amount to avoid oversedation or impaired muscle coordination.

Overdosage

Any medication taken in excess can cause symptoms of overdose. If you suspect an overdose, seek medical attention immediately.

Symptoms of Valium overdose may include:
Coma
Confusion
Diminished reflexes
Sleepiness

Generic name:

VALPROIC ACID

See Depakene, page 177.

Brand name:

VANCENASE

See Beclomethasone Dipropionate, page 57.

Brand name:

VANCERIL

See Beclomethasone Dipropionate, page 57.

Brand name:

VASCOR

Generic name: Bepridil hydrochloride

Why is this drug prescribed?

Vascor, a type of medication called a calcium channel blocker, is prescribed for the treatment of chronic stable angina (chest pain, often accompanied by a feeling of choking, brought on by exertion). Vascor is effective used alone or in combination with beta-blocking drugs and/or nitrates. Calcium channel blockers ease the workload of the heart by slowing down the muscle contractions of the heart and the passage of nerve impulses through the heart. This improves blood flow through the heart and throughout the body, reduces blood pressure, and helps prevent angina pain.

Most important fact about this drug

Vascor can have serious side effects and should be used only if other angina medications have been tried and have not worked. It is very important to see your doctor regularly while taking this medication.

How should you take this medication?

Food does not affect the absorption of Vascor. If the drug upsets your stomach, take it with meals or at bedtime.

Take Vascor exactly as prescribed by your doctor, even if your symptoms have disappeared.

If you miss a dose, take it as soon as you remember. If it is almost time for your next dose, skip the one you missed and go back to your regular schedule. Never take two doses at the same time.

What side effects may occur?

Side effects cannot be anticipated. If any develop or change in intensity, inform your doctor as soon as possible. Only your doctor can determine if it is safe for you to continue taking Vascor.

■ *More common side effects may include:*
Abdominal pain, constipation, difficult or labored breathing, diarrhea, dizziness, drowsiness, dry mouth, flu-like symptoms, hand tremors, headache, inability to sleep, indigestion, loss of appetite, nausea, nervousness, palpitations, respiratory infection, stomach and intestinal discomfort, tingling or pins and needles, tremors, weakness

■ *Less common or rare side effects may include:*
Anxiousness, arthritis, blurred vision, changes in behavior, cough, depression, fainting, fever, fluid retention, gas, high blood pressure, impotence, increased appetite, irregular heartbeat, loss of sex drive, muscle pain and weakness, pain, rapid heartbeat, rash, restlessness, ringing in ears, skin irritation, slow heartbeat, sore throat, stomach inflammation, sweating, taste changes, vertigo

Why should this drug not be prescribed?

Vascor should not be used if you have a history of serious ventricular arrhythmia (irregular heartbeat occurring in a ventricle of the heart).

This medication is not recommended if you have sick sinus syndrome or certain types of heart block (heart disorders which cause heartbeat irregularities) without a pacemaker, or low blood pressure.

If you are sensitive or have ever had an allergic reaction to Vascor or similar drugs, you should not take this medication. Make sure your doctor is aware of any drug reactions you have experienced.

Vascor should not be used with certain medicines for irregular heartbeat. Your doctor will decide if this medication is right for you.

Special warnings about this medication

Vascor can produce serious irregular heartbeats. Your heartbeat should be frequently monitored while taking this medication.

Potassium levels in your blood can affect your heartbeat. If you are taking potassium supplements or potassium-sparing diuretics, such as Moduretic, make sure you take them regularly. Your potassium levels should be monitored while you are taking Vascor.

If you have congestive heart failure, cardiac conduction disorders, or serious liver or kidney disease, this drug should be used with caution.

Vascor can cause a drop in white blood cells. Your doctor should check your blood count regularly.

If you have had a heart attack within the last 3 months, the use of Vascor is not recommended.

This medication can reduce or eliminate angina pain caused by exertion. Be careful not to do too much just because the drug makes you feel well. Be sure to discuss with your doctor how much activity or exercise is safe for you.

Possible food and drug interactions when taking this medication

If Vascor is taken with certain other drugs, the effects of either could be increased, decreased, or altered. It is especially important to check with your doctor before combining Vascor with the following:

Beta-blocking drugs (mainly for blood pressure and cardiac problems) such as Inderal and Tenormin
Digoxin (Lanoxin)
Drugs for depression such as Elavil
Irregular heartbeat drugs such as Quinidex and Procan SR

Special information
if you are pregnant or breastfeeding
The effects of Vascor during pregnancy have not been adequately studied. However, it has affected the development of fetuses in animal studies. If you are pregnant or plan to become pregnant, inform your doctor immediately. Vascor appears in breast milk and may affect a nursing infant. If this medication is essential to your health, your doctor may advise you to discontinue breastfeeding until your treatment is finished.

Recommended dosage

ADULTS

Dosages of this drug should be adjusted by the doctor according to each individual's response and needs.

The usual starting dose of Vascor is 200 milligrams 1 time per day.

After 10 days, the dosage may be adjusted upward depending upon the patient's response—including his or her ability to perform activities of daily living—and the drug's effect on heart rhythms, heart rate, and frequency and severity of angina.

The regular dose of Vascor is usually 300 milligrams, taken 1 time per day; it may not be effective at doses lower than 200 milligrams per day, and daily dosage should not exceed 400 milligrams.

Patients with liver or kidney disorders should use this drug cautiously. Dosages may need to be adjusted accordingly.

CHILDREN

The safety and effectiveness of this medication in children have not been established.

ELDERLY

The starting dose for elderly patients should be the same as for other adults. However, after its effects on the elderly patient are clear, the patient should be more carefully monitored.

Overdosage

Any medication taken in excess can have serious consequences. If you suspect an overdose, seek medical treatment immediately. Observation in a cardiac care facility for at least 48 hours is recommended.

Overdose symptoms of Vascor may include:
Low blood pressure
Rapid heartbeat

Brand name:

VASERETIC

Generic ingredients: Enalapril maleate, Hydrochlorothiazide

Why is this drug prescribed?
Vaseretic is used in the treatment of high blood pressure. It combines an ACE inhibitor with a thiazide diuretic. Enalapril, the ACE inhibitor, works by preventing a chemical in your blood called angiotensin I from converting into a more potent form that increases salt and water retention in your body. Enalapril also enhances blood flow throughout your blood vessels. Hydrochlorothiazide, a diuretic, prompts your body to produce and eliminate more urine, which helps in lowering blood pressure.

Most important fact about this drug
Since blood pressure declines gradually, it may take several weeks for the full effect of Vaseretic to occur. Even if you are feeling well,

you must continue to take the medication. It is needed to maintain control of your blood pressure.

How should you take this medication?
Take this medication exactly as prescribed by your doctor.

If you forget to take a dose, take it as soon as you remember. If it is almost time for your next dose, skip the one you missed and go back to your regular schedule. Never take two doses at the same time.

What side effects may occur?
Side effects cannot be anticipated. If any develop or change in intensity, inform your doctor as soon as possible. Only your doctor can determine if it is safe for you to continue taking Vaseretic.

■ *More common side effects may include:*
Cough, diarrhea, dizziness, drop in blood pressure upon standing up, fatigue, headache, impotence, low potassium levels (leading to symptoms such as dry mouth, excessive thirst, weak or irregular heartbeat, muscle pain or cramps), muscle cramps, nausea, rash, tingling or pins and needles, weakness

■ *Less common or rare side effects may include:*
Abdominal pain, back pain, black stools, blood clots in lungs, blurred vision, bronchitis, chest pain, confusion, conjunctivitis, constipation, decrease in sex drive, depression, disturbances in heart rhythm, dry eyes, dry mouth, excessive sweating, fainting, fluid in lungs, flushing, gas, gout, heart attack, hepatitis, hives, hoarseness, inability to sleep, indigestion, inflammation of mouth, and tongue, inflammation of the pancreas, itching, joint pain, kidney failure, loss of appetite, loss of coordination, loss of hair, low blood pressure, nervousness, rapid heartbeat, restlessness, ringing in ears, runny nose, shortness of breath, sleepiness, sore throat, stroke, tearing, urinary tract infection, vomiting, yellow eyes and skin

Why should this drug not be prescribed?
If you are sensitive to or have ever had an allergic reaction to enalapril, hydrochlorothiazide or similar drugs, or if you are sensitive to other sulfonamide-derived drugs, you should not take this medication. If you have a history of angioedema (swelling of face, extremities, and throat) or inability to urinate, you should not take this medication. Tell your doctor of all allergic reactions you have experienced.

Special warnings about this medication
If you develop swelling of your face, eyes, the area around your lips, tongue or throat, or of arms and legs; or difficulty swallowing, you should contact your doctor immediately. You may need emergency treatment.

If you develop chest pain, a sore throat or fever you should contact your doctor immediately. It could indicate a more serious illness.

If you are taking Vaseretic, a complete assessment of your kidney function should be done. Kidney function should continue to be monitored.

If you have liver disease or collagen vascular disease (a connective tissue disease called lupus erythematosus), Vaseretic should be used with caution.

If you have severe congestive heart failure, you should be carefully watched for low blood pressure.

Excessive sweating, dehydration, severe diarrhea, or vomiting could cause you to lose too much water and cause your blood pressure to become too low. Be careful when exercising and in hot weather.

Vaseretic can cause some people to become drowsy or less alert. If it has this effect on you, driving or operating dangerous machinery or participating in any hazardous activity that requires full mental alertness is not recommended.

If you are diabetic, blood sugar levels should be monitored.

Avoid too much sun due to possible photosensitivity.

Possible food and drug interactions when taking this medication

Vaseretic may intensify the effects of alcohol. Do not drink alcohol while taking this medication.

If Vaseretic is taken with certain other drugs, the effects of either could be increased, decreased, or altered. It is especially important to check with your doctor before combining Vaseretic with the following:

Alcohol
Barbiturates
Certain other antihypertensives
Corticosteroids such as prednisone
Digitalis (Lanoxin)
Insulin
Lithium
Narcotics
Nonsteroidal anti-inflammatory drugs
    such as Naprosyn
Norepinephrine
Oral antidiabetic drugs such as Micronase
Potassium supplements
Potassium-containing salt substitutes
Potassium-sparing diuretics such as Midamor

Special information
if you are pregnant or breastfeeding

Vaseretic can cause birth defects, prematurity, and death to the fetus and newborn. If you are pregnant or plan to become pregnant and are taking Vaseretic, contact your doctor immediately to discuss the potential hazard to your unborn child. Vaseretic appears in breast milk and could affect a nursing infant. If this medication is essential to your health, your doctor may advise you to discontinue breastfeeding until your treatment is finished.

Recommended dosage

ADULTS

Dosages of this drug are always individualized. Your doctor will determine what works best for you. This medication can and may be used in combination with other high blood pressure medications and dosages will be adjusted accordingly. Dosages will also be modified and carefully monitored in patients with reduced kidney function.

Once your doctor has determined that your blood pressure is stable, the usual starting dose is 1 or 2 "10-25" tablets once a day. Maximum daily dosage is 2 tablets.

Diuretic use should, if possible, be stopped before using Vaseretic. If not, your doctor may give an initial dose under his or her supervision before any further medication is prescribed.

CHILDREN

The safety and effectiveness of Vaseretic in children have not been established.

ELDERLY

Dosage should be determined by the particular needs of the elderly patient.

Overdosage

Any medication taken in excess can cause symptoms of overdose. If you suspect an overdose, seek medical attention immediately.

No specific information on treatment of Vaseretic overdose is available.

Symptoms of a Vaseretic overdose may include:
Dehydration
Low blood pressure

Brand name:

VASOTEC

Generic name: Enalapril maleate

Why is this drug prescribed?

Vasotec is a high blood pressure medication known as an ACE inhibitor. It is effective when used alone or in combination with other medications, especially thiazide-type diuretics. It is also used in the treatment of congestive heart failure, usually in combination with diuretics and digitalis.

Most important fact about this drug

You must continue to take Vasotec regularly for it to be effective. Even if you are feeling well, continue to take it. You need the medication to keep your blood pressure under control. Since blood pressure lowers gradually, it may take several weeks for the full effect of Vasotec to occur.

How should you take this medication?

Vasotec can be taken with or without food.

Do not use salt substitutes containing potassium without first consulting your doctor.

Take this medication exactly as prescribed by your doctor.

If you forget to take a dose, take it as soon as you remember. If it is almost time for your next dose, skip the one you missed and go back to your regular schedule. Never take two doses at the same time.

What side effects may occur?

Side effects cannot be anticipated. If any develop or change in intensity, inform your doctor as soon as possible. Only your doctor can determine if it is safe for you to continue taking Vasotec.

■ Side effects may include:

Abdominal pain, anaphylactoid reactions (severe allergic reactions), angina pectoris (chest pain, often accompanied by a feeling of choking or impending death), angioedema (chest pain, swelling of face around lips, tongue and throat, arms and legs, sore throat, fever, chills, difficulty swallowing), asthma, blood clot in lung and tissue loss, blurred vision, breast enlargement in males, bronchitis, confusion, constipation, cough, dark, tarry stool containing blood, decreased urination, depression, diarrhea, difficulty breathing, difficulty sleeping, digestive difficulty and stomach discomfort, dizziness, dizziness on standing, dry eyes, dry mouth, excessive perspiration, fainting, fatigue, flank pain, fluid in lungs, flushing, hair loss, headache, heart fibrillation, heart palpitations, heart rhythm disturbances, hepatitis, herpes zoster, hives, impotence, inflammation of the mouth, inflammation of the tongue, itching, lack of muscle coordination, loss of appetite, loss of sense of smell, low blood pressure, low blood pressure when standing, muscle cramps, nausea, nervousness, pinkeye (conjunctivitis), pneumonia, pounding heartbeat, rapid or slow heartbeat, rash, red skin (like sunburn), ringing in ears, runny nose, sleepiness, sore throat and hoarseness, stroke, taste alteration, tearing, tingling or pins and needles or burning sensation, upper respiratory infection, upset stomach, urinary tract infection, vertigo, vomiting, weakness, wheezing

Why should this drug not be prescribed?

If you are sensitive or have ever had an allergic reaction to Vasotec or similar drugs, or if you have a history of angioedema related to previous treatment with ACE inhibitors, you should not take this medication. Make sure that your doctor is aware of any drug reactions that you have experienced.

Special warnings about this medication

Angioedema, a serious allergic reaction, has occurred with Vasotec and should be reported to your doctor immediately. The symptoms are chest pain; swelling of the face around lips, tongue, and throat; swelling of arms and legs; sore throat; fever; chills; and difficulty swallowing.

If you are taking high doses of diuretics and Vasotec, you may develop excessively low blood pressure. You are at special risk if you have heart disease, kidney disease, or a potassium or salt imbalance.

There have been cases of serious blood disorders reported with the use of Captopril, another ACE inhibitor drug. Your doctor should check your blood regularly while you are taking Vasotec.

ACE inhibitors can cause fetal abnormalities and fetal and newborn deaths when used in pregnancy during the second and third trimesters.

When pregnancy is detected, Vasotec should be discontinued as soon as possible.

If you develop a sore throat or fever, you should contact your doctor immediately. It could indicate a more serious illness.

Excessive sweating, dehydration, severe diarrhea, or vomiting could cause you to lose too much water, causing your blood pressure to drop dangerously. Be careful when exercising or when exposed to excessive heat.

Possible food and drug interactions when taking this medication

If Vasotec is taken with certain other drugs, the effects of either could be increased, decreased, or altered. It is especially important to check with your doctor before combining Vasotec with the following:

Diuretics such as Lasix and HydroDIURIL
Potassium-sparing diuretics such as
   Aldactazide and Moduretic
Potassium supplements such as K-Lyte and
   K-Tab
Potassium-containing salt substitutes
Lithium (Lithobid)

Special information if you are pregnant or breastfeeding

Vasotec can cause birth defects, prematurity, and death to the fetus and newborn. If you are pregnant or plan to become pregnant, inform your doctor immediately. Vasotec may appear in breast milk and could affect a nursing infant. If this medication is essential to your health, your doctor may advise you to stop breastfeeding until your treatment with Vasotec is finished.

Recommended dosage

ADULTS

Hypertension
The usual starting dose for patients not using diuretics is 5 milligrams, taken once a day. Usual regular dose is 10 to 40 milligrams per day, taken as a single dose or divided into 2 smaller doses.

If you are taking a diuretic, your physician may ask you to stop for 2 to 3 days before using Vasotec. Otherwise, he may give an initial dose of 2.5 milligrams of Vasotec under his supervision before any further medication is prescribed.

Patients with kidney disorders must be carefully monitored. Dosages must be adjusted depending on the level of kidney function.

Heart Failure

This medication can be used in conjunction with digitalis and diuretics in heart disease patients. The usual starting dose is 2.5 milligrams once or twice a day.

The usual regular dose is 5 to 20 milligrams each day, given as a single dose or 2 separate doses. The maximum daily dose is 40 milligrams in a single dose or two separate doses.

CHILDREN

The safety and effectiveness of Vasotec in children has not been established.

ELDERLY

Dosage should be determined by the particular needs of the elderly patient.

Overdosage

Any medication taken in excess can have serious consequences. If you suspect symptoms of a Vasotec overdose, seek medical attention immediately.

A sudden drop in blood pressure is the primary effect of a Vasotec overdose.

Brand name:

VEETIDS

See Penicillin V, page 462.

Brand name:

VELOSEF

Generic name: Cephradine
Other brand name: Anspor

Why is this drug prescribed?

Cephradine, a broad-spectrum cephalosporin antibiotic available in capsule or liquid form, is similar to oral penicillin. Cephradine is given to treat certain infections of the upper or lower respiratory tract, including pharyngitis (strep throat) and pneumonia, as well as middle ear, skin, or urinary tract infections.

Most important fact about this drug

Like other antibiotics, cephradine kills some kinds of ordinary intestinal bacteria and allows other kinds to multiply. In some people taking cephradine, overgrowth of certain intestinal bacteria causes diarrhea which has the potential to develop into extremely serious colitis (bowel inflammation). If you get diarrhea while taking cephradine, tell your doctor right away.

How should you take this medication?

Take cephradine exactly as prescribed by your doctor. You usually will be instructed to take a dose every 6 hours or every 12 hours. You may take the medication with meals or between meals.

Do not stop taking cephradine when you start feeling better; it is important to keep taking cephradine on your usual schedule until you have finished all of the medicine.

What side effects may occur?

Side effects cannot be anticipated. If any develop or change in intensity, inform your doctor immediately. Only your doctor can determine if it is safe for you to continue taking cephradine.

Cephradine may cause diarrhea which has the potential to become serious.

■ *Potential side effects include:*
 Abdominal pain, confusion, dizziness, fever, headache, hives, joint pain, loss of appetite, muscle aches, nausea, rash, redness, tightness in the chest, vaginal yeast infection, vomiting

Why should this drug not be prescribed?
You may be at increased risk of an allergic reaction to cephradine if you have a history of allergies, asthma, hay fever, or hives.

If you are allergic to penicillin, be sure to tell your doctor.

If you have impaired kidney function or gastrointestinal disease, your doctor should evaluate your condition before prescribing cephradine.

Special warnings about this medication
You should be aware that cephradine may produce false-positive results on certain urine and blood tests. If your urine tests positive for sugar, protein, or ketosteroids, or if your blood test shows a prolonged prothrombin time, be sure your doctor knows that you are taking cephradine. The test results could actually be negative rather than positive.

Possible food and drug interactions when taking this medication
If cephradine is taken with certain other drugs, the effects of either could be increased, decreased, or altered. It is especially important to check with your doctor before combining cephradine with the following:

Diuretics such as Lasix and Bumex
Other antibiotics
Probenecid (Benemid)

Special information if you are pregnant or breastfeeding
If you are pregnant or plan to become pregnant, inform your doctor immediately. Cephradine should be taken in pregnancy only if clearly needed. Caution is also advised for nursing mothers, since cephradine does appear in breast milk.

Recommended dosage

ADULTS

Respiratory Tract Infections (Other than Lobar Pneumonia) and Skin and Skin Structure Infections
The usual dose is 250 milligrams every 6 hours or 500 milligrams every 12 hours.

Lobar Pneumonia
The usual dose is 500 milligrams every 6 hours or 1 gram every 12 hours.

Urinary Tract Infections
The usual dose is 500 milligrams every 12 hours for uncomplicated urinary tract infections. In more serious urinary tract infections, including prostatitis, 500 milligrams every 6 hours or 1 gram every 12 hours may be given.

Severe or Chronic Infections
Larger doses (up to 1 gram four times a day) may be given for severe or chronic infections. As with antibiotic therapy in general, treatment should be continued for a minimum of 48 to 72 hours after you feel better.

CHILDREN

The usual dose in children over 9 months of age is 25 to 50 milligrams for each 2.2 pounds of body weight per day given in equally divided doses every 6 or 12 hours.

Otitis Media Due to H. influenzae
The recommended dose ranges from 75 to 100 milligrams for each 2.2 pounds of body weight per day, given in equally divided doses every 6 or 12 hours, not to exceed 4 grams per day.

Overdosage
Although no specific information is available regarding overdose, any medication taken in excess can have serious consequences. If

you suspect a cephradine overdose, seek medical attention immediately.

Brand name:

VENTOLIN

See Proventil, page 518.

Generic name:

VERAPAMIL HYDROCHLORIDE

See Calan, page 81.

Brand name:

VERELAN

See Calan, page 81.

Brand name:

VIBRA-TABS

See Doryx, page 216.

Brand name:

VIBRAMYCIN

See Doryx, page 216.

Brand name:

VICODIN

Generic ingredients: Hydrocodone bitartrate, Acetaminophen
Other brand names: Anexia, Lortab, Norcet, Zydone

Why is this drug prescribed?

Vicodin combines a narcotic analgesic (pain killer) and antitussive (cough reliever) with a non-narcotic analgesic for the relief of moderate to moderately severe pain.

Most important fact about this drug

Tolerance and mental and physical dependence can occur with the use of Vicodin when the drug is taken over long periods of time.

How should you take this medication?

Take Vicodin exactly as prescribed by your doctor. Do not increase the amount you take without your doctor's approval. If you miss a dose of this medication, do not double your dosage. Do not take this drug for any other reason other than the one prescribed.

Do not give this drug to others who may have similar symptoms.

What side effects may occur?

Side effects cannot be anticipated. If any develop or change in intensity, inform your doctor as soon as possible. Only your doctor can determine if it is safe for you to continue taking Vicodin.

■ More common side effects may include:
Dizziness
Light-headedness
Nausea
Sedation
Vomiting

If these side effects occur, it may help if you lie down after taking the medication.

■ Less common or rare side effects may include:
Anxiety, constipation, drowsiness, fear, feeling of discomfort, impairment of mental and physical performance, inability to urinate, mental clouding, mood changes, restlessness, sluggishness, troubled, irregular, or slowed breathing

Why should this drug not be prescribed?

If you are sensitive to or have ever had an allergic reaction to hydrocodone, acetaminophen (Tylenol), or drugs of this type, you should not take this medication. Make sure that your doctor is aware of any drug reactions that you have experienced.

Special warnings about this medication

Vicodin may impair the mental and/or physical abilities required for the performance of potentially hazardous tasks such as driving a car or operating machinery.

Use caution in taking Vicodin if you have a head injury. Narcotics tend to increase the pressure of the fluid within the skull, which may be exaggerated by head injuries. Side effects of narcotics can interfere in the treatment of patients with head injuries.

Vicodin should be used with caution if you have a severe liver or kidney disorder, hypothyroidism (underactive thyroid gland), Addison's disease (a disease of the adrenal glands), enlarged prostate, or urethral stricture (narrowing of the urethra).

Narcotics may interfere with the diagnosis and treatment of patients with abdominal conditions.

Hydrocodone suppresses the cough reflex; therefore, Vicodin should be used cautiously after an operation or in patients with a lung disease.

Vicodin contains sodium metabisulfite, a sulfite that may cause an allergic reaction such as an asthma attack, whether life-threatening or less severe. Sensitivity to sulfites is more likely to be seen in asthmatics than in people who do not have asthma.

High doses of hydrocodone may produce troubled, irregular, or slowed breathing; if you are sensitive to this drug, you may experience these effects as well.

Possible food and drug interactions when taking this medication

Hydrocodone is a central nervous system depressant and intensifies the effects of alcohol.

If hydrocodone is taken with certain other drugs, the effects of either may be increased, decreased, or altered. It is especially important to check with your doctor before combining Vicodin with the following:

Antianxiety drugs such as Valium and Librium
Antipsychotics such as Thorazine and Haldol
A class of drugs for severe depression called "MAO Inhibitors," including such drugs as Nardil
Also, depression medications classified as "tricyclic antidepressants," including Elavil and Tofranil
Drugs that control certain muscle contractions such as Cogentin
Other narcotic analgesics such as Demerol and other central nervous system depressants

Special information if you are pregnant or breastfeeding

Do not take Vicodin if you are pregnant or planning to become pregnant unless you are directed to do so by your doctor. Drug dependence occurs in newborns when the mother has taken this drug regularly prior to delivery. Hydrocodone may appear in breast milk and could affect a nursing infant. If this medication is essential to your health, your doctor may advise you to discontinue breastfeeding your baby until your treatment is finished.

Recommended dosage

ADULTS

Your doctor will adjust the dosage according to the severity of the pain and the way the medication affects you.

The dosages given below are for Vicodin and Vicodin ES only. If your doctor prescribes other brands, your daily dose may vary.

The usual dose of Vicodin is 1 or 2 tablets taken every 4 to 6 hours for pain as needed. The total dose should not exceed 8 tablets per day.

The usual dose of Vicodin ES is 1 tablet every 4 to 6 hours for pain as needed. The total dose should not exceed 5 tablets per day.

CHILDREN

The safety and effectiveness of this Vicodin have not been established in children.

ELDERLY

Your doctor will prescribe a dose individualized to suit your needs.

Overdosage

Any medication taken in excess can have serious consequences. If you suspect an overdose, seek emergency medical treatment immediately.

Symptoms of an overdose of Vicodin include: Bluish tinge to skin, cold and clammy skin, coma due to low blood sugar, extreme sleepiness progressing to a state of unresponsiveness, gasping, general feeling of bodily discomfort, heavy perspiration, kidney failure, limp, weak muscles, liver failure, low blood pressure, nausea, slow heartbeat, troubled or slowed breathing, vomiting

In severe overdosage, lack of respiration, shock, heart attack, and death may occur.

Brand name:

VISKEN

Generic name: Pindolol

Why is this drug prescribed?

Visken, a type of medication known as a beta blocker, is used in the treatment of high blood pressure. It is effective alone or combined with other high blood pressure medications, particularly with a thiazide-type diuretic. Beta blockers decrease the force and rate of heart contractions.

Most important fact about this drug

You must take Visken regularly for it to be effective. Even if you are feeling well, you need the medication to keep your blood pressure under control.

How should you take this medication?

Visken can be taken with or without food.

Take this medication exactly as prescribed by your doctor, even if your symptoms have disappeared.

Try not to miss any doses. If this medication is not taken regularly, your condition may worsen.

If you forget to take a dose, take it as soon as you remember. If it's within 4 hours of your next scheduled dose, skip the one you missed and go back to your regular schedule. Never take two doses at the same time.

What side effects may occur?

Side effects cannot be anticipated. If any develop or change in intensity, inform your doctor as soon as possible. Only your doctor can determine if it is safe for you to continue taking Visken.

■ *More common side effects may include:*
Abdominal discomfort, chest pain, dizziness,

fatigue, headache, joint pain, muscle pain or cramps, nausea, nervousness, shortness of breath, strange dreams, swelling due to fluid retention, tingling or pins and needles, trouble sleeping, weakness

■ *Less common or rare side effects may include:*
Anxiety, burning eyes, cold hands and feet, colitis, depression, diarrhea, disorientation, excessive sweating, fainting, fever and sore throat, frequent urination, hair loss, hallucinations, impotence, irregular heartbeat, itching, limping, low blood pressure, memory loss, rapid heartbeat, rash, reversible hair loss, slow heartbeat, sluggishness, vision changes, vomiting, weight gain, wheezing

Why should this drug not be prescribed?
If you have bronchial asthma; severe congestive heart failure; inadequate blood supply to the circulatory system (cardiogenic shock); heart block (conduction disorder); or a severely slow heartbeat, you should not take this medication.

Special warnings about this medication
If you have a history of severe congestive heart failure Visken should be used with caution.

Visken should not be stopped suddenly. It can cause increased chest pain and heart attack. Dosage should be gradually reduced.

If you suffer from asthma, seasonal allergies or other bronchial conditions, coronary artery disease, or kidney or liver disease, this medication should be used with caution.

Ask your doctor if you should check your pulse while taking Visken. This medication can cause your heartbeat to become too slow.

This medication may mask the symptoms of low blood sugar in diabetics or alter blood sugar levels. If you are diabetic, discuss this with your doctor.

Visken may cause you to become disoriented. If it has this effect on you, driving or operating dangerous machinery or participating in any hazardous activity that requires full mental alertness is not recommended.

Notify your doctor or dentist that you are taking Visken if you have a medical emergency, and before you have surgery or dental treatment.

Possible food and drug interactions when taking this medication
If Visken is taken with certain other drugs, the effects of either could be increased, decreased, or altered. It is especially important to check with your doctor before combining Visken with the following:

Catecholamine-depleting drugs such as reserpine
Insulin or oral antidiabetic agents such as Micronase
Thioridazine (Mellaril)

Special information if you are pregnant or breastfeeding
The effects of Visken during pregnancy have not been adequately studied. If you are pregnant or plan to become pregnant, inform your doctor immediately. Visken appears in breast milk and could affect a nursing infant. If this medication is essential to your health, your doctor may advise you to discontinue breastfeeding until your treatment with this medication is finished.

Recommended dosage
ADULTS

Dosage should be individualized.

The usual starting dose is 5 milligrams, 2 times per day, alone or with other high blood pressure medication. Blood pressure reduction is usually seen in 1 to 2 weeks. If blood pressure is not reduced sufficiently within 3 to 4 weeks, your doctor may increase your total daily dosage in 10 milligram increments, at 3 to 4 week intervals, up to a maximum of 60 milligrams a day.

CHILDREN

The safety and effectiveness of Visken have not been established in children.

ELDERLY

Dosage should be determined by the particular needs of the elderly patient.

Overdosage

Any medication taken in excess can cause symptoms of overdose. If you suspect an overdose, seek medical attention immediately.

Symptoms of Visken overdose may include: Bronchospasm (spasm of the air passages) Excessively slow heartbeat Heart failure Low blood pressure

Generic name:

VITAMINS, PRENATAL

See Stuartnatal 1 + 1, page 590.

Generic name:

VITAMINS WITH FLUORIDE

See Poly-Vi-Flor, page 491.

Brand name:

VOLTAREN

Generic name: Diclofenac sodium

Why is this drug prescribed?

Voltaren, a nonsteroidal anti-inflammatory drug, is used to relieve the inflammation, swelling, stiffness, and joint pain associated with rheumatoid arthritis, osteoarthritis (the most common form of arthritis), and ankylosing spondylitis (arthritis and stiffness of the spine). It is also used in the treatment of other kinds of pain.

Most important fact about this drug

You should have frequent check-ups with your doctor if you take Voltaren regularly. Ulcers or internal bleeding can occur without warning.

How should you take this medication?

To minimize stomach upset and related side effects, your doctor may recommend taking Voltaren with food, milk, or an antacid. However, this may delay onset of relief.

Take this medication exactly as prescribed by your doctor.

What side effects may occur?

Side effects cannot be anticipated. If any develop or change in intensity, inform your doctor as soon as possible. Only your doctor can determine if it is safe for you to continue taking Voltaren.

■ *More common side effects may include:* Abdominal bleeding, abdominal pain or cramps, abdominal swelling, constipation, diarrhea, dizziness, fluid retention, gas, headache, indigestion, itching, nausea, peptic ulcer, rash, ringing in ears

■ *Less common or rare side effects may include:*

Abdominal bleeding, abdominal swelling, anaphylaxis (allergic reaction), anemia, anxiety, appetite change, asthma, black stools, bloody diarrhea, blurred vision, changes in taste, colitis, congestive heart failure, decrease in white blood cells, depression, double vision, drowsiness, dry mouth, fluid retention, gas, hair loss, hearing loss, hepatitis, high blood pressure, hives, inability to sleep, inflammation of mouth, inflammation of the pancreas, irritability, kidney failure, low blood pressure, nosebleed, rash, itching, sensitivity to light, skin eruptions, Stevens-Johnson syndrome (a severe form of skin eruption), swelling of eyelids, lips, and tongue, swelling of the throat due to fluid retention, vomiting, yellow eyes and skin

Why should this drug not be prescribed?

If you are sensitive to or have ever had an allergic reaction to Voltaren, aspirin, or similar drugs, or if you have had asthma attacks caused by aspirin or other drugs of this type, you should not take this medication. Make sure that your doctor is aware of any drug reactions that you have experienced.

Special warnings about this medication

Peptic ulcers and bleeding can occur without warning.

This drug should be used with caution if you have kidney or liver disease, and it can cause liver inflammation in some people.

Do not take aspirin or any other anti-inflammatory medications while taking Voltaren, unless your doctor tells you to do so.

If you are taking blood-thinning medication, this drug should be used with caution.

Use with caution if you have heart disease or high blood pressure. This drug can increase water retention.

Possible food and drug interactions when taking this medication

If Voltaren is taken with certain other drugs, the effects of either could be increased, decreased, or altered. It is especially important to check with your doctor before combining Voltaren with the following:

Anticoagulants (blood thinners)
Aspirin
Cyclosporine (Sandimmune)
Digitalis and Digoxin (Lanoxin)
Insulin or oral antidiabetes medications
Lithium (Lithobid)
Methotrexate
Potassium-sparing and other diuretics

Special information if you are pregnant or breastfeeding

The effects of Voltaren during pregnancy have not been adequately studied. If you are pregnant or plan to become pregnant, inform your doctor immediately. Voltaren appears in breast milk and could affect a nursing infant. If this medication is essential to your health, your doctor may advise you to discontinue breastfeeding until your treatment with Voltaren is finished.

Recommended Dosage

ADULTS

Osteoarthritis
100 to 150 milligrams a day in divided doses of 50 milligrams 2 or 3 times a day or 75 milligrams 2 times a day.

Rheumatoid Arthritis
150 to 200 milligrams a day in divided doses of 50 milligrams 3 or 4 times a day or 75 milligrams 2 times a day.

Ankylosing Spondylitis
100 to 125 milligrams a day in divided doses of 25 milligrams 4 times a day, with another 25 milligrams at bedtime if necessary.

The lowest dose that proves beneficial should be used.

CHILDREN

The safety and effectiveness of Voltaren have not been established in children.

ELDERLY

Dosage should be determined by the particular needs of the elderly patient.

Overdosage

Any medication taken in excess can cause symptoms of overdose. If you suspect an overdose, seek medical attention immediately.

The symptoms of Voltaren overdose may include:
Acute kidney failure
Drowsiness
Vomiting

Brand name:

VOSOL

Generic ingredients: Acetic acid (VoSoL), Acetic acid and hydrocortisone (VoSoL HC)

Why is this drug prescribed?

VoSoL and VoSoL HC treat minor infections of the external ear canal. VoSoL is used to treat infection; VoSoL HC is used when there is both an infection and inflammation.

Most important fact about this drug

You may experience a stinging or burning sensation when the VoSoL drops are first placed into your ear.

How should you use this medication?

The "wick" your doctor inserts in your ear should remain in place for at least 24 hours.

What side effects may occur?

Side effects cannot be anticipated. If any develop or change in intensity, notify your doctor as soon as possible. Only your doctor can determine whether it is safe for you to continue using VoSoL and VoSoL HC.

Stinging or burning may occur occasionally. Irritation where the drops touch the skin has occurred very rarely.

Why should this drug not be prescribed?

VoSoL and VoSoL HC should not be used if you are sensitive to or allergic to any of their ingredients, if you have chickenpox or cowpox, or if you have a perforated eardrum.

Special warnings about this medication

Stop using VoSoL or VoSoL HC if you develop any sensitivity or irritation.

To prevent contamination, avoid touching the applicator tip to any surface; keep the container closed.

Possible food and drug interactions when taking this medication

No interactions have been reported.

Recommended dosage

Your doctor will insert a "wick" into your ear saturated with VoSoL or VoSoL HC. The wick should remain in your ear for at least 24 hours and kept moist by adding 3 to 5 drops of VoSoL or VoSoL HC every 4 to 6 hours. The wick can be removed after 24 hours. Continue to place 5 drops of medication in your ear 3 or 4 times a day for as long as your doctor says it is necessary.

Overdosage

Although no specific information is available on VoSoL overdosage, any medication used in excess can have serious consequences.

If you suspect an overdose, seek medical attention immediately.

Generic name:

WARFARIN SODIUM

See Coumadin, page 140.

Brand name:

WELLBUTRIN

Generic name: Bupropion hydrochloride

Why is this drug prescribed?
Wellbutrin, a relatively new oral antidepressant medication that comes in tablet form, is given to help relieve certain kinds of major depression.

Major depression involves a severely depressed mood (for 2 weeks or more) accompanied by sleep and appetite disturbances, agitation or lack of energy, feelings of guilt or worthlessness, decreased sex drive, inability to concentrate, and perhaps thoughts of suicide.

Unlike the more familiar tricyclic anti-depressants, such as Elavil, Tofranil, and others, Wellbutrin tends to have a somewhat stimulant effect.

Most important fact about this drug
Although Wellbutrin occasionally causes weight gain, a more common effect is weight loss: Some 28 percent of people who take this medication lose 5 pounds or more. If depression has already caused you to lose weight, and if further weight loss would be detrimental to your health, Wellbutrin may not be a good choice of antidepressant for you.

How should you take this medication?
Take Wellbutrin exactly as prescribed by your doctor. The usual dosing regimen is 3 equal doses spaced evenly throughout the day. At least 6 hours should elapse between doses. Your doctor will probably start you at a low dosage and gradually increase the dosage; this helps minimize side effects.

If you miss a dose of this medicine, take it as soon as possible. However, if it is within 4 hours of your next dose, skip the missed dose and go back to your regular dosing schedule. Do not take double doses.

Since Wellbutrin may impair your coordination or judgment, do not drive or operate dangerous machinery until you find out how the medication affects you.

If Wellbutrin does work for you, your doctor will probably have you continue taking it for at least several months.

Avoid alcoholic beverages.

What side effects may occur?
Side effects cannot be anticipated. If any develop or change in intensity, inform your doctor as soon as possible. Only your doctor can determine if it is safe for you to continue taking Wellbutrin.

Seizures are perhaps the most worrisome side effect.

- *More common side effects may include:*
  Agitation
  Constipation
  Dizziness
  Dry mouth
  Excessive sweating
  Headache
  Nausea, vomiting
  Skin rash
  Sleep disturbances
  Tremor

- *Other side effects may include:*
  Acne, bed-wetting, blurred vision, breathing

difficulty, chest pain, chills, complete or almost complete loss of movement, confusion, dry skin, episodes of overactivity, elation, or irritability, extreme calmness, fatigue, fever, fluid retention, flu-like symptoms, gum irritation and inflammation, hair color changes, hair loss, hives, impotence, incoordination and clumsiness, indigestion, itching, increased libido, menstrual complaints, mood instability, muscle rigidity, painful ejaculation, painful erection, retarded ejaculation, ringing in the ears, sexual dysfunction, suicidal ideation, thirst disturbances, toothache, urinary disturbances, weight gain or loss

Why should this drug not be prescribed?

Do not take Wellbutrin if you are sensitive to or have ever had an allergic reaction to it.

Since Wellbutrin causes seizures in some people, do not take it if you have any type of seizure disorder.

You should not take Wellbutrin if you currently have, or formerly had, an eating disorder. For some reason, people with a history of anorexia nervosa or bulimia seem to be more likely to experience Wellbutrin-related seizures.

Do not take Wellbutrin if, within the past 14 days, you have taken a monoamine oxidase inhibitor (MAO inhibitor) type of antidepressant, such as Nardil, Marplan, or Parnate. This particular drug combination could cause you to experience a sudden, dangerous rise in blood pressure.

Special warnings about this medication

If you take Wellbutrin, you may be vulnerable to seizures if your dosage is too high or if you ever suffered brain damage or experienced seizures in the past.

Do not take other medications that might help trigger seizures (e.g., antipsychotics, other antidepressants).

If you have been taking Valium or a similar tranquilizer but are ready to stop, taper off gradually rather than quitting abruptly.

Although less stimulating than amphetamines, Wellbutrin does have a slight stimulant effect and thus might hold some appeal for drug abusers.

Possible food and drug interactions when taking this medication

Do not drink alcohol while you are taking Wellbutrin; an interaction between alcohol and Wellbutrin could increase the possibility of a seizure.

If Wellbutrin is taken with certain other drugs, the effects of either could be increased, decreased, or altered. It is especially important to check with your doctor before combining Wellbutrin with the following:

Antipsychotics such as Thorazine
Dilantin
Levodopa (Larodopa and others)
Monoamine oxidase inhibitors such as Nardil
Phenobarbital (Luminal and others)
Tagamet
Tegretol
Tricyclic antidepressants such as Elavil
    and Tofranil

Special information if you are pregnant or breastfeeding

If you are pregnant or plan to become pregnant, notify your doctor immediately. Wellbutrin should be taken during pregnancy only if clearly needed.

Wellbutrin may pass into breast milk and cause serious adverse reactions in a nursing baby; therefore, if you are a new mother, you may need to discontinue breastfeeding while you are taking this medication.

Recommended dosage

No single dose of Wellbutrin should exceed 150 milligrams.

ADULTS

The usual adult dose is 300 milligrams per day given 3 times a day with at least 6 hours between doses. Doses should begin at 200 milligrams per day, given as 100 milligrams 2 times a day.

Based on patient response, this dose may be increased to 300 milligrams per day, given as 100 milligrams 3 times a day, no sooner than 3 days after beginning treatment.

CHILDREN

Safety and effectiveness in children under 18 years old have not been established.

ELDERLY

In general, older patients are known to metabolize drugs more slowly and to be more sensitive to the anticholinergic, sedative, and cardiovascular side effects of anti-depressant drugs.

Overdosage

Any medication taken in excess can have serious consequences. If you suspect symptoms of an overdose of Wellbutrin, seek medical attention immediately.

Symptoms of Wellbutrin overdose may include:
Hallucinations
Heart failure
Loss of consciousness
Rapid heartbeat
Seizures

An overdose that involves other drugs in combination with Wellbutrin may also cause these symptoms:

Breathing difficulties
Coma

Fever
Rigid muscles
Stupor

Brand name:

WYMOX

See Amoxil, page 23.

Brand name:

WYTENSIN

Generic name: Guanabenz acetate

Why is this drug prescribed?

Wytensin is used in the treatment of high blood pressure. It is effective used alone or in combination with a thiazide diuretic. Wytensin begins to lower blood pressure within 60 minutes after taking a single dose and may slow your pulse rate slightly.

Most important fact about this drug

You must take Wytensin regularly for it to be effective. Even if you are feeling well, you must continue to take Wytensin. If you stop, your high blood pressure will return.

How should you take this medication?

Wytensin may be taken with or without food.

Take this medication exactly as prescribed by your doctor.

What side effects may occur?

Side effects cannot be anticipated. If any develop or change in intensity, inform your doctor as soon as possible. Only your doctor can determine if it is safe for you to continue taking Wytensin.

■ *More common side effects may include:*
Dizziness
Drowsiness
Dry mouth

Headache
Weakness

■ *Less common side effects may include:*
Abdominal discomfort, aches in arms and
legs, anxiety, blurred vision, breast
development in males, changes in taste,
chest pain, constipation, decreased sex
drive, depression, diarrhea, fluid retention,
frequent urination, impotence, irregular
heartbeat, itching, lack of muscle
coordination, muscle aches, nausea,
pounding heartbeat, rash, shortness of
breath, sleep disturbances, stomach pain,
stuffy nose, vomiting

■ *Rare side effects may include:*
Cardiac conduction disorders (heart disorder
which causes heartbeat irregularities)

Why should this drug not be prescribed?

Do not take Wytensin if you are sensitive to
it or have ever had an allergic reaction
to it.

Special warnings about this medication

Wytensin can make you drowsy or less alert.
Driving or operating dangerous machinery
or participating in any hazardous activity that
requires full mental alertness is not
recommended until you know how this drug
affects you.

If you have severe heart disease, stroke or
related disorders, or severe liver or kidney
failure, or if you have recently had a heart
attack, this drug should be used with
caution.

Your blood pressure should be carefully
monitored if you have disorders of the
kidney or liver.

Possible food and drug interactions when taking this medication

Wytensin may intensify the effects of alcohol.
Use of alcohol should be avoided.

If Wytensin is taken with certain other drugs,
the effects of either could be increased,
decreased, or altered. It is especially important
to check with your doctor before
combining Wytensin with the following:

Antihistamines (Benadryl)
Phenobarbital
Valium
Xanax

Special information if you are pregnant or breastfeeding

The effects of Wytensin during pregnancy have
not been adequately studied, but it may
affect the fetus. If you are pregnant or plan
to become pregnant, inform your doctor
immediately. Wytensin may appear in breast
milk and could affect a nursing infant.
If this medication is essential to your health,
your doctor may advise you to discontinue
breastfeeding until your treatment is finished.

Recommended dosage

ADULTS

Your doctor will adjust the dosage of this
medication to meet your individual needs.

The usual starting dose is 4 milligrams
2 times per day, whether Wytensin is used
alone or with a thiazide diuretic.

Dosage may be increased in increments of
4 to 8 milligrams per day every 1 to 2
weeks, depending on your response.

The maximum reported dose has been 32
milligrams twice daily, but doses as high
as this are rarely needed.

CHILDREN

The safety and effectiveness of this drug have
not been established in children under 12
years of age.

ELDERLY

This drug should be used with caution in
elderly patients.

Overdosage

Any medication taken in excess can have serious consequences. If you suspect an overdose, seek medical attention immediately.

Symptoms of Wytensin overdose may include:
Excessive contraction of the pupils
Irritability
Low blood pressure
Sleepiness
Slow heartbeat
Sluggishness

Brand name:

XANAX

Generic name: Alprazolam

Why is this drug prescribed?

Xanax is a tranquilizer used in the short-term relief of symptoms of anxiety or the treatment of anxiety disorders. Anxiety disorder is marked by unrealistic worry or excessive fears and concerns.

Xanax is also used in the treatment of panic disorder, which appears as unexpected panic attacks and may be accompanied by avoidance behavior called agoraphobia. Only your doctor can diagnose panic disorder and best advise you about treatment. Anxiety associated with depression is also responsive to Xanax.

Most important fact about this drug

Tolerance and dependence can occur with the use of Xanax. You may experience withdrawal symptoms if you stop using the drug abruptly. Only your doctor should advise you to discontinue or change your dose.

How should you take this medication?

Take this medication exactly as prescribed by your doctor.

Xanax may be taken with or without food.

What side effects may occur?

Side effects cannot be anticipated. If any develop or change in intensity, inform your doctor as soon as possible. Only your doctor can determine if it is safe for you to continue taking Xanax. Your doctor should periodically reassess the need for this drug.

Side effects to Xanax are usually seen at the beginning of treatment and disappear with continued medication.

■ *More common side effects may include:*
Abdominal discomfort, abnormal involuntary movement, abnormal muscle tone, agitation, allergies, anxiety, blurred vision, chest pain, confusion, constipation, decreased or increased sex drive, depression, diarrhea, difficult urination, dizziness, dream abnormalities, drowsiness, dry mouth, fainting, fatigue, fear, fluid retention, headache, hyperventilation (too frequent or too deep breathing), inability to fall asleep, increase or decrease in appetite, increased or decreased salivation, infection, impaired memory, irritability, lack of coordination, light-headedness, low blood pressure, menstrual problems, muscle cramps, muscular twitching, nausea and vomiting, nervousness, palpitations, rapid heartbeat, rash, restlessness, ringing in the ears, sexual dysfunction, skin inflammation, speech difficulties, stiffness, stuffy nose, sweating, talkativeness, tingling sensation, tiredness/sleepiness, tremors, uninhibited behavior, upper respiratory infections, warm feeling, weakness, weight gain or loss

■ *Less common or rare side effects may include:*
Abnormal muscle tone, concentration difficulties, decreased coordination, double vision, fatigue, hallucinations,

irritability, itching, loss of appetite, muscle spasticity, rage, sedation, seizures, sleep disturbances, slurred speech, stimulation, taste alterations, temporary memory loss, urine retention, weakness in muscle and bone, yellow eyes and skin

■ *Side effects due to decrease or withdrawal from Xanax:*
Blurred vision, decreased concentration, decreased mental clarity, diarrhea, heightened awareness of noise or bright lights, impaired sense of smell, loss of appetite, loss of weight, muscle cramps, seizures, tingling sensation, twitching

Why should this drug not be prescribed?

If you are sensitive to or have ever had an allergic reaction to Xanax or similar drugs (other tranquilizers), you should not take this medication. Make sure that your doctor is aware of any drug reactions that you have experienced.

Do not take this medication if you have narrow-angle glaucoma.

Anxiety or tension related to everyday stress usually does not require treatment with Xanax. Discuss your symptoms thoroughly with your doctor.

Special warnings about this medication

Xanax may cause you to become drowsy or less alert; therefore, driving or operating dangerous machinery or participating in any hazardous activity that requires full mental alertness is not recommended.

If you are being treated for panic disorder, you may need to take a higher dose of Xanax than for anxiety alone. High doses of this medication taken for long intervals may cause emotional and physical dependence. It is important that your doctor supervise you carefully when you are using this medication.

Possible food and drug interactions when taking this medication

Xanax may intensify the effect of alcohol. Do not drink alcohol while taking this medication.

If Xanax is taken with certain other drugs, the effects of either could be increased, decreased, or altered. It is important to check with your doctor before combining Xanax with the following:

Cimetidine (Tagamet)
Desipramine (Norpramin)
Imipramine (Tofranil)
Oral contraceptives
Other central nervous system depressants
Other psychotropics

Special information if you are pregnant or breastfeeding

Do not take this medication if you are pregnant or planning to become pregnant. There is an increased risk of respiratory problems and muscular weakness in your baby. Infants may also experience withdrawal symptoms. Xanax may appear in breast milk and could affect a nursing infant. If this medication is essential to your health, your doctor may advise you to stop breastfeeding until your treatment with this medication is finished.

Recommended dosage

ADULTS

Anxiety disorder
The usual starting dose of Xanax is 0.25 to 0.5 milligram taken 3 times a day. The dose may be increased every 3 to 4 days to a maximum daily dose of 4 milligrams, divided into smaller doses.

Panic disorder
You may be given a dose from 1 up to a total of 10 milligrams, according to your needs. The typical dose is 5 to 6 milligrams a day.

The usual starting dose is 0.5 milligram 3 times a day. This dose can be increased by 1 milligram a day every 3 or 4 days.

CHILDREN

Safety and effectiveness have not been established in children under 18 years of age.

ELDERLY

The usual starting dose for an anxiety disorder is 0.25 milligram, 2 or 3 times daily. This dose may be gradually increased if needed and tolerated.

Overdosage

Any medication taken in excess can cause symptoms of overdose. If you suspect an overdose, seek medical attention immediately.

Symptoms of Xanax overdose may include:
Confusion
Coma
Impaired coordination
Sleepiness
Slowed reaction time

Death has occurred with an overdose of Xanax alone or after combining it with alcohol.

Brand name:

YOCON

Generic name: Yohimbine hydrochloride

Why is this drug prescribed?

Yocon is being used to treat male impotence. Its officially approved use is for dilating pupils. It is thought to be an aphrodisiac (a substance that causes sexual excitement).

Most important fact about this drug

Yocon is generally not recommended for women.

How should you take this medication?

Take this medication exactly as prescribed by your doctor.

What side effects may occur?

Side effects cannot be anticipated. If any develop or change in intensity, inform your doctor as soon as possible. Only your doctor can determine if it is safe for you to continue taking Yocon.

■ *Side effects may include:*
Decreased urination, dizziness, flushing, headache, increase in blood pressure, increased heart rate, increased motor activity, irritability, nausea, nervousness, tremor

Why should this drug not be prescribed?

Yocon should not be used if you have kidney disease, or if you are sensitive to or have ever had an allergic reaction to yohimbine. Make sure that your doctor is aware of any drug reactions you have experienced.

Special warnings about this medication

Yocon is generally not recommended for use by children, the elderly, or people with heart and kidney disease who also have a history of gastric or duodenal ulcer. The drug is also not recommended for people being treated for a psychiatric disorder.

Possible food and drug interactions when taking this medication

It is important that you consult with your doctor before taking Yocon with drugs for depression such as Elavil or other drugs that change moods.

Special information if you are pregnant or breastfeeding

Yocon is not recommended for use in women generally and certainly must not be used during pregnancy.

Recommended dosage

ADULTS

Dosages of this drug are based on experimental research in the treatment of male impotence.

This dosage is 1 (5.4-milligram) tablet, 3 times a day.

Occasional side effects reported with this dosage are nausea, dizziness, or nervousness. In the event of side effects, the dosage should be reduced to ½ tablet 3 times a day, followed by gradual increases to 1 tablet 3 times a day.

CHILDREN

This drug is not for use in children.

ELDERLY

This drug should not be used in elderly patients.

Overdosage

Any medication taken in excess can cause symptoms of overdose. If you suspect an overdose, seek medical attention immediately. No specific symptoms of Yocon overdose have been reported.

Generic name:

YOHIMBINE HYDROCHLORIDE

See Yocon, page 691.

Brand name:

ZANTAC

Generic name: Ranitidine hydrochloride

Why is this drug prescribed?

Zantac is prescribed for the short-term treatment (4 to 8 weeks) of active duodenal ulcer and active benign gastric ulcer, and as maintenance therapy for duodenal ulcer, at a reduced dosage, after the ulcer has healed. It is also used for the treatment of hypersecretory conditions, such as Zollinger-Ellison syndrome and systemic mastocytosis, and for gastroesophageal reflux disease (backflow of acid stomach contents).

Most important fact about this drug

Zantac helps reduce the recurrence of duodenal ulcers and aids in more rapid healing of ulcers that occur during maintenance therapy.

How should you take this medication?

Take this medication exactly as prescribed by your doctor.

You can take an antacid for pain while you are taking Zantac.

This medication is available for home use in both tablet and syrup form. There is an injectable form used in hospitals.

Make sure you follow the diet your doctor recommends.

What side effects may occur?

Side effects cannot be anticipated. If any develop or change in intensity, inform your doctor as soon as possible. Only your doctor can determine if it is safe for you to continue taking Zantac.

■ *More common side effects may include:*
Headache, sometimes severe

■ *Less common or rare side effects may include:*
Abdominal discomfort and pain, agitation, changes in blood count (anemia), changes in liver function, constipation, depression, diarrhea, difficulty sleeping, dizziness, hair loss, hallucinations, heart block, hepatitis, hypersensitivity

reactions, inflammation of the pancreas, involuntary movements, irregular heartbeat, joint pain, nausea and vomiting, rapid heartbeat, rash, reduced white blood cells, reversible mental confusion, sleepiness, slow heartbeat, vague feeling of bodily discomfort, vertigo, yellow eyes and skin

If you experience any of these symptoms, notify your doctor immediately.

Why should this drug not be prescribed?
If you are sensitive to or have ever had an allergic reaction to Zantac or similar drugs, you should not take this medication. Make sure that your doctor is aware of any drug reactions that you have experienced.

Special warnings about this medication
A stomach malignancy could be present, even if your symptoms have been relieved by Zantac.

If you have kidney or liver disease, this drug should be used with caution.

Possible food and drug interactions when taking this medication
If Zantac is taken with certain other drugs, the effects of either could be increased, decreased, or altered. It is especially important to check with your doctor before combining Zantac with blood thinners such as warfarin (Coumadin).

Special information if you are pregnant or breastfeeding
The effects of Zantac in pregnancy have not been adequately studied. If you are pregnant or plan to become pregnant, inform your doctor immediately. Zantac appears in breast milk and could affect a nursing infant. If this medication is essential to your health, your doctor may advise you to discontinue breastfeeding until your treatment with this medication is finished.

Recommended dosage

ADULTS

Active Duodenal Ulcer
The usual starting dose is 150 milligrams 2 times a day or 10 milliliters (2 teaspoonfuls) 2 times a day for 4 to 8 weeks. Instead, you may take 300 milligrams or 20 milliliters (4 teaspoonfuls) at bedtime if necessary for your convenience. The dose should be the lowest effective dose. Long-term use should be reduced to a daily total of 150 milligrams or 10 milliliters (2 teaspoonfuls), taken at bedtime.

Other Hypersecretory Conditions (such as Zollinger-Ellison syndrome)
The usual dose is 150 milligrams or 10 milliliters (2 teaspoonfuls) 2 times a day. This dose can be adjusted upwards by your doctor.

Benign Gastric Ulcer and Gastroesophogeal Reflux Disease (GERD)
The usual dose is 150 milligrams or 10 milliliters (2 teaspoonfuls) 2 times a day, for 6 to 8 weeks.

Dosages in patients with reduced kidney function should be adjusted by their doctor.

CHILDREN

The safety and effectiveness of Zantac have not been established in children.

ELDERLY

Dosage should be determined by the particular needs of the elderly patient.

Overdosage
Any medication taken in excess can cause symptoms of overdose. If you suspect an overdose, seek medical attention immediately.

Information concerning Zantac overdosage is limited. However, an abnormal manner of walking, low blood pressure, and exaggerated side effect symptoms may be signs of an overdose.

If you experience any of these symptoms, notify your doctor immediately.

Brand name:

ZAROXOLYN

Generic name: Metolazone
Other brand name: Diulo

Why is this drug prescribed?
Zaroxolyn is a diuretic used in the treatment of high blood pressure and other conditions that require the elimination of excess fluid (water) from the body. These conditions include congestive heart failure and kidney disease. When used for high blood pressure, Zaroxolyn can be used alone or with other high blood pressure medications. Diuretics prompt your body to produce and eliminate more urine, which helps lower blood pressure.

Most important fact about this drug
If you have high blood pressure, you must take Zaroxolyn regularly for it to be effective. Even if you are feeling well, continue to take it. You need the medication to keep your blood pressure under control.

Diuretics can cause your body to lose too much potassium. Ask your doctor for the warning signs of potassium depletion. Also ask whether you should eat specific foods that are rich in potassium or take a potassium supplement to avoid this problem.

Do not interchange Zaroxolyn and other formulations of metolazone such as Diulo. The brands vary in potency of action.

How should you take this medication?
Take Zaroxolyn exactly as prescribed by your doctor. Stopping Zaroxolyn suddenly could cause your condition to worsen.

What side effects may occur?
Side effects cannot be anticipated. If any develop or change in intensity, inform your doctor as soon as possible. Only your doctor can determine if it is safe for you to continue taking Zaroxolyn.

■ *Side effects may include:*
Anemia, bloating of the abdomen, blood clots, blurred vision, chest pain, chills, constipation, depression, diarrhea, dizziness on standing up, dizziness or light-headedness, drowsiness, fainting, fatigue, gout, headache, hepatitis, high blood sugar, hives, impotence, inflammation of the skin, inflammation of the pancreas, joint pain, loss of appetite, low potassium levels (leading to dry mouth, excessive thirst, weak or irregular heartbeat, muscle pain or cramps), low sodium levels in blood, muscle spasms or cramps, nausea, rapid, pounding heartbeat, rash, reddish or purplish spots on the skin, restlessness, sensitivity to light, sugar in the urine, tingling or pins and needles, upset stomach, vertigo, vomiting, weakness, yellow eyes and skin

Why should this drug not be prescribed?
If you are unable to urinate or have severe liver disease, you should not take this medication.

If you are sensitive to or have ever had an allergic reaction to Zaroxolyn or similar drugs, you should not take this medication.

Special warnings about this medication
If you are taking Zaroxolyn, a complete assessment of your kidney function should be done and kidney function should continue to be monitored.

If you have liver disease, diabetes, gout, or lupus erythematosus (a disease of the immune system), Zaroxolyn should be used with caution.

If you have had an allergic reaction to sulfonamide-derived drugs, thiazides, or quinethazone, you may be at greater risk for an allergic reaction to this medication.

Dehydration, excessive sweating, severe diarrhea, or vomiting could deplete your fluids and cause your blood pressure to become too low. Be careful when exercising and in hot weather.

Notify your doctor or dentist that you are taking Zaroxolyn if you have a medical emergency and before you have surgery or dental treatment.

Possible food and drug interactions when taking this medication

Zaroxolyn may intensify the effects of alcohol. Avoid drinking alcohol while taking this medication.

If Zaroxolyn is taken with certain other drugs, the effects of either could be increased, decreased, or altered. It is especially important to check with your doctor before combining Zaroxolyn with the following:

ACTH
Antidiabetic drugs such as Micronase
Barbiturates such as phenobarbital
Corticosteroids such as prednisone
Digitalis glycosides such as Lanoxin
Insulin
Lithium
Loop diuretics, for example furosemide (Lasix)
Methenamine (Mandelamine)
Narcotics such as Percocet
Nonsteroidal anti-inflammatory agents
    such as Naprosyn
Norepinephrine (Levophed)
Other high blood pressure medications
Tubocurarine

Special information if you are pregnant or breastfeeding

The effects of Zaroxolyn during pregnancy have not been adequately studied. If you are pregnant or plan to become pregnant, inform your doctor immediately. Zaroxolyn appears in breast milk and could affect a nursing infant. If this medication is essential to your health, your doctor may advise you to discontinue breastfeeding until your treatment is finished.

Recommended dosage

ADULTS

Dosages of this medication should be adjusted to your individual needs. The lowest possible dose with the maximum effect should be used. The time required for this medication to become effective varies from patient to patient, depending on the diagnosis.

Most starting doses of this medication will be given 1 time per day.

Edema Due to Heart or Kidney Disorders
The usual dosage is 5 milligrams to 20 milligrams 1 time per day.

Mild to Moderate High Blood Pressure
The usual dosage is 2.5 milligrams to 5 milligrams 1 time per day.

CHILDREN

The safety and effectiveness of Zaroxolyn in children have not been established.

ELDERLY

Dosage should be determined by the particular needs of the elderly patient.

Overdosage

Any medication taken in excess can cause symptoms of overdose. If you suspect an overdose, seek medical attention immediately.

Symptoms of Zaroxolyn overdose may include:
Difficulty breathing
Dizziness
Dizziness on standing up
Drowsiness
Electrolyte imbalance
Excessive intestinal movement
Fainting
Irritation of the stomach and intestines
Lethargy leading to coma

Brand name:

ZESTRIL

Generic name: Lisinopril
Other brand name: Prinivil

Why is this drug prescribed?
Lisinopril is used in the treatment of high blood pressure. It is effective when used alone or when combined with other high blood pressure medications. Lisinopril is a type of drug called an ACE inhibitor. It works by inhibiting production of a substance that increases salt and water retention in your body.

Most important fact about this drug
In some patients it may take 2 to 4 weeks for lisinopril to complete the desired reduction in blood pressure.

How should you take this medication?
Lisinopril can be taken with or without food.

Take this medication exactly as prescribed by your doctor. Stopping lisinopril suddenly could cause your blood pressure to rise.

If you forget to take a dose, take it as soon as you remember. If it is almost time for your next dose, skip the one you missed and go back to your regular schedule. Never take two doses at the same time.

What side effects may occur?
Side effects cannot be anticipated. If any develop or change in intensity, inform your doctor as soon as possible. Only your doctor can determine if it is safe for you to continue taking lisinopril.

■ *More common side effects may include:*
Chest pain, cough, diarrhea, difficulty in breathing, dizziness, fatigue, headache, low blood pressure, nausea, rash, vomiting, weakness

■ *Less common or rare side effects may include:*
A drop in white blood cells, abdominal pain, back pain, blurred vision, bronchitis, changes in heart rhythm, confusion, constipation, decreased sex drive, depression, dry mouth, excessive sweating, fever, flushing, gas, gout, heart attack, hepatitis, hives, itching, impotence, inability to sleep, indigestion, inflammation of the pancreas, joint pain, kidney failure, loss of appetite, muscle cramps, nasal congestion, nervousness, prickling, burning sensation, rapid or pounding heartbeat, shoulder pain, sinus inflammation, sleepiness, stroke, urinary tract infection, vertigo, yellow eyes and skin

Why should this drug not be prescribed?
If you are sensitive to or have ever had an allergic reaction to lisinopril or similar drugs, you should not take this medication. Make sure that your doctor is aware of any drug reactions that you have experienced.

Special warnings about this medication
If you develop swelling of your face, lips, tongue or throat, or of your arms and legs, or have difficulty swallowing or breathing, you should contact your doctor immediately. You may need emergency treatment.

If you are taking lisinopril, a complete assessment of your kidney function should be done and kidney function should continue to be monitored.

If you are taking high doses of a diuretic (water pill) and lisinopril, you may develop excessively low blood pressure.

Lisinopril may cause some people to become dizzy, light-headed or faint, especially if they are taking a water pill at the same time. Do not drive, operate dangerous machinery, or participate in any hazardous activity that requires full mental alertness until you are certain lisinopril does not have this effect on you.

If you develop chest pain, sore throat, fever and chills, contact your doctor for medical attention.

Do not use salt substitutes containing potassium without first consulting with your doctor.

Excessive sweating, dehydration, severe diarrhea, or vomiting could cause you to lose too much water and cause your blood pressure to drop dangerously.

Possible food and drug interactions when taking this medication

If lisinopril is taken with certain other drugs, the effects of either could be increased, decreased, or altered. It is especially important to check with your doctor before combining lisinopril with any of the following:

Diuretics such as HydroDIURIL and Lasix
Indomethacin (Indocin)
Lithium
Potassium preparations
Potassium-sparing diuretics

Special information
if you are pregnant or breastfeeding

During the second and third trimester, lisinopril can cause birth defects, prematurity, and death in the fetus and newborn. If you are pregnant or plan to become pregnant and are taking lisinopril, contact your doctor immediately to discuss the potential hazard to your unborn child. Lisinopril may appear in breast milk and could affect a nursing infant. If this medication is essential to your health, your doctor may advise you to discontinue breastfeeding until your treatment with this medication is finished.

Recommended dosage

ADULTS

Hypertension
For patients not on diuretics, the initial starting dose is usually 10 milligrams, taken 1 time a day. After blood pressure is adjusted, dosage is usually 20 to 40 milligrams a day, taken in a single dose.

Diuretic use should, if possible, be stopped before using lisinopril. If not, your physician may give an initial dose of 5 milligrams under his supervision before any further medication is prescribed.

Patients with renal disorders must be carefully monitored, and dosages will be adjusted to the individual patient's needs, depending on kidney function.

CHILDREN

The safety and effectiveness of lisinopril in children have not been established.

ELDERLY

Dosage should be adjusted with caution. It is determined by the particular needs of the elderly patient.

Overdosage

Any medication taken in excess can cause symptoms of overdose. If you suspect an overdose, seek medical attention immediately.

A drop in blood pressure is the primary sign of a lisinopril overdose.

Generic name:

ZIDOVUDINE

See Retrovir, page 540.

Brand name:

ZITHROMAX

Generic name: Azithromycin

Why is this drug prescribed?

Zithromax is a new antibiotic that is related to erythromycin. This drug may be prescribed to treat certain mild to moderate skin infections; upper and lower respiratory tract infections, including pharyngitis (strep throat), tonsillitis, and pneumonia; and sexually transmitted infections of the cervix or urinary tract.

Most important fact about this drug

Zithromax may mask or delay symptoms of syphilis or gonorrhea. Before taking Zithromax to treat a sexually transmitted infection of the cervix or the urinary tract, your doctor should test you for syphilis and gonorrhea. If either test turns out positive, you will need additional medication to treat the syphilis or gonorrhea.

How should you take this medication?

Take Zithromax exactly as prescribed by your doctor. Avoid prolonged exposure to sun while taking this medication.

Take Zithromax at least 1 hour before or 2 hours after a meal. Do not take this medication with food, and do not take it with an antacid that contains aluminum or magnesium, such as Di-Gel, Gelusil, Maalox, and others.

Be sure to take all the Zithromax your doctor prescribes.

What side effects may occur?

Side effects cannot be anticipated. If any develop or change in intensity, inform your doctor as soon as possible. Only your doctor can determine if it is safe for you to continue taking Zithromax.

■ *More common side effects may include:*
Abdominal pain
Diarrhea
Loose stools
Nausea

■ *Less common side effects may include:*
Blood (dark) in the stools, chest pain, dizziness, drowsiness, fatigue, gas, headache, heart palpitations, indigestion, jaundice (yellowing of the skin and the whites of the eyes), light sensitivity, rash, severe allergic reaction including swelling (as in hives), sleepiness, vaginal inflammation, vertigo, vomiting

The single large dose (4 capsules) of Zithromax that is prescribed to treat sexually transmitted infection of the cervix or urinary tract is more likely to cause stomach and bowel side effects than the smaller doses prescribed for a skin or respiratory tract infection.

Why should this drug not be prescribed?

Do not take Zithromax if you have ever had an allergic reaction to it or to another macrolide antibiotic, such as erythromycin (for example, E.E.S., Erythrocin, and others).

If you have pneumonia, you should not be treated with Zithromax if:

Your pneumonia is severe;

You caught the pneumonia in a hospital or nursing home;

You have, or might have, bacteremia (infectious microbes in your blood);

You need to be in a hospital;

You are elderly or run down; or

Your general health is poor because of a damaged immune system.

Special warnings about this medication

Like other antibiotics, Zithromax may cause a potentially life-threatening form of diarrhea called pseudomembranous colitis. Pseudomembranous colitis may clear up spontaneously when the drug is stopped; if it does not, hospital treatment may be required.

If you have a liver problem, your doctor should monitor you very carefully while you arc taking Zithromax.

Possible food and drug interactions when taking this medication

If Zithromax is taken with certain other drugs, the effects of either could be increased, decreased, or altered. It is especially important to check with your doctor before combining Zithromax with the following:

Antacids containing aluminum or magnesium, such as Maalox and Mylanta

Carbamazepine (Tegretol)

Cyclosporine (Sandimmune)

Digoxin (Lanoxin, Lanoxicaps)

Ergot-containing drugs such as Cafergot and D.H.E.

Hexobarbital

Phenytoin (Dilantin)

Theophylline drugs such as Bronkodyl, Slo-Phyllin, Theo-Dur, and others

Triazolam (Halcion)

Warfarin (Coumadin, Panwarfin)

Special information if you are pregnant or breastfeeding

If you are pregnant or plan to become pregnant, inform your doctor immediately. You should take Zithromax during pregnancy only if it is clearly needed. It is not known whether Zithromax can make its way into breast milk. Caution is advised when taking Zithromax while breastfeeding.

Recommended dosage

ADULTS

The usual dose of Zithromax for patients age 16 years and older is 500 milligrams in a single dose the first day. This is followed by 250 milligrams one time each day for the next 4 days. The total amount taken should be 1.5 grams.

For treatment of non-gonococcal urethritis and cervitis (sexually transmitted disease) due to the organism *Chlamydia trachomatis,* take a single gram (1,000 milligrams) one time only.

CHILDREN

This medication is not recommended for children under age 16.

Overdosage

Although no specific information is available, any medication taken in excess can have serious consequences. If you suspect symptoms of an overdose of Zithromax, seek medical attention immediately.

Brand name:

ZOCOR

Generic name: Simvastatin

Why is this drug prescribed?

Zocor is a cholesterol-lowering drug. Your doctor may prescribe Zocor in addition to a cholesterol-lowering diet if your blood cholesterol level is too high, and if you have been unable to lower it by diet alone.

Most important fact about this drug

Before prescribing Zocor, your doctor will try to control your cholesterol level with a specific diet low in cholesterol and saturated fat, exercise, and weight reduction if you are obese. Your doctor will prescribe Zocor only when additional help is needed to lower high cholesterol levels. Zocor is effective only when you follow your prescribed diet and other measures, such as exercise.

How should you take this medication?

If your cholesterol level is too high, you should first try to lower it by diet, exercise, and weight reduction. Your doctor can give you guidelines for an acceptable cholesterol-lowering diet. Follow these guidelines closely.

Take Zocor exactly as prescribed.

Keep following your cholesterol-lowering diet, even when you are taking Zocor. Consider the medication an addition to the diet, not a substitute for the diet.

What side effects may occur?

Side effects cannot be anticipated. If any develop or change in intensity, inform your doctor as soon as possible. Only your doctor can determine whether it is safe for you to continue taking Zocor.

■ *More common side effects may include:*
Abdominal pain
Constipation, diarrhea
Gas
Headache
Muscle pain
Nausea
Upper respiratory infection
Upset stomach
Weakness

■ *Other potential side effects may include:*
Aching joints and muscles, altered sense of taste, anxiety, appetite loss, breast enlargement (in men), depression, difficulty moving eyes or facial muscles, diminished sex drive or sexual performance, dizziness, hepatitis, insomnia, memory loss, nerve pain or palsy, numbness or tingling, pancreatitis, progression of cataracts, tremor, vomiting

Why should this drug not be prescribed?

Do not take Zocor if you have ever had an allergic reaction to it or are sensitive to it.

Do not take Zocor if you have active liver disease.

Do not take Zocor if you are pregnant or plan to become pregnant.

Special warnings about this medication

Because Zocor may damage the liver, your doctor may order a blood test to check your liver enzyme levels before you start taking the drug. Blood tests will probably be done every 6 weeks for the first 3 months of treatment; every 8 weeks for the rest of the first year; and about every 6 months after that. If your liver enzyme levels rise too high, your doctor may tell you to stop taking Zocor.

While you are taking Zocor, your doctor should monitor you very closely if you have ever had liver disease or if you are, or have ever been, a heavy drinker.

Since Zocor may cause damage to muscle tissue, be sure to tell your doctor of any unexplained muscle tenderness or weakness right away, especially if you also have a fever or feel sick. Your doctor may want to do a blood test to check for signs of muscle damage.

To minimize the risk of getting muscle tissue damage from Zocor, you should not take Zocor at the same time as other cholesterol-lowering drugs, such as Atromid-S (clofibrate) or Lopid (gemfibrozil).

If your risk of muscle and/or kidney damage suddenly rises because of major surgery of injury, or a condition such as a severe infection or seizures, your doctor may tell you to stop taking Zocor for a while.

Possible food and drug interactions when taking this medication

If you take Zocor with certain other drugs, the effect of either could be increased, decreased, or altered. It is especially important to check with your doctor before combining Zocor with the following:

Blood-thinning drugs such as Coumadin
    and Dicumarol
Cimetidine (Tagamet)
Clofibrate (Atromid-S)
Cyclosporine (Sandimmune)
Digoxin (Lanoxin, Lanoxicaps)
Erythromycin (PCE and others)
Gemfibrozil (Lopid)
Ketoconazole (Nizoral)
Nicotinic Acid
Spironolactone (Aldactone, Aldactazide)

Special information if you are pregnant or breastfeeding

You must not become pregnant while taking Zocor. This drug lowers cholesterol, and cholesterol is needed for a baby to develop properly. Because of the possible risk of birth defects, your doctor will prescribe Zocor only if you understand this risk and only if you are highly unlikely to get pregnant while taking the drug. If you do become pregnant while taking Zocor, notify your doctor right away. Based on studies of other similar drugs, it is assumed that Zocor could appear in breast milk and could

cause severe adverse effects in a nursing baby. Do not take Zocor while breastfeeding your baby.

Recommended dosage

Patients should be placed on a standard cholesterol-lowering diet for 3 to 6 months before starting treatment with Zocor. Your doctor will determine whether you should continue this diet while using Zocor.

All doses should be adjusted to your individual needs.

ADULTS

The usual starting dose is 5 to 10 milligrams per day, taken as a single dose in the evening. The maximum recommended dose is 40 milligrams per day. Dosage adjustments may be made every 4 weeks, and dose levels should be reduced as cholesterol levels come down.

Patients with severe kidney disease should use Zocor with caution. The recommended dose is 5 milligrams per day with close monitoring.

Zocor may be used with other drugs. Your doctor will determine the proper dose based on your individual needs.

ELDERLY

Reduction of cholesterol in the elderly may be achieved with doses of 20 milligrams per day or less.

Overdosage

Although no specific information about Zocor overdose is available, any medication taken in excess can have serious consequences. If you suspect an overdose of Zocor, seek medical attention immediately.

Brand name:

ZOLOFT

Generic name: Sertraline

Why is this drug prescribed?

Zoloft is a relatively new type of antidepressant medication that is chemically similar to Prozac (fluoxetine).

Your doctor may prescribe Zoloft if you are suffering from major depression. Symptoms of major depression may include a persistent low mood, changes in appetite and sleep patterns, loss of interest in people and activities, concentration problems, guilt, anxiety, feelings of worthlessness, fatigue, agitation or lethargy, and perhaps thoughts of suicide.

Most important fact about this drug

Zoloft is not considered addictive and is not a controlled substance. However, since suicidal thoughts are common in acute depression, some depressed people may contemplate committing suicide by taking an overdose of Zoloft. To minimize the risk of facilitating a deliberate overdosage, your doctor may prescribe only a small amount of Zoloft at a time.

How should you take this medication?

Take Zoloft exactly as prescribed by your doctor: once a day, either in the morning or the evening.

Improvement with Zoloft may not be seen for several days to a few weeks.

Consult your doctor before taking nonprescription or other drugs with Zoloft.

Avoid alcoholic beverages while taking Zoloft.

What side effects may occur?

Side effects cannot be anticipated. If any develop or change in intensity, inform your doctor as soon as possible. Only your doctor can determine if it is safe for you to continue taking Zoloft.

- *More common side effects may include:*
  Confusion, diarrhea or loose stools, difficulty with ejaculation, dizziness, dry mouth, fatigue, headache, increased sweating, indigestion, insomnia, nausea, sleepiness, tremor

- *Less common side effects may include:*
  Abdominal pain, abnormal hair growth, abnormal skin odor, acne, agitation, altered taste, anemia, anxiety, apathy, back pain, bad breath, belching, black stools, breast development in males, bruise-like marks on the skin, chest pain, clumsiness, cold, clammy skin, conjunctivitis (pink eye), constipation, coughing, difficulty breathing, difficulty concentrating, difficulty swallowing, difficulty walking, dilated pupils, double vision, dry eyes, dry skin, earache, enlarged abdomen, eye pain, fainting, feeling faint upon arising from a sitting or lying position, fever, fluid retention, flushing, frequent urination, gas, hair loss, heart attack, hemorrhoids, hernia, hiccups, high blood pressure, hot flushes, increased appetite, increased salivation, inflammation of nose, throat, tongue or mouth, itching, joint pains, lack of coordination, lack of sensation, lethargy, loss of appetite, low blood pressure, menstrual problems, middle ear infection, migraine, muscle cramps or weakness, muscle pain, need to urinate during the night, nervousness, pain upon urination, pounding in chest, racing heartbeat, rash, ringing in the ears, sensitivity to light, skin eruptions or inflammation, sores on tongue, speech problems, stomach and intestinal inflammation, swelling around the eyes, swollen wrists and ankles, thirst, tingling or pins and needles, twitching, urinary

incontinence, urinary trouble, vertigo, vision problems, vomiting, weakness, weight loss or gain, yawning

■ *Zoloft may also cause mental or emotional symptoms such as:*
Abnormal dreams or thoughts, aggressiveness, apathy, delusion, euphoria, depersonalization ("unreal" feeling), hallucinations, memory loss, paranoia, rapid mood shifts, suicidal thoughts or attempted suicide, tooth-grinding, worsened depression

Many people lose a pound or two of body weight while taking Zoloft. This usually poses no problem but may be a concern if your depression has already caused you to lose a great deal of weight.

In a few people, Zoloft may trigger the grandiose, inappropriate, out-of-control behavior called mania or the similar, but less dramatic, "hyper" state called hypomania.

Why should this drug not be prescribed?
There are no known reasons to limit the use of this medication.

Special warnings about this medication
Do not take Zoloft if you have taken an MAO inhibitor type of antidepressant (such as Marplan, Nardil, or Parnate) within the past 14 days.

If you have a kidney or liver disorder, take Zoloft cautiously and under close medical supervision.

You should not drink alcoholic beverages while taking Zoloft.

Possible food and drug interactions when taking this medication
If Zoloft is taken with certain other drugs, the effects of either could be increased, decreased, or altered. It is especially important

to check with your doctor before combining Zoloft with the following:

Diazepam (Valium, Valrelease)
Lithium (Eskalith, Lithobid)
MAO inhibitors (antidepressant drugs such as Nardil, Parnate, and Marplan)
Other psychiatric drugs
Over-the-counter drugs (cold remedies, etc.)
Tolbutamide (Orinase)
Warfarin (Coumadin, Panwarfin)

**Special information
if you are pregnant or breastfeeding**
If you are pregnant or plan to become pregnant, inform your doctor immediately. Zoloft should be taken during pregnancy only if it is clearly needed.

It is not known whether Zoloft can make its way into breast milk. Caution is advised when using Zoloft during breastfeeding.

Recommended dosage

ADULTS

The usual recommended initial dose is 50 milligrams once a day, taken either in the morning or in the evening.

Your doctor may increase your dose depending upon your response. The maximum daily dose is 200 milligrams.

Overdosage
Although no specific information is available, any medication taken in excess can have serious consequences. If you suspect symptoms of an overdose of Zoloft, seek medical attention immediately.

Brand name:

ZOVIRAX

Generic name: Acyclovir

Why is this drug prescribed?
Zovirax capsules, tablets, and liquid are used in the treatment of certain infections with herpes viruses. These include genital herpes, shingles, and chickenpox. This drug may not be appropriate for everyone, and its use should be thoroughly discussed with your doctor. Zovirax ointment is used to treat initial episodes of genital herpes and certain herpes simplex infections of the skin and mucous membranes.

Most important fact about this drug
Zovirax does not cure herpes. However, it does reduce pain and may help the sores caused by herpes to heal faster. Genital herpes is a sexually transmitted disease. Intercourse and other sexual contact should be avoided when visible lesions are present to prevent infecting partners. Your medication should not be shared with others, and the prescribed dose should not be exceeded. Zovirax ointment should not be used in or near the eyes.

How should you take this medication?
Take this medication exactly as prescribed by your doctor.

What side effects may occur?
Side effects cannot be anticipated. If any develop or change in intensity, inform your doctor as soon as possible. Only your doctor can determine if it is safe for you to continue taking Zovirax.

■ *More common side effects may include:*
Confusion, constipation, diarrhea, dizziness, fever, fluid retention, general feeling of bodily discomfort, gland enlargement in the groin, hair loss, hallucinations, headache, hives, itching, medicinal taste, muscle pain, nausea, pain, skin rash, sleepiness, stomach and intestinal problems, tingling sensation, uneasy feeling, visual abnormalities, vomiting

■ *Less common side effects may include:*
Abdominal pain, diarrhea, dizziness, fatigue, gas, inability to sleep, leg pain, loss of appetite, sore throat

■ *Common side effects of Zovirax ointment may include:*
Burning
Itching
Mild pain
Skin rash
Stinging

Why should this drug not be prescribed?
If you are sensitive to or have ever had an allergic reaction to Zovirax or similar drugs, you should not take this medication. Make sure that your doctor is aware of any drug reactions that you have experienced.

Special warnings about this medication
Zovirax capsules, tablets, and liquid are for oral use only. If you are being treated for a kidney disorder, consult with your doctor before taking Zovirax. Although decreased sperm count has been reported in animals given high doses of Zovirax, this effect has not been documented to occur in humans.

Possible food and drug interactions when taking this medication
If Zovirax is taken with certain other drugs, the effects of either could be increased, decreased, or altered. It is important to check with your doctor before combining Zovirax with other medications, especially probenecid (Benemid), an antigout medication.

Special information
If you are pregnant or breastfeeding

The effects of Zovirax during pregnancy have not been adequately studied. If you are pregnant or plan to become pregnant, inform your doctor immediately. Zovirax appears in breast milk and could affect a nursing infant. If this medication is essential to your health, your doctor may advise you to discontinue breastfeeding your baby until your treatment with Zovirax is finished.

Recommended Dosage

ADULTS

For Genital Herpes
The usual dose is one 200-milligram capsule or 1 teaspoonful of liquid every 4 hours, 5 times daily for 10 days. If the herpes is recurrent, the usual adult dose is 400 milligrams (two 200-milligram capsules or 2 teaspoonfuls) 2 times daily for up to 12 months.

If genital herpes is intermittent, the usual adult dose is one 200-milligram capsule or 1 teaspoon of liquid every 4 hours, 5 times a day for 5 days. Therapy should be started at the earliest sign or symptom.

For Herpes Zoster (Shingles)
The usual adult dose is 800 milligrams (four 200-milligram capsules or 4 teaspoonfuls of liquid) every 4 hours, 5 times daily for 7 to 10 days.

If you have a kidney disorder, the dose will need to be adjusted by your doctor.

CHILDREN

The usual dose for chickenpox is 20 milligrams per 2.2 pounds of body weight, not to exceed 800 milligrams, taken orally 4 times daily for 5 days. Therapy should be initiated at the earliest sign or symptom.

The safety and effectiveness of Zovirax have not been established in children under 2 years of age. However, your doctor may decide that the benefits of this medication outweigh the potential risks.

ELDERLY

No special considerations apply.

Overdosage

Zovirax is generally safe; however, there have been cases of kidney disorder.

Any medication taken in excess can cause symptoms of an overdose. If you suspect an overdose, seek medical attention immediately.

Brand name:

ZYDONE

See Vicodin, page 678.

Brand name:

ZYLOPRIM

Generic name: Allopurinol
Other brand name: Lopurin

Why is this drug prescribed?

Allopurinol is used in the treatment of many types of gout, such as acute attacks, tophi (collection of uric acid crystals in the tissues, especially around joints such as the elbow), joint destruction, and uric acid stones. Gout is a form of arthritis characterized by increased blood levels of uric acid. Allopurinol works by preventing the formation of uric acid in the body, thus preventing crystals from forming.

Allopurinol is also used to manage the increased uric acid levels in the blood of patients with certain cancers, such as leukemia. It is also prescribed to manage some types kidney stones.

Most important fact about this drug
Because allopurinol may produce serious side effects, it should not be used for early-stage painless gout (i.e., high levels of uric acid in the blood, but no crystal deposits in the joints).

How should you take this medication?
Take allopurinol exactly as prescribed. Your doctor will probably start you on a low dosage, increasing it gradually each week until you reach the dosage that is best for you.

A typical starting dose is 1 tablet per day. You may want to take allopurinol immediately after a meal to minimize the risk of indigestion.

You should avoid taking large doses of vitamin C because of the increased possibility of kidney stone formation.

While taking allopurinol you should drink plenty of liquids—10 to 12 glasses (8 ounces each per day) unless otherwise prescribed by your doctor.

To help prevent attacks of gout, you should also avoid beer, wine, and purine-rich foods such as anchovies, sardines, liver, kidneys, lentils, and sweetbreads.

If you have been taking colchicine and/or an anti-inflammatory drug, such as Anaprox, Indocin, and others, to relieve your gout, your doctor will probably want you to continue taking this medication while your allopurinol dosage is being adjusted. Later, when you have had no attacks of gout for several months, you may be able to stop taking these other medications.

If you have been taking a drug that promotes the excretion of uric acid in the urine, such as probenecid (Benemid) or sulfinpyrazone (Anturane), to try to prevent attacks of gout, your doctor will probably want to reduce or stop your dosage of this drug while increasing your dosage of allopurinol.

What side effects may occur?
Side effects cannot be anticipated. If any develop or change in intensity, inform your doctor as soon as possible. Only your doctor can determine if it is safe for you to continue taking allopurinol.

Because a skin reaction, the most common side effect of allopurinol, may occasionally become severe or even fatal, you should stop taking Allopurinol if you notice even the beginnings of a rash. Such a rash may be itchy or scaly or may make your skin peel off in sheets; it may be accompanied by chills and fever, aching joints, or jaundice.

■ *More common side effects may include:*
Diarrhea
Nausea
Rash
Acute attack of gout

■ *Less common side effects may include:*
Abdominal pain, bruising, chills, drowsiness, fever, hair loss, headache, hives, indigestion, itching, joint pain, muscle ache, nose bleed, numbness, pins and needles sensation, rare skin condition characterized by severe blisters and bleeding on the lips, eyes, or nose, reddish-brown or purplish spots on skin, stomach upset, taste loss or perversion, tingling, unusual bleeding, vomiting, yellowing of skin and eyes

Why should this drug not be prescribed?
Do not take allopurinol if you have ever had a severe reaction to it in the past.

Special warnings about this medication

If you notice a rash or other signs of an allergic reaction, stop taking allopurinol immediately and consult your doctor. In some people, an allopurinol-induced rash may lead to a serious skin disease, generalized inflammation of a blood or lymph vessel, irreversible liver damage, or even death.

You may experience acute attacks of gout more often in the early stages of allopurinol therapy, even when normal uric acid levels have been attained. These attacks will become shorter and less severe after several months of therapy.

A kidney problem may turn a normal dose of allopurinol into an overdose. If you have a kidney disease, or a condition such as diabetes or high blood pressure that may affect your kidneys, your doctor should prescribe allopurinol cautiously and order periodic blood and urine tests to assess your kidney function.

Because allopurinol may make you drowsy, do not drive or perform hazardous tasks until you know how the medication affects you.

Possible food and drug interactions when taking this medication

If allopurinol is taken with certain other drugs, the effects of either could be increased, decreased, or altered. It is especially important to check with your doctor before combining allopurinol with the following:

Amoxicillin (Amoxil, Larotid, Polymox)
Ampicillin (Amcill, Omnipen, Polycillin, Principen)
Azathioprine (Imuran)
Mercaptopurine (Purinethol)
Sulfinpyrazone (Anturane)
Thiazide diuretics such as HydroDIURIL, Diuril, and others
Blood thinners such as Coumadin
Vitamin C
Drugs for diabetes such as Diabinese and Orinase
Theophylline (Theo-Dur, Slo-Phyllin, and others)

Special information if you are pregnant or breastfeeding

If you are pregnant or plan to become pregnant, notify your doctor immediately. Allopurinol should be taken during pregnancy only if it is clearly needed.

Allopurinol does make its way into breast milk; what effect it may have on a nursing baby is unknown. Caution is advised when allopurinol is taken during breastfeeding.

Recommended dosage

ADULTS

Your doctor will tailor the dosage of allopurinol individually to control the severity of symptoms and to bring the uric acid levels to normal or near normal.

Gout
The recommended initial dose is 100 milligrams once daily. Your doctor may increase your dose by 100 milligrams per day at 1-week intervals until desired results are attained. The usual average dose is 200 to 300 milligrams per day for mild gout and 400 to 600 milligrams daily for moderate to severe gout. The maximum recommended dose is 800 milligrams daily.

Recurrent Kidney Stones
The usual recommended dose is 200 to 300 milligrams daily, divided into smaller doses.

Management of Uric Acid Levels in Certain Cancers
The usual recommended dose is 600 to 800 milligrams daily for 2 to 3 days, together with high fluid intake.

CHILDREN

The usual recommended dose for children 6 to 10 years of age is 300 milligrams daily for the management of uric acid levels in certain types of cancer. Children under 6 years of age are generally given 150 milligrams daily.

Overdosage

Although no specific information is available regarding allopurinol overdosage, any medication taken in excess can have serious consequences. If you suspect symptoms of an overdose of allopurinol, seek medical attention immediately.

Disease Overviews

CHAPTER 1

New Hope
for Heart Patients

Each year heart disease kills twice as many people as cancer and eight times as many people as car accidents or infections. According to the annual National Health and National Nutrition Examination Survey, 43 percent of all deaths recorded each year are caused by heart and other "vascular diseases" such as stroke and kidney failure.

■ Heart disease alone kills more than 940,000 Americans a year.

■ Over 69 million Americans have high blood pressure, coronary heart disease, stroke, or rheumatic heart disease.

■ In 1991, the total U.S. medical costs for heart disease were $108 billion.

But the byword among cardiologists and researchers today is hope, tempered by the knowledge that we can and must do much more. The rate of heart disease in the U.S. is still among the highest in the world, due in part to lack of proper diet and exercise, and other unhealthy personal habits like cigarette smoking. So, the battle to defeat heart disease must be fought on two fronts: the research lab and our homes.

Our attention to changing the way we live—reducing personal stress and seeking early detection and treatment—has helped. From 1979 to 1989 the death rate from heart attacks actually declined 23.4 percent. Much of this progress is also due to a fast-paced revolution in the medicines used to treat and prevent heart attacks, strokes, high blood pressure, and related circulatory diseases that combine to produce high risks of death and disability in many individuals.

Exciting new therapies promise to stop heart attacks even before the patient reaches the hospital, reducing the need for expensive and hazardous coronary artery bypass surgery. Other new treatments promise to dissolve dangerous blood clots and reverse the crippling effects of strokes.

What actually happens when someone suffers a heart attack? What causes high blood pressure or angina (suffocating chest pains)? And why are these particular medicines effective against these and similar conditions?

This chapter and Chapter Two on high blood pressure will help you understand more about your heart medicines and why they can help you if you have heart disease.

What Is a Heart Attack?

The heart is a remarkably effective muscle. Consider that if your heart beats 80 times a minute, in a single year it will pump blood through your body approximately 42 million times. It also pumps blood through itself. Like any muscle, your heart must also receive a supply of blood in order to work properly.

WHAT IS A HEART?

The subject of song and verse, the heart was believed by the ancients to be the seat of the soul and the emotions. Even today we send "heart-shaped" cards (which aren't really shaped anything like hearts) on Valentine's Day and refer to broken-hearted lovers, but modern science tells us that hearts are about as romantic as your car's oil pump. In fact, the heart is a pump—a lumpy mass of muscle about the size of your fist that forces blood first through the lungs to pick up oxygen and then through the body to deliver that oxygen to the body's cells. That's a more mundane job than housing the soul, but vital nonetheless.

The rest of your circulatory system isn't much more difficult

VENA CAVA (Returns oxygen-depleted blood from the body)

AORTA (Delivers oxygenated blood to the body)

PULMONARY ARTERY (Conducts spent blood to the lungs)

RIGHT ATRIUM (Upper pumping chamber)

PULMONARY VEINS (Return oxygen-rich blood to the heart)

RIGHT VENTRICLE (Lower pumping chamber)

to understand than the heart. The arteries and veins are essentially tubing carrying the blood where it's needed around the body. But on closer inspection they turn out to be more than simple hoses.

Veins, for instance, have a series of valves that prevent blood from flowing backward as it returns to the heart. Arteries are really a combination of tubing and pump. The walls of the arteries are made up of layers of muscle that expand with every heartbeat and then rebound between heartbeats, giving the circulation an added boost.

The coronary arteries supply blood directly to the muscle tissue that makes up the heart. Like every other part of the body, the heart needs oxygen, and the coronary arteries' sole purpose is to supply it with oxygen-rich blood. They branch off from the aorta (the main artery that emerges from the heart) and snake along the surface of the heart itself.

To get an idea of how hard your heart works, try clenching and unclenching your fist and see how long you can keep it up. You'll quickly find that your hand and arm soon begin to ache. That ache signals that the muscles are overworked. Yet your heart keeps up that pace 24 hours a day, every day, year after year. So it's vitally important to keep a supply of fresh oxygenated blood coming to the heart through open, unclogged blood vessels. The blood vessels that supply your heart with blood are called coronary arteries.

A heart attack occurs when a portion of the heart muscle dies from lack of oxygen. Usually a problem in the coronary arteries is the cause. These arteries are narrow, and their pathway in the heart follows many twists and turns. For a variety of reasons, they tend to become blocked. When the supply of oxygenated blood they deliver is cut off or reduced, you feel pain, just as you did in your hand and arm. When the pain comes from your heart, it's called angina. You can have angina without having a full-blown heart attack, but angina is a danger signal that can mean serious heart disease.

When your arm got sore from squeezing your fist, you probably stopped and gave it a rest. Unfortunately, your heart can't stop for very long without death as the result. So to try to rest, it starts beating with less force, which results in less blood being circulated throughout the body. This causes some of the symptoms of what is commonly called a heart attack: clammy skin, pallor, and profuse perspiration. Along with the pain from the heart attack, there is general weakness as blood flow to the brain decreases. The person suffering the heart attack may feel dizzy or even lose consciousness. If coronary artery blockage is severe enough, the heart stops beating altogether, and, within a few minutes, death occurs.

Heart attacks can vary greatly in severity. The first attack may be mild, or severe enough to be disabling, or even fatal. Some people never experience a subsequent attack, while others experience several before succumbing to a fatal attack. Having a heart attack does not necessarily mean that you may die any minute of heart disease, but it is a strong signal that help is needed to reduce this possibility. So one of the major areas of cardiac research has been the reduction and prevention of coronary artery disease. As a result, we now have dozens of drugs to prevent and reduce the devastating effects of cardiovascular illnesses.

Your Arteries and Your Heart

What causes the blockages that prevent the heart from working efficiently? How can they be prevented or treated?

Like a system of supply highways running from the suburbs to the central city, the body's arteries are key to the survival of the heart muscle. Each person has miles of veins and arteries that circulate blood to the organs and muscles. Arteries are those blood vessels that carry oxygen-rich blood to the organs and tissues, while veins return blood to the heart. If the highways surrounding the city aren't well maintained, and debris is left along the sides or strewn along the road, traffic is slowed, and the supply system becomes inefficient.

The same problems develop in the body's blood supply system when fatty materials called **cholesterol** start to build up on the walls of the arteries. This narrows the vessels and stiffens their walls, leading to a condition called atherosclerosis. Like any highway with a closed lane, traffic slows to a crawl. But in this case, what is slowed is the life-sustaining flow of oxygen-rich blood, which creeps to a near standstill.

Together, the narrowing and the hardening of the arteries create a risk of high blood pressure, kidney failure, irregular heart rhythms, and stroke. If the blockage isn't treated, the blood flow slows and eventually stops, causing a heart attack. What makes

CLOGGED HIGHWAY TO THE HEART

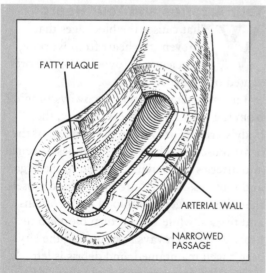

FATTY PLAQUE

ARTERIAL WALL

NARROWED PASSAGE

When fatty deposits of cholesterol and degenerate muscle cells build up on the inside walls of the coronary arteries, heart disease lies ahead. The buildup, known as atherosclerosis, reduces blood flow to the muscles of the heart, ultimately leading to angina. Worse yet, if a blood clot blocks the already narrowed passage, a heart attack may be the result.

matters worse is that the arteries clog gradually and produce few symptoms, if any, until it's too late. Often the presence of atherosclerosis may not be noticed, or diagnosed, until a stroke or a heart attack has occurred.

How We Treat Heart Disease

Beginning in the late 1950s, doctors began to make great strides in the fight against heart disease. In 1959, Swedish doctors implanted the first pacemaker in a 43-year-old man. In 1961, researchers at Johns Hopkins University found that a combination of simple and easily learned resuscitative techniques such as CPR could keep heart-attack victims alive long enough to get them to a hospital and more sophisticated care.

We have learned more about the causes of heart disease and the roles life-style and diet play. In addition, we have now refined surgical techniques like valve replacements and transplants to treat damaged hearts.

Researchers developing medications for heart disease have had a wide range of problems to deal with. We've needed drugs first to forestall heart and vascular disease, then to correct the resulting conditions. Many new drugs have been developed and tested. The first real breakthrough came with the discovery of a surprisingly versatile group of drugs called beta blockers, but we still find extremely useful some drugs discovered more than two centuries ago.

From Garden to Pharmacy: The Discovery of Digitalis

Digitalis (Digitoxin and Digoxin) is a drug class that was first discovered 200 years ago by Dr. William Withering in an ingredient in foxglove, a common flower in English

HEART FACTS

Is it possible to die of a broken heart? Yes, the stress that accompanies the loss of a loved one has, on more than one occasion, triggered a fatal heart attack. Researchers have found that other emotions also can affect the heart. Reducing stress, not only from heart and cardiovascular disease, but also from emotional sources, can be an important factor in improving overall health.

gardens. It was used to treat a condition called **dropsy**, which we know today as **congestive heart failure.** It occurs when an overworked heart can't pump enough blood to meet the body's circulatory needs.

A common symptom of congestive heart failure (and several other problems) is swelling, or edema, as doctors call it. This occurs because the kidneys can't eliminate salt from the body as efficiently as they once could. As salt concentrations build up, the body responds by increasing the amount of water in the blood and other body tissues, which causes swelling and puffiness, particularly in the ankles and feet.

Researchers in the 1930s, working with animals and with heart tissue, learned that digitalis affected the heart muscle by invigorating it and causing it to pump with more force. By beating more powerfully and pumping more blood with each beat, the heart doesn't have to beat as quickly. This also explains the drug's other effects. By strengthening the heartbeat, it almost magically reverses the symptoms of congestive heart failure. Blood passes through the kidneys more quickly, enabling them to eliminate the excess fluid and salt; a heart that has enlarged may shrink back toward its normal

size. The overall result is an improvement of circulation throughout the body.

Digitalis continues to be an extremely useful drug. Nonetheless, there are limits to what it can do. Today this drug and others may be combined in a comprehensive cardiac care program.

Quinidine: Remedy from the Past

Quinidine, another important cardiac drug, was discovered quite by chance. The setting was Vienna, just before the First World War. In 1912, a patient appeared at the office of Viennese physician Karl Wenkebach, complaining of an abnormal heartbeat.

Dr. Wenkebach could offer no cure. But, the man insisted a cure was possible, and he himself could provide it. Wenkebach protested; the man insisted. He would, he said, return the next morning with a regular heart rhythm. True to his word, he was back the next morning, and his heartbeat was normal, thanks to quinine, a drug already in wide use for the treatment of malaria.

That was how the *first* of the "antiarrhythmic" drugs that help restore a normal heartbeat was discovered. Today, doctors prefer to use quinidine—a close relative of quinine—rather than quinine itself, because smaller doses are effective and have fewer side effects.

Nitroglycerin: Help from the Test Tube

Nitroglycerin and related drugs trace their ancestry to the chemist's test tube. Amyl nitrite, first synthesized in 1844, was quickly found to cause flushing of the face due to the relaxation of the tiny blood vessels known as capillaries that connect arteries and veins. Twenty-three years later, a young Scottish medical student by the name of Thomas Lauder Brunton suspected that amyl nitrite might also relieve angina by increasing blood flow to the heart. He was right, as he found when he tried the drug on some of his patients. It wasn't long before nitroglycerin, which is chemically similar to amyl nitrite, was discovered to have a similar effect, relaxing the smooth muscles that make up your veins and arteries and allowing them to dilate. Both drugs are still used for treatment of angina, but nitroglycerin is by far the more common, because it is more easily administered and has fewer side effects.

One new way of delivering nitroglycerin (as well as some other drugs) is by means of a **transdermal patch.** For years doctors have known that nitroglycerin is easily absorbed into the bloodstream through the skin. There are nitroglycerin ointments that can be spread on the skin, tablets that are held under the tongue or in the cheek until they dissolve, and capsules that can be swallowed. The advantage of transdermal patches, which look like big adhesive bandages, is that they regulate the delivery of the drug, providing a constant amount of it for as long as 24 hours at a time.

Other **vasodilators** employed to relax the muscles in the arterial walls are more fully discussed in "Defusing High Blood Pressure," page 721.

There are also drugs used specifically for treating the complications of atherosclerosis elsewhere in the body. One, pentoxifylline (Trental), is known as a hemorrheologic agent and helps reduce the cramping that blocked arteries can cause when blood supply to the legs and feet are cut off.

Beta Blockers:
The First Family of Heart Medicines

Various nerve systems in the body stimulate the activity of the heart. The beta-adrenergic system was discovered to be involved in irregular heartbeats. Scientists began looking for a drug that would block the activity of this system and ended up with a drug that became one of the most valuable medications we have.

Propranolol (Inderal) is the granddaddy of the beta-blocker family, and the first of its class to be approved by the Food and Drug Administration (FDA) for use in the United States. At the time of approval, no one knew that propranolol would someday come to play a starring role in the treatment of heart disease. Few suspected that within 15 years it would become one of the most prescribed drugs in America.

In 1967, its sole approved use was for treatment of irregular heartbeats (arrhythmias). Since then the FDA has expanded the approved uses of the drug to include treatment of angina, high blood pressure, and migraine headaches. Doctors have also researched its value for unapproved uses including anxiety and serious thyroid disease.

These multiple uses would have qualified propranolol as one of the most versatile drugs ever discovered, but its most important use was yet to come.

Despite the technology in modern coronary care units, and advances in treatment, doctors knew that people who'd had one heart attack were at increased risk for a second, which could strike at any time, anywhere, far from the help that had been only seconds away while they were in the hospital. And yet doctors couldn't keep their patients

CPR SAVES THE DAY

Cardiopulmonary resuscitation, or CPR as it's usually called today, has saved countless lives and is taught in high schools, community centers, and company cafeterias. It's also taught to hospital employees and has become a mainstay of "code blue" techniques that bring hospitalized patients back from the threshold of death.

in the hospital, waiting for a subsequent heart attack that might never come.

In 1981, cardiologists conducting a study of propranolol found that it helped prevent second heart attacks, and that it reduced mortality rates among heart patients by 26 percent. They were so excited by this discovery that they ended the study nine months early, believing it would be unethical to withhold the drug from the control group of patients. The study's sponsor, the National Heart, Blood, and Lung Institute, estimated that appropriate use of the drug could save hundreds of thousands of lives a year in the United States alone. Thus, propranolol and other drugs in the beta-blocker class have become extremely useful in reducing the pain and suffering of heart disease.

The Calcium Channel Blockers

When verapamil (Isoptin, Calan), the first calcium channel blocker, was approved by the FDA in 1982, its sole use was for the treatment of arrhythmias (irregular heartbeats), and often it wasn't even the drug of first choice for that condition. If your doctor wanted to give you verapamil, you'd have to be in the hospital to get it, since it was only available in an injectable form. In fact, verapamil was thought to be so unpromising that nobody thought much about how it worked or what beneficial effects it might have other than controlling irregular heartbeats.

This situation changed when cardiologists began to study propranolol and the other beta blockers. Their success with these drugs prompted increased research into other drugs that act upon the heart. When researchers began looking around, they found that verapamil had a lot more potential benefits to offer heart disease victims than anyone had ever guessed.

Your heartbeat is controlled by tiny electrical impulses; that's why doctors sometimes use electronic pacemakers to regulate hearts that don't beat the way they should. Calcium plays a key role in regulating the heart's response to these electrical signals. It flows between the heart cells and surrounding fluid through a sort of chemical revolving door—the calcium channel. The more calcium that gets through the door before the electrical signal comes, the more strongly the heart contracts and the harder it works. Calcium channel blockers, like verapamil and its cousins, don't quite "lock" the revolving door, but they significantly slow it down. This eases the load on a damaged heart and, for many patients, improves heart functioning.

If you suffer from angina, you'll be interested to know that calcium channel blockers have turned out to be among the most effective antianginal medications ever discovered. They help your heart work with less effort; and at the same time, they relax the coronary arteries, improving the supply of oxygen-

THE ROLE OF ADRENALINE

The so-called fight-or-flight response is governed by a complex series of interactions between your mind and body. When your brain perceives a threat, it automatically tells your adrenal glands—small organs that sit atop your kidneys—to start pumping out adrenaline.

The adrenaline, in turn, quickly travels through your bloodstream to all parts of your body, acting as a sort of chemical Paul Revere to warn them that they may soon be called upon to do their best. Your digestive system shuts down, and blood is diverted to the brain, helping you think more quickly. Your muscles are primed to work at peak efficiency—hence the muscular tension that results in shaky knees and twitching muscles—and your breathing becomes faster, bringing more oxygen to the blood. All of this activity is geared to help you either fight or run away. If you decide to fight, the response helps you move and think quickly—to literally stay on your toes. If you decide to run, adrenaline gives you added speed and endurance.

Now let's look specifically at what happens to your heart and cardiovascular system when all that adrenaline hits it.

When you're under stress, your heart starts pounding much harder and faster than usual. That tells you it's working a lot harder, which in turn means it's going to need more oxygen. At the same time, the adrenaline is causing your arteries to squeeze tighter. There are two results. First, your heart has to work that much harder to pump blood through the narrowed arteries, and second, the coronary arteries can't deliver as much oxygen-enriched blood to the heart as usual.

In the normal, healthy person, these effects aren't dangerous, but if the heart is diseased or damaged, they can be disastrous. If the coronary arteries of a diseased heart tighten up, you'll feel pain (angina) which tells you that your heart is starved for oxygen. If they tighten more, or if the heart has to work harder, the oxygen shortage becomes even more severe. The heart falters—parts of it may even die from lack of oxygen—and you experience a heart attack.

enriched blood to the heart itself. The result is almost as if the drug told your heart to sit back, relax, and take a few deep breaths.

Calcium Blockers and the Future

What about the future of this new class of drugs? Researchers are still exploring their potential, and some promising possibilities include the prevention of heart attacks and slowing of atherosclerosis. Other possible uses include treatment of migraine headaches, Raynaud's phenomenon (a condition in which arteries in the extremities spasm, causing pallor), menstrual cramps, and premature labor. Researchers also speculate that calcium channel blockers may someday help

in the treatment of strokes, spinal-cord injuries, certain types of kidney failure, and even cancer.

Cholesterol-Reducing Drugs

One in four Americans is at higher risk for heart disease because of elevated cholesterol levels which are either inherited or acquired due to diet or another disease. Over the past 20 years, physicians and researchers have recognized that high cholesterol levels in both men and women are an important risk factor in cardiovascular diseases. (See your physician to evaluate your own risk levels.) While cholesterol levels can be controlled somewhat by diet alone, adding a medication is the most effective way of lowering them.

Cholesterol-lowering drugs act by preventing the body from manufacturing cholesterol, reducing absorption of dietary cholesterol, or combining with cholesterol to remove it from the bloodstream. Common cholesterol-lowering drugs are niacin, lovastatin (Mevacor), cholestyramine (Questran), gemfibrozil (Lopid), and probucol (Lorelco).

Hope for the Future: Unblocking Clogged Arteries

Heart attacks usually occur because the coronary arteries become clogged by a blood clot, and some of the most promising new drugs work to unclog them directly. These drugs offer an alternative to coronary artery bypass surgery, in which surgeons take lengths of veins from a patient's leg or chest wall and attach them to the coronary arteries to provide a "detour" around blockages.

While bypass surgery can prevent a heart attack, it's no help for patients who come to the hospital in the midst of an acute heart attack. However, three drugs, t-PA (Activase), streptokinase (Streptase), and anistreplase (Eminase), are now being used to open clogged arteries during and after an attack.

These medications work by dissolving blood clots. Blood passing through arteries filled with arterial plaque tends to clot, cutting off the blood supply to tissues downstream.

Depending upon where they create a blockage, blood clots can cause strokes, heart attacks, or life-threatening pulmonary emboli (blockages in the lung). If these clot-dissolving drugs can be given quickly enough, they can reverse these conditions before heart muscle or lung tissue dies from lack of oxygen.

Streptokinase was the first of these drugs to be used. Sometimes it is used in combination with a technique known as percutaneous transluminal coronary angioplasty (PTCA) that reduces blockages.

Tissue-Plasminogen Activator, or t-PA, was the first "genetically engineered" drug to show promise as a post-heart attack treatment. Scientists created this medication by "splicing" genes together. The drug dissolves clots in as little as 10 minutes—a mere fraction of the time streptokinase needs to work. And since t-PA is derived from human cells, not bacteria, it doesn't stimulate the body's immune system.

Studies of these drugs show that the sooner they are administered, the more effective they will be. In the future, these drugs may be used by Emergency Medical Teams when heart attack victims are being transported to the hospital, thus preventing even more deaths. □

CHAPTER 2

Defusing High Blood Pressure

High Blood Pressure or Hypertension is the most common chronic illness in America. The American Heart Association estimates that more than 62 million Americans over the age of six suffer from high blood pressure, and that only a minority of these people have their blood pressure under control. Many don't know they have hypertension, and go untreated, since you can have the disease for years before any symptoms develop. And, because you can be symptom-free, many people think high blood pressure is harmless.

Nothing, in fact, could be further from the truth! Left untreated, hypertension can lead to stroke, heart attack, kidney damage, congestive heart failure, and death.

Uncontrolled mild-to-moderate hypertension will reduce the life expectancy of a typical 35-year-old person by 16 years. Even the mildest form of high blood pressure, "borderline hypertension," can cut your life span by two to four years.

The good news is that more Americans each year are being diagnosed earlier—in routine physicals, workplace screening programs, and health education classes.

Because of extensive research, high blood pressure is actually one of the easiest diseases to diagnose. Breakthroughs in drug treatment described below have saved millions of lives.

What Is Blood Pressure?

Blood pressure is the measure of the force of your blood moving through your body's "circulatory system." This complex network of veins and arteries contains blood vessels that can be as large as a banana or so narrow that blood cells can barely squeeze through them. Ideally, your blood flows through almost 100,000 miles of arteries and veins in a smooth stream—much like water flowing through your home's faucets into the sink or tub.

Within your body, the beats of your heart create a pressure-driven force that sends your blood moving through the body's arterial pathways in a steady, pulsating rhythm. This "force" is measured to determine your blood pressure level.

With each beat, your heart contracts, sending out a "surge" of pressure into the bloodstream. This surge period is called **"systolic"** from a Greek word meaning "to contract." After the pressure surge, your heart rests for a brief time and "expands" to get ready for another beat. The arteries that have received the surge of blood now rebound, forcing it further through the system. This is called the **"diastolic"** or "expansion" period.

Doctors measure your blood pressure during each of these periods. They often say "your pressure is 120 over 80," or some other combination of numbers. This first number is a measure of the "systolic push" of the heartbeat on the blood. The second number is the "diastolic" measurement of the pressure in your arteries as blood continues to flow through the system while the heart is at rest.

Finding this measurement is easy. Anyone can do it with a simple home monitoring device called a *sphygmomanometer* or blood pressure cuff. Your doctor's device may be a little more sophisticated—with a cuff, a stethoscope, and a pressure gauge—but they all work pretty much the same way. When your pressure is measured, this cuff is tightened to cut off the circulation momentarily. The cuff is loosened, and as the blood begins to flow again, the device measures the systolic and diastolic forces. The measurement is expressed in numbers as though they were a fraction (e.g., 140/90).

What Do We Mean by "You have high blood pressure"?

After years of study and research around the world, medical experts have reached certain agreements on "average levels" of blood pressure. If your doctor says you have hypertension, or "high blood pressure," he is actually comparing your blood pressure levels with the "normal" or average blood pressure of people of your age and sex.

LIVING WITH HIGH BLOOD PRESSURE

- Have your pressure monitored frequently—learn to do it yourself.
- Never skip a dose of medication without talking to your doctor. Don't let your prescription run out.
- Report any side effects to your doctor.
- Make your lifestyle changes gradually—but make them.
- Reduce your stress, follow a sensible diet, and get plenty of exercise.

Most physicians agree that in adults, a systolic reading of 100 to 140 and a diastolic reading of 70 to 90 is normal. A reading slightly above those limits—140 to 159 over 90 to 94—is considered mild hypertension. Readings from 160 to 179 over 94 to 114 indicate moderate hypertension. Anything above those limits represents serious high blood pressure. (Blood pressure readings in children vary greatly, and only a physician can determine a "normal" reading for an infant or child.) In general, at least two blood pressure readings should be taken on each of three separate days before a diagnosis of high blood pressure is given.

It's important to remember that high blood pressure is a disease not of the heart but of the arteries. And arterial pressure changes constantly. Normally, blood pressure drops when you sleep and rises when you are subjected to stress, startled by a loud noise, or threatened.

This temporary rise in pressure is the natural result of a complex chemical reaction in the body; and when the events that triggered it subside, your pressure should return to normal. If it doesn't—if it remains high all of the time—it means there is something wrong with your arterial pathways; and you have "hypertension."

What Causes High Blood Pressure?

There are two types of high blood pressure: **primary** (or **"essential"**) **hypertension** and **secondary hypertension**. Although the exact cause of primary hypertension isn't known, contributing factors include heredity, obesity, lack of exercise, diet—including salt intake— cigarette smoking, sex, race, age, and even personality. Over 90 percent of all hypertensives fall into the primary category. Secondary hypertension may be linked to kidney disease, endocrine disorders, the use of oral contraceptives, and excessive use of alcohol.

There is some evidence that continual stress can trigger biochemical changes within the body that raise blood pressure and keep it high. However, the common myth that "nerves" or "a case of the jitters" can bring on hypertension simply isn't true. High blood pressure is a disease; and even though it is often "silent," it must be treated promptly, exactly as directed by your physician.

Changes in the arteries can complicate the problem. Normally the arteries are rather springy; in addition to expanding and contracting in rhythm with the heart, they adjust themselves to the volume of the blood and to other conditions within the body, stretching or tightening up as necessary to raise, lower, or maintain blood pressure. Various factors—stress, for instance—as well as diet, heredity, lifestyle, and aging, have a detrimental effect on the arteries. They become less elastic and thus less able to adjust to changes in the body; and they tend to become coated with arterial cholesterol plaque, a fatty deposit that clogs them, just as deposits in your house's pipes can cause your sink to back up.

This condition, called atherosclerosis, can obstruct coronary arteries, and can lead to a stroke if arteries that supply blood to the brain become blocked.

Drugs That Bring Down Pressure

If high blood pressure is identified early enough, when it is still in its very mildest stages, the first line of defense is an attempt to modify the risk factors associated with it. Of course, we can't do anything about our heredity, age, race, or sex; but we can lose weight, exercise more, stop smoking, and improve our eating habits. We may even be able to alter our personality; your doctor can recommend programs intended to teach Type-A personalities (the hard-driven, success-oriented types who start blowing their horns before the traffic light has changed) how to become easy-going, Type-B personalities.

In most cases, however, the mainstay of treatment is medication. It brings blood pressure down quickly and keeps it down. And although it doesn't cure the disease (if it's discontinued, blood pressure almost always shoots back up), it does prevent the serious and even life-threatening complications that can result if high blood pressure is left untreated.

The first step is usually a prescription for one of four types of medication: a diuretic, a beta blocker, an ACE (angiotensin converting enzyme) inhibitor, or a calcium channel blocker. If these drugs, either alone or in combination, fail to bring blood pressure under control, other classes of drugs may be prescribed.

Here's a closer look at some of these drugs.

Diuretics make it difficult for the kidneys to retain both water and salt, which are then filtered out into the urine. Increasing the amount of urine reduces the amount of fluid in the bloodstream, which in itself reduces blood pressure. It's like turning on a second faucet in your house and watching the water pressure drop in the first—not a subtle mechanism, to be sure, but it works.

Because some important chemicals may be washed out along with the water and salt, a doctor may prescribe supplements—most commonly a potassium supplement—to go with the diuretic.

Beta blockers (discussed in detail in Chapter One) reduce high blood pressure by throttling back the force and speed of the heart. They may also reduce blood pressure by a direct effect on the body's master controls, the central nervous system (CNS).

ACE inhibitors, which include captopril (Capoten), lisinopril (Prinivil), and enalapril (Vasotec), block the production of angiotensin, a chemical the body produces to *raise* blood pressure. Angiotensin's normal role is to maintain equilibrium when blood pressure drops. It acts directly on the arteries, tightening them up to raise the pressure. The angiotensin antagonists can bring blood pressure down quickly but can cause kidney damage and, rarely, a reduction in the number of white blood cells (leading to an increased susceptibility to infection). Thus, they must be used with caution.

Calcium channel blockers (see page 717), like so many of the other drugs used for hypertension, act by relaxing the arteries and reducing resistance to the flow of blood. They have proven to be beneficial not only for high blood pressure, but also for angina and other problems of a weakened heart. Included in this group are drugs such as diltiazem (Cardizem), isradipine (DynaCirc), and verapamil (Calan).

In addition to these four major types of blood pressure medication, there are other potent drugs that work directly on the muscles that make up arterial walls, causing them to relax and thus lower blood pressure. These "vasodilators" are closely related to the alpha adrenergic blocking agents (see below); in fact, there's some overlap between the two groups. There are three classes of oral vasodilators whose specific effects have been found to be most useful: hydralazine (Apresoline), minoxidil (Loniten), and prazosin (Minipress).

Alpha adrenergic blocking agents inhibit both the production and the effect of adrenalin, a potent stimulator released by the body in response to stress. Too much adrenaline can overexcite the circulatory system, causing blood pressure to rise. The most potent effect of alpha blockers is not upon the heart but upon the arteries, causing the muscles in the arterial walls to relax.

Though many of the blood pressure drugs are the result of major scientific breakthroughs, it's all too easy to underestimate their value. There's nothing very magical about the way they work, and they don't, on a day-to-day level, make patients feel demonstrably better. In fact, because hypertension is so often a disease without symptoms, we're usually more aware of the drugs' side effects and inconvenience than of their life-saving properties. But in terms of the number of patients helped, and the number of years added to these patients' lives, these drugs rank among the most important of any in use today. If hypertension is, as it's sometimes called, the "silent killer," then these drugs deserve the title "silent saviors." □

CHAPTER 3

Coping with Arthritis

Arthritis has plagued mankind for millennia. Historians have found references to forms of arthritis in Greek and Roman literature, and some even suspect cavemen suffered from it. Today it's so widespread that one in seven people and one in three families are affected by it. More than 37 million Americans of all ages are victims. Frequently we ignore arthritis, calling it simply the "aches and pains" of old age. Or we self-medicate with painkillers, not bothering to seek professional treatment. But make no mistake: Arthritis is a serious, potentially crippling, and even fatal disease. The early warning signs should never be ignored.

Some Arthritis Facts

■ Women are more likely than men to suffer from arthritis. The disease becomes more prevalent after age 45. Yet it is not a disease exclusively of the elderly, for more than 200,000 children are also affected.

■ Arthritis is a costly disease: It's the leading cause of absenteeism; 45 million work days are lost each year.

■ The estimated yearly cost in lost wages and medical bills is $35 billion (equivalent to one percent of the gross national product).

■ Arthritis patients average eight visits to their doctor each year—twice as many as those suffering from other chronic illnesses like high blood pressure.

■ Approximately six million people are "self-diagnosed" and improperly "self-treated."

What Is Arthritis?

Arthritis" literally means "*inflamed joints.*" It is an umbrella term for more than 100 different forms of joint disease. However, while arthritis primarily affects the joints, it also attacks muscles and connective tissues surrounding organs. Arthritic disease stems from injuries, defects in the immune system, wear and tear on the joints, infections, or genetic predisposition. Whatever the cause, the effect is much the same in all individuals: Where bones meet in the joints, they are actually disintegrating.

Imagine a machine with well-oiled parts working smoothly, all valves pumping, all parts meshing together. Then, for some reason, one part bends, or the lubricating fluid dries up. Over a period of time, the parts begin to wear down or grind together until something gives way. For a variety of reasons, this is what happens in the joints of your arms, legs, hips, and even your back when they become arthritic. Some forms of arthritis do affect other parts of the body—skin, eyes, and various organ systems—and doctors watch for these symptoms in all patients with arthritic disease.

Many people believe that medicine's only answer for arthritis is use of strong prescription painkillers. And so they "self-medicate," follow "alternative diets," or try unproven "miracle" treatments such as copper bracelets or bee stings. Because arthritis is a disease that frequently comes and goes, these non-medical cures often seem to work. In fact, their success is merely a coincidence.

Fortunately, legitimate therapy is *not* limited to a few potent painkillers. There are many safe and effective medications for arthritis that, when combined with physical therapy, some dietary changes, and regular exercise, can enable most patients to lead normal lives.

How Do We Treat Arthritis?

Arthritis treatment is determined by the type you have. In general, however, the front line therapy is an analgesic like *aspirin or acetaminophen* or a member of a group of medications called *nonsteroidal anti-inflammatory drugs, or NSAIDs*. Most arthritis sufferers rely on NSAIDs for daily pain relief. While aspirin is still widely used, NSAIDs have fewer gastric side effects and are longer-acting than aspirin, so you have to take fewer pills each day. Strong anti-inflammatory medications such as corticosteroids or immunosuppressive drugs may also be used.

Here's a rundown of treatments for each form of arthritis:

Osteoarthritis (OA)

Most people will suffer from some form of OA as they grow older, and the joints naturally age through wear and tear. The most notable symptom, a dull aching feeling in the joints, usually appears toward the end of the day. The joints most commonly affected are in the hands, knees, fingers, spine, hips, neck, and feet. OA is a progressive disease and is not usually reversible. However, medication can relieve the symptoms.

Treatment for OA usually starts with a mild drug such as acetaminophen (Tylenol) or aspirin taken every four to six hours as

THE FIVE BASIC TYPES OF ARTHRITIS

1. Osteoarthritis: The most common form, this disease affects 15.8 million Americans (usually over age 45).
2. Rheumatoid Arthritis: Affects more than 2.1 million people, mostly women.
3. Gout: More frequent among men, with an estimated one million victims.
4. Ankylosing Spondylitis (Spinal Arthritis): More than 300,000 patients, also mostly males.
5. Systemic Lupus Erythematosus: Affecting 131,000 people, usually women.
Other, less common forms include Juvenile Rheumatoid Arthritis, Scleroderma and Arthritis Due to Infection.

needed. As the disease progresses, symptoms become more severe, and an NSAID such as ibuprofen (Motrin), indomethacin (Indocin), or naproxen (Naprosyn) may be substituted.

If OA pain becomes especially severe, a doctor will sometimes prescribe a short course of narcotic pain relievers such as Tylenol with Codeine. When joints become inflamed, injections of corticosteroids such as cortisone or prednisone can be effective.

Finally, a real exercise program—swimming, golf, walking, tennis, range-of-motion exercises (such as stretching)—is as valuable as medication in keeping joints flexible and mobile. Weight loss to relieve extra stress on joints is also vital to OA care.

Rheumatoid Arthritis (RA)

Between the ages of 30 and 50, eight times as many women as men develop this crippling form of arthritis. Although we don't know why it develops, researchers suspect that victims have a genetic predisposition.

Unlike OA, RA symptoms are more pronounced in the morning—the joints and muscles tend to stiffen up overnight as you sleep. RA patients may develop swelling in the joints; and this may lead to deformities and, ultimately, total immobility. RA patients may also develop such related symptoms as fever, fatigue, and loss of appetite.

Drug treatment of RA begins with the same types of medications used for OA: aspirin, NSAIDs, and, occasionally, steroids. If these drugs fail to control joint inflammation, other, more potent medications are prescribed. Although we don't know why, an antimalarial drug called hydroxychloroquine (Plaquenil) is known to reduce RA inflamma-

tion. While the drug seems to work well, it has potentially serious side effects that can cause vision problems, so careful monitoring by your physician and eye doctor is important. Gold salts, injected on a weekly or biweekly basis, can reduce joint inflammation, but, again, serious side effects make them impractical for many patients. Another drug—penicillamine (Depen)—works much like gold salts in reducing symptoms and retarding disease in severe cases of RA, and may cause fewer side effects.

Researchers today are exploring the role that immunosuppressive drugs can play in the treatment of RA. One, azathioprine (Imuran), is approved for use in RA cases. A second, methotrexate (Rheumatrex), is now frequently prescribed as well. Immunosuppressants are very powerful drugs and are used only in extremely serious cases where all else has failed. However, the drugs do relieve joint inflammation very effectively, and may even be lifesavers for patients with severe complications.

Like other forms of arthritis, RA should be treated by both medication and physical therapy, which can help restore some of the lost joint function. Surgical procedures such as hip and knee replacements have enabled many patients to return to a more fully functional lifestyle.

Gout

Gout, one of the most painful forms of arthritis, is found primarily in men. While we can't cure it, we do have several highly effective treatments to control it. The symptoms of gout are often centered in the big toe, causing it be become swollen and extremely painful; but any joint may be affected. Pain usually occurs when the body is unable to

HOW ARTHRITIS DISABLES THE JOINTS

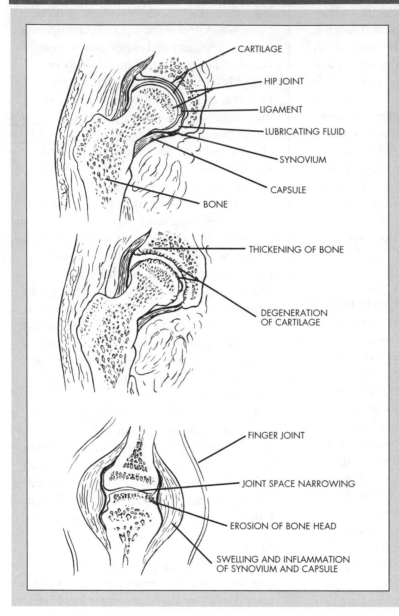

CARTILAGE

HIP JOINT

LIGAMENT

LUBRICATING FLUID

SYNOVIUM

CAPSULE

BONE

THICKENING OF BONE

DEGENERATION
OF CARTILAGE

FINGER JOINT

JOINT SPACE NARROWING

EROSION OF BONE HEAD

SWELLING AND INFLAMMATION
OF SYNOVIUM AND CAPSULE

Normal joint: Where two bones meet, our bodies normally provide a simple and effective lubricating system. Ligaments binding the bones together form a capsule within which a thin membrane called the synovium exudes a fluid lubricant. For good measure, the ends of both bones are cushioned by a smooth layer of cartilage.

Osteoarthritis: In this form of arthritis, trouble begins when the protective cushion of cartilage between the bones slowly degenerates. As it disappears, the synovium and the ends of the bones thicken within the joint, leading to the aching stiffness that characterizes the disease.

Rheumatoid arthritis: The culprit here is the synovium, which for unknown reasons becomes swollen and inflamed, leading to irreversible damage to the joint's capsule and protective cartilage. Eventually the unprotected ends of the bones themselves begin to erode.

eliminate uric acid, a waste product normally in the blood. If your body produces too much uric acid, or your kidneys aren't working properly to excrete it, an acute gout attack can follow.

Through the ages gout was known as the "disease of kings" because it was believed that a rich (man's) diet caused the disease. This myth is partially true. Diets high in purines (organ meats, fish eggs, sardines, anchovies, beer, and wine) can aggravate gout—but only in people who have trouble dealing with uric acid. Likewise, eliminating these foods may help reduce chances of an attack, but won't cure the underlying cause. Alcohol, too, can cause an attack or make one worse. Your diet and drinking habits should be fully discussed with your doctor when you begin treatment.

In general, gout is controlled or prevented by a number of specific medications that reduce the inflammation caused by the crystal-like deposits of uric acid that form in the toe, or other areas, and precipitate an attack.

Colchicine, a drug developed from the crocus plant, is among the best known anti-gout drugs. It provides quick relief during a gout attack and is also used preventively. In addition, there are two types of second-line treatment: Drugs that lower uric acid levels by increasing output, such as probenecid (Benemid) and sulfinpyrazone (Anturane), and drugs like allopurinol (Zyloprim) that prevent uric acid production. These medications are often supplemented with NSAIDs during acute attacks.

Ankylosing Spondylitis (AS)

Ankylosing spondylitis (AS), or spinal arthritis, literally means "fused spine," since its basic symptom is an inability to bend the spinal column. Primarily afflicting men, this form of arthritis usually causes severe pain where the base of the spine connects to the pelvis. During the course of the disease, inflammation actually destroys the flexible joints in the lower spine. A certain genetic marker called HLA B-27 signals an increased risk of AS. Patients first experience pain in the lower back and buttocks, fever, and fatigue. Later, they may develop a stooped-over posture. Inflammation of the eyes and valvular heart disease may also occur.

The good news is that most cases of AS are relatively mild and can be treated with NSAIDs and a regular physical therapy program.

Systemic Lupus Erythematosus (SLE or Lupus)

Though not itself a form of arthritis, lupus is linked to arthritis in more than half the cases. Its victims are teenage girls and young women more often than men. While it is treatable, no cure has been found for this largely hereditary and possibly fatal disease. A less serious form of lupus is discoid lupus erythematosus (DLE).

The main symptom of SLE is inflammation of internal connective tissue. DLE, on the other hand, causes a circular rash on the face or skin. Although we don't know why either form occurs, lupus is classified as an immune system disorder. It can cause the body to attack its own organs, including the kidneys, causing high blood pressure and kidney failure; the lungs, causing pleurisy; or even the central nervous system, causing problems ranging from headache to psychosis. The symptoms wax and wane, reappearing with differing degrees of severity.

Once diagnosed, usually through blood tests or a skin biopsy, lupus is treated mainly by reducing its symptoms. NSAIDs, anti-malarial drugs, and steroids are frequently used. Immunosuppressive drugs are prescribed for difficult cases. Because sunlight can make lupus symptoms worse in many cases, sunblock or sunscreen should always be worn.

While lupus is a serious, life-threatening disease, patient survival rates have steadily improved over the last decade, due to more effective treatment of related kidney disease and other problems.

Other Arthritic Disease

Progressive Systemic Sclerosis, better known as Scleroderma, is a relatively rare disease that causes thickening of the skin and, like lupus, can affect connective tissue in internal organs. While there is no cure, its symptoms are often relieved by high blood pressure medications like vasodilators (see pg. 724), steroids, and immunosuppressive drugs.

Juvenile Rheumatoid Arthritis is also known as Still's Disease, monarticular juvenile arthritis, or polyarticular juvenile arthritis. This disease, which afflicts children and adolescents, usually has symptoms—aching and swollen joints—similar to other forms of arthritis. Treatment includes pain relief with NSAIDs and analgesics. Steroids and other drugs used to treat adult RA may be needed in some juvenile cases.

Infectious arthritis is the name given to arthritis-like symptoms that often occur after severe infections such as Lyme disease or gonorrhea, and viral illnesses such as measles, chickenpox, and mumps. Symptoms usually disappear with treatment of the primary infection by antibiotics or other appropriate drugs.

Living with Arthritis

Many arthritis victims will suffer for prolonged periods, even the rest of their lives. Often simple skills like dressing, eating, and bathing must be relearned. To make life easier, there are many assistive devices that can be installed in the home, such as "grab bars" to help a person get in and out of the bathtub, and other aids such as large-button phones. Any physical therapist or rehabilitation specialist can make a visit to your home to help determine your needs. Often simply removing dangerous electrical cords or other impediments can prevent the falls and other accidents that damage fragile joints. In general, proper use of medications, exercise, rest, and a good diet will do the most to relieve arthritis symptoms.

Over the past three decades, research breakthroughs have helped reduce the suffering of many afflicted with arthritis. We have learned that certain gene patterns mean a susceptibility to arthritis, making early detection possible. There is now evidence that a genetic marker for osteoarthritis may exist. Researchers are closer to understanding which cells trigger the autoimmune forms of arthritis such as lupus, and what these forms may have in common with other diseases such as diabetes and multiple sclerosis. Even the drugs we take for granted today were the result of years of research. And now on the horizon is a new class of medicines called *leumedins* which block inflamed cells from reaching the joints. □

CHAPTER 4

Osteoporosis, Low Back Pain, and Other Bone Disorders

T he human skeleton is an intricate framework of 206 bones that give the body its structure and shape. These bones serve as armor for vital organs and soft tissue, a storehouse for minerals, and a birthplace for blood cells. Together, the bones act in concert with the muscles, ligaments, tendons, and other connective tissue to give humans an amazing range of movement.

Most bone diseases are rare, but a few pose serious health problems. Osteoporosis, for example, is a progressive loss of bone substance that affects 15 to 20 million Americans, mostly postmenopausal Caucasian women. Osteoarthritis, the most common form of arthritis, is widespread among people over 40. (See Chapter 3 on Arthritis.) Low back pain, which often results from slipped vertebrae or disks, is the second most frequent cause of lost work for adults under 45 years of age.

How Bones Are Structured

B ones are made of inorganic salts— including calcium and phosphate— imbedded in collagen fibers. Though solid and seemingly completely formed, bones undergo constant renewal and change. The marrow, or soft center, of certain bones serves as a spawning ground for the many different cells that make up the blood.

There are three types of bones—long, short, and flat or irregular. Long bones include the humerus, radius, and ulna of the arm; the femur, tibia, and fibula of the leg; and the phalanges, metacarpals, and metatarsals of the hand and foot. The tarsal in the foot and the carpal in the wrist are short bones. Flat bones can be found in the head and also include the ribs, breastbone, and collarbone. Irregular bones are located mostly in the spine; certain others are situated in the head.

Osteoporosis

I n osteoporosis a loss of calcium and phosphate salts causes the bones to become porous, brittle, and easily broken. The vertebrae in the spine may compress, causing

OUR 206 BONES

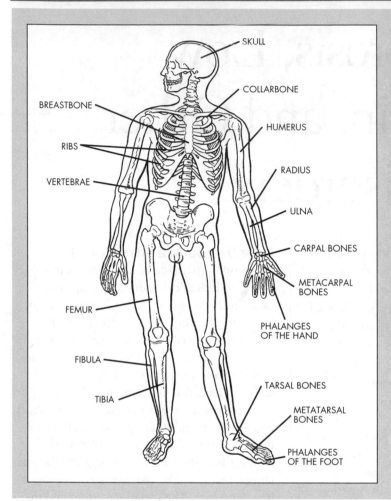

SKULL

COLLARBONE

BREASTBONE

HUMERUS

RIBS

RADIUS

VERTEBRAE

ULNA

CARPAL BONES

METACARPAL BONES

FEMUR

PHALANGES OF THE HAND

FIBULA

TARSAL BONES

TIBIA

METATARSAL BONES

PHALANGES OF THE FOOT

We're conscious of our complex skeletal infrastructure only when something goes awry. The joints are particularly problem-prone; and the spine, with its many joints, gives us the most trouble of all. The effects of osteoporosis may first be seen in the spine. Low back pain arises in the spine. Even neck pain may have its source in the spine. Indeed, where our bones are concerned, back problems are exceeded only by arthritis as a source of pain and suffering.

the back to become bent and resulting in such conditions as kyphosis (round back) or scoliosis (spinal curvature). A deformed spine usually affects other body parts, particularly nearby organs.

Inadequate dietary intake of calcium, hormonal changes associated with aging, and an inactive life-style have all been implicated in the development of osteoporosis. Drug use, alcoholism, lactose intolerance, an overactive thyroid, and faulty calcium absorption may also put people at risk. Other risk factors include premature menopause and the absence or abnormal halt of menstrual periods; a petite, thin build; smoking; a caucasian or oriental background; scoliosis; and a fair complexion.

Menopause, which is accompanied by a sudden, rapid loss of bone minerals, is a particularly critical point in the development of osteoporosis. It's wise to consult a doctor for guidance at this important juncture. Unfortunately, most people learn they have osteoporosis only after the disease has progressed. Indeed, the first signal is often a sharp pain in the lower back while lifting or bending, which usually indicates the collapse of a vertebra. Some people may show signs of increasing deformity, such as a humped back and a loss of height.

Treatment for osteoporosis is aimed at preventing bone mineral loss. It usually includes physical therapy; an exercise regimen; and estrogen, calcium, vitamin D, and in some cases calcitonin.

Low Back Pain

The back is a complex structure comprised of vertebrae (irregular bones), disks (cushions between the vertebrae), the spinal cord, nerves, muscles, and ligaments. Back problems may involve any of these components and are usually very distressing and debilitating. Low back pain is one of the most common complaints, affecting four out of five people at some point in their lives.

Osteoporosis or arthritis may be the cause of low back pain. Scoliosis or slippage of one vertebra onto another vertebra (spondylolisthesis) can also cause severe discomfort in the lower back.

Another common cause of low back pain is ruptured, slipped, or herniated disks. Disks have a soft, gelatinous center (nucleus) surrounded by an outer ring (anulus). Trauma, strain, or degeneration may weaken the outer ring so that the center bulges through and impinges on nerve roots in the spine, or on the spinal cord itself.

Herniated disks usually cause severe lower back pain that radiates to the buttocks, legs, and feet. There may also be a loss of feeling and mobility in the affected areas and ultimately weakness and atrophy of leg muscles.

Treatment of herniated disks usually includes a week or more of bed rest, heat treatments, and exercise. Aspirin or another analgesic is usually recommended; cortisone is prescribed in rare instances. Muscle relaxants, such as methocarbamol (Robaxin) or diazepam (Valium), can also be very helpful. If the pain persists, disk surgery may be necessary.

Neck Pain

Neck pain is another common source of severe discomfort. The neck is less protected than the rest of the spine and thus is more prone to painful and disabling injuries and disorders. As with the lower back, neck pain may result from abnormalities in the muscles, ligaments, and nerves, as well as the joints and bones. Osteoarthritis, rheumatoid arthritis, and cervical degeneration are common causes of pain in this area.

Whiplash injuries, falls, and contact sports can also do real damage to the neck. Careful diagnosis is essential to determine the correct treatment and rehabilitation program. Treatment usually consists of rest, medication, immobilization, exercise, neck braces, and physical therapy. Medications usually

THE CARPAL TUNNEL

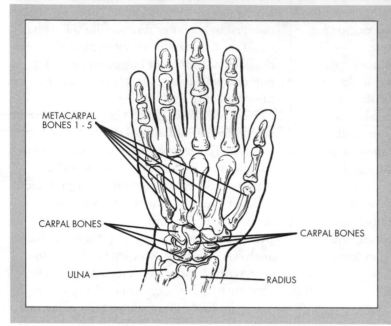

METACARPAL
BONES 1 - 5

CARPAL BONES

CARPAL BONES

ULNA

RADIUS

Within the complex cluster of bones that form the wrist, a collection of ligaments, tendons, blood vessels, and nerves crowd a narrow passage between the arm and the hand. If repeated stress causes swelling within this tunnel, the main nerve will be squeezed against nearby ligaments and tendons. The well-known carpal tunnel syndrome —pain in the wrist, hand, or forearm — then may follow.

include aspirin, nonsteroidal anti-inflammatory drugs (NSAIDs) such as Motrin, other analgesics, and muscle relaxants.

Scoliosis

The spine's normal curves produce the rounding of the shoulders and the inward curve of the lower back. Scoliosis is an abnormal "s" curving of the spine that gives a person the appearance of slumping to one side. Usually first noticed in the teen years, and more prevalent among girls, scoliosis often causes one shoulder blade to protrude and one shoulder to be higher than the other. Hips and ribs can also become misaligned.

The treatment of scoliosis is determined by the severity of the deformity and may include exercise, a brace, surgery, or any combination of these measures.

Carpal Tunnel Syndrome

Carpal tunnel syndrome occurs when the main nerve in the wrist becomes compressed. The compression causes pain and motor difficulties in the hand. The carpal tunnel is a hollow area in the wrist. The median nerve, blood vessels, and flexor tendons of the fingers and thumb all pass through the carpal tunnel. The tunnel is formed by the carpal (wrist) bones and ligaments. Problems arise when the content or structure of the tunnel swells and presses the median nerve against the ligament.

People who use poorly designed tools, assembly-line workers, and typists are prone to carpal tunnel syndrome. This problem can also be brought on by rheumatoid arthritis, pregnancy, kidney failure, acromegaly (a hormonal disorder), menopause, diabetes mellitus, amyloidosis, tuberculosis, myxedema (thyroid hormone disorder), and benign tumors.

Symptoms of carpal tunnel syndrome usually include pain, burning, weakness, tingling, or numbness in one or both hands. Treatment usually consists of wearing braces or splints at night to keep the wrist from bending. NSAIDs and cortisone are often given to reduce swelling. If these methods are not successful, surgery may be required.

Fractures

Broken bones aren't always serious, but a break almost always is debilitating in some way. A fracture usually affects surrounding tissue, so there is often swelling and additional pain as a result of the extra damage. Since most broken bones are caused by trauma of some kind, shock and emotional distress often occur as well.

Broken bones can cause pain, swelling, deformity, discoloration, tenderness, and loss of function in the affected area. Whether the broken bone is in the skull, nose, jaw, rib, hip, or a limb, all fractures and breaks require immediate treatment by a physician. Proper medical care includes treatment of shock and the prevention of blood loss and other serious complications. Realignment of the displaced bones and immobilization with a cast or traction are standard measures.

A local anesthetic such as lidocaine is usually all that's needed to set a broken limb. Analgesics such as meperidine (Demerol) are given to relieve pain; muscle relaxants such as diazepam (Valium) help stretch muscles to make it easier to set the bone. □

CHAPTER 5

Digestive Disorders, Minor and Major

If we are what we eat, then what we are is only as good as our digestion. When it goes awry, it generally affects our total well-being. Whether it's mild nausea, a nasty virus, or a chronic disorder such as irritable bowel syndrome, a disorder of the digestive tract is usually impossible to ignore. If the condition persists, it can undermine our total health, eventually threatening our very lives.

How the Digestive System Works

The gastrointestinal (GI) tract is a long hollow tube stretching from the head to the end of the body, including the mouth, pharynx, esophagus, stomach, small intestine, and large intestine. The salivary glands, liver, gallbladder, and pancreas are also important parts of this far-reaching system.

The main purpose of the GI tract is to break down carbohydrates, fats, and proteins into molecules small enough to be absorbed through cell membranes. In that way, it provides the cells with the necessary energy for life and health.

Digestion begins in the mouth when food is chewed and starch is broken down by ptyalin, an enzyme secreted in saliva. Food then enters the stomach, where it is reduced to tiny particles and further transformed by gastric juices. The solid portion remains in the stomach for one to six hours until it liquefies completely; liquid passes into the duodenum (small intestine), where numerous enzymes produced by the pancreas, along with bile from the liver, break it down further for absorption. When it finally arrives in the large intestine, all nutritional value has been spent, and the only remaining process is the removal of water before final elimination.

Every section of the GI tract is prone to its own unique disorders—some merely annoying, others potentially fatal. Fortunately, for all but a few we now have simple treatments that will, at the very least, relieve the symptoms.

Diseases of the Upper GI Tract

Reflux esophagitis is characterized by heartburn, upper abdominal or chest pain, difficulty swallowing, nausea, or belching that leaves an acid taste. It is caused

MAPPING THE GI TRACT

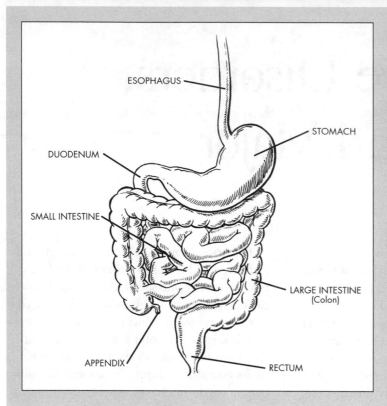

ESOPHAGUS

STOMACH

DUODENUM

SMALL INTESTINE

LARGE INTESTINE
(Colon)

APPENDIX

RECTUM

The digestive tract's convoluted course begins at the mouth, ending yards later at the rectum. In between lie the esophagus, stomach, and small and large intestines. Each segment is vulnerable to a characteristic set of afflictions, ranging from gastritis, gastroenteritis, and ulcers in the upper tract to colitis, diverticulosis, and colon cancer in the lower segments.

by a backflow of acid stomach contents into the esophagus. Symptoms usually occur within an hour after eating, and are most likely to strike when you lie down, bend, or stoop. It is alleviated by taking antacids or sitting up. It may be aggravated by vigorous exercise, and is often associated with hiatal hernia (protrusion of the stomach above the diaphragm). Severe cases can lead to a narrowing of the esophagus requiring medical therapy.

Treatment for this disorder includes short- and long-term approaches. Liquid antacids are effective for immediate relief of heartburn. (If they are unavailable, water often does the trick.) There are also medications available to reduce backflow and acid production. Since almost anything that increases pressure in the abdomen can cause heartburn, long-term therapy involves ways of reducing that pressure. These include losing weight (for those who are overweight); avoiding tight clothing; remembering not to bend or stoop; and elevating the head of the bed by 30 degrees. Eating smaller meals more often can decrease symptoms. It is also wise to avoid lying down for two to three hours after eating and to forgo foods that increase heartburn—such as chocolate, coffee, tea, citrus fruits, alcohol, and those high in fat—as well as smoking.

Gastroenteritis is diarrhea, nausea, vomiting, and abdominal cramping brought on by bacteria, amoebas, parasites, toxins, certain drugs, enzymes, or allergens in foods. Treatment usually includes bed rest, fluids, bismuth-containing products such as Pepto-Bismol, and anti-nausea drugs like trimethobenzamide (Tigan) and prochlorperazine (Compazine).

Chronic gastritis is inflammation of the stomach lining. It is sometimes caused by eating irritating substances. In elderly people, it is associated with pernicious anemia. Some people with this disorder have no symptoms, but many experience vague pain, a feeling of fullness, loss of appetite, belching, nausea and vomiting. Treatment consists of eliminating the irritating foods, avoiding aspirin, and taking antacids if the condition persists. If pernicious anemia is the underlying cause, the doctor may administer vitamin B_{12}. Severe cases may call for other medication.

Ulcers can occur in the lower esophagus, stomach, or any part of the small intestine, and are designated by their location. About 80 percent are **duodenal ulcers**, found in the first segment of the small intestine, mostly in men between 20 and 50. Less common are **gastric ulcers**, located in the stomach and found most often in middle-aged and elderly men and chronic users of aspirin, alcohol, and cigarettes. Both types of ulcer can produce heartburn, pain, nausea, indigestion, and, in gastric ulcer, pain after eating a meal. Weight loss is common with gastric ulcers, while the opposite often happens with duodenal ulcers because patients may eat to relieve discomfort. The cause of ulcers is unknown, though over-secretion of gastric acids and stress have long been regarded as factors. Recent news reports have suggested that bacteria may contribute to the development of ulcers, and that therapy with antibiotics may prove effective.

Therapy includes rest and is generally directed toward buffering stomach acid with antacids, as well as reducing acid production with drugs known as histamine H_2 blockers, including cimetidine (Tagamet), ranitidine

WHERE ULCERS STRIKE

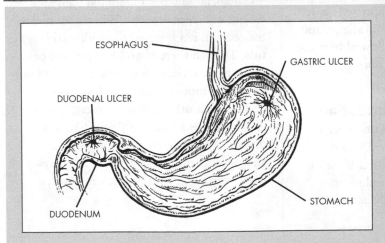

ESOPHAGUS

GASTRIC ULCER

DUODENAL ULCER

STOMACH

DUODENUM

Though we think of ulcers as a stomach problem, the most common variety actually occurs just outside the stomach in the duodenum, or beginning of the small intestine. Others (gastric ulcers) do appear in the stomach; and no part of the intestines is immune to the problem. An ulcer is, essentially, an open sore. We feel pain when stomach acids come in contact with the ulcer's raw, exposed surface.

(Zantac), nizatidine (Axid), and famotidine (Pepcid). The doctor may also prescribe drugs such as sucralfate (Carafate) that coat the ulcer without reducing acid. In the future, so-called protective drugs will be available that can heal ulcers and prevent their recurrence.

Whatever form of therapy is employed, close follow-up by either upper endoscopy or X-rays is required. If an ulcer has not healed after two to three months, surgery may be needed.

Gastric cancer is more common in males than females, especially those over 40. It has a higher incidence in northern industrial areas and a higher mortality in Japan, Iceland, Chile, and Austria. In the U.S., the incidence has decreased 50 percent in the last 25 years. Dietary patterns—such as heavy consumption of pickled, smoked, or salt-preserved foods and those containing nitrates and nitrous compounds—may be implicated in its development. This disease is also more likely in those with Type A blood and those with a history of gastric cancer in their families. The risk may be reduced by a diet including whole milk, fresh vegetables, and vitamin C. Early signs include indigestion and discomfort, followed by weight and appetite loss, a sensation of fullness after eating, fatigue, and anemia. Surgery, sometimes followed by chemotherapy, is currently the only effective treatment.

Diseases of the Large Intestine

Irritable bowel syndrome occurs more frequently in women under age 35, and often begins in late adolescence. It may be related to psychological stress and is commonly marked by an abnormally active—even spastic—lower bowel. Its symptoms are similar to a number of other illnesses, including diverticulosis and lactose intolerance. These symptoms include uncomfortable abdominal sensations and periodic diarrhea or constipation, sometimes occuring alternately. Some patients come to depend on laxatives and even enemas to alleviate the constipation. For others, the only symptom is painless diarrhea. Treatment includes a diet high in fiber and low in fat. Certain gas-producing foods, such as those in the cabbage family, should be avoided, as should any other suspected irritants. For constipation, a bulk-producing product may be recommended; for diarrhea, diphenoxylate (Lomotil) or loperamide (Imodium) are possibilities. As a last resort, antispasmodics such as propantheline (Pro-Banthine) may be prescribed.

Inflammatory bowel disease is a blanket term covering three serious disorders: ulcerative colitis, proctitis, and Crohn's disease.

Ulcerative colitis is an inflammation of the colon that produces ulceration of the inside wall. Its primary symptom is bloody, chronic diarrhea, often containing pus and mucus, and associated with abdominal pain and weight and appetite loss. When confined to the rectum, it's referred to as ulcerative proctitis. Though there is no known cause of ulcerative colitis, it does tend to run in families and is more common in Jews and caucasians than other ethnic or racial groups.

Sometimes known as ileitis, Crohn's disease is an inflammation of the small and/or large intestine, with accompanying pain, cramping, tenderness, gas, fever, nausea, and diarrhea. Though usually mild, bleeding may occur and may sometimes be massive.

Proctitis, an inflammation of the rectum, is characterized by bloody stools, a frequent urge to defecate but inability to do so, and sometimes diarrhea. Possible causes are ulcerative colitis, Crohn's disease, trauma, infection, or radiation.

Ulcerative colitis and Crohn's disease are generally chronic and have no known cures. Treatment usually consists of symptom relief and reduction of inflamation. When there are acute flare-ups, the patient should avoid stimulants such as caffeine, citrus fruits, and foods high in fiber. Medical therapy includes steroids and drugs such as olsalazine (Dipentum), which have both anti-inflammatory and antibacterial properties. These medications can control symptoms and often produce long-term remissions. Steroids should be used only when necessary, and under a physician's guidance, to avoid serious side effects. If attacks of ulcerative colitis become severe enough to be life-threatening, surgical removal of the colon can save the patient's life. Surgery also is sometimes performed for very severe complications of Crohn's disease, but will not cure the disease itself.

Diverticulosis, a condition most common in men over 40, is present in up to as 50 percent of people aged 60. Though generally silent until bleeding and inflammation occur, it can be marked by alternating constipation and diarrhea. The disease occurs when bulging pouches (diverticula) form at weak points in the wall of the colon. If they become inflamed, they can cause severe pain, fever, nausea, and vomiting; if small vessels at the base of the pouch become disrupted, there may be significant intestinal bleeding. When symptoms occur, they can be alleviated by a liquid or bland diet and stool softeners. After symptoms subside, a high-fiber diet is usually effective in preventing recurrence and progression of the disease. When infection is present, treatment includes a broad-spectrum antibiotic and bowel rest.

Intestinal polyps, abnormal growths that may occur anywhere in the GI tract, are most often found in the large intestine. Though they generally cause no symptoms, a major sign is rectal bleeding. Polyps are rare in underdeveloped countries, suggesting that our high-fat, low-fiber diets may be partially responsible. They are more frequent in individuals with a family history of polyps or cancer of the colon. No current treatment is known to prevent recurrence. Reducing the fat content of your diet by 25 percent and consuming fiber-containing foods on a daily basis are both recommended. Because polyps are thought to be precursors of colon cancer, it's important to have them removed. This can be done with colonoscopy on an outpatient basis. An annual examination for polyps is advisable from age 50 onward.

Colon cancer, silent in its earliest stages, becomes evident as it progresses. Symptoms include bleeding, at times invisible to the naked eye, with resultant anemia, as well as a change in bowel habits, often accompanied by pain, weight and appetite loss, weakness, and a general decline in health. The risk for colon cancer increases with age, doubling with each decade after 40. Its exact causes are unknown, but it appears to be related to diets high in fat and low in fiber, and is known to occur more frequently in those with a family history of colon cancer. Surgery, sometimes followed by chemotherapy and radiation, are the current treatments for this type of cancer.

Other GI Problems

Hemorrhoids are dilated veins in the lower rectum and anus. They affect 50 percent of people over age 50. Diets low in fiber are thought to be a major cause. Straining at defecation to evacuate hard stools also seems to promote their development. A high-fiber diet and prompt, strain-free defecation help relieve mildly symptomatic hemorrhoids. Local swelling and pain can be decreased with local anesthetic creams, lotions, or suppositories; astringents; or cold compresses. For those with severe symptoms, rubber band ligation, cryosurgery, injection therapy, or surgical removal may be needed.

Constipation is the term given for infrequent or difficult evacuation of small, hard stools, accompanied by mild abdominal discomfort. When the condition is chronic, it may include nausea, stomach rumbling, appetite loss, and malaise. Constipation is a common condition that affects mostly the very young and the aged. While the number of bowel movements is variable in the general population, a normal individual should have at least three per week, or, ideally, one daily.

Treatment for constipation includes laxatives and enemas, a diet high in fiber, and adequate exercise. If these efforts fail, a doctor should be consulted to rule out causes such as drugs, diabetes, hypothyroidism, or colon problems.

Pancreatitis is an inflammation of the pancreas. It can occur periodically or chronically. The first sign may be a sudden, severe abdominal pain above the navel, which travels through to the back. Accompanying symptoms may include a low-grade fever, nausea, and vomiting. Pancreatitis in men is commonly associated with alcohol use, trauma, and peptic ulcer; in women, with gallstones and disease of the bile duct. In rare instances, a medication may be the cause.

Patients with an acute attack are hospitalized, given intravenous fluids, and administered painkillers. If the symptoms are caused by gallstones, the gallbladder should be removed. If alcohol is the cause, it should be stopped immediately and completely avoided thereafter. Any drugs that might be responsible should be discontinued.

For patients with chronic pancreatitis, analgesics are often used to treat the severe pain. A low-fat diet, along with pancreatic enzymes, is also sometimes part of the treatment regimen.

It's a little-known fact that sexually transmitted diseases may involve not only the genitalia but also the digestive tract. Shigellosis, giardiasis, and amebiasis are the most common of the sexually transmitted digestive diseases. They can also be passed along in food and water contaminated by infected individuals who fail to wash their hands properly. Symptoms generally include watery or even bloody diarrhea associated with severe abdominal pain. Without treatment, an attack may last from days to weeks. Therapy depends on the type of infection. These diseases should always be treated by a physician. □

CHAPTER 6

Defeating the Dangers of Respiratory Disease

We can go without water for days and do without food even longer, but without air we will die in a matter of minutes. Breathing, along with the beating of our hearts, is one of the body's most essential functions, and any disruption can be deadly. Even a minor cold, by affecting our normal intake and outflow of air, can make us feel miserable.

Respiratory problems are common—indeed the most common of all physical complaints. Almost everyone experiences infections of the head, throat, and chest. These infections range from colds to influenza and pneumonia, which can be mildly debilitating or seriously life-threatening.

How The Respiratory System Works

The nose, lungs, and diaphragm are the major respiratory organs. As the diaphragm contracts, the rib cage expands. This action creates negative pressure in the lung cavity, and air is then pulled in through the nose. When the diaphragm stops contracting, the lungs recoil and push the air out. Oxygen is exchanged for carbon dioxide (CO_2) in the blood that flows through the capillaries in any one of the lung's 300 million alveoli. Circulating blood then delivers the oxygen to the body's cells in exchange for CO_2 and metabolic waste. This trade is known as internal respiration. The lungs subsequently exhale CO_2-containing air.

Colds and Flu

The common cold is aptly named: It ranks as the most prevalent infectious disease in humans. Indeed, the common cold accounts for just about as many trips to the drugstore as any other ailment. And although the common cold tends to be benign and brief, this nuisance illness can lead to more serious bacterial infections.

Colds are almost always caused by viral infections of the upper respiratory tract. Many different families of viruses can cause a common cold, and each family has numerous members. The sheer diversity of causative agents is why it has been impossible to develop a vaccine for the common cold.

Different viruses affect different areas of the respiratory tract and may result in fever, chills, malaise, and lethargy. When a virus causes nasal inflammation, you develop stuffiness or runniness, and sometimes post-nasal drip. If the virus travels to the pharynx, you get a sore throat or pharyngitis. If inflammation reaches the vocal cords, you may become hoarse or even lose your voice (laryngitis). If the trachea and main bronchi are involved, you will most likely complain of congestion and coughing, and will also produce sputum. This particular medical condition is called tracheobronchitis or acute bronchitis.

Since there is no cure for colds, treatment focuses on the symptoms. Remedies include aspirin, acetaminophen or ibuprofen, increased fluids, and rest. (Avoid giving aspirin to children. It may be linked with a dangerous condition called Reye's syndrome.) Decongestants, throat lozenges, nasal sprays, cough medicines, and expectorants are all used and may or may not ease the symptoms of a cold. In some instances, antibiotics are needed to wipe out any accompanying bacterial infection. This is often the case with bronchitis.

The **influenza** virus attacks the respiratory tract with particularly debilitating results. Influenza, often called "flu," commonly causes severe aching in the muscles and joints, chills, headache, fever, discomfort, a dry cough, and exhaustion. The virus typically spreads throughout an entire community, often causing serious complications such

A CLOSE-UP VIEW OF OUR AMAZING LUNGS

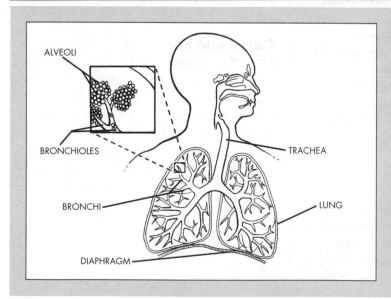

ALVEOLI

BRONCHIOLES

BRONCHI

TRACHEA

LUNG

DIAPHRAGM

Though they fill most of the chest, the lungs perform their crucial task at an almost microscopic level. Starting at the trachea, or windpipe, the air passages within the lungs divide and redivide into ever smaller branches, or bronchioles, finally terminating in 300 million minute air sacs called alveoli. It's within these capillary-laced sacs that the air we inhale meets our circulatory system, passing fresh oxygen to the blood and removing waste CO_2.

as pneumonia, and even death. The good news is that influenza can be prevented if you get an annual vaccination.

The treatment of influenza consists of bed rest, increased fluids, aspirin—or for children, acetaminophen—and an expectorant, such as guaifenesin, to treat the cough. Amantadine, an antiviral agent, has proved helpful in reducing the symptoms and the duration of influenza A, and is also used to help prevent it.

Pneumonia

Pneumonia, an inflammation of the lungs, is usually caused by viruses, bacteria, fungi, protozoa, mycobacteria, mycoplasma, or rickettsia. Pneumonia is a serious matter because the infection may interfere with the lung's very important function of exchanging oxygen and carbon dioxide in the blood.

Common symptoms of pneumonia are fever, shaking chills, pleuritic (lung) pain, cough, and sputum production. In some cases, the resulting sputum may be minimal and off-white in color. Sometimes the patient produces abundant amounts of yellow, green, or brown sputum.

Viral pneumonia is treated symptomatically with adequate liquids and bed rest. Severe cases may require humidified oxygen therapy and mechanical ventilation. The treatment of bacterial pneumonia must also include appropriate antibiotics. There is a vaccine available to prevent the most common bacterial form of this disease.

Chronic Lung Disorders

Chronic obstructive pulmonary disease (COPD), the most common chronic lung disorder, currently afflicts some 17 million Americans. And the incidence of COPD is on the rise. Emphysema, chronic bronchitis, asthma (see chapter on allergies), or any combination of these conditions may result in COPD. Smoking is the most common cause of COPD; recurrent infections and allergies may also predispose an individual to this disorder.

Emphysema actually destroys the lung, causing it to lose its elastic properties. As a result, the lungs have trouble expelling air and thus are unable to move air in and out at a normal rate.

Chronic bronchitis involves an inflammation of the bronchial tubes and is characterized by excessive mucus production. The symptoms of chronic bronchitis are cough and sputum production. The disease begins with a typical smoker's cough. Each morning, coughing helps to clear the excess mucus from the lungs. As the bronchitis progresses, shortness of breath develops and eventually becomes chronic.

People with COPD can live relatively normal lives for years. Sooner or later, though, they will notice a growing inability to exercise or do strenuous work, along with the onset of a productive cough. The symptoms tend to get worse as time goes by, and the individual becomes more and more prone to respiratory infections, shortness of breath, and reduced pulmonary function.

Treatment consists of relieving the symptoms of COPD, preventing complications, educating smokers to stop, and encouraging all patients to eliminate any airborne irritants. Patients are also taught deep breathing exercises to strengthen muscles used in respiration and are trained to cough effectively. Oxygen therapy is sometimes necessary as well. The medications prescribed for COPD are bronchodilators such as theophylline (Theo-Dur), antibiotics for infections, diuretics (water pills) to eliminate the fluid retention, and corticosteroids (for chronic bronchitis and asthma).

The Resurgence of TB

Tuberculosis was declining for many years in America; but, unfortunately, this infection is back and on the rise. Some people who contract tuberculosis fail to take their medication properly. It is this lack of compliance that is often cited as the reason for the increasing spread of this dread disease.

Tuberculosis is a serious, chronic infection. In about five percent of those exposed, tuberculosis develops within one year. However, the infection may also lie dormant for years, emerging as tuberculosis when the person is weakened by another serious illness, such as diabetes, leukemia, or Hodgkin's disease, or when immunity is compromised by immunosuppressive drugs or AIDS. Tuberculosis is transmitted through the air, particularly after an infected person coughs.

The initial infection with TB generally does not produce any symptoms. When symptoms do appear, infected individuals are likely to complain of fever, night sweats, loss of appetite, weight loss, and fatigue. In its reactivated phase, TB may be signaled by a cough with discolored sputum production and sometimes pain in the chest. Patients may also cough up blood. Tuberculosis is caused by *Mycobacterium tuberculosis* and as such is treated with daily oral doses of antibiotics for at least nine months. The drugs used most often are isoniazid and rifampin (Rifadin, Rimactane).

The diagnostic test for tuberculosis is called a Tine test or PPD skin test. A positive reading indicates that a person has been exposed to tuberculosis but does not necessarily predict who will ultimately develop active infection. People with positive skin test results can often prevent subsequent illness by faithfully taking a one-year course of anti-tuberculosis antibiotics.

Childhood Respiratory Diseases

Croup, a childhood disease more common in boys than girls, typically occurs between the ages of three months and three years. This disease usually follows a viral infection and is associated with a harsh, grating, creaking sound upon breathing; hoarse or muffled vocal sounds; labored breathing; and the characteristic sharp, barking cough. Depending on the type of infection, croup may also be accompanied by a sore throat, hoarseness, runny nose, rapid pulse, clammy skin, and breathing marked by sharp inward and outward movement of the spot above the sternum and muscles of the rib cage—like a balloon quickly filling and then losing air.

Treatment for croup usually consists of rest, cool humidification while sleeping, and acetaminophen. If the child has severe respiratory distress, hospitalization and oxygen therapy may be necessary. If a bacterial infection is a factor, the child must also take antibiotics.

Epiglottitis is a disorder in which the epiglottis becomes inflamed—often to the point of blocking breathing. Epiglottis typically strikes children between the ages of two and eight years. It is a critical condition, one that can prove fatal if appropriate emergency treatment is not implemented.

Epiglottitis may begin as a respiratory infection, progressing to complete upper airway obstruction within two to five hours. Symptoms include difficulty in breathing and swallowing, a harsh, grating or creaking sound when breathing, high fever, sore throat, restlessness, irritability, and drooling. Emergency treatment is necessary and includes endotracheal intubation or a tracheotomy, oxygen therapy, and the administration of fluids to prevent dehydration. Patients always receive antibiotics.

For more on childhood diseases, including whooping cough, turn to page 787.

Other Serious Respiratory Illnesses

Legionnaire's disease got its name from the highly publicized outbreak that occurred in 1976 during an American Legion convention in Philadelphia. Legionnaire's disease is usually an acute bronchopneumonia accompanied by diarrhea, malaise, body aches and headaches, loss of appetite, recurrent chills, and a fever that occurs within 12 to 48 hours and rises as high as 105 degrees. Patients subsequently develop a dry cough that may later produce grayish and sometimes blood-streaked sputum. Other possible symptoms of legionnaire's disease include disorientation, vomiting, nausea, mental sluggishness, and mild, temporary amnesia.

As soon as legionnaire's disease is suspected, antibiotics should be administered immediately. Erythromycin, alone or in combination with rifampin, is the preferred treatment for legionnaire's disease. If the patient cannot tolerate erythromycin, doxycycline (alone or with rifampin) may be used instead. Treatment may also consist of aspirin or acetaminophen; drugs that increase blood pressure if necessary; fluid replacement; and oxygen therapy.

Pleurisy is an inflammation of the tissue that lines the lungs and the inner surface of the chest wall. Pleurisy is usually a complication of pneumonia, but may also result from viruses, tuberculosis, chest trauma, rheumatoid arthritis, systemic lupus erythematosus (a collagen vascular disease), cancer, pulmonary infarction (a blood clot in the lungs), and Dressler's syndrome (a complication of heart attack). Pleurisy is characterized by a sharp, stabbing pain that intensifies with breathing. The pain may at times inhibit movement on the affected side. Breathing is labored. Treatment involves anti-inflammatory drugs, painkillers, bed rest, and, in severe cases, a nerve block.

Asthma, a grave respiratory disorder affecting millions, is discussed in the chapter on allergies. See page 797. To learn about lung cancer, turn to page 751. □

CHAPTER 7

Cancer: Improving the Odds of a Cure

Cancer is the scourge of the late 20th century. Few things raise more fear in our hearts than the diagnosis—or even the mere thought—of this dreaded disease. And though cancer has been claiming more lives each year over the past five decades, the news is not entirely grim.

At the turn of the century, almost no one with cancer could expect to live very long. By the 1930s, not even one in five cancer patients was still alive five years after treatment. In the 1940s, the five-year survival rate was one in four; in the 1960s, one in three Americans survived. Today, about four out of 10 cancer patients live for at least five years after the initial diagnosis.

The survival rate increases substantially with early detection. Cancers of the breast, tongue, mouth, colon, rectum, cervix, prostate, testes, and skin account for half of all new cases. Two-thirds of the people diagnosed with these cancers will pass the five-year survival mark. However, the survival rate could climb as high as 89 percent *if* these cancers were diagnosed early through screen-ing and self-examinations *and* were treated promptly. In other words, of the 1,130,000 Americans who will be diagnosed with cancer this year, an additional 100,000 people would survive.

In addition, many cancers are preventable. Researchers say that up to 90 percent of the estimated 600,000 skin cancers diagnosed in 1992 could have been prevented by proper precautions against the sun's rays. All cancers caused by smoking and excessive alcohol use could be prevented entirely. This translates into an estimated 146,000 lung cancer deaths in 1992 and 16,500 cancer deaths related to the heavy consumption of alcohol, often in combination with cigarette use.

What Is Cancer?

The millions of cells that make up the body normally reproduce in an orderly manner, replacing worn-out tissues and repairing injuries to maintain

SOME CANCER FACTS

- Cancer can occur at any age, but mostly appears in people middle-aged and older.
- Cancer causes more deaths in American children aged one to 14 years than any other disease.
- In the 1980s more than 4.5 million Americans died from cancer.
- About 83 million people alive today—or one in three Americans—will eventually get cancer.
- Cancer cost the United States roughly $104 billion in 1990—including medical expenses and loss of work productivity.
- Approximately 520,000 Americans die of cancer each year.

health. However, certain cells may begin to reproduce abnormally, massing together to form tumors.

If a tumor is benign, it will remain self-contained. A malignant—or cancerous—tumor, on the other hand, will invade neighboring tissues, and can spread through the blood and lymphatic systems to distant parts of the body in a process called metastasis.

Cancer is not one disease, but rather many related diseases. Cancer is typed according to the part of the body where it is located and the kind of cells that comprise it. The most common types of cancer cells and their locations are:

Carcinomas originate in skin tissue or tissues that line the body cavities and such internal organs as the lungs, breast, colon, and intestines.

Sarcomas grow in bones and connective tissues between organs and skin, and sometimes spread into the blood or lymphatic system.

Lymphomas are cancers of the lymphatic system, usually occurring in the lymph nodes.

Leukemias form in the blood or circulatory system, particularly in the bone marrow, which is the site of blood cell production.

Myelomas are tumors of bone marrow cells and frequently form simultaneously in many sites, including the ribs, vertebrae, and pelvic bones.

The Latest Advances in Diagnosis and Treatment

Cancer is treated by surgery, chemotherapy, radiation, or a combination of these methods. Diagnoses and treatment have become increasingly individualized in recent years. Early detection and the precise staging of therapies have contributed to higher success rates in the battle against cancer.

Many cancers that only recently had poor prognoses are now considered curable. Potentially curable cancers now include acute lymphocytic leukemia in children, Burkitt's lymphoma, Ewing's sarcoma (a form of bone cancer), Wilm's tumor (a kidney cancer in children), Hodgkin's disease, rhabdomyosarcoma (a cancer of certain muscle tissues), testicular cancer, choriocarcinoma (placental cancer), osteogenic sarcoma, and breast cancer.

Current developments also show the promise of improved treatment for many other forms of cancer. For example, the recently discovered importance of oncogenes—the genes in a tumor cell that are associated with the transformation of normal cells into cancerous ones—promises to help predict which tumors are likely to return after surgery. This knowledge can also help identify family members who are at risk.

It has also been found that cancer cells fused genetically with normal cells produce special antibodies that seek out cancer cells. These monoclonal antibodies are being studied for their potential use in diagnosis and treatment.

There are many other advances, including:

- Adjuvant treatment in which drugs are administered postoperatively in early breast and colon cancers to eradicate remaining cancer cells and thus increase cure rates

- Neoadjuvant chemotherapy in which drugs are given to shrink the cancer before surgery

- Synthetic retinoids (cousins of vitamin A) to prevent cancer in high-risk groups or the recurrence of cancer after surgery

- Removal and replacement of sections of bone in bone cancer instead of amputation of entire limbs

- New high-tech diagnostic imaging techniques (magnetic resonance imaging [MRI] and computerized tomography [CT] scans) instead of exploratory surgery in some cases

- Immunotherapy to enhance the body's disease-fighting capabilities (naturally occurring bodily substances, such as interferon, interleukin-2, and biologic response modifiers, are all in trials for this purpose)

- Bone marrow transplants for the treatment of leukemia

Lung Cancer

The increase in lung cancer largely explains the steady rise in the number of cancer deaths in the United States. Most of the estimated 146,000 deaths caused by lung cancer in 1992 resulted from cigarette smoking. The incidence in men declined from a high of 86.6 per 100,000 in 1984 to 81.5 in 1988. Unfortunately, the rate in women has been rising steadily, reaching a high of 39.8 per 100,000 in 1988. More women are smoking and, as a result, more women now die of lung cancer than breast cancer, which forty years ago was the leading cause of cancer death in women.

The symptoms of lung cancer include a persistent cough, sputum streaked with blood, chest pain, and recurring pneumonia or bronchitis. Additional risk factors include exposure to industrial chemicals (including arsenic, certain organic chemicals, and asbestos); radiation exposure, including possible residential radon exposure (especially for smokers); and for non-smokers, passive exposure to sidestream cigarette smoke.

Unfortunately, early detection of lung cancer is very difficult. Symptoms often don't appear until the disease is in an advanced stage. If smokers quit when early precancerous cellular changes have already damaged bronchial lining tissue, there is a chance that the disease will not progress. Those who continue to smoke often end up with lung cancer.

The treatment of lung cancer depends on the type and stage of the disease and includes surgery, radiation therapy, and chemotherapy. If the cancer is localized, surgery is the best option. However, because only 18 percent of lung cancers are discovered early enough for surgery, radiation and chemotherapy are often necessary.

In small-cell carcinoma, a large percentage of patients achieve remission with chemotherapy—alone or in combination with radiation—instead of surgery. Small-cell carcinomas have responded to the following combinations: cyclophosphamide, doxorubicin, and vincristine; cyclophosphamide, doxorubicin, vincristine, and estoposide; and estoposide and cisplatin.

Experimental immunotherapy for lung cancer uses BCG vaccine, or *Corynebacterium parvulum*. In experimental laser therapy, laser energy is beamed through a bronchoscope to destroy local tumors, which are often the cause of bronchial obstruction and resulting infection.

Colon Cancer

Colon and rectal cancers are the second leading cause of cancer deaths in the United States, claiming the lives of an estimated 58,300 Americans in 1992. People at greatest risk are those with a personal or family history of colon or rectal cancer, or of inflammatory bowel disease. High-fat and/or low-fiber diets are also believed to be risk factors.

Symptoms of colon and rectal cancers include rectal bleeding, blood in the stool, and a change in bowel habits that lasts more than two weeks, such as diarrhea alternating with constipation. Early detection methods include a digital rectal exam, a stool test for occult blood—recommended annually for people over 50—and a proctosigmoidoscopy—an examination of the rectum and colon via a hollow lighted tube, which is recommended every three to five years after age 50.

Colon and rectal cancers are treated by surgery, sometimes in combination with radiation. Patients with metastasis, residual disease, recurrent inoperable tumors, or a high risk of recurrence are candidates for chemotherapy. Drugs used in chemotherapy include 5-fluorouracil, levamisole, mitomycin, lomustine, vincristine, and methotrexate. Colostomies are needed only rarely.

Breast Cancer

An estimated 180,000 new cases of breast cancer were diagnosed in American women in 1992, and approximately 46,300 women died from the disease that same year. The incidence of breast cancer has continued to rise at about three percent a year since 1980, reaching 109.5 cases per 100,000 in 1988.

Every woman is at risk of developing breast cancer. However, women over age 50 and those with a personal or family history are at higher risk. Other risk factors include never having had children and giving birth for the first time after age 30.

Warning signs include persistent breast changes such as a lump, swelling, dimpling, thickening, skin irritations, distortion, retraction, scaliness, pain, discharge, or tenderness of the nipple.

As part of a comprehensive early detection program, every woman should do her own monthly breast examination. Regular clinical examinations are recommended every three

BREAST CANCER: A CLOSER LOOK

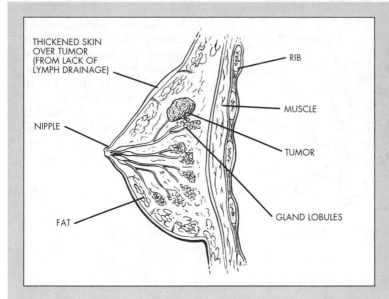

THICKENED SKIN OVER TUMOR (FROM LACK OF LYMPH DRAINAGE)

NIPPLE

FAT

RIB

MUSCLE

TUMOR

GLAND LOBULES

Until fairly sizable, a cancerous breast tumor can easily go unnoticed. That's why monthly self-examinations and regular medical visits are so important: Early treatment can make the difference between a cure and death.

years for women aged 20 to 40 and every year for those over 40. Mammograms can detect cancers too small to feel, and should be done every one or two years for women aged 40 to 49 and every year for women aged 50 and older. Suspicious lumps found on a mammogram should be biopsied for a definitive diagnosis.

Treatment for breast cancer depends on the individual case, and may consist of lumpectomy (local removal of the tumor); mastectomy (surgical removal of the breast); or radiation therapy followed by chemotherapy or hormone manipulation therapy for patients at high risk of metastic disease.

The most common drugs used in the treatment of breast cancer include methotrexate, 5-fluorouracil, cyclophosphamide, and dox-

orubicin. The drugs are usually given in combination. Hormone manipulation therapy may consist of administering progesterone or androgen; anti-estrogen therapy with tamoxifen (Nolvadex); or inhibition of adrenal corticosteroid production with aminoglutethimide (Cytadren).

Prostate Cancer

Prostate cancer claimed an estimated 34,000 lives in 1992, making it the second leading cause of cancer deaths in men. Prostate cancer is also the next-to-most common form of cancer in men (after skin cancer), with some 132,000 new cases reported in 1992.

The incidence of prostate cancer rises with age. More than 80 percent of the cases are diagnosed after the age of 65. Prostate cancer is more prevalent in northwestern Europe and the United States. For some reason,

ANATOMY OF PROSTATE CANCER

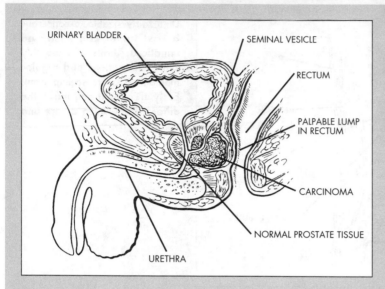

URINARY BLADDER

SEMINAL VESICLE

RECTUM

PALPABLE LUMP
IN RECTUM

CARCINOMA

NORMAL PROSTATE TISSUE

URETHRA

Nestled near the bladder and urethra, the prostate gland is frequently the culprit when urinary problems arise. These difficulties are often due to nothing more than prostate enlargement or infection; but cancer is a possibility. Take any urinary irregularity as a signal to visit your doctor or urologist.

African-Americans currently have the highest incidence of prostate cancer in the world. Dietary fat may be a contributing cause of prostate cancer.

Warning signs appear only after prostate cancer has progressed to an advanced stage. Symptoms include urinary dribbling; inability to urinate; difficulty starting or stopping the urinary stream; frequent urination, especially at night; blood in the urine; pain or burning while urinating; and persistent pain in the lower back, pelvis, or upper thighs. Most of these signs could also be a warning of such benign conditions as infection or prostate enlargement.

As with all cancers, early detection of prostate cancer is essential. Men over 40 are urged to have rectal examinations annually. Through transrectal ultrasound, a new tech

nique, it is now possible to detect cancers too small to show up on physical examination. A blood test for prostate specific antigen (PSA) can also detect the disease at an early stage.

Surgery or radiation is the primary treatment for localized prostate cancer. Hormonal therapy is used for metastic disease. Chemotherapy is tried when other types of therapy cannot be used or have failed. It involves various combinations of anti-cancer agents.

Pancreatic Cancer

In 1992, an estimated 28,300 new cases of pancreatic cancer were reported, while approximately 25,000 Americans died of the disease during the same year, making it the fifth leading cause of cancer deaths.

The incidence of pancreatic cancer rises after age 50, with most cases occurring between the ages of 65 and 79. The risk of pancreatic cancer is twice as high in people who smoke. Other possible predisposing factors include high fat diets, exposure to industrial chemicals, diabetes mellitus, chronic inflammation of the pancreas (pancreatitis), and chronic alcohol abuse.

Pancreatic cancer is a silent disease, producing no symptoms until the advanced stages. The most common warning signs include weight loss, jaundice, abdominal or low back pain, and diarrhea. Others include fever and lesions on the legs. Patients may also experience emotional disturbances such as anxiety and depression, as well as premonitions of life-threatening illness.

Treatment for pancreatic cancer consists of surgery, radiation therapy, and drugs. However, the diagnosis usually comes so late that these therapies are rarely feasible. Drugs used for treating pancreatic cancer are antibiotics, anticholinergics (especially propantheline), antacids, diuretics, insulin, analgesics, and pancreatic enzymes.

Cancer of the Uterus and Cervix

An estimated 45,500 new cases of cancer of the uterus and cervix were diagnosed in 1992. Cervical cancer caused about 4,400 deaths in 1992, with uterine cancer causing some 5,600 deaths. Thanks to regular Pap testing for early detection, the death rate for uterine cancer has shrunk by more than 70 percent in the past 40 years. The incidence of invasive cervical cancer has also decreased steadily, being replaced in frequency by carcinoma in situ, a precancerous condition found mostly in women over the age of 50.

Although all women are at risk for cervical cancer, this type of cancer tends to strike more frequently among women in lower socioeconomic groups. Other risk factors include multiple sex partners, having intercourse at an early age, cigarette smoking, and certain sexually transmitted diseases. Women over 50 are most at risk of getting endometrial cancer, which affects the lining of the uterus.

Warning signs include abnormal vaginal bleeding or an unusual discharge, postcoital pain and bleeding, and for uterine cancer, uterine enlargement.

Treatment consists of surgery and radiation, alone or in combination. Precancerous stages may be treated by cryotherapy, in which cells are destroyed by extreme cold; electrocoagulation, in which tissue is destroyed by intense heat; or by local surgery. Precancerous conditions in the endometrium may be treated with progesterone. Uterine cancer may be treated with doxorubicin, vincristine, cyclophosphamide, and actinomycin D.

Leukemia

Leukemia is a cancer of the blood-forming tissues in which millions of abnormal white blood cells crowd out normal ones. Though usually considered a childhood disease, leukemia struck approximately 25,700 adults in 1992, compared to 2,500 young people. Leukemia caused an estimated 18,200 deaths that same year.

People of all ages and both genders are at risk for leukemia, although those with Down's syndrome and certain other genetic abnormalities tend to experience a higher incidence of this disease. While we don't know what causes leukemia in most cases, excessive exposure to ionizing radiation and certain chemicals are suspected to be contributing factors.

The early warning signs of leukemia include paleness, fatigue, weight loss, a tendency to bruise easily, repeated infections,

CANCER IN CHILDREN

An estimated 7,800 new cases of pediatric cancer were diagnosed in 1992; approximately 1,500 children died of cancer that same year. The cancer mortality rate for this age-group has declined from 8.3 cases per 100,000 in 1950 to 3.3 per 100,000 in 1988.

Unfortunately, pediatric cancers are often difficult to detect. Consequently, regular medical checkups are advised, and parents should be alert to any unusual, persistent symptoms. Warning signs include localized pain or persistent limping; any unusual mass or swelling; unexplained fever, illness, paleness, or loss of energy; frequent headaches, often with vomiting; a sudden tendency to bruise; sudden eye or vision changes; and excessive, rapid weight loss.

The most common childhood cancers include:
- Leukemia
- Osteogenic Sarcoma and Ewing's Sarcoma (bone cancers)
- Neuroblastoma (usually appears in the abdomen with accompanying swelling)
- Rhabdomyosarcoma (cancer of soft tissue in the head and neck area, genitourinary area, trunk, and extremities)
- Brain cancer
- Lymphomas and Hodgkin's Disease (involving the lymph nodes)
- Retinoblastoma (of the eye)
- Wilm's Tumor (kidney cancer)

and hemorrhages such as nosebleeds. Any of these symptoms can appear suddenly in acute leukemia. The progress of chronic leukemia can be slow and produce no symptoms for years.

The treatment of leukemia usually consists of chemotherapy to kill the attacking abnormal blood cells. Treatment varies according to the specific type of leukemia.

Drugs used to treat leukemias include methotrexate, cytarabine, vincristine, prednisone, L-asparaginase, daunorubicin, doxorubicin, thioguanine, cyclophosphamide, amsacrine, 5-azacytidine, and mitoxantrone—alone or in combination.

Treatment of infections associated with the disease may include antifungal, antibacterial, and antiviral drugs. Bone marrow transplants are effective in some cases.

Skin Cancer

Skin cancer is by far the most common of all cancers, with more than 600,000 cases occurring each year. Fortunately, the vast majority of these cancers are highly curable basal cell or squamous cell cancers. A small minority, however, are the extremely dangerous form called melanoma.

Melanoma was diagnosed in an estimated 32,000 people in the United States in 1992. The incidence of melanoma has increased by about four percent a year since 1973.

Excessive exposure to the sun is the greatest risk factor, especially for people with fair complexions. On-the-job exposure to coal tar, pitch, creosote, arsenic compounds, or radium also increases the risk of melanoma.

Early detection is crucial. People should examine their skin regularly for any unusual changes. Any changes in the size or color of a mole or other darkly pigmented spot or growth should be reported to a doctor immediately. Bleeding, scaliness, oozing, or a change in the appearance of a bump or nodule; the spread of pigmentation beyond its border; and any changes in sensation—itchiness, tenderness, or pain—are other warning signals of skin cancer.

Melanoma often begins as a small, mole-like growth that enlarges, changes color, becomes ulcerated, and bleeds easily. A melanoma is usually asymmetrical, has irregular borders and uneven pigmentation, and is larger than six millimeters in diameter.

Skin cancer treatments include surgery; radiation; electrodesiccation, in which the tissue is destroyed by heat; and cryosurgery, in which extreme cold is used to destroy the tissue.

Ovarian Cancer

Ovarian cancer causes more deaths than any other type of cancer affecting the reproductive system. In 1992, an estimated 21,000 women contracted this disease, and approximately 13,000 died from it.

The risk of ovarian cancer increases with age. Women over the age of 60 have the highest incidence. Women who have never given birth are twice as likely to develop ovarian cancer as those who have. Early pregnancy and menopause and the use of oral contraceptives seem to offer protection against ovarian cancer.

Ovarian cancer often shows no symptoms until the later stages. Most commonly, women notice an enlarged abdomen. Other symptoms may include vague, unexplained digestive disturbances.

Treatment is altered according to the stage of the disease and consists of varying combinations of surgery, chemotherapy, and radiation. Drugs useful in treating ovarian cancer include chlorambucil, melphalan, cyclophosphamide, and cisplatin.

Bladder Cancer

Bladder cancer was diagnosed in approximately 51,600 people and caused the deaths of 9,500 Americans in 1992. Bladder cancer strikes many more men than women. It is the fourth most common type of cancer in men and the ninth most common in women.

Smoking is the most serious risk factor for bladder cancer, although people who live in urban areas and those exposed to dye, rubber, or leather products at work are also at higher risk.

The most common symptoms of bladder cancer are blood in the urine and increased frequency of urination.

Treatment consists of surgery—alone or in combination with other therapies. Chemotherapy for bladder cancer often consists of 5-fluorouracil, cisplatin, cyclophosphamide, doxorubicin, methotrexate, and vinblastine.

Other Cancers

Oral cancers killed approximately 7,950 Americans in 1992, with an estimated 30,300 new cases diagnosed that same year. Cigarette, cigar, or pipe smoking, along with the use of smokeless tobacco and excessive alcohol consumption, are the greatest risk factors for this disease.

The warning signs of oral cancer include a sore that bleeds easily and doesn't heal, a persistent red or white patch, and a lump or thickening. As the disease progresses, the individual might also experience difficulty swallowing, chewing, or moving the tongue.

Oral cancers are principally treated by radiation and surgery.

Cancer can develop in any part of any organ in the body. For example, there are malignant brain tumors, pituitary tumors, laryngeal tumors, thyroid cancer, and spinal neoplasms. Cancer can also occur in the stomach, esophagus, kidney, liver, and gallbladder. Cancers of the genitalia include testicular cancer, penile cancer, vaginal cancer, cancer of the vulva, and fallopian tube cancer. People also develop primary malignant bone tumors, multiple myeloma,

Hodgkin's disease (cancer of the lymph nodes), malignant lymphomas, and mycosis fungoides.

Therapy is always determined by the type of cancer, and the extent of its spread at the time of diagnosis. The chance of recovery is largely dependent on the same factors, which is why early detection is so crucially important. Always remember: Finding a cancer before it becomes widespread is the best way of improving your odds of a successful cure. □

CHAPTER 8

New Answers for Pain

Pain is the chief reason that people seek medical care. And whether it is a tooth, ear, stomach, head, or back that aches, people all want the same thing—relief. Since ancient times, humanity has been preoccupied with finding ways to relieve pain. For thousands of years, our ancestors had only a few substances (mainly alcohol, opium, and the coca and hemp plants) to help make the pain go away.

But modern pharmacology changed all that. Today, dozens of drugs mercifully eliminate, or at least greatly reduce, the pain that comes with all types of ailments. However, their effectiveness for chronic pain is a different matter. Treating chronic pain is tricky; great care and caution must be exercised because of the potential for side effects and addiction associated with pain-relieving drugs.

What Is Pain?

Pain is the body's way of telling us that something is wrong. If we place our hand too close to a fire, we feel pain. When a bone is broken or the skin is cut, if we have inflammation from arthritis, or tense muscles from stress, a signal flashes from nerves in the distressed area to a part of the spinal cord where cells called pain receptors are located. These pain receptors send the signal along different tracks in the spinal cord to the brain, where the message of pain is registered.

Pain evokes emotion. Sudden, short-lived pain can cause anxiety; constant, unrelenting pain can leave us seriously depressed. Because of the emotional aspect of pain, treatment may involve much more than common pain-killers, particularly for those in constant distress.

Common Types of Pain

For purposes of treatment, doctors divide pain into the following three basic types:

- Acute pain, which is usually temporary and often the result of injury. Causes of acute pain range from surgery, fractures, infections, and burns to natural events such as childbirth.

THE MYRIAD CAUSES OF CHRONIC PAIN

A list of disorders that can lead to chronic pain would be almost endless; but here is a sample of some common culprits:

- **Lower back problems, slipped disks, and sciatica**
- Arthritis, tendinitis, and bursitis
- Sickle-cell anemia and hemophilia
- **Nerve damage caused by diabetes, kidney failure, and many other problems**

- Chronic pain, which is arbitrarily defined as a pain that persists for more than three to six months and threatens to disrupt the patient's normal activities. Chronic pain is associated with a wide range of long-lasting and permanent disorders (see box).

- Cancer pain syndromes, which can result from either the tumor itself or the surgery, radiation, and chemotherapy used during treatment.

In addition to these three major types of general pain, headaches come in so many forms—and have so many causes—that they are considered a category unto themselves (see box).

Treating Acute Pain

Because this type of pain is often the result of a specific trauma or infection, your doctor's first goal is to eliminate the underlying cause, if at all possible. To relieve the pain while other measures take effect, he or she will draw on a wide array of analgesics, including the following:

- Aspirin, buffered or plain
- Acetaminophen
- Narcotics
- Nonsteroidal anti-inflammatory drugs (NSAIDs), such as Motrin
- Tranquilizers
- Muscle relaxants
- Local anesthetics, applied to the surface or injected

The choice of analgesic varies according to the severity of the pain and the stage of the healing process. Consider, for example, a fracture.

The pain of a fracture results from muscle, nerve, and soft-tissue damage. When the bone is first being set, pain-killing measures vary with the severity of the injury. They can range all the way from general anesthesia to use of a local anesthetic and a narcotic analgesic such as meperidine (Demerol). (A muscle relaxant may be used to help stretch muscles and make it easier to set the bone.)

As the fracture heals, painkillers containing codeine are gradually replaced by milder pain relievers such as aspirin or NSAIDs. Aspirin usually provides sufficient pain relief for strains and sprains. However, if the strain is chronic and doesn't respond to local heat application, muscle relaxants may be necessary.

Likewise, the intense pain typically following surgery and childbirth is treated initially with morphine-based analgesics administered intravenously, intramuscularly, or epidurally (in the spine). These measures may be followed with PCA (patient-controlled intravenous agents), then oral painkillers, and finally milder aspirin and acetaminophen compounds.

Treatment for other forms of acute pain varies with the cause. Depending on the severity, pain from burns is treated with anything from aspirin to narcotic-based painkillers. Though pain occurs with most bacterial infections, the first line of treatment is to cure the infection with antibiotics. Analgesics are given only for specific conditions—in the treatment of certain skin infections, for example. The treatment of viral infections ranges from acetaminophen for the head and muscle aches of the flu to codeine compounds for the uncomfortable itching and pain of shingles.

Treating Chronic Pain

An estimated 80 million Americans suffer from chronic pain. Though narcotic analgesics are extremely effective in easing acute pain, their addictive properties and side effects make these drugs a less desirable choice for long-term use and often undermine the relief they bring. That's why they must be used carefully, if at all, for chronic pain. It is also the reason that other methods have been developed to treat and manage the problem.

HEADACHES

Headaches are the most common pain complaint. Ninety percent of all headaches are caused by tension—muscular, vascular, or a combination of both types. The remaining 10 percent result from underlying intracranial, biological, or psychological disorders. Migraines are severe, throbbing headaches that result from the contraction and expansion of cranial arteries. We don't know what causes migraines, but we do know that they afflict about 10 percent of the population, tend to run in families, and are more prevalent in women.

Most people rely on over-the-counter medications, such as aspirin or acetaminophen, to treat simple headaches. Typically caused by fleeting conditions such as fatigue, emotional strain, menstruation, or environmental stimuli (bright lights, crowds, or noise), these headaches usually subside when the stress ends.

But if a headache persists for more than a few days or recurs over an extended period of time, it should be reported to a physician in order to determine any possible underlying causes. These causes may include glaucoma; diseases of the teeth, scalp, extracranial arteries, external or middle ear; spasms of the shoulder, neck, or face; systemic disease; hypertension; intracranial bleeding; head trauma or tumor; aneurysms; and abscesses. Vasodilators, such as alcohol, histamines, and nitrates, can also cause headaches.

Migraine headaches are characterized by intense localized throbbing that usually spreads. Migraines are often preceded by changes in vision (a flashing blind-spot or the absence of half of the normal field of vision), pins and needles on one side of the body, or impaired speech. The headaches are frequently accompanied by nausea, vomiting, loss of appetite, and sensitivity to light. Sometimes migraines are a symptom of the onset of menopause.

The best treatment for migraines is ergotamine (Cafergot, Bellergal-S), taken alone or with caffeine. Drug treatment is most effective when the medication is used in the early stages of an attack. If nausea and vomiting are present, the drug may be given as a rectal suppository. Propranolol (Inderal) and calcium channel blockers, such as verapamil (Calan, Isoptin) and diltiazem (Cardizem), can help prevent migraines.

The treatment of chronic headaches depends on the type of headache and may include anything from aspirin to codeine or meperidine (Demerol). Acute attacks often respond well to tranquilizers; chronic tension headaches are sometimes alleviated by muscle relaxants. An accurate diagnosis and elimination of underlying causes of the problem are essential. Psychotherapy may be necessary if the headaches are caused by emotional distress.

Indeed, a new medical specialty known as pain management has emerged in recent years. Pain management employs a wide range of therapies to help people learn to live with pain, using only a minimum of drugs. These alternative treatments include exercise, deep-muscle relaxation training, massage, biofeedback, cognitive therapy for pain control, TENS (Transcutaneous Electrical Nerve Stimulation), neural blockade, steroid therapy, and diet counseling. Because chronic pain usually affects a person's psychological well-being and his or her relationships, individual, group, and family therapy are also advised in most cases.

The full spectrum of analgesics and muscle relaxants are prescribed for chronic pain, although morphine-based drugs are generally replaced with NSAIDs to minimize the possibility of addiction. Antidepressants have also been found to be effective for some individuals suffering from long-term pain.

To meet the needs of those with chronic cancer pain, doctors are now using a variety of advanced techniques. Painkillers can be delivered through home intravenous infusion systems or implanted epidural catheters. TENS systems may come into play, and neurolytic (nerve-destroying) neural blockade has proved effective for certain patients.

Despite all these advances, there's still no perfect solution for pain. Many of our current medications present one drawback or another, ranging from gastric side effects to the potential of addiction. Nevertheless, there's no denying we now have more ways of providing effective control of pain than could be imagined just a few decades ago. □

CHAPTER 9

Overcoming Emotional and Psychological Problems

A nyone, at any time, can develop an emotional problem. You begin to feel sad, angry, alone, or just frustrated by the problems of everyday life. You lose sleep, become irritable, or simply want to "pull the covers over your head." Ordinarily, simply "venting"—talking with your spouse or a clergyman, friend, or co-worker—is enough to put you in a better frame of mind.

But if things don't turn around, and your ability to function diminishes each day, you may be suffering from something more than a temporary emotional upset. You may have a condition that needs professional treatment.

If so, you will not be alone. According to the National Institute of Mental Health, more than 41 million Americans—nearly 1 in 5—experience a mental disorder at some point in their lives.

■ More than 7 million children and adolescents suffer from psychological problems such as hyperactivity, autism, and conduct disorders.

■ Severe clinical depression, needing professional treatment, strikes more than 10 million people during the course of their lives.

■ Each year, more than 18 million Americans are affected by the most common of all mental problems: anxiety disorder.

■ Nearly 14 million Americans abuse alcohol or illicit drugs to the point of dependence each year.

■ More than 1.5 million people have schizophrenia and need hospitalization or long-term treatment.

■ Perhaps as many as 14 percent of our elderly suffer from some degree of dementia, or loss of mental function.

Studies conducted by the Institute of Medicine show that direct expenditures on health care for mental illness total $23.4

billion a year; substance abuse adds another $16.9 billion.

But that's only a fraction of the true cost. If mental illness goes undiagnosed, the personal and social consequences can be severe. Suicide is the eighth leading cause of death in the United States and the third leading cause among adolescents and young adults. And the lost workdays, accidents, crime, and reduced productivity that can be traced to untreated mental illness have been estimated to cost us upwards of $250 billion a year.

Much of this suffering and expense could be reduced by early detection and prompt treatment. But unfortunately, as few as one in four who need help seek it. Less than a third of those suffering from depression look for treatment; and less than 10 percent of the children who need help receive it.

Ironically, 80 percent of those suffering from mental illness can be treated effectively with medication and therapy on an outpatient basis.

What Do We Mean by Mental Illness?

Mental illness is a broad, umbrella-term for a wide range of disorders that can strike anyone. Even today, the term "mentally ill" carries with it a heavy burden of social stigma, embarrassment, and fear. The idea of "losing your mind" remains a terrifying thought.

Yet, given today's improved diagnostic and therapeutic techniques, such fears are usually misplaced. With earlier detection, better diagnosis, and faster, more effective treatment, millions of the "mentally ill" are now able to lead satisfying, productive lives.

Amazingly, only 40 years ago more than a half million profoundly ill people were beyond help, languishing in huge mental hospitals where they were managed with restraints, confinement, and sedation. The stigma attached to "mental illness" was enormous—few people would admit that they or any member of their family suffered from any kind of psychiatric disease.

As a result, most of those who were "neurotic" or "phobic" went untreated, leading lives of hidden desperation. For those who did seek help, psychiatric treatment consisted almost entirely of "talk therapy," or psychoanalysis. The most seriously ill psychotic patients were simply warehoused in the hospitals.

In those days, health-care experts predicted that the number of people confined to mental institutions would more than double in the next few decades. Yet by the mid-1970s the number of psychiatric inpatients had actually dropped by half!

What had happened? Why were they wrong?

The answer is simple. For decades, researchers had concentrated on development of medications to cure infections, heart disease, cancer, and other illnesses, while mental disorders were ignored. But in 1952, chlorpromazine (Thorazine) was tried in schizophrenic patients at low doses. People who suffered from delusions, hallucinations, paranoia, and other symptoms improved almost immediately. For the first time, psychiatrists realized that medication could be a partner with other forms of therapy for mental illness. Once the pharmaceutical floodgates opened, psychiatry changed overnight. A new age of "biopsychiatry" was born that led to tremendous strides in the diagnosis and treatment of mental illness.

TEN WARNING SIGNS OF MENTAL ILLNESS

According to the American Psychiatric Association, anyone displaying one or more of these warning signs should be evaluated by a doctor as soon as possible:

1. Marked personality change
2. Inability to cope with problems and daily activities
3. Strange or grandiose ideas
4. Obsessive ideas
5. Prolonged depression and apathy
6. Marked changes in eating or sleeping patterns
7. Thinking or talking about suicide
8. Extreme highs and lows
9. Abuse of alcohol or drugs
10. Excessive anger, hostility, or violent behavior

Major Types of Mental Illness

Today, psychiatrists use everything from blood tests and brain scans to complete physical exams and family histories to aid in the diagnosis of mental disorders. Targeting an emotional disorder for accurate treatment is a complicated task, so mental health professionals have created a unique system to help pin down ambiguous psychiatric problems. Hundreds of types of mental illness are cataloged in a book known as *The Diagnostic and Statistical Manual of Mental Disorders* (DSM-IIIR). Published by the American Psychiatric Association and currently in its third edition, DSM-IIIR, like *Physician's Desk Reference*, is the "bible" of its discipline. Understanding that the mind is, in effect, an organ system like the heart or kidneys and, like these organs, can develop a disease, was an important breakthrough in diagnosis and treatment.

The DSM-IIIR breaks psychiatric illness into 25 major categories and over 100 sub-categories, each with its own unique set of symptoms. When a patient's symptoms fit within the DSM-IIIR criteria, a psychiatrist can pinpoint a specific diagnosis. Among the major categories of mental illness listed in the DSM-IIIR are the following:

- Anxiety Disorders (phobias, panic disorder, post-traumatic stress disorder, obsessive-compulsive disorder)
- Mood Disorders (depression, manic-depressive disorder)
- Schizophrenia
- Developmental Disorders (learning disorders, retardation, autism)
- Disruptive Behavior Disorders (attention deficit hyperactivity disorder, conduct disorder)
- Substance Abuse Disorders (alcoholism, drug dependence)
- Delusional Disorders (delusional paranoia)
- Sexual Disorders
- Sleep Disorders
- Impulse Control Disorders (kleptomania, pyromania)
- Dissociative Disorders (multiple-personality disorder)
- Eating Disorders (anorexia, bulimia)
- Organic Mental Disorders (Alzheimer's disease and other psychiatric diseases that result from metabolic problems in the brain or from substance abuse)

Perhaps the most important step in diagnosing any mental illness is for the patient and the family to actually seek help. As with a physical illness, the earlier an emotional or psychiatric problem is detected, the more likely and the easier is the cure. Unfortunately, psychiatric symptoms are far easier to ignore or misinterpret than physiological symptoms. While the criteria for disorders like cancer, arthritis, and high blood pressure are precisely defined, psychological symptoms (e.g., "the blues") are often ambiguous. Coupled with the stigma or "denial" that is common in questions of mental health, this may make an accurate diagnosis harder to achieve.

Still, the meaning of certain specific sets of symptoms is relatively clear. Here's a closer look at the most prevalent types of mental illness.

Anxiety Disorders

Almost everybody gets anxious. Most of us feel nervous before a test or an important business meeting. The "butterflies" that we all experience from time to time are so common that we tend to ignore them. Yet, for more than 18 million Americans, "anxiety" is so severe that it interferes with their daily functioning.

Actually, a genuine anxiety disorder is marked not by anxiety, but by outright fear. While anxiety is a form of mental tension that we can't really put our finger on, fear is easily recognized. Its symptoms are well known: shakiness, trembling, aching muscles, sweating, chills, dizziness, pounding heart, dry mouth, a lump in the throat.

If you are diagnosed with an anxiety disorder, you suffer from one or more of a group of problems including generalized anxiety disorder, phobias, panic disorders, obsessive-compulsive disorder, and post traumatic stress disorder.

Phobias are the most common of the anxiety disorders. An estimated 5 to 12 percent of the population suffer a psychological and physiological reaction to a place, a situation, or an object that interferes with daily life. The "phobic reaction" is almost a reflex. The victim is filled with dread, horror, and terror. He begins to gasp for breath, shake, and often flees. Some people will go miles out of their way to avoid a phobic situation.

There are hundreds of phobias. For instance, there is "agoraphobia," a phobia that is widely misunderstood. Most think that an "agoraphobic" is simply afraid to leave home. In fact, his real fear is of being alone in public places from which he thinks escape would be difficult or help unavailable if he were hurt or trapped. As a result, agoraphobics stay home rather than risk the terror they've come to expect.

Likewise, people with social phobias aren't antisocial. Rather, they fear that they will do something in a public place that will cause them humiliation. They fear "being watched" while doing almost anything—eating a meal, standing in line at the bank, making small talk at the beach. To some extent, almost everyone has social phobias—nervousness in front of an audience is the most common. However, most of us can cope and get on with it. Someone with a social phobia will, like an agoraphobic, go to any length to avoid placing himself in an "unsafe" situation.

"The Simple Phobias": Make a list of just about anything—dogs, cats, snakes, mice, bats, spiders, insects, dark rooms, heights, closed spaces—and you will find someone with a phobic reaction to it.

Panic Disorder: A panic attack is one of the most frightening of all psychological events.

Imagine that you are walking down the street one day, feeling fine, when, out of the blue, you are overcome by an intense fear and foreboding unlike anything you've ever felt before. You are literally frozen to the sidewalk, unable to move. And then it gets worse. You start to shake, sweat, gasp for air. You are sure you are having a heart attack and that you will die the next instant. People stop and stare; some even offer to help. But you can't move or respond. The weight on your chest is growing heavier, and you are now just waiting to die.

And then, as suddenly as it started, it stops. Gone. Since you feel so good, you carry on, ignoring the event—except that you now avoid the street where it happened.

A week goes by and nothing happens, and then another week. You've almost forgotten about the attack completely when, without warning, it hits you again, this time far more intensely. Your body is tingling. You're overcome with nausea. You are so out of control you think you're going insane. If you don't continue to ignore what's happened and instead call a psychiatrist, chances are you'll be told that you are one of nearly 3 million Americans who suffer from the relatively common form of anxiety called "panic disorder," and that the attacks are every bit as real as they seem.

Panic disorder, many researchers think, may be partly a result of genetics—it does run in families—or may be caused by disturbances of the neurotransmitters that form the brain's chemical messenger system. Panic attacks may also be signs of underlying physiologic illness. Researchers often refer to panic attacks as "impostors," because their symptoms may actually be caused by heart disease, thyroid imbalances, or respiratory problems.

In fact, more than 40 medical problems can cause panic-like symptoms.

Obsessive-Compulsive Disorder: This illness is very much what it sounds like. People who have continual, unwanted thoughts that prevent them from functioning properly are considered "obsessed;" to rid themselves of these nagging ideas, they usually develop "compulsions"—rituals they must go through before they can move on to another activity. Compulsive rituals include repetitious washing, repeating certain phrases, completing steps in a process over and over, counting and recounting, checking and re-checking to make sure something hasn't been forgotten, excessive neatness, and hoarding of useless items.

The cause of OCD, as it's called, has remained a mystery, despite theories that link it to other disorders, such as depression. Research on a physical cause of the disorder is on the rise; and an effective medication (clomipramine) is available.

Post-Tramatic Stress Disorder: PTSD was known for years as shell shock or battle fatigue, but we now know that it's not limited to soldiers who've seen too much of war. PTSD is a disorder that can affect anyone who has survived a severe and unusual trauma, such as a hurricane, tornado, flood, or airplane crash. One psychiatrist calls it "aftershock," which is an apt description, because the symptoms of PTSD may surface months after the actual event.

Veterans do remain the main victims of PTSD. The Department of Veterans Affairs estimates that 700,000 to 800,000 of the

3.5 million Vietnam veterans have experienced PTSD. For these vets and other victims, the symptoms are often a "re-experience of the traumatic event . . . also known as flashbacks." In effect, the person replays the emotions he felt during the traumatic event itself. Some of the afflicted develop insomnia, extreme anger, fear and grief, and even an inability to feel any emotions, which leads to withdrawal from society. Some PTSD patients have "survivor's guilt." Others begin to avoid situations that remind them of the traumatic event (flying, for example).

Treating Anxiety Disorders: Anxiety disorders are often treated with a combination of psychotherapy and drugs. Once medication has reduced the symptoms of the various anxiety disorders, psychiatrists use behavioral therapy, psychotherapy, and other forms of therapy that are tailored to the patient's personal needs.

The most commonly prescribed medications for anxiety are the benzodiazepine class of drugs, such as Valium and Xanax, and other tranquilizers such as Buspar. For panic disorder, tricyclic antidepressants such as Elavil are usually given. Recently some psychiatrists have been using beta blockers such as propranolol (Inderal) to curb certain forms of anxiety and phobias. (For more on beta blockers, see the chapter on heart disease, page 711).

Depression

Depression is not just "the blues." Depression is one of the most serious and common of all mental disorders. It is also one of the most treatable—provided the victim seeks treatment. At any time, more than nine million Americans may be suffering from depression. More than 15 percent of Americans are attacked by depression at some time in their lives.

While we've all felt sad at times, we usually get up, go to work, and try to overcome our general discouragement with life. But when these overwhelming feelings of sadness persist—even if for only a few weeks—you may be suffering from a clinical depression, which means you need some professional treatment. Besides a depressed mood or loss of pleasure, symptoms of clinical depression may include appetite and sleep changes, apathy, fatigue, hopelessness, guilt, loss of concentration, and thoughts of suicide.

There are two major kinds of depression: bipolar and unipolar. In bipolar depression, the patient rides a roller coaster of emotions from high to low, leading to the term "manic depression." Unipolar depression, also known as clinical or major depression, lacks bipolar's "highs."

Treating Depression: The American Psychiatric Association estimates that 80 to 90 percent of all depression can be treated. The first step is an accurate diagnosis. Along with a physical and lab tests to rule out causes such as reduced thyroid activity, a complete psychiatric history should be taken. And because depression and other major psychiatric problems are side effects of many medications, a good work-up will also include a review of the patient's medications and any illicit drug use.

Once a diagnosis is made, the basic medications used for depression today are:

■ **Tricyclic antidepressants** such as Elavil, Tofranil, and Pamelor, and serotonin reuptake blockers such as Prozac: These drugs are prescribed for patients who are in despair, feeling helpless, and unable to feel pleasure.

■ **Monoamine Oxidase (MAO) Inhibitors** like Nardil, Parnate, and Marplan: These medications are usually used when depressive symptoms are accompanied by symptoms of an anxiety disorder.

■ **Lithium**: This is the most effective drug for manic depression. However, it can also be used to prevent recurring episodes of depression.

When one of these medications is prescribed, follow-up and continued medical supervision are critical. Blood tests and other metabolic studies are often performed on a regular basis to determine the effect of the drug on the patient. This can be a drawn-out process, because most drugs for depression don't relieve symptoms instantly. Often it takes four to six weeks for a medication to become effective.

Other forms of therapy for depression include interpersonal psychotherapy to help broken relationships, cognitive behavioral therapy to help reverse the patient's negative view of himself and the world, and traditional psychoanalysis. Electroconvulsive therapy—known as ECT or shock therapy—has been used effectively in patients who cannot tolerate the side effects of today's medications, who cannot wait for the medications to work, or who are unable to take drugs for other reasons. While controversial, ECT has proved to be a good treatment option.

Schizophrenia

One of the most debilitating mental illnesses, schizophrenia often appears first in adolescence. Like alcoholism, diabetes, or high blood pressure, this disease, once it strikes, is usually with the patient for life.

The first signs of schizophrenia may be mild—work performance tails off or the victim stops seeing friends and loved ones. Soon, however, psychotic symptoms surface:

TEN QUESTIONS TO ASK ABOUT ANY INPATIENT TREATMENT PROGRAM

Sometimes mental health problems require hospitalization. This is a serious decision that should not be made without considering the following questions carefully:

1. Is an experienced medical doctor in charge?
2. Does the program provide a total treatment environment, including individual, group, and family therapy?
3. Is a fully qualified staff available, including psychiatrists, psychologists, nurses, and social workers?
4. Does the program use effective diagnostic and laboratory tests to help make correct diagnoses and to evaluate treatment?
5. Does the program provide for family sessions and counseling when necessary? If so, how many family sessions are there?
6. For child and adolescent hospital programs: Does the program offer an accredited school and/or vocational training to prevent children and teens from falling behind in their schoolwork?
7. Are family members encouraged to visit?
8. Are support groups such as Alcoholics Anonymous encouraged?
9. Does the program provide well-defined aftercare through individual or group therapy?
10. How much does the program cost? Will your insurance cover all or part of the treatment, and for how long will your insurance continue?

hallucinations, paranoia, delusions, disordered thinking. At times, the more severe symptoms abate and the patient is left in a sort of withdrawn state. Some people just lose touch and drift off into another reality.

Some experts believe that the causes of schizophrenia are genetic, but lie dormant until adolescence, when the body undergoes changes that produce the combination of chemicals needed to trip off the disease. Other theories suggest that schizophrenia may be an autoimmune disorder in which the immune system turns on the body itself, or that it's the result of a prenatal viral infection. Whatever the cause proves to be, we still know very little about the disease. But we do know how to treat it on some levels.

Treating Schizophrenia: Medications called "antipsychotics," which include Thorazine and Haldol, seem to be effective in reducing symptoms in up to 80 percent of all patients. Despite severe side effects such as tardive dyskinesia, which afflicts 20 to 30 percent of patients with involuntary movements of the mouth and tongue, these medications combat the hallucinations and delusions that are the hallmarks of schizophrenia. As these symptoms subside, psychotherapy and group therapy for the family and patient can create an environment in which the patient can function once again.

Childhood Disorders

Mental illness in children and adolescents is particularly painful. Childhood is supposed to be a time of joy, learning, and growth. But a child hampered by learning disabilities, antisocial behavior or severe depression is robbed of one of the most precious periods of life. The greater tragedy is that of the 7.5 million children suffering from some sort of mental disorder, 70 percent do not receive the kind of treatment they need.

■In the past three decades, mental illness, and particularly clinical depression, has led to a doubling of the suicide rate among adolescents and young adults.

■Between 200,000 and 300,000 children suffer from autism—a developmental disorder that prevents learning and other cognitive growth.

■Three to five percent of all children have Attention Deficit Hyperactivity Disorder (ADHD), also known as minimal brain dysfunction, among other names. Basically, these kids can't concentrate, learn, or behave normally. They can't finish a project, don't seem to listen, and require very close supervision. They can be very bright, yet unable to focus their intelligence. Tragically, many are labeled "troublemakers" and shunted aside in schools and homes that don't understand the problem.

■Conduct Disorders (CD) afflict more adolescent boys and girls than any other emotional illness. As many as nine percent of males and two percent of females are in the grip of violent, socially unacceptable behavior patterns that lead them to destroy property, steal, and make physical or sexual attacks on others. CD may arise from a combination of biological predisposition and environmental influence that is not fully understood. Whatever the cause, CD refers to a specific set of behaviors, not merely to a difficult teenager who's moody and hard to control.

Children also suffer from several forms of anxiety similar to those seen in adults. For example, separation anxiety can lead a child to persistently refuse to leave a parent's side. It may be more apparent when the school years begin, but can strike at any time. Phobias, too are common among children. They include fear of the dark, animals, and certain colors. In fact, according to some estimates, as many as 43 percent of children under age 12 have some sort of exaggerated fear.

Treating Childhood Disorders: Curbing mental illness in children is often controversial, since children are harder to treat effectively on an outpatient basis than are adults. Often their problems stem from sexual or physical abuse, drug addiction, genetic conditions, or dysfunctional family environments. If a child is left in the same destructive environment that caused the problem, medication or therapy may not be effective.

Treatment for children almost always includes the entire family. For some problems, such as depression, anxiety, and phobias, the same medications used in adults can, with close supervision by a doctor, be effective in conjunction with family therapy.

Treatment for ADHD involves medications such as Ritalin, a special educational track that enables the student to remain in school with his peers, and family therapy. Medications enable the child to control his impulsive behavior and perform without loss of attention. The American Psychiatric Association reports that between 70 and 80 percent of ADHD patients "respond to medications when they are properly used." Children with conduct disorders must have treatment that includes behavioral therapy and, when appropriate, medications for underlying depression or ADHD, if present.

There are other mental health problems that affect specific groups such as the elderly (see page 861) or teenage girls (anorexia and bulimia), or that result from organic brain damage, such as mental retardation. If you or a loved one suffers from one of these conditions, you should contact a psychiatrist who specializes in its treatment.

Many people define mental illness as "the absence of mental health." After all, we all know when we do or don't "feel good," both mentally and physically. However, as you can see by the variety of disorders, this definition is too simplistic. A mental illness is a specific problem that causes a sustained disruption of your general well-being, behavior, or mood, and interferes with your normal functioning. It can result in *either* psychological or physiological symptoms. The most important things to remember about mental illness are that it can usually be treated effectively, that it is not a sign of weakness or failure, that it is nobody's fault, and that getting help as soon as possible is a vital part of treatment. □

CHAPTER 10

OB/GYN Disorders: Causes and Treatments

The term OB/GYN stands for **obstetrics and gynecology**. This is the branch of medicine that deals with pregnancy, childbirth, and women's health problems. "Obstetrics" comes from *obstetrix*, the Latin word for midwife; "gynecology" comes from *gune*, the Greek word for woman.

Some OB/GYN specialists limit their practices to obstetrics. They provide health care to women before, during, and after childbirth. Others concentrate on gynecology, diagnosing and treating disorders of the female reproductive and urinary systems. Some OB/GYNs do both.

Good OB/GYN care is important, both to prevent problems and to treat any existing disease or disorder. For example:

■ Pregnant women who do not have regular prenatal checkups run almost double the risk of losing their babies through miscarriage or neonatal (newborn) death.

■ Pelvic inflammatory disease (PID) is diagnosed in more than one million women each year. A high percentage of these women require costly hospitalization; many end up permanently infertile.

Regular OB/GYN checkups could save a great deal of expense and avert much personal tragedy.

Common OB/GYN Disorders and Their Causes

OB/GYN specialists diagnose and treat a wide variety of problems related to menstruation, the urinary tract, the vulva and vagina, the uterus, the ovaries and fallopian tubes, the breasts, and the bone brittleness that sometimes develops after menopause. These physicians also diagnose and treat infertility.

Menstrual Disorders

Dysmenorrhea, or extremely painful menstruation, is a widespread problem, affecting some 10 percent of all women of childbearing age. During menstruation, natural chemicals called prostaglandins make the uterus and its blood vessels contract. Very strong contractions can be painful.

Primary dysmenorrhea occurs when the prostaglandins provoke an overly vigorous uterine response. Secondary dysmenorrhea is caused by such abnormalities as infection, a tumor, or a disorder called endometriosis.

Premenstrual syndrome (PMS) occurs just before a woman's monthly period and consists of physical and mental distress. About one in 10 women has PMS severe enough to create problems at work, at home, and in social relationships.

It was once assumed that PMS was simply the result of an hormonal imbalance. We now know that most women who suffer from PMS have normal hormone levels. A newer theory suggests that PMS may result from an interaction between female hormones and neurotransmitters—chemical messengers manufactured in the brain and nerve cells.

Endometriosis (derived from "endometrium," the lining of the uterus) develops when uterine cells migrate and grow elsewhere in the abdominal cavity. The cells may be found on the outside of the uterus, in the ovaries or fallopian tubes, or on the bowels. During menstruation, the endometrial tissue bleeds into the abdomen and causes inflammation, pain, and scarring.

THE FEMALE URINARY TRACT: COMMON SITE OF INFECTION

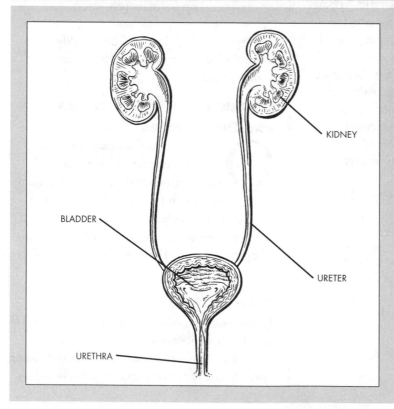

KIDNEY

BLADDER

URETER

URETHRA

A relatively short urethra conspires to increase the risk of urinary tract infections (UTIs) in women. In fact, between the ages of 20 and 50, women suffer 50 times as many UTIs as men. Bacteria traveling up the urethra may attack the bladder or even the kidneys themselves. Infections confined to the bladder are known as cystitis. If bacteria reach the kidneys, a condition called acute bacterial pyelonephritis can result.

Although we don't know what causes endometriosis, there is some evidence that the condition is inherited.

Urinary Tract Disorders

Urinary tract infection (UTI) is an extremely common condition that occurs in the urethra, bladder, or kidneys. UTIs are usually caused by bacteria originating in the bowels. Friction during intercourse sometimes transfers the bacteria from the vulva (external female genitals) into the urethra (passage to the bladder). The urethra is shorter in women than in men, which makes women more susceptible to UTIs.

Urinary incontinence is the chronic leaking of urine. This condition may also involve painful or frequent urination, bedwetting, or the need to urinate frequently throughout the night. Incontinence may be caused by infection, a urinary tract abnormality, estrogen loss after menopause, sagging pelvic muscles, or a neuromuscular disorder.

Disorders of the Vulva and Vagina

Contact dermatitis of the vulva is a chemical irritation of the skin. The dermatitis may be caused by perfumes or dyes in toilet paper, soap, menstrual pads, or feminine hygiene sprays.

Genital warts are caused by the human papillomavirus and are spread through sexual contact. The warts may be flat or raised, painless or painful. **Genital herpes,** an infection caused by the herpes simplex virus, is also transmitted sexually and causes blisterlike sores in the genital area or other parts of the body.

Vulvar intraepithelial neoplasia (VIN), is an abnormality of cell growth on the vulva. Some women have raised, itchy sores; others notice no symptoms at all. Left untreated, the neoplasia may gradually become cancerous. VIN may be caused by infection with the human papillomavirus—the same virus that causes genital warts.

Vaginitis, an inflammation of the vagina, causes redness, itching, discharge, and odor. Some cases of vaginitis stem from infection by bacteria, yeast, or protozoa. Other cases can be traced to antibiotics, birth control pills, frequent douching, tampons, tight or non-breathing pants, obesity, or diabetes.

Disorders of the Uterus

Cervicitis is an inflammation of the cervix, which is the low, narrow end of the uterus. Common in women of childbearing age, it may or may not cause vaginal discharge, pain, tenderness, or slight bleeding between periods.

Some cases of cervicitis are caused by infection with bacteria, protozoa, or a virus; others result from irritation from an IUD or a forgotten tampon. Sometimes the cause is unknown.

Cervical dysplasia is an abnormal growth of the cells of the cervix. Like VIN, this condition may eventually turn cancerous if left untreated.

Women who smoke, have multiple sexual partners, have genital warts, or first had sex before the age of 20 are at special risk of developing cervical dysplasia.

Abnormal uterine bleeding occurs when menstrual periods are irregular, last longer, or are heavier than usual. Bleeding that occurs between periods may also be deemed "abnormal."

Menopause (the "change of life") and hormonal imbalance are the most common causes of irregular periods. Other possible reasons for abnormal or heavy uterine bleeding include miscarriage; infection of the cervix or uterus; tubal pregnancy; abnormal blood clotting; fibroids; polyps in the uterus; abnormal thickening of the uterine lining; thyroid disease; cancer; an intrauterine contraceptive device (IUD); or birth control pills.

Pelvic inflammatory disease (PID) is an infection of the cervix that may spread to the uterus, fallopian tubes, and ovaries. PID affects one woman in seven at some point in life, causing chronic pain and abdominal abscesses. PID is also a leading cause of **tubal pregnancy,** in which the fertilized egg implants in one of the fallopian tubes instead of the uterus. Tubal pregnancy can be a medical emergency. If untreated, a tubal pregnancy may rupture the fallopian tube, causing the embryo to die and possibly endangering the mother's life.

PID usually develops as the result of a sexually transmitted (venereal) disease such as gonorrhea or chlamydial infection. PID may also develop as a result of infection following an abortion, childbirth, or the insertion of an intrauterine contraceptive device (IUD) into the uterus, but such cases are very rare.

KEY ELEMENTS OF THE FEMALE REPRODUCTIVE SYSTEM

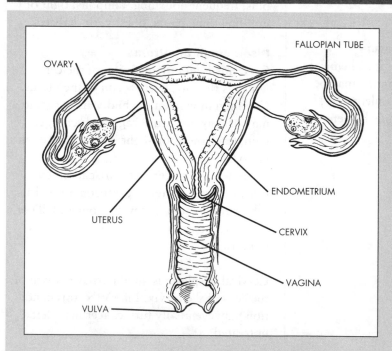

FALLOPIAN TUBE

OVARY

ENDOMETRIUM

UTERUS

CERVIX

VAGINA

VULVA

The female reproductive tract, host to the majority of gynecological disorders, includes the ovaries, uterus, cervix, vagina, and vulva. All are prey to infections; all can fall victim to cancer. Among the most dangerous infections is pelvic inflammatory disease. This condition can lead to a life-threatening tubal pregnancy, in which an egg released from the ovary lodges and develops within the fallopian tube, instead of completing its normal course to the uterus.

FIBROIDS: OFTEN UNNOTICED, SURPRISINGLY COMMON

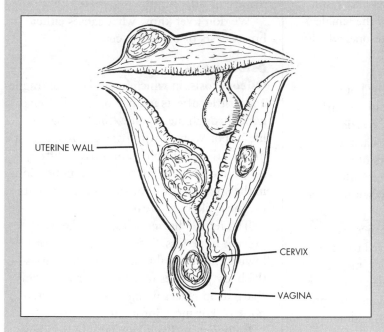

UTERINE WALL

CERVIX

VAGINA

It's estimated that as many as 40 percent of women develop these benign uterine growths by age 40. Few, however, experience any symptoms. If problems such as abnormal bleeding do occur, treatment options include removal of the growths (myomectomy) or the entire uterus (hysterectomy). Fibroids can develop anywhere within the walls of the uterus, or as protrusions attached by a stalk of tissue.

Fibroids (myomas) are noncancerous growths in or on the uterus. One out of every four or five women over the age of 35 has fibroids. These women may experience longer or heavier periods, irregular vaginal bleeding, abdominal or back pain, or frequent urination.

Although we don't know exactly what causes fibroids, we do know that abnormal growths tend to grow larger under the influence of the female hormone estrogen. For instance, fibroids often enlarge during pregnancy, when estrogen levels are high. Fibroids may also get bigger in women who use birth control pills with a relatively high estrogen content.

Uterine cancer most often affects the endometrium, or lining of the uterus. With early detection, the cure rate is more than 90 percent.

A woman is considered to be at increased risk for uterine cancer if her mother or sister has had the disease, or if she has previously had breast, ovarian, or colon cancer. Other risk factors include endometrial hyperplasia (abnormal thickening of the lining of the uterus); cyst-filled ovaries; irregular ovulation; unusually late menopause; and obesity.

Disorders of the Ovaries

Ovarian cysts are blister-like sacs filled with liquid. They may cause pain during intercourse or at other times. Women may also notice feelings of abdominal pressure and fullness. Most ovarian cysts are noncancerous.

Some ovarian cysts form at the time of ovulation, when the ovary releases an egg cell. Other types of ovarian cysts may result from (or cause) an imbalance of the female hormones estrogen and progesterone, which are produced in the ovaries.

Ovarian cancer may affect one or both ovaries. Although the cure rate in the early stages is 85 to 95 percent, early ovarian cancer is "silent" and thus very hard to detect. More than three-quarters of all ovarian cancers go undetected until the advanced stage of the disease, when the cure rate is only 10 to 20 percent.

The exact cause of ovarian cancer is unknown. A woman is considered to be at increased risk if her grandmother, mother, or sister has had the disease. Women who have never had children, are infertile, or have previously had cancer of the breast, endometrium, or colon are also at greater risk.

Disorders of the Breasts

Fibrocystic breast changes are noncancerous cysts that develop within the breasts, usually in women aged 25 to 50. The cysts may be small or large, painful or painless.

Breast cancer is extremely common and affects one woman out of 10. Early-stage breast cancer is usually curable. That's why OB/GYN specialists urge women to examine their own breasts every month for any lumps, thickenings, or other unusual developments.

Most OB/GYNs also advise regular mammograms (breast X-rays) once a woman reaches the age of 40.

We don't yet know what causes either breast cysts or breast cancer.

Osteoporosis

Osteoporosis, in which bones become fragile and brittle, affects many women who have gone through menopause (the "change of life"). For women with osteoporosis, even a minor fall, a light blow, or a trivial lifting action may be enough to break a bone. Bones in the spine, wrist, hip, and upper thigh are the most likely to break.

The female hormone estrogen helps prevent bone loss. After menopause—or following the surgical removal of the ovaries—the body produces much less estrogen. This sharp drop places women at risk for osteoporosis. For more information, turn to "Osteoporosis, Back Pain, and Other Bone Disorders," page 731.

Infertility

Infertility is the inability of a couple to have children. A couple is considered infertile if they fail to conceive after 12 months of trying. About 14 percent of couples in the United States meet this definition. Infertility may be caused by a problem with the man, the woman, or both partners. This is why couples with fertility problems should be diagnosed together.

The common causes of male infertility are sexually transmitted diseases such as gonorrhea or chlamydia; hormonal disorders; damage to the reproductive tract from surgery or disease; certain medications; overheating of the testes from tight clothing, a hot tub, or workplace conditions; and varicose veins in the scrotum.

In women, common causes of infertility are pelvic inflammatory disease (PID); endometriosis; defects or tumors of the uterus; adhesions from past surgery; hormonal imbalance that prevents ovulation; obesity; the use of alcohol, tobacco, or drugs; and the production of antibodies that neutralize the man's sperm.

Thyroid disease, diabetes, or the use of alcohol, tobacco, or marijuana can lead to infertility in both men and women.

Treatments Focus on Comfort and Function

Treatment for an OB/GYN disorder depends on what's wrong. Some conditions require medication, surgery, or both. In any case, the treatment objective is to ease the woman's discomfort and help her body function more normally.

When Surgery Is Needed

Common OB/GYN surgical procedures include:

Dilatation and curettage (D&C) is performed to help control heavy, prolonged, or irregular bleeding from the uterus. In a D&C, the cervix is stretched open and the lining of the uterus is gently suctioned or scraped. A sample of the lining may later be examined for possible tumors.

Laparoscopy is a procedure in which a fiberoptic instrument is inserted through a small incision in the abdomen. The doctor uses an eyepiece to look directly at the uterus, fallopian tubes, and ovaries. During laparoscopy, it is sometimes possible for the doctor to perform a procedure such as draining fluid from an ovarian cyst.

Laser treatment uses a laser (high-intensity beam of light) to destroy abnormal tissue—on the cervix, for example.

Electrosurgical excision involves using an electrified loop made of fine wire to remove growths on the cervix, vagina, or vulva.

Electrosurgery uses heat to destroy abnormal growths.

Cryotherapy uses a probe coated with a freezing agent to destroy abnormal growths.

Myomectomy is an operation to remove fibroids (benign growths) within the uterus.

Hysterectomy is an operation to remove the entire uterus because of abnormal growths.

Oophorectomy is the surgical removal of the ovaries.

When Medication Is Needed

In many cases, **medication** is sufficient to alleviate an OB/GYN problem. For example:

Antibiotics are used to treat reproductive organ or urinary tract infections caused by bacteria or protozoa.

Hormonal therapy typically includes synthetic estrogen and progesterone, the hormones contained in birth control pills. Hormones may also be used to treat dysmenorrhea (painful menstruation), certain types of vaginitis, and endometriosis. Hormonal treatment can also help prevent or halt osteoporosis. Hormones are given to some patients following breast cancer surgery.

Diuretics, or "water pills," help reduce bloating in women who have premenstrual syndrome.

Antiprostaglandins prevent menstrual cramps and menstrual-related nausea, diarrhea, and general achiness.

Antifungal medication is used to treat vaginal infections caused by yeast.

Acyclovir (Zovirax) alleviates the sores and blisters of a genital herpes infection.

Drugs such as **flavoxate (Urispas)**, which control abnormal bladder contractions, are useful in treating certain types of urinary incontinence (inability to hold urine).

Fertility drugs to bring on ovulation are used to treat certain types of infertility in women.

Anticancer drugs are used to treat tumors of the breast, uterus, or ovary, as well as other cancers. □

CHAPTER 11

Birth Control: More Options Than Ever

Over the course of a single year, from 60 to 80 percent of the sexually active women who use no form of birth control will get pregnant. To avoid an unwanted pregnancy, some knowledge of birth control is therefore a virtual necessity.

A wide variety of birth control methods is available. Some are extremely effective. Others are less reliable, but may be more appealing to people with particular beliefs or lifestyles. Several reduce the risk of spreading AIDS and other sexually transmitted diseases; others do not. In this chapter, you'll find the strong points and drawbacks of each.

Birth Control Methods That Work Poorly

Among the least effective techniques for preventing pregnancy is withdrawal, in which the man withdraws before he ejaculates. According to the American College of Obstatrics and Gynecology, of all couples who rely on the withdrawal method, one in five will face pregnancy within a year.

Another form of birth control with a poor track record is fertility awareness. Here the woman avoids having intercourse during the days of the month when she is most likely to get pregnant. To determine which days are "unsafe," she keeps track of her past menstrual periods, or notes changes in her basal body temperature or vaginal secretions. The record for this procedure is no better than withdrawal: Chances of pregnancy are one in five within a year.

Both withdrawal and fertility awareness cost nothing or almost nothing, and are accepted by almost all religions. For most women, however, these benefits are outweighed by several disadvantages: the need for continuous self-monitoring, the potential for sexual frustration, and the relatively low reliability these methods provide.

An Effective—but Irrevocable—Alternative

At the opposite end of the spectrum is surgical sterilization, which, short of total abstinence, is unquestionably the most effective form of birth control (though even surgery is not 100 percent reliable).

PREGNANCY: THE BEGINNINGS

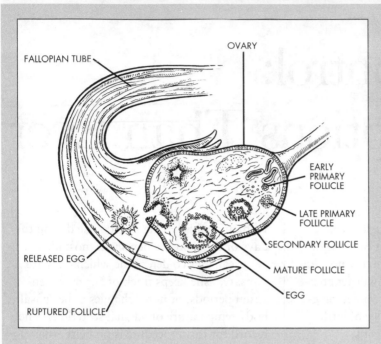

FALLOPIAN TUBE

OVARY

EARLY PRIMARY FOLLICLE

LATE PRIMARY FOLLICLE

SECONDARY FOLLICLE

MATURE FOLLICLE

EGG

RELEASED EGG

RUPTURED FOLLICLE

Human reproduction gets its start in the ovary. Once a month, within one of the two ovaries, a single egg ripens toward maturity. Together with the cells that cluster around it and nourish it, this egg forms a "follicle" moving towards the outer edge. About halfway through the menstrual cycle, the liquid-filled follicle bursts, expelling the mature egg into the fallopian tube. There, if the egg encounters a sperm, conception will take place.

In female sterilization, or tubal ligation, a doctor seals the fallopian tubes, which carry egg cells from the ovaries to the uterus. In male sterilization, or vasectomy, a doctor seals the vasa deferens, the tubes that carry sperm from the testicles to the penis.

Although extremely effective, sterilization is meant to be permanent. If the person later changes his or her mind, the operation may be difficult or even impossible to reverse. Sterilization is therefore not a good choice for anyone who might possibly want to have children someday.

Contraception:
The Other Option

Between withdrawal and sterilization lies contraception, a reversible form of birth control that relies on some kind of equipment, device, or medication. There are three basic kinds of contraception:

(1) **Barrier methods** such as the condom, diaphragm, and cervical cap; or contraceptive foam, jelly, suppositories, and sponges. All of these prevent pregnancy by putting a physical or chemical barrier between the woman's egg and the man's sperm.

(2) **Intrauterine device (IUD)**, a small device left in the woman's uterus. By causing changes in the lining of the uterus, the IUD either prevents the man's sperm from fertilizing the woman's egg, or else prevents a fertilized egg from settling into the wall of the uterus.

(3) **Hormonal methods** such as birth control pills and contraceptive implants and shots. These deliver female hormones that prevent monthly ovulation—the release of a mature egg cell from the woman's ovary. The

pills are generally taken daily at home. Shots are administered every three months at the doctor's office. Implants, which last up to five years, are also administered at the office.

How Does Pregnancy Happen?

To understand how the various contraceptives work, it may be useful to recall some facts about pregnancy.

Every month or so, inside a woman's body, one of the ovaries releases a ripe (mature) egg cell. This is called ovulation. The egg cell travels slowly through the fallopian tube to the uterus—a trip that takes several days. It is only during this time that a woman can become pregnant.

When sexual intercourse occurs, some of the millions of sperm cells in the man's semen travel from the vagina to the woman's uterus, or womb, and on into her fallopian tubes. There, if the sperm meet a ripe egg cell descending from the ovaries, one of the sperm may unite with the egg cell and fertilize it.

When this happens, the fertilized egg cell continues to advance through the fallopian tube and into the uterus, where it settles into the lining and begins to develop, becoming first an embryo and then a fetus. After nine months of pregnancy, the woman gives birth.

Each of the three basic types of contraception—barrier, IUD, and hormonal—disrupts this process at a different point; and each has unique advantages and disadvantages. Let's consider them in turn.

Choosing a Contraceptive: Barrier Methods

Condom: The condom, a latex or natural-membrane sheath that fits over the erect penis, is a physical barrier to conception. During ejaculation, it prevents semen from entering the vagina.

One great advantage of the latex condom is that it offers a measure protection not just against pregnancy, but also against sexually transmitted diseases such as AIDS, hepatitis B, gonorrhea, syphilis, chlamydia, herpes, and genital warts.

What about disadvantages? Occasionally a condom will break, tear, or slip during sex, allowing sperm-laden semen to spill into the vagina (backup protection with a spermicide can be of value here). Also, some men are reluctant to use a condom, claiming it forces an interruption of intercourse or dulls sexual sensation. Couples who rely on condoms alone are at a two to 12 percent risk of accidental pregnancy.

Diaphragm or Cervical Cap: Barrier devices worn by women include the diaphragm, a soft, shallow, rubber cup, and the cervical cap, a small, deep, latex cup shaped like a thimble. After smearing the inside of the diaphragm or cap with contraceptive jelly or cream, the woman inserts the device into her vagina and positions it over her cervix, the opening to her uterus. For the device to be effective she must keep it in place during intercourse and for eight hours afterward.

A diaphragm or cap offers women the advantage of having personal control over contraception. In addition, it can be positioned in advance and need not interrupt love-making. The diaphragm also reduces the risk of pelvic inflammatory disease and certain venereal diseases. And both diaphragm and cap are reusable.

However, as with the condom, these devices do require some preparedness and advance planning. Hence, for women relying on this approach, the risk of accidental pregnancy is six percent to 18 percent.

Spermicides: Chemical barriers to conception include spermicidal (sperm-killing) cream, jelly, and foam. These products are measured into an applicator and inserted into the vagina shortly before intercourse. The contraceptive suppository, which is inserted into the vagina and allowed to dissolve, works on the same principle, and provides protection against pregnancy for roughly an hour. The disposable contraceptive sponge contains a spermicide that becomes active when moistened. Placed against the woman's cervix, it protects against pregnancy for up to 24 hours.

An important advantage of spermicidal chemicals is that they kill not just sperm but also certain microbes, possibly including the AIDS virus. However, they do have drawbacks. Certain brands, in certain people, can cause skin or mucous membrane irritation. And because they taste bad, they can interfere with oral sex. Women who use a spermicide as their sole means of contraception have a three to 21 percent risk of accidental pregnancy.

Combinations: It's worth noting that the combination of a condom for the man **plus** a spermicide for the woman offers excellent protection against both pregnancy and many sexually transmitted diseases. The condom-plus-spermicide combination is the logical form of contraception for anyone who has several sexual partners, or whose sexual partner(s) might be infected with the AIDS virus or some other sexually transmitted microbe.

Choosing a Contraceptive: The Intrauterine Device

The intrauterine device (IUD), a small device that a doctor inserts into a woman's uterus, requires less attention than any other type of contraceptive. Once in place, it provides effortless round-the-clock protection against pregnancy. It deserves consideration by any woman who cannot take birth control pills and is unable or unwilling to use barrier methods consistently.

THE DIAPHRAGM: A BARRIER METHOD FOR WOMEN

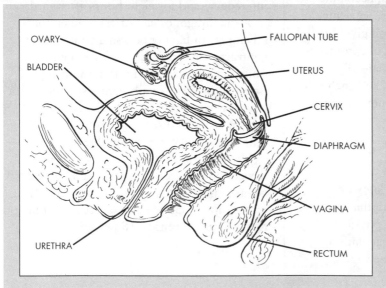

OVARY
BLADDER
FALLOPIAN TUBE
UTERUS
CERVIX
DIAPHRAGM
VAGINA
URETHRA
RECTUM

Stretched across a flexible wire hoop, this shallow rubber cup fits over the cervix, blocking access to the fallopian tubes and the mature egg they may harbor. The device can be inserted prior to love-making, and should be left in place for eight hours afterward. It is usually fitted individually to the woman's vaginal cavity.

EFFORTLESS OPTION: THE INTRAUTERINE DEVICE

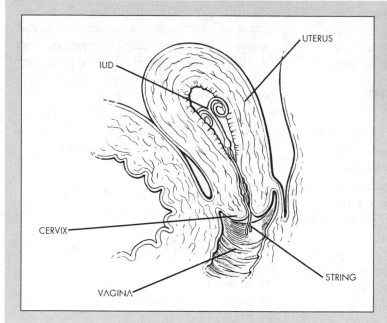

UTERUS

IUD

CERVIX

STRING

VAGINA

The exact reason is unknown, but this small object, when installed in the uterus, prevents conception with better than 95 percent reliability. The device must be inserted by a doctor, but can be left in position for at least a year. The string protruding through the cervix serves to confirm that the IUD has remained properly placed.

With the IUD, maintenance is minimal. All the woman need do is check at least once a month to make sure the device is correctly in place. A string attached to the IUD hangs down through the cervix and into the vagina. If this string can be felt with a fingertip, the IUD is still in position.

Of course, even if the IUD seems to be working fine, it periodically must be replaced: every year for the type containing a slow-release female hormone; every eight years for the type wrapped with copper wire.

Although the IUD sounds beautifully simple, it has a number of distinct disadvantages:

1. Insertion of the IUD may briefly be painful, especially for a woman who has never borne a child.

2. After insertion of the IUD, mild uterine cramps and bleeding may continue for days or even weeks.

3. An IUD may make menstrual periods both heavier and more painful.

4. An IUD increases the risk of a pelvic infection, particularly in women with multiple partners; some such infections can cause permanent sterility.

5. There is some risk that the IUD will damage the wall of the uterus.

6. If a woman gets pregnant despite the IUD, she is at increased risk of an ectopic (tubal) pregnancy, which is a life-threatening emergency.

For all these reasons, a woman should **not** use an IUD if she has multiple sex partners or if she has ever had a pelvic infection, a tubal pregnancy, or unexplained bleeding from the uterus.

Surprisingly, it is still uncertain *how* the IUD prevents pregnancy. It may work by irritating the woman's uterus, changing the uterine lining and secretions in ways that disrupt fertilization.

Women who use an IUD have a two to four percent risk of accidental pregnancy.

Choosing a Contraceptive: Hormonal Methods

Pills: Birth control pills, used by 32 percent of women of reproductive age, contain synthetic versions of two female hormones: estrogen and progesterone. (The so-called minipill contains synthetic progesterone only.) These hormones prevent a woman's ovaries from releasing a ripe egg cell every month.

A woman who uses this method of contraception should take her pill each day at about the same time. With some brands, there is a pill to take every day of the month. With others, a woman takes a pill for 21 days, stops for seven days, then starts over.

Shots: The contraceptive shot (Depo-Provera) works in much the same way as the pill, but need be taken only once every three months. Though Depo-Provera has been in use abroad since 1969, it was not available in the U.S. until 1993.

Implants: The contraceptive implant, also relatively new in the U.S., works on the same hormonal principle. The implant consists of a slow-release female hormone contained in six thin, rubbery capsules. A doctor inserts the capsules beneath the skin on the inside of the woman's upper arm. The gradually released hormone prevents pregnancy round-the-clock for five years before the woman needs a change of implant. If she wants to get pregnant before the five years are up, she can have the implant removed.

Pros and Cons of Hormonal Contraception

High reliability is a major advantage of hormonal contraception: The risk of accidental pregnancy is less than 3 percent. The hormones make for lighter and more regular menstrual periods, and reduce the cramps associated with periods. They also lower the statistical risk of tubal pregnancy, pelvic infections, and certain types of cancer (particularly ovarian cancer).

However, not all women are candidates for hormone-based contraception. A woman should use none of the hormonal methods if she has, or has ever had:

- Breast, uterine, or cervical cancer
- Blood clots in a leg, lung, or eye
- Unusual, unexplained vaginal bleeding
- Angina pectoris (chest pain from a heart condition)
- A liver tumor of any kind
- Jaundice while pregnant or taking the pill

One disadvantage of hormonal contraception is the possibility of nausea and vomiting, the most common side effects. Other possible side effects include breast tenderness, bleeding between periods, missed periods, weight gain or loss, depression, headaches, and blurred vision. In most women, the side effects disappear after a month or two. In others, switching to a different brand may diminish the problems.

Rarely, hormonal contraceptives precipitate a serious medical problem: an internal blood clot, stroke, heart attack (in women aged 40 and over), or liver tumor. Cigarette smoking increases the risk that such a problem will develop. So does the presence of high blood pressure, high cholesterol, or diabetes. For these reasons, it is important for any woman who uses a hormonal contraceptive to have regular medical checkups. □

CHAPTER 12

Handling Familiar Childhood Infections

With all the sore throats, runny noses, intestinal disorders, and allergies that plague our kids, childhood must sometimes seem like a constant blur of illnesses—especially to the parent doing the nursing. But even though these ailments are debilitating and take an enormous toll on the young patient, most of the problems clear up pretty quickly, are not life-threatening, and carry few long-term effects. (See the appropriate chapters for information on these disorders.)

Even so, parents still need to be particularly vigilant about safeguarding their children's health. The recent rise in the incidence of serious diseases—including whooping cough, rubella, measles, mumps, and hepatitis B—makes a compelling case for keeping vaccinations up-to-date. The latest vaccine, now recommended for all newborns, is for hepatitis B, a viral infection that causes an inflamed liver, and may lead to chronic infection and even cancer of the liver.

Routine medical checkups, proper diet, and plenty of rest are also essential to give children the protection they need. When a child falls ill or shows any unexplained or persistent symptoms, prompt medical advice and attention are crucial. This strategy helps keep minor illnesses from getting out of control and ensures early treatment for more serious disorders.

Treating the Diseases of Childhood

Despite great strides in preventive medicine, many familiar diseases of childhood continue to haunt us. Here's a closer look at the most common, and the ways they are treated today.

Chickenpox

Chickenpox remains one of the most prevalent childhood diseases, occurring most frequently in those between two and eight years of age. This highly contagious disease begins with a slight fever, loss of appetite, and malaise. Next, the distinctive itchy, blister-like rash appears, usually on the trunk or scalp at first, later spreading over the body.

Scratching the blisters may result in scarring, impetigo, boils, and other infections. Children mustn't scratch.

Children must be isolated until the blisters are crusted, usually five to seven days from the time of onset. The contagious period starts one or two days before the rash appears, so keep an eye on your child if he or she has been around someone who later broke out in a rash. The time between exposure and onset of the illness is usually 14 to 16 days. Cases have been known to occur as early as 11 or as late as 20 days after exposure.

Treatment of chickenpox consists of acetaminophen (Tylenol) and daily baths with lukewarm water. The doctor may prescribe an antihistamine such as Benadryl to help reduce itching. Trimming the child's fingernails minimizes the possibility of scarring. Medical care generally isn't necessary unless the child's temperature exceeds 102 degrees, or if the fever lasts for more than four days. In severe cases, acyclovir (Zovirax) may be prescribed. If the rash becomes very warm, red, or tender, the child may have a bacterial infection that requires antibiotics, and a physician should be called. Prompt medical treatment is also necessary if a child shows confusion, nervousness, vomiting, convulsions, lack of responsiveness, poor balance, or increasing sleepiness.

A vaccine for chickenpox is currently being tested. For now, though, the only way to protect a child is to avoid exposure.

Measles

There is a vaccine for measles, yet the number of cases in the United States rose from fewer than 1,500 in 1983 to 27,672 cases in 1990. Measles may well be *the* most serious communicable disease of childhood, and it is also becoming more prevalent in

---

VACCINES ESSENTIAL FOR YOUR CHILD'S HEALTH

- Polio
- DPT to protect against diphtheria, pertussis (whooping cough), and tetanus
- MMR to protect against measles, mumps, and rubella (German measles)
- Hemophilus Type B to protect against such serious illnesses as meningitis, epiglottitis (inflammation of the epiglottis), and pneumonia
- Hepatitis B

---

adolescents and young adults who did not respond to vaccination. Authorities now recommend a second measles, mumps, rubella vaccination after age five.

The incubation period for measles lasts from seven to 14 days. The disease is most communicable during the three to five days before the rash appears. Pre-rash symptoms last four to five days and include malaise, loss of appetite, inflamed eyelids, fever, sensitivity to light, hoarseness, runny nose, and a severe cough. Toward the end of this period, tiny, bluish-gray specks encircled by red appear in the mouth. A day or two after their appearance, the temperature shoots up, the oral spots slough off, and an itchy rash appears behind the ears and on the neck and cheeks.

The final stage of measles is marked by a high fever, puffy, red eyes, extensive rash, and a severe cough. Symptoms usually disappear—and communicability ends—five days after the rash begins.

Treatment of measles consists of bed rest and isolation. Vaporizers and a warm room help relieve respiratory symptoms; taking acetaminophen reduces the fever.

Mumps

Mumps, an acute viral disease, is most common in children between the ages of five and nine years. The disease is transmitted in the saliva of an infected person and has an incubation period of 14 to 24 days.

Mumps begins with a headache, muscle pain, low-grade fever, loss of appetite, and malaise. The next wave of symptoms includes an earache, along with swelling and tenderness in the parotid, and, possibly, other salivary glands. Possible complications include swelling and inflammation of the testicles in males past puberty, abdominal pain, nausea, fever, vomiting, and chills. Meningitis develops in about 10 percent of the cases, but does not usually lead to long-term problems.

Treatment for mumps includes acetaminophen to ease the pain and fever and adequate fluid intake. If swallowing is difficult, it may be necessary to replace the fluids intravenously.

Whooping Cough

In the past few years, approximately 4,200 cases of whooping cough (Pertussis) have been reported annually in the United States. Whooping cough may produce shock, seizures, pneumonia, and other serious side effects, especially in children younger than 12 months of age.

Whooping cough is highly contagious, and is marked by sudden fits of coughing followed by a high-pitched whooping sound when the child inhales.

The incubation period for whooping cough is seven to 10 days. The first symptoms include thick mucus, a hacking cough, loss of appetite, sneezing, conjunctivitis, listlessness, and, sometimes, a low-grade fever. The next stage is marked by an increasingly spasmodic cough and possible choking on mucus. The characteristic cough may be triggered by respiratory infections that occur months after this illness subsides. Infants often must be hospitalized for supportive care. Antibiotics such as erythromycin are sometimes administered.

Mononucleosis

Mononucleosis is a viral disease frequently contracted by teenagers. Preschoolers also get mononucleosis, although symptoms may be so mild that the disease is often overlooked. Mononucleosis is caused by the Epstein-Barr virus, which appears intermittently in the mouth of anyone ever infected by it. The disease is usually contracted from someone who is not ill at the time of contact. Symptoms of mononucleosis include fever, sore throat, headache, extreme fatigue, swollen lymph nodes, and possibly a rash. The symptoms tend to subside after six to 10 days, but sometimes may continue for weeks.

Treatment consists of bed rest and acetaminophen. In rare cases, steroids such as Predisone are given if swelling of the tonsils obstructs the airway and makes it hard for the person to breathe.

Other Childhood Diseases

Rubella (German measles) appears most frequently in children between the ages of five and nine years, adolescents, and young adults. The rash is the first sign of disease in children. In adults, the rash, if it develops at all, follows a low-grade fever, loss of appetite, malaise, headache, and swollen glands. In either case, the rash spreads, then disappears rapidly, and usually is completely gone after four to five days. In both children and adults, symptoms may be minimal, or may not appear at all. Treatment includes isolation until the rash disappears plus acetaminophen for pain and fever. Thanks to widespread use of rubella vaccine, the disease is now very rarely seen.

Reye's syndrome is a very rare, but acute and extremely serious childhood disease that usually appears one to three days following a viral illness such as an upper respiratory infection or chickenpox. The child typically recovers from the initial infection only to relapse a few days later with intractable vomiting, mild to severe confusion, agitation, and irritability. The syndrome often progresses to coma and is fatal in 20 percent of the cases. Needless to say, you should contact a doctor immediately if any of these symptoms appear. And, since aspirin increases the risk of Reye's syndrome, give your child acetaminophen instead.

Pinworms are the most common type of worms found in children. Rectal itching at night is the first—and sometimes the only—symptom. The itching can disturb the child's sleep and result in irritability, skin irritation, and scratching. Treatment usually consists of anti-worm medication such as mebendazole (Vermox).

Other childhood diseases include ringworm, lice, and appendicitis. Children also commonly suffer from allergy, dermatitis, middle-ear infections, anemia, asthma, croup, diarrhea, warts, nosebleeds, and impetigo. For more information on these disorders, see the appropriate chapters. □

CHAPTER 13

Ear, Nose and Throat Disorders

Although ear, nose and throat disorders aren't usually fatal, they still can be quite debilitating. Even a minor stuffed nose can make breathing and talking difficult. Ear disorders can disturb our equilibrium or compromise our hearing, impairing our ability to get along in life. Throat ailments can make it hard to eat, breathe and talk.

How the Ear Works

The organ we loosely refer to as the ear consists of a whole array of parts, including the outer ear, the ear canal, the eardrum (tympanic membrane), the middle ear and inner ear (cochlea), the hearing nerve, and the eustachian tube. Hearing occurs when sound waves strike the eardrum, sending vibrations through a set of tiny bones leading to the inner ear. There the sound is transformed into nerve impulses that then travel to the brain.

To maintain health, air in the middle ear must be at the same atmospheric pressure as that outside the ear. Air reaches the middle ear via the eustachian tube, which is connected to the back of the nose. Air passes through this tube to equalize pressure 1,000 times a day.

What the Nose Does

The nose is the main entry point of air for the lungs. Inhaled air is cleansed, moisturized, and warmed by the cilia and mucus that line the nasal passages. In addition, when cilia are touched by air, they send nerve impulses to the olfactory areas of the brain, which register our sense of smell. Mucus is produced in the nose, lungs, and sinuses (air pouches that extend from the inside of the nose to the bones of the face and skull).

A Close Look at the Throat

The throat consists of the pharynx, epiglottis, and larynx. Food travels through the pharynx on the way to the esophagus and stomach. Air passes through the pharynx en route to the trachea and lungs.

INSIDE THE EAR

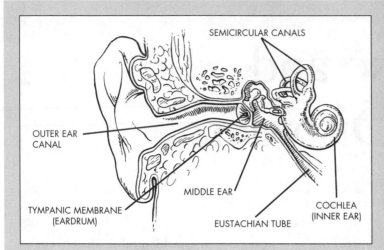

SEMICIRCULAR CANALS

OUTER EAR
CANAL

TYMPANIC MEMBRANE
(EARDRUM)

MIDDLE EAR

EUSTACHIAN TUBE

COCHLEA
(INNER EAR)

The ear boasts two main passageways, one visible, the other hidden. The visible outer ear canal connects the middle and inner ear with the outside world; the hidden eustachian tube travels from the middle ear to the back of the nasal cavity, providing a way to equalize air pressure. Riding atop the inner ear are the semicircular canals, which help us maintain our balance.

When we swallow, food and liquid chewed or manipulated in the mouth is propelled backward by the tongue. It then moves through the pharynx and on to the esophagus and stomach. During this automatic swallowing response, the epiglottis covers the larynx—or voice box—to prevent food from entering the lungs.

With this basic anatomy in mind, let's take a look at the afflictions to which all three of these crucial organs are most prone.

Treating Ear Disorders

Swimmer's ear, or infection of the outer ear canal, is caused by bacteria or fungus that grow when water becomes trapped in that passageway. Symptoms include a feeling of blockage or itching, swelling, pain, foul-smelling discharge, and a temporary partial loss of hearing. Treatment includes acetaminophen (or aspirin for adults) and eardrops containing antibacterial, antifungal, and steroid drugs, such as Cortisporin Otic.

The outer ear canal can also be infected through incorrect use of cotton swabs to clean the ear. Avoid pushing swabs into the canal.

Otitis media, or middle ear infection, is a common reason for childhood visits to the doctor; and adults, too, can be at risk. The condition occurs when the eustachian tube becomes inflamed from a cold, a sinus or throat infection, or an allergic reaction, causing fluid to accumulate in the middle ear. If bacteria or viruses take hold, the resulting infection causes pain, an inflamed eardrum, and a buildup of pus and mucus behind the eardrum.

Common symptoms of otitis media are severe ear pain, fever, a feeling of blockage or pressure, and muffled hearing. (Young babies may tug at their ears.) There may also be signs of an upper respiratory tract infection, nausea, vomiting, and dizziness. On the other hand, there may be no symptoms at all.

Prompt treatment of this condition is vital to prevent it from becoming chronic and causing complications. Therapy consists of antibiotics such as ampicillin, amoxicillin, cefaclor, or co-trimoxazole. Acetaminophen is used for pain. The doctor may also prescribe antihistamines or pain-relieving eardrops. If these measures are not sufficient, a myringotomy (an incision in the ear drum to allow drainage) may be necessary.

If the eardrum ruptures on its own, the pus drains out of the ear, but may be trapped in the middle ear by the swollen eustachian tube. This condition is known as middle ear fluid or effusion, or serous otitis media. It may become chronic, lasting weeks or months past the original infection, and making the individual vulnerable to frequent recurrences of the acute infection.

Mastoiditis is a rare complication of otitis media, usually resulting from the chronic form. It is an infection of the airspace that connects the mastoid sinus to the middle ear. Symptoms include tenderness and a dull ache in the involved area, along with a discharge. This condition requires antibiotics and myringotomy for drainage. If the surrounding bone is diseased, removal of the bones, or mastoidectomy, may be necessary.

A cholesteatoma is an abnormal skin growth in the middle ear behind the eardrum. Often the result of repeated infection, cholesteatomas frequently take the form of a cyst or pouch that sheds layers of old skin,

causing a buildup inside the ear. If a cholesteatoma grows too large, it can destroy the bones of the middle ear. Symptoms include a feeling of pressure, a foul-smelling discharge, earache, and hearing loss. Dizziness and/or muscle weakness on one side of the face are particularly ominous symptoms, signaling the possibility of serious complications. If they occur, seek medical attention immediately. Treatment consists of antibiotics, ear drops, and careful cleansing of the ear. Large cholesteatomas usually necessitate surgery.

A perforated eardrum, often the result of infection or trauma, usually heals spontaneously in a few weeks. If it doesn't, surgery is required. In either circumstance, the eardrum should be observed by a physician and protected from water and trauma.

Ménièrè's disease is a disorder of the inner ear thought to result from an overproduction or malabsorption of the fluids contained therein. Its symptoms are ringing or roaring in the ears, vertigo, and hearing loss. The vertigo is sometimes accompanied by disequilibrium, nausea, and vomiting. Treatment includes meclizine (Antivert) or diazepam (Valium). A low-salt diet and a diuretic may be recommended to reduce frequency of attacks over time.

Treating Nose Disorders

Nosebleeds are usually not serious, especially in children. Often caused by trauma, they can originate either in the front (anterior) or back (posterior) of the nose. In the former instance, the blood flows out of the nostrils. In the latter, it will flow down the back of the nose and throat even while the patient is standing or sitting.

Nosebleeds can also result from acute or chronic infections, polyps, nose-picking, or the inhalation of irritating substances.

Home treatment for an anterior nosebleed includes pinching the nose, pressing firmly toward the face, and holding for five minutes while sitting or lying with head elevated. Ice may also be applied to the nose and cheeks. To prevent re-bleeding, the nose should not be picked or blown, the head should be kept at a level higher than the heart, and the person should not strain or bend down.

If re-bleeding occurs, the nose should be cleared of all clots by gently blowing out through the nose. The involved nostril should be sprayed four times with decongestant spray, and the nose should be pinched and held as described above. In addition, a doctor should be contacted.

Since posterior nosebleeds tend to be more serious, they always require a physician's care. If bleeding continues for 10 minutes after pressure is applied, it is considered severe.

Medical care for nosebleeds may include application of epinephrine to the bleeding site, gauze packing, or a nasal balloon catheter. If packing is needed for longer than 24 hours, antibiotics may be necessary.

A stuffy nose may be a symptom of allergies, upper respiratory infections, or structural abnormalities. Other less common causes of nasal congestion are a chronic condition called vasomotor rhinitis, thyroid disease, emotional stress, and pregnancy. Used correctly, over-the-counter medications can provide relief for most stuffy noses. Products to consider should include antihistamines, decongestants, or a combination of these agents. Surgery is sometimes necessary to correct structural abnormalities such as a deviated septum.

Sinusitis is an infection of the sinuses that may be either acute or chronic. It usually begins with a cold or allergy episode that causes swelling of the mucous membranes

BEHIND THE NOSE

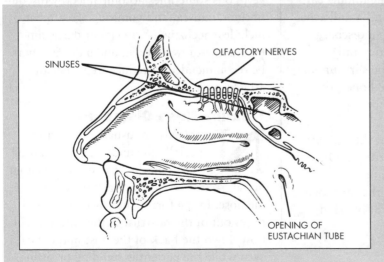

SINUSES

OLFACTORY NERVES

OPENING OF
EUSTACHIAN TUBE

This cut-away view of the nasal cavity reveals a major source of pain and aggravation — the air-filled cavities we call the sinuses. Between the sinuses, hair-like cilia hang from the roof of the nasal cavity, bringing the olfactory nerves in contact with the odors we inhale. Near the juncture of the nasal cavity and the throat below, the entrance of the eustachian tube leads to the middle ear.

WITHIN THE THROAT

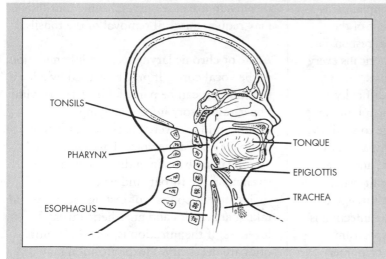

TONSILS

PHARYNX

ESOPHAGUS

TONQUE

EPIGLOTTIS

TRACHEA

The site of numerous trouble-some infections, the throat extends from the back of the nasal cavity downward to the trachea (windpipe) and the esophagus (alimentary canal). Called the pharynx in medical terminology, the throat conducts both food and air to the body below. As food passes down the throat to the esophagus, the epiglottis shuts off access to the nearby windpipe.

and increased production of watery mucus. Because the sinuses are swollen, the mucus tends to build up and become blocked, resulting in the pressure and pain of a sinus headache. The trapped mucus also becomes a breeding ground for bacteria.

Symptoms of sinusitis include characteristic pain in the face, cheeks, forehead and upper teeth; a green or yellow colored and foul-smelling nasal discharge; malaise; fever; and sore throat.

Treatment for sinusitis includes an antibiotic such as amoxicillin, co-trimoxazole, or a cephalosporin; decongestants; and occasionally a topical vasoconstrictor such as phenylephrine. Steam inhalation or heat applications help relieve pain. If sinusitis recurs frequently, it should prompt your doctor to search for an underlying cause, such as structural abnormalities, allergic rhinitis, or immune deficiency.

Postnasal drip, the sensation that mucus is dripping downward from the back of the nose into the throat, results from excessive mucus production due to infection, allergies, irritation, swallowing disorders, or structural abnormalities.

Antibiotics may be required to clear up an underlying infection, while antihistamines, decongestants, inhaled corticosteroids, or immunotherapy might be recommended if allergy is the cause. Structural abnormalities such as a deviated septum or septal spur (sharp projection) may require surgery.

Nasal polyps are associated with chronic allergies, chronic sinusitis, chronic rhinitis, and nasal infections. The primary symptoms are nasal obstruction and loss of the sense of smell. Medical treatment usually includes inhaled corticosteroids, antihistamines and decongestants (for allergy), and antibiotics (for infection). If this fails to provide complete relief, surgery may be considered.

Treating Throat Disorders

Pharyngitis or sore throat, one of the most common medical complaints, is caused by viruses 90 percent of the time. The streptococcus bacteria, responsible for strep throat in one in 10 Americans every year, is a common non-viral cause.

Symptoms include soreness, difficulty swallowing, the feeling of having a lump in the throat, and the constant urge to swallow. The infection may also be accompanied by headache, muscle and joint pain, and fever.

Treatment consists of warm salt-water gargles, mildly anesthetic throat lozenges, fluids, painkillers, and rest. If the infection is bacterial, penicillin or a broad-spectrum antibiotic will be required. (See "Counter-attacking Major Infections," page 813 for more information about strep.)

Acute tonsillitis typically starts out as a mild-to-severe sore throat. Symptoms may then progress to fever, difficulty swallowing, tenderness and swelling of the lymph glands, joint and muscle pain, headache, chills, malaise, and ear pain. In chronic tonsillitis, the sore throat recurs and is usually accompanied by discolored discharge in the area of the tonsils.

Treatment for acute tonsillitis consists of aspirin (for adults) or acetaminophen, rest, and adequate fluid intake. If the infection is bacterial, antibiotics such as penicillin or erythromycin are necessary. Chronic tonsillitis may require surgical removal of the tonsils.

Acute or chronic laryngitis is an inflammation of the vocal cords. It may be caused by a local infection, or can be part of a bacterial or viral upper-respiratory infection. Symptoms include mild to severe hoarseness and even complete loss of the voice. Laryngitis may be accompanied by pain, a dry cough, malaise, swelling in the throat, and fever.

Treatment consists of resting the voice and taking analgesics and anesthetic throat lozenges. If the infection is bacterial, antibiotics are necessary. Hospitalization may be required if acute laryngitis is so severe that the airways become obstructed. □

CHAPTER 14

Relief for Common Allergies

Allergies pose a significant and serious health problem in this country. According to conservative estimates, nearly 15 million Americans are plagued by hay fever and 10 million have asthma. Twelve million more Americans suffer from such allergies as eczema and hives, not to mention allergic reactions to food, drugs, and insect stings. Most of these disorders have a hereditary component and tend to run in families.

What Is An Allergic Reaction?

Basically, an allergic reaction occurs whenever the immune system overreacts to a seemingly harmless substance. Known as allergens, these substances include pollen, mold, house dust, mites, animal saliva and dander (skin shed by cats, dogs, or rabbits), feathers (such as those used in feather pillows), certain foods and drugs, and insect stings.

Allergens are usually absorbed into the body by way of the skin, nasal passages, lungs, or digestive tract. Once inside the body, allergens stimulate the lymphocytes (small white blood cells) to produce what are known as allergic antibodies. The reaction between the allergen and these antibodies, which are attached to certain special cells (mast cells), leads to inflammation of the nose, eyes, lungs, and the digestive tract. A stuffy nose, sneezing, wheezing, skin rash, watery eyes, abdominal cramps, and nausea are some of the most common results.

Asthma

Although asthma is a common condition that affects all age groups, one-third of all cases occur in children under 10 years old. This means that approximately three million children in the fifth grade and below suffer from this disorder. Not surprisingly, asthma accounts for more school absences than any other chronic childhood illness.

The chief symptoms of asthma include coughing, wheezing, and shortness of breath. An asthma attack may be brought on by any of the previously mentioned allergens or by infections in the sinuses or bronchial tubes.

Emotional stress, hormonal changes, irritants such as cigarette smoke, changes in temperature and humidity, and exercise also may trigger an asthmatic episode.

Asthma attacks may begin suddenly with the onset of severe symptoms, or start slowly with a gradually increasing difficulty in breathing. A typical acute asthmatic attack is marked by wheezing, labored breathing, tightness in the chest, and a dry cough. Asthma attacks may produce a feeling of suffocation and an inability to speak without frequent pauses to catch the breath. The victim may also have a rapid pulse, sweat profusely, and turn blue.

Treatment for asthma usually consists of removing the offending allergen or irritant and administering medications that reduce inflammation and open the air passages. For patients with daily symptoms, inhaled steroid drugs such as Azmacort, Beclovent, Vanceril, and AeroBid are frequently prescribed, as are cromolyn sodium (Intal), theophylline (Theo-Dur, Uniphyl), and albuterol (Proventil, Ventolin). For serious attacks, bronchodilators may be given intravenously.

Hay Fever

Allergic rhinitis (hay fever) can be brought on at certain seasons by the airborne pollens of trees, grass, and weeds. Other allergens cause hay fever all year. These year-round troublemakers include molds, dust mites, and animal dander.

Hay fever symptoms include sneezing, watery eyes, runny nose, nasal congestion, and an itchy palate and throat. Hay fever can also be accompanied by conjunctivitis (itchy, swollen eyes), malaise, headache, and sinus pain.

The treatment of hay fever consists of removing the environmental antigen, if possible, and implementing drug therapy and immunotherapy (allergy shots). The newer antihistamines, such as terfenadine (Seldane), cause less drowsiness and dryness. Topical intranasal steroids, such as flunisolide (Nasalide), beclomethasone (Beconase, Vancenase), and triamcinolone (Nasacort), reduce inflammation and may eliminate the need for oral antihistamines and decongestants.

Hives and Angioedema

Hives (urticaria) are itchy, red, swollen patches of skin that appear suddenly. Although they may vanish within one to two hours, they can last as long as two days. They frequently occur in clusters, with new clusters forming as others fade. They do not leave scars.

Hives may have an allergic or non-allergic cause; and the exact culprit usually cannot be determined. They are often triggered by a food or a drug. Common foods that cause hives include nuts, shellfish, peanuts, and eggs. Drugs that typically produce hives include penicillin, sulfa, anticonvulsants, aspirin, and nonsteroidal anti-inflammatory drugs (NSAIDs). Tight-fitting clothing that scratches or rubs the skin, activities that increase the body's temperature (warm baths, hot tubs, exercise, or fever), and exposure to cold or sunlight may all cause hives in susceptible individuals.

Angioedema is a condition like hives that occurs in the deeper layers of the skin, most often in the hands, feet, and face. Certain types of hereditary angioedema may cause fatal swelling of the larynx.

Hives and angioedema are treated by avoiding whatever substance has provoked the outbreak, if it can be identified. Antihistamines such as hydroxyzine (Atarax), diphenhydramine (Benadryl), astemizole (Hismanal), and terfenadine (Seldane) are used to treat daily occurrences. Other types of histamine blockers like cimetidine (Tagamet) and ranitidine (Zantac) may be added next. Oral corticosteroids are considered a last resort.

Dermatitis

Atopic dermatitis is a form of eczema that often begins in early childhood. It is frequently associated with allergic rhinitis or asthma. Half the cases disappear by adulthood.

We don't know what causes atopic dermatitis. The symptoms in infants include itchy red patches on the face, torso, and lower parts of the limbs. These patchy areas crust, scale, and ooze. A child between the ages of two and four may develop clusters of red or flesh-colored scaly patches or bumps on the elbows, knee creases, ankles, neck, wrists, and feet. The rash becomes more concentrated during adolescence, appearing on the sides of the neck, hands, and face, and the skin becomes more thickened.

People with atopic dermatitis are prone to bacterial skin infections that produce itching and redness. Oozing, crusting ulcers may also occur in some cases.

The goal of treatment is to eliminate the itching. Therapeutic measures typically include application of lubricants and moisturizers while the skin is damp after bathing, plus use of topical corticosteroids, such as fluocinolone acetonide (Synalar). Oral antihistamines such as hydroxyzine (Atarax) and diphenhydramine (Benadryl) help ease the itching.

Allergic contact dermatitis may be caused by poison ivy, oak, or sumac, as well as by exposure to nickel, chrome, mercury, certain cosmetics, and drugs applied to the skin.

Poison ivy produces redness, bumps, and blisters, as well as swelling after the initial contact. The blisters burst after a few days, releasing a watery liquid, and healing begins. Treatment includes trying to prevent a rash by promptly washing the affected area with soap and water—within five minutes of contact, if possible. If a rash develops, wet, cold compresses and steroid ointments may be advised. Oral steroids may be necessary for severe cases.

Stings and Anaphylaxis

Stinging insect allergies result when a sensitive individual is stung by a bee, wasp, hornet, yellow jacket, or fire ant. The reaction usually occurs soon after the initial sting and may include wheezing, generalized hives, angioedema, and a sharp drop in blood pressure. The victim may also go into shock and lose consciousness. If not treated immediately, severe reactions may be fatal.

Avoidance is the best strategy for someone with this type of sensitivity. Anyone who has an adverse reaction should consult an allergist for skin testing. Venom immunotherapy could be a lifesaver in the event of a future sting. Sensitive individuals should have injectable epinephrine (EpiPen, Ana-Kit) available in case of an attack.

Anaphylaxis is a severe and potentially life-threatening allergic reaction distinguished by the sudden onset of hives or angioedema, respiratory distress, and a drop in blood pressure. The reaction is caused in susceptible individuals by a variety of allergens, including vaccines; penicillin and other antibiotics; diagnostic chemicals; insect venom; polysaccharides; food (including berries, nuts, seafood, and egg whites); aspirin; and nonsteroidal anti-inflammatory agents. Penicillin is by far the most common culprit. Exercise may also induce anaphylaxis in some people.

Symptoms of anaphylaxis include feelings of impending doom or fright, itching of the skin, nasal congestion and coughing, hives and swelling of tissues in the lips or larynx, wheezing, shortness of breath, low blood pressure, and loss of consciousness. The person's eyes may also itch, swell, and tear. Other symptoms include change of voice, hoarseness, itching of the mouth and throat, sneezing, chest pain and tightness, redness of the skin, cramping of the uterus, a feeling of warmth and flushing, a need to urinate, abdominal cramps, nausea, vomiting, and diarrhea.

Anaphylaxis is an emergency condition that requires an immediate injection of epinephrine. Emergency injection devices such as EpiPen or Ana-Kit could be lifesaving if available for use in an unexpected attack. In any event, if you experience any of these symptoms, seek medical help right away. □

CHAPTER 15

Dealing with Skin Problems

The skin is the body's largest and most visible organ. It reflects a person's general health and performs many important bodily functions. An average-sized person has 20 square feet of skin that serves as the body's front-line defense against injury and bacteria. The skin also regulates body temperature, acts as a sensory and excretory organ, and synthesizes vitamin D when exposed to ultraviolet light. A vast network of blood vessels in the skin provides oxygen and nutrients to sensory and motor nerves and also to skin appendages, including glands, nails, and hair.

Not surprisingly, this complex, exposed organ is vulnerable to many diseases. Each year, as many as seven million people seek medical treatment for newly diagnosed skin diseases. And almost everyone will experience some type of skin problem sooner or later. Skin disorders are usually noticeable and often disfiguring, causing both physical and psychological distress.

Some Other Skin Facts

■ The American Academy of Dermatology reports that one out of four people seeking medical advice about new skin problems is bedridden.

■ Teenagers and young adults account for a significant number of dermatology (skin) patients. In highly urban areas, however, a surprisingly large proportion of patients are adults.

■ Acne is the leading skin disease, occurring in 20 percent of all patients seeking treatment for skin disorders. Contact skin disorders, such as poison ivy and burns or rashes caused by industrial or household chemicals, are the second most common problem.

■ Other common skin disorders include skin cancer, warts, fungal infections, and psoriasis.

- More than three million workdays are lost each year because of skin diseases.
- Chronic skin disease accounts for up to 50 percent of workers compensation claims in some states.
- Skin disease is the fourth largest cause of disability in the Armed Forces, affecting almost seven percent of military personnel.

The Skin's Architecture

The skin has three major layers—the epidermis, the dermis, and the subcutaneous tissue. The epidermis is the outermost layer of skin. Its main function is to produce the keratin that protects the body against harmful environmental substances and controls water loss. Cells in the epidermis also produce melanin, which gives the skin its color.

The next layer of the skin is the dermis. This layer contains a number of important substances such as collagen and reticulin, which prevent the skin from tearing; elastin, which makes the skin resilient; and jellylike substances that make the skin soft and compressible.

The third layer, subcutaneous tissue, is primarily made up of fat, which provides insulation, shock absorption, and calorie reserves. Both the dermis and the subcutaneous tissue contain sensory and motor nerves.

Among the most common causes of skin disorders are infections, overexposure to sunlight, follicle dysfunction, and hormonal

A CLOSER LOOK AT THE LARGEST ORGAN

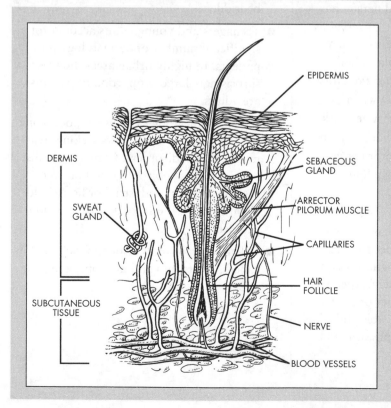

DERMIS

SWEAT GLAND

SUBCUTANEOUS TISSUE

EPIDERMIS

SEBACEOUS GLAND

ARRECTOR PILORUM MUSCLE

CAPILLARIES

HAIR FOLLICLE

NERVE

BLOOD VESSELS

Below the skin's deceptively smooth surface lies a veritable forest of support structures and glands, including nerves, muscles, capillaries, and the sebaceous glands implicated in acne. The epidermis, or top layer, acts as a protective barrier. As its cells are rubbed off and shed, cells in the dermis below are constantly dividing to provide replacements. When this renewal cycle gets out of control, the result is psoriasis.

imbalance. Parasites, external substances, cell dysfunction, genetic factors, stress, and aging also cause skin problems. Here are the most common skin disorders and their treatments:

Acne: The Leading Complaint

Acne typically affects teenagers, occurring during a time of dramatic hormonal shifts and rapid growth. The blackheads, whiteheads, pimples, and boil-like lesions that appear on the face, back, chest, and shoulders are a source of embarrassment and may lead to permanent scarring.

Rising hormone levels during puberty cause the sebaceous glands to enlarge and produce more oil. No one knows why this process causes acne in some people but not in others. However, certain factors are known to contribute to the development of acne. They include oral contraceptives; certain medications, such as steroids, some hormones, iodides, bromides, and lithium; exposure to heavy oils, greases, or tars; trauma or irritation from tight clothing; cosmetics; and emotional stress.

Acne results when small kernels of sebum (oil), skin cells, and bacteria fill up hair follicles, causing blackheads and whiteheads to appear. The sebum ruptures the walls of the follicles, forming pimples and boil-like eruptions in nearby tissue. If the sebum is further altered by bacteria, it may cause even more irritation to the surrounding skin.

Acne is usually treated with an antibacterial agent such as benzoyl peroxide—either alone or in combination with tretinoin (Retin-A). Oral and topical antibiotics such as tetracycline, erythromycin, and topical clindamycin also help alleviate acne. Accutane (oral isotretinoin), inhibits the secretion of sebum, but has severe side effects and must be used cautiously.

Other acne remedies include injecting cortisone directly into the lesions, estrogen therapy for women, and exposure to ultraviolet light. Proper cleansing techniques also are often part of the therapeutic plan.

Rosacea and Rhinophyma

Rosacea is a chronic skin disorder that produces flushing and dilation of the small blood vessels in the face. Tiny pimples also appear. As the disease progresses, small, thin, red lines (telangiectasia) may appear on the skin's surface. In advanced cases—and usually only in men—the nose becomes bulbous and red, the cheeks become puffy, and thick bumps develop on the lower half of the nose and adjacent cheek areas. We don't know what causes this condition, which is called rhinophyma, but the problem may be aggravated by stress, infection, vitamin deficiencies, and glandular upset.

Topical steroids as well as topical and oral antibacterial agents are helpful in the treatment of rosacea. Beta blockers can be used to reduce redness and swelling. The dilated blood vessels of telangiectasias can be closed off with a small needle, a laser, or surgery.

Rhinophyma is usually treated with surgery or dermabrasion. Most people with this disorder are advised to avoid alcohol, spicy foods, hot drinks, and smoking, and to stop using facial products that contain alcohol or other irritants.

Psoriasis: An Array of Treatment Options

Psoriasis affects as many as eight million Americans. Though the cause is unknown, psoriasis results in an over-production of skin cells. The surplus skin leads to thickening and scaling. The resulting silvery plaques generally appear on the scalp, elbows, knees, and lower back. The severity of psoriasis ranges from mild, undetected forms to rare cases in which the scales cover the entire body. Psoriasis may cause pitting of the fingernail surface, thickening and crumbling of the nail plate, and separation of the nail from the nail bed.

Genetic factors apparently cause a biochemical malfunction that triggers the psoriasis. Skin cells mature in three to four days—much faster than the usual 28 to 30 days—resulting in a flaky buildup. Itching, occasional pain, and embarrassment are the chief complaints of psoriasis sufferers.

Treatment of psoriasis consists of removing the scales by softening them with certain preparations, then gently scrubbing the skin with a soft brush in an oatmeal or salt bath. Other treatments include exposure to ultraviolet type B light (UVB), coal tar preparations, steroid creams, methotrexate (an anticancer drug), anthralin, and PUVA (psoralen in conjunction with UVA exposure). Tegison, a synthetic vitamin A derivative, is sometimes used in conjunction with PUVA, UVB, and topical medications. Low-dosage antihistamines may also be prescribed.

Arthritic symptoms often accompany psoriasis. Aspirin and local heat usually relieve these symptoms. Severe cases may require nonsteroidal anti-inflammatory drugs. Psoriasis of the scalp often responds to the use of tar shampoo and steroid lotion.

Psoriasis of the fingernail cannot be treated, but usually clears up when the skin lesions subside.

Dermatitis: Many Forms, Many Remedies

Dermatitis is the general term for any inflammation of the skin. There are many types of dermatitis and many different causes.

Atopic eczema affects about three percent of the United States population and often occurs as an allergic reaction to wool, silk, fur, ointment, detergent, perfume, wheat, milk, or eggs. It produces an intensely itchy rash that blisters, oozes, and crusts. In infants, it appears primarily on the face and scalp. When it occurs in adolescents and young adults, it is usually found in the large folds of the hands and feet; elbow bends and backs of knees; and the face, neck, and upper chest.

Doctors usually treat atopic eczema with topical corticosteroids and petrolatum, sedatives, and antihistamines. Oral antibiotics may be prescribed for a secondary infection; ultraviolet light therapy has been helpful in treating severe cases. Patients are instructed to eliminate or avoid allergens, irritants, extreme temperatures, stress, and other possible aggravating factors.

Seborrheic dermatitis is another common skin disorder. This chronic condition causes red skin covered by yellowish, greasy-appearing scales and usually occurs on the scalp (where it's known as dandruff), sides of the nose, eyebrows, eyelids, skin behind the ears, and the middle of the chest. Treatment with low-strength topical cortisone preparations

WHAT YOU SHOULD KNOW ABOUT SKIN CANCER

Skin cancer is mainly caused by overexposure to ultraviolet light. The rate of skin cancer—the most common of all cancers—is growing at an alarming rate. Recognizing the early signs of the various forms of skin cancer is essential for early detection and successful treatment. All forms of skin cancer are highly curable if caught in time.

usually provides relief. Scalp treatments include frequent shampoos with preparations containing such chemicals as tar, zinc pyrithione, selenium sulfide, sulfur, and/or salicylic acid. Seborrheic dermatitis may be caused or perpetuated by a yeast organism, and antiyeast creams have been used with good results by some people.

Other forms of dermatitis include contact dermatitis, localized neurodermatitis, stasis dermatitis, exfoliative dermatitis, and allergic contact dermatitis (poison ivy, oak, and sumac).

Infections: Common and Surprisingly Stubborn

Athlete's foot may affect as many as 90 percent of Americans. This fungal infection shows up as sores between the toes, or as a blistering rash on the foot. Another type of athlete's foot manifests itself as a very mild inflammation and dry scaling of the entire sole of the foot, along with infection of the toenails. Treatment consists of dressings of tap water or a weak salt solution. Oral antibiotics and topical and oral antifungal medicines are also used. Other fungal infections of the skin include tinea versicolor and dermatophytosis (ringworm).

Other infection-related skin diseases include herpes and warts—both of which are viral infections; impetigo; folliculitis, furunculosis, carbunculosis, and staphylococcal scalded skin syndrome—all bacterial infections; scabies—caused by the itch mite; cutaneous larva migrans—a reaction to infestation by hookworms and roundworms; and pediculosis—caused by parasitic forms of lice.

Also common are such skin conditions as hives, which are treated with antihistamines and the removal of the offending agent; and vitiligo, a condition in which pigment cells are destroyed, which is treated with repigmentation drugs activated by ultraviolet light.

Skin Cancer: The Three Major Types

Basal cell carcinoma is the most common form of skin cancer and affects some 400,000 people each year. The tumors appear as small, fleshy, translucent bumps or nodules on the head, neck, hands, or occasionally, on the trunk of the body. These tumors don't grow quickly and don't metastasize (spread to other organs). If left untreated, however, the tumors begin to bleed, crust over, and then repeat the cycle. If treatment is further delayed, basal cell carcinoma can invade the skin and spread, causing significant damage as it extends.

Squamous cell carcinoma tumors appear as nodules that ulcerate in the center, or as red, scaly patches on the rim of the ear, face, lips, and mouth. The tumors eventually enlarge into sizable masses and can spread via the blood and lymph systems.

A Malignant melanoma is the most virulent of all skin cancers. If untreated, it can be fatal; and in the U.S., the increase in new cases tops all other forms of skin cancer.

Malignant melanoma results from the uncontrolled growth of pigment-producing tanning cells. It resembles an oversized, asymmetrical mole and is characterized by an irregular border and unusual pigmentation. Any mole larger than a pencil eraser that has these characteristics is cause for concern and should be checked.

As with all skin cancers, malignant melanoma is thought to be linked with excessive exposure to the sun. It also tends to run in families. If a relative has had it, extra caution is advisable.

Malignant melanoma may appear suddenly without warning or may begin near a mole or another dark spot on the skin. Additional warning signs include changes in the surface of a mole, oozing, scaliness, bleeding or the appearance of a bump or nodule; spread of pigment from the border of a mole into the surrounding skin; and changes in sensation, such as pain, tenderness, or itching. If detected early enough, melanoma can usually be cured by surgical removal.

Several options are available for treating basal cell and squamous cell carcinomas. Treatment may involve surgical removal; electrodesiccation (destroying cancerous tissue with a high-frequency current transmitted through a needle electrode); cryosurgery (using cold liquid nitrogen to destroy the cancerous tissue); radiation therapy; and topical chemotherapy. □

CHAPTER 16

Correcting Glandular Disorders

The endocrine system is a complex network of glands that acts in concert with the nervous system to control and coordinate the myriad chemical reactions associated with storage and release of energy, growth, maturation, reproduction, and behavior. The sheer complexity of this system makes it vulnerable to breakdown, a fact that is reflected in numerous and varied endocrine disorders. The endocrine system's influence on bodily functions is so profound that many body systems may be affected when any of these glands fails to operate properly.

How Does the Endocrine System Work?

The endocrine system includes the pituitary, thyroid, parathyroid, adrenals, testes, ovaries, pineal, and thymus glands and the islet cells of the pancreas. The endocrine glands function by releasing hormones (or chemical messengers) into the bloodstream. These hormones trigger reactions in specific tissues.

This network of glands is regulated by the hypothalamus—the area at the base of the brain where the endocrine system meets the nervous system—and by the pituitary gland. Together, they generate chemical messages that stimulate the other glands to further activity. When endocrine disorders develop, they usually consist of either hypofunction (underactivity) or hyperfunction (overactivity) of one or more glands. Occasionally, inflammation or development of tumors in a gland leads to trouble as well.

Endocrine hyperfunction and hypofunction may have their source in the hypothalamus, the pituitary, or the target gland itself. Chronic disorders are more common, and generally lead to hypofunction; however, inflammation can cause acute episodic malfunctions. Tumors more commonly occur in the glands themselves, but can appear in other areas of the body, such as the lungs or stomach, where they produce hormones that cause endocrine dysfunction.

Pituitary Disorders

Hypopituitarism is characterized by growth retardation in children, sexual immaturity, and metabolic dysfunction. Hypopituitarism results from a deficiency of the hormones secreted by the anterior pituitary gland. Panhypopituitarism involves a partial or total failure of all this gland's hormones. These two conditions can be caused by tumors; but they may also result from certain chemicals, congenital defects, irradiation, and changes in blood flow.

Symptoms usually develop gradually and may include impotence, the absence of menstrual periods, infertility, decreased sexual drive, and diabetes insipidus (a state of high urinary output unrelated to the more common diabetes mellitus discussed in Chapter 23). Other symptoms are hypothyroidism and adrenal insufficiency (Addison's disease).

Treatment consists of replacement hormones.

Hyperpituitarism results in the extreme overgrowth of the skeleton and is often caused by a tumor. When hyperpituitarism occurs before puberty, the entire body becomes abnormally large. This condition is called gigantism. Post-pubertal hyperpituitarism is called acromegaly and produces bone thickening; this rare condition usually strikes between the ages of 30 and 50.

Other symptoms of hyperpituitarism include oily skin, severe headaches, blurred vision, profuse sweating, a loss of peripheral vision, nervous system impairment, and a rapid metabolism. The head and facial features become enlarged and distorted in hyperpituitarism, and the individual may show symptoms of irritability, hostility, and other psychological disturbances. Treatment consists of removing the tumor, followed by hormone replacement if necessary.

Thyroid Disorders

Hypothryoidism occurs more frequently in women than in men and is diagnosed most often between the ages of 40 and 50. Hypothyroidism, essentially an underproduction of thyroid hormone, can be caused by an insufficiency of the hypothalamus, the pituitary, or the thyroid gland itself.

An underactive thyroid gland may be the result of surgery, inflammation, autoimmune conditions, or insufficient iodine in the diet. Congenital defects may also cause hypothyroidism, and the condition can be a side effect of certain drugs.

The early symptoms of hypothyroidism tend to be vague. They include short-term memory loss, fatigue, lethargy, unexplained weight gain, intolerance to cold, poor wound healing, and constipation. Later signs of hypothyroidism include increased mental instability; puffiness in the face and extremities; thin, dry hair; loss of libido; loss of appetite; hand tremors; and abdominal bloating. If left untreated, hypothyroidism may eventually lead to onset of a life-threatening coma.

Hypothyroidism is treated by replacing the thyroid hormones.

THE MAJOR ENDOCRINE GLANDS AND THEIR FUNCTIONS

■ The pituitary gland, located at the base of the brain, produces several hormones, including antidiuretic hormone (ADH), adrenocorticotrophic hormone (ACTH), thyroid-stimulating hormone (TSH), growth-hormone (GH), follicle-stimulating hormones (FSH), luetinizing hormone (LH), and prolactin. The pituitary has been called the master gland because so many of the hormones it produces control the functions of other glands.

■ The thyroid gland, situated at the front of the throat, secretes thyroxine (T4) and tri-iodothyronine (T3), which are essential for growth and development. These two hormones stimulate metabolism and protein synthesis in most of the body's tissues.

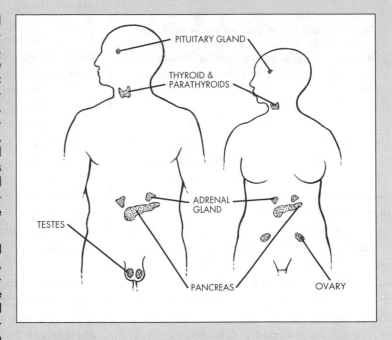

■ The four parathyroid glands are located next to the thyroid glands. The parathyroid glands secrete parathyroid hormone (PTH), which controls phosphorous and calcium metabolism and plays a central role in bone development.

■ The pancreas lies transversely in the abdomen, just behind the stomach. The pancreas secretes digestive juices into the stomach, and two hormones—insulin and glucaugon—into the bloodstream. The hormones regulate glucose metabolism. Insulin promotes use of glucose by the body's cells. Glucagon regulates release of stored glucose into the bloodstream.

■ The adrenal glands sit atop the kidneys and are composed of two separate parts—the outer cortex and the inner medulla. The adrenal cortex, which accounts for 90 percent of the adrenals, secretes aldosterone, which causes the kidneys to excrete potassium and retain sodium; and cortisol, corticos-

terone, and cortisone, which together help the body resist stress; inhibit the immune response; promote normal metabolism of proteins, fats, and carbohydrates; and inhibit inflammation. The adrenal cortex also secretes sex hormones. The adrenal medulla secretes epinephrine and norepinephrine, which produce the body's fight-or-flight response to stress.

■ Men have two testes, which are located in the scrotum outside the abdominal cavity. The testes produce sperm and male hormones—most notably testosterone, which controls the development of the male sex organs.

■ Women have two ovaries, which are situated on either side of the uterus. The ovaries release eggs and secrete female sex hormones. Ovarian hormones include estrogen, which mediates the development of female sex organs and characteristics; and progesterone, which prepares the uterus for pregnancy and readies the breasts for lactation.

THE BEST KNOWN ENDOCRINE PROBLEM

Diabetes mellitus, a dysfunction of the pancreas, is one of the most common endocrine disorders, affecting an estimated 14 million Americans. (For more on diabetes, see Chapter 23.)

Hyperthyroidism is caused by overproduction of thyroid hormone. In Graves' disease, the most common form of hyperthyroidism, patients are likely to have an enlarged thyroid, heat sensitivity, nervousness, difficulty in concentrating, prematurely gray hair, weight loss, increased appetite, diarrhea, palpitations, tremors, sweating, and, in some cases, bulging eyes. Graves' disease is thought to result from an immune-system malfunction that overstimulates the thyroid. The disease may not become apparent until it is triggered by trauma or by a benign tumor of the thyroid gland.

Hyperthyroidism is treated with antithyroid drugs, surgery, and radioactive iodine. The drugs used to treat hyperthyroidism include methimazole (Tapazole) and propylthiouracil (PTU), which reduce thyroid activity. Surgery and radioactive iodine are both aimed at destroying enough thyroid tissue to reduce hormone secretion to more normal levels.

Other thyroid disorders include thyroiditis, an inflammation of the thyroid gland, and goiter, an enlargement of the thyroid glands.

Hypoparathyroidism results from diseased, injured, or congenitally defective parathyroid glands. Injury to the glands most often occurs during surgery involving nearby tissue. Hypoparathyroidism may also be caused by the prolonged, severe magnesium deficiency associated with alcoholism.

Hypoparathyroidism leads to low blood concentrations of calcium, which may cause neuromuscular excitability, including spasms and twitching of the face, hands, and feet; abdominal pain; hair loss; dry skin; and cataracts.

Treatment with vitamin D will usually reverse hypoparathyroidism, although calcium supplementation is sometimes required.

Hyperparathyroidism, usually caused by a benign tumor, can lead to kidney problems, bone abnormalities, brittle bones, and chronic low-back pain. People with hyperparathyroidism also show such signs of gastrointestinal discomfort as pain and ulcers, as well as muscle weakness, constipation, depression, psychosis, stupor, and, sometimes, coma. Treatment consists of surgery to remove the tumor or drugs to correct any abnormalities the condition has caused. In some cases, no specific therapy is required.

Disorders of the Adrenal Glands

Addison's disease (or adrenal insufficiency) usually results from an autoimmune response that destroys the adrenal glands. The symptoms of Addison's disease are loss of appetite, weight loss, fatigue, weakness, vomiting, nausea, and diarrhea. Other signs include a suntanned appearance, intolerance for stress, and a craving for salty food. The treatment of Addison's disease entails lifelong replacement of the steroid hormones produced by the adrenals, usually with hydrocortisone or cortisone. Because serious illness or injury may dramatically increase the body's need for adrenal hormones, patients with Addison's disease should wear an identification bracelet in case of emergency.

Cushing's syndrome results from the oversecretion of adrenal hormones, especially cortisol, or from taking synthetic ACTH or steroids. Excessive cortisol production is, in turn, usually brought on by an oversupply of ACTH, possibly due to a tumor that produces ACTH in another organ.

Common symptoms of Cushing's syndrome include fatty deposits on the face, neck, and trunk, and purple streaking on the skin. This syndrome also produces muscle and bone weakness, poor wound healing, peptic ulcer, irritability, mood swings, difficulty sleeping, high blood pressure, suppressed immune response, diabetes, and changes in the reproductive system.

Treatment for Cushing's syndrome may include radiation, drugs, or surgery. Metyrapone (Metopirone) and aminoglutethimide (Cytadren) are among the medications used to reduce cortisol production. ☐

CHAPTER 17

Counterattacking Major Infections

Our struggle for survival has always entailed a battle against the countless microbes with which we share the earth. Hostile bacteria, viruses, fungi, and parasites invade our bodies and go to war with our immune systems. To fight back, we must call forth all our strength and defenses. Plagues and epidemics are as much a part of our history as any struggle between nations.

Though it may seem hard to believe, prior to the use of penicillin during World War II, physicians had no effective medicines to treat serious infections. Fifty years later, we have more than 100 different antibiotics—including sulfa drugs, synthetic penicillin, and many, many more—to ward off the full spectrum of bacterial diseases. The development of numerous vaccines has virtually wiped out many former killers, both bacterial and viral, in the U.S. and many other developed countries.

Yet infection still plagues us, despite these gains. Many strains of bacteria are now resistant to the drugs that once killed them. Most viruses are impervious to antiviral drugs.

Some microorganisms come in so many different forms that a single vaccine just can't cope with them all. Other microorganisms elude treatment by hiding in hard to reach areas such as the central nervous system and bones. Then too, some people today are simply exposed to a wider range of diseases because of our increased mobility, the use of immunosuppressive drugs, and such invasive procedures as surgery and catheterization.

Consequently, infection is still a serious threat, even in our highly advanced society. In Third World countries, infectious diseases continue to cause widespread mortality.

How Infections Cause Illness

When organisms invade the body, they reproduce and multiply rapidly. In the process, the microorganisms compete with the body's metabolic processes. Some also produce toxins that injure cells. What's more, our own immune response may actually cause even further tissue damage. How sick someone actually gets as a result of the infectious process depends on the type and number of invading organisms and the person's overall health and strength.

Staph Infections

Staphylococcal bacteria produce a wide range of diseases, causing anything from skin eruptions to blood poisoning (bacteremia) and death. Staphylococcal infections include the following conditions:

Bacteremia, the presence of bacteria in the blood, is characterized by a high fever, shaking chills, racing heart, pallor, agitation, and joint pain. It may progress to confusion and stupor, and can be fatal in just 12 hours. Treatment must begin immediately with semisynthetic penicillin (nafcillin or methicillin) or cephalosporins (cefazolin) given intravenously. People who are allergic to penicillin or are infected by penicillin-resistant organisms must be treated with vancomycin.

The symptoms of **staphylococcal pneumonia** are similar to those of other pneumonias—sudden onset of high fever, cough with yellow or bloody sputum, difficulty in breathing, and chest pain. Treatment consists of the same medication used for bacteremia.

The use of some of these drugs, particularly broad-spectrum antibiotics like cephalosporins, sometimes brings on enterocolitis (inflammation of the intestines). This condition is marked by profuse, watery diarrhea; abdominal pain; nausea; vomiting; and dehydration. If a patient develops enterocolitis, the antibiotics must be stopped at once and replaced with a different drug, such as vancomycin.

Osteomyelitis is a bone infection that occurs as a complication of a blood-borne infection, or as a sequel of surgery or trauma. Osteomyelitis may come on rapidly, exhibiting fever, sudden pain, swelling, tenderness, heat, and restricted movement in the affected bone. Its onset can also be insidious, however, with fever as the first warning. Treatment consists of surgery to open and cleanse the wound and large doses of antibiotics for four to eight weeks.

Staphylococcal bacteria are among the most common causes of **food poisoning**. Symptoms of food poisoning include nausea, loss of appetite, diarrhea, vomiting, and abdominal cramps. Since the symptoms typically subside within 18 hours, there's usually no need for treatment unless the person shows signs of dehydration. Full recovery takes one to three days.

Some **skin infections** owe their source to staphylococcal bacteria as well. These infections are manifested by widespread inflammation of soft tissue (cellulitis), and pus-producing or boil-like lesions, sometimes accompanied by fever and discomfort. Treatment includes applying mupirocin ointment (Bactroban), as well as administering oral antibiotics (erythromycin, dicloxacillin, or cloxacillin). Severe infections are treated with intravenous oxacillin, methicillin, or nafcillin. Ointments such as bacitracin-neomycin-polymyxin are used to prevent further infection of broken skin.

Toxic shock syndrome (TSS) is an acute infection that is sometimes associated with tampon use during menstruation. The symptoms of toxic shock syndrome include a high fever, an abrupt episode of shivering and chills, intense muscle pain, profuse watery diarrhea, headache, and vomiting. A dark red rash appears on the palms and soles within a few hours. Shock may develop within 48 hours.

TSS is treated with antibiotics, such as oxacillin, methicillin, and nafcillin, given intravenously.

Strep Infections

A total of 21 species of **streptococcal bacteria** have been identified, but three classes—**Groups A, B, and D**—are responsible for most infections.

Group A bacteria cause the following infections:

Streptococcal pharyngitis accounts for the majority of sore throats caused by bacteria. Children between the ages of five and 10 years get most of these strep throats—mainly from October through April. The symptoms of strep throat may include a fever, severe pain and difficulty swallowing, inflamed tonsils, a sore and red throat, a "strawberry" appearance of the tongue, enlarged lymph nodes, loss of appetite, weakness, malaise, and abdominal discomfort.

Sometimes, however, the symptoms of strep throat are mild, and the infection escapes detection. Left untreated, a strep infection can lead to rheumatic fever.

It is essential that anyone with a strep throat take the full prescription of antibiotics—usually either penicillin or erythromycin. Isolation from others for 24 hours after starting antibiotic therapy is recommended to prevent the disease from spreading.

Scarlet fever may occur along with a strep throat, certain wound infections, and blood poisoning. Children between the ages of two and 10 years are most likely to get scarlet fever. Symptoms include those of strep throat plus a sunburn-like rash that feels like sandpaper to the touch. The rash usually begins on the upper chest and then spreads to the rest of the body. Prompt treatment with an antibiotic is essential.

Erysipelas is another type of strep infection. It usually occurs in infants and in adults over 30 years of age. When erysipelas develops, swollen, red, raised lesions with a raised, firm border suddenly appear and spread. Other symptoms include headache, vomiting, fever, and irritability. An antibiotic should be administered promptly. Cold packs and analgesics, such as aspirin and codeine, can alleviate local pain.

Other infections caused by streptococcal A bacteria include **impetigo** (skin lesions with itching and encrustment) and **lymphadenitis** (red-streaked, painful skin lesions with fever, racing heart, and lethargy.) Both infections require treatment with antibiotics.

Group B streptococcal infections include newborn and adult forms. The adult form usually occurs after women give birth. Both newborn and adult infections are usually treated by penicillin or ampicillin. **Group D streptococcal** bacteria are frequently implicated in endocarditis, an inflammation of the interior of the heart.

Various strains of strep are among the causes of other diseases, including **pneumonia** (see Chapter 6 on respiratory disorders); **otitis media** (fluid in the middle ear); and **meningitis**. All of these infections are treated with penicillin, amoxicillin, or ampicillin.

Meningitis

Meningitis occurs most often in children under five years of age and in people living in crowded conditions such as those found in the military or in institutions. In older patients, meningococcal bacteria are a more likely cause than strep. The symptoms are varied and may include sore throat; stiff neck; a sudden, spiking fever; intense headache; chills; muscle pain in the back and legs; racing heart; and a rash. As many as 20 percent of all cases evolve into a severe form of meningitis marked by extreme prostration, intravascular coagulation, skin lesions, and shock. Left untreated, this particular infection may cause respiratory or heart failure and be fatal in just six to 24 hours.

Meningitis must be treated immediately with large doses of penicillin G, ampicillin, or a cephalosporin, such as ceftriaxone or cefotaxime.

Tetanus

People get tetanus (lockjaw) when a puncture wound becomes contaminated by soil, dust, or animal feces. The incubation period ranges from less than two days in severe cases to three or four weeks in milder cases.

Symptoms include spasms and increased muscle tone near the wound, profuse sweating, and a low-grade fever. Patients also experience an extreme tightening of neck and facial muscles, which produces a grotesque grinning expression; rigidity of abdominal and back muscles; and convulsions.

Treatment must begin within 72 hours after a puncture wound occurs. Patients who have no previous immunization need tetanus immune globulin or tetanus antitoxin for temporary protection, followed by immunization with tetanus toxoid. Those who have not been immunized in the past five years need a booster shot of tetanus toxoid. If tetanus develops, treatment consists of airway maintenance and the use of muscle relaxants, such as diazepam (valium), or a neuromuscular blocker. High doses of antibiotics (preferably penicillin) are also necessary.

Intestinal Infections

Salmonella is an extremely common infection—more than two million new cases are reported in the United States each year. Salmonella bacteria are the cause of typhoid fever, and are often the culprits in gastroenteritis (inflammation of the stomach and intestines). Occasionally, they cause blood poisoning and localized infection.

Gastroenteritis caused by salmonella is usually contracted by eating contaminated or inadequately processed foods—especially eggs, turkey, duck, and chicken. Other sources include contaminated dry milk, chocolate bars, and contact with infected animals or people. Symptoms typically include diarrhea, nausea, abdominal pain, and fever. Though the infection usually clears up on its own, at times it may progress to intervals of high fever, abscesses, dehydration, and blood poisoning. Treatment for uncomplicated cases includes bed rest and fluid and electrolyte replacement.

Typhoid fever is usually contracted by drinking contaminated water, takes three weeks to run its course, and is marked by persistent fever and flu-like symptoms. For this infection, a wide variety of antibiotics may be prescribed.

Infections by *Escherichia coli* and other bacteria living in human intestines cause a great deal of diarrheal illness in American children. These infections are also prevalent among travelers to other countries—particularly those visiting Mexico, South America, and Southeast Asia. People with mild infections recover easily. Those with severe infections, however, require prompt fluid and electrolyte replacement to prevent fatal dehydration. This cautious course is especially important for children, who are highly susceptible to dehydration.

Symptoms include the sudden onset of watery diarrhea, abdominal pain, and cramping. Some forms may produce chills, along with blood and pus in the stools. In small children, the stools may be yellow or green, and the child may experience vomiting, irritability, loss of appetite, and listlessness, possibly progressing to severe dehydration, fever, and shock.

Treatment includes rest and correction of fluid and electrolyte imbalances. Intravenous antibiotics are occasionally needed to treat infections in infants.

Lyme disease

Lyme disease is contracted from the bite of an infected deer tick. A red, enlarging ring is the first sign of infection. This mark may be itchy, but usually causes no irritation. Several days later, a few more lesions may turn up. The blotches last several weeks, and within a few days of their appearance may be joined by a variety of other symptoms including stiff neck, malaise, fatigue, chills, fever, headache, achiness, and muscle pain.

Stage two occurs weeks or months later and may include cardiac and neurologic symptoms such as facial palsy. These symptoms may last for months or become chronic. Stage three can begin weeks or years later and is marked by chronic arthritis-like symptoms.

Early treatment may prevent later complications. The usual treatment for adults is a 10- to 20-day course of oral doxycycline or tetracycline, although penicillin, amoxicillin, or cephalosporins may be used instead. Children under eight years of age usually receive oral penicillin or amoxicillin. In advanced stages of the disease, intravenous penicillin or ceftriaxone may be given for two to four weeks.

The list of infectious diseases goes on—diphtheria, listeriosis, botulism, gas gangrene, actinomycosis, dysentery, cholera, poliomyelitis, Colorado tick fever, Rocky Mountain spotted fever, malaria, giardisis, trichinosis, hookworm—but, happily, most are either rare in this country or easily preventable. If we take full advantage of the immunization measures and advanced antibiotics available today, we now have less to fear than ever before in history. □

CHAPTER 18

Overcoming Kidney Disease

Kidney disease is a major health problem in this country, afflicting some eight million Americans. Kidney and urinary tract diseases together affect an estimated 20 million people, causing more than 95,000 deaths a year and contributing to an additional quarter of a million.

Kidney disorders run the gamut from minor infections to total kidney failure. Kidney disease can cause high blood pressure, anemia, and elevated cholesterol. When chronic, it can lead to depression and sexual dysfunction. Kidney stones, diagnosed in more than one million Americans annually, can be extremely painful and are a significant cause of hospital stays and lost work days. But the picture is not entirely bleak.

Thanks to major medical advances, diagnosis and treatment of kidney problems have improved significantly in the past 30 years. Even people with complete kidney failure can now lead reasonably normal lives because of modern dialysis techniques and new successes in transplantation. Today dialysis keeps alive more than 120,000 Americans who would otherwise perish because of kidney failure. Kidney transplants, first performed in the U.S. some 30 years ago, have saved the lives of thousands more.

Why Are Your Kidneys So Vital?

Called the "master chemists" of the body, the kidneys keep a variety of elements in balance. When the kidneys become damaged, other organs suffer as well.

It's commonly known that the kidneys remove waste products and excess fluids from the body via the urine, and that they maintain a critical balance of salt, potassium and acid. But most people are unaware that kidneys perform other vital functions as well. For example, the kidneys produce a hormone—erythropoietin or EPO—that stimulates the production of red blood cells. Other kidney hormones help regulate blood pressure and calcium metabolism. The kidneys even synthesize the hormones that control tissue growth.

Any time the kidneys' ability to remove and regulate water and chemicals is impaired by disease or blockage, fluids and waste products accumulate, ultimately resulting in extreme swelling and symptoms of uremia (an overload of toxic byproducts) or kidney failure. The kidneys' various functions can each be affected separately, so urine output may be normal despite significant kidney disease.

Kidney diseases, which usually involve both kidneys, are categorized as **hereditary, congenital** or **acquired**.

Inherited kidney disorders usually begin producing symptoms during the teen to adult years, and are often serious.

Congenital kidney diseases typically involve a malformation of the genitourinary tract that can lead to blockages, which, in turn, can cause infection and/or destruction of kidney tissue. Tissue destruction may then lead to chronic kidney failure.

Acquired kidney disorders have numerous causes, including blockages, drugs, and toxins. However, diabetes and high blood pressure are by far the most common culprits.

HOW YOUR AMAZING KIDNEYS WORK

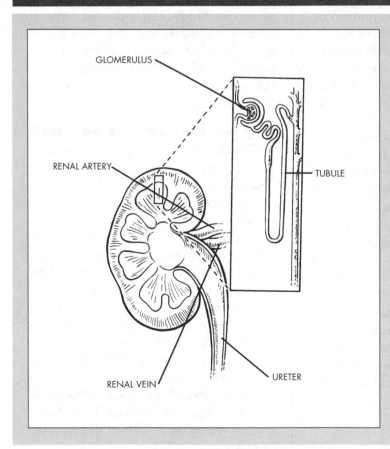

GLOMERULUS

RENAL ARTERY

TUBULE

RENAL VEIN

URETER

The two fist-sized kidneys sit on either side of the spine at the lower end of the rib cage. Each consists of approximately one million nephrons; each nephron contains a filtering apparatus called a glomerulus, which is laced with tiny blood vessels; each glomerulus is attached to a tubule. After blood is filtered in the glomerulus, the remaining fluid passes along the tubule, where chemicals and water are either added or extracted according to the body's needs. The final product of this process is the urine we eliminate.

The kidneys filter and return to the bloodstream about 200 quarts of fluid every 24 hours. Approximately two quarts are eliminated as urine, which flows from the kidneys through the ureter to the bladder, where it is stored for up to eight hours.

Inherited Kidney Diseases

The most common inherited disorder is polycystic kidney disease; others include Alport's syndrome, hereditary nephritis, primary hyperoxaluria, and cystinuria.

Polycystic kidney disease (or PKD) is marked by the formation of fluid-filled cysts in the kidney tubules. These cysts compress functioning kidney tissue, eventually replacing it. In the most common type of the disease (autosomal dominant PKD), almost half of the patients develop chronic kidney failure between the ages of 40 and 60. The rarer form (autosomal recessive PKD) causes kidney failure in early childhood.

In PKD, both kidneys become enlarged. Patients experience back pain, blood in the urine, kidney stones, recurring bladder or kidney infections, and high blood pressure.

Though there is no cure, careful management of high blood pressure and prompt antibiotic treatment of kidney or bladder infections can prolong life. Exercise to help maintain good physical condition is frequently recommended as part of the treatment program. Since PKD is progressive and often leads to kidney failure, patients are counseled, given emotional support, and prepared for the eventuality of dialysis or transplantation.

Congenital Kidney Diseases

There are two types of congenital kidney disease. In one, malformations present at birth usually lead to some type of blockage. This disrupts the normal flow of urine, causing it to back up and exert increasing pressure on the kidneys, ultimately leading to permanent damage. In the other form, the muscles of the bladder fail to contract as they should, due to some abnormality in the muscles or their nerve supply.

Though kidney malformations are common, affecting up to 15 percent of the population, they generally don't cause problems. Blockages that can lead to serious kidney difficulties include the narrowing of the upper urinary tract (**ureteropelvic junction obstruction** or **ureteral stenosis**), congenital contracture of the bladder outlet (**vesical neck contracture**), or narrowing of the channel from the bladder to the outside of the body (**urethral stricture**).

Urinary tract blockages require early diagnosis, ordinarily accomplished by injecting dye into the bloodstream or the bladder so that an X-ray can be taken. Specific diagnostic procedures include intravenous urography and retrograde pyelography. (The latter procedure sometimes actually relieves the blockage, eliminating the need for surgery.) Non-invasive diagnostic techniques include renal scans, ultrasound, and CT scans. Some urinary tract blockages can be treated by abdominal surgery; others can be relieved by surgery through the urethra.

Acquired Kidney Diseases

Inflammation of the kidneys, or nephritis, is the primary characteristic of acquired kidney diseases. In the most common of these, glomerulonephritis (also known as Bright's disease), the glomerulus or filtering part of the kidney becomes inflamed. The disease can be brief and severe, mild and protracted, or rapidly progressive.

Acute post-streptococcal glomerulonephritis typically starts about 10 days after the onset of a strep throat or a skin infection such as impetigo. Though more common in children, it can occur at any age. Most people recover fully, but the few who don't may develop chronic kidney failure within months.

Symptoms include a fall in urine output, "smoke"- or "rust"-colored urine, and a burning sensation when urinating. Swelling of the face, eyelids, and hands due to fluid retention is also common, as are shortness of breath, a cough, and high blood pressure.

Acute post-streptococcal glomerulonephritis usually heals completely within three to 12 months after onset. The only treatment is the relief of symptoms and complications. Accompanying high blood pressure must be treated with an antihypertensive. Fluid retention is controlled with diuretics (water pills), including metolazone (Diulo, Zaroxolyn) or furosemide (Lasix).

Chronic glomerulonephritis is a term used for a wide variety of diseases that cause progressive scarring of the kidneys over a long period of time, often without any initial symptoms. Frequently, the only findings in the early stages of the illness are an abnormal urinalysis and high blood pressure. Edema (fluid retention) and persistent high blood pressure appear as the disease progresses. As with the acute form, the accompanying high blood pressure must be treated with medication. A diet restricting protein, sodium, and potassium is also often part of the treatment plan. Steroids and other drugs have been used to treat this disease; their success depends on the underlying cause.

Rapidly progressive glomerulonephritis (RPGN) is characterized by a decrease in urine output and progressive decline in kidney function over a three to six month period or less. RPGN has no known cause, appears suddenly, and can quickly lead to kidney failure. RPGN is irreversible once kidney function is severely affected, but the kidneys may recover significantly if treatment is begun early enough.

Nephrotic Syndrome: Though not a disease in itself, this condition is often the result of other kidney disorders or more generalized diseases (such as diabetes mellitus and lupus erythematosus). It is marked by heavy loss of protein in the urine, a low protein level in the blood, an increase in blood cholesterol level, and edema (fluid retention). Prognosis is variable and depends on the underlying cause; in some cases, the condition may progress to end-stage kidney failure.

Some forms of nephrotic syndrome respond to corticosteroids, which significantly reduce the amount of protein lost in the urine. In those cases in which steroids do not help, treatment consists of diuretics to control high blood pressure and swelling due to fluid retention.

Acquired Kidney Obstructions: These are generally mechanical in nature. Common causes include an enlarged prostate gland in older men, sagging pelvic muscles in older women, and tumors in the genitourinary organs of both males and females. Kidney stones and scar tissue that develops as a result of infections, X-ray treatment, and surgery may also cause blockage of the urinary tract. Some of these obstructions can be alleviated by surgery and follow-up medical treatment. Tumors are treated with surgery, radiation, and appropriate medications.

Kidney Stones: These hard masses appear when certain chemicals in the urine form crystals that stick together. The crystals can grow into a stone as small as a grain of sand or as large as a golf ball. Small stones are passed out of the body with the urine. The larger ones can block urine flow or irritate the lining of the urinary tract. Some individuals with kidney stones have no symptoms, but most usually experience some of the following: severe pain, nausea, and vomiting; burning and a frequent urge to urinate; fever, chills, and weakness; cloudy or foul-smelling urine; blood in the urine; and a blocked flow of urine. Serious infections can result from a blockage.

Specialized X-rays or sound waves (ultrasound) can be used to diagnose and identify the location and size of kidney stones. Since 90 percent of stones are small enough to pass naturally, treatment usually consists of methods to promote this, such as drinking a lot of liquid. Medications that may be prescribed include antibiotics (if an infection develops) and analgesics such as meperidine (Demerol) for pain. Larger stones are often treated by passing a telescopic device into the ureter or bladder and either removing the stones or breaking them into small fragments with lasers or sound waves. Alternatively, larger stones may be broken down by high-energy shock waves. Only rarely is surgery necessary.

Drinking large amounts of fluids, taking certain medications, and changing the diet may help prevent the formation of new stones.

Treatment of Kidney Failure

As much as 90 to 95 percent of kidney function can be lost before kidney failure becomes apparent. Symptoms include loss of appetite, nausea and vomiting, extreme fatigue, difficulty sleeping, itching and dry skin, muscle cramps, and twitching. Left untreated, the build-up of waste products in the body can lead to coma, seizure, and death.

Many years ago, kidney failure was inevitably fatal. But modern medicine now offers three life-saving treatments.

In **hemodialysis** an artificial kidney machine carries out the vital functions the kidneys can no longer perform. In this procedure, a person is connected to the machine by plastic tubing that attaches to special blood vessels in the arm or leg. The treatment can be done at home or at a dialysis unit.

In **peritoneal dialysis,** waste products from the blood are flushed from the body with fluid instilled and drained through a catheter that has been surgically placed in the abdomen. Once the catheter is in place, this technique is usually done at home.

Since patients with kidney failure are often anemic, many have to take a substance known as EPO (erythropoietin), the synthetic form of a hormone that helps make red blood cells. Iron supplements are also sometimes required.

Though adjusting to kidney failure and dependence on dialysis is difficult, many patients manage to do so, and lead relatively normal lives.

Kidney transplantation, the third option for people with kidney failure, has shown increasing success in recent years. Depending on the quality of the match between donor and recipient, there is an 80 to 90 percent chance that a transplanted organ will still be functioning one year after the operation. The major complication of a transplant, rejection of the organ, is treated with such medications as steroids, azathioprine, and cyclosporine. Many transplant patients also need blood pressure medication, as well as drugs to prevent ulcers and infections. □

CHAPTER 19

Bringing Urinary Disorders under Control

When functioning properly, the urinary tract is a marvel of efficiency. Throughout every 24-hour period, it thoroughly cleanses approximately 200 quarts of fluid, returning most of it to the circulatory system and eliminating the remaining two quarts as urine through the bladder.

As with most parts of the body, however, when this system breaks down, it causes pain and discomfort. And unfortunately, it breaks down quite frequently. Urinary tract infections (UTIs), second only to respiratory infections in frequency, account for 10 million visits to the doctor each year. One in five women will suffer from cystitis, an inflammation of the bladder, at some time in her life. Twenty percent of women who have a UTI will have a second infection, and 30 percent of those will have yet another. In addition, at least 10 million adults suffer from urinary incontinence (an inability to hold urine) to some degree.

Some Facts About Urinary Tract Disorders

■ Women are more prone to UTIs than are men or children.

■ Urinary tract problems increase with menopause.

■ One to two percent of children develop urinary tract infections.

■ Young children have the greatest risk of kidney damage caused by urinary tract infections.

■ Certain people who contract one or more urinary tract infections may need further testing to ensure they do not suffer from other health problems.

The kidneys, ureters, bladder, and urethra are the key components of the urinary tract. The kidneys filter waste from the blood (see "Overcoming Kidney Disease," page 819) and eliminate it in the form of urine. The urine travels from the kidneys to the bladder through narrow tubes called ureters. The bladder, a ball-shaped receptacle in the lower abdomen, stores the urine for anywhere from one to eight hours before it is emptied from the body through the urethra.

TRACING THE COURSE OF THE URINARY TRACT

Originating at the kidneys, the urinary tract conducts waste fluid down the ureters and into the bladder, where it accumulates until expelled through the urethra. Note the striking difference in the lengths of the male and female urethras. This, more than any other factor, accounts for a woman's greater vulnerability to bladder infections.

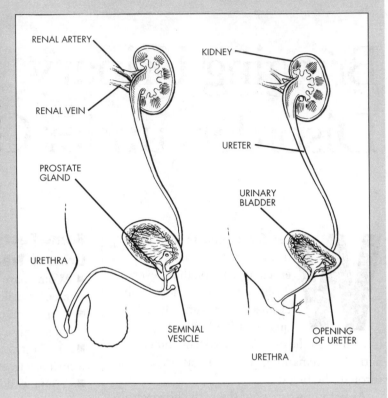

Urinary Tract Infections

Urine contains fluids, salts, and waste products. Normally it is sterile. Trouble starts when microorganisms, usually *Escherichia coli* from the digestive tract, cling to the opening of the urethra and multiply. The type of infection that follows depends on whether the bacteria stay in the urethra or travel to the bladder or even the kidneys themselves. Microorganisms called *Chlamydia* and *Mycoplasma* may also cause UTIs. These infections usually remain limited to the urethra.

The chief causes of UTIs are blockages, changes in hormone levels, prostate enlargement, lowered immunity, catheters, structural abnormalities, and, for some women, sexual intercourse. Women who use a diaphragm are also prone to UTIs.

Symptoms of possible urinary tract infection include:

- A frequent urge to urinate
- A painful, burning sensation in the area of the bladder or urethra during urination
- A feeling of tiredness
- Bladder pain, even when not urinating (caused by pressure above the pubic bone in women and fullness in the rectum in men)

- The passing of only a small amount of urine at a time
- In a few cases, lower back pain, fever, or chills
- Milky or cloudy urine
- Blood in the urine, back pain, or a fever (signs that the infection may have reached the kidneys)
- In children or infants, irritability; loss of appetite; unexplained, persistent fever; incontinence or loose bowels; a change in urinary patterns; or a generally unhealthy appearance

UTIs are treated with antibiotics, usually for seven to 10 days. The regimen may be shorter or longer, however, depending on whether the bladder or kidney is infected. The drugs most commonly used for bladder infections are trimethoprim (Trimpex), trimethoprim/sulfamethoxazole (Bactrim, Septra), amoxicillin (Amoxil, Trimox, Wymox), nitrofurantoin (Macrodantin), and ampicillin. Longer treatments with tetracycline, trimethoprim/sulfamethoxazole or doxycycline are necessary for infections caused by *Chlamydia* or *Mycoplasma*. Lengthier courses of treatment are also usually recommended for men, in part to treat infection of the prostate gland. Women may receive extended treatment to prevent a recurrence. Pregnant women with UTIs should be treated promptly to avoid premature delivery and the risk of high blood pressure (though only certain drugs are safe to use). Severe kidney infections usually require hospitalization and several weeks of antibiotic treatment.

Women who experience recurrent UTIs often respond to one of the following regimens:

- Low doses of an antibiotic such as trimethoprim/sulfamethoxazole or nitrofurantoin daily for six months or longer
- A single dose of an antibiotic after sexual intercourse
- A short course (one or two days) of antibiotics when symptoms first appear

Urinary Incontinence

Though not a natural consequence of the aging process, urinary incontinence is nevertheless a widespread problem among the elderly. It can be caused by age-related changes in the lower urinary tract or by certain illnesses. The good news is that most cases can be cured or improved with proper diagnosis and treatment.

The specific causes of incontinence are numerous. Though many cases do not fit a clear-cut classification, they generally fall into one of three main categories:

PREVENTING UTIs

During treatment of UTIs, and to prevent their recurrence, the following measures are usually recommended:

- Drink plenty of fluids, especially water.
- Drink cranberry juice or take supplements of vitamin C daily to keep urine acidic.
- Do not resist the urge to urinate.
- Wipe from front to back and wash the genital area thoroughly with soap and water after defecating to prevent bacteria from the anal area from entering the vagina
- Cleanse the genital area before having sex, and empty the bladder immediately afterward.
- Take showers instead of baths.
- Avoid using feminine hygiene sprays and scented douches; they may cause irritation of the urethra.

Stress incontinence is the most common type among women. Its hallmark is the involuntary loss of urine during physical activity, sneezing, or coughing. The disorder may have its roots in the unique stress that pregnancy places on the urinary tract. However, symptoms may not be noticed until menopause, when the bladder tissues start to sag due to a drop in estrogen levels. Estrogen supplements often improve the condition. Other remedies include Kegel exercises (rhythmic flexing of the muscles surrounding the vagina, anus, and urethra), and surgery to reposition the bladder.

Urge incontinence is marked by an urgent, and quickly irresistible desire to urinate. In most cases, uninhibited bladder contractions are at fault. They may be a result of damage to the central nervous system from stroke or diseases such as multiple sclerosis, or may be caused by urinary infections or bladder tumors. A variant of this disorder is **reflex incontinence,** in which unintended urination occurs without feelings of urgency.

Overflow incontinence happens when the bladder cannot empty normally and becomes overdistended. This condition usually involves frequent, sometimes nearly constant, urine loss. Causes include neurologic abnormalities such as spinal cord injury and conditions that block outflow such as an enlarged or cancerous prostate or a stricture of the urethra.

Treatment depends on the cause of the problem. Medications prescribed for incontinence include bladder relaxants such as propantheline (Pro-Banthine), flavoxate (Urispas), dicyclomine (Benty), oxybutynin (Ditrupan), calcium channel blockers, and the antidepressant imipramine (Tofranil). Phenylpropanolamine and estrogen replacement are other possibilities. Surgery and behavioral techniques such as pelvic muscle exercises, biofeedback, and bladder training may also be employed.

Other Major Urinary Disorders

Interstitial cystitis occurs when the lining of the bladder becomes scarred or even ulcerated, causing pain when the bladder fills and relief when it empties. This condition is treated by stretching the bladder under anesthesia. It can also be treated by instillations of DMSO (dimethyl sulfoxide) into the bladder through a catheter. Researchers are working on many new treatments for this important and disabling condition.

Bladder cancer accounts for two to four percent of all cancers. It is most prevalent in people over age 50 and more common in men than in women. Approximately one-quarter of the people with this disease have no early symptoms. Most, however, experience blood in the urine. Other symptoms include pain after urination; frequent urination, especially at night; and dribbling.

The causes of bladder cancer are thought to include tobacco, nitrates, and aniline dyes.

Superficial bladder tumors can be removed surgically through the urethra by use of a cystoscope. If a tumor has penetrated the bladder wall, however, partial or even total removal of the bladder may be necessary, depending on the tumor's location. □

CHAPTER 20

Dealing with Liver Disease

The largest internal organ, the liver literally keeps you alive. It performs over 100 separate bodily functions; and its sheer complexity makes it susceptible to almost as many different diseases. Fortunately, most are rare. But there are a few that are all too common, including hepatitis, cirrhosis, liver disorders in children, alcohol-related disorders, and liver cancer.

The American Liver Foundation reports that more than 25 million people are afflicted with liver and gallbladder disease each year. Over 27,000 Americans die from cirrhosis annually, making it the country's third leading cause of death for people between the ages of 25 and 59, and the seventh leading cause of death overall. Viruses, hereditary defects, and reactions to drugs and chemicals are among the known causes of liver breakdown. Though few treatments are effective for life-threatening liver disease, avoiding alcohol and other substances known to cause damage can do a lot to safeguard this important organ. A recently developed vaccine against the hepatitis B virus is now being recommended for children and for adults such as health-care workers who are in danger of exposure. (See section below on viral hepatitis.)

The liver is located behind the lower ribs, right below the diaphragm on the right side of the abdomen. In an average-sized man, it is about the size of a football, weighing a little over three pounds.

A miniature refinery, the liver processes many chemicals necessary for the body's overall functioning. For example, it converts carbohydrates, fats, and proteins into chemicals essential for life and growth. It manufactures and exports to other organs some of the substances they need to function properly, such as the bile used by the intestines during digestion. It modifies drugs taken to treat disease so that they can be used more easily by the body. And it cleanses the blood of toxic substances either ingested or produced by the body itself.

But that's only part of the picture. Below are some of the liver's many other important functions:

- Regulates the blood's ability to clot—governs the transport of fat stores

- Stores extra vitamins, minerals, and sugars to prevent shortages

- Produces quick energy as needed

- Controls the production and excretion of cholesterol

- Breaks down alcohol

- Monitors and maintains the right level of numerous chemicals and drugs in the blood

- Maintains and controls hormone balance

- Helps the body resist infection by producing immune factors and cleansing bacteria from the blood

- Stores iron

The Threat of Viral Hepatitis

Viral hepatitis, a contagious infection of the liver, afflicts more than 70,000 Americans each year. It is usually caused by one of three different organisms.

Hepatitis A, formerly known as infectious hepatitis, can be contracted by consuming contaminated water or food, most notably shellfish. Since the virus is eliminated in the stool, it also spreads through improper hand washing, especially by restaurant workers or anyone else who handles food. Although hepatitis A is seldom serious, in one percent of the cases it can cause severe liver failure and death. It does not cause chronic hepatitis and will not lead to cirrhosis or other long-term liver problems.

Hepatitis B, formerly known as serum hepatitis, is found in blood and other body fluids such as urine, tears, semen, breast milk, and vaginal secretions. It is usually transmitted in blood, via transfusions, or through illicit injectable-drug use. But it also can be contracted through a minor cut or abrasion, or during such everyday acts as toothbrushing, kissing, or having sex. Infants can contract the disease from the mother at birth, or from the mother's breast milk. Dental work, ear piercing, and tattooing are other ways people can get hepatitis B.

Type C hepatitis virus is the cause of a disease known as "non-A, non-B hepatitis," which is also contracted through contact with contaminated blood, or through household or sexual contact with an infected person. It affects approximately 170,000 Americans each year.

Viral hepatitis may produce no symptoms at all. When they occur in type A, they usually begin suddenly and last for several weeks. This period is followed by a convalescent phase of anywhere from two to 12 weeks. Symptoms of viral hepatitis mimic the flu and include mild fever, fatigue, nausea, muscle and joint aches, loss of appetite, vomiting, occasional diarrhea, and vague abdominal pain. Some people also develop a yellow cast to the skin and whites of the eyes known as jaundice, along with dark-colored urine, clay-colored stools, and itching of the skin. The liver may be enlarged and tender.

Patients usually recover completely from hepatitis A and develop a lifelong immunity to it. Immune globulin (Ig) should be administered to anyone exposed to type A hepatitis as soon as possible or within two weeks after

THE GALLBLADDER

The gallbladder stores bile, a substance the liver produces to aid digestion. The most common disorder of the gallbladder is the formation of gallstones. These stones often get stuck in the bile ducts that lead from the gallbladder to the first part of the small intestine, causing the gallbladder to become inflamed. Gallbladder surgery, in which the entire organ is removed, is one of the most common operations in this country. Laparoscopic cholecystectomy, a new procedure that requires only a small incision, has cut down stress and recovery time dramatically. Chenodiol, a recently available drug that dissolves gallstones, is an alternative to surgery. However, due to limited success and troublesome side effects, it is not widely used.

jaundice appears. This medication is 80 to 90 percent effective in preventing the disease. A vaccine for hepatitis A has recently been tested successfully and should be available in a year or two.

Hepatitis B also frequently has no symptoms; but if they do occur, they are similar to those of hepatitis A. The disease follows an unpredictable course, sometimes incapacitating a person for weeks or months and leading to complications, but usually ending in full recovery. Hepatitis C is similar to hepatitis B, but milder. However, like hepatitis B, it may develop into a chronic form in approximately 30 to 50 percent of those who contract it.

The problem with hepatitis B is that five to 10 percent of those who become infected with this disease become chronic carriers who can spread it to others for an indefinite period of time. At present there are more than a million of these silent carriers in this country, and their number is growing by two

to three percent annually. Consequently, authorities recommend that all children and anyone with a high risk of exposure be vaccinated against this dangerous virus.

Chronic carriers usually do not develop chronic hepatitis. If it does develop, however, cirrhosis and primary cancer of the liver can be long-term consequences. An estimated 4,000 people in the United States die from hepatitis B-related cirrhosis annually. Carriers are many times more likely to get liver cancer than are non-carriers.

Treatment for acute hepatitis consists of rest and small, nourishing meals; fluids; and sometimes anti-nausea drugs such as trimethobenzamide (Tigan). Chronic cases of hepatitis B and C are now being treated with interferon, a biotech medicine derived from the human immune system.

Other Diseases of the Liver

In cirrhosis, liver cells are damaged and replaced by scar tissue which, as it accumulates, hardens the liver, diminishes blood flow, and causes even more cells to die. The loss of liver function that accompanies this degenerative condition results in gastrointestinal disturbances, jaundice, enlargement of the liver and spleen, emaciation, and accumulation of fluid in the abdomen and other tissues. Over half of the deaths related to cirrhosis are due to alcohol abuse, hepatitis, and other viruses. Chemicals, poisons, too much iron or copper, and blockages of the bile duct also may cause the disease.

Treatment of cirrhosis usually consists of eliminating the underlying cause, if possible, to avoid further damage, and preventing or treating complications. Care is mostly supportive, often including a specialized diet, diuretics (water pills), vitamins, and abstinence from alcohol. For some patients, a liver transplant is now a feasible option.

Liver abscesses are caused by bacteria, such as *Escherichia coli* (*E. coli*) or staphylococcus (staph), or by *Entamoeba histolytica,* the parasite that causes amebic dysentery. In either case, the offending organisms destroy liver tissue, leaving a cavity that fills with other infectious organisms, white blood cells, and liquefied liver cells. Common symptoms include shoulder and abdominal pain, fever, weight loss, chills, nausea, vomiting, anemia, and, if there is severe liver damage, jaundice. If the offending organism can't be determined, liver abscesses are treated with long-term antibiotics such as aminoglycosides, cephalosporins, clindamycin, or chloramphemicol. If *E. coli* is causing the infection, treatment includes ampicillin; for *Entamoeba histolytica*, emetine, chloroquine, or metronidazole (Flagyl) are included.

Pediatric liver diseases afflict tens of thousands of children in this country annually, and kill hundreds each year. More than 100 different liver diseases are found in infants and children. Most of these disorders are genetic. Among the more common are:

Biliary atresia, an inadequate bile duct, often fatal but sometimes relieved by surgery;

Chronic active hepatitis, in which scar tissue forms and destroys the liver;

Wilson's disease, in which an abnormally large buildup of copper in the liver is treated with vitamin B_6 and d-penicillamine, or, in some cases, corticosteroids such as prednisone;

Reye's syndrome, an acute, often fatal disease secondary to flu or other infections in which fat accumulates in the liver and the patient lapses into coma.

Other serious diseases of the liver, fortunately seen less frequently than these discussed above, include fatty liver, hepatic coma, and liver cancer. □

CHAPTER 21

Facing Up to Sexually Transmitted Disease

S exually transmitted disease (STD) constitutes a staggering public health problem in the U.S. According to the government's Centers for Disease Control, nearly 12 million new cases are diagnosed annually. Young people aged 15 to 29 have the highest rates of infection. By the age of 21, almost one American in five requires treatment for a disease acquired through sexual contact. Among teenagers who are sexually active, the infection rate is a whopping one in four.

Sexually transmitted diseases are more than just a nuisance. Some of these diseases may be fatal, particularly to women and their unborn babies. Other STDs cause pelvic inflammatory disease, tubal pregnancy, sterility, certain types of cancer, or blindness. Babies whose mothers are infected with STDs may suffer from birth defects or mental retardation.

Although the rates of disease and disability from sexually acquired illnesses are highest among the poor, the impact of STDs on health care spending touches all income levels. Indeed, STDs cost Americans more than $3.5 billion a year. Almost 75 percent of this amount goes to treat pelvic inflammatory disease and its consequences, which include tubal pregnancy and female infertility.

During the 1970s, the government monitored just five sexually transmitted diseases—syphilis, gonorrhea, chlamydial infection/nongonococcal urethritis, pelvic inflammatory disease, and genital herpes/warts.

In the 1980s, however, the mounting AIDS epidemic triggered an explosion of research into and monitoring of diseases that were transmitted sexually. The painstaking study of AIDS taught scientists a great deal about other STDs; and today the federal government recognizes some 50 types of sexually transmitted infection.

Thanks to public awareness campaigns, many people now know how to protect themselves from the AIDS virus by avoiding injection drug use and by faithfully using "safer sex" techniques. Fortunately, this same approach also protects them from the many other disease agents transmitted through sexual contact or some other transfer of bodily fluids.

Basic Facts About Sexually Transmitted Diseases

Here are a few basic facts everyone should know for his or her own protection:

- STDs are easily spread through any person-to-person transfer of bodily fluids such as semen, vaginal secretions, or blood.

- When someone has a sexually transmitted disease, anyone who has sex with that person stands a good chance of becoming infected. Thus, having sex with multiple partners carries a greater risk of disease than staying faithful to a spouse or long-term partner. Even a monogamous relationship isn't necessarily risk-free, however, since one partner could be carrying an infection picked up during a prior sexual encounter.

- Many sexually transmitted diseases are highly contagious. For example, if a man has gonorrhea, a woman who has sex with him **just once** stands a 40 to 50 percent chance of getting infected. If the man has gonorrhea plus chlamydia, as frequently happens, the woman could be infected with both diseases at the same time.

AIDS: IN A CLASS OF ITS OWN

AIDS, although definitely an STD, has become such an overriding public health concern that it is discussed separately in this book. Turn to Chapter 22.

- Vaginal intercourse is the classic route of STD infection. However, other important routes include anal sex (among men or man-to-woman), oral sex, sexual abuse of children, and mother-to-baby infection during childbirth.

- Sexually transmitted diseases weaken the immune system, so a person infected with one STD has a greater risk of acquiring other infections. Unfortunately, recovering from an STD does not make a person immune. Anyone who has had a particular STD is still at risk of getting it again.

- Men are more likely to show clear symptoms of STDs. Symptoms in women may not be as obvious, and the problem could be misdiagnosed.

- Many women infected with certain types of STDs have no early symptoms at all and may unknowingly infect sexual partner(s).

- In the past, gay men have tended to have an above-average rate of infection with STDs. This is largely attributed to promiscuity and may have declined in response to the AIDS epidemic. Additionally, some men are secretly bisexual. If a man picks up an STD from a homosexual encounter, he may then pass the infection on to unsuspecting heterosexual partners.

- Lesbians have a lower-than-average risk for STDs, since most sexually acquired diseases are not easily spread from woman to woman.

Preventive Measures

It is important to distinguish between birth control and prevention of STDs. While birth control pills and IUDs help prevent pregnancy, neither measure offers any worthwhile protection against disease.

Practicing "safer sex" is the most reliable way for sexually active people to protect themselves against STDs. Using a latex condom with a contraceptive foam or jelly is an excellent option. The chemical in the foam or jelly kills some infectious microorganisms along with the sperm. (Warning: People who reach for a tube of contraceptive jelly during sex should make sure they do not accidentally grab a tube of simple lubricating jelly, which has no sperm- or germ-killing ingredients.) It's also wise to think about a partner's sexual history, and avoid intimate contact with people at high risk of infection, such as those with multiple sexual partners.

People who even suspect they might have acquired a sexually transmitted disease should stop having sex until they consult a doctor and find out for sure. If test results show an infection, it is essential to notify *all* sexual partners so they can be tested, too. It is vitally important to follow the treatment exactly as prescribed and to abstain from sexual contact until receiving a clean bill of health.

How Sexually Transmitted Disease Is NOT Spread

In most cases, people do NOT pick up sexually transmitted diseases from doorknobs, toilet seats, or towels. That's because the microorganisms that cause STDs thrive in a warm, moist environment such as the mucous membranes of the genitals or the mouth. Many of these organisms die soon after being exposed to dry air. (The virulent hepatitis B virus is a notable exception.)

Common Sexually Transmitted Diseases

As we've seen, the government currently monitors about 50 sexually transmitted diseases. Here is a brief overview of some common STDs (excluding AIDS).

Gonorrhea

Gonorrhea is an infection caused by the *Gonococcus* bacterium. In men, it is marked by a thick, white discharge from the penis and a burning pain when urinating.

In women, gonorrhea may infect the cervix. There may be mild pain and a discharge. If the urethra is infected, there may be a burning sensation during urination. However, women's symptoms are most often mild or simply unnoticeable. Even so, it is important to treat the infection because gonorrhea can lead to pelvic inflammatory disease (see below).

When gonorrhea is transmitted during anal or oral sex, painful infection of the rectum or throat may occur in both men and women.

Chlamydia

Infection by the *Chlamydia trachomatis* bacterium is the leading cause of nongonococcal urethritis in men. This condition consists of pain or burning during urination, a thin discharge from the penis, and staining on underwear. Chlamydial infection may also inflame the sperm-collecting tubules in the scrotum and eventually cause sterility. A man infected with Chlamydia may be infected simultaneously with *Ureaplasma urealyticum*, which also causes urethritis.

In women, a chlamydial infection may cause a thin vaginal discharge, pain during urination, or pain in the lower abdomen about 10 to 20 days after exposure. However, women often do not notice any early symptoms. Chlamydia may also lead to pelvic inflammatory disease.

Pelvic Inflammatory Disease

Pelvic inflammatory disease (PID) is an infection of the uterus, fallopian tubes, or ovaries and usually results from either gonorrhea or chlamydial infection.

The disease typically develops in two stages. First the infection attacks the cervix (the lower part of the uterus). It then spreads to the uterus, fallopian tubes, and ovaries. Sometimes PID starts directly within the uterus when germs gain entry following

CERVICAL CANCER: A DEADLY STD

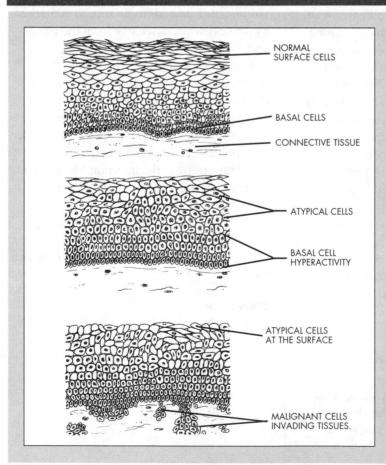

NORMAL SURFACE CELLS

BASAL CELLS

CONNECTIVE TISSUE

Normal cervix: Like skin, the surface of the cervix is constantly being replaced with new cells from below. Generated by division of the basal cells, these new cells rise as older ones are shed from the surface.

ATYPICAL CELLS

BASAL CELL HYPERACTIVITY

Cervical dysplasia: Triggered by an HPV infection, the cervical basal cells may go into overdrive, producing an excessive number of new — but malformed — replacement cells. These cells are not cancerous, but signal the danger of cancer to come.

ATYPICAL CELLS AT THE SURFACE

MALIGNANT CELLS INVADING TISSUES.

Invasive cancer of the cervix: As the condition progresses, truly malignant cells develop and migrate downward into underlying tissues. Unchecked, the disease can be fatal.

childbirth, abortion, or the insertion of an intrauterine contraceptive device (IUD). This, however, is rare.

Since PID causes scar tissue to form, there is up to a 40 percent risk of infertility. PID is also the single most common cause of tubal pregnancy, in which a fertilized egg begins to grow while still in the fallopian tube, instead of the uterus. If the tube bursts, the woman could die.

Genital Warts

Genital warts (condyloma) are caused by the human papillomavirus (HPV) and look much like other warts. They usually occur near the tip of the penis in men. In women, the warts appear on the vulva, in the vagina, on the cervix of the uterus, or near the anus.

Genital warts are flat, hard, and painless when they first appear. If allowed to grow, however, they develop a "cauliflower" appearance and hurt when pressed. Genital warts tend to get bigger during pregnancy. In rare instances, very large warts may interfere with childbirth, making a Caesarean section necessary.

There are several types of HPV. Some types can cause precancerous cell changes in the tissues of a woman's vulva, anus, cervix, or vagina. An invasive cervical cancer can be fatal, which is why women with genital warts should have a Pap test at least once a year.

Vaginitis

Vaginitis, or inflammation of the vagina, is an extremely common gynecological problem. Some types of vaginitis occur because of irritation from tampons, tight clothing, or frequent douching. Other types develop as a side effect of birth control pills or treatment with antibiotics, which may encourage fungal infections.

Two types of vaginitis, however, can be transmitted sexually: Bacterial vaginosis is caused by an overgrowth of several bacteria; trichomoniasis is caused by a one-celled organism called a protozoon. Although these infections do not carry dire consequences, they do cause burning, itching, discharge, and odor, and should certainly be treated.

In either case, it is important for both sexual partners to be treated at the same time. Men may harbor these organisms without showing any symptoms. Unless both partners are cured, the couple could keep passing the problem back and forth.

Genital Herpes

Infection by the *Herpes simplex* virus causes red bumps. These bumps change to watery blisters and then rupture, leaving little hollow spots that may ooze or bleed. The first attack is often accompanied by high fever and swollen lymph nodes in the groin.

In men, genital herpes sores may develop on the penis, scrotum, buttocks, anus, or thighs. The sores can also develop inside the urethra (urinary passage), remaining invisible but possibly causing a thin discharge and painful urination.

Women develop herpes sores on the outer genital area, buttocks, or thighs, or in the vagina or cervix. The sores may cause vaginal discharge, pain during urination, inflammation of the vulva, and aching or pain in the entire genital region.

Herpes sores usually scab over and heal within a week to 10 days, even without treatment. However, because the virus continues to live inside the body, the outbreaks of sores may recur periodically. A tingling sensation in the genitals often announces the development of a new outbreak.

Pregnant women infected with herpes are at risk for miscarriage or premature delivery. A woman may pass herpes on to her baby during childbirth. This happens rarely, but can cause blindness, brain damage, and infant death.

Syphilis

The spirochete bacterium *Treponema pallidum* causes syphilis. The infection develops in distinct stages:

The first symptom is often a painless but highly infectious sore called a chancre. The sore develops from nine to 90 days after exposure and is sometimes accompanied by swollen lymph glands in the groin. Chancres may occur on the genitals or on the mouth, lips, breast, anus, or even the fingertips. The chancre often goes unnoticed in women because it develops inside the vagina. Some infected people never do get a chancre sore. Although a chancre disappears within one to five weeks, the syphilis bacteria remain in the body.

Stage two starts a week to six months later and involves a rash, mouth sores, and/or flu symptoms (headache, mild fever, aching joints). By this time, the bacteria have multiplied and spread, and the disease can be transmitted just by kissing.

Stage three, the latent stage, begins approximately a year after initial infection and lasts 10 to 20 years. There are no noticeable signs of the disease during this period, and after several years the disease is no longer contagious. However, the syphilis bacteria may be silently invading the heart, brain, or other organs.

Stage four is the late stage. Depending on which organs have been attacked, the accumulated damage may cause heart disease, blindness, mental illness, or crippling.

If syphilis is not treated during pregnancy, the mother-to-be may pass the disease on to her baby, and the infant could be born dead, deformed, or diseased.

Before syphilis was curable, it was the most dreaded of the sexually transmitted diseases. The advent of penicillin in the 1940s brought a large and gratifying drop in the syphilis rate. The case load plummeted from 575,600 in 1943 to fewer than 68,000 cases in 1985. Unfortunately, rampant prostitution among crack cocaine users has now driven the syphilis rate back up to its highest level since the early 1950s.

Hepatitis B

Like AIDS, hepatitis B is caused by a virus and can be transmitted via sexual contact, bodily secretions, or blood. But unlike the virus that causes AIDS, hepatitis B is a hardy virus and can remain infectious for quite a while, even in dried blood, saliva, or other secretions.

Hepatitis B begins with flu-like symptoms that disappear as jaundice, the second stage, sets in. The person infected with hepatitis B is thin, weak, lethargic, and irritable and has an enlarged, painful liver. The resulting liver damage is often permanent, and one-fourth of those with hepatitis B eventually die of liver failure.

People who know about hepatitis B fear the virus because it is so easy to catch—especially when compared to AIDS. A hepatitis B vaccine is available, and medical personnel must be inoculated. Unfortunately, the very people most likely to get hepatitis B—intravenous drug users, prostitutes, and sexual partners of infected individuals—generally don't bother to get vaccinated or simply don't know the vaccine exists. That's why the incidence of this serious disease has been rising since 1982.

Treating Sexually Transmitted Diseases

Once again, the best way to handle sexually transmitted disease is to prevent its spread by faithfully following safety precautions, including "safer sex" techniques.

If an STD does develop, it may be treated with medications, surgical procedures, or possibly both.

For a given STD, it is important to take the right medication exactly as prescribed. For example, even though gonorrhea and chlamydial infections often occur together, they require different medications. Never try to treat a sexually transmitted disease without a doctor's supervision. Using the wrong medication could do more harm than good.

By far the most common group of medications used to treat sexually transmitted diseases are the antibiotics that are available in ever-increasing variety. Sometimes a disease-causing organism "learns" to outwit a given antibiotic, at which point a different one is required. To cope with this ongoing problem, pharmaceutical companies are constantly striving to develop new antibiotics.

Metronidazole, a different type of antimicrobial medication, is used to combat STDs caused by anaerobic (non-oxygen-dependent) bacteria or protozoa.

Various caustic creams, ointments, and solutions are used to shrink genital warts. Dry ice can be used to freeze and remove them. Laser surgery is also employed.

Although not a cure, acyclovir helps prevent or reduce the severity of genital herpes sores. To remove growths on or in the vagina, cervix, or uterus, electrosurgical excision is an option. □

CHAPTER 22

The Facts about AIDS

No disease is so widely misunderstood or so controversial as Acquired Immunodeficiency Syndrome, better known as AIDS. Myth and controversy swirl around AIDS because it is primarily a sexually transmitted disease, has only recently been identified, and has caused a seemingly sudden surge of fatalities among certain high-risk groups in this country. While it affects far fewer people than high blood pressure, cancer, or heart disease, it has captured our attention because of its abrupt apocalyptic appearance and its almost certain fatal outcome.

AIDS is simple in neither cause nor effect. Basically, it is a life-threatening disruption of the immune system by the Human Immunodeficiency Virus (HIV). This virus progressively weakens the body's ability to fight off disease, opening it to severe infections with both common and exotic organisms, as well as various forms of cancer. In the United States, most cases of AIDS have been traced to the virus called HIV-1.

HIV is particularly dangerous because it can lie hidden for years. Someone infected by HIV may not yet have AIDS, and, in fact, may have no symptoms at all. As symptoms related to the viral infection do begin to appear, the term AIDS-Related Complex (ARC) is often used to describe the situation. Only when the immune system nears total collapse, or specific infections or cancers develop, is a patient said to have AIDS.

HIV has sparked tremendous fear and controversy, not only because of whom it attacks and the way it is transmitted, but because of its hidden nature and lethal results. No virus since polio has garnered so much scientific attention. Researchers have yet to find a cure; but their efforts have paid off with a growing number of medicines that can slow the progress of the infection and prolong the patient's life.

Our Status Today

AIDS was not recognized until the early 1980s, when frequent reports of unusual lung infections with *Pneumocystis carinii* and a rapidly spreading form of cancer called Kaposi's sarcoma, found primarily in homosexual men, reached the Centers for Disease Control in Atlanta, Georgia. The fact that these previously rare diseases were clustered in a single group of people led scientists to suspect that some sort of underlying infection was involved. As more and more people developed the exotic diseases now known to be symptoms of AIDS, it became clear that a "new" illness had surfaced in the U.S. HIV, the virus responsible for AIDS, was first identified by French and American research groups in 1984, and since that time, both public and private organizations have committed considerable resources to combat this disease.

By the end of 1989, there were 115,000 reported cases of AIDS in the United States. For 1993, the U.S. Department of Health and Human Services has estimated that the total will rise to between 390,000 and 480,000 reported cases, and that 285,000 to 340,000 people will have died from the disease.

All told, there are an estimated million to a million and a half people infected with HIV in the United States. While only 10 to 20 percent per year will develop the AIDS group of symptoms, all are believed to be capable of transmitting and spreading the virus.

When the AIDS epidemic struck, it first spread within the homosexual community, whose sexual practices put them at especially high risk. Today, AIDS among heterosexuals is also on the rise, with a 30 percent increase from 1989 to 1990.

We now know that women who have had sexual relations with bisexuals, as well as injection drug users and certain other populations, are also at high risk for infection. In 1985, only seven percent of AIDS cases were women; now the proportion is almost 13 percent. AIDS is the leading cause of death in women between ages 25 and 44 in New York City. Urban teenagers, according to the American Foundation for AIDS Research, are the next group that will develop widespread HIV infection. HIV infections among urban teens admitted to hospitals rose by 250 percent from 1987 to 1991.

Total annual costs of AIDS were projected at between $5 and $13 billion by the end of 1992. AIDS is now the seventh leading cause of death in the U.S. and is the leading cause of death among injection drug users and hemophiliacs.

According to the Department of Health and Human Services, "Despite the uncertainty about the incidence of HIV infection and the ultimate magnitude of the problem, HIV and AIDS are a growing threat to the health of the nation and will continue to make major demands on health and social systems for many decades."

The Virus and What It Does

In order to understand AIDS, it's important to know a few basic facts about the "germs" we call viruses. These tiny invaders are especially difficult to repel. While infections by bacteria can be treated with common antibiotics, a viral infection cannot.

Viruses are minute microorganisms that commandeer the machinery of the body's own cells to survive and reproduce. They can take hold in many parts of the body, but under ordinary circumstances are eventually eradicated—or at least held in check—by the immune system. HIV is scientifically termed a *retrovirus*. What makes it so deadly is the fact that it attacks certain key cells of the immune system itself.

These cells, known as "helper" or T-4 lymphocytes, play a central role in the body's defense against infections. But as they are themselves infected and destroyed by HIV, their number declines, and the chance of successful attack by other germs steadily rises. Treatment with an anti-retroviral drug such as zidovudine (AZT, Retrovir) can, at least temporarily, halt this decline. In fact, physicians often monitor a patient's helper lymphocyte count to gauge the success of therapy.

Other cells of the immune system are also liable to HIV attack. Called monocytes and macrophages, these cells may serve to transport the virus to the brain. They may also act as a long-term reservoir of infection.

How Do You Get AIDS?

Most researchers now agree that HIV is the main cause of AIDS. They also agree that, unlike airborne or animal-transmitted viruses, HIV's primary method of transmission is via a substance that contains the virus or infected cells. In most cases, the vehicle seems to have been male seminal fluid, which enters the body through mucous membranes that become torn during anal or vaginal intercourse. AIDS may also be transmitted in infected transfused blood or menstrual blood, on used needles shared among drug users, through deep puncture wounds in healthcare workers, from mother to baby, and possibly by some other unknown routes.

Fortunately, HIV is not spread through routine social interaction. AIDS is not passed on through casual non-sexual contact—shaking hands, attending school with an HIV-positive person, hugging, or even sharing the same plates and utensils. In

PREVENTION OF AIDS IS THE BEST CURE

The spread of AIDS can be stopped only by eliminating the behaviors that spread the disease, including high-risk sexual practices and injection drug use. Health-care institutions, such as blood banks and hospitals, have taken steps to protect the blood supply and to reduce risk among health-care workers. However, the most important line of defense against AIDS must come from the people most at risk. Since we are relatively sure of the way AIDS is spread, it is comparatively easy to identify what needs to be done. For your personal safety, always remember the three key precautions:

■ Avoid high-risk behavior such as injection drug abuse, sexual promiscuity, and sexual contact with anyone you believe has indulged in such activities. Make certain you know a partner's sexual history. Remember that someone can appear perfectly healthy, yet still be harboring HIV.

■ All people who are at risk (i.e. have multiple sexual contacts or a partner with multiple contacts) must practice "safer sex." This means no sexual contact should be unprotected. Latex condoms and spermicidal jellies that can kill the virus should always be used. Sexual practices such as unprotected anal intercourse should be avoided. If you suspect you're at risk, get tested for HIV periodically. Remember that it may take up to six months—or even a year—for the virus to show up. Do not donate blood if unsure of your status.

■ Although the blood supply is generally safe in the U.S., you may want to consider banking your own blood prior to elective surgery.

general, HIV is passed from men to men or men to women during intercourse, but less readily from women to men.

It is this fact that has mislead many people to believe that AIDS is simply a "gay" or "drug addict's" disease. But as we have seen, this is increasingly untrue. And because the infection can go undetected for years, an unsuspecting carrier can pass on the virus to sexual partners unknowingly, until symptoms finally appear.

What Are the Symptoms of AIDS?

HIV infection poses a difficult diagnostic problem because the blood tests most commonly used don't identify the virus itself, but rather, the presence of antibodies that the body gradually develops to fight the infection. The first test, often referred to as an ELISA (enzyme-linked immunosorbent assay), will, when positive, usually lead to a second test called the Western blot. However, if conducted too soon after exposure, both tests may fail to detect any antibodies—even though the person is already infected and capable of transmitting the virus. For this reason, experts recommend repeat testing for six months (or up to one year) after known or suspected exposure.

When first infected with HIV, a person may experience the same symptoms seen in many other viral infections—fever, sore throat, headache, rash, or a mononucleosis-type illness. For the majority of those infected, however, there may be no symptoms at all.

After this first flare-up, if it occurs, there are usually no symptoms for an extended period—typically five to six years. There is some evidence, however, that for those infected through blood transfusions, the time is much shorter.

While this period wears on, some patients develop shingles, itchy skin lesions, tuberculosis, fungal infections of the mouth (thrush), night sweats, fatigue, or swollen lymph nodes. Then, as damage to the immune system increases, additional problems may appear, including bacterial infections of the blood and lungs, a severe form of pneumonia caused by *Pneumocystis carinii*, various cancers such as lymphoma, severe herpes infections of the genitals or mouth, a fungal form of meningitis, toxoplasmosis involving the brain, and severe diarrhea. Also possible in the more advanced stages of the disease are sight-threatening cytomegalovirus infections of the eyes; generalized infection with *Mycobacterium avium-intracellulare*, or "MAI" (an organism resembling the cause of tuberculosis); and numerous neurological disorders, including progressive dementia.

Finally, in addition to the many bizarre infections that strike only those with failing immune systems, HIV patients are subject to all the more common infections as well, often in their severest forms.

How Is HIV Infection Treated?

There is still no cure for HIV; but we do have ways of delaying its progress and fighting the "opportunistic" infections that can seize hold in its wake. To control the virus itself, we now have several anti-retroviral drugs. To fend off opportunistic infections, there are potent antibiotics. And, for the future, work continues on a vaccine to fight the virus in those already infected.

Treatment with anti-retroviral drugs is difficult for several reasons. First, the virus usually has time to become well established before any symptoms appear. Second, a drug must be able to attack the virus *within* infected cells, while preventing infection of additional cells. Third, because the drugs currently in use also affect healthy cells, they tend to produce significant side effects. These unwanted side effects impose unavoidable limits on the way the drugs can be used.

In developing anti-retroviral drugs, scientists have taken advantage of critical steps in HIV's life cycle. For example, the three currently available drugs for treating HIV infection—zidovudine (AZT, Retrovir), didanosine (ddI, Videx) and zalcitabine (ddC, Hivid)—all act by inhibiting an enzyme (transcriptase) that the virus uses to reproduce. Unfortunately, the effectiveness of these drugs seems to decrease with prolonged use; and laboratory studies have shown that the virus can develop resistance to each. Most AIDS researchers today believe a multi-pronged attack with drugs that fight the virus in several different ways will ultimately prove more effective. Numerous other compounds, including interferons, are currently under study.

To prevent the life-threatening infections that can break through the HIV-weakened immune system, doctors use a variety of antibiotics. For example, the development of the serious pneumonia caused by *Pneumocystis carinii* can be prevented or delayed by medications such as oral trimethoprim-sulfamethoxazole (Bactrim, Septra) or aerosolized pentamadine (Pentam, NebuPent). The same drugs, usually administered intravenously, are often used to treat the infections once they take hold. For some infections, medication may be continued for life because of the high risk of recurrence. Unfortunately, the use of these drugs too may be limited by significant side effects.

Because all of these drugs can, in fact, improve the lives of those with HIV infections, anyone at risk of AIDS owes it to him- or herself to get an HIV test. □

CHAPTER 23

Keeping Diabetes under Control

Diabetes is a chronic disease marked by an abnormally high level of sugar in the blood. It develops when the body loses its normal ability to use sugar for energy. Diabetes is by no means a rare condition. In the U.S. some 14 million people have diabetes; more than 50,000 new cases are diagnosed each year.

To date, there is no cure for the disease. Left untreated, it can eventually cause blindness, heart problems, kidney malfunction, foot infections leading to gangrene, or even death. However, excellent treatment exists to control diabetes, enabling most people with the disease to lead full, essentially normal lives.

What Is Diabetes?

When doctors say that diabetes involves the body's response to "sugar," this means more than just refined white table sugar. Healthful foods such as fruits, vegetables, milk, grains, and pasta all contain naturally occurring sugars of various types.

During digestion these different kinds of sugars are broken down into a simpler form, glucose, which is the body's normal source of fuel. The bloodstream carries glucose throughout the entire body, providing an energy source to every cell. A constant supply of glucose is crucial to life; it is needed for everything from thinking to moving to pumping blood.

But in order for glucose to leave the blood and enter the cells, another important substance is required: the hormone insulin. Produced in a gland called the pancreas, insulin has three functions:

1. It helps glucose pass from the blood into the cells, where it is used for energy.

2. It keeps the blood from getting overloaded with too rich a supply of glucose.

3. It prevents the body from breaking down its own fat cells and muscle cells as sources of energy.

In Diabetes, What Goes Wrong?

In diabetes, glucose from digested food enters the bloodstream as usual—but because of a lack or malfunction of insulin, the glucose does not find its way into the cells. When this happens, it triggers a series of increasingly dangerous events.

At the outset, the unused glucose builds up in the blood. The medical term for this state of too-high blood sugar is hyperglycemia. While a normal sugar level is 60 to 110 milligrams per 100 milliliters of blood, people with diabetes may have from 150 to 500 milligrams or more per 100 milliliters.

Because mild or moderate hyperglycemia may cause no symptoms, it is possible for a person to have diabetes for some time without being aware of it. However, if hyperglycemia becomes more severe, people begin to experience continual thirst and a need to urinate frequently, even at night. This condition results when the kidneys, in response to a buildup of sugar in the blood, filter out as much of it as possible and dump it into the urine. (Glucose begins to spill over into the urine when the blood sugar level exceeds 180.) At the same time, the kidneys draw large amounts of water out of the body to prevent the sugar-rich urine from becoming too thick. This constant depletion of water perpetuates a cycle of urination and thirst.

If severe hyperglycemia continues unchecked, it can next lead to **ketoacidosis**—a buildup of ketones and fatty acids in the blood that results in further complications. This is what happens:

Sensing that its glucose-starved cells need energy, the body begins to break down its own muscle and fat tissue. This produces backup energy sources known as ketones and fatty acids. Without insulin to regulate the flow, however, excess ketones and fatty acids accumulate in the blood, causing nausea, vomiting, rapid breathing, and—as in hyperglycemia—increased urination and thirst.

As ever more water leaves the body, it washes out various minerals needed for normal body function. If no treatment is given, the person goes into shock and eventually lapses into a coma. In the days before effective therapy was available, this was how people died from diabetes.

Isn't There More Than One Kind of Diabetes?

Yes, there are two main types of diabetes.

In **Type I (insulin-dependent) diabetes,** the pancreas loses its ability to make insulin.

In **Type II (non-insulin-dependent) diabetes,** the pancreas can still make insulin, but either it makes too little or the body has difficulty using it—or both. Type II is the more common form of diabetes. Of the 14 million diabetics in the U.S., almost 13 million have Type II.

In addition to Type I and Type II diabetes, there are three less common conditions also related to high blood sugar:

Impaired glucose tolerance involves blood sugar levels higher than normal, but not high enough to count as diabetic. This is not technically a type of diabetes. However, people with impaired glucose tolerance may go on to develop diabetes.

Gestational diabetes is high blood sugar that first develops during pregnancy. Although it usually disappears after the baby is born, the woman may eventually develop diabetes. If she does, it will probably be Type II.

Secondary diabetes is caused by damage to the pancreas—from cancer, for example, or from diseases of other glands, or harmful chemicals.

What Causes Diabetes?

Doctors still do not know what causes diabetes, but scientists now believe the tendency to develop the disorder is genetic—in other words, it is present in the individual even before birth.

Type I diabetes is thought to involve a physical malfunction called an autoimmune reaction. Normally the body's immune system forms antibodies to kill invaders such as viruses. Sometimes, however, the immune system mistakenly attacks some of the body's own tissues—such as the pancreas cells that make insulin. It's possible that a virus may trigger the onset of Type I diabetes. However, Type I diabetes is not contagious.

Type II diabetes seems to be caused by overweight—80 to 90 percent of people with this form of diabetes carry excess pounds. Their basic problem is not a shortage of insulin, but an inability to use it properly.

DIAGNOSING DIABETES

When diabetes is suspected, the person may undergo a fasting blood glucose test. A blood sample is taken in the morning before breakfast. If the glucose level is over 140, and a repeat test gives the same reading, the patient has diabetes.

If the reading is between 115 and 140, however, a further test is necessary: the glucose tolerance test. The person swallows a sugary liquid that produces temporary high blood sugar. Then blood samples are taken 30 minutes, one hour, two hours, and three hours later; and the glucose level is measured in each sample. The results show how quickly the person's body was able to bring the blood sugar level back down to normal. The glucose tolerance test helps diagnose Type II diabetes.

Their excess fat tissue somehow seems to prevent the insulin in their bodies from doing its job.

Who Gets Diabetes?

Type I diabetes most often occurs in children and young adults, but can develop at any age.

People who have Type I diabetes almost always suspect they are ill. Their symptoms, which usually develop rapidly and "out of the blue," include: excessive thirst and frequent urination; unusual hunger; sudden weight loss; weakness; fatigue; irritability; and nausea or vomiting.

By contrast, Type II diabetes most often occurs in adults.

People who have Type II diabetes may not know about their condition for weeks, months, or even years, because the symptoms usually develop gradually. Symptoms of Type II diabetes may include any of the symptoms of Type I diabetes and/or: slow-healing; infections of the bladder, gums, or skin; itching; numb or tingling hands or feet; blurred vision; and drowsiness.

About six million Americans have Type II diabetes but do not know it. People at highest risk for Type II diabetes are more than 40 years old, need to lose weight, and have close blood relatives (grandparents, parents, or siblings) who are diabetic. Anyone corresponding to this description should be tested regularly for diabetes.

Can Diabetes Be Prevented?

As yet there is no known way to prevent Type I diabetes, although research is under way.

On the other hand, people who know they are at risk for Type II diabetes—because of age, overweight, and a family history of non-insulin-dependent diabetes—can often prevent the onset of the disease by losing weight and keeping fit.

Treatment: Blood Sugar Control

Treatment of diabetes aims at **control** of the amount of sugar in the blood. The object is to keep blood sugar levels within a safe range. Research results suggest that tight control of blood sugar may prevent, or at least delay, the long-term complications of diabetes.

Type I (insulin-dependent) diabetes is treated with daily **injections of insulin,** plus **regular exercise** and wholesome, **balanced meals**.

Insulin injections are not as bad as they sound. Because the needles are short and sharp, the needle prick is almost painless. Even diabetic children can learn to administer their own injections.

While food raises blood sugar, insulin lowers it. Unfortunately, too much insulin causes a problem of its own—low blood sugar, or hypoglycemia. This unpleasant condition, also known as an insulin reaction or insulin shock, may develop even after an ordinary dose of insulin if the person eats too little food, eats later than usual, or does an unusual amount of exercise.

Hypoglycemia can make the person feel weak, shaky, cold, very hungry, nervous, irritable, or confused. It may cause a headache or bizarre behavior. The remedy for hypoglycemia is a quick dose of sugar-rich food, which brings the blood sugar level back up to normal.

Untreated hypoglycemia eventually causes unconsciousness, which can progress to coma and permanent brain damage. When this happens, an injection of glucose or glucagon, a prescription drug that raises blood sugar, can be a lifesaver. Because of the danger of hypoglycemia, anyone taking medicine for diabetes should be sure to wear an identification tag.

To maintain steady blood sugar levels, it's necessary to eat frequently and at regular, fixed intervals: three meals a day, plus two or three snacks. Insulin should also be taken at fixed times of day. Many people with Type I diabetes find it easier to control their blood sugar level if they take two or more injections of insulin a day, rather than one big dose.

Type II (non-insulin-dependent) diabetes is first treated with an individualized, low-sugar, **weight-loss diet** plus a regimen of **regular exercise.** If diet and exercise do not improve the body's ability to use its own insulin, the doctor may prescribe **pills** to increase both the production and the effectiveness of insulin. If blood sugar levels are still hard to control, **insulin injections** may be needed. However, diet and exercise remain important.

How Do People with Diabetes Know What Their Blood Sugar Level Is?

The original way to test for diabetes was to measure sugar levels in the urine. But sugar does not even start to appear in the urine until the blood sugar level tops 180. This means urine testing is not very sensitive. The person may have abnormally high blood sugar for hours before it shows up in a urine test.

Today, many doctors recommend that diabetics perform frequent home blood tests. This test, which is simple and easy, shows the blood sugar level at the exact moment of testing. It is done by pricking the finger and smearing a single drop of blood onto a chemically treated testing strip. The amount of sugar in the blood determines what color the strip will turn.

People with Type I diabetes are often advised to test their own blood sugar levels up to four times a day. Those with Type II diabetes may need to test less often. Results of the blood tests should be recorded faithfully in a notebook. They serve as guides for adjusting food and insulin intake.

In addition, many doctors recommend a glycohemoglobin test every three to six months. This blood test, which must be done by a laboratory, shows the average blood sugar level over the preceding 30 to 60 days. Here is how it works:

Because glucose is sticky, it adheres to hemoglobin, the oxygen-carrying part of each red blood cell. The sugar-coated hemoglobin (known as glycosylated hemoglobin or, more simply, glycohemoglobin) will stay in the blood for many weeks before it is replaced by new hemoglobin. A high level of glycohemoglobin means the person had hyperglycemia (high blood sugar) at some point during the preceding month or two. This tells the doctor that further work is needed to bring the person's blood sugar level under tighter control.

The Drugs that Bring Blood Sugar under Control

Here is a look at some of the drugs used in managing diabetes:

Beef insulin and **pork insulin,** which are taken from the pancreases of animals, are given by injection to treat Type I (insulin-dependent) diabetes. They may also be given to patients with Type II (non-insulin-dependent) diabetes whose blood sugar is not suffi-

LIVING WITH DIABETES

Because it is a chronic disease that cannot be cured, diabetes is stressful for the person who has it—and sometimes for that person's family, too.

Children with diabetes fear other youngsters may reject them for being different. Parents of diabetic children feel uncertain and guilty: "Did my child inherit this from me? Did I do something wrong?"

Adults with diabetes chafe at having to maintain a regular schedule for meals and medication. Spouses of diabetics may resent the illness for its demands on time and energy, or may live in fear of its long-term consequences.

Denial, guilt, and anger are common, normal responses to diabetes. Support groups and professional counselors are available to assist diabetic patients and their families. Education about diabetes is helpful. Dread often stems from misconceptions.

ciently controlled by diet, exercise, and antidiabetic medicine. These insulins come in fast-acting, intermediate-acting, and slow-acting forms. What kind to take, and when, depends on the person's schedule and lifestyle. At the beginning of treatment, doctor and patient need to work together to customize the insulin regimen.

Human insulin, which was developed through genetic engineering, is a manufactured product identical to the insulin produced by a normal human pancreas. It has largely supplanted animal-derived insulin. It can be injected through an ordinary syringe or through a cartridge device designed to look like a ballpoint pen.

Antidiabetic medications, also known as oral hypoglycemic drugs, are pills used in treating Type II diabetes. They should be used to supplement, not replace, a low-sugar diet. These medications stimulate the pancreas to produce more insulin, and may also make insulin work more efficiently. Included in this group are DiaBeta, Diabinese, Glucotrol, Micronase, Orinase, and Tolinase.

Glucagon, like insulin, is a hormone produced by the pancreas. It acts on the liver, causing the blood sugar level to rise. A person with diabetes who becomes uncon-scious because of insulin shock may be treated with either glucagon or intravenous dextrose.

Testing strips are chemically treated paper strips for urine or blood tests. The strips turn a particular color according to the concentration of sugar in the urine or blood. Some urine-testing strips show levels of both sugar and ketones. □

CHAPTER 24

Correcting Disorders in the Blood

Fortunately, though disorders of the blood are common, most are not serious. Frequently they are caused by infections or deficiencies, both of which can be corrected by appropriate treatment. Even some of the more severe, malignant, or life-threatening blood disorders often respond well to treatment, which can prolong life or even produce a complete cure.

Common causes of blood disorders include trauma, malnutrition, infection, drugs, chronic diseases, surgery, exposure to toxins and radiation, and congenital or genetic abnormalities—all of which undermine blood production and functioning.

What Does Blood Do?

Blood serves as the body's primary transportation, emergency, and communication network. It brings oxygen and nutrients to each cell, removes waste, and literally keeps us alive. By marshaling the body's immune responses, it helps us fend off the invaders that threaten us every day. Because the blood carries important hor-

mones that regulate various bodily functions, it also plays a vital role in keeping the various systems in balance and harmony with each other. What's more, the blood helps regulate acid-base and fluid balances, not to mention body temperature.

The average person has 10 and one-half pints of blood constantly circulating throughout his or her vessels. The blood consists of two major parts: The plasma, or liquid portion, transports nutrients and antibodies to tissues and removes waste. Suspended in the plasma are the cellular elements of blood (erythrocytes, thrombocytes, and leukocytes). These blood cells are formed in bone marrow throughout the body, but are primarily manufactured in the core bones, such as the breastbone, ribs, vertebrae, and pelvis.

The majority of blood cells are red cells (erythrocytes), which carry oxygen and carbon dioxide back and forth between the lungs and the tissues. Red cells get their coloring from the hemoglobin that carries oxygen to the tissues. The thrombocytes (platelets) regulate the blood's ability to clot. If the number of platelets declines, bleeding from even a minor injury will be prolonged. The leukocytes (white blood cells or WBCs) come in five different types, the most numerous being granulocytes and lymphocytes. The main function of WBCs is to defend the body against infection, foreign substances, trauma, and tissue damage. Granulocytes engulf and kill invading bacteria. Lymphocytes produce the antibodies that prepare invaders for destruction.

Red cells outnumber white blood cells 500 to one. The red blood cells (RBCs) are smaller than the white blood cells and survive for an average of 120 days. Platelets last seven to 10 days; granulocytes survive for only six to 10 hours. Lymphocytes, on the other hand, can survive for many months.

Treating the Many Forms of Anemia

Anemia is any deficiency in the number of red blood cells. The most common types of anemia are as follows:

Iron Deficiency Anemia
Iron deficiency anemia affects 10 to 30 percent of the adults in the United States. This type of anemia results from poor diet, iron malabsorption, abnormal chronic blood loss, and pregnancy. Iron deficiency anemia is most common in premenopausal women, infants, children, and adolescents.

Symptoms of iron deficiency anemia include shortness of breath, pallor, listlessness, fatigue, difficulty in concentrating, headache, and irritability.

Treatment entails taking oral iron supplements in combination with vitamin C to enhance absorption. Correcting the underly-

ing cause of chronic blood loss—such as a peptic ulcer—is mandatory.

Pernicious Anemia
People with pernicious anemia experience decreased production of hydrochloric acid and an intestinal secretion called the *intrinisic factor* that is necessary for the absorption of Vitamin B_{12}. The vitamin deficiency, in turn, causes a decrease in formation of all blood cells (particularly red blood cells), and nerve cells.

Typically found in people of northern European ancestry, pernicious anemia tends to appear between the ages of 50 and 60. The disease usually is unnoticed at first, but eventually results in a sore tongue, weakness, and tingling and numbness in the extremities. The tongue, gums, and lips are pale; and the skin may be jaundiced (yellow). People with pernicious anemia sometimes become very susceptible to infections, particularly infections of the genitourinary tract. Other symptoms of pernicious anemia include nausea, vomiting, diarrhea, loss of appetite, weight loss, constipation, bleeding gums, and tongue inflammation. The impaired nerve function that accompanies pernicious anemia can lead to a number of neurological difficulties, such as weakness in the extremities, light-headedness, impaired coordination, blurred vision, loss of bladder and bowel control, and impotence. The resulting decrease in red blood cells can lead to cardiovascular difficulties, such as angina (crushing chest pain) and congestive heart failure (palpitations, labored breathing, and breathlessness).

Vitamin B_{12} injections will often minimize the complications and reverse the disease.

The B_{12} shots may also prevent permanent-nerve damage if it has not progressed too far. Once the patient starts to improve, monthly B_{12} shots are then given indefinitely to prevent a recurrence.

If hemoglobin is extremely low, blood transfusions may be needed to tide the patient over during the one to two weeks needed for the B_{12} injections to take effect. However, bed rest is usually preferred. Treatment of cardiac problems may be necessary.

Folic Acid Deficiency Anemia

Folic acid is another vitamin needed for blood cell production. Folic acid deficiency anemia appears most frequently in infants, adolescents, pregnant and lactating women, the elderly, alcoholics, and individuals with serious intestinal disorders or malignancies. Folic acid anemia progresses slowly, but eventually exhibits such symptoms as palpitations, shortness of breath, headache, irritability, fatigue, sore tongue, weakness, appetite loss, fainting, nausea, slight jaundice, pallor, and forgetfulness. Unlike pernicious anemia, it does not cause nerve damage.

Treatment consists of folic acid supplementation and dietary counseling.

Aplastic Anemia

Aplastic anemia arises because production of blood cells by the bone marrow is somehow defective or has been halted by drugs, toxins, or radiation. In aplastic anemia the normal production of all blood cells is inhibited since all are produced in the marrow.

The symptoms of aplastic anemia include fatigue and weakness, pallor, and headache. Other symptoms that may be seen are bruises, small red spots on the skin, and excessive bleeding in the nose, gums, rectum, vagina, and into the retina. Patients may also develop severe infections.

Bone marrow transplants are increasingly used to treat aplastic anemia. Transplants are successful in approximately half of the cases. If the disease is mild, treatment options include the use of corticosteroids, marrow-stimulating substances such as androgen, immunosuppressive drugs, and antithymocyte globulin (ATG).

Other Major Disorders

Thalassemia refers to a group of hereditary anemias characterized by a deficiency of hemoglobin. These disorders occur worldwide, but are most commonly found in the Mediterranean countries and in Southeast Asia. Thalassemia major, also known as Cooley's anemia, usually develops soon after birth and is characterized by severe anemia, failure to thrive, bone abnormalities, and potentially fatal complications. Symptoms of thalassemia include pallor, jaundice, frequent infections, and appetite loss. Treatment is essentially supportive and includes repeated transfusions and folic acid supplements, along with antibiotics for infections and iron-removal therapy to correct the iron overload that comes from frequent transfusions.

Sickle cell anemia is a congenital disease that occurs mostly in Black people. Defective hemoglobin molecules make red blood cells rough and sickle-shaped. These abnormal cells disrupt circulation in small blood vessels and die off too quickly, which leads to chronic health problems. Sickle cell anemia is marked by serious complications and periodic crises. Half of the victims will die before reaching their late twenties. Fortunately, while about 78 percent of African-Americans have the sickle cell trait, only one in 650 develops anemia.

Symptoms of sickle cell anemia include abnormal heart rhythms and murmurs, an enlarged heart, breathlessness upon exertion, chronic fatigue, swollen joints, pallor, aching bones, jaundice, chest pain, leg ulcers, and increased susceptibility to infections.

Acetaminophen is the painkiller of choice for treating the mild pain crises of sickle cell anemia. Codeine is usually given for severe episodes. In some cases, stronger analgesics, such as meperidine (Demerol), hydromorphone (Dilaudid), or oxycodone (Percodan), are necessary.

Hemorrhagic disorders involve an impairment of the coagulation process. The most common cause of these disorders is a deficiency of platelets. The deficiency, known as thrombocytopenia, may be congenital or acquired, and is known to be a side effect of certain medications, such as quinidine, sulfa drugs, and oral antidiabetic medicines. The abnormal bleeding in the gastrointestinal, genitourinary, or respiratory tract that results from hemorrhagic disorders causes fatigue, malaise, and lethargy. Shortness of breath, a racing heart, loss of consciousness, and death may also result. Treatment consists of removing the offending agent when appropriate and, depending on the cause, administering corticosteroids, immunosuppresive drugs, or intravenous immunoglobulins. Removal of the spleen, an organ that retires aging blood cells from circulation, is often requried.

Hemophilia is the most common X-linked genetic disease, and occurs only in males. A bleeding disorder that results from deficiencies of specific clotting factors in the blood, hemophilia produces abnormal bleeding that may be mild, moderate, or severe. The milder form of hemophilia may go unnoticed until adulthood, when the person experiences a trauma or undergoes surgery. In severe cases, profuse bleeding occurs after only a minor injury, and patients may bleed internally as well as externally. In such cases, hemophilia can cause nerve damage, pain, muscle atrophy, gangrene, shock, and even death.

During bleeding episodes, hemophiliacs require replacement of the clotting factors they lack. Replacement products include cryoprecipitate, lyophilized factor VIII or IX, and fresh frozen plasma. Hemophiliacs may also take acetaminophen, propoxyphene (Darvon), codeine, or meperidine (Demerol) for pain. Aspirin is always contraindicated, because it increases the likelihood of bleeding.

Though not yet curable, hemophilia does respond to corrective treatment, which can prevent the development of crippling deformities and prolong life. □

CHAPTER 25

Relief for Troubled Feet

The human foot is a masterpiece of design and functionality. Despite its small size, each foot contains 26 bones, and together, the feet account for one quarter of the bones in the body. In addition, each foot has 33 joints; a network of more than 100 tendons, muscles, and ligaments; and a vast system of blood vessels and nerves. Indeed, so many nerves converge in the foot that ancient therapies often included daily massage of this extremity in order to insure total health and well-being. The foot's complex network of nerves and their relation to other body parts also explains why when our feet hurt, we tend to feel bad all over.

Foot ailments are very common health problems, affecting 75 percent of Americans to some degree at some time in their lives.

Because most people tend to accept sore feet as a necessary evil, few seek the treatment they need. This is unfortunate, since proper medical care from a trained orthopedist or podiatrist can go a long way toward alleviating foot problems and preventing chronic conditions.

How Do Our Feet Break Down?

Our feet are subjected to enormous stress. In an average day's walking, they sustain repeated force totaling several hundred tons. No wonder feet are injured more frequently than any other body part! In addition, poor-fitting shoes, corns and calluses, conditions such as unequal leg lengths, and simply standing for hours at a time all take their toll on our tender feet.

The symptoms of several more general diseases such as diabetes, circulatory disorders (particularly clogged blood vessels), anemia, and kidney problems first appear in the feet. Arthritis, particularly rheumatoid arthritis and gout, also is often first seen in the joints of the feet.

How We Treat Foot Problems

Athlete's foot is a fungal skin disorder. It usually begins between the toes, but can spread to other parts of the foot and body. The dry skin, itching, scaling, inflammation, and blisters of this disease can be prevented by careful hygiene. Daily washing with soap and water, thorough drying (especially between the toes), changing shoes and hose regularly, and dusting with foot powder to reduce moisture can do a lot to deter fungal growth.

Medications for athlete's foot include fungicides and fungistatic drugs, taken orally or applied to the skin. If a bacterial infection develops, antibiotics may be prescribed.

Corns and calluses occur when the foot's surface is subjected to constant friction or pressure, such as that from an ill-fitting shoe or a bone spur. Corns and calluses cause pain by putting pressure on underlying tissue. They occur most frequently on the big toe, the fifth toe, and under the ends of the foot bones.

Corns are more sharply defined than calluses and have a hard central core. They are usually more painful than calluses and may require surgical removal. Both corns and calluses can be treated by applying salicylic acid plasters, which soften them, making them easier to remove by rubbing with a pumice stone or even a towel.

Never remove corns or calluses with a sharp instrument. See your doctor for treatment. If surgical abrasion is required, a local anesthetic is usually administered.

Heel pain usually results from gait abnormalities (faulty styles of walking), which can cause excessive stress on the heel bone and attached soft tissues. Common causes of heel pain include heel spurs (bony growths on the front underside of the heel bone), plantar fasciitis (inflammation of the band of connective tissue that runs along the bottom of the foot), and excessive pronation (abnormal inward motion of the arch upon walking).

THE HUMBLE FOOT: TOUGH, SOPHISTICATED, COMPLEX

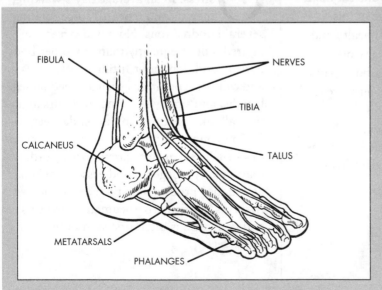

FIBULA

NERVES

TIBIA

CALCANEUS

TALUS

METATARSALS

PHALANGES

Given the complexity of this extraordinary aggregation of bones, muscles, blood vessels, and nerves, it's a wonder that more doesn't go wrong. Even so, disorders of the feet have given rise to a profession unto themselves. Podiatrists, or foot doctors, are not M.D.s, but must complete a four-year course devoted entirely to feet before receiving a license.

Most cases of heel pain improve spontaneously. Stretching exercises are often all that's needed to relieve the pain. Sometimes medication is used to reduce swelling of the foot's soft tissues. Shoe inserts may also be used. For persistent pain, steroid injections may be necessary. Plantar fasciitis can be relieved by surgery. However, only in extreme, chronic cases of heel pain is surgery recommended.

Neuromas are abnormal, benign nerve growths that usually appear between the third and fourth toes. They are caused by abnormally shaped bones and ill-fitting shoes that rub against and irritate the nerve. Treatment may include orthotic devices (arch supports) and/or cortisone injections. The problem is also sometimes alleviated by wearing wider shoes or a pad on the sole of the foot to spread the bones. In difficult cases, surgical removal of the growth may be necessary.

Plantar warts are warts that appear on the sole or plantar surface of the foot. Because of the weight placed on the foot while standing, these warts grow inward.

Plantar warts are caused by a virus, often disappear spontaneously, and usually require no treatment. Those that do persist can be treated by electrodesiccation and curettage (heat and surgical removal), cryotherapy (extreme cold), acid therapy (such as 40 percent salicylic acid plasters), or by application of a compound of 25 percent podophyllum and tincture of benzoin. The use of antiviral drugs for the treatment of warts is under investigation.

Nail problems may seem of little consequence unless, of course, you have them. **Ingrown toenails** can cause intense pain, irritation, and swelling. They are caused by incorrect nail trimming, shoe pressure, bacterial or fungal infection, injury, poor foot structure, and heredity. Ingrown nails should be treated by a physician.

Fungal infections of the toenails can also be painful. Nails that show thickening, discoloration, crumbling, and separation from the nail bed are typical of such infections. If treatment with antifungal medications or antibiotics doesn't yield results, removal of the nail may be necessary.

Changes in the toenails may also be manifestations of other diseases. Pitting of nails and increased thickness may indicate the presence of psoriasis. When the nails become concave—rounded inward instead of outward—it may signal impending iron deficiency anemia. When tissue beneath the rear of the nail turns red, it may foretell heart failure.

Other foot disorders include **bunions** (deformities of the joint at the base of the big toe) and **hammer toes** (in which the joints of the toes curl in a clawlike fashion). Treatment for both of these conditions ranges from shoe modifications to surgery.

When foot problems are the result of diabetes, arthritis, or poor circulation, therapy involves treatment of the underlying disorder. □

CHAPTER 26

Drugs and the Elderly

When it comes to medications, the elderly are just like everyone else—only more so. They have more health problems, take more medicines, get more side effects, and sustain more deaths from improper use. In fact, some two-thirds of all people over age 65 take medication regularly. The elderly spend upwards of $10 billion per year on drugs, about 25 percent of the national pill bill, though they comprise only about 12 to 15 percent of the population. Today more elderly live longer, better lives than ever because of the many new medicines that keep jumpy hearts in line, arteries unclogged, aging bones from breaking, and eyesight from diminishing.

In fact, those over age 65 are among the main beneficiaries of the revolutionary advances in medicine during the twentieth century. Three key developments have especially helped the aging population have healthier and more productive lives: heart and high blood pressure medications, medicines that treat pain and injuries, and medica-

tions that overcome the mental health problems encountered in the aged. Medications that fight diabetes and kidney problems have also benefited the elderly.

Along with better nutrition and low cholesterol, low salt diets, the development of drugs that help us as we age has reduced death rates from heart attacks, strokes, and suicides significantly in the past few decades. But medications used by any aging person are truly the proverbial double-edged sword, since as many as 80 percent of the elderly are on confusing multiple-drug regimens. Indeed, some studies show that less than 30 percent of the aged use their drugs properly.

What Do We Mean By Aging?

Aging isn't just "getting old." It's a process that involves biological, emotional, social, and even financial changes that affect a person's overall health. Disease and mental attitude are the wild cards that affect the speed of the aging process. Certainly, we all know people over age 65 who differ widely in their ability to get around. Some run marathons in their eighties and beyond, and others are so debilitated by illness that just getting up in the morning is a major effort. How do we explain this disparity among older people? Age is less a chronological marker than a combination of factors that determine the overall functioning of people in their mid-sixties and beyond.

First, genetics plays an important part in the aging process. Aging is associated with the development of chronic diseases such as high blood pressure that contribute to wear and tear on the body. Most of us who develop a chronic condition do so because we have a genetic predisposition to the disorder. High cholesterol, heart disease, cancer, diabetes, and other problems "run in families," just as eye color and hair color do. Some experts feel that our body's immune system is also affected by aging, gradually losing its ability to recognize outside threats—a virus, for example—and hence putting us at greater risk of disease.

Emotional and psychological issues have a major impact on overall health and the aging process. Even though an older person is well physically, he may still be at risk for mental illnesses such as Alzheimer's disease, depression, and anxiety. According to the American Psychiatric Association, 15 to 25 percent of the elderly in the U.S. suffer from "significant symptoms of mental illness." The aged—especially elderly men—are more likely to commit suicide than the rest of the population (some 6,000 do each year), but most do not seek professional help. Despite the fact that over one million elderly have some sort of abnormal memory loss (senility or dementia), they are often too embarrassed or too ill to seek help.

Social and financial changes are commonly overlooked as part of the aging process, but they can contribute to both physical and mental illness in the elderly. First of all, many elderly live on fixed budgets. If their income is modest, then every fluctuation in the economy, change in interest rates and cutback in government care has an impact on their lives. This can affect their nutrition (the elderly often skip meals to save money), which can lead to reduced body weight and, in turn, a change in the effects of medications they are taking. If their budget problems are too severe, they may even skip doses or stop their medications entirely.

Many older people also suffer severe stress from radical changes in life-style. Frequently this happens to aging widows who outlive their spouses. Retirement itself can be a source of stress for the elderly, whether financially secure or not. Some who have worked all their lives have no idea how to "slow-down" or may find it hard to adjust to full-time life with their spouses. These massive changes, when added to a heart condition, for example, increase stress on already inefficient organ systems.

How Does Aging Affect Medication Use?

Despite the eternal search for the "fountain of youth," there are no medications that prevent or "cure" aging. The drugs used by the elderly are the same as those that a younger person might take—yet they can have a far different effect. It doesn't matter whether a person has heart disease or arthritis, osteoporosis, or high blood pressure, the story is the same: Because our organ systems tend to function less efficiently as we age, medications are handled differently by our bodies. Here are some of the most common changes affecting our health and our response to medicines:

- Our stomachs may not absorb food and medication as well as they did before.

- Our kidneys and livers don't eliminate fluids and toxins in the same efficient manner.

- Skin "dries up," making us more vulnerable to bruises.

- Our lung capacity diminishes, which increases risk of pneumonia and diseases caused by smoking or air pollution (emphysema).

- Muscles and joints weaken and wear out, making injury to hips, legs, and wrists more likely from even a simple fall.

- The heart and circulatory system loose peak efficiency.

- The senses we depend on—hearing, sight, taste—change subtly and affect mobility (driving a car) or pleasure (sexuality).

- The body's weight and composition changes, so that "usual" doses of medication require adjustments.

- Our immune systems decline, making us more prone to both infection and cancer.

- Our memories may deteriorate as chemical changes or clogged arteries cause brain cell damage.

All of the above contribute to the potential harm that medications can cause in the aging body. If a kidney can't eliminate a drug after it has done its work, it remains in the body longer, perhaps causing an overdose or an adverse effect. If someone forgets to take a medication that regulates the heart or blood pressure, a stroke or heart attack could be the result.

Any person over the age of 65 who is taking medications in the following categories should be aware of the potential for increased side effects, overdose, and diminished efficacy:

- Antibiotics
- Antihistamines
- Antihypertensives
- Antiulcer medicines
- Blood thinners
- Bronchodilators
- Calcium or potassium supplements
- Cardiac medications
- Corticosteroids
- Estrogens
- Over-the-counter drugs containing alcohol (cough and cold medications) or caffeine (diet aids)
- Pain relievers (nonsteroidal anti-inflammatories such as Motrin, narcotic analgesics)
- Psychiatric medications (antidepressants, tranquilizers)
- Skin medications and creams

Aging, Mental Health and Medications—a Special Note

Among the first signs that a drug may not be working properly in an older person is a change in mood, energy, attitude, or memory. Too often, these alterations are overlooked, ignored, or chalked off to "old age" or senility. Older people may themselves feel that their blue mood is caused by something external such as the death of a friend or simply by boredom. Nothing could be farther from the truth. Virtually every heart medication, blood pressure drug, sleeping pill, and tranquilizer has been known to trigger depressive symptoms.

When a psychological symptom appears in an older person, examine his or her medication or drug use first. Consider, too, factors like alcohol intake, poor nutrition, and hormone imbalance. And never dismiss the possibility that a real psychological problem has developed and may itself require medication. Any older person with feelings of hopelessness, worthlessness, unexplained crying, thoughts of suicide and similar symptoms could be among the five percent of the elderly who have a treatable, reversible depression.

Likewise, up to 15 percent of the aging population suffer from the symptoms of dementia: memory loss, disorientation, and confusion. Dementia can be a side effect of medicines. It may also be related to high blood pressure or conditions like Huntington's disease (a genetic disorder), Parkinson's disease (involuntary tremors), or Creutzfeldt-Jakob disease (a viral infection). Treatment of these can, to a small extent, reverse the dementia. However, some 60 percent of those with symptoms of dementia have Alzheimer's disease, a slow, progressive mental deterioration that, so far, can't be cured.

Alzheimer's disease is a particularly tragic disorder. It can affect people in their forties, but is more common among the elderly. Among the first signs of Alzheimer's are loss of short-term or recent memory—forgetting to shut off a light or the stove, or pick up the kids on time. As the disease gets worse, the person tends to become lost more easily and begins to forget how to do simple tasks like adding up numbers or reading the newspaper. Later on, all mental functions deteriorate, although the body is usually spared.

Scientists know almost nothing about the cause of Alzheimer's. Some feel it may be caused by a virus or a deficit of chemicals or metals in the brain.

Treatment today consists largely of keeping the patient nourished, reducing agitation through tranquilizers, and helping the family cope through support groups. Several potentially helpful medications are under investigation, but none is currently available.

Safe Medication Use for the Aged

Safe medication use for the elderly requires vigilance on the part of the older person and those assisting him. It is especially important to keep track of maintenance drugs and make sure they are taken regularly. For a chronic condition such as high blood pressure, these medications are a key to maintaining good health.

Rember, too, that perfectly ordinary medications really can lead to unexpected results—especially in the elderly. Be alert for gradual changes that may signal an unwanted side effect. And guard against harmful drug interactions by making sure the doctor knows about all the medicines the older person is taking, including those prescribed by other doctors and any over-the-counter drugs. □

PART THREE

Color Photo Section

ACEBUTOLOL HCI

SECTRAL
WYETH-AYERST

200 MG

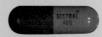

400 MG

ACETAMINOPHEN/ CODEINE PHOSPHATE

PHENAPHEN W/CODEINE NO. 2
A. H. ROBINS

325 MG / 15 MG

PHENAPHEN W/CODEINE NO. 3
A. H. ROBINS

325 MG / 30 MG

PHENAPHEN W/CODEINE NO. 4
A. H. ROBINS

325 MG / 60 MG

TYLENOL W/CODEINE NO. 1
McNEIL PHARMACEUTICAL

300 MG / 7.5 MG

TYLENOL W/CODEINE NO. 2
McNEIL PHARMACEUTICAL

300 MG / 15 MG

TYLENOL W/CODEINE NO. 3
McNEIL PHARMACEUTICAL

300 MG / 30 MG

TYLENOL W/CODEINE NO. 4
McNEIL PHARMACEUTICAL

300 MG / 60 MG

ACETAMINOPHEN/ HYDROCODONE

LORCET PLUS
UAD LABORATORIES

650 MG / 7.5 MG

ACETAZOLAMIDE

DIAMOX
LEDERLE

125 MG   250 MG

DIAMOX SEQUELS
LEDERLE

500 MG

ACYCLOVIR

ZOVIRAX
BURROUGHS WELLCOME

200 MG

800 MG

ALBUTEROL SULFATE

PROVENTIL
SCHERING

2 MG   4 MG

PROVENTIL REPETABS
SCHERING

4 MG

ALLOPURINOL

LOPURIN
BOOTS

300 MG   100 MG

ZYLOPRIM
BURROUGHS WELLCOME

100 MG   300 MG

ALPRAZOLAM

XANAX
UPJOHN

0.25 MG   0.5 MG

1 MG

2 MG

AMANTADINE HCI

SYMMETREL
DU PONT

100 MG

AMILORIDE HCI/ HYDROCHLOROTHIAZIDE

MODURETIC
MERCK & CO.

5 MG / 50 MG

AMITRIPTYLINE HCI

GENERIC
GENEVA

10 MG   25 MG

50 MG   75 MG

100 MG

150 MG

ELAVIL
STUART

10 MG   25 MG

50 MG   75 MG

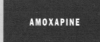

100 MG

150 MG

AMOXAPINE

ASENDIN
LEDERLE

25 MG   50 MG

100 MG   150 MG

AMOXICILLIN

AMOXIL
SMITHKLINE BEECHAM

250 MG

500 MG

AMOXIL CHEWABLE
SMITHKLINE BEECHAM

125 MG

250 MG

POLYMOX
APOTHECON

250 MG

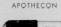

500 MG

WYMOX
WYETH-AYERST

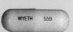

250 MG

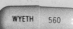

500 MG

AMOXICILLIN/ CLAVULANATE POTASSIUM

AUGMENTIN
SMITHKLINE BEECHAM

250 MG / 125 MG

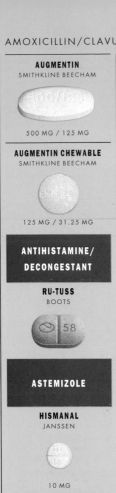

AUGMENTIN
SMITHKLINE BEECHAM

500 MG / 125 MG

AUGMENTIN CHEWABLE
SMITHKLINE BEECHAM

125 MG / 31.25 MG

**ANTIHISTAMINE/
DECONGESTANT**

RU-TUSS
BOOTS

ASTEMIZOLE

HISMANAL
JANSSEN

10 MG

ATENOLOL

TENORMIN
ICI PHARMA

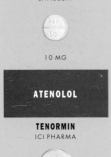

100 MG

**ATENOLOL /
CHLORTHALIDONE**

TENORETIC
ICI PHARMA

50 MG / 25 MG

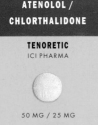

100 MG / 25MG

AURANOFIN

RIDAURA
SMITHKLINE BEECHAM

3 MG

**AZATADINE MALEATE/
PSEUDOEPHEDRINE
SULFATE**

TRINALIN
KEY PHARMACEUTICALS

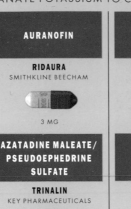

1 MG / 120 MG

AZITHROMYCIN

ZITHROMAX
PFIZER

250 MG

**BELLADONNA ALKALOIDS/
PHENOBARBITAL**

DONNATAL
A. H. ROBINS

16.2 MG+

16.2 MG+

BENAZEPRIL HCI

LOTENSIN
CIBA

LOTENSIN   LOTENSIN

5 MG   10 MG

LOTENSIN   LOTENSIN

20 MG   40 MG

BENZONATATE

TESSALON
FOREST

100 MG

**BENZTROPINE
MESYLATE**

COGENTIN
MERCK & CO.

0.5 MG

1 MG

2 MG

BEPRIDIL HCI

VASCOR
McNEIL PHARMACEUTICAL

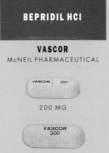
VASCOR   200

200 MG

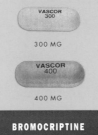
VASCOR
300

300 MG

VASCOR
400

400 MG

**BROMOCRIPTINE
MESYLATE**

PARLODEL
SANDOZ

2.5 MG

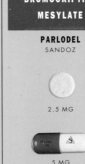

5 MG

BUMETANIDE

BUMEX
ROCHE

0.5 MG   1 MG

BUMEX
2

2 MG

BUPROPION HCI

WELLBUTRIN
BURROUGHS WELLCOME

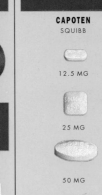

75 MG   100 MG

BUSPIRONE HCI

BUSPAR
MEAD JOHNSON

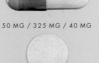
MJ 5   MJ 10

5 MG   10 MG

**BUTALBITAL/
ASPIRIN/
CAFFEINE**

FIORINAL
SANDOZ

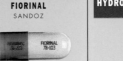
FIORINAL
78-103

50 MG / 325 MG / 40 MG

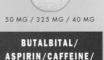

50 MG / 325 MG / 40 MG

**BUTALBITAL/
ASPIRIN/CAFFEINE/
CODEINE**

FIORINAL W/CODEINE #3
SANDOZ

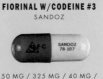
SANDOZ
78-107

50 MG / 325 MG / 40 MG /
30 MG

CALCITRIOL

ROCALTROL
ROCHE

0.25 MCG

0.5 MCG

CAPTOPRIL

CAPOTEN
SQUIBB

12.5 MG

25 MG

50 MG

100 MG

**CAPTOPRIL/
HYDROCHLOROTHIAZIDE**

CAPOZIDE
SQUIBB

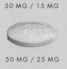

25 MG / 15 MG

25MG / 25 MG

50 MG / 15 MG

50 MG / 25 MG

CARBAMAZEPINE

TEGRETOL
BASEL

200 MG

TEGRETOL CHEWABLE
BASEL

100 MG

CARBINOXAMINE MALEATE/ PSEUDOEPHEDRINE HCl

RONDEC
ROSS LABORATORIES

4 MG / 60 MG

CARISOPRODOL

SOMA
WALLACE

350 MG

CARTEOLOL HCl

CARTROL FILMTAB
ABBOTT

2.5 MG   5 MG

CEFACLOR

CECLOR
LILLY

250 MG

500 MG

CEFADROXIL MONOHYDRATE

DURICEF
PRINCETON PHARMACEUTICALS

500 MG

CEFIXIME

SUPRAX
LEDERLE

400 MG

CEFUROXIME AXETIL

CEFTIN
ALLEN & HANBURYS

125 MG

250 MG

500 MG

CEPHALEXIN

GENERIC
BIOCRAFT

250 MG

500 MG

KEFLEX
DISTA

250 MG

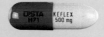

500 MG

CEPHALEXIN HCl

KEFTAB
DISTA

250 MG

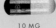

500 MG

CEPHRADINE

VELOSEF
APOTHECON

250 MG

500 MG

CHLORDIAZEPOXIDE/ AMITRIPTYLINE HCl

LIMBITROL
ROCHE

5 MG / 12.5 MG

LIMBITROL DS
ROCHE

10 MG / 25 MG

CHLORDIAZEPOXIDE HCl

GENERIC
RUGBY

5 MG

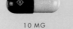

10 MG

GENERIC
RUGBY

25 MG

LIBRIUM
ROCHE

5 MG

10 MG

25 MG

CHLOROTHIAZIDE

DIURIL
MERCK & CO.

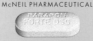

500 MG

CHLORPHENIRAMINE/ PHENINDAMINE/ PHENYLPROPANOLAMINE

NOLAMINE
CARNRICK

4 MG / 24 MG / 50 MG

CHLORPROMAZINE HCl

THORAZINE
SMITHKLINE BEECHAM

25 MG   50 MG

CHLORPROPAMIDE

DIABINESE
PFIZER

100 MG   250 MG

CHLORTHALIDONE

HYGROTON
RHÔNE-POULENC RORER

100 MG

25 MG   50 MG

CHLORZOXAZONE

PARAFON FORTE DSC
McNEIL PHARMACEUTICAL

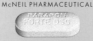

500 MG

CHOLINE MAGNESIUM TRISALICYLATE

TRILISATE
PURDUE FREDERICK

500 MG

CIMETIDINE

TAGAMET
SMITHKLINE BEECHAM

200 MG   300 MG

400 MG

800 MG

CIPROFLOXACIN HCl

CIPRO
MILES

250 MG

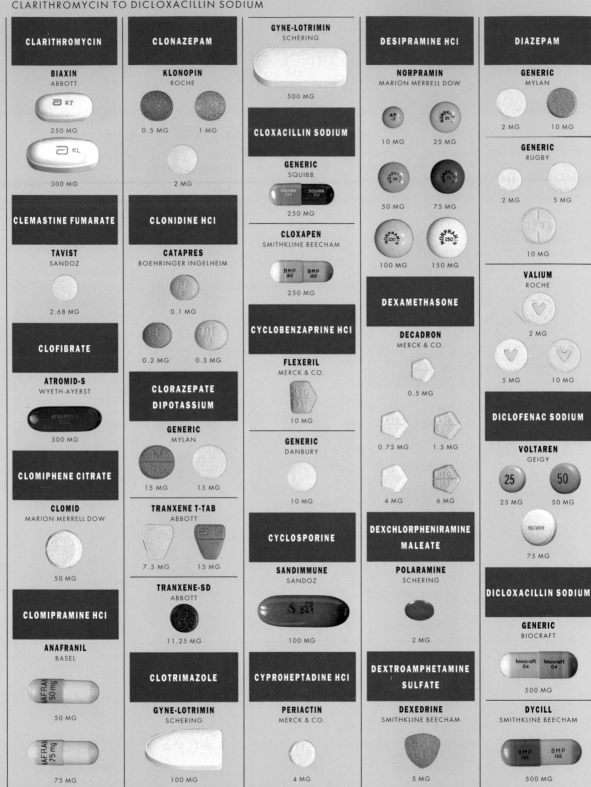

CLARITHROMYCIN

BIAXIN
ABBOTT

250 MG

500 MG

CLEMASTINE FUMARATE

TAVIST
SANDOZ

2.68 MG

CLOFIBRATE

ATROMID-S
WYETH-AYERST

500 MG

CLOMIPHENE CITRATE

CLOMID
MARION MERRELL DOW

50 MG

CLOMIPRAMINE HCl

ANAFRANIL
BASEL

50 MG

75 MG

CLONAZEPAM

KLONOPIN
ROCHE

0.5 MG   1 MG

2 MG

CLONIDINE HCl

CATAPRES
BOEHRINGER INGELHEIM

0.1 MG

0.2 MG   0.3 MG

CLORAZEPATE DIPOTASSIUM

GENERIC
MYLAN

15 MG   15 MG

TRANXENE T-TAB
ABBOTT

7.5 MG   15 MG

TRANXENE-SD
ABBOTT

11.25 MG

CLOTRIMAZOLE

GYNE-LOTRIMIN
SCHERING

100 MG

GYNE-LOTRIMIN
SCHERING

500 MG

CLOXACILLIN SODIUM

GENERIC
SQUIBB

250 MG

CLOXAPEN
SMITHKLINE BEECHAM

250 MG

CYCLOBENZAPRINE HCl

FLEXERIL
MERCK & CO.

10 MG

GENERIC
DANBURY

10 MG

CYCLOSPORINE

SANDIMMUNE
SANDOZ

100 MG

CYPROHEPTADINE HCl

PERIACTIN
MERCK & CO.

4 MG

DESIPRAMINE HCl

NORPRAMIN
MARION MERRELL DOW

10 MG   25 MG

50 MG   75 MG

100 MG   150 MG

DEXAMETHASONE

DECADRON
MERCK & CO.

0.5 MG

0.75 MG   1.5 MG

4 MG   6 MG

DEXCHLORPHENIRAMINE MALEATE

POLARAMINE
SCHERING

2 MG

DEXTROAMPHETAMINE SULFATE

DEXEDRINE
SMITHKLINE BEECHAM

5 MG

DIAZEPAM

GENERIC
MYLAN

2 MG   10 MG

GENERIC
RUGBY

2 MG   5 MG

10 MG

VALIUM
ROCHE

2 MG

5 MG   10 MG

DICLOFENAC SODIUM

VOLTAREN
GEIGY

25   50

25 MG   50 MG

75 MG

DICLOXACILLIN SODIUM

GENERIC
BIOCRAFT

500 MG

DYCILL
SMITHKLINE BEECHAM

500 MG

DICYCLOMINE

BENTYL
MARION MERRELL DOW

10 MG

DIETHYLPROPION HCI

TENUATE
MARION MERRELL DOW

25 MG

TENUATE DOSPAN
MARION MERRELL DOW

75 MG

DIFLUNISAL

DOLOBID
MERCK & CO.

250 MG

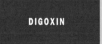

500 MG

DIGOXIN

LANOXIN
BURROUGHS WELLCOME

0.125 MG

0.25 MG

0.5 MG

DILTIAZEM HCI

CARDIZEM SR
MARION MERRELL DOW

60 MG

90 MG

120 MG

DIPHENHYDRAMINE HCI

BENADRYL
PARKE-DAVIS

50 MG

DIPHENOXYLATE HCI/ ATROPINE SULFATE

LOMOTIL
SEARLE

2.5 MG / 0.025 MG

DIPYRIDAMOLE

GENERIC
GENEVA

GG 49 — 25 MG   GG 45 — 50 MG

GG 464 — 75 MG

PERSANTINE
BOEHRINGER INGELHEIM

BI — 25 MG

BI — 50 MG   BI — 75 MG

DISOPYRAMIDE PHOSPHATE

NORPACE CR
SEARLE

150 MG

DIVALPROEX SODIUM

DEPAKOTE
ABBOTT

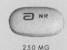

125 MG

NR — 250 MG

NS — 500 MG

DEPAKOTE SPRINKLE
ABBOTT

125 MG

DOCUSATE SODIUM

COLACE
APOTHECON

50 MG

100 MG

DOXAZOSIN MESYLATE

CARDURA
ROERIG DIVISON

1 MG   2 MG

CARDURA
ROERIG DIVISON

4 MG

8 MG

DOXEPIN HCI

GENERIC
MYLAN

MYLAN 3125 — 25 MG

MYLAN 4250 — 50 MG

MYLAN 5375 — 75 MG

MYLAN 6410 — 100 MG

SINEQUAN
ROERIG

ROERIG 534 — 10 MG

 ROERIG 535 — 25 MG

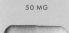 ROERIG 536 — 50 MG

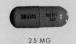 ROERIG 539 — 75 MG

 ROERIG 538 — 100 MG

 ROERIG 537 — 150 MG

DOXYCYCLINE HYCLATE

GENERIC
MYLAN

MYLAN 145 — 50 MG

MYLAN 148 — 100 MG

100 MG

DORYX
PARKE-DAVIS

100 MG

VIBRA-TABS
PFIZER

100 MG

VIBRAMYCIN
PFIZER

VIBRA PFIZER 094 — 50 MG

 VIBRA PFIZER 095 — 100 MG

ENALAPRIL MALEATE

VASOTEC
MERCK & CO.

10 MG

ENALAPRIL MALEATE/ HYDROCHLOROTHIAZIDE

VASERETIC
MERCK & CO.

10 MG / 25 MG

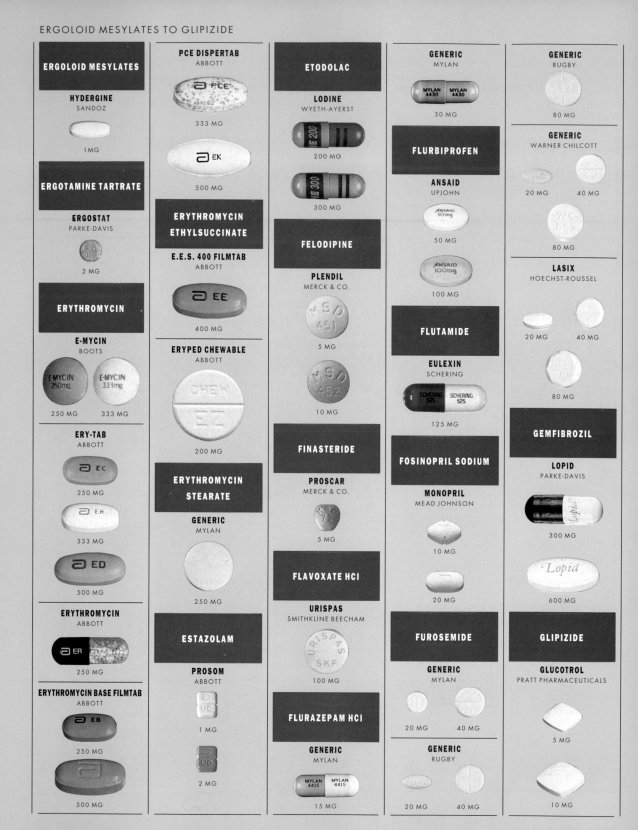

ERGOLOID MESYLATES

HYDERGINE
SANDOZ

1 MG

ERGOTAMINE TARTRATE

ERGOSTAT
PARKE-DAVIS

2 MG

ERYTHROMYCIN

E-MYCIN
BOOTS

E-MYCIN 250mg | E-MYCIN 333mg

250 MG | 333 MG

ERY-TAB
ABBOTT

250 MG

333 MG

500 MG

ERYTHROMYCIN
ABBOTT

250 MG

ERYTHROMYCIN BASE FILMTAB
ABBOTT

250 MG

500 MG

PCE DISPERTAB
ABBOTT

333 MG

500 MG

ERYTHROMYCIN ETHYLSUCCINATE

E.E.S. 400 FILMTAB
ABBOTT

400 MG

ERYPED CHEWABLE
ABBOTT

200 MG

ERYTHROMYCIN STEARATE

GENERIC
MYLAN

250 MG

ESTAZOLAM

PROSOM
ABBOTT

1 MG

2 MG

ETODOLAC

LODINE
WYETH-AYERST

200 MG

300 MG

FELODIPINE

PLENDIL
MERCK & CO.

5 MG

10 MG

FINASTERIDE

PROSCAR
MERCK & CO.

5 MG

FLAVOXATE HCl

URISPAS
SMITHKLINE BEECHAM

100 MG

FLURAZEPAM HCl

GENERIC
MYLAN

15 MG

GENERIC
MYLAN

30 MG

FLURBIPROFEN

ANSAID
UPJOHN

50 MG

100 MG

FLUTAMIDE

EULEXIN
SCHERING

125 MG

FOSINOPRIL SODIUM

MONOPRIL
MEAD JOHNSON

10 MG

20 MG

FUROSEMIDE

GENERIC
MYLAN

20 MG | 40 MG

GENERIC
RUGBY

20 MG | 40 MG

GENERIC
RUGBY

80 MG

GENERIC
WARNER CHILCOTT

20 MG | 40 MG

80 MG

LASIX
HOECHST-ROUSSEL

20 MG | 40 MG

80 MG

GEMFIBROZIL

LOPID
PARKE-DAVIS

300 MG

600 MG

GLIPIZIDE

GLUCOTROL
PRATT PHARMACEUTICALS

5 MG

10 MG

GLYBURIDE

DIABETA
HOECHST-ROUSSEL

1.25 MG

2.5 MG   5 MG

MICRONASE
UPJOHN

1.25 MG

2.5 MG   5 MG

HALOPERIDOL

HALDOL
McNEIL PHARMACEUTICAL

2 MG   5 MG

10MG   20 MG

HYDRALAZINE HCl / HYDROCHLOROTHIAZIDE

APRESAZIDE
CIBA

25 MG / 25 MG

50 MG / 50 MG

100 MG / 50 MG

APRESOLINE-ESIDRIX
CIBA

25 MG / 15 MG

HYDROCHLOROTHIAZIDE

GENERIC
RUGBY

25 MG   50 MG

ESIDRIX
CIBA

25 MG   50 MG

HYDRODIURIL
MERCK & CO.

25 MG   50 MG

100 MG

ORETIC
ABBOTT

25 MG   50 MG

HYDROCODONE BITARTRATE / ACETAMINOPHEN

CO-GESIC
CENTRAL

5 MG / 500 MG

HYDROCET
CARNRICK

5 MG / 500 MG

VICODIN
KNOLL

5 MG / 500 MG

HYDROMORPHONE HCl

DILAUDID
KNOLL

1 MG   2 MG

3 MG   4 MG

GENERIC
ROXANE

2 MG   4 MG

HYDROXYCHLOROQUINE SULFATE

PLAQUENIL
SANOFI WINTHROP

200 MG

HYDROXYZINE HCl

ATARAX
ROERIG

10 MG   25 MG

50 MG   100 MG

GENERIC
RUGBY

10 MG

25 MG   50 MG

HYOSCYAMINE SULFATE

LEVSIN
SCHWARZ

0.125 MG

LEVSIN/SL
SCHWARZ

0.125 MG

IBUPROFEN

GENERIC
BOOTS

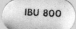

IBU 400

400 MG

IBU 600

600 MG

IBU 800

800 MG

MOTRIN
UPJOHN

300 MG

400 MG

600 MG

800 MG

IMIPRAMINE HCl

JANIMINE
ABBOTT

10 MG   25 MG

50 MG

TOFRANIL
GEIGY

10 MG   25 MG

50 MG

INDAPAMIDE

LOZOL
RHÔNE-POULENC RORER

2.5 MG

INDOMETHACIN

INDOCIN
MERCK & CO.

25 MG

50 MG

INDOCIN-SR
MERCK & CO.

75 MG

IODINATED GLYCEROL

ORGANIDIN
WALLACE

30 MG

ISOMETHEPTENE MUCATE/ DICHLORALPHENAZONE +

MIDRIN
CARRICK

65 MG / 100 MG +

ISOSORBIDE DINITRATE

GENERIC
RUGBY

10 MG   20 MG

ISORDIL
WYETH-AYERST

20 MG   30 MG

40 MG

ISORDIL SUBLINGUAL
WYETH-AYERST

2.5 MG   10 MG

ISORDIL TITRADOSE
WYETH-AYERST

5 MG   10 MG

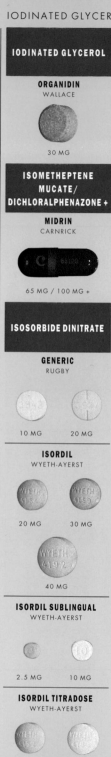

SORBITRATE
ICI PHARMA

20 MG

SORBITRATE CHEWABLE
ICI PHARMA

5 MG

SORBITRATE ORAL
ICI PHARMA

5 MG   10 MG

30 MG   40 MG

SORBITRATE ORAL SA
ICI PHARMA

40 MG

SORBITRATE SUBLINGUAL
ICI PHARMA

2.5 MG   10 MG

ISOTRETINOIN

ACCUTANE
ROCHE

10 MG

20 MG

40 MG

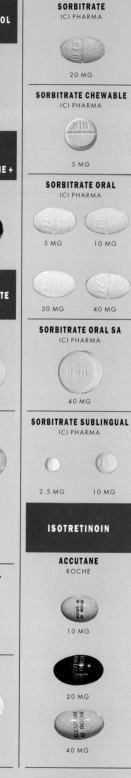

ISRADIPINE

DYNACIRC
SANDOZ

2.5 MG

5 MG

KETOCONAZOLE

NIZORAL
JANSSEN

200 MG

KETOPROFEN

ORUDIS
WYETH-AYERST

25 MG

50 MG

75 MG

LABETALOL HCl

NORMODYNE
SCHERING

100 MG   200 MG

300 MG

TRANDATE
ALLEN & HANBURYS

100 MG

200 MG

300 MG

LEVODOPA

LARODOPA
ROCHE

100 MG   250 MG

500 MG

LEVOTHYROXINE SODIUM

LEVOTHROID
FOREST

0.1 MG

SYNTHROID
BOOTS

0.025 MG   0.05 MG

0.075 MG   0.088 MG

0.1 MG   0.112 MG

0.125 MG   0.15 MG

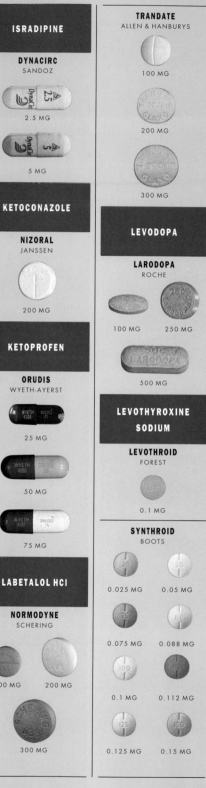

SYNTHROID
BOOTS

0.175 MG   0.2 MG

0.3 MG

LIOTRIX

EUTHROID
PARKE-DAVIS

0.5 GR   1 GR

2 GR   3 GR

THYROLAR
FOREST

¼   ½

1

2   3

LISINOPRIL

PRINIVIL
MERCK & CO.

5 MG   10 MG

20 MG   40 MG

ZESTRIL
STUART

10 MG   20 MG

40 MG

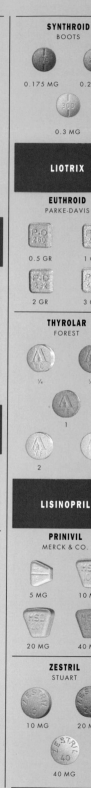

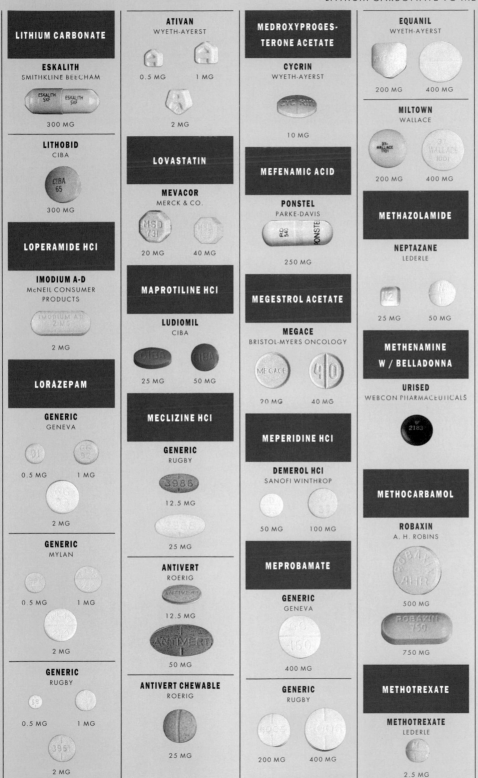

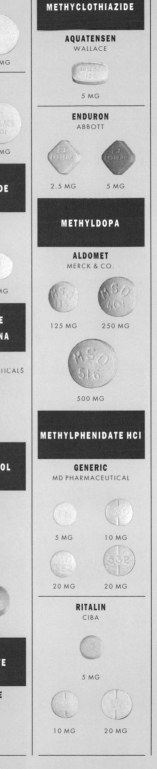

LITHIUM CARBONATE

ESKALITH
SMITHKLINE BEECHAM

300 MG

LITHOBID
CIBA

300 MG

LOPERAMIDE HCl

IMODIUM A-D
McNEIL CONSUMER PRODUCTS

2 MG

LORAZEPAM

GENERIC
GENEVA

0.5 MG   1 MG

2 MG

GENERIC
MYLAN

0.5 MG   1 MG

2 MG

GENERIC
RUGBY

0.5 MG   1 MG

2 MG

ATIVAN
WYETH-AYERST

0.5 MG   1 MG

2 MG

LOVASTATIN

MEVACOR
MERCK & CO.

20 MG   40 MG

MAPROTILINE HCl

LUDIOMIL
CIBA

25 MG   50 MG

MECLIZINE HCl

GENERIC
RUGBY

3986

12.5 MG

25 MG

ANTIVERT
ROERIG

12.5 MG

50 MG

ANTIVERT CHEWABLE
ROERIG

25 MG

MEDROXYPROGES-TERONE ACETATE

CYCRIN
WYETH-AYERST

10 MG

MEFENAMIC ACID

PONSTEL
PARKE-DAVIS

250 MG

MEGESTROL ACETATE

MEGACE
BRISTOL-MYERS ONCOLOGY

20 MG   40 MG

MEPERIDINE HCl

DEMEROL HCl
SANOFI WINTHROP

50 MG   100 MG

MEPROBAMATE

GENERIC
GENEVA

400 MG

GENERIC
RUGBY

200 MG   400 MG

EQUANIL
WYETH-AYERST

200 MG   400 MG

MILTOWN
WALLACE

200 MG   400 MG

METHAZOLAMIDE

NEPTAZANE
LEDERLE

25 MG   50 MG

METHENAMINE W / BELLADONNA

URISED
WEBCON PHARMACEUTICALS

METHOCARBAMOL

ROBAXIN
A. H. ROBINS

500 MG

750 MG

METHOTREXATE

METHOTREXATE
LEDERLE

2.5 MG

METHYCLOTHIAZIDE

AQUATENSEN
WALLACE

5 MG

ENDURON
ABBOTT

2.5 MG   5 MG

METHYLDOPA

ALDOMET
MERCK & CO.

125 MG   250 MG

500 MG

METHYLPHENIDATE HCl

GENERIC
MD PHARMACEUTICAL

5 MG   10 MG

20 MG   20 MG

RITALIN
CIBA

5 MG

10 MG   20 MG

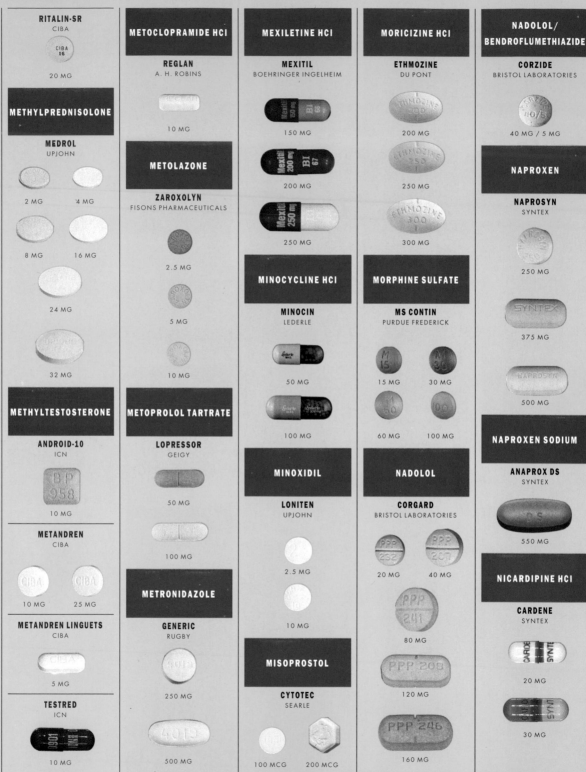

RITALIN-SR
CIBA

20 MG

METHYLPREDNISOLONE

MEDROL
UPJOHN

2 MG   4 MG

8 MG   16 MG

24 MG

32 MG

METHYLTESTOSTERONE

ANDROID-10
ICN

BP 958

10 MG

METANDREN
CIBA

CIBA 10 MG   CIBA 25 MG

METANDREN LINGUETS
CIBA

5 MG

TESTRED
ICN

10 MG

METOCLOPRAMIDE HCl

REGLAN
A. H. ROBINS

10 MG

METOLAZONE

ZAROXOLYN
FISONS PHARMACEUTICALS

2.5 MG

5 MG

10 MG

METOPROLOL TARTRATE

LOPRESSOR
GEIGY

50 MG

100 MG

METRONIDAZOLE

GENERIC
RUGBY

250 MG

500 MG

MEXILETINE HCl

MEXITIL
BOEHRINGER INGELHEIM

150 MG

200 MG

250 MG

MINOCYCLINE HCl

MINOCIN
LEDERLE

50 MG

100 MG

MINOXIDIL

LONITEN
UPJOHN

2.5 MG

10 MG

MISOPROSTOL

CYTOTEC
SEARLE

100 MCG   200 MCG

MORICIZINE HCl

ETHMOZINE
DU PONT

200 MG

250 MG

300 MG

MORPHINE SULFATE

MS CONTIN
PURDUE FREDERICK

M 15   M 30

15 MG   30 MG

M 60   100

60 MG   100 MG

NADOLOL

CORGARD
BRISTOL LABORATORIES

PPP 232   PPP 207

20 MG   40 MG

PPP 241

80 MG

PPP 208

120 MG

PPP 246

160 MG

NADOLOL/ BENDROFLUMETHIAZIDE

CORZIDE
BRISTOL LABORATORIES

40/5

40 MG / 5 MG

NAPROXEN

NAPROSYN
SYNTEX

250 MG

SYNTEX 375 MG

NAPROSYN 500 MG

NAPROXEN SODIUM

ANAPROX DS
SYNTEX

DS 550 MG

NICARDIPINE HCl

CARDENE
SYNTEX

20 MG

30 MG

NIFEDIPINE

PROCARDIA
PFIZER

10 MG

20 MG

PROCARDIA XL
PFIZER

 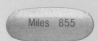

30 MG   60 MG

NIMODIPINE

NIMOTOP
MILES

30 MG

NITROFURANTOIN

MACRODANTIN
PROCTER & GAMBLE

25 MG

50 MG

100 MG

NITROGLYCERIN

NITRO-BID PLATEAU CAP
MARION MERRELL DOW

2.5 MG

NITRO-BID PLATEAU CAP
MARION MERRELL DOW

6.5 MG

9 MG

NIZATIDINE

AXID
LILLY

150 MG

NORFLOXACIN

NOROXIN
MERCK & CO.

400 MG

NORTRIPTYLINE HCl

PAMELOR
SANDOZ

50 MG

NYSTATIN

MYCOSTATIN
APOTHECON

500,000 UNITS

MYCOSTATIN PASTILLES
SQUIBB

200,000 UNITS

OFLOXACIN

FLOXIN
ORTHO

200 MG

300 MG

400 MG

OMEPRAZOLE

PRILOSEC
MERCK & CO.

20 MG

ORPHENADRINE CITRATE

NORFLEX
3M PHARMACEUTICALS

100 MG

OXAZEPAM

SERAX
WYETH-AYERST

10 MG

15 MG

15 MG

SERAX
WYETH-AYERST

30 MG

OXTRIPHYLLINE

CHOLEDYL
PARKE-DAVIS

100 MG

200 MG

CHOLEDYL SA
PARKE-DAVIS

400 MG

600 MG

OXYCODONE HCl/ ACETAMINOPHEN

PERCOCET
DU PONT

5 MG / 325 MG

TYLOX
McNEIL PHARMACEUTICAL

5 MG / 500 MG

PANCRELIPASE

PANCREASE
McNEIL PHARMACEUTICAL

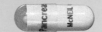

PANCREASE MT 4
McNEIL PHARMACEUTICAL

PANCREASE MT 10
McNEIL PHARMACEUTICAL

PANCREASE MT 16
McNEIL PHARMACEUTICAL

PEMOLINE

CYLERT
ABBOTT

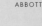

18.75 MG   37.5 MG

75 MG

PENICILLIN V POTASSIUM

GENERIC
BIOCRAFT

250 MG

500 MG

GENERIC
WARNER CHILCOTT

250 MG

500 MG

BEEPEN-VK
SMITHKLINE BEECHAM

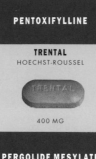

250 MG

500 MG

LEDERCILLIN VK
LEDERLE

250 MG

PEN-VEE K
WYETH-AYERST

250 MG

V-CILLIN K
LILLY

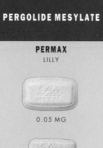

125 MG

250 MG

500 MG

PENTAZOCINE HCl / NALOXONE HCl

TALWIN NX
SANOFI WINTHROP

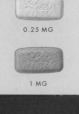

50 MG / 0.5 MG

PENTOBARBITAL SODIUM

NEMBUTAL
ABBOTT

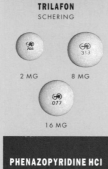

100 MG

PENTOXIFYLLINE

TRENTAL
HOECHST-ROUSSEL

400 MG

PERGOLIDE MESYLATE

PERMAX
LILLY

0.05 MG

0.25 MG

1 MG

PERPHENAZINE

TRILAFON
SCHERING

2 MG   8 MG

16 MG

PHENAZOPYRIDINE HCl

PYRIDIUM
PARKE-DAVIS

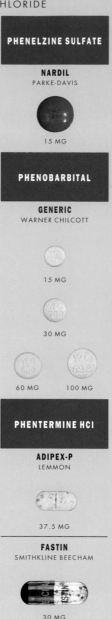

100 MG

200 MG

PHENELZINE SULFATE

NARDIL
PARKE-DAVIS

15 MG

PHENOBARBITAL

GENERIC
WARNER CHILCOTT

15 MG

30 MG

60 MG   100 MG

PHENTERMINE HCl

ADIPEX-P
LEMMON

37.5 MG

FASTIN
SMITHKLINE BEECHAM

30 MG

IONAMIN
FISONS PHARMACEUTICALS

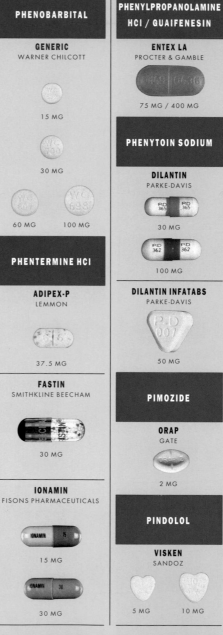

15 MG

30 MG

PHENYLEPHRINE/ CHLORPHENIRAMINE / PYRILAMINE TANNATE

RYNATAN
WALLACE

25 MG / 0 MG / 25 MG

PHENYLPROPANOLAMINE HCl / GUAIFENESIN

ENTEX LA
PROCTER & GAMBLE

75 MG / 400 MG

PHENYTOIN SODIUM

DILANTIN
PARKE-DAVIS

30 MG

100 MG

DILANTIN INFATABS
PARKE-DAVIS

50 MG

PIMOZIDE

ORAP
GATE

2 MG

PINDOLOL

VISKEN
SANDOZ

5 MG   10 MG

PIROXICAM

FELDENE
PFIZER

10 MG

20 MG

POTASSIUM CHLORIDE

K-DUR 10
KEY PHARMACEUTICALS

10 MEQ

K-DUR 20
KEY PHARMACEUTICALS

20 MEQ

KLOR-CON 10
UPSHER-SMITH

10 MEQ

KLOR-CON 8
UPSHER-SMITH

18 MEQ

MICRO-K 10
WYETH-AYERST

10 MEQ

MICRO-K EXTENCAPS
WYETH-AYERST

8 MEQ

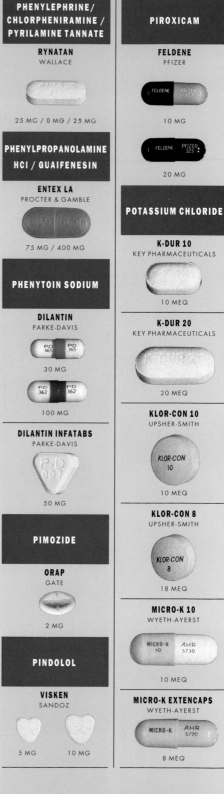

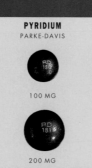

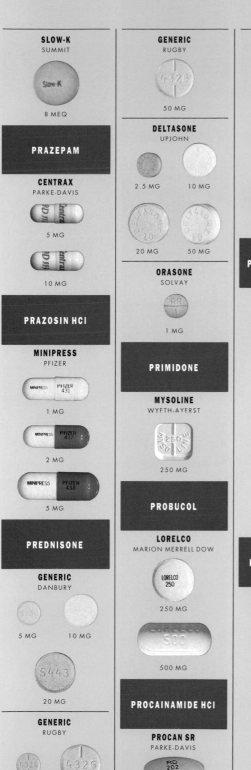

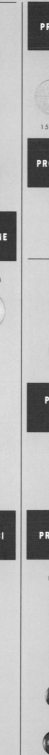

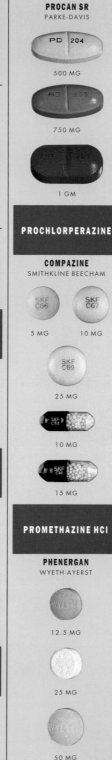

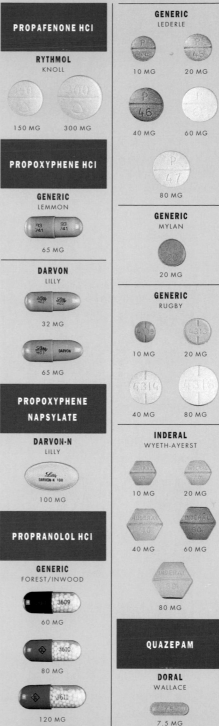

SLOW-K
SUMMIT

8 MEQ

PRAZEPAM

CENTRAX
PARKE-DAVIS

5 MG

10 MG

PRAZOSIN HCl

MINIPRESS
PFIZER

1 MG

2 MG

5 MG

PREDNISONE

GENERIC
DANBURY

5 MG   10 MG

20 MG

GENERIC
RUGBY

5 MG   20 MG

GENERIC
RUGBY

50 MG

DELTASONE
UPJOHN

2.5 MG   10 MG

20 MG   50 MG

ORASONE
SOLVAY

1 MG

PRIMIDONE

MYSOLINE
WYETH-AYERST

250 MG

PROBUCOL

LORELCO
MARION MERRELL DOW

250 MG

500 MG

PROCAINAMIDE HCl

PROCAN SR
PARKE-DAVIS

250 MG

PROCAN SR
PARKE-DAVIS

500 MG

750 MG

1 GM

PROCHLORPERAZINE

COMPAZINE
SMITHKLINE BEECHAM

5 MG   10 MG

25 MG

10 MG

15 MG

PROMETHAZINE HCl

PHENERGAN
WYETH-AYERST

12.5 MG

25 MG

50 MG

PROPAFENONE HCl

RYTHMOL
KNOLL

150 MG   300 MG

PROPOXYPHENE HCl

GENERIC
LEMMON

65 MG

DARVON
LILLY

32 MG

65 MG

PROPOXYPHENE NAPSYLATE

DARVON-N
LILLY

100 MG

PROPRANOLOL HCl

GENERIC
FOREST/INWOOD

60 MG

80 MG

120 MG

160 MG

GENERIC
LEDERLE

10 MG   20 MG

40 MG   60 MG

80 MG

GENERIC
MYLAN

20 MG

GENERIC
RUGBY

10 MG   20 MG

40 MG   80 MG

INDERAL
WYETH-AYERST

10 MG   20 MG

40 MG   60 MG

80 MG

QUAZEPAM

DORAL
WALLACE

7.5 MG

15 MG

QUINIDINE SULFATE

QUINIDEX EXTENTAB
A. H. ROBINS

300 MG

QUININE SULFATE

QUINAMM
MARION MERRELL DOW

260 MG

RAMIPRIL

ALTACE
HOECHST-ROUSSEL

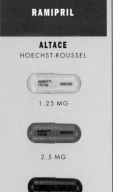

1.25 MG

2.5 MG

5 MG

10 MG

RANITIDINE HCl

ZANTAC
GLAXO

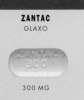

300 MG

RIFAMPIN

RIMACTANE
CIBA

300 MG

RITODRINE HCl

YUTOPAR
ASTRA PHARMACEUTICAL
PRODUCTS

10 MG

SALSALATE

DISALCID
3M PHARMACEUTICALS

500 MG

500 MG

750 MG

SECOBARBITAL SODIUM

SECONAL SODIUM
LILLY

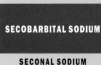

100 MG

SELEGILINE HYDROCHLORIDE

ELDEPRYL
SOMERSET

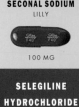

5 MG

SIMVASTATIN

ZOCOR
MERCK & CO.

10 MG   20 MG

SODIUM FLUORIDE

LURIDE-SF LOZI-TABS
COLGATE-HOYT

1 MG

SPIRONOLACTONE

ALDACTONE
SEARLE

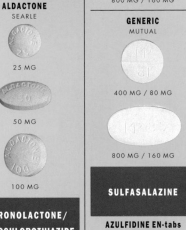

25 MG

50 MG

100 MG

SPIRONOLACTONE/
HYDROCHLOROTHIAZIDE

ALDACTAZIDE
SEARLE

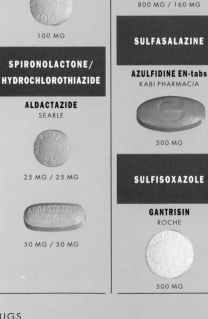

25 MG / 25 MG

50 MG / 50 MG

SUCRALFATE

CARAFATE
MARION MERRELL DOW

1GM

SULFAMETHOXAZOLE/
TRIMETHOPRIM

GENERIC
DANBURY

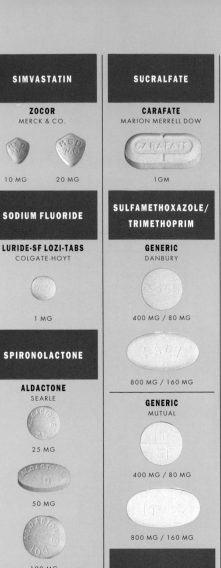

400 MG / 80 MG

800 MG / 160 MG

GENERIC
MUTUAL

400 MG / 80 MG

800 MG / 160 MG

SULFASALAZINE

AZULFIDINE EN-tabs
KABI PHARMACIA

500 MG

SULFISOXAZOLE

GANTRISIN
ROCHE

500 MG

SULINDAC

CLINORIL
MERCK & CO.

150 MG

200 MG

TAMOXIFEN

NOLVADEX
ICI PHARMA

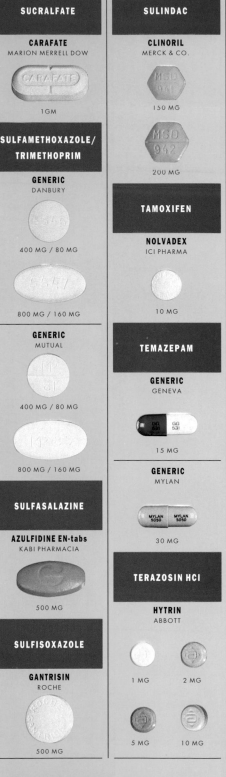

10 MG

TEMAZEPAM

GENERIC
GENEVA

15 MG

GENERIC
MYLAN

30 MG

TERAZOSIN HCl

HYTRIN
ABBOTT

1 MG   2 MG

5 MG   10 MG

TERFENADINE

SELDANE
MARION MERRELL DOW

60 MG

TETRACYCLINE HCl

ACHROMYCIN V
LEDERLE

250 MG

500 MG

TETRACYCLINE HCl
WYETH-AYERST

250 MG

500 MG

THEOPHYLLINE

SLO-BID
RHÔNE-POULENC RORER

75 MG

100 MG

125 MG

200 MG

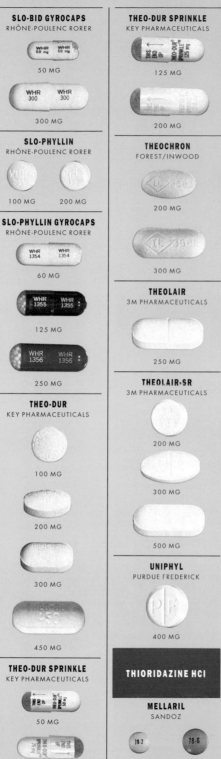

SLO-BID GYROCAPS
RHÔNE-POULENC RORER

50 MG

300 MG

SLO-PHYLLIN
RHÔNE-POULENC RORER

100 MG   200 MG

SLO-PHYLLIN GYROCAPS
RHÔNE-POULENC RORER

60 MG

125 MG

250 MG

THEO-DUR
KEY PHARMACEUTICALS

100 MG

200 MG

300 MG

450 MG

THEO-DUR SPRINKLE
KEY PHARMACEUTICALS

50 MG

75 MG

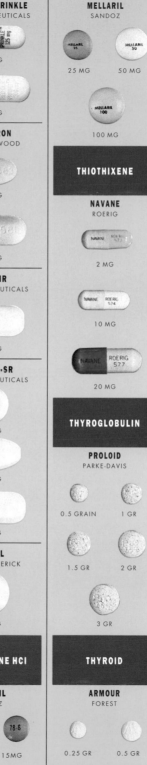

THEO-DUR SPRINKLE
KEY PHARMACEUTICALS

125 MG

200 MG

THEOCHRON
FOREST/INWOOD

200 MG

300 MG

THEOLAIR
3M PHARMACEUTICALS

250 MG

THEOLAIR-SR
3M PHARMACEUTICALS

200 MG

300 MG

500 MG

UNIPHYL
PURDUE FREDERICK

400 MG

THIORIDAZINE HCl

MELLARIL
SANDOZ

10 MG   15MG

MELLARIL
SANDOZ

25 MG   50 MG

100 MG

THIOTHIXENE

NAVANE
ROERIG

2 MG

10 MG

20 MG

THYROGLOBULIN

PROLOID
PARKE-DAVIS

0.5 GRAIN   1 GR

1.5 GR   2 GR

3 GR

THYROID

ARMOUR
FOREST

0.25 GR   0.5 GR

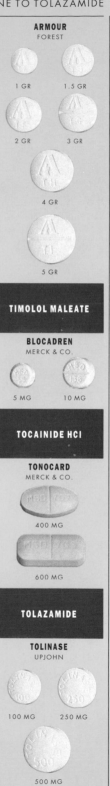

ARMOUR
FOREST

1 GR   1.5 GR

2 GR   3 GR

4 GR

5 GR

TIMOLOL MALEATE

BLOCADREN
MERCK & CO.

5 MG   10 MG

TOCAINIDE HCl

TONOCARD
MERCK & CO.

400 MG

600 MG

TOLAZAMIDE

TOLINASE
UPJOHN

100 MG   250 MG

500 MG

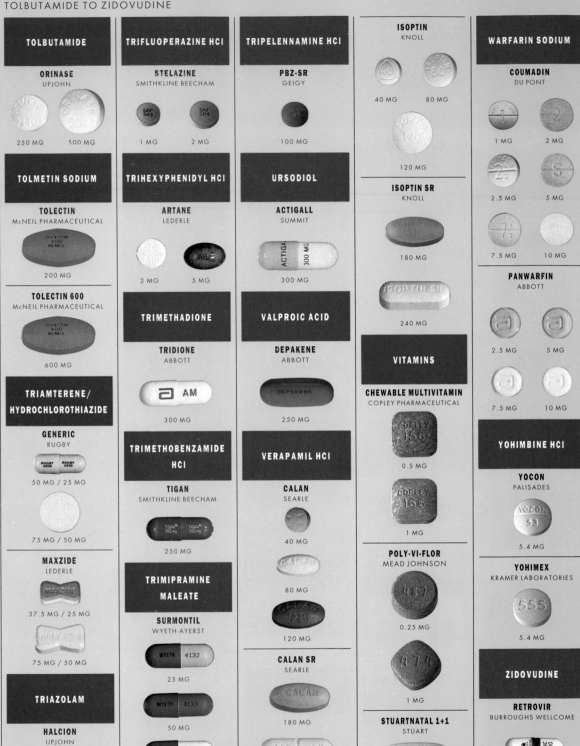

TOLBUTAMIDE

ORINASE
UPJOHN

250 MG   500 MG

TOLMETIN SODIUM

TOLECTIN
McNEIL PHARMACEUTICAL

200 MG

TOLECTIN 600
McNEIL PHARMACEUTICAL

600 MG

**TRIAMTERENE/
HYDROCHLOROTHIAZIDE**

GENERIC
RUGBY

50 MG / 25 MG

75 MG / 50 MG

MAXZIDE
LEDERLE

37.5 MG / 25 MG

75 MG / 50 MG

TRIAZOLAM

HALCION
UPJOHN

0.125 MG

TRIFLUOPERAZINE HCl

STELAZINE
SMITHKLINE BEECHAM

SKF
503   SKF
504

1 MG   2 MG

TRIHEXYPHENIDYL HCl

ARTANE
LEDERLE

2 MG   5 MG

TRIMETHADIONE

TRIDIONE
ABBOTT

AM

300 MG

**TRIMETHOBENZAMIDE
HCl**

TIGAN
SMITHKLINE BEECHAM

TIGAN 250 mg   TIGAN 250 mg

250 MG

**TRIMIPRAMINE
MALEATE**

SURMONTIL
WYETH-AYERST

WYETH 4132

25 MG

WYETH 4133

50 MG

WYETH 4158

100 MG

TRIPELENNAMINE HCl

PBZ-SR
GEIGY

100 MG

URSODIOL

ACTIGALL
SUMMIT

ACTIGALL 300 MG

300 MG

VALPROIC ACID

DEPAKENE
ABBOTT

DEPAKENE

250 MG

VERAPAMIL HCl

CALAN
SEARLE

40 MG

CALAN SR

80 MG

CALAN
120

120 MG

CALAN SR
SEARLE

CALAN

180 MG

CALAN

240 MG

ISOPTIN
KNOLL

40 MG   80 MG

ISOPTIN
120

120 MG

ISOPTIN SR
KNOLL

ISOPTIN
SR

180 MG

ISOPTIN SR

240 MG

VITAMINS

CHEWABLE MULTIVITAMIN
COPLEY PHARMACEUTICAL

COPLEY
158

0.5 MG

COPLEY
166

1 MG

POLY-VI-FLOR
MEAD JOHNSON

487

0.25 MG

474

1 MG

STUARTNATAL 1+1
STUART

Stuart
021

WARFARIN SODIUM

COUMADIN
DU PONT

1 MG   2 MG

2.5 MG   5 MG

7.5 MG   10 MG

PANWARFIN
ABBOTT

2.5 MG   5 MG

7.5 MG   10 MG

YOHIMBINE HCl

YOCON
PALISADES

YOCON
53

5.4 MG

YOHIMEX
KRAMER LABORATORIES

555

5.4 MG

ZIDOVUDINE

RETROVIR
BURROUGHS WELLCOME

100 MG

Appendix one: Safe medication use

Using medications safely is largely a matter of common sense and caution. Remember that the effects of a drug can vary from one person to another, so don't rely on others for drug information. Seek the advice of trained professionals such as your doctor or pharmacist before making any changes in the way you take a medication. The following are general guidelines for most situations:

You and your doctor

■Always tell your doctor everything about your medical history, including reactions to medications you've used in the past. In fact, it may be a good idea to keep a family medication log to help your doctor.

■Tell the doctor about any medications you are using now, even if they are over-the-counter drugs like antacids or cold medications. They may contain ingredients that could cause a reaction with the drugs your doctor prescribes.

■Keep track of your reactions to a medication—both positive and negative—and report them to your doctor at a follow-up visit.

■Ask your doctor what you can or cannot do when given a new drug. For example, are there any foods to avoid when taking the drug? Should you avoid alcohol? Is it safe to drive a car? Is it allright to go out in bright sunlight?

■Never change your dose schedule unless your doctor tells you to do so.

■Ask about the addiction or dependence potential of any new drug.

■Don't be shy—ask your doctor ANY question you may have in mind and report any side effect, even if it seems trivial or embarrassing.

You and your pharmacist

■Your pharmacist is a medication specialist. Don't be afraid to ask questions you might have forgotten to ask your doctor. See if there are any written instructions that you can take with you.

■Ask the pharmacist to explain clearly when and how to take the drug, or to translate into plain English any information you don't understand, such as "milliliters" or "kilograms."

■Check the ingredients of over-the-counter drugs you may be [subsequently] taking to ensure that your prescription doesn't interact with them.

■If you are starting a new medication, ask your pharmacist to fill only half the prescription in case you have an adverse reaction and the drug is stopped.

■ Ask how long the medication remains effective. Don't take it after its expiration date.

■ If you are going on a vacation, make sure your drug can be used in different climates.

You and your medications
■ Never take someone else's medication; and don't share your own medicines with anyone else.

■ Check the label each time you take a drug. Don't take a drug in the dark.

■ Keep your medications in a dry, safe spot.

■ Avoid confusion: If the label falls off, tape it back on or replace it. Keep each medicine in the bottle from the drug store. Don't mix medicines together in a single bottle.

■ If you think you are pregnant or plan to become pregnant, consult with your doctor before using any medication.

■ Destroy any unused portions of a drug and throw out the bottle.

■ If you need a certain medicine (for instance, insulin) in case of emergency, carry the information with you or obtain a special bracelet from an organization such as Medic Alert. This will help a paramedic or emergency room doctor treat you properly.

Your medicines and your children
■ Keep all medications in a locked cabinet or in a spot that is well out of the reach of children.

■ Ask the pharmacist to use child-proof safety bottles.

■ To ensure that you're giving the proper dose, be alert and awake when giving a child medication.

■ Make sure that children know medications are only to be taken when sick and can be dangerous if misused.

■ Keep antidotes such as Syrup of Ipecac on hand.

■ Keep the numbers of your EMS and poison control centers handy.

Your medicines and the elderly
■ The elderly are no different than anyone else when it comes to safe medication use. They are, however, more likely to suffer a side effect or adverse reaction if proper dosing is not followed. The elderly should always be aware of any potential side effects from a medication and should report them to a doctor or family member whenever they occur.

Appendix two: Sugar-free products

The following is a selection of products that contain no sugar. Remember, however, that some may contain sorbitol, alcohol, or other sources of carbohydrates. If you are diabetic or carefully watching your weight, read the product label carefully for a listing of all the ingredients. Make sure your doctor and your pharmacist know that you cannot take prescription or over-the-counter products that contain sugar.

Analgesics (pain relievers)
Bufferin AF Nite Time
Children's Myapap Elixir
Children's Panadol Drops
Children's Panadol Liquid
Children's Panadol Tablets, Chewable
Dolanex Elixir
Extra Strength Tylenol PM
Methadone HCl Intensol
Myapap Drops
St. Joseph Aspirin-Free Liquid
St. Joseph Aspirin-Free Drops
Tempra Tablets, Chewable

Antacids and anti-gas products
Alamag Suspension
Aluminum Hydroxide Concentrated Suspension
Aludrox Suspension
Calglycine Tablets
Camalox Suspension
Citrocarbonate Granules
Di-Gel Liquid
Dimacid
Eno Powder
Gaviscon Liquid
Gelusil Liquid

Gelusil II Suspension
Gelusil-M Suspension
Kolantyl Gel
Maalox Suspension
Maalox Plus, Extra Strength Suspension
Maalox Therapeutic Concentrate
Magnesia and Alumina Oral Suspension USP
Mallamint Tablets, Chewable
Marblen Suspension
Marblen Tablets
Milk of Magnesia USP
Mylanta Liquid
Mylanta II Liquid
Mylicon Drops
Nephrox Suspension
Pepto-Bismol Liquid
Pepto-Bismol Tablets
Phosphaljel Suspension
Riopan Suspension
Riopan Plus Suspension
Titracid Tablets
Titralac Plus Liquid
Titralac Tablets
WinGel Liquid
WinGel Tablets

Anticonvulsants
Mysoline Suspension

Antidiarrhea products
Diasorb Liquid
Kaolin with Pectin
 Suspension
Konsyl Powder
Lomotil Liquid
Paregoric USP
Pepto-Bismol Liquid
Pepto-Bismol Tablets

Antihistamines/ decongestants (drugs for allergies or congestion)
Dimetane Decongestant
 Elixir
Dimetapp Elixir
Hay-Febrol Liquid
Naldecon Pediatric Drops
Naldecon Pediatric Syrup
Naldecon Syrup
Novahistine Elixir
Phenergan Syrup
Phenergan Fortis Syrup
Ryna Liquid
Tavist Syrup
Trind Liquid

Anti-infective medications
Augmentin Suspension
Furadantin Suspension
Furoxone Suspension

Humatin
Mandelamine Suspension
 Forte
Minocin Suspension
NegGram Suspension

Antimanic products (drugs used to treat mania)
Cibalith-S Syrup
Lithium Citrate Syrup

Asthma medications (for asthma and other breathing problems)
Aerolate Liquid
Elixophyllin Elixir
Elixophyllin-GG Liquid
Lufyllin Elixir
Metaprel Syrup
Mucomyst Solution
Mudrane-GG Elixir
Organidin Solution
Slo-Phyllin 80 Syrup
Theo-Organidin Elixir

Blood modifiers/iron preparations
Amicar Syrup
Geritol Complete Tablets
Geritonic Liquid
Iberet Liquid
Incremin with Iron Syrup
Kovitonic Liquid
Niferex Elixir
Nu-Iron Elixir

Corticosteroids
Decadron Elixir
Dexamethasone Solution
Dexamethasone Intensol
 Solution
Pediapred Oral Liquid

Cough/cold preparations
Anatuss Syrup
Cerose-DM
Chlorgest HD
Codegest Expectorant
Codiclear DH Syrup
Codimal-DM Syrup
Colrex Expectorant
Conex with Codeine Syrup
Contac Jr. Liquid
Day-Night Comtrex
Decorel Forte
Dexafed Cough Syrup
Dimetane-DC Cough Syrup
Dimetane-DX Cough Syrup
Elixir Terpin Hydrate with
 Codeine
Entuss Expectorant Syrup
Fedahist Expectorant Syrup
Fedahist Expectorant
 Pediatric Drops
Histafed Pediatric Liquid
Hycomine Syrup
Hycomine Pediatric Syrup
Lanatuss Expectorant

Naldecon-DX Adult Liquid
Naldecon-DX Pediatric
  Drops
Naldecon-EX Syrup
Non-Drowsy Comtrex
Organidin Solution
Potassium Iodide Solution
Robitussin-CF Liquid
Robitussin Night Relief
  Liquid
Ryna Liquid
Ryna-C Liquid
Ryna-CX Liquid
Scot-Tussin DM Cough
  Chasers
S-T Decongestant Liquid
S-T Forte SF Liquid
Scot-Tussin Expectorant
Scot-Tussin DM Syrup
Silexin Cough Syrup
Tolu-Sed Cough Syrup
Tolu-Sed DM Elixir
Trind-DM Liquid
Tussar SF Syrup
Tussi-Organidin Liquid
Tussionex Extended-Release
  Suspension
Tussirex Sugar Free Liquid
Tuss-Ornade Liquid

Gastrointestinal drugs
Dipentum
Paregoric
Reglan Syrup
Tagamet Liquid

Laxatives
Agoral Marshmallow
  Emulsion
Agoral Plain Emulsion
Agoral Raspberry Emulsion
Cascara Sagrada Fluid
  Extract
Castor Oil
Colace Liquid
Disonate Liquid
Doxinate Solution
Emulsoil
Fiberall Powder
Haley's M-O
Hydrocil Instant Powder
Kondremul Plain Emulsion
Konsyl Powder
Magnesium Citrate Solution
Metamucil Sugar Free
  Powder
Metamucil Instant Mix,
  lemon-lime or orange
Milk of Magnesia
  Suspension
Milkinol Emulsion
Mineral Oil
Neoloid Liquid
Nu-LYTELY

Miscellaneous
Artane Elixir
Bicitra Solution
Colestid
Duvoid
Digoxin Elixir
Lipomul Liquid
Nicorette Chewing Gum
Polycitra-K Solution
Polycitra-LC Solution

Mouthwash and oral care
Anbesol Gel
Anbesol Liquid
Babee Teething Lotion
Baby Orajel
Chloraseptic
  Mouthwash/Gargle
Moi-Stir Solution
Mycinettes Lozenges
N'ice Lozenges
Orabase with Benzocaine
Orabase-O
Orabase Plain
Orajel Brace-Aid Gel
Ora-Jel D Gel
Orajel Mouth-Aid Gel
Peroxyl Gel
Peroxyl Mouthrinse
Point-Two Rinse
Rid-A-Pain Drops
Rid-A-Pain Gel
Salivart Solution
Sucrets Maximum Strength
  Mouthwash/Gargle
Tanac Liquid
Tanac Stick
Tanac Roll-On Liquid
Xero-Lube Solution

Potassium Supplements
Cena-K Solution
K-G Elixir
Kaochlor-Eff Tablets for
  Solution
Kaochlor S-F
Kaon Elixir
Kaon-Cl 20% Solution
Kay Ciel Elixir
Kay Ciel Powder
Klor-Con Powder
Klor-Con/EF Tablets

Klorvess Effervescent
Granules
Klorvess Tablets for
Solution
Kolyum Powder
Kolyum Solution
Potasalan Liquid
Potassium Chloride Oral
Liquid USP
Potassium Gluconate
Elixir NF
Rum-K Solution
Tri-K Liquid

**Psychotropics/sedatives
(drugs that alter mood)**
Butabarbital Elixir
Butisol Elixir
Haldol Concentrate
Loxitane C Drops
Permitil Concentrate
Solution
Serentil Concentrate
Solution

Vitamins/minerals
Aquasol A Capsules
Bugs Bunny Chewable
Tablets
Bugs Bunny Plus Iron
Chewable Tabs
Bugs Bunny with Extra C
Chewable Tabs
Bugs Bunny Plus Minerals
Chewable Tabs
Calciferol Drops
Caltrate 600 Tablets
Cod Liver Oil
Decagen Tablets
DHT Solution
DHT Intensol Solution
Flintstones Complete
Chewable Tablets
Flintstones Plus Iron
Chewable Tablets
Flintstones with extra C
Chewable Tablets
Fluorinse
Gel-Kam
Incremin with Iron Liquid
Karidium Drops
Karidium Tablets
Karigel
Karigel-N
Luride Drops
Luride Lozi-tabs
Luride-SF Lozi-tabs
Luride 0.25 Lozi-tabs
Luride 0.5 Lozi-tabs

Oyst-Cal 500 Tablets
Pediaflor Drops
Phos-Flur Rinse
Poly-Vi-Flor Drops
Poly-Vi-Sol Infant Drops
Poly-Vi-Sol with Iron Drops
Posture Tablets
Spider-Man Children's
Chewable Vitamin
Tablets
Spider-Man Plus Iron
Tablets
Stop Gel
Theragran Jr. Children's
Chewable Tablets
Tri-Vi-Flor Drops
Tri-Vi-Flor with Iron Drops
Tri-Vi-Sol Drops
Tri-Vi-Sol with Iron Drops
Vi-Daylin Drops
Vi-Daylin ADC Drops
Vi-Daylin/F Drops
Vi-Daylin/F ADC Drops
Vi-Daylin plus Iron Drops
Vi-Daylin plus Iron ADC
Drops
Vitalize SF Liquid

Appendix three: Alcohol-free products

Many medicines contain alcohol. If you must avoid alcohol or other substances that have a sedative-like effect (i.e. sleeping pills, tranquilizers), the following is a representative list of liquid preparations, both over the counter and prescription, that are alcohol-free. For easy identification, the drugs are listed by category. Before you take any drug, it's wise to check with your doctor or pharmacist about ingredients.

Analgesics (pain-relievers)
Arthropan Liquid
Bufferin AF Nite Time
Children's Panadol Drops
Children's Panadol Liquid
Demerol Syrup
Extra Strength Tylenol PM
Infants' Anacin-3 Drops
Liquiprin Drops
Methadone HCL Intensol
No Drowsiness Tylenol
PediaProfen Suspension
Roxanol Concentrated Oral
    Solution
St. Joseph Aspirin-Free
    Infant Drops
St. Joseph Aspirin-Free
    Liquid for Children
Tempra Drops
Tempra Syrup

Antacids
Aludrox Suspension
Amphojel Suspension
Camalox Suspension
Di-Gel suspension
Gelusil Liquid
Maalox Suspension
Mylanta Liquid
Riopan Suspension
Titralac Liquid

Anticonvulsants
Mysoline Suspension
Tridione Solution
Zarontin Syrup

Antidiarrhea products
Kaodene Non-Narcotic
    Suspension
Kaodene with Paregoric
    Suspension
Kaopectate Suspension
Pepto Bismol Suspension

Antiemetics (drugs that control nausea and vomiting)
Emetrol

Antihistamines/ decongestants (drugs for allergies or congestion)
Hayfebrol

Anti-infective medications
E.E.S. 400 Suspension
Furoxone Liquid
Gantanol Oral Suspension
Ilosone Suspension
Mandelamine Oral
   Suspension
Negram Suspension
Symmetrel Syrup

Asthma Medications
Aerolate Oral Solution
Alupent Syrup
Choledyl Pediatric Syrup
Dilor G Liquid
Elixophyllin-GG Liquid
KIE Syrup
Metaprel Syrup
Slo-Phyllin 80 Syrup
Slo-Phyllin GG Syrup
Tedral Suspension
Theolair Solution

Cough/cold preparations
Actifed Syrup
Bromfed-DM Cough Syrup
Chlorgest HD
Codegest Expectorant
Codimal Expectorant
Conar Expectorant Syrup
Congespirin Syrup for
   Children
CoTylenol Liquid
   (Children's)
Deconamine Syrup
Delsym Liquid
Dorcol Children's
   Decongestant Liquid
Dorcol Children's Cold
   Formula Liquid
Fedahist Decongestant
   Syrup
Fedahist Expectorant Syrup
Hycodan Syrup
Hycomine Pediatric Syrup
Ipsatol Cough Formula
   Liquid for Children
KIE Syrup
Kolephrin GG/DM
   Expectorant
Lanatuss Expectorant
Non-Drowsy Comtrex
Noratuss II Expectorant
Noratuss II Liquid
PediaCare Infants'
   Decongestant

PediaCare Cough-Cold
   Liquid
Ryna Liquid
Rynatuss Pediatric
   Suspension
Scot-Tussin Original Cold
   Formula Syrup
Scot-Tussin DM Liquid
Sudafed Liquid, Children's
Triaminic Expectorant
   Liquid
Triaminic DM Syrup
Tussar DM Cough Syrup
Tussirex Sugar Free Liquid

Electrolytes (e.g. calcium, sodium, potassium)
Klor-10%
Kolyum Liquid

Iron preparations
Feostat Drops
Feostat Suspension
Troph-Iron Liquid

Laxatives

Agoral Emulsion
Colace Liquid
Disonate Liquid
Disonate Syrup
Haley's M-O
Kondremul Plain
Milkinol Emulsion
Neo-Cultol
Neoloid Emulsion
Nu-LYTELY

Miscellaneous

Dayto Himbin Liquid
Glandosane

Mouthwash and oral care

Chloraseptic Liquid
Gel-Kam
Gly-Oxide Liquid
Orabase with Benzocaine
Orabase HCA
Orabase-O orthodontic gel
Orabase Plain
Ora Fresh Mouthwash
  (cinnamon)
Ora Fresh Mouthwash
  (peppermint)
Phos-Flur
Proxigel
ST-37

Psychotropics (drugs that affect mood)

Haldol Concentrate
Stelazine Concentrate
Taractan Concentrate
Thorazine Syrup

Vitamins/minerals

Abdec Baby Vitamin Drops
Abdec with Fluoride
Adeflor Drops
Aquasol A Drops
Cecon Solution
Clusivol Syrup
Drisdol Liquid
Lederplex Liquid
Livitamin Liquid
Neo-Calglucon Syrup
Poly-Vi-Sol Drops
Theragran Liquid
Tri-Vi-Sol Drops
Vitalize

Appendix four: Drugs that may cause a reaction to sunlight

Some people may have what is known as a "photosensitivity reaction" when taking certain drugs. This means they may suffer an allergic reaction if exposed to bright sunlight. The effects may be as mild as itching, scaling and rash, or as severe as skin cancer, premature skin aging, skin and eye burns, cataracts, reduced immunity, blood vessel damage, and other toxic reactions. The following list is not all-inclusive, and shows only a representative brand name for each generic drug. When in doubt, always check specific product labeling or consult with your doctor or your pharmacist.

Generic name	Representative Brand
Acetazolamide	Diamox
Amiloride/hydrochlorothiazide	Moduretic
Amiodarone	Cordarone
Amitriptyline	Elavil
Amoxapine	Asendin
Astemizole	Hismanal
Atenolol/chlorthalidone	Tenoretic
Auranofin	Ridaura
Azatadine	Optimine
Azatadine/pseudoephedrine	Trinalin
Benzthiazide	Exna
Bromodiphenhydramine	Ambenyl
Captopril	Capoten
Captopril/hydrochlorothiazide	Capozide
Carbamazepine	Tegretol
Chlordiazepoxide/amitriptyline	Limbitrol
Chlorothiazide	Diuril
Chlorpheniramine	Chlorpheniramine
Chlorpheniramine/D-pseudoephedrine	Deconamine
Chlorpheniramine/phenylpropanolamine	Ru-Tuss II
Chlorpromazine	Thorazine
Chlorpropamide	Diabinese
Chlorprothixene	Taractan
Chlorthalidone	Hygroton
Chlorthalidone/reserpine	Regroton
Ciprofloxacin	Cipro
Clemastine	Tavist
Clofazime	Lamprene
Clonidine/chlorthalidone	Combipres
Coal tar	Estar Gel
Contraceptive, oral	Ortho-Novum
Cromolyn	Intal inhaler
Cyclobenzaprine	Flexeril
Cyproheptadine	Periactin

Dacarbazine	DTIC-Dome
Danazol	Danocrine
Demeclocycline	Declomycin
Desipramine	Norpramin
Dexchlorpheniramine	Polaramine
Diclofenac	Voltaren
Diflunisal	Dolobid
Diltiazem	Cardizem
Diphenhydramine	Benadryl
Diphenylpyraline	Hispril
Doxepin	Sinequan
Doxycycline	Vibramycin
Doxycycline hyclate	Doryx
Enalapril	Vasotec
Enalapril/hydrochlorothiazide	Vaseretic
Erythromycin ethylsuccinate/sulfisoxazole	Pediazole
Estrogens	Oral contraceptives
Ethionamide	Trecator-SC
Etretinate	Tegison
Floxuridine	FUDR Injectable
Flucytosine	Ancobon
Fluorouracil	Adrucil
Fluphenazine	Prolixin
Flurbiprofen	Ansaid
Flutamide	Eulexin
Furosemide	Lasix
Gentamicin	Garamycin
Glipizide	Glucotrol
Glyburide	Micronase
Gold salts (compounds)	Solganal
Gold sodium thiomalate	Myochrysine
Griseofulvin	Fulvicin U/F
Griseofulvin ultramicrosize	Grisactin ultra
Guanethidine/hydrochlorothiazide	Esimil
Haloperidol	Haldol
Hexachlorophene	Phisohex
Hydralazine/hydrochlorothiazide	Apresazide
Hydrochlorothiazide	HydroDIURIL
Hydrochlorothiazide/deserpidine	Oreticyl
Hydrochlorothiazide/triamterene	Dyazide
Hydroflumethiazide	Diucardin
Hydroflumethiazide/reserpine	Salutensin
Ibuprofen	Motrin
Imipramine	Tofranil
Indapamide	Lozol
Interferon ALFA-2B	Intron A
Isocarboxazid	Marplan
Isotretinoin	Accutane
Ketoprofen	Orudis
Labetalol	Normodyne
Labetalol/hydrochlorothiazide	Trandate HCT
Lisinopril/hydrochlorothiazide	Prinzide
Lovastatin	Mevacor
Maprotiline	Ludiomil
Merperidine/promethiazine	Mepergan
Mesoridazine	Serentil
Methacycline	Rondomycin
Methazolamide	Neptazane
Methdilazine	Tacaryl
Methotrexate	Rheumatrex
Methyclothiazide	Aquatensin
Methyclothiazide/deserpidine	Enduronyl
Methyclothiazide/reserpine	Diutensin-R
Methyldopa/hydrochlorothiazide	Aldoril
Methyldopa/chlorothiazide	Aldoclor
Metolazone	Diulo
Metoprolol/hydrochlorothiazide	Lopressor HCT
Minocycline	Minocin
Minoxidil	Rogaine
Nabilone	Cesamet
Nadolol/bendroflumethiazide	Corzide
Nalidixic acid	NegGram
Naproxen	Naprosyn
Nifedipine	Procardia
Norfloxacin	Noroxin
Nortriptyline	Pamelor
Oxytetracycline	Terramycin
Perphenazine	Trilafon
Perphenazine/amitriptyline	Triavil
Phenylbutazone	Butazolidin
Phenylpropanolamine/pheniramine/pyrilamine	Triaminic TR
Piroxicam	Feldene
Polythiazide	Renese
Prazosin/polythiazide	Minizide
Prochlorperazine	Compazine
Promethazine	Phenergan
Propranolol/hydrochlorothiazide	Inderide
Protriptyline	Vivactil
Pyrazinamide	Pyrazinamide
Quinethazone	Hydromox
Quinidine gluconate	Quinaglute Dura-Tabs
Quinidine sulfate	Quindex Extentabs
Quinine	Quinamm

Rauwolfia Serpentina/bendroflumethiazide .....Rauzide
Reserpine/chlorothiazide.............................Diupres
Reserpine/hydrochlorothiazide...............Serpasil-Esidrix
Reserpine/hydralazine/hydrochlorothiazide ..Ser-Ap-Es
Selegiline ....Eldepryl
Spironolactone/hydrochlorothiazide ....Aldactazide
Sulfadoxine/pyrimethamine.........................Fansidar
Sulfamethizole/phenazopyridine ....Thiosulfil-A
Sulfamethoxazole................................Gantanol
Sulfamethoxazole/phenazopyridine ....Azo Gantanol
Sulfapyridine..(generic only)
Sulfasalazine ....Azulfidine
Sulfinpyrazone..Anturane
Sulfasoxazole...Gantrisin
Sulfasoxazole/phenazopyridine ....Azo Gantrisin
Sulfone..Dapsone
Sulindac..Clinoril
Terfenadine ....Seldane
Tetracycline ....Achromycin
Thioridazine...Mellaril
Thiothixene..Navane
Timolol/hydrochlorothiazide.......................Timolide

Tolazamide..Tolinase
Tolbutamide..Orinase
Tretinoin ....Retin-A
Triamterene...Dyrenium
Trifluoperazine..Stelazine
Triflupromazine...Vesprin
Trimeprazine..Temaril
Trimethoprim..Trimpex
Trimethoprim/sulfamethoxazole.......................Bactrim
Trimipramine...Surmontil
Tripelannamine..PBZ
Triprolidine...Actidil
Triprolidine/pseudoephedrine ....Actifed
Vinblastine...Velban

Adapted from *Medications that Increase Sensitivity to Light: a 1990 Listing*, prepared by Jerome I. Levine, M.S., R.Ph., U.S. Department of Health and Human Services, Public Health Service/Food and Drug Administration Center for Devices and Radiological Health.

Appendix five: Poison control centers

If there is one phone number that no home should be without, it is the nearest poison control center. Perhaps you will never need to use it, but if someone in your home accidentally swallows a household chemical or takes too much medication, having this number might mean the difference between life and death. Place the phone number inside the door of your medicine cabinet or in some other convenient place where it can be easily located in case of emergency. You should also have on hand a bottle of Syrup of Ipecac, a drug that causes vomiting within 20 minutes. With certain poisons, you may need to induce vomiting to remove the substance from the body. Call the poison control center to make sure whether this should be done.

The following is a list of regional centers that are certified members of the American Association of Poison Control Centers. To be certified, they must be supervised by a medical director; have pharmacists and nurses available to answer questions you may have; be open 24 hours a day; and be accessible by direct dialing or a toll-free number. The staffs at these centers are trained to help you treat the poison victim at home or refer you to a hospital if necessary.

These regional centers have a wide variety of resources, including a computer data bank with information on over 350,000 substances updated 4 times a year. They also provide educational services and information to the community. Write or call to learn how you can "poison-proof" your home, what plants are dangerous for children or pets, what to do if a poisoning occurs. The

Poison Control Center will guide you through any action they recommend.

The Centers below are organized by region and are listed alphabetically by name.

FAR WEST

Fresno Regional Poison Control Center
Fresno Community Hospital
Medical Center
2823 Fresno St.
Fresno, CA 93715
(800) 346-5922 (CA only)

Los Angeles County Regional Poison Control Center
1925 Wilshire Blvd.
Los Angeles, CA 90057
(213) 484-5151

Oregon Poison Center
Oregon Health Sciences
University
3181 S.W. Sam Jackson
Park Rd.
Portland, OR 97201
(503) 494-8968 (Local)
(800) 452-7165 (OR only)

**San Diego Regional
Poison Center**
U.C.S.D. Medical Center
225 West Dickinson St.
San Diego, CA 92103
(619) 543-6000
(800) 876-4766
(619 area code only)

**San Francisco Bay Area
Regional Poison
Control Center**
San Francisco General
Hospital
1001 Potrero Ave.,
Room 1E86
San Francisco, CA 94110
(415) 476-6600
(800) 523-2222
(415, 707 area codes only)

**Santa Clara Valley
Medical Center**
Regional Poison Control
Center
751 S. Bascom Ave.
San Jose, CA 95128
(408) 299-5112, 5113, 5114
(800) 662-9886, 9887 (CA
only)

**UCDMC Regional Poison
Control Center**
2315 Stockton Blvd.,
Room 1511
Sacramento, CA 95817
(916) 734-3692
(800) 342-9293 (CA only)

GREAT LAKES

**Blodgett Regional
Poison Center**
1840 Wealthy St. S.E.
Grand Rapids, MI 49506
(616) 774-2963
(800) 632-2727 (MI only)
(800) 356-3232 (TTY for
deaf)

**Central Ohio
Poison Center**
Columbus Children's
Hospital
700 Children's Dr.
Columbus, OH 43205
(614) 228-1323
(800) 682-7625 (MI only)
(614) 228-2272 (TTY for
deaf)

Indiana Poison Center
Methodist Hospital
1701 N. Senate Blvd.
Indianapolis, IN 46206
(317) 929-2323
(800) 382-9097
(317) 929-2336 (TTY for
deaf)

Poison Control Center
Children's Hospital of
Michigan
3901 Beaubien Blvd.
Detroit, MI 48201
(313) 745-5711
(800) 462-6642 (MI only)

**Regional Poison
Control System**
Cincinnati Drug and Poison
Information Center
231 Bethesda Ave.,
M.L. #144
Cincinnati, OH 45267-0144
(513) 558-5111
(800) 872-5111

GREAT PLAINS

Cardinal Glennon Children's Hospital Regional Poison Center
1465 S. Grand Blvd.
St. Louis, MO 63104
(314) 772-5200
(800) 366-8888
(314) 577-5336 (TTY for deaf)

Hennepin Regional Poison Center
Hennepin County
Medical Center
701 Park Ave. S.
Minneapolis, MN 55415
(612) 347-3141
(612) 337-7474 (TTY for deaf)

Mid Plains Poison Control Center
Children's Memorial
Hospital
8301 Dodge St.
Omaha, NE 68114
(402) 390-5400
(800) 955-9119 (NE, ID, IA, KS, MO, SD only)

Minnesota Regional Poison Center
St. Paul-Ramsey
Medical Center
640 Jackson St.
St. Paul, MN 55101
(612) 221-2113
(800) 222-1222 (MN only)

MIDDLE ATLANTIC

The Poison Control Center
(serving the greater Philadelphia metropolitan area)
One Children's Center
34th and Civic Center Blvd.
Philadelphia, PA 19104
(215) 386-2100

Long Island Regional Poison Control Center
Nassau County
Medical Center
2201 Hempstead Tpk.
East Meadow, NY 11554
(516) 542-2323

New Jersey Poison Information and Education System
Newark Beth Israel
Medical Center
201 Lyons Ave.
Newark, NJ 07112
(201) 923-0764
(800) 962-1253 (NJ only)
(201) 926-8008 (TTY for deaf)

New York City Poison Control Center
455 First Ave., Room 123
New York, NY 10016
(212) 340-4494
(212) POISONS

Pittsburgh Poison Center
3705 Fifth Ave.
at DeSoto St.
Pittsburgh, PA 15213
(412) 681-6669

MID-SOUTH

Regional Poison Control Center
Children's Hospital
of Alabama
1600 Seventh Ave. S.
Birmingham, AL 35233-1711
(205) 939-9201
(800) 292-6678 (AL only)

Kentucky Regional Poison Center of Kosair Children's Hospital
315 East Broadway
Louisville, KY 40232-5070
(502) 629-7275
(800) 722-5725 (KY only)

NEW ENGLAND

Massachusetts Poison Control System
The Children's Hospital
300 Longwood Ave.
Boston, MA 02115
(617) 232-2120
(800) 682-9211 (MA only)

**Rhode Island
Poison Center**
593 Eddy St.
Providence, RI 02902
(401) 277-5727

ROCKY MOUNTAINS

**Arizona Poison and Drug
Information Center**
University of Arizona
Health Sciences Center
Rm. 3204K
1501 N. Campbell Ave.
Tucson, AZ 85724
(602) 626-6016
(800) 362-0101 (AZ only)

**Intermountain Regional
Poison Control Center**
50 N. Medical Dr.,
Building 428
Salt Lake City, UT 84132
(801) 581-2151
(800) 456-7707 (UT only)

**New Mexico Poison and
Drug Information Center**
University of New Mexico
Albuquerque, NM 87131
(505) 843-2551
(800) 432-6866 (NM only)

**Rocky Mountain Poison
and Drug Center**
645 Bannock St.
Denver, CO 80204
(303) 629-1123
(800) 332-3073 (CO only)

**Samaritan Regional
Poison Center**
Good Samaritan
Medical Center
1130 E. McDowell Rd.,
Suite A-5
Phoenix, AZ 85006
(602) 253-3334SOUTH
ATLANTIC

SOUTH ATLANTIC

**Florida Poison
Information Center**
Tampa General Hospital
P.O. Box 1289
Tampa, FL 33601
(813) 253-4444
(800) 282-3171 (FL only)

**Georgia Regional Poison
Control Center**
Grady Memorial Hospital
80 Butler St. S.E.
Atlanta, GA 30335-3801
(404) 589-4400
(800) 282-5846 (GA only)
(404) 525-3323 (TTY for
deaf)

Maryland Poison Center
20 N. Pine St.
Baltimore, MD 21201
(301) 528-7701
(800) 492-2414 (MD only)

**National Capital
Poison Center**
Georgetown University
Hospital
3800 Reservoir Rd. N.W.
Washington, DC 20007
(202) 625-3333
(202) 784-4660 (TTY for
deaf)

**West Virginia
Poison Center**
West Virginia University
Health Sciences
Center/Charleston Division
3110 MacCorkle Ave. S.E.
Charleston, WV 25304
(304) 348-4211
(800) 642-3625 (WV only)

SOUTH

**North Texas
Poison Center**
P.O. Box 35926
Dallas, TX 75235
(214) 590-5000
(800) 441-0040 (TX only)

Sources

CHAPTERS ONE AND TWO

New Hope for Heart Patients

Defusing High Blood Pressure

Gold, Mark S, Boyette, Michael.
Wonder Drugs: How They Work.
New York: Pocket Books, Simon & Schuster, Inc.;
1987.

Solomon, Harold S, Chilnick LD.
Beat the Odds.
New York: Villard Books; 1986.

Solomon, Harold S.
Interview.
Boston, Mass: Brigham and Women's Hospital;
February-April, 1992.

CHAPTER THREE

Coping with Arthritis

Arthritis Foundation.
Arthritis Fact Book for the Media.
Atlanta, Ga.; 1991.

Arthritis Foundation.
Arthritis Facts.
Atlanta, Ga.; 1991.

Arthritis Foundation.
Arthritis Today.
Dallas, Tex.; 1991.

CHAPTER FOUR

**Osteoporosis, Back Pain,
and Other Bone Disorders**

American Academy of Orthopaedic Surgeons.
Carpal Tunnel Syndrome.
Park Ridge, Ill.: 1990; 200M1190.

American Academy of Orthopaedic Surgeons.
Common Foot Problems.
Park Ridge, Ill.: 1991; 50M0191.

American Academy of Orthopaedic Surgeons.
Fractures.
Park Ridge, Ill.: 1988; 25M0491.

American Academy of Orthopaedic Surgeons.
Low Back Pain.
Park Ridge, Ill.: 1991; 80M0891.

American Academy of Orthopaedic Surgeons.
Neck Pain.
Park Ridge, Ill.: 1989; 200M0289.

American Academy of Orthopaedic Surgeons.
Osteoporosis.
Park Ridge, Ill.: 1988; 300M1287.

American Academy of Orthopaedic Surgeons.
Scoliosis.
Park Ridge, Ill.: 1988; 200M1287.

American Academy of Orthopaedic Surgeons.
Sprains and Strains.
Park Ridge, Ill.: 1991; 100M1091.

American Podiatric Medical Association.
Footwear (Your Podiatrist Talks About).
Bethesda, Md.: 1992; F150M.

CHAPTER FIVE

Digestive Disorders, Minor and Major

DeCross, Arthur J, Peura, David A.
Role of H pylori in peptic ulcer disease.
Contemporary Gastroenterology.
May, 1992; 18–26.

Health Information Services, Merck Sharp & Dohme.
Acid Related G.I. Disease.
West Point, Penn.: 1989; 19486.

Kolata, Gina.
New study backs ulcer-cure theory.
New York Times.
May 6, 1992; C14.

Lewis, Ricki.
The gallbladder; an organ you can live without.
FDA Consumer.
May 1991; 13–15.

National Digestive Diseases Information
Clearinghouse.
IBD and IBS: Two Very Different Problems.
Bethesda, Md.: November 1989; No. 90-3079.

National Digestive Diseases Information
Clearinghouse.
What is Irritable Bowel Syndrome?
Bethesda, Md.: October 1989; No. 90-693.

Springhouse Corporation.
Professional Guide to Diseases; Third Edition.
Springhouse, Penn.: 1990.

Steinhart, Melvin J.
**Irritable bowel syndrome; how to relieve
symptoms enough to improve daily function.**
Postgraduate Medicine.
May 1992; 91:6.

U.S. Department of Health and Human Services.
Cirrhosis of the Liver.
Bethesda, Md.: November 1991; Fact Sheet 92-1134.

U.S. Department of Health and Human Services.
Constipation.
Bethesda, Md.: March 1992; Fact Sheet 92-2754.

U.S. Department of Health and Human Services.
Diverticulosis and Diverticulitis.
Bethesda, Md.: October 1991; Fact Sheet 92-1163.

U.S. Department of Health and Human Services.
Facts and Fallacies About Digestive Diseases.
Bethesda, Md.: 1991; Fact Sheet 92-2673.

U.S. Department of Health and Human Services.
Heartburn.
Bethesda, Md.: March 1992; Fact Sheet 92-882.

U.S. Department of Health and Human Services.
Hiatal Hernia.
Bethesda, Md.: October 1991; Fact Sheet 92-498.

U.S. Department of Health and Human Services.
Lactose Intolerance.
Bethesda, Md.: February 1991; Fact Sheet 91-2751.

U.S. Department of Health and Human Services.
Pancreatitis.
Bethesda, Md.: September 1991; Fact Sheet 91-1596.

U.S. Department of Health and Human Services.
Stomach Ulcers.
Bethesda, Md.: October 1991; Fact sheet 92-676.

U.S. Department of Health and Human Services.
Ulcerative Colitis.
Bethesda, Md.: April 1992; Fact Sheet 92-1597.

CHAPTERS SIX AND THIRTEEN

Defeating the Dangers of Respiratory Disease

Ear, Nose and Throat Disorders

Alexander Graham Bell Association for the Deaf.
Hearing Alert!
Washington, D.C.: 1984.

American Academy of Otolaryngology-Head and
Neck Surgery, Inc.
**Antihistamines, Decongestants, and "Cold"
Remedies.**
Alexandria, Va.: 1991.

American Academy of Otolaryngology-Head and Neck Surgery, Inc.
Assistive Communication Devices.
Alexandria, Va.: 1989.

American Academy of Otolaryngology-Head and Neck Surgery, Inc.
Cholesteatoma: A Serious Ear Condition.
Alexandria, Va.: 1989.

American Academy of Otolaryngology-Head and Neck Surgery, Inc.
Cochlear Implant: A Device to Help the Deaf Hear.
Alexandria, Va.: 1990.

American Academy of Otolaryngology-Head and Neck Surgery, Inc.
Dizziness and Motion Sickness.
Alexandria, Va.: 1992.

American Academy of Otolaryngology-Head and Neck Surgery, Inc.
"Doctor, What Causes the Noise in My Ears?"
Alexandria, Va.: 1992.

American Academy of Otolaryngology-Head and Neck Surgery, Inc.
Earache and Otitis Media.
Alexandria, Va.: 1991.

American Academy of Otolaryngology-Head and Neck Surgery, Inc.
Ears, Altitude, and Airplane Travel.
Alexandria, Va.: 1990.

American Academy of Otolaryngology-Head and Neck Surgery, Inc.
Earwax: What to Do About It.
Alexandria, Va.: 1991.

American Academy of Otolaryngology-Head and Neck Surgery, Inc.
Facial Nerve Problems.
Washington, D.C.: 1989.

American Academy of Otolaryngology-Head and Neck Surgery, Inc.
5 Minute Hearing Test.
Washington, D.C.: 1989.

American Academy of Otolaryngology-Head and Neck Surgery, Inc.
Hay Fever, Summer Colds, and Allergies.
Alexandria, Va.: 1991.

American Academy of Otolaryngology-Head and Neck Surgery, Inc.
Head and Neck Cancer: Know What the Warning Signs Are.
Alexandria, Va.: 1992.

American Academy of Otolaryngology-Head and Neck Surgery, Inc.
Is My Baby's Hearing Normal?
Alexandria, Va.: 1991.

American Academy of Otolaryngology-Head and Neck Surgery, Inc.
Laser Surgery in Otolaryngology.
Alexandria, Va.: 1992.

American Academy of Otolaryngology-Head and Neck Surgery, Inc.
Ménière's Disease.
Alexandria, Va.: 1992.

American Academy of Otolaryngology-Head and Neck Surgery, Inc.
Noise, Ears and Hearing Protection.
Alexandria, Va.: 1992.

American Academy of Otolaryngology-Head and Neck Surgery, Inc.
Nose Bleeds.
Alexandria, Va.: 1991.

American Academy of Otolaryngology-Head and Neck Surgery, Inc.
Pain and the TMJ (Temporo-Mandibular Joint).
Alexandria, Va.: 1991.

American Academy of Otolaryngology-Head and Neck Surgery, Inc.
Perforated Eardrum.
Alexandria, Va.: 1992.

American Academy of Otolaryngology-Head and Neck Surgery, Inc.
Post-Nasal Drip.
Alexandria, Va.: 1991.

American Academy of Otolaryngology-Head and Neck Surgery, Inc.
Salivary Glands: What's Normal, What's Abnormal?
Alexandria, Va.: 1992.

American Academy of Otolaryngology-Head and Neck Surgery, Inc.
Sinus: Pain, Pressure, Drainage.
Alexandria, Va.: 1992.

American Academy of Otolaryngology-Head and Neck Surgery, Inc.
Skull Base Surgery: A Ray of Hope for Advanced Head and Neck Cancer.
Alexandria, Va.: 1990.

American Academy of Otolaryngology-Head and Neck Surgery, Inc.
Smell & Taste Disorders.
Alexandria, Va.: 1990.

American Academy of Otolaryngology-Head and Neck Surgery, Inc.
Smokeless Tobacco.
Alexandria, Va.: 1991.

American Academy of Otolaryngology-Head and Neck Surgery, Inc.
Smoking: the Hows and Whys of Quitting.
Alexandria, Va.: 1991.

American Academy of Otolaryngology-Head and Neck Surgery, Inc.
Snoring: Not Funny, Not Hopeless.
Alexandria, Va.: 1992.

American Academy of Otolaryngology-Head and Neck Surgery, Inc.
Sore Throats: Causes and Cures.
Alexandria, Va.: 1991.

American Academy of Otolaryngology-Head and Neck Surgery, Inc.
Swallowing Disorders.
Alexandria, Va.: 1992.

American Academy of Otolaryngology-Head and Neck Surgery, Inc.
Swimmer's Ear, Itchy Ears, and Ear Fungus.
Alexandria, Va.: 1991.

American Academy of Otolaryngology-Head and Neck Surgery, Inc.
The Environment: Our Mutual Concern.
Alexandria, Va.: 1991.

American Academy of Otolaryngology-Head and Neck Surgery, Inc.
Tonsils & Adenoids.
Alexandria, Va.: 1991.

American Academy of Otolaryngology-Head and Neck Surgery, Inc.
Travel Tips for Hearing Impaired People.
Washington, DC: 1989.

American Academy of Otolaryngology-Head and Neck Surgery, Inc.
What is an Otolaryngologist-Head and Neck Surgeon?
Alexandria, Va.: 1991.

American Academy of Otolaryngology-Head and Neck Surgery, Inc.
You and Your Stuffy Nose.
Alexandria, Va.: 1989.

American Academy of Otolaryngology-Head and Neck Surgery, Inc.
Your Medical Bills and Insurance Benefits.
Alexandria, Va.: 1990.

American Academy of Otolaryngology-Head and Neck Surgery, Inc.
Your Thyroid Gland.
Alexandria, Va.: 1992.

National Cancer Institute, US Department of Health and Human Services.
Chew or Snuff is Real Bad Stuff.
Bethesda, Md.: 1991.

CHAPTER SEVEN

Cancer: Improving the Odds of a Cure

American Cancer Society.
Cancer Facts and Figures - 1992.
Elizabeth, N.J.: 1992; 92-425M-No.5008.92-LE.

American Cancer Society.
Chemotherapy (What It Is; How It Helps).
Elizabeth, N.J.: 1990; 90-100-M-No.4512.

American Cancer Society.
Living with Cancer.
Elizabeth, N.J.: 1988; 88-25M-No.3480.07-PE.

U.S. Department of Health and Human Services.
Chemotherapy and You (A Guide To Self-Help During Treatment.
Third Edition. Bethesda, Md.: 1991.

U.S. Department of Health and Human Services.
Radiation Therapy and You (A Guide To Self-Help During Treatment).
Revised 1990. Bethesda, Md.: 1992.

CHAPTER EIGHT

New Answers for Pain

Makarowski, William S.
Living With Pain.
Washington, DC: Rehab Hospital Services Corporation; 1990.

Professional Guide to Diseases.
Second Edition, Revised. Loeb, Stanley, ed.
Springhouse, Pa.: Springhouse Corporation; 1987.

CHAPTER NINE

Overcoming Emotional and Psychological Problems

American Psychiatric Association.
Anxiety Disorders.
Washington, D.C.: 1990.

American Psychiatric Association.
Childhood Disorders.
Washington, D.C.: 1988.

American Psychiatric Association.
Choosing a Psychiatrist.
Washington, D.C.: 1991.

American Psychiatric Association.
Depression.
Washington, D.C.: 1989.

American Psychiatric Association.
Manic-Depressive Disorder.
Washington, D.C.: 1988.

American Psychiatric Association.
Mental Health of the Elderly.
Washington, D.C.: 1988.

American Psychiatric Association.
Mental Illness—There Are a Lot of Troubled People.
Washington, D.C.: 1990.

American Psychiatric Association.
Obsessive-Compulsive Disorder.
Washington, D.C.: 1988.

American Psychiatric Association.
Panic Disorder.
Washington, D.C.: 1989.

American Psychiatric Association.
Phobias.
Washington, D.C.: 1988.

American Psychiatric Association.
Post-Traumatic Stress Disorder.
Washington, D.C.: 1988.

American Psychiatric Association.
Schizophrenia.
Washington, D.C.: 1990.

American Psychiatric Association.
Spread the Words.
Washington, D.C.: 1992.

American Psychiatric Association
Teen Suicide.
Washington, D.C.: 1988.

CHAPTERS TEN AND TWENTY-ONE

OB/GYN Disorders:
Causes and Treatments

Facing Up to Sexually Transmitted Diseases

Centers for Disease Control, U.S. Department of Health and Human Services.
Resource List for Informational Materials on Sexually Transmitted Diseases (STDs) and HIV/AIDS.
Atlanta, Ga.: 1991; 00-4730.

Centers for Disease control, U.S. Department of Health and Human Services.
Sexually Transmitted Diseases.
Atlanta, Ga.: 1991; 00-5925.

The American College of Obstetricians and Gynecologists.
Abnormal Uterine Bleeding.
Washington, D.C.: 1991.

The American College of Obstetricians and Gynecologists.
Cancer of the Ovary.
Washington, D.C.: 1992.

The American College of Obstetricians and Gynecologists.
Cancer of the Uterus.
Washington, D.C.: 1992.

The American College of Obstetricians and Gynecologists.
Contraception.
Washington, D.C.: 1990.

The American College of Obstetricians and Gynecologists.
Detecting and Treating Breast Problems.
Washington, D.C.: 1987.

The American College of Obstetricians and Gynecologists.
Diseases of the Vulva.
Washington, D.C.: 1990.

The American College of Obstetricians and Gynecologists.
Disorders of the Cervix.
Washington, D.C.: 1992.

The American College of Obstetricians and Gynecologists.
Dysmenorrhea.
Washington, D.C.: 1985.

The American College of Obstetricians and Gynecologists.
Genital Herpes.
Washington, D.C.: 1990.

The American College of Obstetricians and Gynecologists.
Genital Warts (Condyloma).
Washington, D.C.: 1987.

The American College of Obstetricians and Gynecologists.
Gonorrhea and Chlamydial Infections.
Washington, D.C.: 1991.

The American College of Obstetricians and Gynecologists.
How to Prevent Sexually Transmitted Diseases.
Washington, D.C.: 1991.

The American College of Obstetricians and Gynecologists.
Important Facts About Endometriosis.
Washington, D.C.: 1986.

The American College of Obstetricians and Gynecologists.
Infertility: Causes and Treatments.
Washington, D.C.: 1992.

The American College of Obstetricians and Gynecologists.
Ovarian Cysts.
Washington, D.C.: 1987.

The American College of Obstetricians and Gynecologists.
Pain During Intercourse.
Washington, D.C.: 1991.

The American College of Obstetricians and Gynecologists.
Pelvic Inflammatory Disease (PID).
Washington, D.C.: 1991.

The American College of Obstetricians and Gynecologists.
Pelvic Support Problems.
Washington, D.C.: 1991.

The American College of Obstetricians and Gynecologists.
Premenstrual Syndrome.
Washington, D.C.: 1985.

The American College of Obstetricians and Gynecologists.
Preventing Cancer.
Washington, D.C.: 1992.

The American College of Obstetricians and Gynecologists.
Preventing Osteoporosis.
Washington, D.C.: 1991.

The American College of Obstetricians and Gynecologists.
Understanding Hysterectomy.
Washington, D.C.: 1991.

The American College of Obstetricians and Gynecologists.
Urinary Incontinence.
Washington, D.C.: 1990.

The American College of Obstetricians and Gynecologists.
Urinary Tract Infections.
Washington, D.C.: 1991.

The American College of Obstetricians and Gynecologists.
Uterine Fibroids.
Washington, D.C.: 1987.

The American College of Obstetricians and Gynecologists.
Vaginitis: Causes and Treatments.
Washington, D.C.; 1986.

CHAPTER ELEVEN

Birth Control: More Options Than Ever

Planned Parenthood Federation of America, Inc.
Facts About Birth Control.
New York, N.Y.: 1989.

Planned Parenthood Federation of America, Inc.
You & the Pill.
New York, N.Y.: 1985.

Private Line.
"No!" and Other Methods of Birth Control.
Kenilworth, Ill.: 1991.

Rutgers Student Health Service.
Common Questions about Birth Control Pills.
New Brunswick, N.J.: 1991.

Rutgers Student Health Service.
Condoms and Foam.
New Brunswick, N.J.: 1991.

Rutgers Student Health Service.
Diaphragm.
New Brunswick, N.J.: 1989.

Rutgers Student Health Service.
Natural Family Planning and Awareness Method.
New Brunswick, N.J.: 1988.

Rutgers Student Health Service.
Spermicidal Vaginal Suppository.
New Brunswick, N.J.: 1986.

Rutgers Student Health Service.
The Pill–Oral Contraceptive.
New Brunswick, N.J.: 1986.

Rutgers Student Health Service.
Vaginal Contraceptive Sponge.
New Brunswick, N.J.: 1991.

Wyeth-Ayerst Laboratories.
Birth Control Options.
Philadelphia, Penn.: 1991.

CHAPTER TWELVE

Handling Familiar Childhood Infections

American Academy of Pediatrics.
Authors explain recent hepatitis B recommendation.
AAP News.
May 1992.

American Academy of Pediatrics.
Caring For Your Adolescent: Ages 12 to 21.
Elk Grove Village, Ill.: 1991.

American Academy of Pediatrics.
Diptheria, Tetanus, and Pertussis.
Elk Grove Village, Ill.: 1992.

American Academy of Pediatrics.
Facts on Immunizations.
Elk Grove Village, Ill.

American Academy of Pediatrics.
Haemophilus Influenzae Type B; What Parents Need to Know.
Elk Grove Village, Ill.: 1992.

American Academy of Pediatrics.
Haemophilus Influenzae Type B Conjugate Vaccines: Immunization of Children 2 to 15 Months of Age.
Elk Grove Village, Ill.: 1991; RE9203.

American Academy of Pediatrics.
Health Resources.
Elk Grove Village, Ill.: 1992.

American Academy of Pediatrics.
Hepatitis B; What Parents Need to Know.
Elk Grove Village, Ill.: 1992.

American Academy of Pediatrics.
Immunization Protects Children.
Elk Grove Village, Ill.: 1992.

American Academy of Pediatrics.
Measles: recessment of the current immunization policy.
Pediatrics.
1989; 84:6: 1110-13.

American Academy of Pediatrics.
Parent Resource Guide.
Elk Grove Village, Ill.: 1992.

American Academy of Pediatrics.
Report of the Committee on Infectious Disease.
Elk Grove Village, Ill.: 1991.

American Academy of Pediatrics.
Universal Hepatitis B Immunization.
Pediatrics.
April 1992: 89:4.

American Academy of Pediatrics.
You and Your Pediatrician; Common Childhood Problems.
Elk Grove Village, Ill.: 1991.

CHAPTER FOURTEEN

Relief for Common Allergies

American Academy of Allergy and Immunology.
Adverse Reactions to Food Additives.
Milwaukee, Wisc.: 1987; No. 13.

American Academy of Allergy and Immunology.
Allergic Contact Dermatitis.
Milwaukee, Wisc.: 1986; No. 7.

American Academy of Allergy and Immunology.
Allergies to Animals.
Milwaukee, Wisc.: 1992; No. 14.

American Academy of Allergy and Immunology.
Anaphylaxis.
Milwaukee, Wisc.: 1989; No. 18.

American Academy of Allergy and Immunology.
Atopic Dermatitis.
Milwaukee, Wisc.: 1987; No. 15.

American Academy of Allergy and Immunology.
Helpful Hints for the Allergic Patient.
Milwaukee, Wisc.: 1985.

American Academy of Allergy and Immunology.
Hives.
Milwaukee, Wisc.: 1987; No. 10.

American Academy of Allergy and Immunology.
Removing House Dust and Other Allergic Irritants From Your Home.
Milwaukee, Wisc.: 1992; No. 2.

American Academy of Allergy and Immunology.

Stinging Insect Allergy.
Milwaukee, Wisc.: 1991.

American Academy of Allergy and Immunology.
The Role of the Trained Allergist and Clinical Immunologist in Cost Effective Patient Care.
Milwaukee, Wisc.: 1992.

American Academy of Allergy and Immunology.
Understanding the Pollen and Mold Season.
Milwaukee, Wisc.: 1992; No. 8.

American Academy of Allergy and Immunology.
What Every Patient Should Know About Asthma and Allergy Medications.
Milwaukee, Wisc.: 1987; No. 12.

American Academy of Allergy and Immunology.
What Is an Allergic reaction?
Milwaukee, Wisc.: 1986; No. 5.

CHAPTER FIFTEEN

Dealing with Skin Problems

American Academy of Dermatology.
Acne.
Evanston, Ill.: 1991; TPAM02 9/91.

American Academy of Dermatology.
Allergic Contact Rashes.
Evanston, Ill.: 1990; TPAM15 6/90.

American Academy of Dermatology.
Athlete's Foot.
Evanston, Ill.: 1990; TPAM-19.

American Academy of Dermatology.
Atopic Eczema/Dermatitis.
Schaumburg, Ill.: 1992; TPAM07.

American Academy of Dermatology.
Common Sense About Moles.
Evanston, Ill.: 1991; TPAM-04 3/91.

American Academy of Dermatology.
Dermatologic Survey.
Schaumburg, Ill.: 1992; TPAM23 4/92.

American Academy of Dermatology.
Facts About Black Skin.
Schaumburg, Ill.: 1986; TPAM18 4/92.

American Academy of Dermatology.
Hair Loss.
Evanston, Ill.: 1991; TPAM21.

American Academy of Dermatology.
Hand Eczema.
Evanston, Ill.: 1991; TPAM09-9/91.

American Academy of Dermatology.
Herpes Simplex.
Evanston, Ill.: 1991; TPAM20-8/91.

American Academy of Dermatology.
Lifelong Healthy Skin.
Evanston, Ill.: 1991; TPAM28 5/88.

American Academy of Dermatology.
**Melanoma/Skin Cancer;
You can Recognize the Signs.**
Schaumburg, Ill.: 1990; TPAM14-2/92.

American Academy of Dermatology.
Permanent Hair Replacement—Transplantation of Hair to Correct Baldness.
Schaumberg, Ill.: 1988; TPAM31 5/92.

American Academy of Dermatology.
Pityriasis Rosea.
Schaumburg, Ill.: 1987; TPAM26-4/92.

American Academy of Dermatology.
Psoriasis.
Schaumburg, Ill.: 1991; TPAM13.

American Academy of Dermatology.
Reactions to Cosmetics.
Evanston, Ill.: 1987; TPAM 17-9/87.

American Academy of Dermatology.
**Resources for Dermatology:
Patient Education and Support Groups.**
Schaumburg, Ill.: 1992.

American Academy of Dermatology.
Rosacea.
Schaumburg, Ill.: 1990; TPAM 36 3/92.

American Academy of Dermatology.
Scabies.
Evanston, Ill.: 1991; TPAM37 10/91.

American Academy of Dermatology.
Seborrheic Dermatitis.
Schaumburg, Ill.: 1991; TPAM24.

American Academy of Dermatology.
Skin Cancer Fact Sheet.
Schaumburg, Ill.: 1992.

American Academy of Dermatology.
Skin Care Under the Sun—The Importance of Sun Protection.
Evanston, Ill.: 1988; TPAM30 7/91.

American Academy of Dermatology.
Skin Conditions Related to AIDS and Human Immunodeficiency Virus (HIV) Infection.
Evanston, Ill.: 1988; TPAM08 1/88.

American Academy of Dermatology.
Spider Vein, Varicose Vein Therapy.
Schaumburg, Ill.: 1991; TPAM16 2/92.

American Academy of Dermatology.
Sun Protection for Children; A Parent's Guide.
Schaumburg, Ill.: 1989; TPAM33 4/92.

American Academy of Dermatology.
The Sun and Your Skin.
Evanston, Ill.: 1990; TPAM06.

American Academy of Dermatology.
Tinea Versicolor.
Schaumburg, Ill.: 1991; TPAM27 4/92.

American Academy of Dermatology.
Uticaria—Hives.
Schaumburg, Ill.: 1992; TPAM22.

American Academy of Dermatology.
Vascular Birthmarks.
Evanston, Ill.: 1986; TPAM10 4/86.

American Academy of Dermatology.
Vitiligo.
Schaumburg, Ill.: 1992; TPAM07 4/92.

American Academy of Dermatology.
Warts.
Evanston, Ill.: 1991; TPAM03-5/91.

American Academy of Dermatology.
What's in a Scar.
Evanston, Ill.: 1991; TPAM35 2/91.

American Academy of Dermatology.
Your Skin and Your Dermatologist.
Evanston, Ill.: 1987: TPAM01 8/88.

Brody, Jane E.
The sun: an attractive menace for the skin that is exacting an ever-worsening toll.
Personal Health.
June 19, 1991.

CHAPTER SIXTEEN

Correcting Glandular Disorders

Nurses Clinical Library.
Endocrine Disorders.
Springhouse, Penn.: Nursing 84 Books, Springhouse Corporation; 1984.

CHAPTER SEVENTEEN

Counterattacking Major Infections

Benenson, Abram S.
Control of Communicable Diseases in Man.
15th Ed. Washington, D.C.: American Public Health Association; 1990; ISBN 0-87553-170-9.

CHAPTER EIGHTEEN

Overcoming Kidney Disease

The National Kidney Foundation, Inc.
About Kidney Stones.
New York, N.Y.: 1990; 08-047.

The National Kidney Foundation, Inc.
About Organ and Tissue Donation.
New York, N.Y.: 1991; 14449AD-9-90.

The National Kidney Foundation, Inc.
About Urinary Tract Disorders.
New York, N.Y.: 1990; 12880D-7-88.

The National Kidney Foundation, Inc.
Coping Effectively—A Guide for Patients and Families.
New York, N.Y.: 1989; 0871.

The National Kidney Foundation, Inc.
Diabetes and Kidney Disease.
New York, N.Y.: 1991; 02-09-PP.

The National Kidney Foundation, Inc.
Dialysis.
New York, N.Y.: 1991; 03-01-PP.

The National Kidney Foundation, Inc.
Dining out with Confidence (A Guide For Renal Patients).
New York, N.Y.: 1992; 04-05MP.

The National Kidney Foundation, Inc.
EPO: Treating Anemia in Chronic Renal Failure.
New York, N.Y.: 1991; 03-05-CP.

The National Kidney Foundation, Inc.
Family Focus . . . The Renal Community's Newspaper.
New York, N.Y.: 1991; Vol. 3 No. 1.

The National Kidney Foundation, Inc.
Fitness after Kidney Failure—Building Strength Through Exercise.
New York, N.Y.: 1990; 08-58.

The National Kidney Foundation, Inc.
Glomerulonephritis.
New York, N.Y.: 1987; 08-67-87 50M.

The National Kidney Foundation, Inc.
High Blood Pressure & Your Kidneys.
New York, N.Y.: 1990; 08-38.

The National Kidney Foundation, Inc.
How Common is Kidney Disease in the USA?
New York, N.Y.

The National Kidney Foundation, Inc.
Kidney Transplant—A New Lease on Life.
New York, N.Y.: 1991; 03-04-CP.

The National Kidney Foundation, Inc.
New Technique for Treating Kidney Stones.
New York, N.Y.: 1987; 08-68-87 50M/4-87.

The National Kidney Foundation, Inc.
Nutrition and Changing Kidney Function.
New York, N.Y.: 1990; 08-55.

The National Kidney Foundation, Inc.
Nutrition and Hemodialysis.
New York, N.Y.: 1990; 08-57.

The National Kidney Foundation, Inc.
Nutrition and Peritoneal Dialysis.
New York, N.Y.: 1990; 08-62.

The National Kidney Foundation, Inc.
Nutrition and Transplantation.
New York, N.Y.: 1990; 08-66.

The National Kidney Foundation, Inc.
Peritoneal Dialysis—An Alternative to Hemodialysis.
New York, N.Y.: 1986; 08-64.

The National Kidney Foundation, Inc.
Polycystic Kidney Disease.
New York, N.Y.: 1990; 08-45.

The National Kidney Foundation, Inc.
Sexuality and Chronic Kidney Failure.
New York, N.Y.: 1991; 05-04-PP.

The National Kidney Foundation, Inc.
Social Work Service for the Patient with Chronic Renal Failure.
New York, N.Y.: 1991; 08-01-PP.

The National Kidney Foundation, Inc.
Statistics and Facts.
New York, N.Y.

The National Kidney Foundation, Inc.
Sun—Summer Newsletter.
New York, N.Y.: 1992; 9:1.

The National Kidney Foundation, Inc.
The Health Care Team.
New York, N.Y.: 1991; 08-22-PP.

The National Kidney Foundation, Inc.
The Organ Donor Program.
New York, N.Y.: 1988; 08-37.

The National Kidney Foundation, Inc.
Treating Impotence: A Sexual Problem in Men.
New York, N.Y.: 1991; 02-13-CP.

The National Kidney Foundation, Inc.
Urinary Incontinence: Treating Loss of Urine Control.
New York, N.Y.: 1991; 02-02-CP.

The National Kidney Foundation, Inc.
Urinary Tract Infections.
New York, N.Y.: 1990; 08-53.

The National Kidney Foundation, Inc.
Urinary Tract Obstructions.
New York, N.Y.: 1986; 08-39-86 50M.

The National Kidney Foundation, Inc.
What Everyone Should Know About Kidneys and Kidney Disease.
New York, N.Y.: 1992; No. 11593.

The National Kidney Foundation, Inc.
Working with Kidney Disease.
New York, N.Y.: 1990; 08-54.

U.S. Department of Health and Human Services.
Medicare—Coverage of Kidney Dialysis and Kidney Transplant Services.
Baltimore, Md.: 1991; No.HCFA 10128.

CHAPTER NINETEEN

Bringing Urinary Disorders under Control

Bowe, Claudia.
Body briefing: The urinary tract.
Lears.
Sept. 1989.

National Institutes of Health Consensus Development Conference Statement.
Urinary Incontinence in Adults.
Bethesda, Md.: October 3-5, 1988; Vol. 7, No. 5.

The Bladder Health Council.
Answers to Your Questions About Urinary Tract Infections.
Baltimore, Md.: 1992.

U.S. Department of Health and Human Services.
Urinary Tract Infection in Adults.
Bethesda, Md.: 1991; No. 91-2097.

CHAPTER TWENTY

Dealing with Liver Disease

American Liver Foundation.
Alcohol and the Liver; Myths vs. Facts.
Cedar Grove, N.J.: 1989.

American Liver Foundation.
Cirrhosis.
Cedar Grove, N.J.: 1991.

American Liver Foundation.
Hepatitis A, B, and C—Liver Diseases You Should Know About.
Cedar Grove, N.J.: 1992.

American Liver Foundation.
Your Liver Lets You Live.
Cedar Grove, N.J.: 1992.

CHAPTER TWENTY-TWO

The Facts about AIDS

American Foundation for AIDS Research (AMFAR).
AIDS/HIV Treatment Directory.
;New York, N.Y.: 1992; Vol. 5, No. 4, ISSN 0898-5030.

Centers For Disease Control; U.S. Department of Health and Human Services.
AIDS and You.
Atlanta, Ga.: 1991; DO56.

Centers For Disease Control; U.S. Department of Health and Human Services.
HIV Infection.
Atlanta, Ga.: 1991; No. 18, 00-5923.

Centers for Disease Control; U.S. Department of Health and Human Services.
Morbidity and Mortality Weekly Report.
Atlanta, Ga.: 36:31: 509-26.

Centers For Disease Control, U.S. Department of Health and Human Services.
Surgeon General's Report on Acquired Immune Deficiency Syndrome.
Atlanta, Ga.: 1991.

Norwood, Chris.
Advice For Life: A Woman's Guide to AIDS Risks and Prevention.
New York: Pantheon Books; 1987.

Switching drugs is found to help in AIDS cases.
The New York Times National.
August 27, 1992; B7.

CHAPTER TWENTY-THREE

Keeping Diabetes under Control

American Diabetes Association.
Month of Meals.
Alexandria, Va.: 1990.

American Diabetes Association.
1992 Product Catalog.
McLean, Va.: 1992.

American Diabetes Association.
What You Need to Know About Diabetes (an Introduction).
Alexandria, Va.: 1984; 12/91-200M.

Becton Dickinson Consumer Products.
Blood Glucose Testing.
Franklin Lakes, N.J.: 1985; Cat.9941.

Becton Dickinson Consumer Products.
Controlling Low Blood Sugar Reaction.
Franklin Lakes, N.J.: 1989; Cat.9948.

Becton Dickinson Consumer Products.
Drawing and Injection Insulin.
Franklin Lakes, N.J.: 1989; Cat.9902.

Becton Dickinson Consumer Products.
Exercise and its Benefits.
Franklin Lakes, N.J.: 1989; Cat.9943.

Becton Dickinson Consumer Products.
Mixing Insulins.
Franklin Lakes, N.J.: 1985; Cat.9903.

Becton Dickinson Consumer Products.
Vacations, Travel, and Diabetes.
Franklin Lakes, N.J.: 1985; Cat.9945.

Diabetes Center of New Jersey.
Bringing Diabetes Education to You.
Plainfield, N.J.: 1988.

Eli Lilly and Company.
Basic Meal Planning.
Indianapolis, Ind.: 1991; 60-HI-2722-0.

Eli Lilly and Company.
High Blood Sugar.
Indianapolis, Ind.: 1991; 60-HI-2725-0.

HDI-Home Diagnostics Inc.
Blood Sugar Testing System.
Eatontown, N.J.: 1991; U1020 1291.

Mandel, Ellen D.
Nutritionally Speaking; The Diabetic Diet: A Model for Americans.
Chatham, N.J.: The Nutrition Counseling Center.

Metro Drugs.
Diabetes Control Center—Products and Supplies.
N.J.

Squibb Novo.
Type II Diabetes Mellitus.
1989: 269-050B.

CHAPTER TWENTY-FOUR

Correcting Disorders in the Blood

Aplastic Anemia Foundation of America.
The Blood System: Erythrocytes, Platelets, Leukocytes and the Immune System.
Baltimore, Md.: 1990.

Bank, A. Blood Disorders. In: Fubak-Sharpe, Genell, ed.
The Columbia University College of Physicians and Surgeons Complete Home Medical Guide.
New York: Crown; 1989: 536-539.

Benedict, CR, Mueller S, Anderson, HV, Willerson, JT.
Thrombolytic therapy: a state of the art review.
Hospital Practice.
June 15, 1992: 61-72.

Bithell, TC. Disorders of Platelets. In:
Fundamentals of Clinical Hematology (Fifth edition).
Philadelphia: W.B. Saunders Company; 1987: 792-819.

Bone Marrow Failure. In:
Fundamentals of Clinical Hematology (Fifth edition).
Philadelphia: W.B. Saunders Company; 1987:
364-372.

Braman, AM, Schwartz, KA.
Platelet disorders.
Laboratory Medicine.
December, 1989: 831-835.

Disorders of Blood Coagulation. In: Fubak-Sharpe,
Genell, ed.
**The Columbia University College of Physicians and
Surgeons Complete Home Medical Guide.**
New York: Crown; 1989: 545-46.

Gaston, M,
Sickle Cell Anemia.
Bethesda, Md.: U.S. Department of Health and
Human Services; June 1990.

Giardina, PJ, Hilgartner, MW.
Thalassemia: practical points.
Hospital Medicine.
June 1985: 162-205.

Runge, MS.
The future of thrombolytic therapy.
Heart Disease and Stroke.
January/February, 1992: 39-42.

U.S. Department of Health and Human Services.
**Cooley's Anemia: Prevention Through
Understanding.**
Bethesda, Md.: 1980.

U.S. Department of Health and Human Services.
Management and Therapy of Sickle Cell Disease.
Charache, S, Lubin, B, Reid, CD, eds. Bethseda, Md.:
1992.

CHAPTER TWENTY-FIVE

Relief for Troubled Feet

American Academy of Orthopaedic Surgeons.
Common Foot Problems.
Park Ridge, Ill.: 1991.

American Podiatric Medical Association.
Aging.
Bethesda, Md.: 1991.

American Podiatric Medical Association.
Arthritis.
Bethesda, Md.: 1992.

American Podiatric Medical Association.
Athlete's Foot.
Bethesda, Md.: 1990.

American Podiatric Medical Association.
Careers in Podiatric Medicine.
Bethesda, Md.: 1991.

American Podiatric Medical Association.
Children's Feet.
Bethesda, Md.: 1992.

American Podiatric Medical Association.
Diabetes.
Bethesda, Md.: 1992.

American Podiatric Medical Association.
Foot and Ankle Injuries.
Bethesda, Md.: 1990.

American Podiatric Medical Association.
Foot Health.
Bethesda, Md.: 1990.

American Podiatric Medical Association.
Foot Surgery.
Bethesda, Md.: 1991.

American Podiatric Medical Association.
Heel Pain.
Bethesda, Md.: 1991.

American Podiatric Medical Association.
High Blood Pressure.
Bethesda, Md.: 1991.

American Podiatric Medical Association.
Medicare.
Bethesda, Md.: 1990.

American Podiatric Medical Association.
Nail Problems.
Bethesda, Md.: 1991.

American Podiatric Medical Association.
On-the-Job Foot Health.
Bethesda, Md.: 1990.

American Podiatric Medical Association.
Orthoses (Arch Supports).
Bethesda, Md.: 1991.

American Podiatric Medical Association.
Podiatric Medicine (the Physician, the Profession, the Practice).
Bethesda, Md.: 1990.

American Podiatric Medical Association.
Walking.
Bethesda, Md.: 1991.

American Podiatric Medical Association.
Warts.
Bethesda, Md.: 1990.

CHAPTER TWENTY-SIX

Drugs and the Elderly

Barnhart, Edward R.
PDR 1991 Physicians' Desk Reference for Nonprescription Drugs,
12th ed. Montvale, N.J.: Medical Economics Data; 1991.

Gould, Mark A.
A Consumer's Guide to Psychiatric Diagnosis.
Summit, N.J.: The PIA Press; 1989.

Graedon, Teresa, Graedon, Joe.
50+; The Graedons' People's Pharmacy for Older Adults.
New York: Bantam Books; 1988.

Intermed Communications, Inc.
Professional Guide to Drugs.
Second Ed. Springhouse, Penn.: 1982.

Jarvik, Lissy, Small, Gary.
Parentcare: A Compassionate, Commonsense Guide for Children and Their Aging Parents.
New York: Bantam Books; 1990.

Schwartz, Arthur N.
Survival Handbook for Children of Aging Parents.
Chicago: Follett Publishing Company; 1977.
Silverstone, Barbara, Hyman, Helen Kandel.
You and Your Aging Parent.
New York: Pantheon Books, a Division of Random House, Inc.; 1976.

The American Psychiatric Association.
Diagnostic and Statistical Manual of Mental Disorders.
Third Ed., Revised. Washington, D.C.: 1987.

The Boston Women's Health Book Collection.
The New Our Bodies, Ourselves.
New York, Simon & Schuster Inc.; 1992.

Uris, Auren.
The Definitive Guide to the Best Years of Your Life Over 50.
New York: Bantam Books; 1981.

GENERAL REFERENCE

Brace, Edward R., Anderson, Kenneth.
The New Pediatric Guide to Drugs and Vitamins.
Tucson, Ariz.: The Stonesong Press; 1987.

Chilnick, LD, ed.
The Pill Book.
Fifth Edition. New York: Bantam Books; 1992.

Chilnick, LD, ed.
The Pill Book of Anxiety and Depression.
New York: Bantam Books; 1986.

Chilnick, LD, ed.
The Pill Book of Arthritis Drugs & Treatment.
New York: Bantam Books; 1985.

Chilnick, LD, ed.
The Pill Book of Heart Disease Drugs & Treatment.
New York: Bantam Books; 1985.

Chilnick, LD, ed.
The Pill Book of High Blood Pressure.
New York: Bantam Books; 1985.

Extein, Irl.
Guide to the New Medicines of the Mind.
Summit, N.J.: The PIA Press; 1988.

Gold, Mark S.
The Facts About Drugs and Alcohol.
Third Edition, revised. New York: Bantam Books;
1988.

Gold, Mark S.
**The Good News About Drugs and Alcohol; Curing,
Treating and Preventing Substance Abuse in the
New Age of Biopsychiatry.**
New York: Villard Books; 1991.

Gold, Mark S, Boyette, Michael.
Wonder Drugs: How They Work.
New York: Pocket Books of Simon & Schuster Inc.:
1987.

Gould, Mark A.
A Consumer's Guide to Pschiatric Diagnosis
Summit, N.J.: PIA Press; 1989.

Graedon, Teresa, Graedon, Joe.
**50+; The Graedons' People's Pharmacy for Older
Adults.**
New York: Bantam Books; 1988.

Intermed Communications, Inc.
Professional Guide to Drugs.
Second Edition. Springhouse, Pa.: 1982.

Jarvik, Lissy, Small, Gary.
**Parentcare; A Commpassionate, Commonsense
Guide for Children and Their Aging Parents.**
New York: Bantam Books; 1990.

Langley, Beryl W., Stapp, Joyce E.
For Women Only; A Guide to Emotional Well-Being.
New York: Berkley Books; 1990.

Long, James W.
The Essential Guide to Prescription Drugs.
New York: Harper Collins Publishers, Inc.; 1992.

ME Data Company.
1992 Drug Topics Red Book.
Montvale, N.J.: 1992.

ME Data Company.
**PDR 1993 Physicians' Desk Reference for
Nonprescription Drugs.**
14th Edition. Montvale, N.J.: 1993.

Othmer, Ekkehard, Othmer, Sieglinde C.
**Life on a Roller Coaster; Coping With the Ups and
Downs of Mood Disorders.**
Summit, N.J.: The PIA Press; 1989.

Schwartz, Arthur N.
Survival Handbook for Children of Aging Parents.
Chicago: Follett Publishing Company; 1977.

Silverstone, Barbara; Hyman, Helen Kandel.
You and Your Aging Parent.
New York: Pantheon Books, a Division of Random
House, Inc.; 1976.

Solomon, Harold S, Chilnick, L.D.
Beat the Odds.
New York: Villard Books; 1986.

The American Medical Associaltion; Clayton, Charles
B, ed.
Home Medical Encyclopedia.
New York: Random House; 1989.

The American Psychiatric Association.
**Diagnostic and Statistical Manual of Mental
Disorders.**
Third Edition, Revised. Washington, D.C.: 1987.

The Boston Women's Health Book Collection.
The New Our Bodies, Ourselves.
New York: Simon & Schuster Inc.: 1992.

Uris, Auren.
**The Definitive Guide to the Best Years of Your Life
Over 50.**
New York: Bantam Books; 1981.

Vickery, Donald M, Fries, James F.
**Take Care of Yourself; A Consumer's Guide to
Medical Care.**
Sixth Edition, Revised. Reading, Mass.: Addison-
Wesley Publishing Company, Inc.; 1984. □

Disease and Disorder Index

Use this index to find the various drugs prescribed for a specific medical problem. Both brand and generic names are listed; the generic names are shown in italics. Only those brands covered in the drug profiles are included.

Acne
Accutane.................................1
Achromycin V 3
A/T/S....................................242
Benzac W.............................181
Benzagel 181
BenzaShave...........................181
Benzamycin 63
Benzoyl Peroxide....................181
Cleocin T..............................113
Clindamycin Phosphate..........113
Desquam-E............................181
Doryx...................................216
Doxycycline Hyclate..............216
Erycette 242
Erythromycin, Oral 239
Erythromycin with Benzoyl
    Peroxide..............................63
Isotretinoin..............................1
Minocin................................385
Minocycline Hydrochloride ...385

Retin-A................................538
Sumycin..................................3
T-Stat 242
Tetracycline Hydrochloride 3
Theroxide.............................181
Tretinoin 538
Vibramycin...........................216

Adrenal gland tumors
Inderal.................................290
Propanolol Hydrochloride.....290

Adrenal hormone deficiency
Decadron Tablets 165
Deltasone.............................172
Dexamethasone.....................165
Medrol 361
Methylprednisolone 361
Orasone................................172
Pediapred.............................457
Prednisolone Sodium
    Phosphate 457
Prednisone............................172

AIDS and AIDS-related infections
See Infections, HIV

Alcohol withdrawal
Chlordiazepoxide
    Hydrochloride 320
Diazepam 667
Libritabs 320
Librium 320
Valium 667

Allergies, severe
Cyproheptadine
    Hydrochloride..................467
Decadron Tablets..................165
Deltasone.............................172
Dexamethasone 165
Medrol 361
Methylprednisolone 361
Orasone 172
PBZ-SR................................448
Pediapred.............................457
Periactin..............................467
Prednisolone Sodium
    Phosphate 457
Prednisone 172
Tripelennamine
    Hydrochloride..................448

Allergies, symptomatic relief of,
Astemizole 279
Atarax 42
Azatadine Maleate and
    Pseudoephedrine Sulfate....656
Benadryl 59
Clemastine Fumarate 606
Cyproheptadine
    Hydrochloride..................467
Dexchlorpheniramine
    Maleate 489
Diphenhydramine
    Hydrochloride....................59
Hismanal 279
Hydroxyzine Hydrochloride ...42
PBZ-SR................................448
Periactin 467
Phenergan 474
Polaramine............................489

Promethazine
  Hydrochloride 474
Seldane 571
Tavist...................................606
Terfenadine.........................571
Trinalin Repetabs 656
Tripelennamine
  Hydrochloride...................448

Angina

Atenolol...............................616
Bepridil Hydrochloride 669
Calan 81
Calan SR..................................81
Cardene 91
Cardizem 94
Corgard 135
Diltiazem Hydrochloride 94
Inderal 290
Isoptin 81
Isoptin SR 81
Isosadil 303
Isosorbide Dinitrate..............303
Lopressor..............................337
Metoprolol Tartrate..............337
Nadolol 135
Nicardipine Hydrochloride 91
Nifedipine 505
Nitro-Bid 420
Nitro-Dur 420
Nitroglycerin 420
Nitrolingual Spray 420
Nitrostat Tablets....................420
Procardia 505
Propranolol Hydrochloride...290
Sorbitrate 303
Tenormin 616
Transderm-Nitro....................420
Vascor 669
Verapamil Hydrochloride 81
Verelan 81

Anxiety disorders

Alprazolam 689
Atarax 42
Ativan 44
BuSpar 74
Buspirone Hydrochloride........74
Centrax..................................105
Chlordiazepoxide
  Hydrochloride 320
Clorazepate Dipotassium 644
Compazine 132
Diazepam 667
Equanil 382
Hydroxyzine Hydrochloride .420
Lorazepam..............................44
Librium.................................320
Meprobamate 382
Miltown 382
Oxazepam 575
Prazepam.............................105
Prochlorperazine..................132
Serax 575
Stelazine 588
Tranxene 644
Trifluoperazine
  Hydrochloride 588
Valium 667
Xanax 689

Arthritis

Anaprox 27
Ansaid 31
Aspirin...................................40
Auranofin 542
Butazolidin 76
Choline Magnesium
  Trisalicylate.......................654
Clinoril 115
Decadron Tablets..................165
Deltasone 172
Dexamethasone 165
Diclofenac Sodium...............682
Diflunisal.............................208
Disalcid.................................204
Dolobid 208
Empirin.................................40
Etodolac 331
Feldene 250

Fenoprofen Calcium 398
Flurbiprofen...........................31
Genuine Bayer 40
Hydroxychloroquine Sulfate .485
Ibuprofen.............................393
Indocin 295
Indomethacin 295
Ketoprofen............................445
Lodine 331
Meclofenamate Sodium.........359
Meclomen 359
Medrol 361
Methotrexate 368
Methylprednisolone 361
Motrin Tablets.......................393
Nalfon 398
Naprosyn 402
Naproxen 402
Naproxen Sodium...................27
Orudis 445
Pediapred 457
Phenylbutazone 76
Piroxicam 250
Plaquenil 485
Prednisolone Sodium
  Phosphate 457
Prednisone 172
Ridaura 542
Salsalate 204
Sulindac 115
Tolectin 636
Tolmetin Sodium 636
Trilisate 654
Voltaren................................682

Asthma

AeroBid 9
Albuterol Sulfate 518
Alupent 20
Atrovent 46
Beclomethasone Dipropionate 57
Beclovent Inhalation Aerosol ..57
Brethine 69
Bricanyl 69
Bronkometer...........................71

Choledyl 107
Cromolyn Sodium................144
Decadron Turbinaire 167
Decadron Tablets................165
Deltasone 172
Dexamethasone 165
Flunisolide 9
Intal 144
Ipratropium Bromide..............46
Isoetharine 71
Medrol 361
Metaproterenol Sulfate............20
Methylprednisolone 361
Oxtriphylline 107
Pediapred 457
*Prednisolone Sodium
    Phosphate* 457
Prednisone 172
Proventil 518
Terbutaline Sulfate................69
Theophylline 622
Theo-Dur 622
Vanceril 57
Ventolin............................518

Athletes foot
See Infections, fungal

**Attention-deficit disorders
with hyperactivity**
Cylert..................................150
Dexedrine 184
Dextroamphetamine Sulfate..184
*Methylphenidate
    Hydrochloride*..................546
Pemoline 150
Ritalin................................546

Baldness
Minoxidil............................552
Rogaine 552

Bed-wetting
DDAVP 156
Desmopressin Acetate..........156
Imipramine Hydrochloride ...633
Janimine 633
Tofranil 633

**Behavior problems
in children, severe**
Chlorpromazine..................625
Haldol 277
Haloperidol 277
Thorazine 625

Bleeding, postpartum
Methergine 367
Methylergonovine Maleate....367

Bleeding, uterine, abnormal
*Medroxyprogesterone
    Acetate* 521
Provera 521

Blood pressure, high
See High blood pressure

Blood clotting abnormalities
Coumadin..........................140
Dipyridamole......................472
Persantine 472
Warfarin Sodium 140

Bowel cleansing
Colyte 130
*Polyethylene Glycol with
    Electrolytes* 130

Breast milk suppression
Bromocriptine Mesylate........455
Parlodel 455

Bursitis
See Inflammatory diseases

Burns
Silvadene Cream 577
Silver Sulfadiazine................577

Calcium levels, high
Calcimar 84
Calcitonin-Salmon 84

Calcium levels, low
Calcitriol............................550
Rocaltrol............................550

Cancer
Android 29
Cyclophosphamide 154
Cytoxan..............................154
Diethylstilbestrol..................193
Efudex 224
Estrogens, Conjugated 498

Eulexin 245
Fluorouracil 224
Flutamide 225
Megace 363
Megestrol Acetate 363
Methotrexate 368
Methyltestosterone................29
Nolvadex 425
Premarin 498
Tamoxifen Citrate................425

Candidiasis
Butoconazole Nitrate 252
Femstat 252
Miconazole Nitrate 390
Monistat 3 390
Terazol 3 620
Terconazole 620

Chickenpox
Acyclovir 704
Zovirax................................704

Cholera
Doryx 216
Doxycycline Hyclate 216
Minocin 385
Minocycline Hydrochloride ..385
Vibramycin 216

Cholesterol levels, high
Cholestyramine Resin 528
Colestid 126
Colestipol Hydrochloride......126
Gemfibrozil 335
Lopid 335
Lorelco 340
Lovastatin 371
Mevacor 371
Pravachol............................494
Pravastatin Sodium 494
Probucol 340
Questran 528
Simvastatin 699
Zocor................................699

Circulation, impaired
Also see Leg cramps
Pentoxifylline 646
Trental 646

Colds
See Coughs and Colds

Colitis
Azulfidine 51
Decadron Tablets 165
Deltasone 172
Dexamethasone 165
Dipentum 202
Medrol 361
Mesalamine 556
Methylprednisolone 361
Olsalazine Sodium 202
Orasone 172
Pediapred 457
Prednisolone Sodium
  Phosphate 457
Prednisone 172
Rowasa 556
Sulfasalazine 51

Collagen diseases
Decadron Tablets 165
Deltasone 172
Dexamethasone 165
Medrol 361
Methylprednisolone 361
Orasone 172
Pediapred 457
Prednisolone Sodium
  Phosphate 457
Prednisone 172

Constipation
Chronulac Syrup 110
Colace 123
Docusate Sodium 123
Duphalac 110
Lactulose 110

Contraception
Demulen 437

Levlen 437
Loestrin 437
Lo/Ovral 437
Modicon 437
Nordette 437
Norethin 437
Norinyl 437
Ortho-Novum 437
Ovcon 437
Ovral 437
Ovrette 437
Triphasil 437

Coughs and colds
Azatadine Maleate and
  Pseudoephedrine Sulfate 656
Benadryl 59
Benzonatate 621
Cyproheptadine
  Hydrochloride 467
Deconamine 170
Dimetane-DC 200
Diphenhydramine
  Hydrochloride 59
Entex LA 237
Iodinated Glycerol with
  Dextromethorphan 658
Nolamine 424
PBZ-SR 448
Periactin 467
Phenergan with Codeine 476
Phenylpropanolamine with
  Guaifenesin 237
Promethazine with Codeine ..476
Ru-Tuss Tablets 558
Rynatan 560
Tessalon 621

Trinalin Repetabs 656
Tripelennamine
  Hydrochloride 448
Tussionex 659
Tussi-Organidin DM 658

Depression
Adapin 581
Amitriptyline Hydrochloride .226
Amoxapine 38
Asendin 38
Aventyl 450
Bupropion Hydrochloride 685
Chlordiazepoxide with
  Amitriptyline
  Hydrochloride 324
Desipramine Hydrochloride ..435
Desyrel 182
Doxepin Hydrochloride 581
Elavil 226
Endep 226
Fluoxetine Hydrochloride 523
Imipramine Hydrochloride ...633
Janimine 633
Limbitrol 324
Ludiomil 348
Maprotiline Hydrochloride ...348
Nardil 404
Norpramin 435
Nortriptyline Hydrochloride .450
Pamelor 450
Perphenazine and Amitryptyline
  Hydrochloride 648
Phenelzine Sulfate 404
Prozac 523
Sertraline Hydrochloride 702
Sinequan 581
Surmontil 593
Tofranil 633
Trazodone Hydrochloride 182
Triavil 648
Trimipramine Maleate 593
Wellbutrin 685
Zoloft 702

Diabetes
Chlorpropamide 187
Diabeta 377
Diabinese 188
Glipizide 270
Glucotrol 270
Glyburide 377
Humulin 297
Iletin I 297
Iletin II 297
Insulatard 297
Insulin 297
Insulin, NPH......................297
Insulin, Regular 297
Micronase 377
Mixtard 297
Novolin 297
Orinase 442
Tolazamide 638
Tolbutamide 442
Tolinase 638
Velosulin...........................297

Diabetes, insipidus
DDAVP 156
Desmopressin Acetate 156

Diarrhea
Diphenoxylate with Atropine
    Sulfate 333
Donnagel-PG 210
Imodium 288
Lomotil 333
Loperamide Hydrochloride ...288

Diarrhea, infectious
Bactrim 53
Cipro 111
Ciprofloxacin
    Hydrochloride 111
Colistin Sulfate 128
Coly-Mycin S Oral...............128
Cotrim 53
Doryx 216
Doxycycline Hyclate 216
Septra 53

Trimethoprim with
    Sulfamethoxazole 53
Vibramycin 216

Dysentery
Doryx 216
Doxycycline Hyclate 216
Flagyl...............................259
Metronidazole.....................259
Minocin 385
Minocycline Hydrochloride ..385
Vibramycin 216

Earache
Antipyrine and Benzocaine
    in Glycerin 48
Auralgan............................48

Edema
See Fluid retention

Emphysema
See Asthma

Epilepsy
Acetazolamide Sodium..........190
Atretol 608
Carbamazepine 608
Clonazepam 308
Depakene 177
Depakote 178
Diamox..............................190
Diazepam 667
Dilantin 195
Divalproex Sodium 178
Epitol................................608
Klonopin 308
Mysoline 396
Phenobarbital 478
Phenytoin Sodium................195
Primidone 396
Tegretol 608
Tridione 652
Trimethadione 652
Valium...............................667
Valproic Acid.......................177

Eye, infections
See Infections, eye

Eye, inflammation of
See Inflammatory diseases
    of the eye

Fever
Acetaminophen 661
Aspirin 40
Aspirin Free Anacin 661
Empirin 40
Genuine Bayer 40
Panadol.............................661
Tylenol 661

Flu prevention or treatment
Amantadine Hydrochloride ..595
Symadine 595
Symmetrel..........................595

Fluid retention
Acetazolamide Sodium..........190
Bumetanide.........................72
Bumex 72
Chlorothiazide 206
Chlorthalidone 284
Diamox..............................190
Diuril...............................206
Dyazide.............................219
Esidrix 281
Furosemide 314
HydroDIURIL......................281
Hydrochlorothiazide.............281
Hygroton 284
Indapamide.........................347
Lasix................................314
Lozol 346
Maxzide............................357
Thalitone 284
Triamterene with
    Hydrochlorothiazide ..219,357

Fluoride deficiency
Luride 351
Sodium Fluoride 351

Gallstones
Actigall 7
Ursodiol............................7

Gingivitis
Chlorhexidine Gluconate 469
Peridex................................469

Glaucoma
Acetazolamide Sodium...........190
Betagan.................................65
Betaxolol Hydrochloride
    (Ophthalmic) 66
Betoptic 66
Diamox................................190
Dipivefrin Hydrochloride 513
Echothiophate Iodide 481
Isopto-Carpine.....................483
Levobunolol Hydrochloride....65
Methazolamide 412
Neptazane............................412
Phospholine Iodide 481
Pilocar 483
Pilocarpine Hydrochloride 483
Propine 513
Timolol Maleate
    (Ophthalmic) 630
Timoptic 630

Gonorrhea
See Sexually transmitted diseases

Gout
Allopurinol 705
Anaprox 27
ColBENEMID.......................124
Col-Probenecid 124
Naprosyn.............................402
Naproxen 402
Naproxen Sodium.................402
Probenecid with
    Colchicine 124
Zyloprim 705

Hay fever
Astemizole 279
Azatadine Maleate and
    Pseudoephedrine Sulfate....656
Beclomethasone
    Dipropionate.....................57
Beconase 57
Beconase AQ Nasal Spray.......57
Benadryl 59

Carbinoxamine and
    Pseudoephedrine
    Hydrochloride 57
Clemastine Fumarate 606
Decadron Turbinaire 167
Deconamine 170
Dexamethasone 165
Dexchlorpheniramine
    Maleate 489
Diphenhydramine
    Hydrochloride 59
Hismanal 279
Nasalcrom 144
Nolamine 424
PBZ-SR 448
Phenergan 474
Polaramine...........................489
Promethazine
    Hydrochloride 474
Rondec 554
Ru-Tuss Tablets....................558
Rynatan 560
Seldane 571
Tavist..................................606
Terfenadine.........................571
Trinalin Repetabs 656
Tripelennamine
    Hydrochloride 448
Vancenase AQ 57
Vancenase Pockethaler............57

Headache, migraine
Cafergot................................79
Ergotamine Tartrate
    with Caffeine......................79
Inderal 290
Methysergide Maleate 565
Midrin 381
Propranolol Hydrochloride...290
Sansert 565

Headache, simple
See Pain

Headache, tension
Butalbital, Acetaminophen, and
    Caffeine...........................253
Butalbital, Aspirin,
    and Caffeine 255

Butalbital, Codeine,
    Aspirin, and Caffeine 257
Esgic 253
Fioricet 253
Fiorinal 255
Fiorinal with Codeine 257
Isollyl.................................255

**Heart attack, prevention of
recurrence**
Atenolol..............................616
Inderal 290
Lopressor 337
Metoprolol Tartrate 337
Propranolol Hydrochloride...290
Tenormin............................616

**Heartburn and related
stomach problems**
Metoclopramide
    Hydrochloride 534
Reglan 534

Heart failure, congestive
See also Fluid retention
Acetazolamide Sodium..........190
Amiloride Hydrochloride with
    Hydrochlorothiazide 388
Bumetanide 72
Bumex 72
Capoten 85
Captopril 90
Diamox...............................190
Digoxin 310
Enalapril Maleate 674
Esidrix 281
Furosemide 314
HydroDIURIL.....................281
Hydrochlorothiazide 281
Lanoxin 310
Lasix 314
Moduretic...........................388
Vasotec 674

Heart rhythms, abnormal
Acebutolol Hydrochloride 569
Calan 81
Calan SR...81
Digoxin 310
Disopyramide Phosphate 433
Ethmozine......................................243
Flecainide Acetate 604
Inderal 290
Isoptin 81
Isoptin SR 81
Lanoxin 310
Mexiletine Hydrochloride 373
Mexitil...373
Moricizine Hydrochloride.....243
Norpace..433
Procainamide
    Hydrochloride 503
Procan SR 503
Propafenone Hydrochloride..561
Propranolol Hydrochloride...290
Quinidex Exentabs 530
Quinidine Sulfate...................530
Rythmol..561
Sectral...569
Tambocor 604
Tocainide Hydrochloride 640
Tonocard 640
Verapamil Hydrochloride 81
Verelan 81

Herpes simplex
Acyclovir 704
Zovirax..704

Herpes zoster
See Shingles

High blood pressure
Acebutolol Hydrochloride 569
Aldactazide 11
Aldactone 13
Aldomet...15
Altace..18

Amiloride Hyrochloride with
    Hydrochlorothiazide 388
Atenolol..616
Atenolol/Chlorthalidone 614
Benazepril Hydrochloride 342
Calan 81
Calan SR...81
Capoten 85
Capozide..87
Captopril 85
Captopril with
    Hydrochlorothiazide 87
Cardizem 94
Cardura 95
Carteolol Hydrochloride 97
Cartrol...97
Catapres 99
Chlorothiazide 206
Chlorthalidone...........................284
Clonidine Hydrochloride 99
Corgard 135
Corzide 138
Diltiazem Hydrochloride 94
Diulo 694
Diuril..206
Doxazosin Mesylate................95
Dyazide...219
DynaCirc 221
Enalapril Maleate 674
Enalapril Maleate and
    Hydrochlorothiazide 671
Enduron...235
Esidrix 281
Felodipine 487
Fosinopril Sodium.................391
Furosemide 314
Guanabenz Acetate 687
Guanfacine Hydrochloride ...612
HydroDIURIL..............................281
Hydrochlorothiazide...............281
Hygroton 284
Hytrin...286
Indapamide..................................346
Inderal 290
Inderide 293
Isoptin 81
Isoptin SR 81
Isradipine......................................221

Labetalol Hydrochloride.......429
Lasix 314
Lisinopril 696
Lopressor 337
Lotensin 342
Lozol 346
Maxzide 357
Methyclothiazide.......................235
Methyldopa 15
Metolazone 694
Metoprolol Tartrate 337
Minipress.......................................383
Moduretic 388
Monopril 391
Nadolol 135
Nadolol/
    Bendroflumethiazide 138
Nifedipine 505
Normodyne 429
Pindolol 680
Plendil..487
Prazosin Hydrochloride 383
Procardia XL 507
Propranolol Hydrochloride...290
Propranolol/
    Hydrochlothiazide.............293
Ramipril 18
Reserpine, Hydralazine, and
    Hydrochlorothiazide 573
Sectral..569
Ser-Ap-Es.....................................573
Spironolactone.........................13
Spironolactone with
    Hydrochlorothiazide 11
Spirozide..11
Tenex...612
Tenoretic 614
Tenormin.......................................616
Terazosin Hydrochloride 286
Thalitone 284

Triamterene with
    Hydrochlorothiazide ..219,357
Vaseretic 671
Vasotec 674
Verapamil Hydrochloride 81
Verelan 81
Visken..................................680
Wytensin..............................687
Zaroxolyn.............................694
Zestril...................................696

Hives
See Skin inflammations,
    swelling and redness

Hyperactivity
See Attention-deficit disorder
    with hyperactivity

Impetigo
Bactroban 56
Mupirocin...............................56

Impotence
Yocon 691
Yohimbine Hydrochloride 691

Infections, bone and joint
Cephalexin............................306
Cephalexin Hydrochloride 306
Cipro 111
Ciprofloxacin
    Hydrochloride...................111
Flagyl..................................259
Keflex 305
Keftab.................................306
Metronidazole.......................259

Infections, central nervous system
Flagyl..................................259
Metronidazole.......................259
Rifadin................................544
Rifampin..............................544
Rimactane............................544

Infections, dental
Pen Vee-K............................462
Penicillin V 462
V-Cillin K 462
Veetids.................................462

Infections, ear
Amoxicillin 23
Amoxicillin/Clavulanate
    Potassium...........................47
Amoxil....................................23
Anspor.................................676
Augmentin 47
Bactrim..................................53
Ceclor 102
Cefaclor...............................102
Ceftin...................................103
Cefixime 591
Cefuroxime Axetil.................103
Cephradine 676
Colistin Sulfate, Neomycin,
    and Hydrocortisone 129
Coly-Mycin S Otic 129
Cotrim...................................53
E.E.S....................................239
ERYC 239
Erythrocin............................239
Erythromycin, Oral...............239
Erythromycin Ethylsuccinate
    with Sulfisoxazole Acetyl...460
Hydrocortisone with
    Acetic Acid 684
Ilosone 239
PCE 239
Pediazole..............................460
Pen Vee-K............................462
Penicillin V 462
Polymox 23
Septra 53
Suprax 591
Trimethoprim with
    Sulfamethoxazole 53
Trimox 23
V-Cillin K 462
Veetids.................................462
Velosef.................................462
VoSoL...................................684
Wymox...................................23

Infections, eye
Achromycin V............................3
Bleph-10 583
Cortisporin Ophthalmic.........137
Doryx 216
Doxycycline Hyclate.............216
Garamycin Ophthalmic...........269
Gentacidin 269
Gentamicin Sulfate 269
NeoDecadron 410
Neomycin and
    Dexamethasone................410
Sodium Sulamyd 583
Sulfacetamide Sodium 583
Sumycin 3
Tetracycline Hydrochloride.......3
Tobramycin 632
Tobrex..................................632
Vibramycin 216

Infections, fungal
Butoconazole Nitrate 252
Ciclopirox Olamine 339
Clotrimazole 344
Clotrimazole with
    Betamethasone
    Dipropionate......................345
Econazole Nitrate 586
Femstat 252
Fulvicin P/G 273
Griseofulvin 273
Gris-PEG 273
Ketoconazole 423
Loprox..................................339
Lotrimin 344
Lotrisone 345
Mycelex................................344
Myco-Triacet II.....................395
Mycolog II............................395
Mytrex..................................395
Nizoral 423
Nystatin with
    Triamcinolone...................395
Oxiconazole Nitrate 447
Oxistat Cream 447
Spectazole Cream...................586

Infections, gynecologic
Flagyl.................................259
Metronidazole...................259

Infections, heart
E.E.S..................................239
ERYC................................239
Erythrocin..........................239
Erythromycin, Oral..............239
Ilosone..............................239
PCE..................................239
Pen Vee-K..........................462
Penicillin V.......................462
V-Cillin K.........................462
Veetids..............................462

Infections, HIV
Retrovir.............................540
Zidovudine.......................540

**Infections,
lower respiratory tract**
Achromycin V.......................3
Amoxicillin........................23
*Amoxicillin/Clavulanate
Potassium*.......................47
Amoxil................................23
Anspor..............................676
Augmentin..........................47
Azithromycin.....................698
Biaxin................................68
Ceclor...............................102
Cefaclor...........................102
Cefixime...........................591
Ceftin...............................103
Cefuroxime Axetil................103
Cephalexin........................305
Cephalexin Hydrochloride....306
Cephradine.......................676
Cipro................................111
*Ciprofloxacin
Hydrochloride*...................111
Clarithromycin....................68
Dicloxacillin Sodium............223
Doryx...............................216
Doxycycline Hyclate............216
Dynapen...........................223

E.E.S..................................239
ERYC................................239
Erythrocin..........................239
Erythromycin, Oral..............239
Flagyl...............................259
Floxin...............................263
Ilosone..............................239
Keflex...............................305
Keftab...............................306
Metronidazole...................259
Minocin.............................385
Minocycline Hydrochloride..385
Ofloxacin..........................263
PCE..................................239
Pen Vee-K..........................462
Penicillin...........................462
Polymox..............................23
Sumycin................................3
Suprax...............................591
Tetracycline Hydrochloride.......3
Trimox.................................23
V-Cillin K...........................462
Veetids..............................462
Velosef..............................676
Vibramycin.........................216
Wymox................................23
Zithromax...........................698

Infections, rickettsiae
Doryx...............................216
Doxycycline Hyclate............216
Minocin.............................385
Minocycline Hydrochloride..385
Vibramycin.........................216

Infections, sinuses
*Amoxicillin/Clavulanate
Potassium*.......................47
Augmentin..........................47
Biaxin................................68
Clarithromycin....................68
Dicloxacillin Sodium............223
Dynapen...........................223

Infections, skin
Amoxicillin........................23
*Amoxicillin/Clavulanate
Potassium*.......................47

Amoxil................................23
Anspor..............................676
Augmentin..........................47
Azithromycin.....................698
Biaxin................................68
Ceclor...............................102
Cefaclor...........................102
Cefadroxil Monohydrate......218
Ceftin...............................103
Cefuroxime Axetil................103
Cephalexin........................305
Cephalexin Hydrochloride....306
Cephradine.......................676
Cipro................................111
*Ciprofloxacin
Hydrochloride*...................111
Clarithromycin....................68
Dicloxacillin Sodium............223
Doryx...............................216
Doxycycline Hyclate............216
Duricef..............................218
Dynapen...........................223
E.E.S..................................239
ERYC................................239
Erythrocin..........................239
Erythromycin, Oral..............239
Flagyl...............................259
Floxin...............................263
Ilosone..............................239
Keflex...............................305
Keftab...............................306
Metronidazole...................259
Minocin.............................385
Minocycline Hydrochloride..385
Ofloxacin..........................263
PCE..................................239
Pen Vee-K..........................462
Penicillin V.......................462
Polymox..............................23
Trimox.................................23
Ultracef.............................218
V-Cillin K...........................462
Veetids..............................462
Velosef..............................676

Vibramycin 216
Wymox 23
Zithromax 698

Infections, upper respiratory tract
Achromycin V 3
Amoxicillin 23
Amoxil 23
Anspor 676
Azithromycin 698
Bactrim 53
Biaxin 68
Ceclor 102
Cefaclor 102
Cefadroxil Monohydrate 218
Cefixime 591
Ceftin 103
Cefuroxime Axetil 103
Cephradine 676
Clarithromycin 68
Cotrim 53
Doryx 216
Doxycycline Hyclate 216
Duricef 218
E.E.S. 239
ERYC 239
Erythrocin 239
Erythromycin, Oral 239
Ilosone 239
Minocin 385
Minocycline Hydrochloride ..385
PCE 239
Pen Vee-K 462
Penicillin V 462
Polymox 23
Septra 53
Sumycin 3
Suprax 591
Tetracycline Hydrochloride 3
*Trimethoprim with
    Sulfamethoxazole* 53

Trimox 23
Ultracef 218
V-Cillin K 462
Veetids 462
Velosef 676
Vibramycin 216
Wymox 23
Zithromax 698

Infections, urinary tract
Achromycin V 3
*Amoxicillin/Clavulanate
    Potassium* 47
Anspor 676
Augmentin 47
Bactrim 53
Ceclor 102
Cefaclor 102
Cefadroxil Monohydrate 218
Ceftin 103
Cefuroxime Axetil 103
Cephalexin 305
Cephalexin Hydrochloride 306
Cephradine 676
Cipro 111
*Ciprofloxacin
    Hydrochloride* 111
Cotrim 53
Doryx 216
Doxycycline Hyclate 216
Duricef 218
E.E.S. 239
ERYC 239
Erythrocin 239
Erythromycin, Oral 239
Flagyl 259
Floxin 263
Gantrisin 267
Ilosone 239
Keflex 305
Keftab 306
Macrobid 354
Macrodantin 354
*Methenamine and Belladonna
    Alkaloids* 664
Metronidazole 259
Minocin 385
Minocycline Hydrochloride ..385
Nitrofurantoin 354

Norfloxacin 431
Noroxin 431
Ofloxacin 263
PCE 239
Septra 53
Sulfisoxazole 267
Sumycin 3
Tetracycline Hydrochloride 3
*Trimethoprim with
    Sulfamethoxazole* 53
Ultracef 218
Urised 664
Velosef 676
Vibramycin 216

Infertility, female
Clomid 117
Clomiphene Citrate 117
Serophene 117

Inflammatory diseases
Decadron Tablets 165
Deltasone 172
Dexamethasone 165
Medrol 361
Methylprednisolone 361
Orasone 172
Pediapred 457
*Prednisolone Sodium
    Phosphate* 457
Prednisone 172

Inflammatory diseases of the eye
Cromolyn Sodium 144
FML S.O.P. 248
Fluorometholone 248
Naphazoline Pheniramine 400
Naphcon-A 400
Opcon A 400
Opticrom 144
Pred Forte 496
Prednisolone Acetate 496

Insomnia
Dalmane 157
Doral 214
Estazolam 516
Flurazepam Hydrochloride ...157
Halcion 275
Nembutal..............................409
Pentobarbital Sodium 409
ProSom 516
Quazepam 214
Restoril 537
Secobarbital Sodium 567
Seconal 567
Temazepam 537
Triazolam 275

**Intestinal disorders,
inflammatory**
See Colitis

Irritable bowel syndrome
See Spastic colon

Jock itch
See Infections, fungal

Juvenile arthritis
See Arthritis

Kidney stones
Allopurinol 705
Zyloprim 705

Leg cramps
See also Circulation, impaired
Quinamm...............................533
Quinine Sulfate 533

Legionnaires' disease
E.E.S. 239
ERYC 239
Erythrocin.............................239
Erythromycin, Oral...............239
Ilosone 239
PCE 239

Lupus
Decadron Tablets..................165
Deltasone 172
Dexamethasone 165
*Hydroxychloroquine
  Sulfate* 361
Medrol 361
Methylprednisolone 361
Orasone 172
Pediapred 457
Plaquenil 485
*Prednisolone Sodium
  Phosphate* 457
Prednisone 172

Lyme disease
See Infections, rickettsiae

Malaria
*Hydroxychloroquine
  Sulfate* 485
Plaquenil 485

Manic-depressive illness
Lithium Carbonate 328
Lithobid 328

Meningitis
*See Infections,
  central nervous system*

Menopause
Estrogens, Conjugated 498
Premarin 498

Menstrual cramps
Acetaminophen 661
Anaprox 27
Aspirin Free Anacin 661
Ibuprofen.............................393
Ketoprofen...........................445
Meclofenamate Sodium.........359
Meclomen 359
Mefenamic Acid....................492
Motrin Tablets......................393
Naproxen Sodium..................27
Orudis 445
Panadol...............................661
Ponstel 492
Rufen 393
Tylenol 661

**Menstrual periods,
regulation of**
*Medroxyprogesterone
  Acetate* 521
Provera 521

**Mental capacity,
decline in**
Ergoloid Mesylates 280
Hydergine 280

Migraine headache
See Headache, migraine

Motion sickness
Antivert................................33
Benadryl 59
*Diphenhydramine
  Hydrochloride*......................59
Meclizine Hydrochloride.........33
Phenergan 474
Promethazine Hydrochloride 474

Mountain sickness
Acetazolamide Sodium..........190
Diamox................................190

Muscle spasm
Atrofen 326
Baclofen..............................326
Dantrium 159
Dantrolene Sodium 159
Lioresal...............................326

**Muscular discomfort due
to sprain, strain, or injury**
Carisoprodol.........................585
Chlorzoxazone......................454
*Cyclobenzaprine
  Hydrochloride*.....................261
Diazepam 667
Flexeril...............................261
Methocarbamol 368
Norgesic Forte 427
Parafon Forte DSC................454
Robaxin...............................549
Soma...................................585
Valium................................667

Narcolepsy
Dexedrine 184
Dextroamphetamine Sulfate..184
Methylphenidate
Hydrochloride 546
Ritalin..................................546

Nasal polyps
Beclomethasone Dipropionate 57
Beconase 57
Beconase AQ............................57
Decadron Turbinaire 167
Dexamethasone 165
Vancenase AQ 57
Vancenase Pockethaler............57

Nausea
See Vomiting and Nausea

Neuralgia, trigeminal
Atretol 608
Carbamazepine 608
Epitol 608
Tegretol 608

Neurological deficiencies
Nimodipine...........................419
Nimotop 419

Obesity
Diethylpropion
Hydrochloride 618
Fastin...................................249
Ionamin 301
Phentermine Hydrochloride ..249
Phentermine Resin 301
Tenuate................................618

**Obsessive-compulsive
disorder**
Anafranil 25
Clomipramine
Hydrochloride 25

Organ rejection
Cyclosporine 563
Sandimmune.........................563

Osteoarthritis
See Arthritis

Osteoporosis
Calcimar 84
Calcitonin-Salmon 84
Estrogens, Conjugated 498
Premarin 498

Paget's disease
Calcimar 84
Calcitonin - Salmon 84

Pain
Acetaminophen 661
Acetaminophen
with Codeine 662
Anaprox 27
Ansaid 31
Aspirin...................................40
Aspirin Free Anacin 661
Aspirin with Codeine 232
Choline Magnesium
Trisalicylate 654
Clinoril 115
Darvocet-N 161
Darvon 163
Demerol................................175
Diclofenac Sodium................682
Diflunisal.............................208
Dilaudid................................198
Dolobid.................................208
Empirin..................................40
Empirin with Codeine 232
Etodolac 331
Feldene 250
Fenoprofen Calcium 398
Flurbiprofen............................31
Genuine Bayer 40
Hydrocodone with
Acetaminophen 678
Hydromorphone
Hydrochloride 198
Indocin 295
Indomethacin........................295
Ketoprofen............................445
Lodine 331
Lortab...................................678
Meclofenamate Sodium..........359
Meclomen..............................359
Meperidine Hydrochloride 175
Morphine Sulfate 352

MS Contin 352
Nalfon 398
Naprosyn 402
Naproxen 402
Naproxen Sodium..................402
Norcet 678
Orudis 445
Oxycodone with
Acetaminophen 465
Panadol 661
Pentazocine Hydrochloride ...602
Percocet 465
Phenaphen with Codeine 662
Piroxicam 250
Propoxyphene
Hydrochloride 163
Propoxyphene Napsylate
with Acetaminophen 161
Roxicet 465
Sulindac 115
Synalgos-DC 597
Talwin Compound................602
Tolectin 636
Tolmetin Sodium 636
Trilisate 654
Tylenol 661
Tylenol with Codeine............662
Tylox 465
Vicodin 678
Voltaren 682
Zydone 678

Painful twitch
See Neuralgia, trigeminal

Pancreatic enzyme deficiency
Pancrease 453
Pancrelipase...........................453

Panic disorder
Alprazolam 689
Xanax...................................689

Parkinson's disease
Amantadine Hydrochloride ..595
Artane....................................36
Benadryl 59
Benztropine Mesylate............122

Bromocriptine Mesylate 455
Caridopa/Levodopa 578
Cogentin 122
Diphenhydramine
    Hydrochloride 59
Eldepryl 229
Larodopa 312
Levodopa/Carbidopa 578
Parlodel 455
Pergolide Mesylate 467
Permax 470
Selegiline Hydrochloride 229
Sinemet CR 578
Symadine 595
Symmetrel 595
Trihexyphenidyl
    Hydrochloride 36

Pertussis
See Whooping cough

Pharyngitis
See Infections,
    upper respiratory tract

Pinkeye
See Infections, eye

Pneumonia
See Infections,
    lower respiratory tract

Poison ivy
See Skin inflammation,
    swelling and redness

Potassium deficiency
Klor-Con 376
Micro-K 376
Potassium Chloride 376
Slow-K 376

Prostate enlargement, benign
Finasteride 515
Proscar 515

Psoriasis
Methotrexate 368

Psychotic disorders
Chlorpromazine 625
Clozapine 119
Clozaril 119
Compazine 132
Fluphenazine Hydrochloride .157
Haldol 277
Haloperidol 277
Mellaril 365
Navane 407
Perphenazine with
    Amitriptyline 648
Prochlorperazine 132
Prolixin 510
Stelazine 588
Thioridazine Hydrochloride ..365
Thiothixene 407
Thorazine 625
Triavil 648
Trifluoperazine
    Hydrochloride 588

Rheumatic fever
E.E.S. 239
ERYC 239
Erythrocin 239
Erythromycin, Oral 239
Ilosone 239
PCE 239
Pen Vee-K 462
Penicillin V 462
V-Cillin K 462
Veetids 462

Rheumatoid arthritis
See Arthritis

Ringworm infections
See Infections, fungal

Rocky Mountain spotted fever
See Infections, rickettsiae

Sedation
See also Anxiety and Insomnia
Atarax 42
Hydroxyzine Hydrochloride .485
Phenergan 474
Phenobarbital 478
Promethazine
    Hydrochloride 474

Seizure disorders
See Epilepsy

Sex hormone
deficiency, female
Estrogens, Conjugated 498
Premarin 498

Sex hormone deficiency, male
Android 29
Methyltestosterone 29

Sexually transmitted diseases
Achromycin V 3
Acyclovir 704
Amoxicillin 23
Amoxil 23
Azithromycin 698
Ceftin 103
Cefuroxime Axetil 103
Doryx 216
Doxycycline Hyclate 216
E.E.S. 239
ERYC 239
Erythrocin 239
Erythromycin, Oral 239
Flagyl 259
Floxin 263
Ilosone 239
Metronidazole 259
Metryl 259
Minocin 385
Minocycline Hydrochloride ..385
Norfloxacin 431
Noroxin 431
Ofloxacin 263
PCE 239
Polymox 23
Sumycin 3
Tetracycline Hydrochloride 3
Trimox 23
Vibramycin 216
Vibra-Tabs 216
Wymox 23
Zithromax 698
Zovirax 704

Shingles
Acyclovir 704
Zovirax..................................704

**Skin inflammation,
swelling and redness**
Aclovate.....................................5
Alclometasone Dipropionate.....5
Amcinonide 148
Benadryl 59
Betamethasone
    Dipropionate.....................203
Clobetasol Propionate 611
Cutivate 147
Cyclocort 148
Desonide..................................650
DesOwen 650
Desoximetasone.....................642
Diflorasone Diacetate 525
Diphenhydramine
    Hydrochloride.....................59
Diprolene...............................203
Elocon 231
Fluocinonide 322
Fluticasone Propionate 147
Lidex 322
Psorcon...................................525
Temovate................................611
Topicort..................................642
Tridesilon 650

Sleep attacks, recurrent
See Narcolepsy

Sleep difficulties
See Insomnia

Smoking cessation
Habitrol...............................275
Nicoderm.............................416
Nicorette..............................413
Nicotine 416
Nicotine Polacrilex 418
Nicotrol 416
Prostep.................................416

Sore throat symptoms
See Coughs and colds

Sore throat treatment
See Infections,
    upper respiratory tract

Spastic colon
Anaspaz 316
Bentyl 61
Chlordiazepoxide
    Hydrochloride with
        Clidinium Bromide............319
Clindex 319
Dicyclomine Hydrochloride 61
Donnatal...............................212
Hyoscyamine Sulfate.............316
Levsin 316
Librax...................................319
Phenobarbital with
    Belladonna Alkaloids 212

Syphilis
See Sexually transmitted diseases

Thyroid hormone deficiency
Armour Thyroid 34
Euthroid 246
Levothroid 598
Levothyroxine Sodium...........598
Levoxine 598
Liotrix 246
Proloid 511
Synthroid 598
Thyroglobulin 51
Thyroid Hormones 34

Tic fevers
See Infections, rickettsiae

Tics
Haldol 277
Haloperidol 277
Orap 440
Pimozide 440

Tonsillitis
See Infections,
    upper respiratory tract

Trachoma
See Infections, eyes

Tremors, hereditary
Inderal 290
Propranolol Hydrochloride...290

Tuberculosis
Rifadin.................................544
Rifampin...............................544
Rimactane.............................544

Typhus fever
See Infections, rickettsiae

Ulcers, peptic
Axid 50
Carafate 90
Cimetidine 600
Cytotec 152
Famotidine 464
Misoprostol 152
Nizatidine 50
Omeprazole 501
Pepcid 464
Prilosec 501
Ranitidine Hydrochloride 692
Sucralfate 90
Tagamet...........................600
Zantac 692

Urinary tract pain
Flavoxate Hydrochloride 666
*Methenamine and
    Belladonna Alkaloids* 664
*Phenazopyridine
    Hydrochloride* 527
Pyridium 527
Urised 664
Urispas.............................666

Vaginal yeast infection
See Candidiasis

**Vitamins and
fluoride deficiency**
Poly-Vi-Flor 491
Vitamins with Fluoride 491

**Vitamins and minerals,
prenatal**
Stuartnatal 1+1 590
Vitamins, Prenatal 590

Vomiting and nausea
Compazine 132
*Metoclopramide
    Hydrochloride* 534
Phenergan 474
Prochlorperazine................132
*Promethazine
    Hydrochloride* 474
Reglan 534
Tigan 628
*Trimethobenzamide
    Hydrochloride* 628

Wheezing
See Asthma

Whooping cough
E.E.S. 239
ERYC 239
Erythrocin..........................239
Erythromycin, Oral 239
Ilosone 239
PCE 239

General Index

L isted in this index are the drugs, diseases, and other key subjects mentioned in the Disease Overview chapters. Also shown, with page numbers in bold type, are the products described in the Drug Profile section. Drugs and diseases mentioned within the profiles are not included in the index.

A

Abdomen, enlarged, as symptom of ovarian cancer, 757
Abdominal bloating, as symptom of hypothyroidism, 808
Abdominal pain, as symptom
anaphylaxis, 800
E. coli infections, 817
enterocolitis, 814
food poisoning, 814
gastroenteritis, 739
mumps, 789
pancreatic cancer, 755
pancreatitis, 742
salmonella, 816
STDs in digestive tract, 742
Abortion, PID and, 838
Abscess. *See also* Liver, abscess of
abdominal, PID and, 776
migraine and, 761
salmonella and, 816
Accutane, **1-3**
for acne, 803
Acebutolol hydrochloride. *See* Sectral
ACE inhibitors, to control hypertension, 723-724
Acetaminophen. *See also* Darvocet-N; Fioricet; Midrin; Percocet; Tylenol; Tylenol with Codeine; Vicodin
for acute pain, 760
for arthritis, 726
for common cold, 744
for croup, 746
for headaches, 761
for hemophilia, 856

for influenza, 745
for Legionnaire's disease, 747
for measles, 788
for mononucleosis, 789
for mumps, 789
for otitis media, 793
replacing aspirin in children, 790
for rubella, 790
for sickle cell anemia, 856
for swimmer's ear, 792
for tonsillitis, 796
for viral infections, 761
Acetazolamide. *See* Diamox
Acetic acid. *See* VoSoL
Acetonide. *See* Mycolog-II
Achromycin V Capsules, **3-5**
Acid therapy
for corns and calluses, 858
for plantar warts, 859
Aclovate, **5-7**
Acne, 801, 803
Acquired immune deficiency syndrome (AIDS), 833-834, 841-845. *See also* Human immunodeficiency virus (HIV)
condom and, 783
preventing, 843
statistics, 842
transmission of, 843-844
tuberculosis and, 746
Acromegaly, 808
carpal tunnel syndrome and, 735
ACTH. *See* Adrenocorticotrophic hormone (ACTH)

Actigall, **7-8**
Actinomycin D, for uterine cancer, 755
Activase, for dissolving blood clots, 719
Acute bacterial pyelonephritis, 774 (fig.)
Acute pain, treating, 760-761
Acyclovir. *See also* Zovirax
for genital herpes, 839
Adalat. *See* Procardia
Adapin. *See* Sinequan
Addiction. *See also* Alcohol abuse; Substance abuse
drug treatments for chronic pain and, 761
Addison's disease, 811
hypopituitarism and, 808
ADH (Antidiuretic hormone), 809
ADHD (Attention-deficit hyperactivity disorder), 770-771
Adjuvant treatment, for cancer, 751
Adolescents
acne and, 803
AIDS and, 842
Adrenal cortex, 809
Adrenal glands, 718, 809
disorders of, 811
Adrenaline
function of, 718
hypertension and, 724
Adrenal medulla, 809
Adrenocorticotrophic hormone (ACTH), 809
Cushing's syndrome and, 811
Advil. *See* Motrin Tablets
AeroBid, **9-11**
for asthma, 798
African-Americans. *See also* Sickle-cell anemia
prostate cancer among, 754
Agoraphobia, 766
AIDS. *See* Acquired immune deficiency syndrome (AIDS)
AIDS-related complex (ARC), 841
Albuterol sulfate. *See* Proventil
Alclometasone dipropionate. *See* Aclovate

Alcohol abuse
cancer and, 749
cirrhosis and, 831
depression in elderly and, 864
hypertension and, 723
oral cancer and, 757
pancreatic cancer and, 755
pancreatitis and, 742
Aldactazide, **11-13**
Aldactone, **13-15**
Aldomet, **15-18**
Aldosterone, 809
Allergens, 797, 800
Allergic contact dermatitis, 799, 805
Allergic reaction, defined, 797
Allergic rhinitis. *See* Hay fever
Allergies
and postnasal drip, 795
treating, 797-800
Allopurinol. *See* Zyloprim
Alpha adrenergic blocking agents, in treating hypertension, 724
Alport's syndrome, 821
Alprazolam. *See* Xanax
Altace, **18-20**
Alupent, **20-22**
Alzheimer's disease, 862, 864
Amantadine hydrochloride. *See also* Symmetrel
for influenza, 745
Amcinonide. *See* Cyclocort
Amebiasis, 742
Amebic dysentery, 832
Amiloride. *See* Moduretic
Aminoglutethimide
for Cushing's syndrome, 811
in treating breast cancer, 753
Aminoglycosides, for liver abscess, 832
Amitriptyline hydrochloride. *See* Elavil; Limbitrol; Triavil
Amnesia, as symptom, Legionnaire's disease, 747
Amoxapine. *See* Asendin
Amoxicillin. *See also* Amoxil; Augmentin
for bladder infections, 827
for Lyme disease, 817
for otitis media, 793

for sinusitis, 795
for strep infections, 815
Amoxil, **23-24**
Ampicillin
for bladder infections, 827
for liver abscess, 832
for meningitis, 816
for otitis media, 793
for strep infections, 815
Amsacrine, for leukemia, 756
Amyl nitrite, 715
Amyloidosis, carpal tunnel syndrome and, 735
Anafranil, **25-27**
Ana-Kit. *See* Epinephrine, injectable
Analgesics. *See also* Acetaminophen; Aspirin
for acute pain, 760
for pancreatic cancer, 755
for pancreatitis, 742
Anaphylaxis, 800
Anaprox, **27-29**
Anaspaz. *See* Levsin
Androgen
in treating aplastic anemia, 855
in treating breast cancer, 753
Android, **29-31**
Anemia. *See also* Pernicious anemia
early symptoms in feet, 857
treating, 854-855
Anemia, as symptom
colon cancer, 741
gastric cancer, 740
liver abscess, 832
Aneurysms, migraine and, 761
Anexia. *See* Vicodin
Angina
calcium channel blockers and, 717-718, 724
defined, 713
hormonal contraceptives and, 786
Inderal and, 716
nitroglycerin and, 716
stress and, 718
Angioedema, 799
sting allergies and, 799
Angiotensin, 724. *See also* ACE inhibitors
Anistreplase. *See* Eminasse
Ankylosing spondylitis, 726, 729
Anorexia, 771
Ansaid, **31-33**
Anspor. *See* Velosef
Antacids
for pancreatic cancer, 755
for reflux esophagitis, 738
for ulcers, 739
Anthralin, for psoriasis, 804
Antibiotics. *See also particular antibiotics*
for atopic eczema, 804

elderly and, 863
for HIV infections, 845
infection and, 813
for OB/GYN disorders, 779
for pancreatic cancer, 755
for staph infections, 814
for STDs, 839
in treating kidney stones, 823
for ulcers, 739
for UTIs, 827
Anticholinergics, for pancreatic cancer, 755
Anticonvulsants, allergic reactions from, 798
Antidepressants. *See also* Tricyclic antidepressants
elderly and, 863
for treating pain, 762
Antidiuretic hormone (ADH), 809
Antifungal medications, for vaginal yeast infections, 780, 839
Antihistamines. *See also particular antihistamine drugs*
for atopic eczema, 804
for chickenpox, 788
elderly and, 863
for hay fever, 798
for hives, 799, 805
for nasal polyps, 795
for nasal problems, 794
for otitis media, 793
for postnasal drip, 795
for psoriasis, 804
Antimalarial drugs, for SLE, 729
Antiprostaglandins, for OB/GYN disorders, 780
Antipyrine. *See* Auralgan
Antithymocyte globulin, for aplastic anemia, 855
Antithyroid drugs, for hyperthyroidism, 810
Antivert, **33-36**
for Ménière's disease, 793
Anturane. *See* Sulfinpyrazone
Anxiety disorders, 763, 766-767
in children, 771
treating, 768
Aplastic anemia, 855
Appetite increase, as symptom, Graves' disease, 810
Appetite loss, as symptom
Addison's disease, 811
chickenpox, 787
constipation, 742
E. coli infections, 817
folic acid deficiency anemia, 855
food poisoning, 814
gastric cancer, 740
gastritis, 739
hypothyroidism, 808
Legionnaire's disease, 747

measles, 788
migraine, 761
mumps, 789
pernicious anemia, 854
rheumatoid arthritis, 727
rubella, 789
streptococcal pharyngitis, 815
thalassemia, 855
tuberculosis, 746
viral hepatitis, 830
whooping cough, 789
Apresoline (hydralazine hydrochloride), 724. *See also* Ser-Ap-Es
ARC (AIDS-related complex), 841
Armour Thyroid, **34-36**
Arrhythmia
drugs for, 715
Inderal and, 716
quinidine and, 715
in sickle cell anemia, 856
verapamil and, 717
Artane, **36-38**
Arthritis, 760
defined, 725
foot problems and, 857, 859
psoriasis and, 804
statistics, 725
treating, 725-730
Arthritis-like symptoms, Lyme disease and, 817
Artificial kidney machine, 823
Asendin, **38-40**
L-asparaginase, for leukemia, 756
Aspirin, **40-42**. *See also* Empirin, with Codeine; Fiorinal; Fiorinal with Codeine; Norgesic Forte; Synalgos-DC; Talwin Compound
for acute pain, 760
for arthritis, 726
for arthritis with psoriasis, 804
for chronic headaches, 761
for common cold, 744
for erysipelas, 815
for headaches, 761
hemophilia and, 856
for influenza, 745
for Legionnaire's disease, 747
for neck pain, 734
Reye's syndrome and, 790
for rheumatoid arthritis, 727
for slipped disk, 733
for swimmer's ear, 792
for tonsillitis, 796
Aspirin Free Anacin. *See* Tylenol
Astemizole. *See* Hismanal
Asthma, 747, 797-798
COPD and, 745
Atarax, **42-44**
for atopic dermatitis, 799

for hives, 799
Atenolol. *See* Tenoretic; Tenormin
ATG. *See* Antithymocyte globulin
Atherosclerosis, 714, 714 (fig.), 723
drugs for, 716
Athlete's foot, 805, 857-858
Ativan, **44-45**
Atopic dermatitis, 799
Atopic eczema, 804
Atretol. *See* Tegretol
Atrofen. *See* Lioresal
Atropine sulfate. *See* Donnagel-PG; Donnatal; Lomotil; Ru-Tuss Tablets; Urised
Atrovent, **46-47**
A/T/S. *See* Erythromycin, topical
Attention-deficit hyperactivity disorder (ADHD), 770-771
Augmentin, **47-48**
Auralgan, **48-49**
Auranofin. *See* Ridaura
Auroto Otic. *See* Auralgan
Autism, 763, 770
Autoimmune disorders. *See* Immune system disorders
Autoimmune reaction, diabetes as, 849
Aventyl. *See* Pamelor
Axid, **50-51**
for ulcers, 740
5-Azacytidine, for leukemia, 756
Azatadine maleate. *See* Trinalin Repetabs
Azathioprine
with kidney transplants, 824
for rheumatoid arthritis, 727
Azithromycin. *See* Zithromax
Azmacort, for asthma, 798
Azulfidine, **51-53**

B

Bacitracin-neomycin-polymixin ointment, 814
Back pain, 732 (fig.). *See also* Low back pain
Baclofen. *See* Lioresal
Bacteremia, 814
Bactrim, **53-56**
for bladder infections, 827
for *Pneumocystis carinii* pneumonia, 845
Bactroban, **56-57**
for skin infections, 814
Basal cell carcinoma, of skin, 805
Bayer. *See* Aspirin
BCG vaccine, for small-cell carcinoma of lung, 752
Beclomethasone dipropionate, **57-59**

for asthma, 798
for hay fever, 798
Beclovent Inhalation Aerosal.
See Beclomethasone dipropi-
onate
Beconase AQ Nasal Spray. *See*
Beclomethasone dipropi-
onate
Beconase Inhalation Aerosol.
See Beclomethasone dipropi-
onate
Beef insulin, for Type I dia-
betes, 851
Beepen VK. *See* Penicillin V
Belching, as symptom
gastritis, 739
reflux esophagitis, 737
Benadryl, 59-61
for atopic dermatitis, 799
for chickenpox, 788
for hives, 799
Benazepril hydrochloride. *See*
Lotensin
Bendroflumethiazide. *See*
Corzide
Benty, for urinary inconti-
nence, 828
Bentyl, 61-63
Benzac-W. *See* Desquam-E
Benzagel. *See* Desquam-E
Benzamycin, 63-64
BenzaShave. *See* Desquam-E
Benzocaine. *See* Auralgan
Benzodiazepines, for anxiety
disorders, 768
Benzoic acid. *See* Urised
Benzonatate. *See* Tessalon
Benzoyl peroxide. *See also*
Benzamycin; Desquam-E
for acne, 803
Benztropine mesylate. *See* Co-
gentin
Bepridil hydrochloride. *See*
Vascor
Beta-adrenergic system, 716
Beta-blockers. *See also* Inderal
for anxiety disorders, 768
for hypertension, 723-724
for rosacea, 803
Betagan, 65-66
Betamethasone dipropionate.
See Diprolene; Lotrisone
Betapen-VK. *See* Penicillin V
Betaxolol hydrochloride. *See*
Betoptic
Betoptic, 66-68
Biaxin, 68-69
Bile duct, diseases of, and pan-
creatitis, 742
Biliary atresia, 832
Biofeedback
in treating pain, 762
in treating urinary inconti-
nence, 828
Biologic response modifiers, in
cancer treatment, 751
Biopsychiatry, 764

Bipolar depression, 768
Birth control methods. *See*
Contraception
Birth control pills, 786
fibroids and, 777
STDs and, 835
uterine bleeding and, 777
vaginitis and, 837
Birth defects
genital herpes and, 838
STDs and, 833
Bladder
cancer of, 757, 828
drugs for infections of, 827
exercises for urinary incontinence, 828
malformations of, 821
at menopause, 828
pain, as symptom of UTI,
827
relaxants, 828
Bleeding, intracranial, migraine and, 761
Bleeding, as symptom
aplastic anemia, 855
of bowel, in Crohn's disease,
740
leukemia, 756
Bleph-10. *See* Sodium Sulamyd
Blindness
STDs and, 833
syphilis and, 838
Blisters, as symptom, genital
herpes, 837
Blood clots
dissolving, 719
hormonal contraception
and, 786
Blood disorders
causes, 853
correcting, 853-856
Blood poisoning, salmonella
and, 816
Blood pressure. *See also* Hypertension
defined, 721-722
measuring, 722
sting allergies and, 800
Blood sugar, 848. *See also* Hyperglycemia; Hypoglycemia
controlling, 850-851
testing level of, 850
Blood test, for diabetes, 850
Blood thinners, elderly and,
863
Blood transfusions, AIDS and,
843
Body fluids
spread of hepatitis B
through, 830
spread of STDs through,
834
Body temperature, hives and,
798
Bones
abnormalities of, and thalassemia, 855

disorders of, 731-735
function of, 731
staph infections of, 814
tumors of, 758
Bone cancer, surgical techniques, 751
Bone marrow, 853
function of, 731
tumors of. *See* Myelomas
Bone marrow transplants
for aplastic anemia, 855
for leukemia, 751, 756
Brain cancer, in children, 756
Breast, disorders of, 778
Breast cancer, 750, 752-753,
753 (fig.), 778
hormonal therapy for, after
surgery, 779
Breast milk, transmission of
hepatitis B through, 830
Brethaire. *See* Brethine
Brethine, 69-70
Bricanyl. *See* Brethine
Bright's disease. *See* Glomeru-
lonephritis
Bromides, acne and, 803
Bromocriptine mesylate. *See*
Parlodel
Brompheniramine maleate. *See*
Dimetane-DC
Bronchitis
acute, 744
chronic, 745
recurring, as symptom of
lung cancer, 751
Bronchodilators
for asthma, 798
elderly and, 863
Bronkometer, 71-72
Bronkosol, 71-72
Bruising, as symptom
aplastic anemia, 855
childhood cancers, 756
leukemia, 755
Brunton, Thomas Lauder, 716
Bulimia, 771
Bumetanide. *See* Bumex
Bumex, 72-74
Bunions, 859
Bupropion hydrochloride. *See*
Wellbutrin
Burkitt's lymphoma, 750
Burns, treating pain from, 761
Bursitis, 760
BuSpar, 74-76
for anxiety disorders, 768
Buspirone hydrochloride. *See*
BuSpar
Butalbital. *See* Fioricet; Fiori-
nal; Fiorinal with Codeine
Butazolidin, 76-79
Butoconazole nitrate. *See* Fem-
stat

C

Caesarian section, genital
warts and, 837
Cafergot, 79-80
for migraine, 761
Calan, 81-83
for arrhythmia, 717
for hypertension, 724
for migraine, 761
Calan SR. *See* Calan
Calcimar, 84-85
Calcitonin, for osteoporosis,
733
Calcitonin-Salmon. *See* Calcimar
Calcitriol. *See* Rocaltrol
Calcium
hypoparathyroidism and levels of, 810
for osteoporosis, 733
role in regulating heart action, 717
Calcium channel blockers,
717-718
for hypertension, 723-724
for urinary incontinence,
828
Calcium supplements, elderly
and, 863
Calluses (foot), 858
Cancer. *See also particular organs*
advances in treatment, 749-
758
and AIDS, 844
calcium channel blockers
and, 718
defined, 749-750
drug treatment of, 780
gastrointestinal tract, 740
hormonal contraceptives
and, 786
pain associated with, 760
pleurisy and, 747
statistics, 750, 756
STDs and, 833
survival rates, 749
treating chronic pain of. 760
See also Antidepressants
Capillaries, amyl nitrite and,
715-716
Capoten, 85-87
for hypertension, 724
Capozide, 87-90
Captopril. *See* Capoten;
Capozide
Carafate, 90-91
for ulcers, 740
Carbamazepine. *See* Tegretol
Carbidopa. *See* Sinemet CR
Carbinoxamine maleate. *See*
Rondec
Carbunculosis, 805
Carcinoma, 750
of cervix, 755
small-cell, of lung, 752

Cardene, 91-93
Cardiac arrhythmia. See Arrhythmia
Cardiopulmonary resuscitation (CPR), 714, 717
Cardiovascular disease, pernicious anemia and, 854
Cardizem, 94-95,
  for hypertension, 724
  for migraine, 761
Cardura, 95-97
Carisoprodol. See Soma
Carpal tunnel, 734 (fig.)
Carpal tunnel syndrome, 734-735
Carteolol hydrochloride. See Cartrol
Cartilage, 728 (fig.)
Cartrol, 97-99
Catapres, 99-102
Ceclor, 102-103
Cefaclor. See also Ceclor
  for otitis media, 793
Cefadroxil monohydrate. See Duricef
Cefazolin, for bacteremia, 814
Cefixime. See Suprax
Cefotaxime, for meningitis, 816
Ceftin, 103-105
Ceftriaxone
  for Lyme disease, 817
  for meningitis, 816
Cefuroxime axetil. See Ceftin
Cellulitis, 814
Centrax, 105-106
Cephalexin. See Keflex
Cephalexin hydrochloride. See Keftab
Cephalosporin
  for liver abscess, 832
  for Lyme disease, 817
  for meningitis, 816
  side effects, 814
  for sinusitis, 795
Cephradine. See Velosef
Cervical cancer, 755, 836 (fig.)
  and genital warts, 837
Cervical cap, 782-783
Cervical dysplasia, 775-776, 836 (fig.)
Cervicitis, 775
Cervix
  disorders of, 775-776
  normal, 836 (fig.)
Chancre, 838
Chenodiol, for gallstones, 831
Chest pain, as symptom. See also Lungs, pain as symptom
  anaphylaxis, 800
  lung cancer, 751
  reflux esophagitis, 737
  staphylococcal pneumonia, 814
Chest trauma, pleurisy and, 747
Chickenpox, 787-788

infectious arthritis and, 730
Childbirth. See also Pregnancy; Premature labor
  PID and, 837
  treating pain associated with, 760
Children
  arthritis in, 730
  aspirin and, 744
  asthma in, 797
  cancer in, 756
  diabetes in, 849
  liver diseases of, 832
  mental illness in, 763, 770-771
  respiratory diseases in, 746-747
  treating common infections in, 787-790
  UTIs in, 825, 827
Chlamydia, 833, 835-836
  condoms and, 783
  gonorrhea and, 834, 839
  UTIs and, 826-827
Chlamydia trachomatis, 835
Chlorambucil, for ovarian cancer, 757
Chloramphemicol, for liver abscess, 832
Chlordiazepoxide. See Librium; Limbitrol
Chlordiazepoxide hydrochloride. See Librax
Chlorhexidine gluconate. See Peridex
Chloroquine, for liver abscess, 832
Chlorothiazide. See Diuril
Chlorpheniramine maleate. See Deconamine; Nolamine; Ru-Tuss Tablets
Chlorpheniramine polistirex. See Tussionex
Chlorpheniramine tannate. See Rynatan
Chlorpromazine. See Thorazine
Chlorpropamide. See Diabinese
Chlorthalidone. See Hygroton; Tenoretic
Chlorzoxazone. See Parafon Forte DSC
Choledyl, 107-109
Cholesteatoma, 793
Cholesterol
  atherosclerosis and, 714
  heart disease and, 718
  high levels and hormonal contraceptive risk, 786
  increase in, and nephrotic syndrome, 822
Cholesterol-reducing drugs, 718-719
Cholestyramine. See Questran
Choline magnesium. See Trilisate

Choriocarcinoma, 750
Chronic diseases, genetic factor in, 862
Chronic obstructive pulmonary disease (COPD), 745-746
Chronic pain
  causes, 760
  narcotic analgesics for, 761
  treating, 760
Chronulac Syrup, 110
Cibalith-S (lithium citrate). See Lithobid
Ciclopirox olamine. See Loprox
Cilia, 791
Cimetidine. See Tagamet
Cipro, 111-113
Ciprofloxacin hydrochloride. See Cipro
Circulatory problems. See also Heart disease
  foot problems and, 857, 859
Circulatory system, 712, 712 (fig.). See also Blood pressure
Cirrhosis, 831
  hepatitis B and, 831
Cisplatin
  for bladder cancer, 757
  for ovarian cancer, 757
  for small-cell carcinoma of lung, 752
Clarithromycin. See Biaxin
Clavulanate potassium. See Augmentin
Clemastine fumarate. See Tavist
Cleocin T, 113-114
Clindamycin
  for acne, 803
  for liver abscess, 832
Clindamycin phosphate. See Cleocin T
Clindex. See Librax
Clinidium bromide. See Librax
Clinoril, 115-117
Clobetasol propionate. See Temovate
Clomid. See Clomiphene citrate
Clomiphene citrate, 117-119
Clomipramine hydrochloride. See also Anafranil
  for obsessive-compulsive disorder, 767
Clonazepam. See Klonopin
Clonidine. See Catapres
Clorazepate dipotassium. See Tranxene
Clotrimazole. See Lotrimin; Lotrisone
Cloxacillin, for skin infections, 814
Clozapine. See Clozaril
Clozaril, 119-121

Coagulation, intravascular, as symptom of meningitis, 816
Coal tar preparations, for psoriasis, 804
Cochlea, 791
Codeine. See also Dimetane-DC; Empirin with Codeine; Fiorinal with Codeine; Phenergan with Codeine; Tylenol with Codeine
  for chronic headaches, 761
  for erysipelas, 815
  for hemophilia, 856
  for shingles, 761
  for sickle cell anemia, 856
Cogentin, 122-123
Cognitive therapy, for treating pain, 762
Colace, 123-124
ColBENEMID, 124-126
  for gout, 729
Colchicine. See also ColBENEMID
  gout and, 729
Cold intolerance, as symptom of hypothyroidism, 808
Cold packs, for erysipelas, 815
Cold temperatures, hives and, 798
Colestid, 126-128
Colestipol hydrochloride. See Colestid
Colistin sulfate. See Coly-Mycin S Oral; Coly-Mycin S Otic
Collagen, 802
Colon, constipation as symptom of problems, 742
Colon cancer, 741-742, 752
Colonoscopy, 741
Colostomy, 752
Col-Probenecid. See ColBENEMID
Coly-Mycin S Oral, 128-129
Coly-Mycin S Otic, 129-130
Colyte, 130-132
Coma, diabetic, 848
Common cold, 743-744
Compazine, 132-135
  for gastroenteritis, 739
Computerized tomography (CT), 751, 821
Condoms, 782-783
  AIDS prevention and, 843
  STDs and, 835
Conduct disorders, 763, 770
Condyloma. See Genital warts
Confusion, as symptom
  bacteremia, 814
  hypoglycemia, 850
  Reye's syndrome, 790
Congestive heart failure, 714-715
Conjugated estrogens. See Premarin
Conjunctivitis, as symptom
  hay fever, 798

whooping cough, 789
Constipation, 742
Constipation, as symptom
  colon cancer, 752
  diverticulosis, 741
  hyperparathyroidism, 810
  hypothyroidism, 808
  irritable bowel syndrome, 740
  pernicious anemia, 854
Contact dermatitis, 805
  of vulva, 775
Contraceptive foam/jelly. *See* Spermicides
Contraceptive implant, 786
Contraceptives. *See* Oral Contraceptives
Convulsions, as symptom, tetanus, 816
Cooley's anemia. *See* Thalassemia
Copper, in liver. *See* Wilson's disease
Corgard, **135-136**
Corns (foot), 858
Coronary arteries, 712, 712 (fig.), 714 (fig.)
  clot-dissolving drugs, 719
  diseases of, 713
  reducing need for bypass surgery, 711, 719
Corticosteroids
  for aplastic anemia, 855
  for atopic dermatitis, 799
  for atopic eczema, 804
  for COPD, 746
  elderly and, 863
  for hives, 799
  for nasal polyps, 795
  for nephrotic syndrome, 822
  for postnasal drip, 795
  for thrombocytopenia, 856
Corticosterone, 809
Cortisol
  Cushing's syndrome and, 811
  reducing, 811
Cortisone, 809
  for acne, 803
  for Addison's disease, 811
  for carpal tunnel syndrome, 735
  for neuromas, 858
  for osteoarthritis, 727
  for slipped disk, 733
Cortisporin Ophthalmic Suspension, **137-138**
Cortisporin Otic, for swimmer's ear, 792
Corynebacterium parvulum, 752
Corzide, **138-140**
Cotrim. *See* Bactrim
Cotton swabs, ear infections and, 792
Cough, as symptom
  asthma, 797

chronic bronchitis, 745
croup, 746
laryngitis, 796
Legionnaire's disease, 747
lung cancer, 751
measles, 788
staphylococcal pneumonia, 814
whooping cough, 789
Coumadin, **140-144**
CPR (cardiopulmonary resuscitation), 714, 717
Creutzfeldt-Jakob disease, 864
Crohn's disease, 740-741
  proctitis and, 741
Cromolyn sodium, **144-147**
Croup, 746
Cryoprecipitate, 856
Cryosurgery
  for hemorrhoids, 742
  for OB/GYN disorders, 779
  for plantar warts, 859
  for precancerous uterine or cervical conditions, 755
  for skin cancer, 757, 806
Curettage, for plantar warts, 859
Cushing's syndrome, 811
Cutaneous larva migrans, 805
Cutivate, **147-148**
Cyclobenzaprine hydrochloride. *See* Flexeril
Cyclocort, **148-150**
Cyclophosphamide. *See also* Cytoxan
  for bladder cancer, 757
  for breast cancer, 753
  for leukemia, 756
  for ovarian cancer, 757
  for small-cell carcinoma of lung, 752
  for uterine cancer, 755
Cyclosporine. *See also* Sandimmune
  with kidney transplants, 824
Cylert, **150-151**
Cyproheptadine. *See* Periactin
Cystinuria, 821
Cystitis, 774 (fig.), 825. *See also* Interstitial cystitis
Cystoscope, 828
Cysts, ovarian, and uterine cancer, 777-778
Cytadren. *See* Aminoglutethimide
Cytarabine, for leukemia, 756
Cytomegalovirus infections, and AIDS, 844
Cytotec, **152-154**
Cytoxan, **154-156**

D

Dalmane, **157-159**
D&C (dilatation and curettage), 779

Dandruff. *See* Seborrheic dermatitis
Dantrium, **159-161**
Dantrolene sodium. *See* Dantrium
Darvocet-N, **161-163**
Darvon, **163-165**
  for hemophilia, 856
Darvon Compound 65. *See* Darvon
Darvon-N. *See* Darvocet-N
Daunorubicin, for leukemia, 756
DDAVP, **156-157**
ddC. *See* Zalcitabine
ddI. *See* Didanosine
Decadron Respihaler, **167-170**
Decadron Tablets, **165-167**
Decadron Turbinaire, **167-170**
Deconamine, **170-172**
Decongestants
  for common cold, 744
  for nasal polyps, 795
  for nasal problems, 794
  for nosebleeds, 794
  for postnasal drip, 795
  for sinusitis, 795
Deformity, as symptom, fracture, 735
Dehydration
  enterocolitis and, 814
  from intestinal infections, 816-817
  salmonella and, 816
  staph infections and, 814
Deltasone, **172-175**
Delusions, as symptom of schizophrenia, 770
Dementia, 864
  and AIDS, 844
Demerol, **175-177**
  for chronic headaches, 761
  for fractures, 735, 760
  for hemophilia, 856
  for kidney stones, 823
  for sickle cell anemia, 856
Demulen. *See* Oral contraceptives
Depakene, **177-178**
Depakote, **178-180**
Depen. *See* Penicillamine
Depo-Provera, 786
Depression, 763, 768-769. *See also* Antidepressants
  among elderly, 862
  as side effect of medication, 863-864
  treating, 768-769
Dermabrasion, for rhinophyma, 803
Dermatitis. *See also* Allergic contact dermatitis; Atopic dermatitis; Contact dermatitis
  treating, 804-805
Dermatophytosis, 805
Dermis, 802

DES. *See* Diethylstilbestrol (DES)
Desipramine hydrochloride. *See* Norpramin
Desmopressin acetate. *See* DDAVP
Desonide. *See* Tridesilon
DesOwen. *See* Tridesilon
Desoximetasone. *See* Topicort
Desquam-E, **181**
Desyrel, **182-183**
Deviated septum, surgery for, 794-795
Dexamethasone. *See* Decadron Tablets
Dexamethasone sodium phosphate. *See* Decadron Respihaler; Decadron Turbinaire; Neodecadron Ophthalmic Ointment and Solution
Dexchlorpheniramine maleate. *See* Polaramine
Dexedrine, **184-187**
Dextroamphetamine sulfate. *See* Dexedrine
Dextromethorphan hydrobromide. *See* Tussi-Organidin DM
Diabeta. *See* Micronase
Diabetes, 730
  chemical processes occurring in, 848
  consequences of, 847
  constipation and, 742
  controlling, 847-852
  Cushing's syndrome and, 811
  diagnosing, 849
  foot problems and, 857, 859
  hormonal contraceptives and, 786
  infertility and, 779
  lifestyle management and, 851
  oral medications and thrombocytopenia, 856
  tuberculosis and, 746
  Type 2 (non-insulin-dependent), 848
  Type 1 (insulin-dependent), 848
Diabetes insipidus, as symptom of hypopituitarism, 808
Diabetes mellitus, 810
  carpal tunnel syndrome and, 735
  nephrotic syndrome and, 822
  pancreatic cancer and, 755
Diabinese, **187-190**
  for diabetes, 852
Diagnostic and Statistical Manual of Mental Disorders (DSM-IIIR), 765
Dialysis, 819. *See also* Hemodialysis; Peritoneal dialysis

Diamox, **190-192**
Diaphragm (body part), 743
Diaphragm (contraception), 782-783, 784 (fig.)
Diarrhea, as symptom
  Addison's disease, 811
  AIDS, 844
  anaphylaxis, 800
  colon cancer, 752
  Crohn's disease, 741
  diverticulosis, 741
  E. coli infection, 817
  enterocolitis, 814
  food poisoning, 814
  gastroenteritis, 739
  Graves' disease, 810
  irritable bowel syndrome, 740
  Legionnaire's disease, 747
  pancreatic cancer, 755
  proctitis, 741
  salmonella, 816
  STDs in digestive tract, 742
  toxic shock syndrome, 815
  ulcerative colitis, 740
  viral hepatitis, 830
Diastolic pressure, 722
Diazepam. *See* Valium
Dichloralphenazone. *See* Midrin
Diclofenac sodium. *See* Voltaren
Dicloxacillin sodium. *See also* Dynapen
  for skin infections, 814
Dicyclomine hydrochloride. *See* Bentyl
Didanosine, for HIV infection, 845
Diet
  colon cancer and, 741, 752
  gastric cancer and, 741-42
  gout and, 728-729
  hypertension and, 723
  mood changes in elderly and, 864
  osteoporosis and, 732
Diet, in treatment
  chronic bowel problems, 741-742
  chronic glomerulonephritis, 822
  cirrhosis, 832
  diabetes, 850
  pancreatitis, 742
  reflux esophagitis, 737-738
  rhinophyma, 803
Dietary fat
  pancreatic cancer and, 754-755
  prostate cancer and, 754
Diet counseling, for treating pain, 762
Diethylpropion hydrochloride. *See* Tenuate
Diethylstilbestrol (DES), **193-194**

Diflorasone diacetate. *See* Psorcon
Diflunisal. *See* Dolobid
Digestion, process of, 847-848
Digestive system, disorders of. *See* Gastrointestinal tract, disorders of
Digitalis, for congestive heart failure, 714-715
Digitoxin, for congestive heart failure, 714
Digoxin. *See also* Lanoxin
  for congestive heart failure, 714
Dihydrocodeine bitartrate. *See* Synalgos-DC
Dilantin, **195-198**
Dilatation and curettage (D&C), 779
Dilaudid, **198-200**
  for sickle cell anemia, 856
Diltiazem hydrochloride. *See* Cardizem
Dimetane-DC, **200-201**
Dimethyl sulfoxide. *See* DMSO
Dipentum, **202**
  for chronic bowel disease, 741
Diphenhydramine hydrochloride. *See* Benadryl
Diphenoxylate hydrochloride. *See* Lomotil
Diphtheria, vaccine for, 788
Dipivefrin hydrochloride. *See* Propine
Diprolene, **203-204**
Dipyridamole. *See* Persantine
Disalcid, **204-206**
Discharge, as symptom
  cholesteatoma, 793
  sinusitis, 795
  swimmer's ear, 792
Discoid lupus erythematosus (DLE), 729
Discoloration, as symptom, fracture, 735
Disk, slipped, 731, 733, 760
Disopyramide phosphate. *See* Norpace
Disorientation, as symptom, Legionnaire's disease, 747
Ditrupan. *See* Oxybutynin
Diulo. *See* Zaroxolyn
Diuretics
  for cirrhosis, 832
  to control hypertension, 723-724
  for COPD, 746
  for Ménière's disease, 793
  for nephrotic syndrome, 822
  for OB/GYN disorders, 779
  for pancreatic cancer, 755
Diuril, **206-208**
Divalproex sodium (Valproic acid). *See* Depakote
Diverticulosis, 741

irritable bowel syndrome and, 740
Dizziness, as symptom. *See also* Vertigo
  cholesteatoma, 793
  heart attack, 713
  otitis media, 793
DLE. *See* Discoid lupus erythematosus (DLE)
DMSO, for interstitial cystitis, 828
Docusate sodium. *See* Colace
Dolobid, **208-210**
Donnagel-PG, **210-212**
Donnatal, **212-213**
Doral, **214-215**
Doryx, **216-217**
Douching
  UTIs and, 827
  vaginitis and, 837
Down's syndrome, leukemia and, 755
Doxazosin mesylate. *See* Cardura
Doxepin hydrochloride. *See* Sinequan
Doxorubicin
  for bladder cancer, 757
  for breast cancer, 753
  for leukemia, 756
  for small-cell carcinoma of lung, 752
  for uterine cancer, 755
Doxycycline. *See also* Doryx
  for bladder infections, 827
  for Legionnaire's disease, 747
  for Lyme disease, 817
DPT vaccine, 788
Dressler's syndrome, pleurisy and, 747
Drooling, as symptom, epiglottitis, 747
Dropsy. *See* Congestive heart failure
Drowsiness, as symptom, diabetes, 849
Drug abuse. *See* Alcohol abuse; Substance abuse
Drugs, allergic reactions from, 798
Duodenal ulcers, 938
Duphalac. *See* Chronulac Syrup
Duricef, **218-219**
Dyazide, **219-221**
DynaCirc, **221-223**
  for hypertension, 724
Dynapen, **223-224**
Dysmenorrhea, 773-774
  hormonal therapy for, 779

E

Ear, nose and throat disorders, 791-796
Earache, as symptom

cholesteatoma, 793
  mumps, 789
  tonsillitis, 796
Ear canal, 791
  infections of outer, 792
Eardrops, for swimmer's ear, 792
Eardrum
  perforated, 793
  rupture of, 793
Echothiophate iodide. *See* Phospholine Iodide
Econazole nitrate. *See* Spectazole Cream
Ecotrin. *See* Aspirin
Ectopic pregnancy, 776 (fig.), 786
  IUD and, 785
  PID and, 776, 837
  STDs and, 833
  uterine bleeding and, 776
Eczema. *See* Atopic dermatitis; Atopic eczema
Edema, as symptom
  chronic glomerulonephritis, 822
  congestive heart failure, 715
  fracture, 735
  nephrotic syndrome, 822
E.E.S. *See* Erythromycin
Efudex, **224-226**
Elastin, 802
Elavil, **226-229**
  for depression, 768
  for panic disorder, 7688
Eldepryl, **229-230**
Elderly, medication use by, 861-864
Electrocoagulation, for precancerous uterine or cervical conditions, 755
Electroconvulsive therapy (ECT), for depression, 769
Electrodesiccation, for skin cancer, 757, 806
Electrodessication, for plantar warts, 859
Electronic pacemakers, 717
Electrosurgery. *See also* Electrocoagulation; Electrodesiccation
  for OB/GYN disorders, 779
  for STD growths, 839
ELISA test for AIDS, 844
Elocon, **231-232**
Emaciation, as symptom, cirrhosis, 831
Emetine, for liver abscess, 832
Eminase, for dissolving blood clots, 719
Emphysema, 745
  among elderly, 863
Empirin. *See* Aspirin
Empirin with Codeine, **232-234**
E-Mycin. *See* Erythromycin
Enalapril maleate. *See* Vaseretic; Vasotec

Endep. See Elavil
Endocarditis, Group D strep-
tococcal infections and, 815
Endocrine disorders, hyperten-
sion and, 723
Endocrine system, function of,
807, 809
Endometrial cancer, 755
Endometrial hyperplasia, and
uterine cancer, 777
Endometriosis, 774-775
hormonal therapy for, 779
infertility and, 779
Endometrium, treating precan-
cerous conditions, 755
Endoscopy, for monitoring ul-
cers, 740
Endotracheal intubation, for
epiglottitis, 747
Enduron, 235-237
Enemas, 740, 742
Entamoeba histolytica, liver
abscess and, 832
ENT disorders. See Ear, nose
and throat disorders
Enterocolitis, as side effect of
antibiotics, 814
Entex LA, 237-238
Epidermis, 802
Epidural catheters, for deliver-
ing painkilling drugs, 762
Epiglottis, 791-792
Epiglottitis, 747
vaccine for, 788
Epinephrine, 809
for anaphylaxis, 800
for nosebleeds, 794
for sting allergies, 800
Epitol. See Tegretol
EPO. See Erythropoietin
(EPO)
Epstein-Barr virus, mononu-
cleosis and, 789
Equanil. See Miltown
Ergoloid mesylates. See Hy-
dergine
Ergotamine tartrate. See
Cafergot
ERYC. See Erythromycin, Oral
Erycette, See Erythromycin,
topical
Erysipelas, 815
Ery-Tab. See Erythromycin, Oral
Erythrocin. See Erythromycin,
Oral
Erythrocytes, 853-854
Erythromycin, See also Benzamycin
for acne, 803
for Legionnaire's disease, 747
for skin infections, 814
for streptococcal pharyngi-
tis, 815
for tonsillitis, 796
oral, 239-242
topical, 242-243
for whooping cough, 789

Erythromycin ethylsuccinate.
See Pediazole
Erythropoietin (EPO), 819
for anemia, 824
Escherichia coli, 817
liver abscess and, 832
UTIs and, 826
Esgic. See Fioricet
Esidrix. See HydroDIURIL;
Ser-Ap-Es
Estazolam. See ProSom
Estoposide, for small-cell car-
cinoma of lung, 752
Estrogen, 809
in birth control pills, 786
bone loss and, 778
conjugated. See Premarin
elderly and, 863
fibroids and, 777
urinary incontinence and,
775
Estrogen, as treatment
acne, 803
OB/GYN disorders, 779
osteoporosis, 733
urinary incontinence, 828
Ethmozine, 243-245
Etodolac. See Lodine
Eulexin, 245-246
Eustachian tube, 791
infections, 792
Euthroid, 246-247
Ewing's sarcoma, 750, 756
Exfoliative dermatitis, 805
Expectorants, for common
cold, 744
Eyes. See also Conjunctivitis
bulging, as symptom of
Graves' disease, 810
inflammation of, and ankylosing spondylitis, 729
inflammation of, as symp-
tom of measles, 788

F

Face, muscle weakness and
cholesteatoma, 793
Facial palsy, as symptom,
Lyme disease, 817
Failure to thrive, as symptom,
thalassemia, 855
Fainting, as symptom
folic acid deficiency anemia,
855
thrombocytopenia, 856
Famotidine. See Pepcid
Fastin, 249-250
Fasting blood glucose test, 849
Fatty acids, 848
Fatty deposits, as symptom,
Cushing's syndrome, 811
Fatty liver, 832
Feldene, 250-252
Felodipine. See Plendil
Feminine hygiene sprays, UTIs
and, 827

Femstat, 252-253
Fenoprofen calcium. See Nal-
fon
Fertility awareness, for pre-
venting pregnancy, 781
Fertility drugs, 780
Fibrocystic breast changes,
778
Fibroids, 777, 777 (fig.)
and uterine bleeding, 776
Fight-or-flight response. See
Adrenaline
Finasteride. See Proscar
Fioricet, 253-255
Fiorinal, 255-257
with Codeine, 257-259
Flagyl, 259-261
for liver abscess, 832
Flavoxate hydrochloride. See
Urispas
Flecainide acetate. See Tambo-
cor
Flexeril, 261-263
5-Flourouracil, for bladder
cancer, 757
Floxin, 263-266
Fluid replacement, for Legion-
naire's disease, 747
Flunisolide. See AeroBid
for hay fever, 798
Fluocinolone acetonide, for
atopic dermatitis, 799
Fluocinonide. See Lidex
Fluoride. See Poly-Vi-Flor
Fluorometholone. See FML
S.O.P.
Fluorouracil. See Efudex
for breast cancer, 753
for colon cancer, 752
Fluoxetine hydrochloride. See
Prozac
Fluphenazine hydrochloride.
See Prolixin
Flurazepam hydrochloride. See
Dalmane
Flurbiprofen. See Ansaid
Flutamide. See Eulexin
Fluticasone propionate. See
Cutivate
FML S.O.P., 248-249
Folic acid. See also Poly-Vi-
Flor
for folic acid deficiency ane-
mia, 855
for thalassemia, 855
Folic acid deficiency anemia,
855
Follicle-stimulating hormones
(FSH), 809
Folliculitis, 805
Food poisoning, staph-caused,
814
Forgetfulness, as symptom,
folic acid deficiency anemia,
855
Fosinopril sodium. See Mono-
pril

Fractures, 735
analgesics for, 760
FSH (follicle-stimulating hormone), 809
Fulvicin P/G. See Gris-PEG
Fungal infections. See also
Athlete's foot
of foot, 858
with HIV virus, 844
of skin, 805
of toenail, 859
Fungicides, for athlete's foot,
858
Fungistatic drugs, for athlete's
foot, 858
Furosemide. See Lasix
Furunculosis, 805

G

Gait abnormalities, foot prob-
lems and, 858
Gallbladder, 831
Gallstones, 831
pancreatitis and, 742
Gantrisin, 267-268
Garamycin Ophthalmic, 269
Gastric cancer, 740
Gastric ulcers, 739
Gastritis, chronic, 739
Gastroenteritis, 739, 816
Gastrointestinal tract, 738
(fig.)
cancers of, 758
disorders of, 737-742
functions of, 737
infections of, 817
Gemfibrozil. See Lopid
Genetics, aging and, 862
Genital herpes, 775, 833, 837-
838
condoms and, 783
treating, 839
Zovirax for, 780
Genital warts, 775, 833, 837
condoms and, 783
treating, 839
Gentacidin. See Garamycin
ophthalmic
Gentamicin sulfate. See
Garamycin ophthalmic
German measles, 789
Gestational diabetes, 848
GH (growth hormone), 809
Giardiasis, 742
Gigantism, 808
Glaucoma, migraine and, 761
Glipizide. See Glucotrol
Glomerulonephritis
chronic, 822
following strep infection,
822
rapidly progressive, 822
Glomerulus, 820 (fig.)
Glucagon, 809
for diabetes, 852
for hypoglycemic coma, 850

Glucose
  for hypoglycemic coma, 850
  impaired tolerance for, 848
  insulin production and, 847-848
Glucose tolerance test, 849
Glucotrol, 270-272
  for diabetes, 852
Glyburide. *See* Micronase
Glycerin. *See* Auralgan
Glycohemoglobin, testing, 851
Glycohemoglobin test, for diabetes, 851
Goiter, 810
Gold salts, for rheumatoid arthritis, 727
Gonococcus, 835
Gonorrhea, 833-835
  chlamydia and, 839
  condoms and, 783
  infectious arthritis and, 730
Gout, 726, 729
Granulocytes, 854
Graves' disease, 810
Grisactin. *See* Gris-PEG
Griseofulvin. *See* Gris-PEG
Gris-PEG, 273-274
Growth hormone (GH), 809
Growth retardation, hypopituitarism and, 808
Guaifenesin. *See* Entex LA
  for influenza, 745
Guanabenz acetate. *See* Wytensin
Guanfacine hydrochloride. *See* Tenex
Gums, bleeding, as symptom, pernicious anemia, 854

H

Habitrol. *See* Nicotine Patches
Hair, premature graying, and Graves' disease, 810
Halcion, 275-277
Haldol, 277-279
  for schizophrenia, 770
Hallucinations, as symptom, schizophrenia, 770
Haloperidol. *See* Haldol
Hammer toe, 859
Hand
  pain in, and carpal tunnel syndrome, 735
  tremors, as symptom of hypothyroidism, 808
Hay fever, 798
  sinusitis and, 795
Headache, 760-761
Headache, as symptom
  aplastic anemia, 855
  erysipelas, 815
  folic acid deficiency anemia, 855
  hay fever, 798
  hyperpituitarism, 808
  hypoglycemia, 850

iron deficiency anemia, 854
Legionnaire's disease, 747
Lyme disease, 817
meningitis, 816
mononucleosis, 789
mumps, 789
rubella, 789
SLE, 729
tonsillitis, 796
toxic shock syndrome, 815
Head trauma, migraine and, 761
Hearing, ear and, 791
Hearing loss, as symptom
  cholesteatoma, 793
  ear problems, 792
  Ménière's disease, 793
  otitis media, 792
Hearing nerve, 791
Heart attack, defined, 713
Heartburn, as symptom, reflux esophagitis, 737
Heart disease, 711-719
  ankylosing spondylitis and, 729
  congestive heart failure, 715
  panic attacks and, 767
  statistics, 711
  syphilis and, 838
  toenail changes as indicator of, 859
  treating, 714-719
Heart failure, meningitis and, 816
Heat sensitivity, as symptom, Graves' disease, 810
Heat treatment, for slipped disk, 733
Heel pain, causes, 858
Heel spurs, 858
Hemodialysis, 823
Hemophilia, 856
  chronic pain and, 760
Hemophilus Type B vaccine, 788
Hemorrhage. *See* Bleeding
Hemorrhagic disorders, 856
Hemorrheologic agents, 716
Hemorrhoids, 742
Hepatic coma, 832
Hepatitis A, 830
Hepatitis B, 831
  chronic carriers of, 831
  condoms and, 783
  transmission of, 835, 838
  vaccine for, 788
Hepatitis Type C, 830
Herniated disk. *See* Disk, slipped
Herpes infections, 806. *See also* Genital herpes and AIDS, 844
Herpes simplex, 775, 837
Hiatal hernia, reflux esophagitis and, 738
High blood pressure. *See* Hypertension

Hip replacment surgery, 727
Hismanal, **279-280**
  for hives, 799
Histamine H_2 blockers, for ulcers, 739
HIV. *See* Human immunodeficiency virus (HIV)
Hives, 798-799, 805
  sting allergies and, 799
Hivid. *See* Zalcitabine
HLA B-27 genetic marker, 729
Hodgkin's disease, 750, 758
  in children, 756
  tuberculosis and, 746
Home intravenous infusion systems, for treating cancer pain, 762
Homosexuals
  AIDS and, 842
  STDs and, 834
Hookworms, 805
Hormonal disorders, infertility and, 778
Hormonal therapy
  for breast cancer, 753
  for metastatic prostate cancer, 754
  for OB/GYN disorders, 779
Hormones. *See also* Contraception, hormonal methods; Endocrine system
  acne and, 803
  female, in contraception, 782-783, 786
  imbalance of, and depression in elderly, 864
  imbalance of, and ovarian cysts, 778
  imbalance of, and uterine bleeding, 776
  PMS and, 774
  sex, 809
Human immunodeficiency virus (HIV)
  effects of, 841
  statistics, 842
  structure, 843
  treating, 844-845
Human insulin, for Type I diabetes, 851
Human papillomavirus (HPV), 837
  genital warts and, 775
Humulin. *See* Insulin
Hunger, unusual, as symptom, diabetes, 849
Huntington's disease, dementia and, 864
Hydergine, **280-281**
Hydrochlorothiazide. *See* Aldactazide; Capozid; Dyazide; HydroDIURIL; Inderide; Maxzide; Moduretic; Vaseretic
Hydrocodone bitartrate. *See* Vicodin

Hydrocodone polistirex. *See* Tussionex
Hydrocortisone. *See also* Cortisporin Ophthalmic Suspension; VoSoL
  for Addison's disease, 811
Hydrocortisone acetate. *See* Coly-Mycin S Otic
HydroDIURIL, **281-283**
Hydromorphone hydrochloride. *See* Dilaudid
Hydroxychloroquine sulfate. *See* Plaquenil
Hydroxyzine hydrochloride. *See* Atarax
Hygroton, **284-286**
Hyoscyamine. *See* Urised
Hyoscyamine sulfate. *See* Donnagel-PG; Donnatal; Levsin; Ru-Tuss Tablets
Hyperactivity, 763
Hyperglycemia, testing for, 851
Hyperoxaluria, 821
Hyperparathyroidism, 810
Hyperpituitarism, 808
Hypertension
  causes of, 723
  with chronic glomerulonephritis, 822
  consequences of uncontrolled, 721
  coronary artery disease and, 714
  Cushing's syndrome and, 811
  defined, 722
  dementia and, 864
  drugs to control, 723-724
  hormonal contraceptives and, 786
  Inderal and, 716
  living with, 722
  migraine and, 761
  polycystic kidney disease (PKD) and, 821
  with post-strep glomerulonephritis, 822
  treating, 721-724
  treating in elderly, 863
Hyperthyroidism, 810
Hypoglycemia, 850
Hypoparathyroidism, 810
Hypopituitarism, 808
Hypothalamus, 807
Hypothyroidism, 808
  constipation and, 742
  hypopituitarism and, 808
Hysterectomy, 777 (fig.), 779
Hytrin, **286-287**

I

Ibuprofen. *See also* Motrin Tablets
  for common cold, 744
Identification bracelet

for Addison's disease sufferers, 811
for diabetics, 850
Ileitis. *See* Crohn's disease
Iletin *See* Insulin
Ilosone. *See* Erythromycin, Oral
Imipramine hydrochloride. *See* Tofranil
Immune globulin (IG), for viral hepatitis, 830
Immune system
changes with aging, 862-863
deficiency in, and sinusitis, 795
disorders of. *See* Acquired immune deficiency syndrome (AIDS); Arthritis; Schizophrenia; Systemic lupus erythematosus (SLE)
HIV and, 841, 843
STDs and, 834
Immunosuppressive drugs
for aplastic anemia, 855
for scleroderma, 730
for SLE, 729
for thrombocytopenia, 856
tuberculosis and, 746
Immunotherapy
for cancer, 751
for hay fever, 798
for postnasal drip, 795
for small-cell carcinoma of lung, 752
Imodium, 288-290
for diarrhea, 740
Impetigo, 805, 815
glomerulonephritis and, 822
Implant, contraceptive, 786
Impotence
pernicious anemia and, 854
as symptom of hypopituitarism, 808
Imuran. *See* Azathioprine
Incontinence, pernicious anemia and, 854
Incontinence, urinary, 825, 827-828
Urispas for, 780
in women, 775
Indapamide. *See* Lozol
Inderal, 290-292. *See also* Inderide
for anxiety disorders, 768
for arrhythmia, 716
for migraine, 761
Inderide, 293-295
Indigestion, as symptom, gastric cancer, 740
Indocin, 295-297
for osteoarthritis, 727
Indomethacin. *See* Indocin
Infection
illness and, 813-814
treating, 813-817
Infectious arthritis, 730
Infertility, 778-779
ovarian cancer and, 778

as symptom of hypopituitarism, 808
Inflammatory bowel disease, 740-741, 752
Ingrown toenail, 859
Injection therapy, for hemorrhoids, 742
Inner ear, 791
disorders of, 793
Insomnia, as symptom
Cushing's syndrome, 811
kidney failure, 823
Insulatard NPH. *See* Insulin
Insulatard NPH Human. *See* Insulin
Insulin, 297-301, 809
for diabetes, 850
functions of, 847
for pancreatic cancer, 755
types of, 851
Insulin shock, 850
Intal, for asthma, 798
Intal Aerosol Spray. *See* Cromolyn sodium
Intal Capsules. *See* Cromolyn sodium
Intal Solution. *See* Cromolyn sodium
Interferon
in cancer treatment, 751
for hepatitis B, 831
for HIV infection, 845
Interleukin-2, in cancer treatment, 751
Interstitial cystitis, 828
Intestinal bleeding, as symptom, diverticulosis, 741
Intrauterine contraceptive device (IUD), 782, 784-786, 785 (illus.)
PID and, 837
STDs and, 835
and uterine disorders, 776
Intravenous urography, 821
Intrinsic factor, pernicious anemia and, 854
Iodides, acne and, 803
Iodinated glycerol. *See* Tussi-Organidin DM Liquid
Iodine
radioactive, for hyperthyroidism, 810
thyroid disorders and, 808
Ionamin, 301-302
Ipratropium bromide. *See* Atrovent
Iron deficiency anemia, 854
toenail changes and, 859
Iron-removal therapy, for thalassemia, 855
Iron supplements, for anemia, 824, 854
Irritable bowel syndrome, 740
Isoetharine mesylate. *See* Bronkometer/Bronkosol
Isollyl. *See* Fiorinal

Isometheptene mucate. *See* Midrin
Isoniazid, for tuberculosis, 746
Isoptin. *See* Calan
Isoptin SR. *See* Calan
Isopto-Carpine. *See* Pilocar
Isordil, 303-305
Isosorbide dinitrate. *See* Isordil
Isotretinoin. *See* Accutane
Isradipine. *See* DynaCirc
Itching, as symptom
anaphylaxis, 800
diabetes, 849
kidney failure, 823
IUD. *See* Intrauterine contraceptive device (IUD)

J

Janimine. *See* Tofranil
Jaundice, hormonal contraceptives and, 786
Jaundice, as symptom
cirrhosis, 831
folic acid deficiency anemia, 855
hepatitis B, 838
liver abscess, 832
pancreatic cancer, 755
pernicious anemia, 854
sickle cell anemia, 856
thalassemia, 855
viral hepatitis, 830
Joint pain, as symptom
bacteremia, 814
viral hepatitis, 830
Joints, normal, 728 (fig.)
Joint swelling, as symptom
rheumatoid arthritis, 727
sickle cell anemia, 856
Juvenile rheumatoid arthritis, 730

K

Kaolin. *See* Donnagel-PG
Kaposi's sarcoma, 842
Keflex, 305-306
Keftab, 306-308
Kegel exercises, 828
Keratin, 802
Ketoacidosis, 848
Ketoconazole. *See* Nizoral
Ketones, 848
Ketoprofen. *See* Orudis
Kidney disease
acquired, 820, 823
congenital, 820
early symptoms in feet, 857
hypertension and, 723
inherited, 820
statistics, 819
treating, 819-824
Kidney failure
calcium channel blocker and, 718

carpal tunnel syndrome and, 735
coronary artery disease and, 714
treating, 823-824
Kidney stones, 819, 823
polycystic kidney disease (PKD) and, 821
Kissing
transmission of hepatitis B by, 830
transmission of syphilis by, 838
Klonopin, 308-310
Klor-Con. *See* Micro-K
Knee replacement surgery, 727
Kyphosis, 732

L

Labetalol hydrochloride. *See* Normodyne
Lactose intolerance, irritable bowel syndrome and, 740
Lactulose. *See* Chronulac Syrup
Lanoxin, 310-312
Laparoscopic cholecystectomy, 831
Laparoscopy, for OB/GYN disorders, 779
Large intestine, diseases of, 740-742
Larodopa, 312-314
Larotid. *See* Amoxil
Laryngitis, 744, 796
Larynx, 791-792
angioedema and, 799
Laser therapy
for genital warts, 839
for kidney stones, 823
for OB/GYN disorders, 779
for small-cell carcinoma of lung, 752
for telangiectasias, 803
Lasix, 314-316
for post-strep glomerulonephritis, 822
Laxatives, 740, 742
Legionnaire's disease, 747
Lente Insulin. *See* Insulin
Lesbians, STDs and, 834
Lesions, as symptom
AIDS, 844
erysipelas, 815
impetigo, 815
Lyme disease, 817
lymphadenitis, 815
meningitis (severe form), 816
pancreatic cancer, 755
sickle cell anemia, 856
staph skin infections, 814
Leukemia, 750, 755-756
acute lymphocytic, 750
bone marrow transplants, 751

in children, 756
tuberculosis and, 746
Leukocytes, 853-854
ACE inhibitors and, 724
Leumedins, for arthritis. *See also* Arthritis
Levamisole, for colon cancer, 752
Levlen. *See* Oral contraceptives
Levobunolol hydrochloride. *See* Betagan
Levodopa. *See* Larodopa; Sinemet CR
Levothroid. *See* Synthroid
Levothyroxine. *See* Synthroid
Levoxine. *See* Synthroid
Levsin, 316-319
LH (luetinizing hormone), 809
Libido, loss of, in endocrine disorders, 808
Librax, 319-320
Libritabs. *See* Librium
Librium, 320-322
Lidex, 322-324
Lidocaine, for fractures, 735
Lifestyle, heart disease and, 711
Ligaments, 728 (fig.)
Light sensitivity, as symptom
measles, 788
migraine, 761
Limbitrol, 324-326
Limping, persistent, as symptom, childhood cancers, 756
Lioresal, 326-328
Liotrix. *See* Euthroid
Lisinopril, 724. *See* Zestril
Lithium. *See also* Lithobid
acne and, 803
for bipolar depression, 769
Lithobid, 328-331
Liver. *See also* Hepatitis
abscess of, 832
diseases of, 829-832
functions, 829-830
transplantation of, 832
Liver cancer, hepatitis B and, 831
Liver tumor, hormonal contraceptives and, 786
Local anesthetics, for acute pain, 760
Lockjaw. *See* Tetanus
Lodine, 331-332
Loestrin. *See* Oral contraceptives
Lomotil, 333-335
for diarrhea, 740
Lomustine, for colon cancer, 752
Lo/Ovral. *See* Oral contraceptives
Loperamide hydrochloride. *See* Imodium
Lopid, 335-337
for reducing cholesterol, 719

Lopressor, 337-339
Loprox, 339-340
Lopurin. *See* Zyloprim
Lorazepam. *See* Ativan
Lorelco, 340-341
for reducing cholesterol, 719
Lortab. *See* Vicodin
Lotensin, 342-344
Lotrimin, 344
Lotrisone, 345-346
Lovastatin. *See* Mevacor
Low back pain, 731, 732 (fig.), 733, 760
Low back pain, as symptom, polycystic kidney disease (PKD), 821
Lozol, 346-348
Lubricating jelly, 835
Ludiomil, 348-350
Luetinizing hormone (LH), 809
Lump, as symptom, breast cancer, 752
Lumpectomy, 753
Lung cancer, 751-752
Lungs. *See also* Pneumonia
chronic disorders of, 745-746
diminished capacity with age, 863
function of, 743
pain as symptom of pleurisy, 747
pain as symptom of pneumonia, 745
structure of, 744 (fig.)
Lupus. *See* Systemic lupus erythematosus (SLE)
Luride, 351-352
Lyme disease, 817
infectious arthritis and, 730
Lymphadenitis, 815
Lymph glands, swollen, as symptom
AIDS, 844
genital herpes, 837
mononucleosis, 790
rubella, 789
streptococcal pharyngitis, 815
syphilis, 838
tonsillitis, 796
Lymphocytes, 854. *See also* T-4 lymphocytes
Lymphomas, 750, 756, 758
Lyophilized blood factor, 856

M

Macrobid. *See* Macrodantin
Macrodantin, 354-357
for bladder infections, 827
Macrophages, HIV and, 843
Magnesium deficiency, hypoparathyroidism and, 810
Magnetic resonance imaging (MRI), 751

Malignant melanoma, 806
Mammograms, 753, 778
Manic depression. *See* Bipolar depression
MAO inhibitors. *See* Monoamine oxidase (MAO) inhibitors
Maprotiline hydrochloride. *See* Ludiomil
Marplan, for depression, 768
Massage, for treating pain, 762
Mast cells, 797
Mastectomy, 753
Mastoidectomy, 793
Mastoiditis, 793
Maxzide, 357-359
Measles, 788
infectious arthritis and, 730
vaccine for, 788
Mebendazole, for worms, 790
Meclizine hydrochloride. *See* Antivert
Meclofenamate sodium. *See* Meclomen
Meclomen, 359-361
Medrol, 361-363
Medroxyprogesterone acetate. *See* Provera
Mefanamic acid. *See* Ponstel
Megace, 363-364
Megestrol acetate. *See* Megace
Melanin, 802
Melanoma, 756-757
Mellaril, 365-367
Melphalan, for ovarian cancer, 757
Memory loss
among elderly, 862-863
hypothyroidism and, 808
Ménière's disease, 793
Meningitis, 816
and AIDS, 844
mumps and, 789
strep and, 815
vaccine for, 788
Menopause
carpal tunnel syndrome and, 735
irregular menstruation and, 776
late, and uterine cancer, 778
migraine headaches and, 761
osteoporosis and, 733, 778
ovarian cancer and, 757
stress incontinence and, 828
UTIs and, 825
Menstruation
absence of as symptom of hypopituitarism, 808
causes of irregular, 776
disorders of, 773-774
IUD and, 785
painful, calcium channel blockers and, 718

painful, medications for, 780
Mental illness
among elderly, 862
defined, 764
diagnostic difficulties, 765
hyperparathyroidism and, 810
major categories, 765
statistics, 763
syphilis and, 838
warning signs, 765
Mental retardation, 771
STDs and, 833
Meperidine hydrochloride. *See* Demerol
Meprobamate. *See* Miltown
Mesalamine. *See* Rowasa
Metabolic dysfunction, hypopituitarism and, 808
Metaprel. *See* Alupent
Metaproterenol sulfate. *See* Alupent
Metastasis, 750
Methazolamide. *See* Neptazane
Methenamine. *See* Urised
Methergine, 367-368
Methicillin
for bacteremia, 814
for skin infections, 814
for toxic shock syndrome, 815
Methimazole, for hyperthyroidism, 810
Methocarbamol. *See* Robaxin
Methotrexate, 368-370
for bladder cancer, 757
for breast cancer, 753
for colon cancer, 752
for leukemia, 756
for psoriasis, 804
for rheumatoid arthritis, 727
Methyclothiazide. *See* Enduron
Methyldopa. *See* Aldomet
Methylene blue. *See* Urised
Methylergonovine maleate. *See* Methergine
Methylphenidate hydrochloride. *See* Ritalin
Methylprednisolone, *See* Medrol
Methyltestosterone. *See* Android
Methysergide maleate. *See* Sansert
Metoclopramide hydrochloride. *See* Reglan
Metolazone. *See* Zaroxolyn
Metopirone. *See* Metyrapone
Metoprolol tartrate. *See* Lopressor
Metronidazole. *See* Flagyl
for STDs, 839
Metryl. *See* Flagyl

Metyrapone, for Cushing's syndrome, 811
Mevacor, 371-373
  for cholesterol reduction, 719
Mexiletine hydrochloride. See Mexitil
Mexitil, 373-376
Miconazole nitrate. See Monistat 3
Micro-K, 376-377
Micronase, 377-380
  for diabetes, 852
Middle ear, 791
  infections of, 792-793
Midrin, 381-383
Migraine headaches, 761
  calcium channel blockers and, 718
  Inderal and, 716
Miltown, 382-383
Minipress, 383-385, 724
Minocin, 385-387
Minocycline hydrochloride. See Minocin
Minoxidil, 724. See also Rogaine
Miscarriage, and uterine bleeding, 776
Misoprostol. See Cytotec
Mitomycin, for colon cancer, 752
Mitoxantrone, for leukemia, 756
Mixtard 70/30. See Insulin
Mixtard Human 70/30. See Insulin
MMR vaccine, 788
Modicon. See Oral contraceptives
Moduretic, 388-390
Mole, changes in as symptom of melanoma, 756-757, 806
Mometasone furoate. See Elocon
Monistat 3, 390-391
Monoamine oxidase (MAO) inhibitors, for depression, 769
Monoarticular juvenile arthritis. See Juvenile rheumatoid arthritis
Monoclonal antibodies, in cancer treatment, 751
Monocytes, HIV and, 843
Mononucleosis, 789
Monopril, 391-393
Moricizine hydrochloride. See Ethmozine
Morphine-based analgesics, 760
  addiction and, 762
Morphine sulfate. See MS Contin
Motrin Tablets, 393-395
  for acute pain, 760
  for neck pain, 734

for osteoarthritis, 727
Mouth sores, as symptom of oral cancer, 757
MS Contin, 352-354
Mucous membranes, in sinusitis, 794-795
Mucus
  blocked, in sinusitis, 795
  role in respiratory system, 791
  in whooping cough, 789
Multiple myeloma, 758
Multiple sclerosis, 730
  urge incontinence and, 828
Mumps, 789
  infectious arthritis and, 730
  vaccine for, 788
Mupirocin. See Bactroban
Muscle pain, as symptom
  kidney failure, 823
  Lyme disease, 817
  meningitis, 816
  mumps, 789
  toxic shock syndrome, 815
Muscle relaxants
  for acute pain, 760
  for chronic headaches, 761
  for neck pain, 734
Muscle rigidity, as symptom, tetanus, 816
Mycelex. See Lotrimin
Mycobacterium avium-intracellulare, and AIDS, 844
Mycobacterium tuberculosis, 746
Mycolog II, 395-396
Mycoplasma, UTIs and, 826-827
Mycosis fungoides, 758
Myco-Triacet II. See Mycolog II
Myelomas, 750
Mykrox. See Zaroxolyn
Myomas. See Fibroids
Myomectomy, 777 (fig.), 779
Myringotomy, 793
Mysoline, 396-398
Mytrex. See Mycolog II
Myxedema, carpal tunnel syndrome and, 735

N

Nadolol. See Corgard; Corzide
Nafcillin
  for bacteremia, 814
  for skin infections, 814
  for toxic shock syndrome, 815
Nalfon, 398-400
Naphazoline hydrochloride. See Naphcon-A
Naphcon-A, 400-402
Naprosyn, 402-404
  for osteoarthritis, 727
Naproxen sodium. See Anaprox; Naprosyn

Narcotic analgesics, elderly and, 863
Narcotics, for acute pain, 760
Nardil, 404-407
  for depression, 768
Nasacort. See Triamcinolone
Nasal balloon catheter, 794
Nasalcrom Nasal Solution. See Cromolyn sodium
Nasalide. See AeroBid
Nasal polyps, 795
Nasal sprays, for common cold, 744
Natural thyroid hormones T$_3$ and T$_4$. See Armour Thyroid
Nausea, as symptom
  Addison's disease, 811
  anaphylaxis, 800
  constipation, 742
  diabetes, 848-849
  diverticulosis, 741
  enterocolitis, 814
  folic acid deficiency anemia, 855
  food poisoning, 814
  gastritis, 739
  gastroenteritis, 739
  kidney failure, 823
  kidney stones, 823
  Legionnaire's disease, 747
  liver abscess, 832
  Ménière's disease, 793
  migraine, 761
  mumps, 789
  otitis media, 792
  pancreatitis, 742
  pernicious anemia, 854
  reflux esophagitis, 737
  salmonella, 816
  viral hepatitis, 830
Navane, 407-408
NebuPent. See Pentamidine
Neck pain, 733-734
Neck stiffness, as symptom
  Lyme disease, 817
  meningitis, 816
Nembutal Sodium Capsules, 409-410
Neoadjuvant chemotherapy, for cancer, 751
Neodecadron Ophthalmic Ointment and Solution, 410-412
Neomycin sulfate. See Coly-Mycin S Otic; Cortisporin Ophthalmic Suspension; Neodecadron Ophthalmic Ointment and Solution
Nephritis, 821-822
Nephron, 820 (fig.)
Nephrotic syndrome, 822
Neptazane, 412-413
Nerve blockers, for pleurisy, 747
Nerve damage, chronic pain and, 760

Nervous system
  hyperpituitarism and, 808
  SLE and, 729
Neural blockade, for treating pain, 762
Neuroblastoma, in children, 756
Neurodermatitis, 805
Neurological difficulties, pernicious anemia and, 854
Neuromas (foot), 859
Neuromuscular blocker, for tetanus, 816
Neurotransmitters, PMS and, 774
Niacin, 718. See also Poly-Vi-Flor
Nicardipine hydrochloride. See Cardene
Nicoderm. See Nicotine Patches
Nicorette, 413-416
Nicotine Patches, 416-418
Nicotine polacrilex. See Nicorette
Nicotrol. See Nicotine Patches
Nifedipine. See Procardia; Procardia XL
Night sweats, as symptom
  AIDS, 844
  tuberculosis, 746
Nimodipine. See Nimotop
Nimotop, 419-420
Nipple soreness, as symptom, breast cancer, 752
Nitro-Bid. See Nitroglycerin
Nitro-Dur. See Nitroglycerin
Nitrofurantoin. See Macrodantin
Nitroglycerin, 420-422
  heart disease and, 715-716
Nitrolingual Spray. See Nitroglycerin
Nitrostat Tablets. See Nitroglycerin
Nizatidine. See Axid
Nizoral, 423-424
Nolamine, 424-425
Nolex LA. See Entex LA
Nolvadex, 425-427
  for breast cancer, 753
Nonsteroidal anti-inflammatory drugs (NSAIDs)
  for acute pain, 760
  allergic reactions from, 798
  for ankylosing spondylitis, 729
  for arthritis, 726-727
  for arthritis with psoriasis, 804
  for carpal tunnel syndrome, 735
  elderly and, 863
  for gout, 729
  for juvenile rheumatoid arthritis, 730
  for rheumatoid arthritis, 727

for SLE, 729
for treating pain, 762
Norcet. *See* Vicodin
Nordette. *See* Oral contraceptives
Norepinephrine, 809
Norethin. *See* Oral contraceptives
Norfloxacin. *See* Noroxin
Norgesic. *See* Norgesic Forte
Norgesic Forte, 427-428
Norinyl. *See* Oral contraceptives
Normodyne, 429-430
Noroxin, 431-433
Norpace, 433-435
Norpramin, 435-437
Nortriptyline hydrochloride. *See* Pamelor
Nosebleeds, 793-794
Novolin. *See* Insulin
NPH Iletin I. *See* Insulin
Nutrition. *See* Diet
Nystatin. *See* Mycolog II

O

Obesity
  Type II diabetes and, 849
  and uterine cancer, 778
Obsessive-compulsive disorder, 767
Ofloxacin. *See* Floxin
Olsalazine sodium. *See* Dipentum
Omeprazole. *See* Prilosec
Oncogenes, 751
Oophorectomy, 779
Opcon-A. *See* Naphcon-A
Opium, powdered. *See* Donnagel-PG
Opticrom Ophthalmic Solution. *See* Cromolyn sodium
Oral cancer, 757-758
Oral contraceptives, 437-440
  acne and, 803
  hypertension and, 723
  ovarian cancer and, 757
Orap, 440-442
Orasone. *See* Deltasone
Organidin (iodinated glycerol). *See* Tussi-Organidin DM
Organ transplantation
  bone marrow, 751, 756, 855
  heart, 714
  kidney, 819, 824
  liver, 832
Orinase, 442-445
  for diabetes, 852
Orphenadrine citrate. *See* Norgesic Forte
Ortho-Novum. *See* Oral contraceptives
Orthotic devices, for neuromas, 859
Orudis, 445-447

Osteoarthritis (OA), 726-727, 728 (fig.), 731
  genetic marker for, 730
  neck pain and, 733
Osteomyelitis, 814
Osteoporosis, 731-733, 732 (fig.), 778
  hormonal therapy for, 779
Otitis media, 792-793
  strep and, 815
Ovarian cancer, 757, 778
  hormonal contraceptives and, 786
Ovaries
  disorders of, 778
  hormones from, 809
  removal of, and osteoporosis, 778
Ovcon. *See* Oral contraceptives
Overflow incontinence, 828
Ovral. *See* Oral contraceptives
Ovulation, 782 (fig.), 783
  irregular, and uterine cancer, 778
  ovarian cysts and, 777-778
Oxacillin
  for skin infections, 814
  for toxic shock syndrome, 815
Oxazepam. *See* Serax
Oxiconazole nitrate. *See* Oxistat Cream
Oxistat Cream, 447-448
Oxtriphylline. *See* Choledyl
Oxybutynin, for urinary incontinence, 828
Oxycodone hydrochloride. *See* Percocet
Oxygen, in blood supply, 713-714, 718
Oxygen therapy
  for COPD, 746
  for croup, 746
  for epiglottitis, 747
  for Legionnaire's disease, 747
  for pneumonia, 745

P

Pacemakers, 714
Packing, for nosebleeds, 794
Pallor, as symptom
  aplastic anemia, 855
  bacteremia, 814
  childhood cancers, 756
  folic acid deficiency anemia, 855
  heart attack, 713
  iron deficiency anemia, 854
  leukemia, 755
  sickle cell anemia, 856
  thalassemia, 855
Palpitations, as symptom
  bacteremia, 814

folic acid deficiency anemia, 855
Graves' disease, 810
meningitis, 816
thrombocytopenia, 856
Pamelor, 450-452
  for depression, 768
Panadol. *See* Tylenol
Pancreas, 809-810. *See also* Diabetes mellitus; Endocrine system
  insulin production in, 847-848
Pancrease, 453
Pancreatic cancer, 754-755
Pancreatic enzymes, in treating pancreatic cancer, 755
Pancreatitis, 742
  pancreatic cancer and, 755
Pancrelipase. *See* Pancrease
Panhypopituitarism, 808
Panic disorder, 766-767
  treating, 768
Pap test, 755, 837
Parafon Forte DSC, 454-455
Paranoia, as symptom, schizophrenia, 770
Parasites, skin infections from, 805
Parathyroid glands, 809-810
Parathyroid hormone (PH), 809
Parkinson's disease, dementia and, 864
Parlodel, 455-457
Parnate, for depression, 768
Parotid, swelling in, and mumps, 789
Patient-controlled intravenous agents (PCA), 760
PBZ-SR, 448-450
PCA, 760
PCE. *See* Erythromycin, oral
Pectin. *See* Donnagel-PG
Pediapred, 457-460
Pediazole, 460-461
Pediculosis, 805
Pelvic infections
  hormonal contraceptives and, 786
  IUD and, 785
Pelvic inflammatory disease (PID), 773, 776 (fig.), 783, 836-837
  infertility and, 779
  STDs and, 833
  and uterine bleeding, 776
Pelvic muscle exercises, in treating urinary incontinence, 828
Pemoline. *See* Cylert
Penicillamine
  for rheumatoid arthritis, 727
  for Wilson's disease, 832
Penicillin
  allergic reactions from, 798
  for bacteremia, 814

for Lyme disease, 817
for pharyngitis, 796
for strep infections, 815
for streptococcal pharyngitis, 815
synthetic, 813
for syphilis, 838
for tetanus, 818
for tonsillitis, 796
Penicillin G, for meningitis, 816
Penicillin V, 462-463
Penis, discharge as symptom of STDs, 835-836
Pentam. *See* Pentamadine
Pentamadine, for *Pneumocystis carinii* pneumonia, 844
Pentazocine hydrochloride. *See* Talwin Compound
Pentobarbital sodium. *See* Nembutal Sodium Capsules
Pentoxifylline. *See* Trental
Pen-Vee K. *See* Penicillin V
Pepcid, 464-465
  for ulcers, 740
Peptic ulcer
  anemia and, 854
  Cushing's syndrome and, 811
  pancreatitis and, 742
Pepto-Bismol, for gastroenteritis, 739
Percocet, 465-467
Percodan, for sickle cell anemia, 856
Percutaneous transluminal coronary angioplasty (PTCA), 719
Pergolide mesylate. *See* Permax
Periactin, 467-469
Peridex, 469-470
Peritoneal dialysis, 823-824
Permax, 470-472
Pernicious anemia, 854-855
  gastritis and, 739
Perphenazine. *See* Triavil
Persantine, 472-473
Personality, and hypertension, 723
Pertussis. *See* Whooping cough
Petrolatum, for atopic eczema, 804
Pharyngitis, 744, 796. *See also* Streptococcal pharyngitis
Pharynx, 791. *See also* Throat
Phenaphen with Codeine. *See* Tylenol with Codeine
Phenazopyridine hydrochloride. *See* Pyridium
Phenelzine sulfate. *See* Nardil
Phenergan, 474-476
  with Codeine, 476-478
Phenindamine tartrate. *See* Nolamine
Pheniramine maleate. *See* Naphcon-A

Phenobarbital, 478-481. *See
also* Donnatal
Phentermine hydrochloride.
See Fastin
Phentermine resin. *See* Ion-
amin
Phenylbutazone. *See* Butazo-
lidin
Phenylephrine, for sinusitis,
795
Phenylephrine hydrochloride.
See Ru-Tuss Tablets
Phenylephrine tannate. *See* Ry-
natan
Phenylpropanolamine hy-
drochloride. *See also*
Dimetane-DC; Entex LA;
Nolamine; Ru-Tuss Tablets
for urinary incontinence,
828
Phenyl salicylate. *See* Urised
Phenytoin sodium. *See* Dilan-
tin
Phobias, 766
in children, 771
Phospholine Iodide, 481-483
PH (parathyroid hormone),
809
Physical therapy
for ankylosing spondylitis,
729
for osteoporosis, 733
PID. *See* Pelvic inflammatory
disease (PID)
Pilocar, 483-484
Pilocarpine hydrochloride. *See*
Pilocar
Pimozide. *See* Orap
Pindolol. *See* Visken
Pinworms, 790
Piroxicam. *See* Feldene
Pituitary gland, 807, 809
disorders of, 808
PKD, 821
Plantar fasciitis, 858
Plantar warts, 859
Plaquenil, 485-487
for rheumatoid arthritis, 727
Plasma
defined, 853
fresh-frozen, for hemophilia,
856
Platelets. *See* Thrombocytes
Plendil, 487-489
Pleurisy, 747
SLE and, 729
PMS (premenstrual syn-
drome), 774
Pneumocystis carinii, 842, 844
Pneumonia, 745. *See also*
Staphylococcal pneumonia
pleurisy and, 747
recurring, as symptom of
lung cancer, 751
strep and, 815
vaccine for, 788
whooping cough and, 789

Podophyllum-benzoin com-
pound, for plantar warts,
859
Poison control centers, 879-
882
Poison ivy. *See also* Allergic
contact dermatitis
dermatitis caused by, 799
Poison oak. *See* Allergic con-
tact dermatitis
Poison sumac. *See* Allergic
contact dermatitis
Polaramine, 489-491
Poliomyelitis, vaccine for, 788
Polyarticular juvenile arthritis.
See Juvenile rheumatoid
arthritis
Polycystic kidney disease
(PKD), 821
Polyethylene glycol. *See* Colyte
Polymixin B sulfate. *See* Cor-
tisporin Ophthalmic Suspen-
sion
Polymox. *See* Amoxil
Polyps
intestinal, 741
nasal, 795
in uterus, and abnormal
bleeding, 776
Poly-Vi-Flor, **491-492**
Ponstel, **492-494**
Pork insulin, for Type I dia-
betes, 851
Postnasal drip, 744, 795
Post-traumatic stress disorder
(PTSD), 767-768
Potassium chloride. *See*
Colyte; Micro-K
Potassium supplements
elderly and, 863
in treating hypertension,
723-724
PPD skin test for tuberculosis,
746
Pravachol, **494-496**
Pravastatin sodium. *See* Pravachol
Prazepam. *See* Centrax
Prazosin hydrochloride. *See*
Minipress
Pred Forte, **496-498**
Prednisolone. *See* Pediapred
Prednisolone acetate. *See* Pred
Forte
Prednisone. *See also* Deltasone
for leukemia, 756
for mononucleosis, 789
for osteoarthritis, 727
for Wilson's disease, 832
Pregnancy. *See also* Childbirth
carpal tunnel syndrome and,
735
early, ovarian cancer and,
757
genital herpes and, 838
genital warts and, 837
gestational diabetes in, 848

IUD use and, 786
preventing. *See* Birth control
methods
process of, 783
stuffy nose and, 794
syphilis and, 838
UTIs and, 827
Premarin, **498-501**
Premature labor, calcium
channel blockers and, 718
Premenstrual syndrome
(PMS), 774
Prenatal examinations, impor-
tance of, 773
Pressure, as symptom
cholesteatoma, 793
otitis media, 792
Prilosec, 501-503
Primidone. *See* Mysoline
Prinivil. *See* Zestril
Pro-Banthine. *See* Propanthe-
line
Probenecid. *See* ColBENEMID
Probucol. *See* Lorelco
Procainamide hydrochloride.
See Procan SR
Procan SR, 503-505
Procardia, 505-507
Procardia XL, 507-509
Prochlorperazine. *See* Com-
pazine
Proctitis, 741
Proctosigmoidoscopy, 752
Progesterone, 809
in birth control pills, 786
for OB/GYN disorders, 779
for precancerous endome-
trial conditions, 755
in treating breast cancer,
753
Progressive systemic sclerosis.
See Scleroderma
Prolactin, 809
Prolixin, **510-511**
Proloid, **511-513**
Promethazine hydrochloride.
See Phenergan; Phenergan
with Codeine
Pronation, excessive, 858
Propafenone hydrochloride.
See Rythmol
Propanolol hydrochloride. *See*
Inderal; Inderide
Propantheline
for diarrhea, 740
for pancreatic cancer, 755
for urinary incontinence,
828
Propine, 513-514
Propoxyphene hydrochloride.
See Darvon
Propoxyphene napsylate. *See*
Darvocet-N
Propylthiouracil, for hyperthy-
roidism, 810
Proscar, **515-516**
ProSom, **516-518**

Prostaglandins, 774
Prostate
enlarged, and kidney ob-
struction, 823
enlarged, and overflow in-
continence, 828
treating infections of, 827
Prostate cancer, 754 (fig.),
753-754
Prostate specific antigen (PSA),
test for, 754
Prostep. *See* Nicotine Patches
Prostitution, syphilis rate and,
838
Protamine, Zinc and Iletin. *See*
Insulin
Protein loss, in nephrotic syn-
drome, 822
Proventil, 518-521
for asthma, 798
Provera, 521-523
Prozac, 523-525
for depression, 768
Pseudoephedrine hydrochlo-
ride. *See* Deconamine; Ron-
dec
Pseudoephedrine sulfate. *See*
Trinalin Repetabs
Psoralen, for psoriasis, 804
Psorcon, 525-527
Psoriasis, 802 (fig.), 804
toenail pitting and, 859
Psychoanalysis, 764
Psychological problems. *See*
Emotional problems; Mental
illness
Psychosis, as symptom, SLE,
729
Psychotherapy
for chronic headaches, 761
for depression, 769
PTSD (post-traumatic stress
disorder), 767-768
PTU. *See* Propylthiouracil
Pulmonary disease. *See* Lungs,
chronic disorders of
Pulmonary embolism, 719
Pulmonary infarction, pleurisy
and, 747
PUVA, for psoriasis, 804
Pyridium, 527-528
Pyrilamine tannate. *See* Rynatan

Q

Quazepam. *See* Doral
Questran, 528-530
for lowering cholesterol, 719
Quinamm, 533-534
Quinidex Extentabs, 530-532
Quinidine
for arrhythmia, 715
thrombocytopenia and, 856
Quinidine sulfate. *See*
Quinidex Extentabs
Quinine, arrhythmia and, 715
Quinine sulfate. *See* Quinamm

R

Radiation therapy
  for breast cancer, 753
  for colon cancer, 752
  for Cushing's syndrome, 811
  for lung cancer, 752
  for oral cancer, 758
  for ovarian cancer, 757
  for prostate cancer, 754
  for skin cancer, 757, 806
  for small-cell carcinoma of
    lung, 752
  for uterine and cervical can-
    cer, 755
Ramipril. See Altace
Ranitidine hydrochloride. See
  Zantac
Rapidly progressive glomerulonephritis (RPGN), 822
Rash, as symptom
  athlete's foot, 805
  atopic dermatitis, 799
  chickenpox, 787
  DLE, 729
  HIV infection, 843
  measles, 788
  meningitis, 816
  mononucleosis, 789
  rubella, 789
  scarlet fever, 815
  syphilis, 838
  toxic shock syndrome, 815
Raynaud's phenomenon, calcium channel blockers and,
  718
Rectal bleeding, as symptom
  colon cancer, 752
  intestinal polyps, 741
Rectal itching, as symptom,
  worms, 790
Rectum, STD infections, 835
Red blood cells. See Erythrocytes
Reflex incontinence, 828
Reflux esophagitis, 737-738
Reglan, **534-536**
Regular Insulin. See Insulin
Relaxation training, for treating pain, 762
Respiration, internal, 743
Respiratory disease, 743-747
Respiratory failure, meningitis
  and, 816
Respiratory infections, COPD
  and, 745
Respiratory problems. See also
  Lungs; Shortness of breath
  panic attacks and, 767
Respiratory problems, as
  symptom
  allergy, 797
  anaphylaxis, 800
  croup, 746
  epiglottitis, 747
  hay fever, 798
  measles, 788

Restoril, **537-538**
Reticulin, 802
Retin-A, **538-540**
  for acne, 803
Retinoblastoma, in children,
  756
Retrograde pyelography, 821
Retrovir, **540-542**
  for AIDS, 843
  for HIV infection, 844
Retroviruses, 843
  drugs against, 844
Reye's syndrome, 744, 790,
  832
Rhabdomyosarcoma, 750, 756
Rheumatic fever, streptococcal
  pharyngitis and, 815
Rheumatoid arthritis (RA),
  726-728, 728 (fig.)
  carpal tunnel syndrome and,
    734
  neck pain and, 733
  pleurisy and, 747
Rheumatrex. See Methotrex-
  ate
Rhinophyma, 803
Rhythm method. See Fertility
  awareness
Riboflavin. See Poly-Vi-Flor
Ridaura, **542-544**
Rifadin, **544-546**
  for Legionnaire's disease,
    747
  for tuberculosis, 746
Rifampin. See Rifadin
Rimactane. See Rifadin
Ringing in ears, as symptom,
  Ménière's disease, 793
Ringworm. See Dermatophy-
  tosis
Ritalin, **546-549**
  for ADHD in children, 771
Robaxin, **549-550**
  for slipped disk, 733
Rocaltrol, **550-552**
Rogaine, **552-554**
Rondec, **554-556**
Rosacea, 803
Roundworms, 805
Rowasa, **556-558**
Roxicet. See Percocet
Rubber band ligation, for he-
  morrhoids, 742
Rubella, 790
  vaccine for, 788
Rufen. See Motrin Tablets
Ru-Tuss Tablets, **558-560**
Rynatan, **560-561**
Rythmol, **561-563**

S

Safe sex practices, 835, 843
Salicylic acid, for dandruff,
  805
Salicylic acid plasters, 858-859

Salivary glands. See also
  Parotid
Salmonella, 816
Salsalate. See Disalcid
Salt. See also Low-salt diet
  edema from buildup of, 715
Salt craving, as symptom, Ad-
  dison's disease, 811
Salt solution, for athlete's foot,
  805
Salt-water gargles, for pharyn-
  gitis, 796
Sandimmune, **563-565**
Sansert, **565-567**
Sarcoma, 750
  osteogenic, 750, 756
Scabies, 805
Scalp
  psoriasis of, 804
  treating dandruff, 804-805
Scarlet fever, 815
Schizophrenia, 763, 769-770
Sciatica, 760
Scleroderma, 726, 730
Scoliosis, 732, 734
Scopolamine hydrobromide.
  See Donnagel-PG; Donnatal;
  Ru-Tuss Tablets
Scratching, in chickenpox, 788
Scrotum, varicose veins in, and
  infertility, 778
Seborrheic dermatitis, 804
Sebum, 803
Secobarbital sodium. See Sec-
  onal
Seconal, **567-569**
Sectral, **569-571**
Sedatives, for atopic eczema,
  804
Seldane, **571-573**
  for hay fever, 798
  for hives, 799
Selegiline hydrochloride. See
  Eldepryl
Selenium sulfide, for dandruff,
  805
Semilente Insulin. See Insulin
Separation anxiety, in chil-
  dren, 771
Septal spur, surgery for, 795
Septra. See Bactrim
Ser-Ap-Es, **573-575**
Serax, **575-577**
Serophene. See Clomiphene
  citrate
Serotonin reuptake blockers,
  for depression, 768
Serous otitis media, 793
Serpasil (reserpine). See Ser-
  Ap-Es
Sertraline. See Zoloft
Sex hormones, 809
Sexual immaturity, hypopitu-
  itarism and, 808
Sexually transmitted diseases
  (STDs), 833-839
  condoms and, 783

  of digestive tract, 742
  infertility in men and, 778
  PID and, 776
  preventing, 835
  statistics, 833
  transmission of, 834-835
  treating, 839
Shampoos, for dandruff, 804
Shigellosis, 742
Shingles
  AIDS and, 844
  codeine compounds for, 760
Shock
  from broken bones, 735
  meningitis (severe form)
    and, 816
Shortness of breath, as symptom
  folic acid deficiency anemia,
    855
  iron deficiency anemia, 854
  sickle cell anemia, 856
  thrombocytopenia, 856
Sickle-cell anemia, 855-856
  chronic pain and, 760
Silvadene Cream 1 %, **577-
578**
Silver sulfadiazine. See Sil-
  vadene Cream 1 %
Simvastatin. See Zocor
Sinemet CR, **578-581**
Sinequan, **581-583**
Sinus, 794 (fig.)
  infection of. See Mastoiditis;
    Sinusitis
  pain, as symptom of hay
    fever, 798
Sinusitis, 794-795
Skeleton, 732 (fig.)
Skin cancer, 756-757, 805-806
Skin color. See also Jaundice
  Addison's disease and, 811
  purple streaking and Cush-
    ing's syndrome, 811
Skin problems
  statistics, 801-802
  treating, 801-806
SLE. See Systemic lupus ery-
  thematosus (SLE)
Slow-K. See Micro-K
Smell, loss of sense of, nasal
  polyps and, 795
Smoking
  bladder cancer and, 757
  cancer and, 749
  COPD and, 745
  heart disease and, 711
  hormonal contraceptives
    and, 786
  hypertension and, 723
  lung cancer and, 751
  oral cancer and, 757
  pancreatic cancer and, 754
Social phobias, 766
Sodium bicarbonate. See
  Colyte
Sodium chloride. See Colyte

Sodium fluoride. *See* Luride
Sodium Sulamyd, **583-585**
Sodium sulfate. *See* Colyte
Soma, **585-586**
Sorbitrate. *See* Isordil
Sores. *See also* Lesions
  from genital herpes, 838
  from syphilis, 838
Sore throat. *See* Pharyngitis
Sore throat, as symptom
  epiglottitis, 747
  HIV infection, 844
  meningitis, 816
  mononucleosis, 789
  sinusitis, 795
  tonsillitis, 796
Spasms, as symptom, tetanus, 816
Spectazole Cream, **586-587**
Speech impairment, as symptom, migraine, 761
Spermicides, 782-783
  AIDS prevention and, 843
  STDs and, 835
Sphygmomanometer, 722
Spinal arthritis, 729. *See also* Ankylosing spondylitis
Spinal cord injury
  calcium channel blocker and, 718
  and overflow incontinence, 828
Spine
  compression by osteoporosis, 731-732
  deformities of, 731-732
  as source of pain, 732 (fig.)
Spironolactone. *See* Aldactazide; Aldactone
Spirozide. *See* Aldactazide
Spleen, removal of, for hemorrhagic disorders, 856
Spondylolisthesis, 733
Sputum, as symptom
  chronic bronchitis, 745
  pneumonia, 745
Sputum, bloody, as symptom
  lung cancer, 751
  staphylococcal pneumonia, 814
  tuberculosis, 746
Squamous cell carcinoma, 805
Staphylococcal infections, 814-815
Staphylococcal pneumonia, 814
Staphylococcal scalded skin syndrome, 805
Staphylococcus, liver abscess and, 832
Stasis dermatitis, 805
STDs. *See* Sexually transmitted diseases (STDs)
Steam inhalation, for sinusitis, 795
Stelazine, **588-590**
Sterility

PID and, 837
STDs and, 833, 836
Sterilization, surgical, 781-782
Steroids
  acne and, 803
  for allergic contact dermatitis, 799
  for asthma, 798
  for chronic bowel disease, 741
  for chronic glomerulonephritis, 822
  for juvenile rheumatoid arthritis, 730
  for kidney transplants, 824
  for psoriasis, 804
  for rheumatoid arthritis, 727
  for rosacea, 803
  for scleroderma, 730
  for SLE, 729
  for treating pain, 762
Still's disease. *See* Juvenile rheumatoid arthritis
Stings, allergies caused by, 799
Stool color, *E. coli* infections, 817
Stools, bloody, as symptom, proctitis, 741
Stool softeners, for diverticulosis, 741
Stool test, 752
Strep infections. *See* Streptococcal infections
Streptase, for dissolving blood clots, 719
Strep throat. *See* Streptococcal pharyngitis
Streptococcal infections, 815
  glomerulonephritis following, 822
  Group B, 815
  Group D, 815
Streptococcal pharyngitis, 815
Streptococcus bacteria. *See also* Streptococcal infections
  pharyngitis and, 796
Streptokinase. *See* Streptase
Stress incontinence, 828
Stroke, urge incontinence and, 828
Stuartnatal 1 + 1, **590**
Subcutaneous tissue, 802
Substance abuse, 763. *See also* Alcohol abuse
  infertility and, 779
Sucralfate. *See* Carafate
Sugar-free products, 869-872
Suicide, 764, 770
  among elderly, 862
Sulfacetamide sodium. *See* Sodium Sulamyd
Sulfa drugs, 813
  allergic reactions from, 798
  thrombocytopenia and, 856
Sulfamethoxazole. *See* Bactrim
Sulfasalazine. *See* Azulfidine
Sulfinpyrazone, for gout, 729

Sulfisoxazole. *See* Gantrisin; Pediazole
Sulfur, for dandruff, 805
Sulindac. *See* Clinoril
Sumycin. *See* Achromycin V Capsules
Sunblock, for SLE sufferers, 729
Suprax, **591-593**
Surgery
  for colon cancer, 741-742, 752
  for Crohn's disease, 741
  for Cushing's syndrome, 811
  for gastric cancer, 740
  for hyperthyroidism, 810
  for kidney obstructions, 823
  for lung cancer, 752
  for nasal problems, 794
  for OB/GYN disorders, 779
  for oral cancer, 758
  for osteomyelitis, 814
  for ovarian cancer, 757
  for prostate cancer, 754
  for rhinophyma, 803
  for skin cancer, 757, 806
  for telangiectasias, 803
  in treating hyperparathyroidism, 810
  treating pain associated with, 760
  for urinary incontinence, 828
  for urinary tract blockages, 822
  for uterine and cervical cancer, 755
Surmontil, **593-594**
Sweating, as symptom. *See also* Night sweats
  heart attack, 713
  hyperpituitarism, 808
  tetanus, 816
Swelling. *See* Edema
Swimmer's ear, 792
Symadine. *See* Symmetrel
Symmetrel, **595-597**
Synalar. *See* Fluocinolone acetonide
Synalgos-DC, **597-598**
Synovium, 728 (fig.)
Synthetic retinoids, in cancer treatment, 751
Synthroid, **598-600**
Syphilis, 833, 838
  condom and, 783
Systemic lupus erythematosus (SLE), 726, 729-730
  nephrotic syndrome and, 822
  pleurisy and, 747
Systolic pressure, 722

T

Tagamet, **600-602**
  for hives, 799
  for ulcers, 739

Talwin Compound, **602-604**
Tambocor, **604-606**
Tamoxifen citrate. *See* Nolvadex
Tampons
  vaginitis and, 837
  yeast infections and, 775
Tapazole. *See* Methimazole
Tardive dyskinesia, as side-effect of antipsychotic medications, 770
Tar preparations, for dandruff, 805
Tavist, **606-608**
Tegison, for psoriasis, 804
Tegretol, **608-610**
Telangiectasia, rosacea and, 803
Temazepam. *See* Restoril
Temovate, **611-612**
Tendinitis, 760
Tenex, **612-614**
Tenoretic, **614-616**
Tenormin, **616-618**
Tension, headaches and, 761
TENS (transcutaneous electrical nerve stimulation), 762
Tenuate, **618-620**
Terazol 3, **620-621**
Terazosin hydrochloride. *See* Hytrin
Terbutaline sulfate. *See* Brethine
Terconazole, *See* Terazol 3
Terfenadine. *See* Seldane
Tessalon, **621-622**
Testes, 809
  cancer of, 750
  inflammation of, and mumps, 789
  overheating of, and infertility, 778
Testing strips, for urine and blood tests, 852
Testosterone, 809
Tetanus, 816
  vaccine for, 788
Tetracycline. *See also* Achromycin V Capsules
  for acne, 803
  for bladder infections, 827
  for Lyme disease, 817
Thalassemia, 855
Thalitone. *See* Hygroton
Theo-Dur, **622-625**
  for asthma, 798
  for COPD, 746
Theophylline. *See* Theo-Dur
Theroxide. *See* Desquam-E
Thiamine. *See* Poly-Vi-Flor
Thioguanine, for leukemia, 756
Thioridazine hydrochloride. *See* Mellaril
Thiothixene. *See* Navane
Thirst, as symptom
  diabetes, 849

hyperglycemia, 848
Thonzonium bromide. *See* Coly-Mycin S Otic
Thorazine, 625-628
for schizophrenia, 764, 770
Thrombocytes, 854
Thrombocytopenia, as side effect of medications, 856
Thyroglobulin. *See* Proloid
Thyroid, 809
imbalance of, and panic attacks, 767
Thyroid disease, 810
Inderal for, 716
infertility and, 779
stuffy nose and, 794
and uterine bleeding, 776
Thyroid hormones T_3 and T_4. *See* Armour Thyroid
Thyroiditis, 810
Thyroid-stimulating hormone (TSH), 809
Thyroxine (T_4), 809
Ticks, Lyme disease and, 817
Tigan, 628-630
for gastroenteritis, 739
for hepatitis B, 831
Timolol maleate. *See* Timoptic Ophthalmic Solution
Timoptic Ophthalmic Solution, 630-632
Tinea versicolor, 805
Tine test for tuberculosis, 746
Tingling, as symptom
carpal tunnel syndrome, 735
herpes outbreaks, 838
migraine, 761
pernicious anemia, 854
Tissue-Plasminogen Activator. *See* Activase
T-4 lymphocytes, 843
Tobramycin. *See* Tobrex
Tobrex, 632-633
Tocainide hydrochloride. *See* Tonocard
Toe, swollen joints as symptom of gout, 727
Tofranil, 633-636
for depression, 768
for urinary incontinence, 828
Tolazamide. *See* Tolinase
Tolbutamide. *See* Orinase
Tolectin, 636-638
Tolinase, 638-640
for diabetes, 852
Tolmetin sodium. *See* Tolectin
Tongue, `strawberry` appearance and streptococcal pharyngitis, 815
Tongue soreness, as symptom
folic acid deficiency anemia, 855
oral cancer, 757-758
pernicious anemia, 854
Tonocard, 640-642
Tonsillitis, acute, 796

Tonsils
inflammation of, and strep throat, 815
swelling of, in mononucleosis, 789
Topicort, 642-643
Toxic shock syndrome (TSS), 815
Toxoplasmosis, and AIDS, 844
t-PA. *See* Activase
Tracheobronchitis, 744
Tracheotomy, for epiglottitis, 747
Trandate. *See* Normodyne
Tranquilizers
for acute pain, 760
for Alzheimer's disease patients, 864
for anxiety disorders, 768
for chronic headaches, 761
elderly and, 863
Transcriptase, inhibition by anti-retroviral drugs, 845
Transcutaneous Electrical Nerve Stimulation (TENS), 762
Transdermal patch (nitroglycerin), 716
Transderm-Nitro. *See* Nitroglycerin
Transrectal ultrasound, 754
Tranxene, 644-645
Tranxene-SD. *See* Tranxene
Tranxene-SD Half-Strength. *See* Tranxene
Trauma, pancreatitis and, 742
Trazodone hydrochloride. *See* Desyrel
Trental, 646-647
for atherosclerosis, 716
Treponema pallidum, 838
Tretinoin. *See* Retin-A
for acne, 803
Triamcinolone. *See* also Mycolog-II
for hay fever, 798
Triamterene. *See* Dyazide; Maxzide
Triavil, 648-650
Triazolam. *See* Halcion
Trichomoniasis, 837
Tricyclic antidepressants
for depression, 768
for panic disorder, 768
Tridesilon, 650-651
Tridione, 652-653
Trifluoperazine hydrochloride. *See* Stelazine
Trihexyphenidyl hydrochloride. *See* Artane
Triiodothyronine (T_3), 809
Trilisate, 654-655
Trimethadione. *See* Tridione
Trimethobenzamide hydrochloride. *See* Tigan
Trimethoprim. *See* Bactrim

for bladder infections, 827
Trimipramine maleate. *See* Surmontil
Trimox. *See* Amoxil
Trimpex. *See* Bactrim
Trinalin Repetabs, 656-658
Tripelennamine hydrochloride. *See* PBZ-SR
Triphasil. *See* Oral contraceptives
Trisalicylate. *See* Trilisate
TSH (thyroid-stimulating hormone), 809
T-Stat. *See* Erythromycin, topical
Tubal ligation, 782
Tubal pregnancy. *See* Ectopic pregnancy
Tuberculosis, 746-747
AIDS and, 844
carpal tunnel syndrome and, 735
pleurisy and, 747
Tumor
benign, carpal tunnel syndrome and, 735
bladder, removing, 828
bladder, urge incontinence and, 828
common locations, 758
endocrine malfunction and, 807
hyperparathyroidism and, 810
kidney obstruction and, 823
menstrual disorders and, 774
pituitary disorders and, 808
Tussionex, 659-661
Tussi-Organidin DM 658-659
Twitching, as symptom, kidney failure, 823
Tylenol, 661-662
for chickenpox, 788
with Codeine, 662-664
Tylenol with codeine, for osteoarthritis, 727
Tylox. *See* Percocet
Tympanic membrane, 791
Typhoid fever, 816

U

Ulcerative colitis, 740
proctitis and, 741
Ulcerative proctitis, 740
Ulcers, 739-740
hyperparathyroidism and, 810
treating in elderly, 863
typical locations, 739 (fig.)
Ultracef. *See* Duricef
Ultralente Insulin. *See* Insulin
Ultrasound
for diagnosing kidney stones, 823
for urinary tract blockages, 821

Ultraviolet light
for acne, 803
for atopic eczema, 804
for psoriasis, 804
for vitiligo, 805
Uniphyl. *See* Theo-Dur
Unipolar depression, 768
Ureaplasma urealyticum, 836
Uremia, 820
Ureteral stenosis, 821
Ureteropelvic junction obstruction, 821
Urethral stricture, 821
and overflow incontinence, 828
Urethritis, 833, 836
Urge incontinence, 828
Uric acid, 727-728
Urinary difficulties, as symptom
bladder cancer, 757
kidney stones, 823
prostate cancer, 754
STDs, 835-836
UTI, 827
Urinary tract
blockage of, 821
disorders of, 825-828
female, 774, 774 (fig.)
female, disorders of, 775
function of, 825-826
structure of, 826 (fig.)
Urinary tract infection (UTI), 774 (fig.), 775
preventing, 827
recurrent, treating, 827
statistics, 825
Urination, frequent, as symptom
diabetes, 849
hyperglycemia, 848
Urine, 820 (fig.)
rust-colored, post-strep glomerulonephritis and, 822
Urine, bloody, as symptom
bladder cancer, 757, 828
polycystic kidney disease (PKD), 821
prostate cancer, 754
UTI, 827
Urine test, for diabetes, 850
Urised, 664-666
Urispas, 666-667
for urinary incontinence, 780, 828
Ursodiol. *See* Actigall
Urticaria. *See* Hives
Uterus
bleeding, abnormal, 776
cancer of, 755, 777-778
D&C for bleeding, 779
disorders of, 775-777
IUD damage to, 785
UTI. *See* Urinary tract infection (UTI)

5/93

V

Vaccination
  for childhood diseases, 787-
    788
  for influenza, 745
Vaccine
  for bacterial pneumonia,
    745
  for chickenpox, 788
  for hepatitis A, 830
  for hepatitis B, 829, 839
  for measles, 788
  for rubella, 790
Vagina, disorders of, 775
Vaginal bleeding, abnormal
  and hormonal contracep-
    tives, 786
  as symptom of uterine and
    cervical cancer, 755
Vaginal secretions, spread of
  STDs through, 834
Vaginitis, 775, 837
  hormonal therapy for, 779
Vaginosis, bacterial, 837
Valium, **667-669**
  for anxiety disorders, 768
  for fractures, 735
  for Ménière's disease, 793
  for slipped disk, 733
  for tetanus, 816
Valproic acid. *See* Depakene
Vancenase. *See* Beclometha-
  sone dipropionate
Vancenase AQ Nasal Spray.
  See Beclomethasone dipropi-
  onate
Vancenase Nasal Inhaler. *See*
  Beclomethasone dipropi-
  onate
Vanceril, for asthma, 798
Vanceril Inhaler. *See* Be-
  clomethasone dipropionate
Vancomycin, for bacteremia,
  814
Vascor, **669-671**
Vasectomy, 782
Vaseretic, **671-673**
Vasodilators
  headaches and, 761
  for hypertension, 716
  for scleroderma, 730
  in treating hypertension, 724
Vasomotor rhinitis, 794
Vasotec, **674-676**
  for hypertension, 724
V-cillin K. *See* Penicillin V
Veetids. *See* Penicillin V
Veins, 712. *See also* Arteries;
  Circulatory system
Velosef, **676-678**
Velosulin. *See* Insulin
Velosulin Human. *See* Insulin
Venom immunotherapy, 799
Ventolin. *See* Proventil
Verapamil hydrochloride. *See*
  Calan

Verelan. *See* Calan
Vermox. *See* Mebendazole
Vertigo, as symptom. *See also*
  Dizziness
  Ménière's disease, 793
Vesical neck contracture, 821
Veterans, PTSD among, 767-
  768
Vibramycin. *See* Doryx
Vibra-Tabs. *See* Doryx
Vicodin, **678-680**
Videx. *See* Didanosine
Vinblastine, for bladder can-
  cer, 757
Vincristine
  for colon cancer, 752
  for leukemia, 756
  for small-cell carcinoma of
    lung, 752
  for uterine cancer, 755
VIN (vulvar intraepithelial
  neoplasia), 775
Viral hepatitis. *See* Hepatitis,
  viral
Viral infections
  treating pain associated
    with, 760
  of upper respiratory tract,
    744
Vision changes, as symptom
  childhood cancers, 756
  migraine, 761
Vision problems, Plaquenil
  and, 727
Vision problems, as symptom
  diabetes, 849
  hyperpituitarism, 808
Visken, **680-682**
Vitamin A. *See* Poly-Vi-Flor
Vitamin and mineral supple-
  ments, maternal. *See* Stuart-
  natal 1+1
Vitamin B$_6$. *See* Poly-Vi-Flor
Vitamin B$_{12}$. *See also*
  Poly-Vi-Flor
  for chronic gastritis, 739
  pernicious anemia and, 854
  for Wilson's disease, 832
Vitamin C. *See also* Poly-Vi-
  Flor
  for anemia, 854
  in treating UTIs, 827
Vitamin D. *See also* Poly-Vi-
  Flor
  for hypoparathyroidism,
    810
  for osteoporosis, 733
Vitamin E. *See* Poly-Vi-Flor
Vitamins, for cirrhosis, 832
Vitiligo, 805
Vocal cords, inflammation of,
  796
Voltaren, **682-684**
Vomiting, as symptom
  Addison's disease, 811
  anaphylaxis, 800
  diabetes, 848-849

diverticulosis, 741
E. coli infections, 817
enterocolitis, 814
erysipelas, 815
food poisoning, 814
gastritis, 739
gastroenteritis, 739
kidney failure, 823
kidney stones, 823
Legionnaire's disease, 747
liver abscess, 832
Ménière's disease, 793
migraine, 761
mumps, 789
otitis media, 793
pancreatitis, 742
pernicious anemia, 854
Reye's syndrome, 790
toxic shock syndrome, 815
viral hepatitis, 830
VoSoL, **684-685**
Vulvar intraepithelial neoplasia (VIN), 775

W

Warfarin sodium. *See*
  Coumadin
Warts, 805
Weight gain, as symptom, hypothyroidism, 808
Weight loss
  in arthritis treatment, 727
  gastric ulcers and, 739
  in reflux esophagitis treat-
    ment, 738
Weight loss, as symptom
  Addison's disease, 811
  childhood cancers, 756
  diabetes, 849
  gastric cancer, 740
  Graves' disease, 810
  leukemia, 755
  liver abscess, 832
  pancreatic cancer, 755
  pernicious anemia, 854
  tuberculosis, 746
Wellbutrin, **685-686**
Wenkebach, Karl, 715
Western blot test for AIDS, 844
Wheezing, as symptom. *See
  also* Respiratory problems
  anaphylaxis, 800
  asthma, 797
  sting allergies, 799
Whiplash injuries, 733
White blood cells. *See* Leuko-
  cytes
Whooping cough, 789
  vaccine for, 788
Wilm's tumor, 750, 756
Wilson's disease, 832
Withering, William, 714
Wrist, 734 (fig.). *See also*
  Carpal tunnel syndrome
Wymox. *See* Amoxil
Wytensin, **687-689**

X

Xanax, **689-691**
  for anxiety disorders, 768

Y

Yeast infections, 775
Yeast organism, seborrheic
  dermatitis and, 805
Yocon, **691-692**
Yohimbine hydrochloride. *See*
  Yocon

Z

Zalcitabine, for HIV infection,
  845
Zantac, **692-694**
  for hives, 799
  for ulcers, 740
Zaroxolyn, **694-696**
  for post-strep glomeru-
    lonephritis, 822
Zestril, **696-698**
Zidovudine. *See* Retrovir
Zinc pyrithione, for dandruff,
  805
Zithromax, **698-699**
Zocor, **699-701**
Zoloft, **701-702**
Zovirax, **704-705**
  for chickenpox, 788
  for genital herpes, 780
Zydone. *See* Vicodin
Zyloprim, **705-708**
  for gout, 729